Clinical Neurology of Aging

Clinical Neurology of Aging

Third Edition

Edited by

Martin L. Albert, MD, PhD
Department of Neurology
Boston University School of Medicine; and
Boston VA Healthcare System
Boston, MA

Janice E. Knoefel, MD, MPH
Departments of Internal Medicine and Neurology
University of New Mexico School of Medicine; and
New Mexico VA Health Care System
Albuquerque, NM

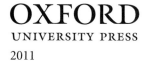

OXFORD
UNIVERSITY PRESS
2011

OXFORD
UNIVERSITY PRESS

Oxford University Press, Inc., publishes works that further
Oxford University's objective of excellence
in research, scholarship, and education.

Oxford   New York

Auckland   Cape Town   Dar es Salaam   Hong Kong   Karachi
Kuala Lumpur   Madrid   Melbourne   Mexico City   Nairobi
New Delhi   Shanghai   Taipei   Toronto

With offices in
Argentina   Austria   Brazil   Chile   Czech Republic   France   Greece
Guatemala   Hungary   Italy   Japan   Poland   Portugal   Singapore
South Korea   Switzerland   Thailand   Turkey   Ukraine   Vietnam

Copyright © 2011 by Oxford University Press, Inc.

Published by Oxford University Press, Inc.
198 Madison Avenue, New York, New York 10016

www.oup.com

Oxford is a registered trademark of Oxford University Press

Library of Congress Cataloging-in-Publication Data
Clinical neurology of aging / edited by Martin L. Albert, Janice E. Knoefel.—3rd ed.
   p. ; cm.
   Includes bibliographical references and index.
   ISBN 978-0-19-536929-8
  1.   Geriatric neurology.   I. Albert, Martin L., 1939– II. Knoefel, Janice E.
   [DNLM: 1.   Nervous System Diseases. 2.   Aged. 3.   Aging—physiology. 4.   Nervous System
Physiological Phenomena.   WL 140 C6406 2011]
   RC346.C54 2011
   618.97'68—dc22   2010010578

This material is not intended to be, and should not be considered, a substitute for medical or
other professional advice. Treatment for the conditions described in this material is highly
dependent on the individual circumstances. And, while this material is designed to offer accurate
information with respect to the subject matter covered and to be current as of the time it was
written, research and knowledge about medical and health issues is constantly evolving and dose
schedules for medications are being revised continually, with new side effects recognized and
accounted for regularly. Readers must therefore always check the product information and
clinical procedures with the most up-to-date published product information and data sheets
provided by the manufacturers and the most recent codes of conduct and safety regulation.
The publisher and the authors make no representations or warranties to readers, express or
implied, as to the accuracy or completeness of this material. Without limiting the foregoing,
the publisher and the authors make no representations or warranties as to the accuracy or efficacy
of the drug dosages mentioned in the material. The authors and the publisher do not accept,
and expressly disclaim, any responsibility for any liability, loss or risk that may be claimed or
incurred as a consequence of the use and/or application of any of the contents of this material.

9 8 7 6 5 4 3 2 1

Printed in the United States of America
on acid-free paper

I wish to dedicate this book to my wife, Phyllis Cohen Albert, who saved my life.

—MLA

I wish to dedicate this volume to my family, Mike and Owen, and to my extended network of family, friends and colleagues who have always supported my efforts on behalf of the elderly. Ultimately it is on our own behalf that we honor and respect the elders, with the hope that someday we will be them.

— JEK

Foreword

Since the first edition of *The Clinical Neurology of Aging* was published twenty-five years ago, the frontiers of our knowledge of aging have advanced beyond previous expectations. We now accept that aging is not a pathological condition, frailty is not inevitable, and that longevity results from a fascinating and complex interaction of genetic endowment, life choices, and environmental influences.

While our knowledge base has progressed, the foundation for a robust clinical infrastructure to apply that knowledge for the improvement of geriatric care has faltered. A key feature of that infrastructure is a well-trained workforce. Not only has the number of clinicians choosing careers in geriatrics not grown in recent years, it has, in fact, dwindled. The reasons for this are multiple—attitudes about aging, inadequate reimbursement rates, among others—and well documented but the outcome remains clear: There are insufficient numbers of clinicians who have the competencies to care for the expanding older population.

Solutions to the workforce shortages will be long-term and incremental. One clear and necessary intermediate step is to infuse geriatric content into training for all clinicians to improve their proficiency in caring for older persons. In no field is this more critical than neurology. The myriad neurological disorders that disproportionately touch the elderly are thoroughly covered in the content of this edition. However, excellence in geriatric care goes well beyond diagnosis and treatment of diseases. The guiding principle of geriatrics is to help the older person remain independent at his or her highest level of functioning for the longest period of time. High quality care, especially for older persons, demands a broad, person-centric approach which is respectful of and responsive to an individual's needs (*Crossing the Quality Chasm*, 2001). By increasing the span of topics covered in this comprehensive volume, with subjects ranging from geriatric assessment to pain management and palliative care, the editors incorporate the geriatric care perspective and a quality-oriented approach to health care. These concepts are essential to providing outstanding care for all elderly. The editors have enlisted an exceptional group of experts in neurology, geriatrics, and clinical research to produce a definitive reference, useful for all clinicians caring for older people and informative to those who set policies that affect research and clinical practice.

The role of the clinician caring for older persons is to understand, anticipate, and, whenever possible, alter the factors that make individuals vulnerable to compromised function. As a physician-educator trained in geriatrics, a former neuroscience researcher, and a health policy professional, I commend this valuable new edition of *The Clinical Neurology of Aging*, which provides state-of-the-art knowledge of neurological conditions with an appreciation of the complexities of aging.

Judith A. Salerno, MD, MS
Washington, DC

Preface to Third Edition

"How old would you be if you didn't know how old you are?"

In this Third Edition of our book, *Clinical Neurology of Aging*, we focus on the wisdom implicit in these words of legendary baseball pitcher Satchel Paige. We understand these words to mean that one may grow older chronologically but remain youthful and vibrant in spirit, vigor, and enthusiasm. A recent article in the *New York Times* carries the headline: "Happiness May Come with Age," and goes on to report "…A large Gallup poll has found that by almost any measure, people get happier as they get older…" To us, the conclusion is clear: the role of the health care provider who deals with an elderly patient is to maximize opportunities for this patient to enjoy life.

In this book we reinforce the clinical emphasis of previous editions in order to help clinicians help older persons maintain joy in their aging years. Of course, we are not blind to the reality of decline. The distinctive field of geriatric neurology responds to the challenge of understanding decline in the context of age-related changes in the nervous system and other organ systems, and in the relation of disease states to these age-related declines. Medical students are often taught the principle of Ockham's razor (the principle of parsimony): to uncover the single disease state that may explain a multiplicity of signs and symptoms. In contrast, in geriatrics and geriatric neurology, as this book demonstrates, the task frequently should be turned around, with a goal of finding the several different medical and neurological conditions that underlie a single sign or symptom.

We have been fortunate in receiving contributions to this edition from many of the world's leading experts. The book consists of eight sections, each comprising several clinically oriented chapters. Major sections cover the following areas: Introduction to Geriatric Neurology; Neurological Assessment in Aging; Cognitive Disorders in Aging; Motor Disorders in Aging; Sensory Disturbance in Aging; Peripheral Neurology in Aging; Disease States in the Elderly; and Neurological Therapeutics. It has been more than fifteen years since the appearance of the *Second Edition* of this book. In bringing the field up-to-date, we have maintained the primary objectives of previous editions: "…to shape a comprehensive text-reference book on the neurology of aging, providing the scientific foundations of clinical practice, together with practical, clinical advice for diagnosis and management of neurological disorders in elderly persons."

MLA
Boston, Massachusetts

JEK
Albuquerque, New Mexico
June 2010

Preface to First Edition

"Let us recognize ourselves in this old man or in that old woman. It must be done if we are to take upon ourselves the entirety of our own humanity."

Simone de Beauvoir

Is growing old worth the effort? Are elderly people doomed to relentless deterioration and consequent suffering? Or is there something that concerned clinicians can offer the older patient that will assist in the maintenance of physical and psychological well-being and the ability to participate comfortably in life's activities. By providing the scientific foundations necessary for diagnosis and treatment of nervous system dysfunction in aging patients, this book is designed to help clinicians help the elderly. Although many books on the neurobiology of aging have been published during the past decade, few have been directed toward the clinician. One major goal of this book is to share with practicing clinicians the experience and knowledge of clinician-scientists who have unusually high levels of expertise in fundamentals of the neurobiology of aging and in the application of these fundamentals to everyday problems of elderly people with neurologic disorders.

In 1970 about 11% of the population of the United States was over age 65. By the year 2030 this percentage is expected to increase to 20%, or about 50 million elderly people in this country alone. Since more than half of the medical incapacitation of people over age 65 is accounted for by neurologic diseases, there is a rapidly increasing need for clinicians to develop a special awareness of the neurology of old age.

The clinical neurology of aging is more than just the practice of general adult neurology within the expanding elderly population. Geriatric neurology, like pediatric neurology before it, is emerging as a distinctive discipline with distinctive clinical and neuroscientific features. Charcot demonstrated in 1867 that the same disease of the nervous system may affect an older patient quite differently from a young adult, and, moreover, that older people are subject to certain neurologic diseases not usually found in younger populations. This book attempts to document the specificity of geriatric neurology by providing a systematic, up-to-date review of the neurobiology of aging as applied to the clinical practice of neurology in the elderly.

No published work of this magnitude could be produced without the practical and moral support of many friends and colleagues. I thank once again the contributors of each chapter for the considerable effort they put into this work. I am also grateful to the two major institutions that supported me while this project was taking shape—Boston University Medical School and the Veterans Administration. At Boston University, Robert Feldman, Chairman of the Department of Neurology, has continually supported and encouraged me; and Dean John Sandson has demonstrated unusual sensitivity and goodwill in his support. Thanks are also due to my associates and colleagues at the Boston VA Medical Center for their encouragement during this project. The Veterans Administration granted me a six-month extended educational leave during which much of the final editorial work on this book was carried out.

Special thanks should be given to Janice Knoefel, geriatric neurologist, and Martha Windrem, philosopher of science and neurolinguist, for their excellent and much appreciated editorial assistance. I am grateful to Jennifer Sandson and Jane Litter for their review of the proofs and to Suzanne Ruscitti, my secretary, for her valuable and reliable assistance.

Much of the editorial work on this book was carried out in Paris while I was visiting the I.N.S.E.R.M. Research Laboratory for Neuropsychological Studies. I thank Pierre Rondot, Director of the Laboratory, for his friendly welcome. Members of the I.N.S.E.R.M. Laboratory for Gerontologic Studies, in particular its former Director, F. Bourlière, and current Director, Y. Courtois, were particularly helpful to me, and I am most appreciative. Our friends Jean and Jan Haegel provided consistent moral and material support which greatly facilitated my task and for which I am grateful.

Thanks are also due to Jeffrey House, editor for medical and scientific publications at Oxford University Press, whose calm and thoughtful advice was always available. I wish especially to thank Phyllis, David, Michael, and Rachel Albert for all their goodwill.

M.L.A.
Boston
October 1, 1983

Acknowledgments

We thank the many participants to the making of this book for their outstanding contributions, and our many colleagues and friends who helped us over the years as we developed our sense of what geriatric neurology might be.

—MLA, JEK

Contents

Section 5 Sensory Disturbance in Aging

Section 6 Peripheral Neurology in Aging

Section 7 Disease States in the Elderly

Section 8 Neurological Therapeutics

Contributors

John C. Adair, MD   Neurology Service, Veterans Medical Center, Department of Neurology, University of New Mexico Health Sciences Center, Albuquerque, NM

Martin L. Albert, MD, PhD   Department of Neurology, Boston University School of Medicine; and, Boston VA Healthcare System, Boston, MA

Alexandra Amen, BA   Department of Neurology, Oregon Health & Science University, Portland, OR

Melissa M. Amick, PhD   Research Service, VA Boston Healthcare System, Boston, MA; Department of Psychiatry, Boston University School of Medicine, Boston, MA

Cynthia Bamford, MD   Neurological Center for Pain, Cleveland Clinic Foundation, Cleveland, OH

Richard J. Barohn, MD   Chair, Department of Neurology, Gertrude and Dewey Ziegler Professor of Neurology, University of Kansas Medical Center, Kansas City, KS

Amanda A. Beck, MD, PhD   Sleep Center, The University of New Mexico Health Sciences Center, Albuquerque, NM

Ron Ben-Yitzhak, MD   Movement Disorders Unit, Department of Neurology, Tel Aviv Sourasky Medical Center, Sackler Faculty of Medicine, Tel Aviv University, Tel Aviv, Israel

David A. Bennett, MD   Rush Alzheimer's Disease Center, Rush University Medical Center, Chicago, IL

Dan R. Berlowitz, MD, MPH   Center for Health Quality, Outcomes and Economic Research, Bedford VA Hospital, Bedford, MA; Boston University Schools of Public Health and Medicine, Boston, MA

David Q. Beversdorf, MD   William and Nancy Thompson Endowed Chair in Radiology, Departments of Radiology, Neurology, and Psychology, Thompson Center for Autism and Neuro-developmental Disorders, University of Missouri-Columbia, Columbia, MO

Don H. Bivins, MD   Good Samaritan Hospice, Roanoke, VA

Christopher B. Brady, PhD   VA Boston Healthcare System; and, Department of Neurology, Boston University School of Medicine, Boston, MA

Richard Camicioli MD, FRCPC   Department of Neurology, University of Alberta, Edmonton, AB

Jessica Campaign, PharmD   Assistant Professor of Pharmacy, The University of New Mexico College of Pharmacy, Albuquerque, NM

Louis R. Caplan, MD, FAAN   Department of Neurology and Stroke Service, Beth Israel Deaconess Medical Center, Boston, MA

Robert Cavaliere, MD   Department of Neurosurgery, Division of Neuro-oncology, The Ohio State University, Columbus, OH

William P. Cheshire, Jr., MD   Professor of Neurology, College of Medicine, Mayo Clinic, Jacksonville, FL

Tanuja Chitnis, MD   Partners Multiple Sclerosis Center, Brigham and Women's Hospital, Harvard Medical School, Boston, MA

Amy Colcher, MD   Clinical Associate Professor of Neurology University of Pennsylvania, Philadelphia, PA

Jody Corey-Bloom, MD, PhD   Department of Neurosciences, University of California, San Diego, CA

Ricardo Cruz, MD   Department of Neurorehabilitation, Weill Medical College of Cornell University, Burke Rehabilitation Hospital, White Plains, NY

Jeffrey L. Cummings, MD   Andre and Joseph Hahn Professor of Neurotherapeutics, Director, Cleveland Clinic Lou Ruvo Center for Brain Health, Cleveland Clinic Neurological Institute, Las Vegas, Nevada and Cleveland, OH

Nabila Dahodwala, MD   Parkinson's Disease and Movement Disorders Center, Department of Neurology, University of Pennsylvania, Philadelphia, PA

Larry E. Davis, MD, FAAN, FACP   Chief Neurology Service, New Mexico VA Health Care System, Albuquerque, NM; Departments of Neurology, Neuroscience, and Molecular Immunology and Microbiology, University of New Mexico School of Medicine, Albuquerque, NM

Mark D'Esposito, MD   Professor of Neuroscience and Psychology Director, Henry H. Wheeler, Jr. Brain Imaging Center, Helen Wills Neuroscience Institute, University of California, Berkeley, CA

Mazen M. Dimachkie, MD   Professor of Neurology, Director of Neuromuscular Section, University of Kansas Medical Center, Kansas City, KS

Melanie A. Dodd, PharmD, PhC, BCPS   Associate Professor of Pharmacy, The University of New Mexico College of Pharmacy, Albuquerque, NM

Richard L. Doty, PhD   Director, Smell & Taste Center; Professor, Department of Otorhinolaryngology: Head and Neck Surgery, University of Pennsylvania School of Medicine, Philadelphia, PA

David A. Drachman, MD   Professor of Neurology, Chairman Emeritus Professor of Physiology, University of Massachusetts Medical School, Worcester, MA

P. James B. Dyck, MD   Head of the Peripheral Nerve Research Laboratory and Peripheral Nerve Section, Mayo Clinic, Rochester, MN

Stanley Fahn, MD   Department of Neurology, Columbia University College of Physician's & Surgeons, New York, NY

K.J. Fiedler, MD   Spinal Cord Injury/Disorders Care Line, New Mexico VA Health Care System; and, Department of Neurology, University of New Mexico, Albuquerque, NM

Michael H. Flores, AuD   Division of Audiology, Veteran Affairs Medical Center; and, Department of Speech and Hearing Sciences, University of New Mexico, Albuquerque, NM

Michael P. Gerardo, DO, MPH   Section of Geriatric Medicine, Rush Medical College, Chicago, IL

Nir Giladi, MD   Movement Disorders Unit, Department of Neurology, Tel Aviv Sourasky Medical Center, Sackler Faculty of Medicine, Tel Aviv University, Tel Aviv, Israel

Molly E. Gilbert, MD   Department of Ophthalmology and Visual Sciences, Section of Neurophthalmology, Illinois Eye and Ear Infirmary, University of Illinois-Chicago, Chicago, IL

Tenielle E. Gofton, MD   Department of Neurology, University of Western Ontario, London Health Sciences Center, London, ON

James Goodwin, MD   Department of Ophthalmology and Visual Sciences, Section of Neurophthalmology, Illinois Eye and Ear Infirmary, University of Illinois-Chicago, Chicago, IL

Mira Goral, PhD   VA Boston Healthcare System, Boston, MA; and, Program in Speech-Language-Hearing Sciences, The Graduate School and University Center and Lehman College, The City University of New York, New York, NY

Neill R. Graff-Radford, MD, MBBCh, FRCP   Department of Neurology, Mayo Clinic, Jacksonville, FL

Laura J. Grande, PhD   Psychology Service, VA Boston Healthcare System, Boston, MA, USA; Department of Psychiatry, Boston University School of Medicine, Boston, MA

Madeleine Grigg-Damberger, MD   Department of Neurology, University of New Mexico School of Medicine, Albuquerque, NM

Katrina Gwinn, MD   Human Motor Control Section, NINDS, NIH, Bethesda, MD

Elizabeth Haberfeld, MD   Gertrude H. Sergievsky Center, Department of Neurology, College of Physicians and Surgeons, Columbia University, New York, NY

Mark Hallett, MD   Human Motor Control Section, NINDS, NIH, Bethesda, MD

Jeffrey M. Hausdorff, PhD   Movement Disorders Unit, Department of Neurology, Tel Aviv Sourasky Medical Center, Sackler Faculty of Medicine, Tel Aviv University, Tel Aviv, Israel

Talia Herman, MSc   Movement Disorders Unit, Department of Neurology, Tel Aviv Sourasky Medical Center, Sackler Faculty of Medicine, Tel Aviv University, Tel Aviv, Israel

Branko Huisa-Garate, MD   Department of Neurology, University of New Mexico Health Sciences Center, Albuquerque, NM

Linda Hunt, PhD, FAOTA, OTR/L   School of Occupational Therapy, Pacific University, Forest Grove, OR

JungMoon Hyun, MS   VA Boston Healthcare System, Boston, MA; and, Program in Speech-Language-Hearing Sciences, The Graduate School and University Center, The City University of New York, New York, NY

Janet L. Jankowiak, MD   Geriatric/Behavioral Neurology Neurorehabilitation, Radius Specialty Hospital, Boston, MA

Scott Y. H. Kim, MD, PhD   Center for Bioethics and Social Sciences in Medicine and Department of Psychiatry, University of Michigan, Ann Arbor, MI

Molly K. King, MD   Neurology Service, New Mexico VA Health System; and, Department of Neurology, University of New Mexico School of Medicine, Albuquerque, NM

Janice E. Knoefel, MD, MPH   Departments of Internal Medicine and Neurology, University of New Mexico Medical School; and, New Mexico VA Health Care System, Albuquerque, NM

Sandeep Kumar, MD   Department of Neurology, Harvard Medical School, Beth Israel Deaconess Medical Center, Boston, MA

Jau-Shin Lou, MD, PhD   EMG Laboratory, Department of Neurology, Oregon Health & Science University, Portland, OR

Elan D. Louis, MD   Gertrude H. Sergievsky Center, Department of Neurology, Taub Institute for Research on Alzheimer's Disease and the Aging Brain, College of Physicians and Surgeons; and, Department of Epidemiology, Joseph P. Mailman School of Public Health, Columbia University, New York, NY

Alan M. Mandell, MD   Departments of Neurology and Psychiatry, Boston University Alzheimer's Disease Research Center, New England GRECC, ENRM VA Medical Center, Bedford, MA

Joseph C. Masdeu, MD, PhD   Section on Integrative Neuroimaging, National Institutes of Health (CBDB-NIMH), Intramural Program, Bethesda, MD; Department of Neurology, New York Medical College, Valhalla, NY

Sachio Matsushita, MD   National Hospital Organization, Kurihama Alcoholism Center, Kanagawa, Japan

Richard Mayeux, MD   The Taub Institute for Research on Alzheimer's Disease and the Aging Brain; The Gertrude H. Sergievsky Center, The Departments of Neurology, Psychiatry, Medicine, College of Physicians and Surgeons, Columbia University, New York, NY; The Department of Epidemiology, School of Public Health, Columbia University, New York, NY

MaryAnn Mays, MD   Neurological Center for Pain, Cleveland Clinic Foundation, Cleveland, OH

Mario F. Mendez, MD, PhD   Director Neurobehavior, VA Greater Los Angeles; Professor of Neurology and Psychiatry & Biobehavioral Sciences, David Geffen School of Medicine at UCLA, Los Angeles, CA

William P. Milberg, PhD   New England GRECC, VA Boston Healthcare System, Boston, MA; Department of Psychiatry, Harvard Medical School, Boston, MA

Masaru Mimura, MD, PhD   Department of Neuropsychiatry, Showa University School of Medicine, Tokyo, Japan

Jennifer R. Molano, MD   Department of Neurology, Mayo Alzheimer's Disease Research Center, Mayo Clinic College of Medicine, Rochester, MN

Loraine K. Obler, PhD   VA Boston Healthcare System; and, Boston University School of Medicine, Boston, MA; Program in Speech-Language-Hearing Sciences, The Graduate School and University Center, The City University of New York, New York, NY

Germaine L. Odenheimer, MD, FAAN   Donald W. Reynolds Department of Geriatric Medicine, Department of Veterans' Affairs, The University of Oklahoma Health Sciences Center, Oklahoma City, OK

Barry S. Oken, MD   Departments of Neurology and Behavioral Neuroscience, Oregon Health & Science University, Portland, OR

David A. Olson, MD   Dekalb Neurology Associates, Dekalb Medical Center, Decatur, GA

Winnie C.W. Pao, MD   Department of Behavioral Neurology, Mayo Clinic College of Medicine, Rochester, MN

Ronald C. Petersen, MD, PhD   Department of Neurology, Mayo Alzheimer's Disease Research Center, Mayo Clinic College of Medicine, Rochester, MN

Bradley P. Pickett, MD   Division of Otolaryngology, Veteran Affairs Medical Center; and, University of New Mexico Health Sciences, Albuquerque, NM

Sarah Pirio Richardson, MD   Department of Neurology, University of New Mexico School of Medicine, Albuquerque, NM

Mary Jo Pugh, PhD, RN   South Texas Veterans Health Care System, VERDICT REAP, University of Texas Health Science Center at San Antonio, Department of Epidemiology and Biostatistics, and Department of Medicine Division of Geriatrics and Gerontology, San Antonio, TX

Michael Rafii, MD, PhD   Director, Memory Disorders Clinic, Assistant Professor of Neurosciences, Associate Medical Director, Alzheimer's Disease Cooperative Study Attending Neurologist, Shiley-Marcos Alzheimer's Disease Research Center University of California, San Diego, CA

Faisal Raja, MD   Neuromuscular Medicine Fellow, Department of Neurology, University of Kansas Medical Center, Kansas City, KS

Frank M. Ralls, MD   Sleep Center, The University of New Mexico Health Sciences Center, Albuquerque, NM

P. Hemachandra Reddy, PhD   Neurogenetics Laboratory, Neuroscience Division, Oregon National Primate Research Center West Campus, Oregon Health and Science University, Beaverton, OR

Mike Reding, MD   Department of Neurorehabilitation, Weill Medical College of Cornell University, Burke Rehabilitation Hospital, White Plains, NY

Christiane Reitz, MD, PhD   The Taub Institute for Research on Alzheimer's Disease and the Aging Brain; The Gertrude H. Sergievsky Center, The Departments of Neurology, College of Physicians and Surgeons, Columbia University, New York, NY

Steven P. Ringel, MD   Department of Neurology, University of Colorado Health Sciences Center, Aurora, CO

Yvonne D. Rollins, MD, PhD   Department of Neurology, University of Colorado Health Sciences Center, Aurora, CO

Gary A. Rosenberg, MD   Departments of Neurology, Neurosciences, and Cell Biology and Physiology, University of New Mexico Health Sciences Center, Albuquerque, NM

Robert L. Ruff, MD, PhD   Neurology Division, Louis Stokes Cleveland Department of Veterans Affairs Medical Center; Departments of Neurology and Neurosciences, Case Western Reserve Medical School; and the Functional Electrical Stimulation Center, Cleveland, OH

Elena Rykhlevskaia, PhD   Department of Psychology, Vista Lab, Stanford University, Stanford, CA

Gabrielle H. Saunders, PhD   National Center for Rehabilitative Auditory Research, Department of Otolaryngology, Oregon Health and Science University, Portland, OR

David Schiff, MD   Neuro-Oncology Center, Departments of Neurology, Neurological Surgery, and Medicine, University of Virginia, Charlottesville, VA

David Schnyer, PhD   Department of Psychology, The University of Texas at Austin, Austin, TX

Patrica Scripko, MD   Neurological Institute, Department of Neurology, Cleveland Clinic Foundation, Cleveland Clinic Lerner College of Medicine, Cleveland, OH

Stephen M. Selkirk, MD, PhD   Spinal Cord Injury Division, Louis Stokes Cleveland Department of Veterans Affairs Medical Center; Department of Neurology, Case Western Reserve Medical School; and the Advanced Platform Technology Center of Excellence, Cleveland VA Medical Center, Cleveland, OH

Krupa Shah, MD, MPH   Instructor in Medicine, Department of Medicine, Division of Geriatrics and Aging, University of Rochester School of Medicine, Rochester, NY

Avron Spiro, III, PhD   VA Boston Health Care System; and, Department of Epidemiology, Boston University School of Public Health, Boston, MA

Matthew B. Stern, MD   Director, Parkinson's Disease and Movement Disorders Center University of Pennsylvania, Philadelphia, PA

Mark Stillman, MD   Neurological Institute, Department of Neurology, Cleveland Clinic Foundation, Cleveland Clinic Lerner College of Medicine, Cleveland, OH

Joan M. Swearer, PhD   Clinical Professor of Neurology and Psychiatry, University of Massachusetts Medical School, Worcester, MA

Jennifer A. Tracy, MD   Consultant, Department of Neurology, Mayo Clinic, Rochester, MN

Gary R. Turner, PhD   Heart and Stroke Foundation Centre for Stroke Recovery, Sunnybrook Health Sciences Centre, Toronto, ON

Anne C. Van Cott, MD, FAAN   Associate Professor, VA Pittsburgh Healthcare System, University of Pittsburgh, Department of Neurology, Pittsburgh, PA

Dennis T. Villareal, MD   Chief, Geriatrics, New Mexico VAHCS, Professor of Medicine, University of New Mexico School of Medicine, NM

Harry V. Vinters, MD   Section of Neuropathology, Departments of Pathology & Lab Medicine and Neurology, David Geffen School of Medicine at UCLA, Los Angeles, CA

Howard L. Weiner, MD   Partners Multiple Sclerosis Center, Brigham and Women's Hospital, Harvard Medical School, Boston, MA

G. Bryan Young, MD, FAAN   Department of Neurology, London health Services Center, London, Canada, ON

1
Introduction to Geriatric Neurology

1 Geriatric Neurology—An Introduction

Janice E. Knoefel and Martin L. Albert

It would be a mistake to assume that all age-related changes are negative or reflect decline. Of a random sample of 106 men and women aged 65 or older who were asked the following question: "What, if anything, gets better as you get older," 62% replied, "I feel calmer than I used to. The world's problems don't bother me as much" (our paraphrase of a typical response. Unpublished data). The remaining 38% initially replied, "Nothing gets better. Everything gets worse." And, then, "Well, now that you mention it, there are some things that do get better—friendships, for example." In a poem written to celebrate the fiftieth anniversary of the Class of 1825 in Bowdoin College, Henry Wadsworth Longfellow offered the following gift:

> But why, you ask me, should this tale be told
> To men grown old, or who are growing old?…
> Cato learned Greek at eighty; Sophocles
> Wrote his grand Oedipus, and Simonides
> Bore off the prize of verse from his compeers,
> When each had numbered more than fourscore years…
> Goethe at Weimar, toiling to the last,
> Completed Faust when eighty years were past.
> What then? Shall we sit idly down and say
> The night hath come; it is no longer day?
> Something remains for us to do or dare;
> Even the oldest tree some fruit may bear;
> For age is opportunity no less
> Than youth itself, though in another dress,
> And as the evening twilight fades away
> The sky is filled with stars, invisible by day.

This third edition of our book, *Clinical Neurology of Aging*, is committed to the optimism and hope (and wise neurological perspective) implicit in the last quatrain:

> For age is opportunity no less
> Than youth itself, though in another dress,
> And as the evening twilight fades away
> The sky is filled with stars, invisible by day.

Our world is flooded with the fear-inducing announcement that American society is witnessing an unprecedented increase in the aging of its population. The U.S. Census Bureau and the Division of Vital Statistics at the Centers for Disease Control and Prevention provide compelling evidence of the demographic shift this country is undergoing. Nearly 39 million people are already over the age of 65, with 15 million waiting to join the ranks during the next 5 years and another 18 million in the 5 years beyond that (U.S. Census Bureau, DP-1 2009). This epidemic of good health and longevity far exceeds the population projections of 25 years ago that predicted "only" 31 million by today.

What accounts for this trend? The age-adjusted death rate for 2006 (the latest year for which such data are available) was 777 deaths per 100,000 standard population—a decrease of 3% from the 2005 rate and, historically, a record low. Age-specific death rates decreased for almost all age groups in 2006 and, most pertinent to this book, included all groups greater than 34 years of age. Life expectancy at birth rose from 69.6 years in 1955 to 75.8 years in 1995, 77.4 years in 2005, 77.7 years in 2006, and to a record 77.9 years in 2007. The declining age-adjusted death rate is the principal contributor to the continuing increases in longevity.

Let us, as neurologists and other health care specialists concerned about the elderly, consider the concept of disability in this aging population. Disability implies the need for environmental intervention and adaptation and, often, assistance from formal and informal caregiving networks. The U.S. Census Bureau measures disability by self-report in the following categories: any disability, sensory disability, physical disability, mental disability, self-care disability and, for the population over the age of 16, a go-outside-the-home disability. Rates of self-reported disability consistently increase with increasing age. For persons over the age of 65, the numbers are staggering. The category of any disability reaches 38%. Those with a sensory disability comprise 15% of the group; a physical disability affects 28%. Mental disabilities are noted by 10% of the population. For those aged 65 and above, 8% have a self-care deficit and nearly 15% have difficulty going outside the home environment (U.S. Census Bureau, S1801 2009).

Aside from neurological conditions, such as migraine headaches, myasthenia gravis, or multiple sclerosis, that peak in incidence in young to middle-aged adults, the vast burden of neurological disease in adults begins squarely in late middle age and inexorably increases in incidence and prevalence until the far reaches of old age (e.g., the dementias, cerebrovascular disease, Parkinson's disease, etc.). This burden of neurological illness in the older population accounts for a disproportionate share of disabilities when compared with other medical and surgical illnesses of equal severity. The medical conditions of heart disease and cancer, for example, while far more likely to be fatal, usually cause little disability until close to the end of life.

This book, then, is designed to help neurologists and other health care specialists understand and manage the neurologic diseases and disabilities of old age. At the same time, it attempts to clarify the distinctions, sometimes fine, between normal neurological changes of aging and pathological changes due to neurological disease or medical disease secondarily affecting the nervous system. As pointed out repeatedly during the past twenty years, "mild changes in neurologic function occur with aging but generally do not substantially interfere with everyday activities unless disease intervenes" (Morris and McManus 1991).

Neurologists are expected, with increasing frequency and regularity, to provide care for older adults. Practitioners of geriatric neurology are defined by their expertise in the diagnosis and treatment of those neurological conditions that affect older individuals. The specialty of geriatric neurology is informed by the unique body of knowledge regarding the aging nervous system, its vulnerability to specific neurological disorders, and its influence on the prevalence and expression of neurological disease.

Maximizing success in clinical care of the elderly requires expertise in geriatric neurology. This includes an understanding of current research regarding the clinical and scientific basis of aging and age-related neurological dysfunction, and the ability to work and communicate effectively with other health care providers. Providing high-quality clinical care suited to the special needs of the elderly with neurological disorders requires screening, diagnostic cognitive and functional evaluation, treatment and management. The practitioner must understand and access support of co-treating specialists, such as primary care providers, rehabilitation therapists, nurses, pharmacists, community and home service providers, supportive counseling therapists, psycho-social intervention specialists, and, ultimately, practitioners of end-of-life care. The most successful providers of high quality neurological care to older adults work routinely with interdisciplinary teams, members of which are all oriented to the care of the elderly.

What do we know about the involvement of specific health disciplines in the care of the geriatric patient? Analysis by the Bureau of Health Professions, National Center for Health Workforce of the U.S. Department of Health and Human Services reports that patients 65 and older currently comprise 28% of the physician workload in primary care, 32% in surgical care, 43% in medical specialty care, and 43% in emergency medical care. Persons over the age of 65 account for 48% of hospital in-patient days.

The need for neurology expertise in the upcoming geriatric tsunami will be even more demanding since, according to current statistics, adult neurologists consult with and care for patients consistently older than those under the care of general surgeons, internists, family medicine doctors, and emergency room care providers. At the present time, few neurologists are trained specifically in geriatrics or geriatric neurology. How will the field of neurology progress from the current "here" of little common geriatric expertise to the future "there" of routine minimum competencies in the care of older individuals?

In an op-ed article for the New York Times, geriatrician Rosanne M. Leipzig writes that

> "Medicare...contributes more than $8 billion a year to support residency training, yet it does not require that part of that training focus on the unique healthcare needs of older adults"
>
> (Leipzig 2009).

Consequently, Medicare beneficiaries receive care from doctors, both trainees and attendings, who likely have had little or no specific training in any aspect of geriatrics. Dr. Leipzig proposes that Medicare money be used for at least some minimal training of residents in care of the elderly. The recently published Consensus on Minimum Geriatrics Competencies for Graduating Medical Students (Leipzig 2009) provides a roadmap of competencies that are needed by a new intern to care adequately for older adults. This consensus is based largely on 10 years of curriculum development activity conducted by the American Geriatrics Society's Education Committee regarding its objectives for medical student education (Education Committee Writing Group of the American Geriatrics Society 2000). The 40 U.S. medical schools participating in this medical school curriculum development effort were funded by the John A. Hartford Foundation specifically for enhanced training in geriatric principles at the medical student level (Anderson 2004). One would imagine, consequently, that

the field of neurology may soon be receiving more assistance from future trainees in its care of aging America than it realizes.

The 2008 Institute of Medicine report "Retooling for an Aging America" furthermore has recommended support for more geriatric training at all levels of health care, resolving that all licensed health care professionals, from physicians to nursing aides, should be required to demonstrate competence in the care of older adults (Institute of Medicine [IOM] 2008). This report resulted from intensive examination and discussion of all aspects of geriatric care by a large, diverse, and interdisciplinary group of educators, clinicians, and industry representatives. The IOM report examines avenues for improving health care of the elderly, concentrating on three main areas: enhancing geriatric competence; increasing recruitment and retention of geriatric health care workers; and improving models of care for the elderly. The report specified that all licensure, certification, and maintenance of certification for health care professionals should include demonstration of competence in the care of older adults as a necessary criterion.

The first edition of this book, appearing 25 years ago, maintained that geriatric neurology embraces all intersecting points between the disciplines of neurology and geriatrics. Charcot was cited as asserting, "The importance of a special study of diseases of old age would not be contested at the present day" (Charcot 1867). The set of clinically focused chapters in this book attests to the accuracy, clarity, and farsightedness of Charcot's claim. He would likely be incredulous at the current state of knowledge of neurological aging and disease.

References

Anderson MB, ed. The AAMC-Hartford Geriatric Curriculum Program: Reports from 40 schools. *Acad Med.* 2004; 79(7 suppl): S1-S226.

Charcot J-M. *Lecons sur les Maladies des Viellards et les Maladies Chroniques.* Paris, Hopital de la Salpetriere, 1867.

Heron M, Hoyert DL, Murphy SL, Xu J, Kochanek KD, Tejada-Vera B. Deaths: Final data for 2006. *National Vital Statistics Reports,* Volume 57, Number 14, April 2009, DHHS Publication No. (PHS) 2009-1120.

Institute of Medicine. Retooling for an aging America: Building the health care workforce. Washington, DC: The National Academies Press; 2008.

Leipzig, RM. The patients doctors don't know. *New York Times* on the Web July 1, 2009. Opinion. www.nytimes.com/2009/07/02/opinion.

Morris JC, McManus DQ. The neurology of aging: normal versus pathologic change. *Geriatrics.* 46: 47–48, 51–54, 1991.

The Education Committee Writing Group of the American Geriatrics Society. Core competencies for the care of older patients: Recommendations of the American Geriatrics Society. *Acad Med.* 2000;75:252–255.

U.S. Census Bureau, DP-1, 2009.

U.S. Census Bureau, S0101, 2009.

U.S. Census Bureau, S1801, 2009.

U.S. Census Bureau, GCT-T4-R, 2009.

U.S. Census Bureau, GCT-T5-R, 2009.

U.S. Department of Health and Human Services, Health Resources and Services Administration, Bureau of Health Processions National Center for Health Workforce Analysis. Exhibit 2.11. Estimated percentage of physician's time spent providing care to patients, by age of patient. In: *Changing Demographics: Implications for Physicians, Nurses, and Other Health Workers. Section 2: Aging of the Population.* Available at: (http://bhpr.hrsa.gov/healthworkforce/reports/changedemo/images/2.11.htm).

2 Epidemiology of Aging and Age-related Neurological Disease

Christiane Reitz and Richard Mayeux

The term "epidemiology" describes the study of the frequency and causes of disease. Accordingly, epidemiological studies are used to define the relationship between a disease and its etiology, or factors that are antecedents to disease or alter its course or its manifestations. Studies of the frequency of disease include estimates of the prevalence and incidence rates and may also include disease-specific mortality rates. Most epidemiological studies are typically observational in nature but can also include other study designs, such as randomized clinical trials. Analytical studies are designed to evaluate specific hypotheses. The null form of the hypothesis is a specific statement such as "compared with disease-free individuals, having diabetes mellitus does not increase the risk of Alzheimer's disease." The "null" implies that there is no relation between the postulated cause and effect, and is in principle refutable. While the hypotheses are stated in qualitative terms, the testing of hypotheses is based on direct measurement in humans. Thus, a central task in epidemiological research is not only to quantify the occurrence of disease in populations, but to identify its antecedents.

Epidemiological studies require the measurement of the association between a risk factor or an exposure and a disease, and it is crucial to consider that observed associations can be due to chance or issues inherent to the study design such as bias or confounding. In this chapter we will address the basic methodological concepts and tools of epidemiological research as applicable for research on aging and age-related neurological disease. We will introduce the commonly used measures of disease frequency, important issues in definition of cases and controls, and the common types of analytical studies. Then we will address the use of biomarkers in research on aging-related disease, commonly used measures of effect and association, and criteria for causal inference. Finally, we will address issues on precision and validity that must be considered when performing epidemiological research.

Measures of Disease Frequency

As described above, the fundamental task in epidemiological research is to quantify the frequency (occurrence) of disease in populations. Crucial when measuring disease occurrence, is to record the number of persons observed, the period of time during which events are counted, and the time elapsed before the disease occurs. The most common measures of disease frequency are "incidence rate," "incidence proportion," and "prevalence."

Incidence is a measure of the risk of developing a new condition within a specific period of time. It is particularly useful when events are studied that are in principle avoidable or that may not occur during the period of observation, leading to the potential that not all events in the population will be observed. Although sometimes simply expressed as the number of new cases occurring during a specific time period, incidence is better expressed as a rate or proportion with a denominator.

Incidence Rate

The incidence rate takes into account the number of individuals in a population that newly develop the disease, and the length of time contributed by all persons during the period they were in the population when events were counted ("person-time at risk"). It has units of inverse time (per year, per month, per day, etc.).

$$\text{Incidence rate} = \frac{\text{Number of disease onsets}}{\sum \text{time spent in populations persons}}$$

When calculating the person-time for the incidence rate, the type of population has to be considered. A closed population adds no new members over time and loses members only to death. As a consequence, a closed cohort ages and becomes smaller over time. In contrast, an open population can gain members through immigration or birth (i.e., individual contributions need not begin at the same time), and can lose members through emigration or death (Figure 1). An open population that has no growth or shrinkage, with a constant number of births and deaths is called "stationary" (i.e., population is in "steady state").

Incidence Proportions and Survival Proportions

When considering a given interval of time, and the population is a "closed population" (i.e., the population size at the beginning of the interval is measured and no one enters or leaves the population after the start of the interval), we can also calculate the proportion of people who become cases among those who entered the interval. Thus, we can calculate the average risk of a specific population to develop the disease.

This quantity is called the "incidence proportion" or "cumulative incidence." Like any other proportion, it ranges from zero to one and is dimensionless. To be interpretable, however, the time period to which it applies must be specified. An incidence proportion of 12%, for example, indicates a very different burden of disease when it refers to a 10-year period than when it refers to a 10-day period. Three useful additional measures of frequency are the "survival proportion," the "incidence odds," and the "incidence density." The survival proportion is the proportion of a closed population at risk that does not experience the disease within the time of observation (for example persons that do not develop a stroke during 5 years of follow-up). The incidence odds is the ratio of the proportion developing the disease to the proportion not developing the disease. Incidence density is the frequency of new events in a given time period. This measure is particularly useful in research of potentially recurrent conditions such as

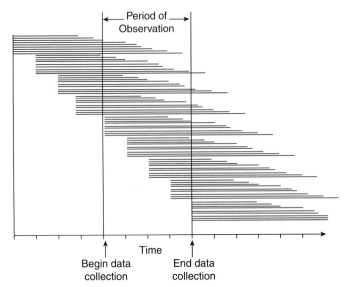

Figure 1 Concept of an open population.

seizures or cerebrovascular events (TIA) (Rothman and Greenland 1998; Johnston 2006).

Prevalence

In contrast to incidence measures, which focus on new events, prevalence (also called "point prevalence," "prevalence proportion," and "prevalence rate") focuses on disease status and is defined as the proportion of the population having the disease at a specific point in time. The prevalence over a specified interval of time such as a calendar year is called "period prevalence."

The subset of the population that has the disease is called the "prevalence pool." Persons exit the prevalence pool by dying from the disease, recovering from the disease, or by emigrating from the population. Consequently, both death and recovery from illness decrease disease prevalence. A disease with high incidence rate, such as cholera, can have low prevalence if it is rapidly fatal. Accordingly, prevalence can also be expressed as the product of incidence rate and duration of disease.

$$\text{Prevalence} = \frac{\text{Number of cases}}{\text{Number of persons in population}}$$
$$= \text{Incidence rate} * \text{Duration of Disease}$$

Other rates. Additional rates of interest are "specific rates," "adjusted/standardized rates," "mortality rate," and the "case-fatality rate." Specific rates are calculated after a population has been categorized into groups with a particular characteristic, e.g. age or sex-specific rates. "Adjusted" or "standardized rates" are crude rates that are modified to control for the effects of age or sex (most frequently) or another characteristic. Standardization can be performed using "direct standardization" (a standard set of weights are applied to a population) or "indirect standardization" (a set of rates from one or more populations (considered as standard) are applied to the population of interest). The comparison between the study population (observed rate) and the standard (adjusted or expected rate) is called "standardized morbidity (mortality) ratio (SMR)." The mortality rate is a measure of the number of deaths (in general, or due to a specific cause) in a population, scaled to the size of that population, per unit

time. It is typically expressed in units of deaths per 1000 individuals per year; thus, a mortality rate of 9.5 in a population of 100,000 would mean 950 deaths per year in that population.

$$\text{Mortality rate} = \frac{\text{number of deaths during a specific time period}}{\text{number of persons in population}}$$

The term case-fatality rate refers to the rate of persons diagnosed as having a specified disease who die as a result of that illness within a given period. This term is often applied to a specific outbreak of acute disease, for example, meningococcal meningitis, in which all patients have been followed for an adequate period of time to include all attributable deaths, or is applied to potentially fatal diseases that, due to their high frequency, play important roles on a public health level. For example, it is a commonly used measure to describe incidence and prognosis of stroke (Sacco, Marini, Toni, Olivieri, and Carolei 2009; Saposnik, Cote, Phillips, et al 2008; Saposnik, Hill, O'Donnell, Fang, Hachinski, and Kapral 2008). Case-fatality rate must be clearly distinguished from the mortality rate.

$$\text{Case-fatality rate} = \frac{\text{Number of death from a disease}}{\text{Number of individuals with the disease}}$$

Definition of Cases and Controls

Crucial to a valid study design is the appropriate definition of disease and health (i.e., definition of cases and controls). When defining a person as a "case" or "control," the definition of presence or absence of disease must take into account degrees of severity. The largest possible case group is a case group that includes mild forms of the disease. However, broad criteria (lack of specificity) can produce misclassification, affect the validity of the study, and can result in an observation of no difference between cases and controls. Severe forms of the disease are less likely to be misclassified and easier to recognize. Restriction of the case group to severe cases only (lack of sensitivity), however, can lead to exclusion of some forms of the illness and to a loss of precision and power by reducing the sample size. In any study, validity should outweigh power and precision concerns. Specificity (and more restrictive case definitions) should outweigh sensitivity (and more inclusive case definitions).

A common bias in case selection is the Berkson's bias, which is the probability of hospitalization among cases with one or more conditions compared with that among cases with only one of the conditions. Hospital cases are different and most likely "sicker" than a group of cases drawn from a general population. They are included in the study because they "came to the clinic." The motivation for coming to the clinic is not measurable and the degree to which this bias affects the outcome of the study is unknown. Selection of cases simply because they reside in a particular place of residence (e.g. community, town, or county) greatly lessens such bias and, in addition, insures a more representative case selection. A good alternative is to include all cases from all regional practitioners. In case selection, it is crucial to ensure that all cases in the population have an equal opportunity to be included.

Additional bias can be induced by a methodological issue called "Neyman's fallacy." This term refers to the use of prevalent versus incident cases in observational studies. Incident cases may die, leaving only a unique subset of individuals as prevalent cases. Thereby, risk factors may identify survivors or non-diseased, and clinical trials that use prevalent cases may represent the more chronic, lingering, less curable forms of disease. A solution to this kind of bias is to include all types of cases including incident or recently diagnosed cases, and cases that represent the whole spectrum of disease. That may mean that individuals with co-morbid illness are included.

Definition of the comparison (control) group. The selection of a control is the most important factor in a clinical investigation. Controls should be selected to reflect the source population; to eliminate potential confounders such as age, ethnic group, or educational background; and should be selected for comparable accuracy to limit recall/reporting bias. Exclusions that apply to cases must also apply to controls. Controls can be a random sample from the population; for example, recruited by random digit dialing; or sampling from health- or service-related data or marketing lists; or a non-random sample such as other hospital patients, neighborhood controls, or spouse controls. In any case, the principle of representativeness must be maintained.

Types of Analytical Studies

Most epidemiological studies are comparative, where groups differing by an exposure of interest (risk factor) are compared for an outcome of interest. The aim of such studies is to assess the effect of the exposure, often expressed as a relative risk or odds ratio (see above). The exposure can be a condition like diabetes, a treatment like donezepil, or a practice like wearing a helmet when doing construction work. The common epidemiological study designs can be broadly divided into two groups: observational studies and experimental studies (Table 1).

Non-experimental studies. The case-control study is essentially retrospective and estimates the odds of having been exposed to a risk factor given the current case-control status. The advantage of a case-control study is its relatively low cost at high efficiency. Cases are selected based on a priori criteria, and matched with healthy controls without the disease from the same source population the cases emerged from. In both cases and controls, the investigator ascertains historical information regarding the type, duration, and means of exposure. The purpose of the control group is to estimate the distribution of exposure in the source population. Therefore, the cardinal requirement of control selection is that the controls must be sampled independent of their exposure status. A serious draw-back of the case-control study design is that disease and exposure status are determined simultaneously. As a consequence, the temporal sequence is

often difficult to establish. One cannot measure absolute incidence rates of disease in those exposed and unexposed to a risk factor, nor calculate attributable risks (risk differences) between those exposed and unexposed. Another problem inherent in the retrospective study design is recall bias affecting the validity of the exposure measure, as cases are more likely than controls to have considered possible explanations for their illness. For example, persons who suffered from a stroke are more likely to recall detection of high blood cholesterol or glucose levels at an earlier doctor's visit than persons who never have had a stroke.

A study that includes as subjects all persons in the population at the time of ascertainment or a representative sample of all such persons, including those who have the disease, is called "cross-sectional study." A cross-sectional study conducted to estimate prevalence is called a "prevalence study." Usually, the exposure information is collected simultaneously with the disease information, so that different exposure subpopulations may be compared with respect to their disease prevalence. A problem of the cross-sectional study can be that the cases in a cross-sectional study will over-represent cases with long duration and under-represent those with short duration of illness. For example, a person contracting the disease of interest at age 30 and living until age 80 can be included in any cross-sectional study during the person's 50 years of disease. In contrast, a person contracting the disease at age 40 and dying within a day has almost no chance of inclusion. Thus, if exposure does not alter disease risk but causes the disease to be very mild if contracted, the prevalence of exposure will be elevated among cases. As a result, a highly significant exposure-disease association will be observed even if exposure has no effect on disease risk. If the exposure causes the disease to be rapidly fatal, the prevalence of exposure will be very low among cases and the exposure-disease association in the population will be very negative.

Cross-sectional studies often deal with exposures that cannot change, such as sex or blood type. For such exposures, current information is useful. For variable exposures, however, current information is often less desirable than etiologically more relevant information from before the case occurred (i.e., exposure history). In a study of the etiology of stroke that compares blood pressure on cases and noncases, current blood pressure levels are not as relevant as their blood pressure histories before the stroke occurred. In fact, use of current blood pressure may even be misleading, as blood pressure can change as a consequence of stroke.

The classic cohort study is a prospective study design in which the exposure status is ascertained before occurrence of disease. This allows calculation of incidence rates in those exposed and unexposed to the risk factors, but it is costly as it requires follow-up of a large number of individuals because risk factor data are collected prior to disease onset. An additional problem of longitudinal follow-up is that investigators are not always able to control confounding variables and maintain high follow-up rates. Adverse outcomes may occur prior to onset of the disease of interest. For example, in a prospective study on Alzheimer's disease, myocardial infarction or stroke are likely to occur at higher frequency ("competing risks"). Another problem with longitudinal follow-up is that the risk factors under observation may become less important during the period of observation. A study on the impact of a diabetes diagnosis on Alzheimer's disease may need to include insulin or glucose levels. If the investigators did not include that information at the baseline interview, it will be difficult to add it at a later visit without biasing the results.

Occasionally, a cohort may have been gathered for a specific investigation and followed for a period. Later, an investigator may want to reconstitute the cohort in order to investigate another disease entity.

Table 1 Common Types of Epidemiologic Study Designs

Study Type	Methodological Approach
Non-experimental studies	
Case-control study	Sampling with respect to disease status
Cross-sectional study	Inclusion of all subjects of a population regardless of exposure or disease status(→ exposure and disease status are assessed at the same point in time)
Cohort study	Sampling with respect to exposure status
Experimental (randomized) studies	
Clinical trial	Individuals are the unit of study

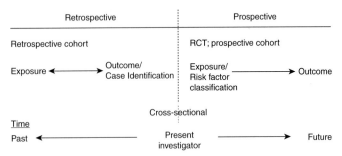

Figure 2 Retrospective, cross-sectional and prospective study design.

The investigator may wish to study factors that were collected previously but will investigate new outcomes or diseases which were not part of the original study goals. This "retrospective" cohort has the design of a prospective cohort but cases are determined in the present time. This type of study is more practical and less costly than prospective cohort studies, but it is often difficult to reconstruct the original cohort and identify other factors accounting for disease occurrence at follow-up, which may affect validity. An alternative, but less often used method is the case-base method in which a random sample of the base or referent population is interviewed for the putative risk factors. Then all incident cases are identified from the entire base population over a specified time period and the frequencies of risk factors in these cases are determined. Because the sampled base yields essentially complete information on the base population, the investigator is able to estimate rates of disease in those exposed and unexposed to the risk factors of interest, assess the attributable risk, and establish risk profiles with considerable economy over the cohort method. However, the problem of temporal direction is difficult to establish in this type of investigation because the same issues that limit the usefulness of case-control studies apply here as well: ascertainment of patient status and risk factors occur at the same time.

In summary, while cross-sectional, case-control and case-base studies are economical and more pragmatic than longitudinal studies, they may only be useful for deriving hypotheses. In most instances, definite analytic studies need to rely on prospective cohort studies of risk factors. Figure 2 shows the different types of analytic studies.

Experimental studies. Experimental studies often use randomization to assign the exposure to study participants. Through randomization, one attempts to ensure that the groups that are being compared are similar in any aspect except for the exposure. The larger the study, the greater the likelihood that randomization will be successful. If the study is small, stratified randomization can ensure balance with respect to other factors known to be related to exposure and the outcome ("confounders"). Under the null hypothesis that the exposure has no effect, randomization allows a probability to be calculated for the observed difference in outcome. Thus, it provides the basis for valid statistical testing.

The clinical trial is an experiment with patients as subjects. The aim of a clinical trial is either to evaluate a potential cure for a disease or to find a preventive of disease consequences such as death or disability. The exposures in a clinical trial, usually drugs of interest, are not primary preventives since they do not prevent occurrence of the initial disease, but they are preventives of the sequelae of the initial disease. For example, intake of donepezil slows progression of Alzheimer's disease.

Subjects whose illness is too mild or too severe to permit the form of treatment being studied should be excluded. In addition to randomized group assignment, clinical trials should attempt to employ

blinding with respect to the treatment assignment. Ideally, the individual who makes the assignment, the patient, and the assessor of the outcome should all be ignorant of the treatment assignment ("triple blind study"). If that is not possible, it is most important to keep the assessor of the outcome blind, especially if the outcome assessment is largely subjective, such as a clinical diagnosis of cognitive impairment or parkinsonism. Patient knowledge of the treatment assignment can affect compliance with the treatment regimen and can bias perception of symptoms that might affect the outcome assessment. Studies in which both the assessor and the patient are blinded as to the treatment assignment are called "double-blind" studies.

If there is no established treatment for the disease being studied, it can be useful to employ a placebo as the comparison treatment. By employing a placebo, an investigator can control for the psychological component of offering treatment and can study the non-psychological benefit of a new intervention. In addition, employing a placebo facilitates blinding if there would otherwise be no comparison treatment. However, when effective treatment is available, the use of placebos may be unethical and the best available treatment should be used as the comparison intervention.

Measures of Effect and Measures of Association

In epidemiology, an effect is the result of a given cause ("exposure"), i.e., the amount of change in a population's disease frequency caused by a specific factor. If disease frequency is measured in terms of incidence rate or proportion, then the effect is the change in incidence rate or proportion brought about by a specific factor. For example, we may say that for persons who have hypertension compared to persons who do not have hypertension, the risk of Alzheimer's disease increases by a certain percent per year. In this case, the percentage per year indicates the effect size of the risk factor. Absolute effects are differences in incidence proportions, incidence rates, prevalences or incidence times. Relative effects are ratios of these measures.

Measures of association can be illustrated using the cohort study design. The cumulative incidence or incidence density of two groups can be compared either on an absolute or relative scale. On an absolute scale, one can calculate a risk or rate difference. On a relative scale, one can take the ratios of two cumulative incidences or incidence densities, called relative risk or relative rate. Relative measures are more frequently used in etiologic research than absolute measures because they indicate the strength of the association. When considering implications of research for an individual patient, however, measurement on an absolute scale is more relevant.

In many case control studies the absolute size of the exposed and non-exposed population at risk cannot be estimated, making it impossible to ascertain a cumulative incidence or incidence density, or to calculate a rate difference. However, a relative risk or rate may be approximated by means of an odds ratio. The odds ratio is obtained by dividing the odds of having the risk factor (number with risk factor/number without risk factor) among the cases, by the odds of having the risk factor (number with risk factor/number without risk factor) among the controls.

It is also possible to calculate other measures of risk such as the attributable risk (i.e., etiologic fraction). These measures, which refer to an exposed group or a total population, are used to estimate the proportion of disease occurrence that is attributable to a specific exposure of interest. All formulas for these measures of association can be derived from a standard 2x2 table and using I_0 = incidence of outcome among the unexposed (baseline risk), I_e = incidence of outcome among the exposed, P_0 = prevalence of outcome among the unexposed (baseline risk), P_e = prevalence of outcome among the exposed:

Outcome (Disease)

		Yes	No	
Exposure	Yes	a	b	a+b
	No	c	d	c+d
		a+c	b+d	

Risk Difference (attributable risk) = a/(a+b) − c/(c+d) = Ie−Io

Risk ratio (RR, CIR) = $\dfrac{a/(a+b)}{c/(c+d)}$ = Ie/Io

Odds ratio (OR) = $\dfrac{a/c}{b/d} = \dfrac{ad}{bc}$

Prevalence ratio = Pe/Po

Attributable risk = a/(a+b) − c/(c+d) = Ie−Io (the same as risk difference)

Causation and Causal Inference

Disease pathway. The concept of the causal disease pathway is a means of demonstrating how and when factors act in the process of the disease (Figure 3). "Etiology" refers to a specific cause, while "pathogenesis" defines the biological process by which the etiology results in disease. The time interval between causal action (etiology) and disease initiation is called the "induction period." The interval between the induction of a disease and its detection is called "latency period" (Rothman and Greenland 1998). While the latent period can be reduced by improvement of disease detection, the true induction period, in contrast, cannot since the disease occurrence marks the end of the induction period. Earlier detection of disease may, however, reduce the apparent induction period: the time between the causal action and the detection of disease.

In neurological disorders or diseases of aging, both the induction period and the latency period are often long. Patterns of associations between factors and disease can indicate where influences act in the disease pathway. For example, risk factors that act during the induction period will most likely have direct effects on risk. For example, traumatic head injury is thought to increase the risk by promoting amyloid beta deposition and tau pathology in the brain. Thus, by acting as an inducer of disease, head injury could increase the risk of dementia.

Studies exploring the effect of exposures during the latency period might in contrast identify risk factors that do not cause, but modify (increase or decrease), the risk associated with the true etiology. They may also identify factors that are in fact a consequence of the disease

("reverse causation"). For example, several studies suggested that high body mass index in late life decreases the risk of Alzheimer's disease, while low body mass index increases disease risk. While it is possible that higher body mass index in fact diminishes the risk, it is also possible that patients lose weight as a result of the disease, for example due to changes in eating behavior or metabolic state during the latency period before the disease is diagnosed. Thus, low body mass index during the latency period might reflect a manifestation of disease rather than a true modifier of disease risk.

Risk factors and causal inference. Risk factors are antecedents that are considered to be components of the disease pathway. They are usually related to the etiology or the cause of the disease or the outcome being investigated. Causal inference from an observed association between a risk factor and a disease is difficult. The investigator needs always to consider the possibility that the association might be due to chance or to some other factor ("confounding"). The "cause" of the disease is an event, condition, or characteristic that plays an essential role in producing an occurrence of the disease. However, it does not have to do so in everyone. For example, while it is clear that smoking "causes" lung cancer, it does not do so in everyone, but only in those susceptible to the effects of smoking. Nonetheless, risk factors, both genetic and environmental, may be considered "causal" by researchers if they are found in a higher proportion in individuals with than without the disease, or if the risk of developing disease over a specified time is greater for those individuals with than without the risk factor. However, it is often difficult to distinguish between a causal and a non-causal association for any given factor and a disease. Epidemiologists rely on the principles of causal inference (Rothman and Greenland 1998). In brief, associations should be strong on the argument that weak associations may be due to confounding or bias. One asks whether the association is a) an artifact of the data collection method, b) indirect due to a measured or unmeasured third variable, and c) due to a causal process operating in the opposite direction ("reverse causation"). Although bias due to an unmeasured variable can never be excluded in an observational study, further steps to assess the likelihood of a causal relationship include consideration of 1) the strength of the association; 2) the consistency of the association in different populations and across different study designs; 3) the specificity of the association; 4) the presence of a dose-response relationship; 5) temporality; and 6) the biologic plausibility of the association.

1. **Strength of the association.** Hill (1965) argued that strong associations are more likely to be causal than weak associations. However, at the same time, he acknowledged that the fact that an association is weak does not rule out a causal connection. A commonly cited example for a weak but causal association is the relation between smoking and cardiovascular disease (point estimates have been consistently between 1.4 and 2.2). As described above, frequently used measures of association are odds ratios, risk ratios, and hazard ratios.

2. **Consistency of the association in different populations and across different study designs.** Hundreds of studies have shown that aging and Alzheimer's disease are associated, and no large, well-designed study has failed to show this association. In contrast, whether estrogen replacement therapy is associated with Alzheimer's disease is uncertain because some studies show an association, but others do not. Meta-analysis is a good method for testing consistency. It summarizes the odds ratios from various studies.

3. **Specificity of the association.** The criterion of specificity requires that a cause leads to a single effect, not multiple effects. This criterion is invalid as causes of a given effect cannot be expected to

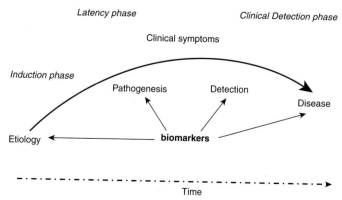

Figure 3 Causal pathway of disease.

lack other effects. A good example for this is "age." Aging is a cause of Alzheimer's disease but also many other age-related diseases such as macular degeneration, osteoarthritis, osteoporosis, and cancer.

4. **Presence of a dose-response relationship**. If a regular gradient of disease risk is found to parallel a gradient in exposure (e.g. persons with slightly elevated insulin levels develop Alzheimer's disease (AD) at a rate intermediate between persons with normal and severely elevated levels) the likelihood of a causal relationship is enhanced. Dose-response is often considered a subcategory of *strength*. However, a biological gradient does not apply to all exposure-disease associations: some causal associations show a threshold effect rather than a monotonic trend, others show a U-shaped or J-shaped association. For example, a study in northern New York City (Luchsinger and Mayeux 2007) found that in younger elderly (65 to 76 years of age), the association between BMI quartiles and AD resembles a U-shaped curve, while in the oldest old (> 76 years), higher BMI is related to a lower AD risk. This study also found that higher waist circumference is related to higher dementia risk in the younger elderly, but not in the oldest. Also, not all associations that show a monotonic trend are causal: confounding can result in a monotonic relation between a risk factor and a disease if the confounding factor itself demonstrates a biologic gradient in its relation with the disease. For example: the non-causal relation between birth rank and Down syndrome shows a biologic gradient that merely reflects the progressive relation between maternal age and Down syndrome occurrence.

5. **Temporality**. Temporality refers to the necessity that the cause precedes the effect in time. This criterion is inarguable, as the putative cause must precede the putative effect. It does not, however, follow that a reverse time order is evidence against the hypothesis that the putative factor can cause the disease.

6. **Biologic plausibility of the association**. This criterion implies that the findings are compatible with pre-existing theory, knowledge, or a reasonable statistical model (e.g. dose-response). For example, several studies have shown that presence of HIV serological markers is associated with greatly elevated rates of encephalitis. That HIV infection is a true cause of HIV encephalitis is also supported by the finding of the unintegrated form of the HIV-1 virus in brain tissues of persons with encephalitis following infection (Trillo-Pazos, Diamanturos, Rislove, et al. 2003).

Using these principles can help establish the type of relationship between exposure and a disease. However, only "temporality" is an irrefutable principle for causality: if the putative cause did not precede the effect, that would be indisputable evidence that the observed association is not causal. Other than that, there is no necessity of sufficient criterion for determining whether an observed association is causal. Besides temporality, consistency and biologic plausibility seem to be the most useful measures.

The use of appropriate statistical tests in addition reduces, but does not eliminate, the possibility that chance alone accounts for the observed association. Subsequent functional studies such as molecular or animal studies can help establish the causal relationship more securely. Simultaneous consideration of an appropriate study design, the principles of causal inference, and systematic bias and confounding are crucial to establish best possible validity of the study when exploring association between the exposure and disease.

Biomarkers

Invaluable tools that can aid in understanding the prediction, cause, diagnosis, progression, regression, or outcome of treatment of disease are "biomarkers." They have been defined as "cellular, biochemical or molecular alterations that are measurable in biological media such as human tissues, cells, or fluids" (Perera and Weinstein 2000). More recently, the definition has been broadened to include biological characteristics that can be objectively measured and evaluated as an indicator of normal biological processes, pathogenic processes, or pharmacological responses to a therapeutic intervention (Naylor 2003). For the nervous system, biomarkers may involve measurements directly on biological media (e.g. blood, brain, muscle, nerve, skin, or cerebrospinal fluid) or measurements, which do not involve direct sampling of biological media but measures on the composition or function of the nervous system such as brain imaging.

Biomarkers have been classified based on the sequence of events from exposure to disease (see disease pathway, Figure 3): biomarkers of exposure that are used in risk prediction and biomarkers of disease that are used in screening and diagnosis and monitoring of disease progression. Their use is well established, and they offer distinct and obvious advantages. The classification of many neurological diseases is based on either standardized clinical criteria or histological diagnosis. Biomarkers have the potential to identify neurological disease at an early stage, provide a method for homogeneous classification of a disease, and extend our knowledge base concerning the underlying disease pathogenesis. In epidemiological (or quasi-experimental) investigations, biomarkers improve validity while reducing bias in the measurement of exposures (or risk factors) for neurological disease. Rather than relying on a history of exposure to a putative risk factor which is often strongly affected by recall bias, direct measurement of the level of exposure or the chromosomal alteration resulting from the exposure lessens the possibility of misclassification of exposure. As discussed above, misclassification does not only produce inaccurate and deceptive results, but also reduces the power of studies to detect effects. Thus, the use of biomarkers improves the sensitivity and specificity of the measurement of the exposures or risk factors. Molecular biomarkers have the additional potential of identifying individuals susceptible to disease (Galasko 2001).

Biomarkers of exposure or antecedent biomarkers. When a disease is suspected of resulting from a toxic exposure, researchers will naturally wish to measure the degree of exposure. External exposure is the measured concentration of the toxin in an individual's immediate environment. While questionnaires offer an historical account of the exposure, direct measurement of the alleged toxin in the air, water, soil, or food can provide accurate information regarding the "dose" of the exposure. Measurement of the external dose provides the basis to understand the relationship to the disease process. However, measurement of the "internal" dose through identification in tissues or body fluids usually provides more accuracy by adding both internal and external validity when examining the effect of the exposure on the outcome. An example is lead exposure. A history of lead exposure can be strengthened by measurement of lead in the environment, but the best indication of the dose of exposure may be determined in blood and tissues (hair, nails, teeth).

Biomarkers are particularly useful in the cross-sectional investigation of acute disease due to the pharmacologic properties of the chemical or toxin. It is, however, very difficult to find biomarkers for exposures that are stable over the long periods required for prospective studies of chronic neurological diseases such as Alzheimer's disease. Banked serum or plasma may be of value in some instances depending on the disorder being investigated and the pharmacologic characteristics of the biomarker. In any case, issues of timing, persistence, dose, and storage site all must be considered for this class of biomarker.

Most adult onset degenerative diseases of the nervous system are likely to be a composite of both genetic and environmental risk factors. The correlated combinations of these features constitute the trait or disease. As a consequence, genetic factors can also be powerful antecedents at any stage of the disease pathway illustrated in Figure 3. They are highly valuable, as they exist before the disease occurs and are independent of other exposures, overcoming the issue of reverse causation. In addition, they improve the precision in the measurement of other associations because they may be synergistic or antagonistic.

For neurological disorders, biomarkers of genetic susceptibility are rapidly becoming more available. Identification of the variant allele in a gene, such as APOE, is quite useful in assessing risk and in providing information regarding the pathogenesis of the Alzheimer's disease. With this information investigators can now examine other genes or environmental risk factors to determine whether they modify (increase or decrease) the risk of Alzheimer's disease. Similarly, variations in several genes appear to influence susceptibility to Parkinson's disease, which has also been related to environmental risk factors. Once established, a specific genotype might be used to predict an association with a particular environmental toxin (Reiber and Peter 2001).

Biomarkers of disease. Biomarkers depicting prodromal signs enable earlier diagnosis or allow for the outcome of interest to be determined at a more primitive stage of disease. In several neurodegenerative diseases, blood, urine, and cerebrospinal fluid provide the necessary biological information for the diagnosis. In these conditions, biomarkers are used as an indicator of a biological factor that represents either a subclinical manifestation, early stage of the disorder, or a surrogate manifestation of the disease. The potential uses of this class of biomarkers include: 1) identification of individuals destined to become affected or who are in the "preclinical" stages of the illness; 2) reduction in disease heterogeneity in clinical trials or epidemiologic studies; 3) reflection of the natural history of disease encompassing the phases of induction, latency, and detection; 4) target for a clinical trial. The improvement in validity and precision far outweigh the difficulty in obtaining such tissues from patients.

Most ethical review boards and the health care systems require adequate follow-up for individuals with and without the disease who screen positive. Also, treatment should be available for those who screen positive and it must be accessible and acceptable.

Precision and Validity in Epidemiologic Studies

There are two sources of error that have to be considered when designing an epidemiologic study: random error leading to lack of precision and systematic error resulting in bias and lack of validity. The two main contributors to random error are error introduced by the selection of study subjects ("sampling variation," "sampling error"), and error introduced by the measurements of key variables. Accordingly, the primary mechanisms to increase precision of statistical estimates are to increase the sample size of the study and to improve the accuracy with which information from the study subjects is obtained. When determining the sample size of the study, it must be considered that a sample size that is too small can make it impossible to discard chance as the explanation for the lack of an effect. A good way to improve the accuracy with which information on biomarkers is obtained is to consider its reliability and repeatability. Kappa statistics

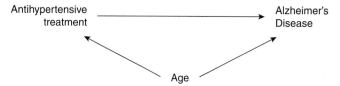

Figure 4 Confounding.

for binary or dichotomous data and intraclass correlation coefficients can help assess test-retest agreement and consistency of laboratory measurements.

The most common types of bias introduced by systematic error are "selection bias," "information bias," and "confounding." Selection bias and information bias can be controlled only during the design phase of a project; confounding can be controlled during the design stage or the data analysis stage.

Selection bias. In particular, selection bias is a major threat to the validity of a case-control study. The primary objective of choosing controls is, as described above, that they be representative of the population from which the cases were drawn. For example, a study on anti-inflammatory treatment and stroke which includes cases who smoke should also include such patients in the control group. On the other hand, if the controls were selected from hospitalized patients and the hospital had an active lung cancer center, smoking patients could be overrepresented among controls. One solution to this problem would be to exclude smokers if they were admitted for treatment related to smoking, but not if they were admitted for other problems such as a broken arm. Alternatively, one could exclude smokers from both the case and the control series. Selection bias may also occur in cohort studies if tracking of subjects for outcome is incomplete. Self-selection bias can occur whenever the group of people being studied has any form of control over whether to participate, and the participants' decision to participate is correlated with traits that affect the study. For example, if an individual is convinced that lead exposure leads to Alzheimer's disease, then individuals with such an exposure may seek to participate in a study on metal exposures and Alzheimer's disease. This self-selection bias might lead to the conclusion from the study that heavy metals are related to the cause of Alzheimer's disease.

Information bias. Information bias can affect ascertainment of exposure and outcome and can be grouped into non-differential and differential misclassification bias. In non-differential misclassification, errors are random and unrelated to exposure or outcome status. An example would be the determination of blood cholesterol levels from a single blood cholesterol measurement in a follow-up study on stroke. Non-differential misclassification tends to dilute the effect, i.e., it makes the size of any observed effect smaller than the true effect. Differential misclassification, which can be caused by recall bias as described above (i.e., cases recall having been exposed to a certain risk factor better than controls), can bias the results towards both a dilution of the effect or a falsely increased effect.

Confounding. Confounding occurs when an extraneous factor is associated with both the exposure and disease, and is not considered a mediator by which the exposure causes the disease. In a study of the relationship between antihypertensive treatment and Alzheimer's disease, age would be considered a confounder (Figure 4). There are various ways to reduce this potential bias. One could match cases and controls (or those exposed and not exposed) for age, one could restrict the age of the study participants to a narrow age range, or one could use statistical adjustment techniques to control for age in the analysis.

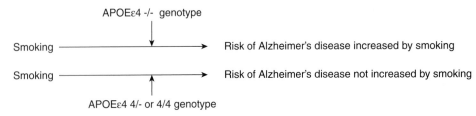

Figure 5 Effect modification of the association between smoking and Alzheimer's disease by APOE genotype.

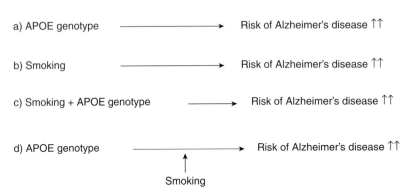

Figure 6 Alternative hypotheses linking smoking and APOE genotype to Alzheimer's disease.

Nonetheless, it has to be considered that the effects of strong confounders such as age, gender, or ethnic group may not be fully eliminated through any statistical model. Compared to a cohort study, an experimental study has the advantage that, through randomization, all potential confounders both known and unknown, can be controlled.

In contrast to confounding, effect modification, a difference in the relationship between exposure and disease outcome according to the value of a third variable (effect modifier, Figure 5), is not a source of bias. Instead, it is a description of the nature of the relationship between exposure and outcome. Nevertheless, if ignored, a misleading measure of overall effect may be obtained. Stratification by the effect modifier can be a good solution in this situation. An example for effect modification is the risk of Alzheimer's disease in smokers. It has been reported by several studies that smoking increases the risk of Alzheimer's disease in persons without but not with the APOEe4 allele (Figure 5). A possible explanation for this is that the APOEe4 allele increases the risk of Alzheimer's disease in such a way that smoking does not increase the risk further.

Figure 6 shows the potential alternative hypotheses linking smoking and APOE genotype to Alzheimer's disease. Both APOE genotype (a) and smoking (b) could be independently associated with Alzheimer's disease. They also could exert an additive effect on Alzheimer's disease (c). Finally, smoking could modify the effect of APOE genotype on risk of dementia (d).

Conclusion

Age-related neurological diseases are a major burden in western societies. Many of these diseases have still largely unknown causes, but in recent years considerable progress has been made in diagnosis, prognosis, and treatment. By combining the tools developed in molecular biology and genetics with large-scale epidemiological approaches, epidemiological research has contributed significantly to this increase in knowledge of the mechanisms underlying these disorders.

When appropriate study design, definition of cases and controls, and the principles of causal inference and systematic bias and confounding are considered, epidemiology is a powerful tool for disentangling the causes underlying age-related disease.

References

Galasko D. New approaches to diagnose and treat Alzheimer's disease: A glimpse of the future. *Clin Geriatr Med* 2001;17(2):393–410.

Hill AB. The environment and disease: Association or causation? *Proc R Soc Med* 1965;58:295–300.

Johnston SC. Preventing cerebrovascular and cardiovascular events after stroke: Eprosartan or nitrendipine? *Nat Clin Pract Neurol* 2006;2(1):24–5.

Luchsinger JA, Mayeux R. Adiposity and Alzheimer's disease. *Curr Alzheimer Res* 2007;4(2):127–34.

Naylor S. Biomarkers: Current perspectives and future prospects. *Expert Rev Mol Diagn* 2003;3(5):525–9.

Perera FP. Weinstein IB. Molecular epidemiology: Recent advances and future directions. *Carcinogenesis* 2000;21(3):517–24.

Reiber H, Peter JB. Cerebrospinal fluid analysis: Disease-related data patterns and evaluation programs. *J Neurol Sci* 2001;184(2):101–22.

Rothman KJ, Greenland S. *Modern epidemiology*. 2nd Ed. New York, NY: Lippincott-Raven, 1998.

Sacco S, Marini C, Toni D, Olivieri L, Carolei A. Incidence and 10-year survival of intracerebral hemorrhage in a population-based registry. *Stroke* 2009;40(2):394–9.

Saposnik G, Cote R, Phillips S, et al. Stroke outcome in those over 80: A multicenter cohort study across Canada. *Stroke* 2008;39(8):2310–7.

Saposnik G, Hill MD, O'Donnell M, Fang J, Hachinski V, Kapral MK. Variables associated with 7-day, 30-day, and 1-year fatality after ischemic stroke. *Stroke* 2008;39(8):2318–24.

Trillo-Pazos G, Diamanturos A, Rislove L, et al. Detection of HIV-1 DNA in microglia/macrophages, astrocytes and neurons isolated from brain tissue with HIV-1 encephalitis by laser capture microdissection. *Brain Pathol* 2003;13(2):144–54.

3 Neurogenetics of Aging

P. Hemachandra Reddy

Introduction

Neurogenetics of aging is the science of neurons in terms of aging and age-related neurological diseases. Several factors are involved in aging, including increased oxidative stress, abnormal energy homeostasis, and accumulation of damaged DNA and proteins. Aging is the primary risk factor in the development of age-related neurodegenerative diseases, such as Alzheimer's (AD), Parkinson's (PD), amyotrophic lateral sclerosis (ALS), and Huntington's (HD). Sirtuins—the biological clocks of aging—are believed to play a large role in aging and age-related diseases (Blander and Guarente 2004; Anekonda and Reddy 2005; Haigis and Guarente 2006). Further, age-related epigenetics factors play a role in the development of each of these diseases. Epigenetics is an emerging frontier of science that involves the study of changes in the regulation of gene activity and expression that are not dependent on DNA sequence. The interactions between selective gene silencing and environmental factors are specific to each of these neurodegenerative diseases. Tremendous progress has been made in understanding neurodegenerative diseases in terms of genetic mutations causing AD, PD, HD and ALS, and the development of cell and animal models to research disease progression in these diseases (Reddy 2008). However, we still do not have clear understanding of causal factors of these diseases. This chapter discusses the role of aging, the longevity of genes—sirtuins, epigenetic factors, and mitochondria—in the progression of age-related neurodegenerative diseases. This chapter also discusses how the science of neurogenetics contributes to the development of therapies to age-related neurodegenerative diseases.

Aging

Aging is the process of gradual and spontaneous change, leading to maturation through childhood, puberty, and young adulthood, and then decline through middle and late ages (Beers and Jones 2004). Healthy aging, a universal and natural phenomenon, has been of particular interest to many researchers who study the mechanisms of aging and age-related diseases.

Physiological aging is a gradual deterioration of physiological function that occurs with age, including a decrease in fecundity (Partridge and Mangel 1999), the inevitable and irreversible loss of viability, and an increase in vulnerability. The human phenotype of aging is any one tissue or organ can fail (Austad 1997; Strehler 1999). Recent studies on individuals who lived over 110 years of age (or centenarians) suggest that they age uniformly, with multiple pathologies (Coles 2004). The number of pathologies increases with age, including diabetes, heart disease, cancer, arthritis, and kidney disease. Some pathologies, like sinusitis, remain relatively constant with age, while others, like asthma, even decline. Overall, aging plays a large role in developing age-related diseases, including neurodegenerative diseases.

In an effort to explain causes for aging, researchers have posited several hypotheses—such as the shortening of telomerase, DNA methylation, reactive oxygen species (ROS) (or free radical theory of aging), mitochondrial abnormalities, epigenetics, and environmental factors (Beckman and Ames 1998; de Carvalho et al. 2000; Mattson 2000; Vijg 2000; Perry et al. 2002). Among them, the free radical theory of aging has been given much attention recently because of its connection with mitochondrial defects and oxidative damage. This theory hypothesizes that ROS, generated by an increase in mitochondria over time, causes defects in the mitochondrial DNA and mitochondrial components, resulting in accelerated cell death and degenerative processes such as AD and PD (Harman 1999; Cadenas and Davies 2000; Biersalski 2002).

Mitochondrial Structure and Physiology

A growing body of evidence suggests that abnormalities in mitochondria are involved in aging, age-related neurodegenerative diseases, cancer, diabetes, and several diseases known to be affected by mitochondria (Lin and Beal 2006; Reddy 2008; DiMauro and Schon 2008). Causal factors for most age-related neurodegenerative diseases, including AD, PD, and ALS are largely unknown. Genetic defects are reported to cause a small number of neurodegenerative diseases (Table 1), but cellular, molecular, and pathological mechanisms of disease progression and selective neuronal cell death are not well understood in these diseases. However, based on several cellular, molecular, and animal model studies of AD, PD, ALS, cancer, and diabetes, aging appears to play a large role in cell death (Table 1) (Beal 2005; Manczak et al. 2005). Age-dependent, mitochondrially-generated ROS has been identified as an important factor that is responsible for disease progression and cell death, particularly in late-onset diseases, in which genetic mutations are not causal factors of disease progression (Swerdlow and Khan 2004; Beal 2005; Lin and Beal 2006; Reddy and Beal 2008; Reddy 2008).

Mitochondria are cytoplasmic organelles essential for life and death. They perform several cellular functions, including: 1) intracellular calcium regulation, 2) ATP production, 3) the release of proteins that activate the caspase family of proteases, 4) alteration of the reduction-oxidation potential of cells, and 5) free-radical scavenging (Reddy 2007, 2008). Mitochondria are compartmentalized into two lipid membranes: the outer mitochondrial membrane and the inner mitochondrial membrane. The outer membrane is porous and allows the passage of low molecular-weight substances between the cytosol and the inter-membrane space. The inner membrane provides a highly efficient barrier to ionic flow, houses the mitochondrial respiratory chain or electron transport chain (ETC), and covers the mitochondrial matrix, which contains tricarboxylic acid (TCA) and beta-oxidation (see Figure 1). Mitochondria are transmitted maternally. However, in rare situations, paternal inheritance and a recombination of mitochondrial DNA (mtDNA) have been reported (reviewed in Reddy and Beal 2005).

Mitochondria are controlled by both nuclear and mitochondrial genomes. mtDNA consists of a 16,571 base-pair, double-stranded, circular DNA molecule (Anderson et al. 1981). A mitochondrion contains 2–10 copies of mtDNA (Reddy 2008). mtDNA contains 13 polypeptide genes that encode essential components of the ETC. mtDNA also encodes the 12S and 16S rRNA genes and the 22 tRNA genes required for mitochondrial protein synthesis (Reddy and Beal 2005). Nuclear genes encode the remaining mitochondrial proteins, metabolic enzymes, DNA and RNA polymerases, ribosomal proteins, and mtDNA regulatory factors, such as mitochondrial transcription factor A.

Nuclear mitochondrial proteins are synthesized in the cytoplasm and are subsequently transported into mitochondria.

Mitochondrial ATP is generated via oxidative phosphorylation (OXPHOS) within the inner mitochondrial membrane (Figure 1). Free radicals are generated as a byproduct of OXPHOS. In the respiratory chain, complexes I and III leak electrons to oxygen, producing primarily superoxide radicals. The superoxide radicals are dismutated by manganese superoxide dismutase (Mn-SOD), generating H_2O_2 and oxygen. Complex I generates only toward the mitochondrial matrix, but complex III generates toward both the inter-membrane space and the matrix. In addition, the components of tricarboxylic acid, including α-ketoglutarate dehydrogenase, generate superoxide radicals in the

Table 1 Major Diseases that Involve Aging and Mitochondria

Age-related Diseases	Prevalence	Mitochondrial Abnormalities
Aging	Aging is involved in several diseases that involve mitochondrial dysfunction and decreased expression of sirtuins.	DNA defects in the mitochondrial genome are responsible for aging and senescence. Somatic accumulation of DNA defects is responsible for increased ROS production and oxidative damage in aged tissues. Age-dependent, decreased expression of sirtuins is another critical factor for age-related diseases.
Cancer	Most common in persons over 60 years old.	Tumor cells accumulate mitochondrial DNA defects, and their mitochondria decrease in respiration and ATP synthesis. Cancer cells up-regulate enzymes of glycolysis and adapt to decreased oxygen tension, a characteristic of most solid tumors.
Diabetes	Worldwide, 8% of the population suffers from diabetes.	Hyperglycemia causes pathological features of type 1 and 2 diabetes. Increased free-radical production is found in hyperglycemia. Pancreatic beta cells disrupt glucose-stimulated insulin secretion.
Alzheimer's disease	Worldwide, 5% of persons 65 years of age, and 50% of persons 85 years of age and older suffer from AD. Two percent of the total number of AD patients has genetic mutations in APP, PS1, and PS2 genes.	APP and Aβ are found in mitochondrial membranes and in the matrix of neurons affected by AD. Mitochondria APP and Aβ induce free radicals, decrease cytochrome oxidase activity, and inhibit ATP production. N-terminal ApoE4 causes mitochondrial oxidative damage. Aging plays a major role in the progression and pathogenesis of AD.
Parkinson's disease	Worldwide, 0.5 to 1% of persons 65 to 69 years of age suffer from PD.	Both wild-type and mutant α-synuclein are found in mitochondrial membranes and cause mitochondrial dysfunction. DJ1 is a redox sensor protein, localized to mitochondrial inter-membrane space and the mitochondrial matrix. PINK1 is a nuclear-encoded, mitochondrial kinase protein. Over-expression of PINK1 causes reduced mitochondrial membrane potential. Parkin is a gene product of Ubiquitin E3 ligase and is associated with the outer mitochondrial membrane. Parkin induces free radical production. LRRK2 is associated with the outer mitochondrial membrane and may induce free radicals. OMI/HTRA2 are pro-apoptotic serine proteases, which are found in the mitochondrial inter-membrane space.
Huntington's disease	Four to 10 persons per 100,000 (mainly Caucasians) suffer from HD.	Mutant huntingtin binds to the outer mitochondrial membrane and induces free-radical production and oxidative damage. The abnormal interaction between mitochondrial proteins and mutant huntingtin disrupts mitochondrial movements and axonal transport, and causes selective neuronal damage.
Amyotrophic lateral sclerosis	One to 2 persons per 100,000 (variety of ethnic groups) suffer from ALS. Ten percent of all ALS patients have genetic defects.	SOD1 is a cytosolic ROS scavenging enzyme. Mutant SOD1 aggregates have been found in the outer mitochondrial membrane, the inner mitochondrial membrane space, and the mitochondrial matrix. Mutant SOD1 induces free radicals and mitochondrial dysfunction in ALS patients.

matrix. These mitochondrially-generated free radicals and superoxide radicals are carried to the cytoplasm via voltage-dependent anion channels and participate in lipid peroxidation, and protein and DNA oxidation. Mitochondria are critical in the metabolism of all mammalian cells, including brain neurons, and abnormalities in mitochondrial structure and function may lead to age-related neurodegenerative diseases.

Mitochondria and Aging

Mitochondrial dysfunction has been well documented in aging and age-related neurodegenerative diseases (Lin and Beal 2006; Reddy 2008). In aging, mitochondrial dysfunction is caused by an accumulation of mtDNA defects and an increased production of ROS. Mitochondrial ETC is responsible for the transfer of electrons from NADH or FADH, to electron acceptors, and to oxygen, the final transfer of which leads to the production of H_2O. These biochemical events lead to a small amount (0.5–5%) of electron leakage and, subsequently, to ROS production (Reddy 2008).

mtDNA is localized close to the source of ROS production and may be vulnerable to DNA damage. Oxidized guanosine levels are higher in mtDNA relative to nuclear DNA (Richer et al. 1988). It has been reported that several DNA repair mechanisms may operate within mitochondria, but one such repair mechanism—nucleotide excision repair—may be absent in mtDNA, leaving mtDNA vulnerable to a number of DNA changes (Larsen et al. 2005). mtDNA defects that reduce the accuracy of electron transfer may increase the production of ROS and decrease the production of ATP. An increase in the production of ROS may further damage mtDNA.

Further, an age-dependent increase of Ca^{2+} has been found to induce ROS production within mitochondria (Brown et al. 2004). Recently, Brown and colleagues studied Ca^{2+} influx and ROS production in mitochondria isolated from Fischer 344 rats, ranging in age from 4 to 25 months. Mitochondria isolated from the cortex of the 25-month-old rat brain exhibited greater rates of ROS production and mitochondrial swelling in response to increasing Ca^{2+} loads than did mitochondria isolated from younger (4- and 13-month) animals, suggesting that increased mitochondrial swelling may be indicative of the opening of the mitochondrial permeability transition pore in aged animals (Brown et al. 2004).

Changes in mtDNA are responsible for aging phenotypes (Cooper et al. 1992; Trifunovic et al. 2004; Kujoth et al. 2005). Many tissues from aged rodents have lower respiratory function compared to those from younger individuals (Cooper et al. 1992). Both mtDNA single-nucleotide mutations and deletions are highly prevalent in aged cells. There is evidence that DNA damage is more prevalent in aged tissues (Lu et al 2004; Wang et al. 2008; Hoeijmakers 2009).

To help elucidate the role of mitochondrial mutations in aging, two investigators independently created mouse lines containing a point mutation in the proofreading region of DNA polymerase gene, the catalytic subunit of mtDNA polymerase (Trifunovic et al. 2004; Kujoth et al. 2005). The mutant DNA polymerase-γ mice had normal DNA polymerase activity but lacked the exonuclease activity necessary for proofreading. Homozygous mutant mice showed a 3- to 8-fold increase in mtDNA point mutations in several tissues. These homozygous mutated mice had reduced life spans and experienced an early onset of age-associated features, including weight loss, reduction in subcutaneous fat, hair loss, curvature of the spine, and osteoporosis. The findings from these studies suggest that mtDNA changes are critical in the aging process (Trifunovic et al. 2004; Kujoth et al. 2005).

Further, a recent mitochondrially targeted catalase transgenic mice study supports the involvement of mitochondria in aging process and longevity (Schriner et al. 2005). To determine the protective effects of catalase (antioxidant), Schriner et al. created transgenic mouse lines that over-express human catalase localized to peroxisomes, nuclei, and

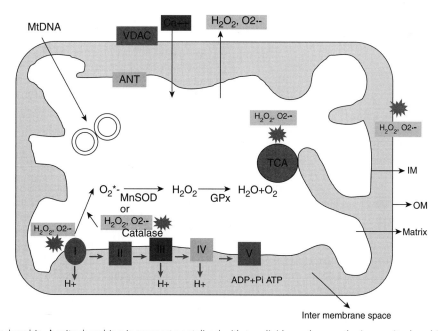

Figure 1 Structure of mitochondria. A mitochondrion is compartmentalized with two lipid membranes: the inner mitochondrial membrane and the outer mitochondrial membrane. The inner mitochondrial membrane houses the mitochondrial respiratory chain and provides a highly efficient barrier to ionic flow. In the ETC, complexes I and III leak electrons to oxygen, producing primarily superoxide radicals. Superoxide radicals are dismutated by manganese superoxide dismutase and produce H_2O_2. In addition, ETC involves H_2O_2 reducing to H_2O and O_2 by catalase or glutathione peroxidase-accepting electrons donated by NADH and $FADH_2$ and then yielding energy to generate ATP from adenosine diphosphate and inorganic phosphate. Free radicals are also generated by tricarboxylic acid in the matrix.

mitochondria. Catalase is found mainly in peroxisomes, and rapidly converts toxic H_2O_2 into H_2O and O_2. Schriner and colleagues found that the transgenic mice showed about a 20% increase in median and maximal life span (on average, 5.5 months) compared to the life span of non-transgenic, age-matched wild-type littermates. The ability of catalase to increase longevity was most apparent when the enzyme was targeted to mitochondria. Nuclear catalase (NCAT) expression (in NCAT mice) had no effect on either the median or the maximal life span of the mice.

Overall, findings from these aging studies suggest that mtDNA mutations are involved in the aging phenotype and that mitochondrially generated ROS (including H_2O_2 and superoxide radicals) are critical factors affecting longevity.

Mitochondria and Alzheimer's Disease

Alzheimer's disease is a late-onset, progressive, age-dependent neurodegenerative disease, characterized by the progressive decline of memory, cognitive functions, and changes in behavior and personality (Selkoe 2001; Mattson 2004; Reddy 2006a, 2006b; Reddy and Beal 2008). Two major pathological features have been observed in postmortem brains from AD patients: 1) intracellular neurofibrillary tangles and 2) extracellular amyloid beta (Aβ) deposits in the regions of the brain that are responsible for learning and memory. AD is also associated with the loss of synapses, synaptic function, mitochondrial abnormalities, inflammatory responses, and neuronal loss (Selkoe 2001; Mattson 2004; Reddy et al. 2005; Reddy and Beal 2008). Genetic mutations in APP, PS1, and PS2 genes cause about 2% of all AD cases; however, causal factors are still unknown for a vast majority of AD patients. Several factors—including lifestyle, diet, environmental exposure, apolipoprotein allele E4, and a genetic variant in sortilin-related receptor 1 gene, clusterin, and complement component receptor 1—may contribute to late-onset AD (Reddy and Beal 2008; Harold et al. 2009; Lambert et al. 2009).

The prevalence of AD is high among aged persons: 13% of individuals 65 years old have AD and 50% of individuals 85 years of age and older have AD (Reddy and McWeeney 2006). In addition to the personal and family hardships that AD creates, these numbers translate into extremely high health care costs. Although AD pathogenesis involves a large number of molecular and cellular events, two events that occur early in AD development are: 1) synaptic damage and 2) mitochondrial dysfunction (Selkoe 2002; Nunomura et al. 2001; Reddy and Beal 2008; Reddy 2009). These events are likely caused by mutant APP/ amyloid beta (Aβ) and aging. It is generally accepted that an age-dependent accumulation of Aβ at synapses and in synaptic mitochondria interferes with synaptic activities, including the release of vesicles and neurotransmitters, and the production of ATP at the synapses. For normal communication across neurons, and normal cognitive and memory functions, it is critical that synaptic activities and ATP supply are normal (Reddy and Beal 2008). However, it is these events that are interrupted more and more frequently in elderly individuals and in AD patients. In addition, mitochondrial trafficking is largely interrupted in neurons affected by AD. In normal, healthy neurons, mitochondria move from cell body to axons, dendrites, and synapses by an anterograde mechanism, supplying ATP at nerve terminals. Mitochondria then travel back to the cell body from synapses through a retrograde mechanism. In AD neurons, these mechanisms are believed to be abnormal primarily due to defective or functionally inactive mitochondria (Reddy 2007; Reddy 2009). Recently, mitochondrial abnormalities have been identified in AD patients: Changes in mitochondrial DNA, decreased mitochondrial enzyme activities, abnormal mitochondrial gene expressions, increased mitochondrial fragmentation, and decreased

mitochondrial fusion (Reddy 2009). These events occur very early in the development and progression of AD and are described below.

Mitochondrial dysfunction has been observed in AD postmortem brains, in platelets from AD patients, in AD transgenic mice, and in cell lines that express mutant APP and/or cells treated with Aβ (Reddy 2009). Several lines of evidence suggest that mitochondrial abnormalities play a large role in AD pathogenesis: Studies of mitochondrial enzyme activities found decreased levels of cytochrome oxidase activity, pyruvate dehydrogenase, and α-ketodehydrogenase in fibroblasts, lymphoblasts, and postmortem brains from AD patients, compared to neurons, fibroblasts, and lymphoblasts from age-matched healthy subjects (reviewed in Reddy and Beal 2008).

Several studies found increased free radical production, lipid peroxidation, oxidative DNA damage, oxidative protein damage, decreased ATP production, and decreased cell viability in postmortem AD brains compared to brains from age-matched healthy subjects (Gibson et al. 1998; Parker et al. 1990; Maurer et al. 2000; Smith et al. 1996; Devi et al. 2006). Mitochondrial DNA changes were found increased in postmortem brain tissue from AD patients and aged-matched healthy subjects, compared to DNA changes in postmortem brain tissue from young, healthy subjects, suggesting that the accumulation of mitochondrial DNA in AD pathogenesis is age-related (Lin et al. 2002; Coskun et al. 2004).

Several groups investigated mitochondrial gene expressions in postmortem AD brains and in brain specimens from AD transgenic mice (Chandrasekharan et al. 1994; Reddy et al. 2004; Manczak et al. 2005). They found mitochondrially encoded genes abnormally expressed in the brains of AD patients and AD mice. A recent, time-course global gene expression study in Tg2576 mice and age-matched non-transgenic littermates revealed an up-regulation of mitochondrial genes in the Tg2576 mice, suggesting that mitochondrial metabolism is impaired by mutant APP/Aβ and that the up-regulation of mitochondrial genes may be a compensatory response to mutant APP/Aβ (Reddy et al. 2004). Further, Manczak et al. found an abnormal expression of mitochondrially-encoded genes in postmortem AD brains compared to the brains of healthy subjects (Manczak et al. 2004), suggesting impaired mitochondrial metabolism in AD. Further, several recent studies found that Aβ and APP are localized to mitochondrial membranes, and mitochondrial Aβ induce free radical production, disrupt mitochondrial function, inhibit ATP production and damage neurons affected by AD (Manczak et al. 2006; Reddy and Beal 2008; Reddy 2009).

Overall, mitochondria are dysfunctional in AD patients and critically involved in the progression and development of AD.

Mitochondria and Parkinson's Disease

Parkinson's disease is a degenerative disorder characterized by muscle rigidity, tremors, a slowing of physical movement, and, in extreme cases, a loss of physical movement. Morphological and pathological changes of PD are the loss of dopaminergic neurons in the pars compacta region of the substantia nigra and the presence of cytoplasmic inclusions, or Lewy bodies, containing α-synuclein (Gandhi and Wood 2005; Abeliovich and Beal 2006; Martin 2006; Thomas and Beal 2007). PD is both chronic and progressive. It is now well-established that both genetic and environmental toxins are involved in the development of PD (Reddy 2008).

In the last decade, genetic discoveries in PD patients have revealed DNA mutations linked to PD. These include: α-synuclein (autosomal dominant form of PD) (Polymeropoulos et al. 1997), Parkin (autosomal recessive juvenile form of PD) (Kitada et al. 1998), DJ1 (an autosomal recessive early-onset form of PD) (Bonifati et al. 2003), PTEN-induced kinase 1 (an autosomal-recessive form of PD)

(Valenti et al. 2004), OMI/HTRA2 (Strauss et al. 2005), leucine rich repeat kinase LRRK2 (a late-onset autosomal dominant form of PD) (Zimprich et al. 2004), and ubiquitin carboxy-terminal esterase L1 (Leroy et al. 1998).

Human exposure to the environmental toxin 1-methyl-4-phenyl-1,2,3,6-tetrahydropyridine (MPTP) results in permanent PD syndrome (Langston et al. 1983). Thus, MPTP is used as a model for PD as it can rapidly induce PD symptoms in human beings and other animals, of any age. Other toxin-based models employ PCBs, paraquat (an herbicide) in combination with maneb (a fungicide), rotenone (an insecticide), and specific organochlorine pesticides, including dieldrin and lindane. MPTP administered to laboratory animals destroys the substantia nigra and induces Lewy body formation in aged chimpanzees. Other studies have found that MPTP is converted into the active neurotoxic metabolite N-mentyl-4-phenylpyridinium ion and accumulates, via a dopamine transporter, in dopaminergic neurons where MPTP inhibits complex I. The chronic administration of rotenone (ETC complex I inhibitor) also produces an animal model that reproduces the loss of dopaminergic nigral neurons, the PD phenotype, and α-synuclein inclusions that have been seen in humans with PD.

Mutations in mtDNA are known to cause PD. A point mutation in the mitochondrial 12SrRNA has been found in patients with PD, and the G11778A mutation in the complex I gene (ND4) has been found in a PD family associated with Leber's optic neuropathy (Simon et al. 1999). Mutations in nuclear-encoded mtDNA polymerase-γ gene impair mtDNA replication and result in multiple mtDNA deletions, typically causing chronic progressive external opthalmoplegia and myopathy. In those PD families, polymerase-γ gene mutations cosegregate with PD.

The inhibition of complex 1, found in PD patients, induces the generation of free radicals that cause oxidative stress and the depletion of ATP (Figure 2) (Gandhi and Wood 2005). Elevated levels of lipid peroxidation markers (4-hydroxynonenal and malondialdehyde) and protein nitration have been found in the substantia nigra and Lewy bodies (Andersen 2004). Reduced levels of glutathione and oxidized glutathione, which act as antioxidants, are the earliest marker of nigral cell loss in the brains of PD patients (Sian et al. 1994). Furthermore, complex 1 activity was found to be reduced by 30% in brain and muscle tissues and in platelets of idiopathic PD patients (Schapira et al. 1990; Parker et al. 1989). Support for a primary role of oxidative stress has emerged from the study of rare familial forms of PD.

A variety of missense, truncating, splice site, and deletion mutations have been identified in the gene DJ-1 (Bonifati et al. 2003), which causes an autosomal recessive form of PD. The precise function of DJ-1 is unclear, but the over-expression of DJ-1 appears to protect cells against mitochondrial complex 1 inhibitors and oxidative damage induced by H_2O_2. This protective effect appears to be abrogated by DJ-1 mutations (Canet-Aviles et al. 2004) or by DJ-1 knockdown using siRN (Taira et al. 2004). DJ-1 may be able to act directly as an antioxidant because it can be oxidized at the cysteine residue C106. Moreover, it has been demonstrated that endogenous DJ-1 is localized to the mitochondrial matrix and the mitochondrial intermembrane space, in addition to its cytoplasmic pool (Zhang et al. 2005). Interestingly, a quantitative proteomic study of the substantia nigra of mice treated with MPTP revealed a significant increase in the protein DJ-1 in mitochondrial fraction of the substantia nigra. Together, this evidence suggests that DJ-1 may play an important role in neuroprotection against oxidative damage caused by mitochondrial toxins.

Missense and truncating mutations of the PINK1 gene were found to cause autosomal recessive PD, and analysis of the PINK1 protein revealed that PINK 1 has a highly conserved kinase domain and a motif that targets mitochondria. The presence of the N-terminal mitochondrial-targeting domain, combined with transfected cells, is interesting (Beilina et al. 2005). As with the other genes that cause autosomal recessive PD, PINK1 has been suggested to have neuroprotective properties against a variety of cellular stresses, a function that is not found in neurons with the mutation G309D that has been identified in certain PD families (Valente et al. 2004).

Overall, these studies suggest that mitochondria play a large role in PD, and treating mitochondria is one possible option to treat patients with PD.

Mitochondria and Huntington's Disease

Huntington's disease (HD) is an autosomal, dominantly inherited neurodegenerative disease. It is characterized by chorea, seizures, involuntary movements, dystonia, cognitive decline, intellectual impairment, and emotional disturbances (Vonsattel et al. 1985; Folstein 1990; Bates 2005; Lin and Beal 2006; Montoya et al. 2006). HD occurs in 4 to 10 per 100,000 persons mainly of Caucasian origin. In patients with HD, selective medium spiny neuronal loss has been observed in the caudate and putamen of the striatum of basal ganglia, in pyramidal neurons of the cerebral cortex and, to lesser extent, in hippocampal and subthalamus neurons (Byers et al. 1973; Vonsattel et al. 1985; Spargo et al. 1993). Up to 80% neuronal loss has been found in patients with severe HD (Vansettal et al. 1985). Reactive astrogliosis has also been observed in the affected brain regions of HD patients. In addition, mutant huntingtin (Htt) protein aggregates or intraneuronal inclusions have been found in pathological sites in HD postmortem brain specimens and brain specimens from HD mouse models (Mangiarini et al. 1996; DiFiglia et al. 1997; Davies et al. 1997; Reddy et al. 1998, 1999; Schilling et al. 1999; Hodgson et al. 1999; Levine et al. 1999; Wheeler et al. 1999; Yamamoto et al. 2000).

In the last 20 years, tremendous progress has been made in HD research in terms of: 1) discovering the HD gene, 2) understanding the expanded polyglutamine repeat containing the mutant Htt protein, 3) developing HD celland animal models (which now include HD-fly, -worm, and -mouse models) and nonhuman primate models of HD (Mangiarini et al. 1996; Reddy et al. 1998; Jackson et al. 1998; Schilling et al. 1999; Kim et al. 1999; Hodgson et al. 1999; Levine et al. 1999; Yamamoto et al. 2000; Wheeler et al. 1999; Faber et al. 1999; Marsh et al. 2000; Romero et al. 2008; Lin et al. 2001; Laforet et al. 2001; Yang et al. 2008), 4) decreasing the expression of the expanded polyglutamine repeat allele that has been found to damage or kill medium spiny neurons in HD patients (Harper et al. 2005; DiFiglia et al. 2007; Van Bilen et al. 2008; Zhang et al. 2009; Boudreau et al. 2009), and 5) developing therapeutics to reduce symptoms of HD in HD animal models and HD patients.

HD is a purely genetic disease, unlike AD and PD (Reddy 2007, 2008). In 1983, the HD gene was mapped to the p arm of chromosome 16 (Gusella et al. 1983), and after ten years of intense research using state-of-the-art molecular-biology techniques and collaborations among several labs across the world, the HD gene was identified in 1993 (The Collaborative Research Group, 1993). The discovery of the HD gene ('CAG repeat or polyglutamine repeat expansion as a mutation') opened the door for the identification of mutant genes associated with another eight brain diseases with expanded polyglutamine repeats. HD is caused by a genetic mutation that results in an expanded polyglutamine encoding repeat, within exon 1 of the HD gene. In persons affected by HD, the number of polyglutamine repeats ranges from 36–120, whereas in unaffected persons it ranges from only 6–35 (Reddy et al. 1999). Polyglutamine repeats are highly polymorphic in general, and their length increases in every generation when expanded polyglutamine repeats are inherited through males. This phenomenon is referred to as genetic anticipation (Reddy et al. 1999). Epidemiological and genetic data suggest that the onset of HD inversely correlates with the length of the polyglutamine repeats in the HD gene.

Htt, the product of the HD gene, is a 350 kDa protein ubiquitously expressed in the brain and peripheral tissues (see reviews of Reddy et al. 1999; Li and Li 2006; Bates 2005; Orr and Zoghbi 2007). In the brain, Htt is primarily localized in the cytoplasm of neurons (see reviews of Reddy and Tagle 1999; Li and Li 2005; Bates 2005; Orr and Zoghbi 2007). However, several recent studies have reported a small portion of mutant polyglutamine Htt in several subcellular organelles, including the nucleus, plasma membrane, mitochondria, lysosomes, and endoplasmic reticulum; and they have found that the translocated Htt protein impairs organelle function (Kegel et al. 2002, 2005; Panov et al. 2002; Choo et al. 2004; Truant et al. 2006; Strehlow et al. 2007; Atwal et al. 2007; Orr et al. 2008). Mutant Htt interacts with a large number of brain proteins. The extent of this interaction depends on its number of expanded polyglutamine repeats (see review of Borell-Pages et al. 2006). This interaction among mutant proteins ultimately leads to the Htt gene gaining function during disease progression.

Both mutant and wild-type Htt are expressed ubiquitously in the brain, and the selective, premature death of striatal projection neurons has been reported in HD patients and HD transgenic mice (Vonsattel et al. 1985; Folstein 1990; Reddy et al. 1998; Reddy and Tagle 1999; Hodgson et al. 1999; Schilling et al. 1999; Van Raamsdonk et al. 2007). Causes of this neuronal loss are not well understood, and how the mutant Htt causes HD progression is also unclear. Several mechanisms and pathways have been proposed to explain HD progression, including: transcriptional dysregulation, the interaction of expanded polyglutamine repeat Htt proteins and other proteins in the central nervous system (see review of Borell-Pages 2006; Sayer et al. 2005), caspase activation (Rigmonte et al. 2000; Jana et al. 2001; Hermel et al. 2004; Zhang et al. 2006; Majumdar et al. 2007; Warby et al. 2008), NMDAR activation (Sun et al. 2001; Centoze et al. 2001; Lee and Chang 2004; Fernandes et al. 2007), calcium dyshomeostasis (Panov et al. 2002, 2005; Oliveira et al. 2006; Milakovic et al. 2006; Oliveira et al. 2007; Fernandes et al. 2007; Gellerich et al. 2008; Lim et al. 2008; Oliveira and Goncalves 2009), and abnormal mitochondrial bioenergetics and axonal trafficking (Browne and Beal 2004, 2006; Trushina et al. 2004; Li and Li 2006; Chang et al. 2006; Orr et al. 2008).

Several lines of evidence suggest that abnormal mitochondrial bioenergetics is involved in HD progression. Body weight loss is a major factor in the progression of HD that is reported in patients with HD and mouse models of HD (Kirkwood et al. 2001; Mahant et al. 2003; Hamilton et al. 2004; Phan et al. 2009; Aziz et al. 2008).

Studies using magnetic resonance imaging of postmortem brains of HD patients revealed a progressive atrophy of the striatum compared to brain images of age-matched control subjects (Bamford et al. 1989; Aylward et al. 1994). Several other studies found atrophy in the caudate nucleus, putamen, globus pallidus and thalamus (Jernigan et al. 1991; Aylward et al. 1997). Reduced volume of the frontal and temporal cortical lobes in patients with HD has also been reported, and this reduction in volume may reflect white-matter loss (Aylward et al. 1998; Dierks et al. 1999). Findings from these imaging studies suggest that neuronal loss occurs in the striatum and cortical regions known to be affected in HD progression, and that white matter loss is involved in HD progression.

Using positron emission tomography in functional studies of the brains of HD patients and control subjects, researchers found a marked decrease in glucose utilization in the striatum of patients (Kuhl et al. 1982; Young et al. 1986; Kuwert et al. 1990; Berent et al. 1998; Powers et al. 2007). Decreased glucose metabolism was shown to correlate with several performance tasks in HD patients, including immediate recall memory, verbal associative learning, and executive functions, suggesting that cerebral glucose metabolism is defective in HD patients.

Biochemical studies of mitochondria in striatal neurons from late-stage HD patients revealed reduced activity of several components of oxidative phosphorylation, including complexes II, III, and IV of the electron transport chain (Browne et al. 1997; Tabrizin et al. 1999; Senatorov et al. 2003; Browne and Beal 2004; Fukui and Moraes 2007). Further, in studies of HD transgenic and knockin mice and in experimental HD rodent models, decreases in enzyme activities of complexes I, II, III, and IV were found in brain tissues (Pandey et al. 2008), suggesting that mitochondria are involved in HD pathogenesis.

Recently, Fukui and Moreas investigated mitochondrial respiratory function using human osteosarcoma 143B cells expressing mutant Htt in an inducible manner (Fukui and Moreas 2007). They found that cells expressing mutant Htt but not wild-type Htt exhibited a reduced activity of complex III and an increased activity of complex IV. In these studies, they also conversely found that pharmacological treatments inhibited complex III activity and significantly promoted the formation of Htt aggregates. This complex III-mediated modulation of Htt aggregates was observed in a neuronal progenitor RN33B cell line transduced by lentivirus carrying a mutant Htt. This effect of complex III inhibition on Htt aggregates appeared to be mediated by the inhibition of proteasome activity, but not by the depletion of ATP or the production of ROS. Accordingly, complex III mutant cells also showed a decrease in proteasome activity. These results suggest a feedback system in the HD brain, connecting the mitochondrial respiratory complex III and Htt aggregates.

Recently, Solans et al. (2006) investigated mitochondrial respiration activity in yeast cells using an expanded polyglutamine repeat protein that they labeled with a green fluorescence protein. They found that in yeast cells expressing 103 polyglutamine repeats, cell respiration progressively reduced after 4–6 h of induction with galactose, and after 10 h of induction it further reduced to 50% of the control. The production of ROS was also found significantly enhanced in yeast cells expressing 103 polyglutamines. The quenching of ROS with resveratrol partially prevented defects in cell respiration. Mitochondrial morphology and distribution were also altered in cells expressing 103 polyglutamines; this may have resulted from the interaction of aggregates and portions of the mitochondrial web and from a progressive disruption of the actin cytoskeleton. Interactions of misfolded aggregated polyglutamine domains with the mitochondrial and actin networks led to disturbances in mitochondrial distribution and function and to an increase in ROS production. Oxidative damage could preferentially affect the stability and function of enzymes containing iron-sulfur clusters, such as complexes II and III. Findings from this yeast mitochondrial study further support that mitochondrial dysfunction may be involved in HD.

Recent studies of HD knock-in striatal cells and lymphoblasts from HD patients revealed that expanded polyglutamine repeats are associated with low mitochondrial ATP and decreased mitochondrial ADP-uptake, suggesting that in HD, mutations in the HD gene may be associated with functional defects in mitochondria (Seong et al. 2005).

Biochemical studies of HD cell lines in HD mice revealed that calcium-induced mitochondrial permeability is a major factor in HD pathogenesis (Panov et al. 2002, 2005). This evidence is the strongest among all pathomechanisms reported in HD pathogenesis thus far and has been replicated in a large number of studies (Milakovic et al. 2006; Oliveira et al. 2006; Lim et al. 2008; Fernandes et al. 2007; Oliveira et al. 2007; Gellerich et al. 2008; Oliveira and Goncalves 2009). Recent studies of mitochondrial trafficking in HD cortical neurons revealed that mutant Htt aggregates impair the movement of mitochondria (Trushina et al. 2004; Chang et al. 2006; Orr et al. 2008).

The shape, structure, and morphology of mitochondria are maintained by two opposing forces: mitochondrial fission and mitochondrial fusion (Chan et al. 2006; Reddy 2007, 2009; Wang et al. 2009). In a healthy neuron, fission and fusion mechanisms balance equally. Through mitochondrial trafficking, mitochondria alter their shape and size to move from the cell body to the axons, dendrites, and synapses, and back to the cell body. Fission and fusion are controlled by evolutionary conserved, large GTPases belonging to the dynamin family. Fission is controlled and regulated by the dynamin-related protein Drp1 and the mitochondrial fission 1 protein Fis1, the latter of which is localized to the outer membrane of mitochondria (Reddy 2007). Most of the Drp1 protein is localized in the cytoplasm, but a small part punctates the outer membrane, which promotes mitochondrial fragmentation. The increase in mitochondrial free radicals activates Fis1, which is also critical for mitochondrial fission.

Mitochondrial fusion is controlled by three GTPase proteins: two outer-membrane localized proteins Mfn1 and Mfn2, and one inner-membrane localized protein Opa (Reddy 2007). The C-terminal part of Mfn1 mediates oligomerization between Mfn1 molecules of adjacent mitochondria and facilitates mitochondrial fusion. In HD neurons, mitochondrially generated free radicals activate Fis1 and promote an increase in mitochondrial fragmentation, which in turn produces defective mitochondria that ultimately damage neurons.

Mitochondrial fusion protects cells from the toxic effects of mitochondrial DNA and from mitochondrial mutant Htt by allowing functional complementation of mitochondrial DNA, proteins, and metabolites. Cell hybrids resulting from the fusion of parental cells carrying pathogenic mutations have been found to restore mitochondrial ETC activity (Ono et al. 2001). Increased mitochondrial fission may be due to the association of mutant Htt in HD neurons, which may decrease mitochondrial fusion activity and subsequently damage HD neurons.

Treating mitochondria with mitochondrially targeted antioxidants is an important option to treat patients with HD.

Mitochondria and Amyotrophic Lateral Sclerosis

ALS is a progressive, invariably fatal neurological disease that attacks the neurons responsible for controlling voluntary muscles. In ALS, both the upper and lower motor neurons degenerate or die, ceasing to send messages to muscles. Unable to function, the muscles gradually weaken, twitch, and waste away. Eventually, the brain loses its ability to control voluntary movement (Martin 2006; Hervias et al. 2006). Individuals with ALS lose strength and ultimately the ability to move, speak, swallow and breath. ALS has an incidence of 1–2 in 100,000, with fairly uniform distribution worldwide and equal representation among racial groups (Boillee et al. 2006). The incidence of

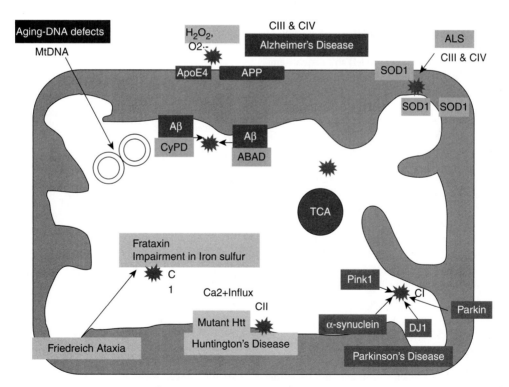

Figure 2 Mutant proteins and mitochondria. In AD, Aβ peptides enter mitochondria and interact with mitochondrial proteins, induce free radicals, decrease cytochrome oxidase activity, and inhibit ATP generation. In AD brains, APP is transported to outer mitochondrial membranes, blocks the import of nuclear cytochrome oxidase proteins to mitochondria, and may be responsible for decreased cytochrome oxidase activity. In HD neurons, mutant Htt binds to the outer mitochondrial membrane and induces free radical production. Free radicals may interrupt with calcium uptake. In PD neurons, mutant proteins of α-synuclein, parkin, PINK1, and DJ1 are associated with mitochondria and cause mitochondrial dysfunction. Complex I activity is inhibited in PD neurons. In ALS, mutant SOD1 is localized to the inner and outer mitochondrial membranes and matrix, and induces free radical production and oxidative damage. Impairment of complexes II and IV are associated with ALS. Frataxin is a mitochondrial protein responsible for heme biosynthesis and the formation of iron-sulfur clusters. In Friedriech ataxia, mutant frataxin facilitates the accumulation of iron in mitochondria and induces free radicals.

ALS is greatest in persons aged 50–70 years. The male:female ratio is about 1.5:1. Genetic studies have identified several missense mutations in the gene encoding Cu/Zn superoxide dismutase (SOD1) on the long arm of chromosome 21 as the cause of the disease in about one-fifth of autosomal-dominant cases. The genetic causes of ALS are known for only about 10% of total ALS cases.

Cytoplasmic SOD1 protein aggregates have been observed in both sporadic and familial ALS cases, as well as in mutant SOD1 transgenic mice (Bruijn et al. 1998; Gurney et al. 1994; Watanabe et al. 2001; Wong et al. 1995). It has been used to define accumulations of detergent-insoluble forms of SOD1, that were detected by immunoblotting of filter-trappable material (Deng et al. 2006; Furukawa et al. 2006). The detergent-insoluble forms were detectable only in affected tissues of mutant SOD1 mice and were most prominent at symptomatic stages of disease progression (Furukawa et al. 2006; Jonsson et al. 2006). The most misfolded unstable SOD1 mutants are most prone to aggregation.

A common feature of many neurodegenerative diseases is damage to mitochondria that contributes to the degenerative phenotype. Mitochondria have been implicated as a target of toxicity in ALS by histopathological observations of vacuolated and dilated mitochondria with disorganized cristae and membranes in the motor neurons of ALS patients (Hirano et al. 1984). Mitochondrial defects have been reported in spinal cords and muscle biopsies of patients, with such defects ranging from impaired mitochondrial respiration to increased levels of uncoupling proteins (Chung and Suh 2002; Dupuis et al. 2003).

Mitochondrial abnormalities have been observed in the motor neurons of mice that develop ALS from an accumulation of dismutase active mutants (Wong et al. 1995) and hSOD1G93A mice (Higgins et al. 2003) prior to any detectable motor neuron loss or other observable damage (Higgins et al. 2003; Wong et al. 1995). A proportion of the predominantly cytosolic SOD1 localizes to mitochondria in certain contexts, in brain samples from ALS rodent models and patient samples. In these samples, mutant SOD1 was present in fractions enriched for mitochondria that were derived from affected tissues, but not from unaffected tissues (Bergemalm et al. 2006; Deng et al. 2006; Liu et al. 2004; Vijayvergiya et al. 2005). Mitochondrial localization of SOD1 has been confirmed by electron microscopy in both isolated mitochondria (Liu et al. 2004) and motor neurons in situ (Higgins et al. 2002). SOD1 mutants that cause disease at the lowest accumulated levels (hSOD1G85R and hSOD1G127X) have the highest relative proportions that are mitochondrially associated (Liu et al. 2004). Mutant SOD1 has been reported in the intermembrane space and the matrix, as well as both in the inner and outer membranes of the spinal cord and brain mitochondria (Figure 2) (Bergemalm et al. 2006; Deng et al. 2006; Higgins et al. 2002; Liu et al. 2004; Vijayvergiya et al. 2005).

Overall, mitochondrial dysfunction is involved in patients with ALS and therapeutic approaches targeting mitochondriamay be an important option to treat patients with ALS.

Mutant Proteins Association and Mitochondria

Several recent molecular, cellular, biochemical, and animal model studies of inherited neurodegenerative diseases revealed that mutant proteins—such as amyloid beta in AD, mutant Htt in HD, mutant SOD1 in ALS, mutant parkin, mutant DJ1 and mutant α-synuclein in PD, and frataxin in FRDA—are localized to mitochondrial membranes, leading to an increased production of free radicals, a low production of cellular ATP, and ultimately cell death (Beal 2005; Reddy 2008) (Figure 2). Evidence from molecular, cellular, biochemical, and animal model studies suggests that mitochondrial dysfunction is an age-dependent common cellular change in the disease progression of several neurodegenerative diseases (listed in Table 1).

The Biological Clocks of Aging—Sirtuins

Silent information regulator two (Sir2) protein is evolutionarily conserved protein found in organisms ranging from bacteria to humans (Anekonda and Reddy 2005; Haiges and Guarente 2006). Sir2 was discovered in yeast, and researchers found that an extra copy of Sir2 extends the lifespan of yeast by 50% and that deleted Sir2 shortens lifespan (Haigis and Guarente 2006). Sir2 is responsible for cellular regulation in yeast, and sirtuins regulate important biological pathways in eubacteria, archaea, and eukaryotes. The exploration of sirtuins is conducted extensively in lower organisms such as yeast and worms; however, research is in the early stages in higher organisms such as rodents and humans.

Table 2 summarizes biological functions of Sir2 homologues in rodents and humans that have been extensively investigated. Sirtuins perform multiple cellular functions, including: increasing cell survival, reducing DNA damage, deacetylation, and apoptosis; they prevent axonal degeneration; and regulate cell structure, intracellular transport, and cell cycle (Anekonda and Reddy 2005; Haigis and Guarente 2006). Seven mammalian sirtuins have been found to express ubiquitously across different types of tissues. Molecular phylogenetic analyses of 60 sirtuins from prokaryotes and eukaryotes suggest that the biological structure of sirtuins has been evolutionarily conserved and that sirtuins participate in important cellular functions (Frye 1999 and 2000; Anekonda and Reddy 2005).

SIRT1 and deacetylation. SIRT1 is closely related to Sir2 and is implicated in the lifespan extension of lower organisms such as yeast to mammals as mouse. Functions of SIRT1 are rapidly being identified in the current literature. SIRT1 interacts and deacetylates histones H1-Lys26, H3-Lys9, Lys14, and H4-Lys16, and reduces methylation of histone H3-Lys79 (Imai et al. 2000; Vaquero et al. 2004). SIRT1 also deacetylates and represses the activities of p53 (Vaziri et al. 2001), a forkhead transcription factor 3a (FOXO3a), FOXO1, and FOXO4 (Motta et al. 2004; Yang et al. 2005). Under oxidative stress, SIRT1 increases the ability of FOXO3 to induce cell cycle or to withstand oxidative stress, and SIRT1 reduces the apoptotic ability of FOXO3 (Brunet et al. 2004). The overexpression of SIRT1 in clonal PC12 cells has been found to reduce the cellular consumption of O_2 by ~25% and to deacetylate and interact with peroxisome proliferator-activated receptor-gamma coactivator-1a (PGC-1a), a master regulator of the cellular gluconeogenic pathway (Nemoto et al. 2005). SIRT1 physically associates with the human Hairy-related bHLH repressor proteins HES1 and HEY2 both *in vitro* and *in vivo* (Takata et al. 2003). In studies of SIRT1-deficient mice, they were small and showed developmental defects in the retina and heart, and the SIRT1-deficient cells of these mice showed p53 hyperacetylation after DNA damage (Cheng et al. 2003). Mice with Sir2a or SIRT1 null alleles were also smaller and died early during the postnatal period, suggesting that the SIRT1 protein may be essential for embryogenesis and reproduction (McBurney et al. 2003).

SIRT1 and disease pathologies. SIRT1 in promyelocytic leukemia protein nuclear bodies deacetylates and negatively regulates PML-induced p53 transactivation and prevents premature cellular senescence (Langley et al. 2002). In human non-small-cell lung cancer cells, SIRT1 physically interacts with the Rel/p65 subunit of NF-kB, deacetylates it at Lys310, and inhibits NF-kB transcription (Yeung et al. 2004). NF-kB up-regulates genes essential for cell survival. Treatment with resveratrol was found to potentiate SIRT1 proteins in

Table 2 Mammalian Sirtuins: their Localizations, Interactions, and Cellular Functions

Sirtuins	Localization	Interaction	Molecular and Cellular Functions	References
SIRT1	Nucleus	P53	Repression; reduced DNA damage; increased cell survival	Vaziri et al. 2001; Langley et al. 2002; Cheng et al. 2003; Howitz et al. 2003; Motta et al. 2004; Nemoto et al. 2004, Michishita et al. 2005
		TAF_I68	Repression; regulation of rRNA synthesis	Muth et al. 2001
		Histones H1, H3; H4	Deacetylation and reduced methylation	Imai et al. 2000; Vaquero et al. 2004
		CTIP2	Repression	Senawong et al. 2003
		HES1 & HEY2	Repression	Takata et al. 2003
		FOXO1; FOXO3a; FOXO4	Repression; increased resistance to stress; increased cell cycle or reduced apoptosis	Motta et al. 2004; Yang et al. 2005; Brunet et al. 2004; Nemoto et al. 2004
		Ku70	Reduced apoptosis	Cohen et al. 2004
		NF-kB	Increased apoptosis	Yeung et al. 2004
		PPAR-g	Increased lypolysis of triglycerides	Picard et al. 2004
		PGC-1a	Reduced cellular O_2 consumption	Nemoto et al. 2005
		HIV Tat	Regulates HIV transcription	Pagans et al. 2005
		BCL11A	Repression	Senawong et al. 2005
		(Sir2a/SIRT1 allele)	Essential for embryogenesis and reproduction	McBurney et al. 2003; Cheng et al. 2003
		(Nmat1 activity)	Increases; prevented axonal degeneration	Araki et al. 2004
		(HdhQ11 KO)	Rescued neurons from polyQ toxicity	Parker et al. 2005
SIRT2	Cytoplasm	a-tubulin	Cell structure, intracellular transport, and cell motility	North et al. 2003, Michishita et al. 2005
		HOXA10	Mammalian development	Bae et al. 2004
		(G2/M proteins)	Controls mitotic cell cycle exit	Dryden et al. 2003
SIRT3	Mitochondria	(G477T marker)	Associated with human longevity	Rose et al. 2003, Michishita et al. 2005
		(SIRT3 intron 5 VNTR polymorphism)	Survival at the oldest age	Bellizi et al. 2005
		PGC-1a;UCP-1	Reduced ROS production; increased respiration rates in adipose tissue	Shi et al. 2005
SIRT4	Mitochondria	Expressed ubiquitously; exhibits no histone deacetylase activity	Involved in the functions of insulin degrading enzyme	North et al. 2003; Shi et al. 2005; Michishita et al. 2005; Ahuja et al. 2007
SIRT5	Mitochondria	Expressed ubiquitously; deacetylates carbamoyl phosphate synthetase 1 (CPS1) is an enzyme that is the first and rate-limiting step of urea cycle.	Involved in urea cycle	North et al. 2003; Shi et al. 2005; Michishita et al. 2005; Nakagawa et al. 2009

Continued

Table 2 Continued

Sirtuins	Localization	Interaction	Molecular and Cellular Functions	References
SIRT6	Nucleus	Expressed ubiquitously	ADP-ribosyltransferase activity; SIRT6 is implicated in fundamental biological processes in aging, including maintaining telomere integrity, fine-tuning aging-associated gene expression programs, preventing genomic instability, and maintaining metabolic homeostasis.	Liszt et al. 2005; Tennin et al. 2010
SIRT7	Nucleus	Expressed ubiquitously	Inhibits cell growth and proliferation; involved in ribosomal DNA transcription	North et al. 2003; Shi et al. 2005; Michishita et al. 2005; Vakhrusheva et al. 2008; Grob et al. 2009

the promoter region of cIAP-2, which correlated with a loss of NF-kB expression and TNF-a-induced apoptosis (Yeung et al. 2004). SIRT1 was also found to interact with and deacetylate the human immunodeficiency virus Tat protein and to act as a transcriptional coactivator during Tat transactivation (Pagans et al. 2005). In addition, SIRT1 interacts directly with and represses B cell leukemia 11A protein (Senawong et al. 2005). The overexpression of Ezh2, a histone-lysine methyltransferase, in a cell-culture model for prostate cancer promotes the formation of polycomb repressive complex 4 (PRC4) that contains SIRT1 and the PRC2 isoform, Eed2 (Kuzmichev et al. 2005). The four and a half LIM2 protein in prostate cancer cells enhances the interaction of FOXO1 and SIRT1 (Yang et al. 2005). These studies strongly implicate SIRT1 functions to important pathological pathways that are, as yet, to be studied and understood.

Caloric restriction (CR) and SIRT1. Nutritional stress in PC12 cells and in mice induced a FOXO3a-dependent increase in SIRT1 expression through the interaction of SIRT1 with p53 (Nemoto et al. 2004). CR in FVB mice activated SIRT1 in white adipose tissue, and SIRT1 in turn triggered fat mobilization, enhanced lipolysis of triglycerides, released free fatty acid, and inhibited the peroxisome proliferator-activated receptor-gamma? (Picard et al. 2004). In the liver of fasted C57BL/6 mice, the levels of SIRT1, PGC-1a, phosphoenol-pyruvate kinase, pyruvate, and NAD+ increased and lactate levels decreased, suggesting that SIRT1 controls the regulation of gluconeogenic and glycolytic genes (Rodgers et al. 2005). CR and IGF-I/insulin mechanisms in the liver tissues of GHRKO mice and bGH Tg mice were distinct but overlapped, suggesting a major role for the Akt/FOXO1 pathway in the regulation of aging (Al-Regaiey et al. 2005). Resveratrol treatment also increased cell and animal survival by stimulation of the SIRT1-dependent deacetylation of p53 (Howitz et al. 2003). CR and resveratrol in Fisher 344 rats increased SIRT1 expression, deacetylated Ku70, and suppressed Ku70-Bax-mediated apoptosis (Cohen et al. 2004). Thus CR and resveratrol treatments increase SIRT1 expression, deacetylase several transcription proteins and protect cells from apoptotic death.

Sirtuins 2-7. Relatively little is known about the remaining six mammalian sirtuins (SIRT2-7). SIRT2 was found to be an NAD+-dependent a-tubulin deacetylase that colocalizes with the cytoplasmic tubulin network (North et al. 2003), increases expression during the M phase of mitotic cell cycle, controls mitotic exit (Dryden et al. 2003), and also interacts with the homeobox transcription factor HOXA10 (Bae et al. 2004) (Table 2). SIRT3 localized to the inner membrane and matrix of mitochondria and showed NAD+-dependent protein deacetylation in mitochondria (Onyango et al. 2002; Schwer et al. 2002). In the brown adipose tissue of C57BL/6 mice, CR enhanced the expression of SIRT3,

PGC-1a, the uncoupling protein 1, COX II, COX IV, and ATP synthase. Further, SIRT3 stimulated CREB phosphorylation, reduced ROS production, and increased the respiration rates of the mice (Shi et al. 2005), strongly indicating SIRT3 roles in mitochondrial functions. Although expressed ubiquitously, SIRT4, SIRT5, SIRT6, or SIRT7 failed to deacetylate ^{3}H-labeled acetylated histone H4 (North et al. 2003), perhaps suggesting these proteins may have other unknown cellular functions. In a recent study, SIRT6 localized to the nucleus and also failed to show deacetylation activity, but showed a mono-ADP-ribosyltransferase activity in vitro (Liszt et al. 2005).

Sirtuins and Neuronal Protection in Neurodegenerative Diseases

Recent molecular, cellular, and animal model studies revealed that sirtuins play a key role in protecting neurons from neurodegenerative diseases—particularly Alzheimer's (Anekonda 2006; Reddy 2007, 2008). Interestingly, in mouse models of AD, CR has also been found to diminish AD symptoms (Patel et al. 2005; Mattson et al. 2003), and in a primate model, to increase neurotrophic factors and attenuate behavioral deficits (Maswood et al. 2004), suggesting a potential therapeutic value of CR via Sirt1 for AD patients. Resveratrol—which was found to extend the lifespan of mice through the overexpression of SIRT1 (Bordone and Guarente 2005; review by Anekonda 2006) and which has been epidemiologically linked to longer life in humans (Luchsinger and Mayeux 2004; Panza et al. 2004)—also protects cells against Aβ-induced ROS production and DNA damage in vitro (Jang and Surh 2003; Russo et al. 2003; Savaskan et al. 2003). In a rat model of sporadic AD, resveratrol also prevented cognitive impairment in intracerebroventricular streptozotocin (Sharma and Gupta 2002). It is still unknown how the expression of intracellular sirtuins, triggered by CR or CR mimetics, could mitigate any intracellular accumulation of Aβ.

Insulin/IGF-1 is known to protect neurons against AD by facilitating the clearance of Aβ from the brain or preventing tau hyperphosphorylation (Gasparini and Xu 2003). Lifespan extension studies have found that a decrease in insulin/IGF-1 levels increases SIRT1 expression and that SIRT1 is a primary causal factor for longevity (Cohen et al. 2004). One explanation given to this apparent paradox between lifespan extension and neuronal protection is that insulin/IGF-1 is an upstream signal and its impact on downstream signals might be context dependent (Tang 2005a). Therefore, although SIRT1 in liver, kidney, and adipose tissues may contribute to lifespan extension, its role in the CNS may be different. In addition, SIRT1, found to trigger by CR, flavonoids, and non-steroidal anti-inflammatory drug treatments that suppress GTPase Rho and Rho-associated kinase, might promote non-amyloidogenic or non-pathogenic pathways in APP processing (Tang 2005b). The current literature suggests that the intracellular accumulation of soluble Aβ causes axonopathy and transport deficits about a year before the formation of Aβ deposits (Stokin et al. 2005) and that such deficits may ultimately lead to cognitive deficits and early onset of AD (Billings et al. 2005). Intracellular Aβ42 stimulated the overexpression of the tumor suppressor and transcription factor p53 and causes apoptosis in AD neurons; Aβ40 also causes apoptosis, but less severely (Culmsee and Mattson 2005; Ohyagi et al. 2004).

Two recent studies have highlighted the neuroprotective roles of SIRT1 in disorders of the central nervous system. In Wallerian-degeneration slow mice, SIRT1 was found to increase the activity of the nicotinamide adenine dinucleotide biosynthetic enzyme 1, which in turn protects axons from injury and degeneration (Araki et al. 2004). Further, in this study, resveratrol treatment prior to axotomy also decreased axonal degeneration. Resveratrol-induced SIRT1 in neurons from HdhQ111 knock-in mice and Sir2 in the neurons of polyQ mutant Tg *C. elegans* (both models for Huntington's disease) rescued neuronal dysfunction caused by polyQ toxicity (Parker et al. 2005).

Overall, sirtuins play a big role in healthy longevity of lower organisms and even rodents and humans.

Epigenetic Factors in Aging and Neurodegenerative Diseases

In both AD and PD, there are no pathological differences between early-onset familial patients and late-onset patients. The only difference is that in late-onset patients, pathological changes occur later than in the early-onset patients. In early-onset cases, genetic mutations accelerate the disease process. In late-onset patients, in the absence of genetic mutations, age-related cellular changes control disease progression, which is why late-onset AD and PD patients take more time to exhibit pathological features. As described above, age-related mitochondrial abnormalities contribute to disease progression in late-onset AD and PD. However, if age-dependent mitochondrial abnormalities and oxidative stress are likely factors affecting the development of AD and PD (and possibly even affecting cancer and diabetes in aged individuals), it is still unclear what makes some aged persons susceptible to PD development and others, to AD. Epigenetic factors and lifestyle activities may contribute to age-dependent susceptibility to these diseases.

Epigenetic factors play a major role in developing late-onset brain diseases, including AD, PD, and ALS. Epigenetics factors likely involved in transcriptional silencing of genes important in free radical scavenging, such as *MnSOD*, have been observed (Hitchler et al. 2006). An increase in free radicals and superoxide radicals likely affects antioxidant enzymes, including catalase and glutathione, and these decreased antioxidant enzymes may lead to DNA methylation in cells. Antioxidant enzymes have been shown to decrease with aging. Increased antioxidant enzyme production influences epigenetic processes including DNA and histone methylation by limiting the availability of S-adenosylmethionine, which is a cofactor utilized during epigenetic control of gene expression by DNA and histone methyltransferases (Hitchler et al. 2006). It is possible that additional free radical- related mechanisms involving hydrogen peroxide that can lead to further changes of the chromatin structure.

Lifestyle activities and environmental factors play a key role in aging and late-onset neurodegenerative diseases. Daily diet is an important factor that may contribute to a healthy brain. A recent longitudinal epidemiological study revealed that intake of a Mediterranean diet delayed AD (Panza et al. 2004). Environmental factors, including metals, pesticides, solvents, electromagnetic fields, brain injuries, and inflammation may lead to development of late-onset brain diseases in humans (Migliore and Coppede 2009).

Therapeutic Approaches to Treat Aging and Neurodegenerative Diseases

As discussed above, mitochondrial dysfunction has been reported in early pathogenic events associated with aging, neurodegenerative diseases, cancer, and diabetes. It may be possible to treat these pathogenic events by developing molecules that affect mitochondria (by targeting ROS). These molecules could decrease free radical production and oxidative damage, and boost overall mitochondrial function, which ultimately increases synaptic branching of neurons. Caloric-restricted diet is another option to extend health or treat patients with neurodegenerative diseases.

Given the huge involvement of mitochondrial dysfunction in aging and neurodegenerative diseases, it is reasonable to treat or supplement diet with antioxidants in patients with neurodegenerative diseases such as AD, PD, and HD. However, recent studies of intake of natural antioxidants in AD patients gave mixed results. Some epidemiologic studies suggest that the increased intake of antioxidant vitamins (including vitamin E, vitamin C, and beta carotene) might reduce the risk of developing AD or PD, while other studies did not (Reddy and Beal 2008). Currently, available antioxidant approaches are not effective in treating neurodegenerative diseases because naturally occurring antioxidants, such as vitamins E and C, do not cross the blood-brain barrier and so cannot reach the relevant sites of free radical generation. To overcome these problems and to better assess whether antioxidant approaches may be valuable therapeutic treatments, improved delivery of antioxidants to the brains of patients with neurodegenerative diseases is needed.

In the last decade, considerable progress has been made in developing mitochondrially targeted antioxidants. To increase the delivery of antioxidants into mitochondria, several antioxidants have been developed: the triphenylphosphonium-based antioxidants (MitoQ, MitoVitE, and MitoPBN), the cell-permeable, small peptide-based antioxidant SS31, and mitochondrial permeability transition pore inhibitors such as Dimebon (Szeto 2008; Murphy and Smith 2007; Reddy 2008; Doody et al. 2008). The application of these mitochondrially targeted agents to neurodegenerative diseases is at its early stages and is focused on animal models of AD, PD, and ALS. Recent clinical studies of AD treatments conducted in Russia found that Dimebon significantly improved the clinical course of mild-to-moderate AD and may be safe and well-tolerated (Doody et al. 2008). Further research is needed to test the efficacies of mitochondrially targeted molecules using animal models of aging and neurodegenerative diseases.

Concluding Remarks

Tremendous progress has been made in understanding the science of neurogenetics and its role in aging and age-related neurodegenerative diseases. It is now clear that mitochondria play a large role in age-related diseases, including cancer, diabetes, and neurodegenerative diseases. Age-dependent accumulation of mitochondrial abnormalities and mutant proteins lead to both structural and functional changes in neuronal function and to cell death. In addition to aging, epigenetic factors and lifestyle activities may likely contribute to neurodegeneration and cell death. Through studies that are elucidating the role of mitochondria in disease onset and development, investigators have begun to focus research efforts on developing therapies, such as molecules that target and protect mitochondria and neurons from the toxicity of aging and mutant proteins. Tremendous progress is being made in this research, and optimism is running high that significant steps can continue, taking us much closer to a future time when such devastating diseases as AD, PD and ALS can be controlled.

Acknowledgments

The research presented in this chapter was supported by grants from American Federation for Aging Research and National Institutes of Health (AG020872, RR00163, and AG025061), Alzheimer Association IIRG grant −09-92429.

References

Abeliovich, A. and Beal, M. F. 2006. Parkinsonism genes: Culprits and clues. *J Neurochem* 99, 1062–1072.

Ahuja, N. Schwer, B. Carobbio, S. et al. 2007. Regulation of insulin secretion by SIRT4, a mitochondrial ADP-ribosyltransferase. *J Biol Chem* 282, 33583–33592.

Al-Regaiey, K.A., Masternak, M.M., Bonkowski M. and Sun L, Bartke A. 2005. Long-lived growth hormone receptor knockout mice: Interaction of reduced insulin-like growth factor i/insulin signaling and caloric restriction. *Endocrinology* 146, 851–860.

Andersen, J. K. 2004. Iron dysregulation and Parkinson's disease. *J Alzheimers Dis* 6, S47–52.

Anderson, S., Bankier, A.T., Barrell, B.G., et al. 1981 Sequence and organization of the human mitochondrial genome. *Nature* 290, 457–465.

Anekonda, T.S. and Reddy, P.H. 2005. Can plants provide a new generation of drugs for treating Alzheimer's disease? *Brain Res Rev* 50, 361–376.

Anekonda, T.S. and Reddy, P.H. 2006. Neuronal protection by sirtuins in Alzheimer's disease. *J Neurochem* 96, 305–313.

Anekonda, T. 2006. Resveratrol—a boon for treating Alzheimer's disease? *Brain Res Rev* 52, 316–326.

Araki, T., Sasaki, Y. and Milbrandt, J. 2004 Increased nuclear NAD biosynthesis and SIRT1 activation prevent axonal degeneration. *Science* 305, 1010–1013.

Atwal, R.S., Xia, J., Pinchev, D., Taylor, J., Epand, R.M., Truant, R. 2007. Huntingtin has a membrane association signal that can modulate huntingtin aggregation, nuclear entry and toxicity. *Hum Mol Genet* 16, 2600–2615.

Austad, S. N. 1997a. *Why we age: What science is discovering about the body's journey through life.* New York: JohnWiley & Sons.

Aylward, E.H., Brandt, J., Codori, A.M., et al. 1994. Reduced basal ganglia volume associated with the gene for Huntington's disease in asymptomatic at-risk persons. *Neurology* 44, 823–828.

Aziz, N.A., van der Burg, J.M., Landwehrmeyer, G.B., Brundin, P., Stijnen, T., EHDI Study Group., Roos, R.A., 2008. Weight loss in Huntington disease increases with higher CAG repeat number. *Neurology* 71, 1506–1513.

Bae, N.S., Swanson M.J., Vassilev A. and Howard B.H. 2004. Human histone deacetylase SIRT2 interacts with the homeobox transcription factor HOXA10. *J Biochem* (Tokyo) 135, 695–700.

Bamford, K.A., Caine, E.D., Kido, D.K., et al. 1989. Clinical-pathologic correlation in Huntington's disease: a neuropsychological and computed tomography study. *Neurology* 39, 796–801.

Bates, G.P. 2005. History of genetic disease: the molecular genetics of Huntington disease—a history. *Nat Rev Genet* 6, 766–773.

Beal, M.F. 2005. Mitochondria take center stage in aging and neurodegeneration. *Ann Neurol* 58, 495–505.

Beckman, K. B. and Ames, B. N. 1998. The free radical theory of aging matures. *Physiol Rev* 78, 547–581.

Beers, M. and Jones, T. V. 2004. *Merck manual of health and aging.* Merck.

Beilina, A., Van Der Brug, M., Ahmad, R., et al. 2005. Mutations in PTEN-induced putative kinase 1 associated with recessive parkinsonism have differential effects on protein stability. *Proc Natl Acad Sci USA* 102, 5703–5708.

Bellizzi, D., Rose, G., Cavalcante, P., et al. 2005. A novel VNTR enhancer within the SIRT3gene, a human homologue of SIR2, is associated with survival at oldest ages. *Genomics* 85, 258–263.

Berent, S., Giordani, B., Lehtinen, S., et al. 1998. Positron emission tomographic scan investigations of Huntington's disease: cerebral metabolic correlates of cognitive function. *Ann Neurol* 23, 541–546.

Bergemalm, D., Jonsson, P. A., Graffmo, K. S., et al. 2006. Overloading of stable and exclusion of unstable human superoxide dismutase-1 variants in mitochondria of murine amyotrophic lateral sclerosis models. *J Neurosci* 26, 4147–4154.

Biersalski, H. K. 2002. Free radical theory of aging. *Curr Opin Clin Nutr Metab Care* 5, 5–10.

Billings, L.M., Oddo, S., Green, K.N., McGaugh, J.L. and Laferla, F.M. 2005. Intraneuronal Abeta causes the onset of early Alzheimer's disease-related cognitive deficits in transgenic mice. *Neuron* 45, 675–688.

Blander, G. and Guarente, L. 2004. The Sir2 family of protein deacetylases. *Annu Rev Biochem* 73, 417–435.

Boillee, S., Vande Velde, C. and Cleveland, D.W. 2006. ALS: A disease of motor neurons and their nonneuronal neighbors. *Neuron* 52, 39–59.

Bonifati, V., Rizzu, P., van Baren M. J., et al. 2003. Mutations in the DJ-1 gene associated with autosomal recessive early-onset Parkinsonism. *Science* 299, 256–259.

Bordone, L. and Guarente, L. 2005. Calorie restriction, SIRT1 and metabolism: Understanding longevity. *Nat Rev Mol Cell Biol* 6, 298–305.

Borrell-Pagès, M., Zala, D., Humbert, S., Saudou, F., 2006. Huntington's disease: From huntingtin function and dysfunction to therapeutic strategies. *Cell Mol Life Sci* 63, 2642–2660.

Boudreau, R.L., McBride, J.L., Martins, I., et al. 2009. Nonallelespecific silencing of mutant and wild-type huntingtin demonstrates therapeutic efficacy in Huntington's disease mice. *Mol Ther* 2009 Feb 24. [Epub ahead of print].

Brown, M.R., Geddes, J.W., Sullivan, P.G. 2004. Brain region-specific, age-related, alterations in mitochondrial responses to elevated calcium. *J Bioenerg Biomembr* Aug;36(4):401–6.

Browne, S.E., Beal, M.F., 2006. Oxidative damage in Huntington's disease pathogenesis. *Antioxid Redox Signal* 8, 2061–2073.

Browne, S.E., Beal, M.F. 2004. The energetics of Huntington's disease. *Neurochem Res* 29, 531–546.

Browne, S.E., Bowling, A.C, MacGarvey, U., et al.1997. Oxidative damage and metabolic dysfunction in Huntington's disease: selective vulnerability of the basal ganglia. *Ann Neurol* 41, 646–653.

Bruijn, L.I., Houseweart, M.K., et al. 1998. Aggregation and motor neuron toxicity of an ALS-linked SOD1 mutant independent from wild-type SOD1. *Science* 281, 1851–1854.

Brunet A., Sweeney L.B., Sturgill J.F., et al. 2004. Stress-dependent regulation of FOXO transcription factors by the SIRT1 deacetylase. *Science* 303, 2011–2015.

Byers, R.K., Gilles, F.H. and Fung, C. 1973. Huntington's disease in children. Neuropathologic study of four cases. *Neurology* 23, 561–569.

Cadenas, E. and Davies, K. J. 2000. Mitochondrial free radical generation, oxidative stress, and aging. *Free Radic Biol Med.* 29, 222–230.

Canet-Avilés, R.M., Wilson, M.A., Miller, D.W., et al. 2004. The Parkinson's disease protein DJ-1 is neuroprotective due to cysteine-sulfinic acid-driven mitochondrial localization. *Proc Natl Acad Sci USA.* Jun 15;101(24):9103–8.

Centonze, D., Gubellini, P., Picconi, B., et al. 2001. An abnormal striatal synaptic plasticity may account for the selective neuronal vulnerability in Huntington's disease. *Neurol Sci* 22, 61–62.

Chan, D.C. 2006. Mitochondrial fusion and fission in mammals. *Annu Rev Cell Dev Biol* 22, 79–99.

Chang, D.T., Rintoul, G.L., Pandipati, S. and Reynolds, I.J. 2006. Mutant huntingtin aggregates impair mitochondrial movement and trafficking in cortical neurons. *Neurobiol Dis* 22, 388–400.

Chandrasekaran, K., Giordano, T., Brady, D.R., Stoll, J., Martin, L.J. and Rapoport, S.I. 1994. Impairment in mitochondrial cytochrome oxidase gene expression in Alzheimer disease. *Brain Res Mol Brain Res* 24, 336–340.

Cheng H.L., Mostoslavsky R., Saito S., et al. 2003. Developmental defects and p53 hyperacetylation in Sir2 homolog (SIRT1)-deficient mice. *Proc Natl Acad Sci USA* 100, 10794–10799.

Choo, Y.S., Johnson, G.V., MacDonald, M., Detloff, P.J. and Lesort, M. 2004. Mutant huntingtin directly increases susceptibility of mitochondria to the calcium-induced permeability transition and cytochrome c release. *Hum Mol Genet* 13, 1407–1420.

Chung, M. J. and Suh, Y. L. 2002. Ultrastructural changes of mitochondria in the skeletal muscle of patients with amyotrophic lateral sclerosis. *Ultrastruct Pathol* 26, 3–7.

Cohen, H.Y., Miller, C., Bitterman K.J., et al. 2004. Calorie restriction promotes mammalian cell survival by inducing the SIRT1 deacetylase. *Science* 305, 390–392.

Coles, L.S. 2004. Demographics of human supercentenarians and the implications for longevity medicine. *Ann NY Acad Sci* 1019:490–495.

Cooper, J.M., Mann, V.M and Schapira, A.H. 1992. Analyses of mitochondrial respiratory chain function and mitochondrial DNA deletion in human skeletal muscle: effect of ageing. *J Neurol Sci* 113, 91–98.

Coskun, P.E., Beal, M.F. and Wallace, D.C. 2004. Alzheimer's brains harbor somatic mtDNA control-region mutations that suppress mitochondrial transcription and replication. *Proc Natl Acad Sci USA* 101, 10726–10731.

Culmsee, C. and Mattson, M.P. 2005. p53 in neuronal apoptosis. *Biochem Biophys Res Commun* 331, 761–777.

Davies, S.W., Turmaine, M., Cozens, B.A., et al. 1997. Formation of neuronal intranuclear inclusions underlies the neurological-dysfunction in mice transgenic for the HD mutation. *Cell* 90, 537–548.

de Carvalho, C. V., Payao, S. L. and Smith, M. A. 2000. DNA methylation, ageing and ribosomal genes activity. *Biogerontology* 1, 357–361.

Deng, H.X., Shi, Y., Furukawa, Y., Zhai H., et al. 2006. Conversion to the amyotrophic lateral sclerosis phenotype is associated with intermolecular linked insoluble aggregates of SOD1 in mitochondria. *Proc Natl Acad Sci USA* 103, 7142–7147.

Devi, L., Prabhu, B. M., Galati, D.F., Avadhani, N.G. and Anandatheerthavarada, H.K. 2006. Accumulation of amyloid precursor protein in the mitochondrial import channels of human Alzheimer's disease brain is associated with mitochondrial dysfunction. *J Neurosci* 26, 9057–9068.

Dierks, T., Linden, D.E., Hertel, A., et al. 1999. Multimodal imaging of residual function and compensatory resource allocation in cortical atrophy: a case study of parietal lobe function in a patient with Huntington's disease. *Psychiatry Res* 90, 67–75.

DiFiglia, M., Sapp, E., Chase, K.O., et al. 1997. Aggregation of huntingtin in neuronal intranuclear inclusions and dystrophic neurites in brain. *Science* 277, 1990–1993.

DiMauro, S. and Schon, E.A. 2008.Mitochondrial disorders in the nervous system. *Annu Rev Neurosci* 31, 91–123.

Ding, Q., Cecarini, V. and Keller, J.N. 2007. Interplay between protein synthesis and degradation in the CNS: physiological and pathological implications. *Trends Neurosci* 30, 31–36.

Doody, R.S., Gavrilova, S.I., Sano, M., et al. and Dimebon Investigators. 2008. Effect of dimebon on cognition, activities of daily living, behaviour, and global function in patients with mild-to-moderate Alzheimer's disease: A randomised, double-blind, placebo-controlled study. *Lancet* 372 (9634):207–15.

Dryden, S.C., Nahhas, F.A., Nowak, J.E., Goustin, A.S. and Tainsky, M.A. 2003. Role for human SIRT2 NAD dependent deacetylase activity in control of mitotic exit in the cell cycle. *Mol Cell Biol* 23, 3173–3185.

Dupuis, L., di Scala, F., Rene, F., et al. 2003. Up-regulation of mitochondrial uncoupling protein 3 reveals an early muscular metabolic defect in amyotrophic lateral sclerosis. *FASEB J* 17, 2091–3.

Faber, P.W., Alter, J.R., MacDonald, M.E. and Hart, A.C., 1999. Polyglutamine-mediated dysfunction and apoptotic death of a Caenorhabditis elegans sensory neuron. *Proc Natl Acad Sci USA* 96, 179–84.

Fernandes, H.B., Baimbridge, K.G., Church, J., Hayden, M.R. and Raymond, L.A. 2007. Mitochondrial sensitivity and altered calcium handling underlie enhanced NMDA induced apoptosis in YAC128 model of Huntington's disease. *J Neurosci* 27, 13614–13623.

Folstein, S.E. 1990. *Huntington's disease.* Johns Hopkins University Press.

Frye, R.A. 1999. Characterization of five human cDNAs with homology to the yeast SIR2 gene: Sir2-like proteins (sirtuins) metabolize NAD and may have protein ADP-ribosyltransferase activity. *Biochem Biophys Res Commun* 260, 273–279.

Frye, R.A. 2000. Phylogenetic classification of prokaryotic and eukaryotic Sir2-like proteins. *Biochem Biophys Res Commun* 273, 793–798.

Fukui, H. and Moraes, C.T. 2007. Extended polyglutamine repeats trigger a feedback loop involving the mitochondrial complex III, the proteasome and huntingtin aggregates. *Hum Mol Genet* 16,783–797.

Furukawa, Y., Fu, R., Deng, H.X., Siddique, T. and O'Halloran, T.V. 2006. Disulfide cross-linked protein represents a significant fraction of ALS-associated Cu, Zn-superoxide dismutase aggregates in spinal cords ofmodel mice. *Proc Natl Acad Sci USA* 103, 7148–7153.

Gandhi, S. and Wood, N.W. 2005. Molecular pathogenesis of Parkinson's disease. *Hum Mol Genet* 14 Spec No. 2, 2749–2755.

Gasparini, L. and Xu, H. 2003. Potential roles of insulin and IGF-1 in Alzheimer's disease. *Trends Neurosci* 26, 404–406.

Gellerich, F.N., Gizatullina, Z., Nguyen, H.P., et al. 2008. Impaired regulation of brain mitochondriaby extramitochondrial Ca2+ in transgenic Huntington disease rats. *J Biol Chem* 283, 30715–30724.

Gibson, G.E., Sheu, K.F., and Blass, J.P. 1998. Abnormalities of mitochondrial enzymes in Alzheimer disease. *J Neural Transm* 105, 855–870.

Grob, A., Roussel, P., Wright, J.E., McStay, B., Hernandez-Verdun, D. and Sirri V. 2009. Involvement of SIRT7 in resumption of rDNA transcription at the exit from mitosis. *J Cell Sci* 122, 489–498.

Gurney, M.E., Pu, H., Chiu, A.Y., et al. 1994. Motor neuron degeneration in mice that express a human Cu,Zn superoxide dismutase mutation. *Science* 264, 1772–1775.

Gusella, J.F., Wexler, N.S., Conneally, P.M., et al. 1983. A polymorphic DNA marker genetically linked to Huntington's disease. *Nature* 306, 234–238.

Haigis, M.C. and Guarente, L.P. 2006. Mammalian sirtuins—emerging roles in physiology, aging, and calorie restriction. *Genes Dev* 20, (21):2913–21.

Hamilton, J.M., Wolfson, T., Peavy, G.M., Jacobson, M.W., Corey-Bloom, J; Huntington Study Group. 2004. Rate and correlates of weight change in Huntington's disease. *J Neurol Neurosurg Psychiatry* 75, 209–212.

Harman, D. 1999. Aging: Minimizing free radical damage. *J Anti-Aging Med* 2, 15–36.

Harold, D., et al. 2009. Genome-wide association study identifies variants at CLU and PICALM associated with Alzheimer's disease. *Nat Genet* 41(10):1088–93. Epub (2009) Sep 6.

Harper, S.Q., Staber, P.D., He, X., et al. 2005. RNA interference improves motor and neuropathological abnormalities in a Huntington's disease mouse model. *Proc Natl Acad Sci USA* 102, 5820–5805.

Hermel, E., Gafni, J., Propp, S.S., et al. 2004. Specific caspase interactions and amplification are involved in selective neuronal vulnerability in Huntington's disease. *Cell Death Differ* 11, 424–438.

Hervias, I., Beal, M. F and Manfredi, G. 2006. Mitochondrial dysfunction and amyotrophic lateral sclerosis. *Muscle Nerve* 33, 598–608.

Higgins, C.M., Jung, C. and Xu, Z. 2003. ALS-associated mutant SOD1G93A causes mitochondrial vacuolation by expansion of the intermembrane space and by involvement of SOD1 aggregation and peroxisomes. *BMC Neurosci* 4, 16.

Hirano, A., Donnenfeld, H., Sasaki, S. and Nakano, I. 1984. Fine structural observations of neurofilamentous changes in amyotrophic lateral sclerosis. *J Neuropathol Exp Neurol* 43, 461–470.

Hitchler, M.J., Wikainapakul, K., Yu, L., Powers, K., Attatippaholkun, W. and Domann, F.E. 2006. Epigenetic regulation of manganese superoxide dismutase expression in human breast cancer cells. *Epigenetics* 1(4):163–71.

Hodgson, J.G., Agopyan, N., Gutekunst, C.A., et al. 1999. A YAC mouse model for Huntington's disease with full-length mutant huntingtin, cytoplasmic toxicity, and selective striatal neurodegeneration. *Neuron* 23, 181–192.

Hoeijmakers, J.H. 2009. DNA damage, aging, and cancer. *N Engl J Med* 361, (15):1475–1485.

Howitz, K.T., Bitterman, K.J., Cohen, H.Y., et al. 2003. Small molecule activators of sirtuins extend Saccharomyces cerevisiae lifespan. *Nature* 425, 191–196.

Imai, S., Armstrong, C.M., Kaeberlein, M. and Guarente, L. 2000. Transcriptional silencing and longevity protein Sir2 is an NAD-dependent histone deacetylase. *Nature* 403, 795–800.

Jackson, G.R., Salecker, I., Dong, X., et al. 1998. Polyglutamine-expanded human huntingtin transgenes induce degeneration of Drosophila photoreceptor neurons. *Neuron* 21, 633–642.

Jana, N.R., Zemskov, E.A., Wang, G.H. and Nukina, N., 2001. Altered proteasomal function due to the expression of polyglutamine-expanded truncated N-terminal huntingtin induces apoptosis by caspase activation through mitochondrial cytochrome c release. *Hum Mol Genet* 10, 1049–1059

Jang, J.H. and Surh, Y.J. 2003. Protective effect of resveratrol on beta-amyloid-induced oxidative PC12 cell death. *Free Radic Biol Med* 34, 1100–1110.

Jernigan, T.L., Salmon, D.P., Butters, N, et al. 1991. Cerebral structure on MRI, part II: Specific changes in Alzheimer's and Huntington's diseases. *Biol Psychiatry* 29, 68–81.

Jonsson, P.A., Graffmo, K.S., Andersen, P.M., et al. 2006. Disulphide-reduced superoxide dismutase-1 in CNS of transgenic amyotrophic lateral sclerosis models. *Brain* 129, 451–464.

Kegel, K.B., Meloni, A.R., Yi, Y., et al. 2002. Huntingtin is present in the nucleus, interacts with the transcriptional corepressor Cterminal binding protein, and represses transcription. *J Biol Chem* 277, 7466–7476.

Kegel, K.B., Sapp, E., Yoder, J., et al. 2005. Huntingtin associates with acidic phospholipids at the plasma membrane. *J Biol Chem* 280, 36464–36473.

Kim, M., Lee, H.S., LaForet, G., et al. 1999. Mutant huntingtin expression in clonal striatal cells: dissociation of inclusion formation and neuronal survival by caspase inhibition. *J Neurosci* 19, 964–973.

Kirkwood, S.C., Su, J.L., Conneally, P. and Foroud, T. 2001. Progression of symptoms in the early and middle stages of Huntington disease. *Arch Neurol* 58, 273–278.

Kitada, T., Asakawa, S., Hattori, N., et al. 1998. Mutations in the parkin gene cause autosomal recessive juvenile parkinsonism. *Nature* 392, 605–608.

Kuhl, D.E., Phelps, M.E., Markham, C.H., et al. 1982. Cerebral metabolism and atrophy in Huntington's disease determined by 18FDG and computed tomographic scan. *Ann Neurol* 12, 425–434.

Kujoth, G.C., Hiona, A., Pugh, T.D., et al. 2005. Mitochondrial DNA mutations, oxidative stress, and apoptosis in mammalian aging. *Science* 309, 481–448.

Kuwert, T., Lange, H.W., Langen, K.J., et al. 1990. Cortical and subcortical glucose consumption measured by PET in patients with Huntington's disease. *Brain* 113, 1405–23.

Kuzmichev, A., Margueron, R., Vaquero, A., et al. 2005. Composition and histone substrates of polycomb repressive group complexes change during cellular differentiation. *Proc Natl Acad Sci USA* 102, 1859–1864.

Kwong, J.Q., Beal, M.F. and Manfredi, G. 2006. The role of mitochondria in inherited neurodegenerative diseases. *J Neurochem* 97, 1659–1675.

Laforet, G.A., Sapp, E., Chase, K., et al. 2001. Changes in cortical and striatal neurons predict behavioral and electrophysiological abnormalities in a transgenic murine model of Huntington's disease. *J Neurosci* 21, 9112–9123.

Lambert, J.C., et al. 2009. Genome-wide association study identifies variants at CLU and CR1 associated with Alzheimer's disease. *Nat Genet* 41(10):1094–9.

Langley, E., Pearson, M., Faretta, M., et al. 2002. Human SIR2 deacetylates p53 and antagonizes PML/p53-induced cellular senescence. *EMBO J* 21, 2383–2396.

Langston, J.W., Ballard, P., Tetrud, J.W. and Irwin, I. 1983. Chronic parkinsonism in humans due to a product of meperidine-analog synthesis. *Science* 219, 979–980.

Larsen, N.B., Rasmussen, M., and Rasmussen, L.J. 2005. Nuclear and mitochondrial DNA repair: Similar pathways? *Mitochondrion* 5(2):89–108.

Lee, W.T. and Chang, C., 2004. Magnetic resonance imaging and spectroscopy in assessing 3-nitropropionic acidinduced brain lesions: An animal model of Huntington's disease. *Prog Neurobiol* 72, 87–110.

Leroy, E., Boyer, R, Auburger, G. et al. 1998. The ubiquitin pathway in Parkinson's disease. *Nature* 395, 451–452.

Levine, M.S., Klapstein, G.J., Koppel, A., et al. 1999. Enhanced sensitivity to N-methyl- D-aspartate receptor activation in transgenic and knockin mouse models of Huntington's disease. *J Neurosci Res* 58, 515–532.

Li, S. and Li, X.J. 2006. Multiple pathways contribute to the pathogenesis of Huntington disease. *Mol Neurodegener* 1, 19.

Lim, D., Fedrizzi, L., Tartari, M., et al. 2008. Calcium homeostasisand mitochondrial dysfunction in striatal neurons of Huntington disease. *J Biol Chem* 283, 5780–5789.

Lin, C.H., Tallaksen-Greene, S., Chien, W.M., et al. 2001. Neurological abnormalities in a knock-in mouse model of Huntington's disease. *Hum Mol Genet* 10(2):137–44.

Lin, M.T. and Beal, M.F. 2006. Mitochondrial dysfunction and oxidative stress in neurodegenerative diseases. *Nature* 443, 787–795.

Lin, M.T., Simon, D.K., Ahn, C.H., Kim, L.M. and Beal, M.F. 2002. High aggregate burden of somatic mtDNA point mutations in aging and Alzheimer's disease brain. *Hum Mol Genet* 11, 133–145.

Liszt, G., Ford, E., Kurtev, M. and Guarente, L. 2005. Mouse Sir2 homolog SIRT6 is a nuclear ADPribosyltransferase. *J Biol Chem* Mar 28; [Epub ahead of print]

Liu, J., Lillo, C., Jonsson, P.A., et al. 2004. Toxicity of familial ALS-linked SOD1 mutants from selective recruitment to spinal mitochondria. *Neuron* 43, 5–17.

Lu, T., Pan, Y., Kao, S.Y., et al. 2004. Gene regulation and DNA damage in the ageing human brain. *Nature* 429, 883–891.

Luchsinger, J.A. and Mayeux, R. 2004. Dietary factors and Alzheimer's disease. *Lancet Neurol* 3, 579–587.

Maswood, N., Young, J., Tilmont, E. et al. 2004. Caloric restriction increases neurotrophic factor levels and attenuates neurochemical and behavioral deficits in a primate model of Parkinson's disease. *Proc Natl Acad Sci USA* 101, 18171–18176.

Lustbader, J.W., Cirilli. M., Lin, C., et al. 2004. ABAD directly links Abeta to mitochondrial toxicity in Alzheimer's disease. *Science* 304, 448–452.

Mahant, N., McCusker, E.A., Byth, K., Graham, S.; Huntington Study Group. 2003. Huntington's disease: clinical correlates of disability and progression. *Neurology* 61,1085–1092.

Majumder, P., Raychaudhuri, S., Chattopadhyay, B. and Bhattacharyya, N.P. 2007. Increased caspase-2, calpain activations and decreased mitochondrial complex II activity in cells expressing exogenous huntingtin exon 1 containing CAG repeat in the pathogenic range. *Cell Mol Neurobiol* 27, 1127–1145.

Manczak, M., Jung, Y., Park, B.S., Partovi, D. and Reddy, P.H. 2005. Time-course of mitochondrial gene expressions in mice brains: Implications for mitochondrial dysfunction, oxidative damage, and cytochrome c in aging. *J Neurochem* 92, 494–504.

Manczak, M., Anekonda, T.S., Henson, E., Park, B.S., Quinn, J. and Reddy, P.H. 2006. Mitochondria are a direct site of A beta accumulation in Alzheimer's disease neurons: Implications for free radical generation and oxidative damage in disease progression. *Hum Mol Genet* 15, 1437–1449.

Manczak, M., Park, B.S., Jung, Y. and Reddy, P.H. 2004. Differential expression of oxidative phosphorylation genes in patients with Alzheimer's disease: Implications for early mitochondrial dysfunction and oxidative damage. *Neuromolecular Med* 5, 147–162.

Mangiarini, L., Sathasivam, K., Seller, M., et al. 1996. Exon 1 of the HD gene with an expanded CAG repeat is sufficient to cause a progressive neurological phenotype in transgenic mice. *Cell* 87, 493–506.

Marsh, J.L., Walker, H., Theisen, H., et al. 2000. Expanded polyglutamine peptides alone are intrinsically cytotoxic and cause neurodegeneration in Drosophila. *Hum Mol Genet* 9, 13–25.

Martin, L. J. 2006. Mitochondriopathy in Parkinson disease and amyotrophic lateral sclerosis. *J Neuropathol Exp Neurol* 65, 1103–1110.

Mattson, M. P. 2000. Emerging neuroprotective strategies for Alzheimer's disease: Dietary restriction, telomerase activation, and stem cell therapy. *Exp Gerontol* 35, 489–502.

Mattson, M.P. 2003. Methylation and acetylation in nervous system development and neurodegenerative disorders. *Ageing Res Rev* 2, 329–342.

Mattson, M.P., Duan, W. and Guo, Z. 2003. Meal size and frequency affect neuronal plasticity and vulnerability to disease: cellular and molecular mechanisms. *J Neurochem* 84, 417–431.

Mattson, M.P. 2004. Pathways towards and away from Alzheimer's disease. *Nature* 430, 631–639.

Maurer, I. Zierz, S. and Moller, H.J. 2000. A selective defect of cytochrome c oxidase is present in brain of Alzheimer disease patients. *Neurobiol Aging* 21, 455–462.

McBurney, M.W., Yang X., Jardine K., et al. 2003. The mammalian SIR2alpha protein has a role in embryogenesis and gametogenesis. *Mol Cell Biol* 23, 38–54.

Michishita, E., Park, J.Y., Burneskis, J.M., Barrett, J.C. and Horikawa, I. 2005. Evolutionarily conserved and nonconserved cellular localizations and functions of human SIRT proteins. *Mol Biol Cell* 16, 4623–4635.

Migliore, L. and Coppedè, F. 2009. Environmental-induced oxidative stress in neurodegenerative disorders and aging. *Mutat Res* 674, (1-2):73–84.

Milakovic, T., Quintanilla, R.A. and Johnson, G.V. 2006. Mutant huntingtin expression induces mitochondrial calcium handling defects in clonal striatal cells: functional consequences. *J Biol Chem* 281, 34785–34795.

Montoya, A., Price, B.H., Menear, M. and Lepage, M., 2006. Brain imaging and cognitive dysfunctions in Huntington's disease. *J Psychiatry Neurosci* 31, 21–29.

Motta, M.C., Divecha, N., Lemieux, M., et al. 2004. Mammalian SIRT1 represses forkhead transcription factors. *Cell* 116, 551–563.

Murphy, M.P. and Smith, R.A. 2007. Targeting antioxidants to mitochondria by conjugation to lipophilic cations. *Annu Rev Pharmacol Toxicol* 47, 629–656.

Nakagawa, T., Lomb, D.J., Haigis, M.C. and Guarente, L. 2005. SIRT5 Deacetylates carbamoyl phosphate synthetase 1 and regulates the urea cycle. *Cell* 137, 560–570.

Nemoto, S., Fergusson, M.M. and Finkel, T. 2004. Nutrient availability regulates SIRT1 through a forkheaddependent pathway. *Science* 306, 2105–2108.

Nemoto, S., Fergusson, M.M. and Finkel, T. 2005. SIRT1 functionally interacts with the metabolic regulator and transcriptional coactivator PGC-1a. *J Biol Chem* 280, 16456–16460.

North, B.J. and Verdin, E. 2005. Sirtuins: Sir2-related NAD-dependent protein deacetylates. *Genome Biol* 5, 224.

North, B.J., Marshall, B.L., Borra, M.T., Denu, J.M. and Verdin, E. 2003. The human Sir2 ortholog, SIRT2, is an NAD+ dependent tubulin deacetylase. *Mol Cell* 11, 437–444.

Nunomura, A., Perry, G., Aliev, G., et al. 2001. Oxidative damage is the earliest event in Alzheimer disease. *J Neuropathol Exp Neurol* 60, 759–767.

Ohyagi, Y., Asahara, H., Chui, D.H., et al. 2005. Intracellular Abeta42 activates p53 promoter: a pathway to neurodegeneration in Alzheimer's disease. *FASEB J* 19, 255–257.

Oliveira, J.M., Chen, S., Almeida, S., et al. 2006. Mitochondrial-dependent Ca2+ handling in Huntington's disease striatal cells: Effect of histone deacetylase inhibitors. *J Neurosci* 26, 11174–11186.

Oliveira, J.M. and Gonçalves, J. 2009. In situ mitochondrial Ca2+ buffering differences of intact neurons and astrocytes from cortex and striatum. *J Biol Chem* 284, 5010–5020.

Oliveira, J.M., Jekabsons, M.B., Chen, S., et al. 2007. Mitochondrial dysfunction in Huntington's disease: The bioenergetics of isolated and in situ mitochondria from transgenic mice. *J Neurochem* 101, 241–249.

Ono, T., Isobe, K., Nakada, K., Hayashi, J.I. 2001. Human cells are protected from mitochondrial dysfunction by complementation of DNA products in fused mitochondria. *Nat Genet* 28(3):272–5.

Onyango, P., Celic, I., McCaffery, J.M., Boeke, J.D. and Feinberg, A.P. 2002. SIRT3, a human SIR2 homologue, is an NAD-dependent deacetylase localized to mitochondria. *Proc Natl Acad Sci USA* 99, 13653–13658.

Orr, A.L., Li, S., Wang, C.E., et al. 2008. N-terminal mutant huntingtin associates with mitochondria and impairs mitochondrial trafficking. *J Neurosci* 28, 2783–2792.

Orr, H.T. and Zoghbi, H.Y. 2007. Trinucleotide repeat disorders. *Ann Rev Neurosci* 30, 575–621.

Pagans, S., Pedal, A., North, B.J., et al. 2005. SIRT1 regulates HIV transcription via Tat deacetylation. *PLoS Biol* 3, e41.

Panov, A.V., Gutekunst, C.A., Leavitt, B.R., et al. 2002. Early mitochondrial calcium defects in Huntington's disease are a direct effect of polyglutamines. *Nat Neurosci* 5, 731–736.

Panov, A.V., Lund, S. and Greenamyre, J.T., 2005. Ca2+-induced permeability transition in humanlymphoblastoid cell mitochondria from normal and Huntington's disease individuals. *Mol Cell Biochem* 269, 143–52.

Panza, F., Solfrizzi, V., Colacicco, A.M., et al. 2004. Mediterranean diet and cognitive decline. *Public Health Nutr* 7, 959–963.

Parker, W.D. Jr, Filley, C.M. and Parks, J.K. 1990. Cytochrome oxidase deficiency in Alzheimer's disease. *Neurology* 40, 1302–1303.

Parker, J.A., Arango, M., Abderrahmane, S., et al. 2005. Resveratrol rescues mutant polyglutamine cytotoxicity in nematode and mammalian neurons. *Nat Genet* 37, 349–350.

Partridge, L. and Mangel, M. 1999. Messages from mortality: the evolution of death rates in the old. *Trends in Ecology and Evolution* 14(11):438–442.

Patel, N.V., Gordon, M.N., Connor, K.E., et al. 2005. Caloric restriction attenuates Abeta-deposition in Alzheimer transgenic models. *Neurobiol Aging* 26, 995–1000.

Perry, G., Nunomura, A., Hirai, K., et al. 2002. Is oxidative damage the fundamental pathogenic mechanism of Alzheimer's and other neurodegenerative diseases? *Free Radic Biol Med* 1, 1475–1479.

Phan, J., Hickey, M.A., Zhang, P., Chesselet, M.F. and Reue, K. 2009. Adipose tissue dysfunction tracks disease progression in two Huntington's disease mouse models. *Hum Mol Genet* 18(6): 1006-16.

Picard, F., Kurtev, M., Chung, N., et al. 2004. Sirt1 promotes fat mobilization in white adipocytes by repressing PPAR-gamma. *Nature* 429, 771–776. Erratum in: Nature. 430, 921.

Polymeropoulos, M.H., Lavedan, C., Leroy, E., et al. 1997. Mutation in the alpha-synuclein gene identified in families with Parkinson's disease. *Science* 276, 2045–2047.

Powers, W.J., Videen, T.O., Markham, J., et al. 2007. Selective defect of in vivo glycolysis in early Huntington's disease striatum. *Proc Natl Acad Sci U S A* 104, 2945–2949.

Reddy, P.H. 2008. Mitochondrial medicine for aging and neurodegenerative diseases. *Neuromolecular Med* 10, 291–315.

Reddy, P.H. 2009. Amyloid beta, mitochondrial structural and functional dynamics in Alzheimer's disease. *Exp Neurol* 218, 286–292.

Reddy, P.H. and Beal, M.F. 2005. Are mitochondria critical in the pathogenesis of Alzheimer's disease? *Brain Res Rev* 49, 618–632.

Reddy, P.H. and Beal, M.F. 2008. Amyloid beta, mitochondrial dysfunction and synaptic damage: implications for cognitive decline in aging and Alzheimer's disease. *Trends Mol Med* 14(2):45–53.

Reddy, P.H., Mani, G., Park, B.S., et al. 2005. Differential loss of synaptic proteins in Alzheimer's disease: Implications for synaptic dysfunction. *J Alzheimers Dis* (2):103-17; discussion 173–180.

Reddy, P.H., Mao, P. and Manczak, M. 2009. Mitochondrial structural and functional dynamics in Huntington's disease. *Brain Res Rev* 61, 33–48.

Reddy, P.H. and McWeeney, S. 2006. Mapping cellular transcriptosomes in autopsied Alzheimer's disease subjects and relevant animal models. *Neurobiol Aging* 27, 1060–1077.

Reddy, P.H., McWeeney, S., Park, B.S., et al. 2004. Gene expression profiles of transcripts in amyloid precursor protein transgenic mice: upregulation of mitochondrial metabolism and apoptotic genes is an early cellular change in Alzheimer's disease. *Hum Mol Genet* 13, 1225–1240.

Reddy, P. H., Williams, M. and Tagle, D.A. 1999. Recent advances in understanding the pathogenesis of Huntington's disease. *Trends Neurosci* 22, 248–255.

Reddy, P.H. 2006a. Amyloid precursor protein-mediated free radicals and oxidative damage: Implications for the development and progression of Alzheimer's disease. *J Neurochem* 96, 1–13.

Reddy, P.H. 2006b. Mitochondrial oxidative damage in aging and Alzheimer's disease: Implications for mitochondrially targeted antioxidant therapeutics. *J Biomed Biotechnol* 31372 (13 pages).

Reddy, P.H. 2007. Mitochondrial dysfunction in aging and Alzheimer's disease: Strategies to protect neurons. *Antioxidants & Redox Signaling* 9, 1647–1658.

Reddy, P.H. and Tagle, D.A., 1999. Biology of trinucleotide repeat disorders. In Mark P. Mattson, ed. *Genetic Aberrancies and Neurodegenerative Disorders, Vol 3: Advances in cell aging and gerontology.* Stanford, CT: Jai Press Inc.

Reddy, P.H., Charles, V., Williams, M., et al. 1999. Transgenic mice expressing mutated full-length HD cDNA: A paradigm for locomotor changes and selective neuronal loss in Huntington's disease. *Philos Trans R Soc Lond B Biol Sci* 354, 1035–1045.

Reddy, P.H., Williams, M. and Tagle, D.A. 1999. Recent advances in understanding the pathogenesis of Huntington's disease. *Trends Neurosci* 22, 248–255.

Reddy, P.H., Williams, M., Charles, V., et al. 1998. Behavioural abnormalities and selective neuronal loss in HD transgenic mice expressing mutated full-length HD cDNA. *Nat Genet* 20, 198–202.

Richter, C., Park, J.W. and Ames, B.N. 1988. Normal oxidative damage to mitochondrial and nuclear DNA is extensive. *Proc Natl Acad Sci U S A* 85, 6465–6467.

Rigamonti, D., Bauer, J.H., De-Fraja, C., et al. 2000. Wild-type huntingtin protects from apoptosis upstream of caspase-3. *J Neurosci* 20, 3705–3713.

Rodgers J.T., Lerin C., Haas W., Gygi S.P., Spiegelman B.M. and Puigserver P. 2005. Nutrient control of glucose homeostasis through a complex of PGC-1alpha and SIRT1. *Nature* 434, 113–118.

Romero, E., Cha, G.H., Verstreken, P., et al. 2008. Suppression of neurodegeneration and increased neurotransmission caused by expanded full-length huntingtin accumulating in the cytoplasm. *Neuron* 57, 27–40.

Rose, G., Dato, S., Altomare, K., et al. 2005. Variability of the SIRT3gene, human silent information regulator Sir2 homologue, and survivorship in the elderly. *Exp Gerontol* 38,1065–1070.

Russo, A., Palumbo, M., Aliano, C., Lempereur, L., Scoto, G. and Renis, M. 2003. Red wine micronutrients as protective agents in Alzheimer-like induced insult. *Life Sci* 72, 2369–2379.

Savaskan, E., Olivieri, G., Meier, F., Seifritz, E., Wirz-Justice, A. and Muller-Spahn, F. 2003. Red wine ingredient resveratrol protects from beta-amyloid neurotoxicity. *Gerontology* 49, 380–383.

Sayer, J.A., Manczak, M., Akileswaran, L., Reddy, P.H. and Coghlan, V.M. 2005. Interaction of the nuclear matrix protein NAKAP with HypA and huntingtin: Implications for nuclear toxicity in Huntington's disease pathogenesis. *Neuromolecular Med* 7, 297–310.

Schapira, A.H., Cooper, J.M., Dexter, D., Clark, J.B., Jenner, P. and Marsden, C.D. 1990. Mitochondrialcomplex I deficiency in Parkinson's disease. *J Neurochem* 54, 823–827.

Schilling, G., Becher, M. W., Sharp, A. H., et al. 1999. Intranuclear inclusions and neuritic aggregates in transgenic mice expressing a mutant N-terminal fragment of huntingtin. *Hum Mol Genet* 8, 397–407.

Schilling, G., Coonfield, M.L., Ross, C.A. and Borchelt, D.R. 2001. Coenzyme Q10 and remacemide hydrochloride ameliorate motor deficits in a Huntington's disease transgenic mouse model. *Neurosci Lett* 315, 149–153.

Schriner, S.E., Linford, N.J., Martin, G.M., et al. 2005. Extension of murine lifespan by overexpression ofcatalase targeted to mitochondria. *Science* 308, 1909–1911.

Schwer, B., North, B.J., Frye, R.A., Ott, M. and Verdin, E. 2002. The human silent information regulator (Sir)2 homologue hSIRT3 is a mitochondrial nicotinamide adenine dinucleotide-dependent deacetylase. *J Cell Biol* 158, 647–657.

Selkoe, D.J. 2001. Alzheimer's disease: genes, proteins, and therapy. *Physiol Rev* 81, 741–766.

Selkoe, D.J. 2002. Alzheimer's disease is a synaptic failure. *Science* 298, 789–791.

Senatorov, V.V., Charles, V., Reddy, P.H., Tagle, D.A. and Chuang, D.M. 2003. Overexpression and nuclear accumulation of glyceraldehyde-3-phosphate dehydrogenase in a transgenic mouse model of Huntington's disease. *Mol Cell Neurosci* 22, 285–297.

Senawong, T., Peterson, V.J. and Leid, M. 2005. BCL11A-dependent recruitment of SIRT1 to a promoter template in mammalian cells results in histone deacetylation and transcriptional repression. *Arch Biochem Biophys* 434, 316–325.

Senawong, T., Peterson, V.J., Avram, D., et al. 2003. Involvementof the histone deacetylase SIRT1 in chicken ovalbumin upstream promoter transcription factor (COUP-TF)interacting protein 2-mediated transcriptional repression. *J Biol Chem* 278, 43041–43050.

Seong, I. S., Ivanova, E., Lee, J. M., et al. 2005. HD CAG repeat implicates a dominant property of huntingtin in mitochondrial energy metabolism. *Hum Mol Genet* 14, 2871–2880.

Sharma, M. and Gupta, Y.K. 2002. Chronic treatment with trans resveratrol prevents intracerebroventricular streptozotocin induced cognitive impairment and oxidative stress in rats. *Life Sci* 71, 2489–2498.

Shi, T., Wang, F., Stieren, E. and Tong, Q. 2005. SIRT3, a mitochondrial sirtuin deacetylase, regulates mitochondrial function and thermogenesis in brown adipocytes. *J Biol Chem* 280, 13560–13567.

Sian, J., Dexter, D.T., Lees, A.J., et al. 1994. Alterations in glutathione levels in Parkinson's disease and other neurodegenerative disorders affecting basalganglia. *Ann Neurol* 36, 348–355.

Simon, D.K., Pulst, S.M., Sutton, J.P., Browne, S.E., Beal, M.F. and Johns, D.R. 1999. Familial multisystem degeneration with parkinsonism associated with the 11778 mitochondrial DNA mutation. *Neurology* 53(8):1787–93.

Smith, M.A, Perry, G., Richey, P.L., et al. 1996. Oxidative damage in Alzheimer's. *Nature* 382, 120–121.

Solans, A., Zambrano, A., Rodríguez, M. and Barrientos, A. 2006. Cytotoxicity of a mutant huntingtin fragment in yeast involves early alterations in mitochondrial OXPHOS complexes II and III. *Hum Mol Genet* 15(20):3063–81.

Spargo, E., Everall, I.P. and Lantos, P.L. 1993. Neuronal loss in the hippocampus in Huntington's disease: A comparison with HIV infection. *J Neurol Neurosurg Psychiatry* 56(5):487–91.

Stokin, G.B., Lillo, C., Falzone, T.L., et al. 2005. Axonopathy and transport deficits early in the pathogenesis of Alzheimer's disease. *Science* 307, 1282–1288.

Strauss, K.M., Martins, L.M., Plun-Favreau, H., et al. 2005. Loss of function mutations in the gene encodingOmi/HtrA2 in Parkinson's disease. *Hum Mol Genet* 14, 2099–2111.

Strehler, B. L. 1999. *Time, cells, and aging.* Larnaca: Demetriades Brothers.

Strehlow, A.N., Li, J.Z. and Myers, R.M. 2007. Wild-type huntingtin participates in protein trafficking between the Golgi and the extracellular space. *Hum Mol Genet* 16(4):391–409.

Sun, Y., Savanenin, A., Reddy, P.H. and Liu, Y.F. 2001. Polyglutamine-expanded huntingtin promotes sensitization of N-methyl-D-aspartate receptors via post-synaptic density 95. *J Biol Chem* 276, 24713–24728.

Swerdlow, R.H. and Khan, S.M. 2004. A "mitochondrial cascade hypothesis" for sporadic Alzheimer's disease. *Med Hypotheses* 63, 8–20.

Szeto, H.H. 2008. Development of mitochondria-targeted aromatic-cationic peptides for neurodegenerativediseases. *Ann NY Acad Sci* 1147,112–121.

Tabrizin, S. J., Cleeter, M. W., Xuereb, J., Taanman, J. W., Cooper, J. M. and Schapira, A. H. 1999. Biochemical abnormalities and excitotoxicity in Huntington's disease brain. *Ann Neurol* 45, 25–32.

Taira, T., Saito, Y., Niki, T., Iguchi-Ariga, S.M., Takahashi, K. and Ariga, H. 2004. DJ-1 has a role inantioxidative stress to prevent cell death. *EMBO Rep* 5, 213–218.

Takata, T. and Ishikawa, F. 2003. Human Sir2-related protein SIRT1 associates with the bHLH repressors HES1 and HEY2 and is involved in HES1- and HEY2-mediated transcriptional repression. *Biochem Biophys Res Commun* 301, 250–257.

Tang, B.L. 2005a. SIRT1, neuronal cell survival and insulin/IGF-1 aging paradox. *Neurobiol Aging* In Press.

Tang, B.L. 2005b. Alzheimer's disease: Channeling APP to non-amyloidogenic processing. *Biochem Biophysb Res Commun* 331, 375–358.

Tennen, R.I., Berber, E. and Chua, K.F. 2010. Functional dissection of SIRT6: Identification of domains that regulate histone deacetylase activity and chromatin localization. *Mech Ageing Dev* Feb 1.

The Huntington's Disease Collaborative Research Group. 1993. A novel gene containing a trinucleotide repeat that is expanded and unstable on Huntington's disease chromosomes. *Cell* 72, 971–983.

Thomas, B. and Beal, M.F. 2007. Parkinson's disease. *Hum Mol Genet* 16 Spec No. 2:R183–94.

Trifunovic, A.; Wredenberg, A., Falkenberg, M. et al. 2004. Premature ageing in mice expressing defectivemitochondrial DNA polymerase. *Nature* 429, 417–423.

Truant, R., Atwal, R. and Burtnik, A. 2006. Hypothesis: Huntingtin may function in membrane association and vesicular trafficking. *Biochem Cell Biol* 84(6):912–7.

Trushina, E., Dyer, R.B., Badger, J.D. 2nd., et al. 2004. Mutant huntingtin impairs axonal trafficking in mammalian neurons in vivo and in vitro. *Mol Cell Biol* 24, 8195–8209.

Vakhrusheva, O., Braeuer, D., Liu, Z., Braun, T. and Bober, E. 2008. Sirt7-dependent inhibition of cell growth and proliferation might be instrumental to mediate tissue integrity during aging. *J Physiol Pharmacol* 9, 201–212.

Valente, E.M., Abou-Sleiman, P.M., Caputo, V. et al. 2004. Hereditary early-onset Parkinson's disease caused by mutations in PINK1. *Science* 304, 1158–1160.

van Bilsen, P.H., Jaspers, L., Lombardi, M.S., Odekerken, J.C., Burright, E.N. and Kaemmerer, W.F., 2008. Identification and allele-specific silencing of the mutant huntingtin allele in Huntington's disease patientderived fibroblasts. *Hum Gene Ther* 19, 710–719.

Van Raamsdonk, J.M., Metzler, M., Slow, E., et al. 2007. Phenotypic abnormalities in the YAC128 mouse model of Huntington disease are penetrant on multiple genetic backgrounds and modulated by strain. *Neurobiol Dis* 26, 189–200.

Vaquero, A., Scher, M., Lee, D., Erdjument-Bromage, H., Tempst, P. and Reinberg, D. 2004. Human SirT1 interacts with histone H1 and promotes formation of facultative heterochromatin. *Mol Cell* 16, 93–105.

Vaziri, H., Dessain, S.K., Ng Eaton, E., et al. 2001. hSIR2(SIRT1) functions as an NAD-dependent p53 deacetylase. *Cell* 107, 149–159.

Vijayvergiya, C., Beal, M.F., Buck, J. and Manfredi, G. 2005. Mutant superoxide dismutase 1 formsaggregates in the brain mitochondrial matrix of amyotrophic lateral sclerosis mice. *J Neurosci* 25, 2463–2470.

Vijg, J. 2000. Somatic mutations and aging: A re-evaluation. *Mutat Res* 447, 117–135.

Vonsattel, J.P., Myers, R.H., Stevens, T.J, Ferrante, R.J., Bird, E.D. and Richardson, E.P.Jr. 1985. Neuropathological classification of Huntington's disease. *J Neuropathol Exp Neurol* 44, 559–577.

Wang, A.L., Lukas, T.J., Yuan, M. and Neufeld, A.H. 2008. Age-related increase in mitochondrial DNA damage andloss of DNA repair capacity in the neural retina. *Neurobiol Aging* Dec 10.

Wang, H., Lim, P.J., Karbowski, M. and Monteiro, M.J. 2009. Effects of overexpression of huntingtin proteins on mitochondrial integrity. *Hum Mol Genet* 18, 737–752.

Warby, S.C., Doty, C.N., Graham, R.K., et al. 2008. Activated caspase-6 and caspase-6-cleaved fragments of huntingtin specifically colocalize in the nucleus. *Hum Mol Genet* 17, 2390–2404.

Watanabe, M., Dykes-Hoberg, M., Culotta, V.C., Price, D.L., Wong, P.C. and Rothstein, J.D. 2001. Histological evidence of protein aggregation in mutant SOD1 transgenic mice and in amyotrophic lateral sclerosis neural tissues. *Neurobiol Dis* 8, 933–941.

Wheeler, V.C., Auerbach, W., White, J.K., et al. 1999. Length-dependent gametic CAG repeat instability in the Huntington's disease knock-in mouse. *Hum Mol Genet* 8, 115–122.

Wong, P.C., Pardo, C.A., Borchelt, D.R., et al. 1995. An adverse property of a familial ALS-linked SOD1 mutation causes motor neuron disease characterized by vacuolar degeneration of mitochondria. *Neuron* 14, 1105–1116.

Yamamoto, A., Lucas, J.J. and Hen, R. 2000. Reversal of neuropathology and motor dysfunction in a conditional model of Huntington's disease. *Cell* 101, 57–66.

Yang, Y., Hou, H., Haller, E.M., Nicosia, S.V. and Bai, W. 2005. Suppression of FOXO1 activity by FHL2 through SIRT1-mediated deacetylation. *EMBO J* 24, 1021–1032.

Yang, S.H., Cheng, P.H., Banta, H., et al. 2008. Towards a transgenic model of Huntington's disease in a non-human primate. *Nature* 453, 921–924.

Yeung, F., Hoberg, J.E., Ramsey, C.S., et al. 2004. Modulation of NF-kappaB-dependent transcription and cell survival by the SIRT1 deacetylase. *EMBO J* 23, 2369–2380.

Young, A.B., Penney, J.B., Starosta-Rubinstein, S., et al. 1986. PET scan investigations of Huntington's disease:cerebral metabolic correlates of neurological features and functional decline. *Ann Neurol* 20, 296–303.

Zhang, L., Shimoji, M., Thomas, B., et al. 2005. Mitochondrial localization of the Parkinson's disease related protein DJ-1: implications for pathogenesis. *Hum Mol Genet* 14(14):2063–73.

Zhang, Y., Engelman, J. and Friedlander, R.M. 2009. Allele-specific silencing of mutant Huntington's disease gene. *J Neurochem* 108, 82–90.

Zhang, Y., Leavitt, B.R., van Raamsdonk, J.M., et al. 2006. Huntingtin inhibits caspase-3 activation. *EMBO J* 25, 5896–5906

Zimprich, A., Biskup, S., Leitner, P. et al. 2004. Mutations in LRRK2 cause autosomal-dominant parkinsonism with pleomorphic pathology. *Neuron* 44, 601–607.

4   Special Aspects of Research in Aging

Dan R. Berlowitz, Mary Jo Pugh, and Michael P. Gerardo

Medical research encompasses a broad field of scientific inquiry that aims to develop generalizable knowledge regarding the pathogenesis, progression, detection, prevention, and treatment of disease. The subject of inquiry may range from the subcellular level, through the individual patient to complex health care systems. Causal pathways are often examined that aim to understand how specific factors such as genetics, behaviors, medications, sociodemographics, or health system organization impact on outcomes of interest. The knowledge generated through this process may reduce uncertainty and enhance clinical decision-making. The ultimate goal of this endeavor is to improve outcomes for individuals and the population.

In order to accomplish this, rigorous methodologies have been developed and are widely used in clinical research which,(as opposed to basic science) will be the focus of this chapter. These methodologies are described in many standard textbooks addressing topics such as randomized clinical trials, epidemiology, and health services research. Underlying these methodologies are a number of standard assumptions regarding the pathogenesis and treatment of disease that are often based on experiences gained in studying younger patients. Yet, it has long been recognized that these assumptions may not be appropriate for older patients and that as a result, studies performed in younger patients cannot be blindly applied to frail older patients with multiple comorbidities (Zimmer et al. 1985; Applegate and Curb, 1990; Avorn, 1997). Consequently, clinicians caring for older patients require evidence that is based on research studies that not only include large numbers of older patients, but that were designed so as to consider the unique challenges inherent in studying this population.

This need for evidence is especially true in neurology, where clinicians must make decisions every day regarding the management of elderly patients with complex medical presentations. The evidence base to guide these clinical decisions is limited and much of the evidence that is available is based on research studies performed in younger and healthier patients. To interpret evidence, and to understand how research designs may be strengthened, clinicians need to appreciate some of the unique aspects of research in older adults. We now describe why research in older patients is required and discuss some of the methodologic difficulties inherent in studying this population. It is expected that this information will be useful to clinicians evaluating research studies to gain guidance on how best to manage older patients with specific neurological conditions. Additionally, this chapter will provide insights on likely challenges that will be encountered by investigators planning future studies in the elderly.

Issues in Research Design
Defining the Research Question

Most research begins with a well-defined research question or hypothesis. It is essential to have a clear conception as to what is being evaluated and to whom the study results will be applicable. This requires an understanding of the current state of medical knowledge, where there are important gaps in knowledge, and how resources should be directed to best address these gaps. This will help ensure that the study is of sufficient importance so that results influence clinical practice or policies. This need for a well-defined research question is no different when studying older patients.

However, operationalizing the research question through a well-designed and executed study will be more difficult in older adults. In developing a question, most research studies consider a tradeoff between external validity, the ability to generalize the results to a larger population, and internal validity with its more focused study sample, so as to maximize chances of detecting a positive impact of the intervention. Usually, the decision is made to tilt in the direction of internal validity and study a relatively homogeneous population with a well-defined medical condition. The goal is to identify a particular group of patients with a similar pathologic process in whom the efficacy of an intervention can be tested. To accomplish this, strict eligibility requirements define who has the disease of interest and may enter the research study. Such efforts at balancing internal and external validity are challenging in the elderly because of the different presentation of disease, the presence of multiple comorbidities, and the focus on different outcomes. The net result is that many research studies exclude older patients. This underrepresentation of the elderly in clinical trials has been extensively demonstrated for non-neurological conditions, including cardiac disease and cancer (Hutchins et al. 1999; Lee et al. 2001), and the mean age of people enrolled in clinical trials may be twenty years younger than the age of the population with the disease (Heiat et al. 2002).

Disease Presentation in Older Adults

To maximize internal validity, researchers will typically study a well-defined disease or syndrome that is characterized by a particular group of signs and symptoms and that usually reflects a single underlying cause. The underlying cause represents an external stress to the system that has overwhelmed the homeostatic and regulatory mechanisms that humans have developed for protection. Through the process of diagnostic evaluation, clinicians aim to uncover this single underlying cause and then subsequently initiate appropriate therapeutic interventions.

In older adults, this direct correspondence between a single underlying cause and a specific pattern of signs and symptoms is a less common presentation of disease. For example, pulmonary, urinary, or other infections, as well as many other diseases may present similarly with neural dysfunction characterized by delirium rather than signs of disease in the affected organ. In one study involving over 140 patients presenting for geriatric evaluation, only 40% fit the "traditional" disease model that is typically seen in younger patients (Fried et al. 1991).

Atypical presentations reflect the fact that aging is often characterized by a decline in organ capacity and a reduced compensatory ability to respond to external stresses. Consequently, disease may develop in a number of different ways in the elderly (Studenski et al. 2008). First, reflecting the reduced organ capacity, milder external stresses may produce disease. Second, multiple mild processes may interact to contribute to a single presentation. Third, the failure of a widely-used compensatory mechanism may result in the simultaneous presentation of several conditions.

Not only is the presentation of disease in older adults different, there are also different "diseases" that may be the subject of research. The interaction of multiple processes with a general decline in compensatory mechanisms is associated with the development of "geriatric syndromes" such as falls, incontinence, pressure ulcers, and delirium (Inouye et al. 2007). These highly prevalent conditions have been defined as "multifactorial health conditions that occur when the accumulated effects of impairments in multiple systems render a person vulnerable to situational changes" (Tinetti et al. 1995). Research on these conditions must recognize that they develop in response to the interaction of many different precipitating factors. A further implication for research is that interventions to prevent geriatric syndromes must also be multifactorial (Tinetti et al. 1994; Inouye et al. 1999; Allore et al. 2005); no single intervention is likely to work in the majority of patients.

The final common pathway of disease in many older patients is frailty and disability. These are distinct concepts and researchers should explicitly consider the inclusion of these patients in studies. Disability, representing difficulty or dependence in performing activities necessary for independent living, may be present in as many as 30% of community-living elderly (Fried et al. 2004). Frailty is a biologic syndrome of decreased reserve resulting from declines in multiple physiologic systems (Fried et al. 2001). Frailty is characterized by weight loss, sarcopenia, weakness, poor endurance, and slowness. Specific criteria for identifying patients with frailty have been developed, unique challenges to performing research in this population have been described, and a detailed research agenda has been published (Ferrucci et al. 2004; Walston et al. 2006).

Presence of Multiple Comorbidities

To enhance internal validity of research, it is also often desirable to exclude patients with multiple comorbidities. In part, this reflects the desire to create as "pure" a test as possible of the effect of the intervention on the target condition without the confounding influence of competing diseases. The presence of such competing diseases could lead to greater heterogeneity in treatment response so that the same treatment produces different results in patients with different comorbidities (Kravitz et al. 2004). Moreover, many comorbid diseases may also be relative contraindications to the intervention of interest. For example, in a randomized clinical trial of depression care in the elderly, major or minor medical contraindications to antidepressant therapy existed in over 90% of depressed patients (Koenig et al. 1989). Yet the presence of multiple comorbidities is the norm in the elderly. Studies suggest that 62% of people over age 65 have two or more chronic conditions that persist for a year or more and require ongoing medical attention (Anderson and Horvath 2004).

Once the decision is made to include patients with multiple comorbidities in a research study, it often becomes necessary to describe the comorbidity burden. While a simple yes/no categorization could be used for each diagnosis, this approach may be difficult to operationalize given the large number of different diagnoses present in older adults. As a consequence, a variety of different measures have been developed that intend to describe the extent of comorbidities. Among the oldest and most widely used approaches is the Charlson Index, which consists of a weighted measure considering the presence of 17 different diseases (Charlson et al. 1987). Increasingly though, the Elixhauser Index (Elixhauser et al. 1998), which considers the presence of diseases in 30 different categories, is being used by researchers due to reports of improved performance in predicting outcomes when compared to the Charlson Index (Southern et al. 2004). Several measures have been developed specifically for use in the elderly, including the Cumulative Illness Rating Scale (Waldman and Potter 1992) and the High-Risk Diagnoses for the Elderly Scale (Desai et al. 2002) but there is less experience with their use. Proprietary systems initially developed to predict resource utilization based on ICD-9-CM codes contained in administrative databases, including Adjusted Clinical Groups (ACGs) (Weiner et al. 1991) and Diagnosis Cost Groups (DCGs) (Ellis et al. 1996) are also beginning to be used in research applications. Selection and use of a comorbidity index for research purposes should be based on a clear conceptualization of the likely association between comorbidities and the outcome of interest. Is it expected that all comorbidities will equally impact the outcome, that some will be more important than others, or that different comorbidities will impact the outcome in opposite directions? While it is not always evident which comorbidity measure should be used, it is clear that different methods will vary in their ability to predict these outcomes (Berlowitz et al. 2008).

The large number of comorbidities suggests that older patients will be on many different medications. Studies have shown this to be the case, with 44% of men and 57% of women over age 65 on five or more medications (Kaufman et al. 2002). To avoid potential drug-drug interactions, such patients are often excluded from clinical trials, enhancing internal validity at the expense of external validity. This may be particularly true in neurology as many of the commonly used medications for neurological diseases such as epilepsy (e.g. phenytoin, carbamazepine) are potent inducers of hepatic enzymes and have potential interactions with drugs commonly used to treat hypercholesterolemia, hypertension, psychiatric disease, and other diseases common in older adults. Thus, the elderly are disproportionately excluded from randomized controlled trials designed for drug approval.

Selection of Appropriate Outcome Measures

The heterogeneity of older adults also ensures that the selection of appropriate outcome measures will be considerably more complex. In younger patients with single diseases, research typically focuses on "hard" outcomes that are relatively easy to measure such as development of disease complications, survival, or remission. However, with aging and in many neurological conditions, these hard outcomes may become less important as multiple disease processes interact to reduce physical and emotional function. People then may focus more on issues such as preserving function or ameliorating the decline, sometimes at the expense of length of survival. This function must be captured through assessments of multiple domains, many of which are subjective, that may include activities of daily living, mobility, cognitive function, and mood (Katz et al. 1963). More global measures that describe concepts such as health-related quality of life may also be used (Ware and Sherbourne 1992). Patient-centered outcomes that capture patient and family goals for care may be especially desirable in research studies but are challenging to operationalize (Bradley et al. 2000).

Reflecting their decreased reserve and altered pharmacokinetics, older adults are more prone to adverse drug reactions and other complications of interventions. Outcome measures then may also need to focus on the development of complications. One creative approach that has been used is to combine efficacy and tolerability into a single measure. Thus, a recent randomized clinical trial of different medications for epilepsy therapy in the elderly used as its primary outcome measure the ability to stay on the study drugs for up to twelve months, capturing both seizure control and presence of severe side affects (Rowan et al. 2005).

Complicating the selection of outcomes is the fact that older patients will have very different preferences for specific outcomes and for enduring present risk in exchange for future benefits. In many situations, trade-offs will exist between benefits such as enhanced survival versus ongoing side effects from the intervention. A variety of different techniques are available for eliciting these preferences including standard gamble, time trade-off, and conjoint analysis. As one example, a recent study using conjoint analysis found that only 50% of hypertensive elderly favored increased medications to reduce cardiovascular events if it came at the expense of fall injuries and other adverse medication effects (Tinetti et al. 2008). These results emphasize how significant effort may be required in research studies when selecting outcomes relevant to the individual.

Each outcome measure used in a research study should be carefully evaluated. Criteria for such an evaluation have been described for instruments used in assessing geriatric depression and are likely appropriate for other conditions (Rigler et al. 1998). Key issues include understanding the purpose for which the instrument was developed and why it was selected for the study, determining whether reliability and validity have been demonstrated in the study population, identifying what is a clinically meaningful change in the outcome, and ensuring that the study time-frame is of sufficient duration so that meaningful changes in the outcome can occur. Special consideration must be given to floor and ceiling effects with all instruments. It is also important to recognize that in working with an older population, death will not be an uncommon occurrence. How deaths are accounted for with each outcome measure must be considered.

Selection of Study Design

This tension between internal and external validity is also present in the study design selected for a given research project. Depending upon the focus of the study, a number of different options may exist. Some designs, like the randomized clinical trial, provide high internal validity in that the design allows one to test the efficacy of a treatment or intervention in controlled conditions. Because participants are randomly assigned to a treatment or control group, we assume that known and unknown sources of confounding are randomly distributed between the groups. Thus, it may not be necessary to control for individual demographic and clinical characteristics in analyses. However, it is critical that the allocation of participants to treatment or control groups remains blinded to assure unbiased data collection and results (Schulz and Grimes, 2002). As emphasized above, the major limitation of randomized clinical trials in a geriatric population is that generalizability is limited by the extent to which study participants are similar to patients in clinical practice. Moreover, randomized clinical trials are expensive to conduct, particularly in a population that may have a high rate of attrition due to mortality and increasing physical or cognitive disability.

Observational studies, on the other hand, examine treatments or interventions in real world conditions, thus maximizing external validity. They are particularly useful to examine the effectiveness of different treatments in actual clinical conditions. Because few elderly persons are included in randomized clinical trials, and those who are included are often dissimilar to patients treated in clinical practice (Zetin and Hoepner 2007; Gilliam 2003), the effect of many treatments in older

patients with multiple comorbid conditions will not be well understood without observational studies. Fall risk for elderly people on psychoactive medications will be underestimated if only the "healthier" people enrolled in clinical trials are evaluated. Moreover, observational studies allow one to examine questions that would not be ethical to pursue using randomized clinical trials. For instance, it would be unethical to induce a stroke in humans to determine the extent to which such an event may be associated with dementia, epilepsy, or other subsequent medical or psychiatric conditions.

Observational studies may encompass a variety of different designs. They can be retrospective, using pre-existing data to study treatments and outcomes that have already occurred, or prospective. Prospective studies may also use pre-existing data, following the same patient over time, or they may collect new data from the onset of disease or treatment and observing variations in outcomes. Cross-sectional designs have often been used for observational studies in the elderly. Cross-sectional studies take data collected at a single time point and examine associations among variables. The impact of aging on the outcome of interest is then assessed by comparing younger to older people. These studies are limited, though, by the fact that timing of the variables is not examined, so that it is impossible to examine issues of cause and effect (Bowling and Iliffe 2006; Maxwell and Cole 2007; JRank.org 2009). Thus, study differences by age are identified, but they cannot infer that the observed variation is due to aging because the observations are not from the same individuals at different ages (Aldwin and Gilmer 2003). Rather, the variation may be associated with a cohort effect, where there may be differences in a disease state due to variation in exposures for individuals born at a similar time. Cross-sectional studies may be best considered as hypothesis generating or for use when data are needed which can be leveraged to conduct additional clinical research studies that are more focused.

Thus, longitudinal study designs that follow the same individuals over a period of time are generally preferred for aging research. When changes occur over time in measures such as memory or disease states, it is easier to associate those changes with aging. Longitudinal observational studies are the most helpful in understanding the temporal relationship between variables. Such a study could be used to examine the relationship of a specific drug treatment and subsequent patient outcomes over an extended period of time. For instance, it is hypothesized that use of enzyme-inducing antiepileptic drugs induce osteoporosis and are associated with hip fractures. A clinical trial or cross-sectional study would not be able to assess this relationship adequately since it may take two to five years for osteoporosis to develop (Ensrud et al. 2003). Longitudinal observational studies are also useful in examining the temporal relationship between different diseases. For instance, if individuals with a history of psychoses are more likely than those without psychoses to develop new-onset epilepsy in old age, one might posit a causal link that could be explored more closely in subsequent research.

Longitudinal observational studies in the elderly also have some weaknesses. In particular, they may suffer from survivor effects (Aldwin and Gilmer, 2003; Diehr et al. 2003). Over time, participants may be lost to follow-up due to death, disability, or address change. Those lost to follow-up tend to be individuals with poor health; those remaining tend to be healthier, wealthier, and better educated (Aldwin and Gilmer 2003; Diehr et al. 2003). Thus, a longitudinal study may find that memory improves with age if those with poor memory are more likely to drop out of the analyses. Special techniques may be required to account for missing data due to attrition (Hardy et al. 2009).

While observational studies have many benefits, they are complicated in older adults due to the presence of multiple comorbidities and polypharmacy, as described above. While the generalizability is better than a randomized clinical trial, the internal validity may suffer due to confounding—the distortion of the effect of one risk factor by the presence of another. Confounding occurs when two risk factors for a disease are also related, but independently act on the disease or outcome of interest. For instance, stroke and hypertension may both be associated with epilepsy when examined in separate analyses. Because hypertension is a risk factor for stroke, the effect of hypertension may be attenuated or disappear when included in an analysis with stroke. Confounding by indication is another critical issue in observational studies comparing treatments in the elderly. Because treatment is not randomized, a variety of patient characteristics (sex, age, race, disease severity, concomitant medications, symptoms, and patient preferences), and the clinician's attitudes and prognosis for the patient may affect treatment choice (Signorello et al. 2002; Walker and Stampfer 1996). Consequently, groups receiving different treatments will vary on baseline characteristics such as disease severity, and comparisons on outcomes will be difficult. If patients with the most severe disease are treated with different agents than patients with less severe disease, comparisons of the groups will indicate higher mortality or more symptoms related to the treatment—a finding that is due primarily to pre-existing differences rather than the treatment itself.

Because we do not randomly assign individuals in an observational study, confounders are not distributed randomly between the groups. However, confounding can be controlled by restriction (excluding those who meet certain criteria), by matching on the confounding variable or by including it in the statistical analysis (Klein-Geltink et al. 2007). For confounding by indication, propensity score analysis may be used to control for the relationship between a more severe disease state and treatment with a specific drug (Psaty et al. 1999). Typically, in determining a propensity score, logistic regression analysis is used to model the probability of receiving the treatment of interest based on demographic and clinical characteristics available. That analysis yields a propensity score (probability) for each participant. One can then use that propensity score in an overall regression model to control for confounding, stratify patients into groups (typically quintiles) and run analyses by quintile, or match patients exposed or unexposed to the treatment based on the propensity score (McMahon 2003).

Conduct of Research Studies in Older Adults

Not only are there unique considerations in the design of research studies for older patients, there are many practical issues that must be considered in the conduct of the research. Research practices that work well in younger patients may not sufficiently meet the special needs of an older population. Ultimately, how well a research study addresses these practical issues may determine the success or failure of a research project.

Data Sources

Traditionally, research has relied on data collected from four different sources; administrative data, medical record reviews, surveys, or direct observations and testing. The selection of a data source will often be dictated by the research question and study design. While medical records and administrative data make use of existing information, surveys and direct observations and testing involve the primary collection of data. Each of these approaches has their unique strengths and weaknesses and there may be special considerations when working with an older population.

Administrative data has been defined as large, computerized data files generally compiled in billing for health care services. They are typically used in observational studies assessing the quality and

effectiveness of care across large populations or geographic areas. Given the central role of government agencies in financing care for the elderly, files maintained by the Centers for Medicare and Medicaid Services such as the Medicare Standard Analytic Files are particularly useful for studying people over age 65. Among the chief advantages of administrative data is the ability to study large numbers of patients, often totaling thousands or millions of people. This may then be the only way to easily study certain groups such as centenarians or individuals with rare neurologic conditions. Because of their size, it is also possible to detect small differences in outcomes and infrequent events. Additionally, they are relatively easy and cost-effective to use and are non-intrusive. The main disadvantages are that the accuracy of the data is often uncertain and clinically detailed information critical in appreciating disease severity is lacking. The lack of information on functional status in hospitals, but not long-term care settings, may be especially problematic in older adults.

Medical record reviews can provide the more detailed and clinically nuanced information particularly necessary for research in older adults. It also may be the best source of data on providers' thoughts. However, medical record reviews are often time consuming and expensive and it is rarely possible to collect data on more than several hundred people. Information that might be of interest is often missing. Additionally, care for older patients may be especially fragmented and they are likely to see multiple providers; collecting records from these multiple sources may be difficult.

Surveys performed by mail, telephone, in-person, or by other means, are typically the best way to get information on patient attitudes, beliefs, and perceptions. They can be used to collect information on large numbers of people. For example, the Large Survey of Veterans collected information on health-related quality of life and health behaviors on close to a million enrollees of the Department of Veterans Affairs hospitals using a mail survey (Selim et al. 2004). It is important to recognize that older people will have more difficulty and require more time in completing the survey due to auditory, visual, or cognitive deficits. Survey design and methods will want to take this into account. Missing or erroneous data may also be more likely in older patients, so special imputation techniques may be required to help address potential bias (Hardy et al. 2009). Overall response rates have been reported as lower in the elderly and the time to complete surveys will likely be longer.

Direct observation or testing of patients, usually following highly standardized protocols, can provide the most specific data required for a research study. Close attention to the special needs of older patients is often required to ensure the success of these protocols. Along with the previously mentioned concerns regarding hearing, vision, and cognition, limited mobility is common, so study protocols may need to be adapted to decrease the burden associated with study participation. The decline in homeostatic reserve associated with aging may result in more complications from testing. This could alter the balance of benefits and risks associated with the research and needs to be considered throughout the informed consent process.

Increasingly, the sharp distinction between administrative data and more clinically detailed data sources is becoming irrelevant. The growing availability of electronic medical records and new data mining techniques should make it possible to combine the advantages of administrative data, in terms of easily studying large numbers of patients, with the availability of detailed clinical information. This will facilitate a wide variety of research efforts.

Additional Issues with Primary Data Collection

Recruitment of elderly subjects is often more difficult. Travel costs, discomfort, limited mobility, and the need for help from others may all limit interest in participating in a research study. Care must be taken with the sites from where elderly patients are being recruited. If these sites are mostly used by the "healthy" elderly, concerns with external validity will remain. Once enrolled in a research study, the same issues that made recruitment difficult will make retention more difficult. Research protocols will need to be flexible in their scheduling, staff should be aware of special considerations in working with the elderly, and budgets may need to be higher in recognition of these difficulties. Close monitoring of recruitment and retention are essential and case-management strategies may be employed to maximize study involvement. Additionally, dropouts will be more common due to the increased mortality of older adults. This emphasizes that sample size requirements will often be higher in studies with many elderly people. Strategies for maximizing recruitment and retention in studies with older adults have been recently reviewed (Mody et al. 2008).

Setting-specific Issues

Research involving older adults typically must consider a broader range of settings including hospitals, outpatient clinics, nursing homes, home care, hospice, and acute rehabilitation. There are unique issues with conducting research within each of these settings. For example, in hospitals, timely access to research subjects is a major difficulty due to demands from medical care staff, off-unit tests, illness severity, and shorter hospital stays (Berkman et al. 2001). It may be difficult to interview the patient during the hospital stay, delays and difficulties should be anticipated, and effective patient-tracking systems are essential. In nursing homes, where strong academic connections may be weak and resources can be especially constrained, it is essential to enlist support from management and staff. Finding patients is often less of an issue in nursing homes but significant time is often required for personal care and meals, which may limit availability for research interviews (Zermansky et al. 2007). Design issues surrounding the unit of randomization are especially critical in clinical trials involving nursing homes. Often, all patients on a single unit are randomized to receive an intervention. This will reduce power and unless this clustering effect is considered, bias may be introduced (Hahn et al. 2005).

Regardless of initial research setting, it will be important to be aware of transitions between care settings. These transitions are themselves often worth studying and could serve as a study outcome or a predictor for future events. Alternatively, transitions may just complicate the study design as collecting data from patients and dealing with Institutional Review Boards at all these different sites may be difficult.

Informed Consent

The informed consent process is central to the conduct of research but this process may be difficult for individuals with neurological diseases resulting in cognitive impairment. Key components of the informed consent process that should be considered when dealing with cognitively impaired research participants include describing the study to eligible participants and obtaining their voluntary consent to participate in the project. An appropriate study description includes the study purpose, benefits, risks, participation requirements, alternative procedures, confidentiality measures, contact information of the researchers, and the voluntary nature of participation in the study. The decision a subject makes to participate in the study relies not only on understanding this information but also on the reasoned judgment of the subject to participate in the study (e.g. being able to identify whether the benefits of study participation outweigh the risks). The decisional capacity of cognitively impaired individuals may be limited in part because they are unable to understand the information about the study as it is provided to them.

Cognitive impairment, therefore, poses a unique problem to participation in clinical research since the subject's decision-making capacity is affected by their own disease process. Established guidelines state that individuals with impaired capacity may participate in research that does not pose adverse effects to the health status of the study subject or caregiver (Sachs 2009; American Psychiatric Society 2009). Individuals with either very mild or mild dementia exhibit the ability to understand the study (Buckles et al. 2003; Hirschman et al. 2005). As the disease severity worsens, however, the aptitude to understand the study and take part in the decision-making process decreases (Kim et al. 2002). In addition, the motivation a cognitively impaired patient has to partake in the study declines as the invasiveness and risk of the procedure increases (Kim et al. 2002; Sachs 1994). This last observation may be important with regard to studies that focus on identifying novel approaches in therapeutics such as immunotherapy. Even with riskier treatment, most individuals feel that they would trust a family member to perform proxy consent (Kim et al. 2005).

Proxy consent as permitted by federal regulations is a common consideration for research, perhaps most importantly when an individual's cognitive status is at the transition to loss of decision-making capacity (Kim and Kieburtz 2006). While individuals with mild to moderate disease may have the capacity to participate in treatment decisions, as the severity of disease worsens the capacity to participate in the decision-making process declines and the proxy plays a greater role in the process. The proxy, however, is fixed between balancing the risks and benefits of participation in the study for not only the study subject, but also themselves.

In addition to impaired reasoned judgment, various factors have been shown to influence the ability of cognitively impaired individuals to comprehend the study information—including print size of the written materials, use of a third party facilitation, and readability of the written materials (Tymchuket al.1986; Stiles et al. 2001). The investigative team should make every effort to identify and remedy these alternative issues prior to obtaining informed consent (e.g. use of audio amplifiers in those with hearing impairment).

There is no consensus on the appropriate instrument used to determine decisional capacity. Various instruments have been described in the literature, including MacArthur Competency Assessment Tool for Clinical Research (MacCAT-CR), Mini Mental Status Exam (MMSE), Mini-Cog, and Clinical Dementia Rating Scale (CDR) (Buckles et al. 2003; Kim et al. 2001). Most authorities agree that while a gold standard has yet to be identified, it is imperative that the investigative team outline measures to determine the decisional capacity of both the patient and proxy. Researchers should also be aware that decisional capacity will change over time and the potential for change in decisional capacity over time is particularly concerning for trials of longer duration. The investigative team should also be aware that the proxy may also suffer from multiple comorbidities, including cognitive impairment. These comorbidities in and of themselves may limit an individual's ability to understand the informed consent process.

The problem of selection bias is introduced by proxy-based informed consent. Selection bias occurs when the study conclusions are distorted due to the method of selecting study participants. For example, individuals who agree to participate in research may carry less burden of disease or less time spent in care giving. The burden of the decision to participate in research is often dependent on severity of dementia, risk and nature of the study, extent to which the subjects are able to participate in the study, and duration of trial (Kim et al. 2002; Beattie 2007).

This selection effect may influence study conclusions such as health service use or health status. For example, a study may falsely conclude fewer adverse outcomes (e.g. disability, fragility, or death) among a study sample of participants with less severe cognitive impairment. Selection bias may also affect the generalizability of the results of a therapeutic trial because generalization to the public depends on the degree to which the study subjects represent the general population.

The proxy should be made aware of their role in the research process: Observing for adverse events, including those that must be reported immediately to the investigators such as delirium secondary to study medication, as well as less urgent ones such as resolved non-specific symptoms (e.g. nausea or headache); ensuring that the subject take study medication; reporting any change in medications or other co-morbidities including new drugs that may have drug-drug interactions; reporting the identification of new co-morbid illnesses that may exclude the patient from study participation; observing the benefits of medications; and observing for subjective measures of disease efficacy such as caregiver stress/burden.

Conclusions

The challenge for research today is to provide evidence-based information that can help guide clinical practice. Given the prevalence of older adults in most clinical settings, there is a particular need for this research to specifically address the unique challenges inherent in studying this population. Critical is balancing the need for an internally valid study while producing results that are applicable to the patients typically seen in neurology practices. Only when this is successfully done will clinicians get the type of information that will lead to improved patient outcomes.

References

Aldwin, C.M. and Gilmer, D.F.: "Health, illness, and optimal aging: Biological and psychosocial perspectives." California: Sage Publications, 2003.

Allore, H.G., Tinetti, M.E., Gill, T.M., et al.: Experimental designs for multicomponent interventions among persons with multifactorial geriatric syndromes. *Clinical Trials* 2: 13–21, 2005.

American Psychiatric Association: *Informed consent: Office of Healthcare Systems and Financing, June 2001.* Available at: http://www.psych.org/Departments/HSF/ECPBook/InformedConsent.aspx. Accessed May 28, 2009.

Anderson, G. and Horvath, J.: The growing burden of chronic disease in America. *Public Health Reports* 119:263–270, 2004.

Applegate, W.B. and Curb, J.D.: Designing and executing randomized clinical trials involving elderly people. *J Am Geriatr Soc* 38: 943–950, 1990.

Avorn, J. Including elderly people in clinical trials. *BMJ* 315:1033–1034, 1997.

Beattie, B.: Consent in Alzheimer's disease research: Risk/benefit factors. *Canadian Journal of Neurological Sciences* 34: S27–S31, 2007.

Berkman, C.S., Leipzig, R.M., Greenberg, S.A., et al.: Methodologic issues in conducting research on hospitalized older people. *J Am Geriatr Soc* 49:172–178, 2001.

Berlowitz, D.R., Hoenig, H., Cowper, D.C., et al.: Impact of comorbidities on stroke rehabilitation outcomes: Does the method matter? *Arch Phys Med Rehabil* 89:1903–1906, 2008.

Bowling, A. and Iliffe, S.: Which model of successful ageing should be used? Baseline findings from a British longitudinal survey of ageing. *Age Ageing* 35:607–14, 2006.

Bradley, E.H., Bogardus, S.T., van Doorn, C., et al.: Goals in geriatric assessment: Are we measuring the right outcomes? *Gerontologist* 40: 191–196, 2000.

Buckles, V.D., Powlishta, K.K., Palmer, J.L., et al.: Understanding of informed consent by demented individuals. *Neurology* 61: 1662–1666, 2003.

Charlson, M.E., Pomperi, E.P., Ales, K.L., et al.: A new method of classifying prognostic comorbidity in longitudinal studies: Development and validation. *J Chronic Dis* 40:373–383, 1987.

Diehr, P., Patrick, D.L., McDonell, M.B., et al.: Accounting for deaths in longitudinal studies using the SF-36: The performance of the Physical Component Scale of the Short Form 36-item health survey and the PCTD. *Med Care* 41:1065–73, 2003.

Desai, M.M., Bogardus, S.T., Williams, C.S., et al.: Development and validation of a risk-adjustment index for older patients: The High-Risk Diagnoses for the Elderly Scale. *J Am Geriatr Soc* 50: 474–481, 2002.

Elixhauser, A., Steiner, C., Harris, D., et al.: Comorbidity measures for use with administrative data. *Med Care* 36:8–27, 1998.

Ellis, R.P., Pope, G.C., Iezzoni, L., et al.: Diagnosis-based risk adjustment for Medicare capitation payments. *Health Care Finance Rev* 17:101–128, 1996.

Ensrud, K.E., Blackwell, T.L., Mangione, C.M., et al.: Central nervous system-active medications and risk for falls in older women. *J Am Geriatr Soc* 50:1629–1637, 2002.

Ferrucci, L., Guralnik, J., Studenski, S., et al.: Designing randomized, controlled trials aimed at preventing or delaying functional decline and disability in frail, older persons: A consensus report. *J Am Geriatr Soc* 53:625–634, 2004.

Fried, L., Storer, D., King, D., et al.: Diagnosis of illness presentation in the elderly. *J Am Geriatr Soc* 39:117–123, 1991.

Fried, L., Tangen, C., Walston, J. et al.: Frailty in older adults: Evidence for a phenotype. *J Gerontol Med Sci* 56A: M146–M156, 2001.

Fried, L., Ferrucci, L., Darer, J., et al.: Untangling the concepts of disability, frailty, and comorbidity: Implications for improved targeting and care. *J Gerontol Med Sci* 59:255–263, 2004.

Gilliam, F.: What we don't learn from clinical trials in epilepsy. *Epilepsia* 44:51–54, 2003.

Hahn, S., Puffer, S., Torgerson, D.J., et al.: Methodologic bias in cluster randomized trials. *BMC Medical Research Methodology* 5:10, 2005.

Hardy, S.E., Allore, H., and Studenski, S.A.: Missing data: A special challenge in aging research. *J Am Geriatr Soc* 57: 722–729, 2009.

Heiat, A., Gross, C. and Krumhotz, H.: Representation of the elderly, women, and minorities in heart failure clinical trials. *Arch Intern Med* 162:1682–1688, 2002.

Hirschman, K., Joyce, C., James, B., et al.: Do Alzheimer's disease patients want to participate in a treatment decision, and would their caregivers let them? *Gerontologist* 45: 381–388, 2005.

Hutchins, L., Unger, J., Crowley, J., et al.: Underrepresentation of patients 65 years of age or older in cancer-treatment trials. *N Engl J Med* 341:2061–2067, 1999.

Inouye, S., Bogardus, S., Charpentier, P., et al.: A multicomponent intervention to prevent delirium in hospitalized older patients. *N Engl J Med* 340:669–676, 1999.

Inouye, S., Studenski, S., Tinetti, M., et al.: Geriatric syndromes: Clinical, research, and policy implications of a core geriatric concept. *J Am Geriatr Soc* 55:780–791, 2007.

JRank.org. *Methods of studying children—longitudinal versus cross-sectional studies.* 2009. http://social.jrank.org/pages/411/Methods-Studying-Children-Longitudinal-versus-Cross-Sectional-Studies.html. Accessed July, 7, 2009.

Katz, S., Ford, A.B., Moskowitz, R.W., et al.: Studies of illness in the aged: The index of ADL, as standardized measure of biological and psychosocial function. *JAMA* 185: 914–919, 1963.

Kaufman, D.W., Kelly, J.P., Rosenberg, L., et al.: Recent patterns of medication use in the ambulatory adult population of the United States. *JAMA* 287:337–344, 2002.

Kim, S., Caine, E.D., Currier, G.W., et al.: Assessing the competence of persons with Alzheimer's disease in providing informed consent for participation in research. *American Journal of Psychiatry* 159: 712–717, 2001.

Kim, S., Cox, C., and Caine, E.: Impaired decision-making ability in subjects with Alzheimer's disease and willingness to participate in research. *American Journal of Psychiatry* 159: 797–802, 2002.

Kim, S., Kim, H., McCallum, C., et al.: What do people at risk for Alzheimer disease think about surrogate consent for research? *Neurology* 65: 1395–1401, 2005.

Kim, S. and Kieburtz, K.: Appointing a proxy for research consent after one develops dementia: The need for further study. *Neurology* 66: 1298–1299, 2006.

Klein-Geltink, J.E., Rochon, P.A., Dyer, S., Laxer, M., and Anderson, G.M. Readers should systematically assess methods used to identify, measure and analyze confounding in observational cohort studies. *J Clin Epidemiol* 60:766.e1–766.e11, 2007.

Koenig, H., Goli, V., Shelp, F., et al.: Antidepressant use in elderly medical inpatients: Lessons from attempted clinical trial. *J Gen Intern Med* 4:498–505, 1989.

Kravitz, R.L., Duan, N., and Braslow, J.: Evidence-based medicine, heterogeneity of treatment effects, and the trouble with averages. *Millbank Quarterly* 82:661–687, 2004.

Lee, P., Alexander, K., and Hammill, B.: Representation of elderly persons and women in published randomized trials of acute coronary syndromes. *JAMA* 286:708–713, 2001.

Maxwell, S.E., and Cole, D.A. Bias in cross-sectional analyses of longitudinal mediation. *Psychol Methods* 12:23–44, 2007.

McMahon, A.D.: Approaches to combat with confounding by indication in observational studies of intended drug effects. *Pharmacoepidemiol Drug Saf* 12:551–558, 2003.

Mody L., Miller, D., McGloin, J., et al. Recruitment and retention of older adults in aging research. *J Am Geriatr Soc* 56:2340–2348, 2008.

Psaty, B.M., Koepsell, T.D., Lin D., et al.: Assessment and control for confounding by indication in observational studies. *J Am Geriatr Soc* 47:749–54, 1999.

Rigler, S.K., Studenski, S., and Duncan, P.W.: Pharmacologic treatment of geriatric depression: Key issues in interpreting the evidence. *J Am Geriatr Soc* 46: 106–110, 1998.

Rowan, A.J., Ramsay, R.E., Collins, J.F., et al.: New onset geriatric epilepsy: A randomized study of gabapentin, lamotrigine, and carbamazepine. *Neurology* 64: 1868–1873, 2005.

Sachs, G.A.: Advanced consent for dementia research. *Alzheimer's disease and Associated Disorders* 8: S19–S27, 1994.

Sachs, G.A.: *Position Statement Informed Consent for Research on Human Subjects with Dementia AGS Ethics Committee: American Geriatrics Society, 2007.* Available at: http://www.americangeriatrics.org/products/positionpapers/infconsent.shtml. Accessed May 28, 2009.

Schulz, K.F. and Grimes, D.A.: Allocation concealment in randomised trials: Defending against deciphering. *Lancet* 359:614–618, 2002.

Selim, A.J., Berlowitz, D.R., Fincke, G., et al.: The health status of elderly veteran enrollees in the Veterans Health Administration. *J Am Geriatr Soc* 52: 1271–1276, 2004.

Signorello, L.B., McLaughlin, J.K., Lipworth, L., et al.: Confounding by indication in epidemiologic studies of commonly used analgesics. *Am J Ther* 9:199–205, 2002.

Southern, D.A., Quan, H., and Ghali, W.A.: Comparison of the Elixhauser and Charlson/Deyo methods of comorbidity measurement in administrative data. *Med Care* 42:355–360, 2004.

Stiles, P.G., Poythress, N.G., Hall, A., et al.: Improving understanding of research consent disclosures among persons with mental illness. *Psychiatric Services* 52: 780–785, 2001.

Studenski, S., Ferrucci, L., and Resnick, N.M.: Geriatrics. In *Clinical and Translational Science: Principles of Human Research.* (Robertson, D. and Williams, G.H., Eds.) London: Academic Press, 2008, pp 477–495.

Tinetti, M., Baker, D., McAvay, G., et al.: A multifactorial intervention to reduce the risk of falling among elderly people living in the community. *N Engl J Med* 331:821–827, 1994.

Tinetti, M., Inouye, S., Gill, T., et al.: Shared risk factors for falls, incontinence, and functional dependence. *Unifying the approach to geriatric syndromes. JAMA* 273:1348–1353, 1995.

Tinetti, M.E., McAvay, G.J., Fried, T.R., et al.: Health outcome priorities among competing cardiovascular, fall injury, and medication-related symptom outcomes. *J Am Geriatr Soc* 56: 1409–1416, 2008.

Tymchuk, A.J., Ouslander, J.G., and Rader, N.: Informing the elderly. A comparison of four methods. *J Am Geriatr Soc* 34: 818–822, 1986.

Waldman, E. and Potter, J.: A prospective evaluation of the Cumulative Illness Rating Scale. *Aging Clin Exp Res.* 4:171–178, 1992.

Walker, A.M. and Stampfer, M.J.: Observational studies of drug safety. *Lancet* 348: 489, 1996.

Walston, J., Hadley, E.C., Ferrucci, L., et al.: Research agenda for frailty in older adults: Toward a better understanding of physiology and etiology: Summary from the American Geriatrics Society/National Institute on Aging Research Conference on Frailty in Older Adults. *J Am Geriatr Soc* 54:991–1001, 2006.

Ware, J.E. and Sherbourne, C.E.: The MOS 36-item short-form health survey (SF-36). I. Conceptual framework and item selection. *Med Care* 30: 473–483, 1992.

Weiner, J.P., Starfield, B.H., Steinwachs, D.M., et al.: Development and application of a population-oriented measure of ambulatory care case-mix. *Med Care* 29:452–472, 1991.

Zermansky, A.G., Alldred, D.P., Petty, D.R., et al.: Striving to recruit: The difficulties of conducting clinical research on elderly home care residents. *J R Soc Med* 100: 258–261, 2007.

Zetin, M. and Hoepner, C.T.: Relevance of exclusion criteria in antidepressant clinical trials: A replication study. *J Clin Psychopharmacol* 27:295–301, 2007.

Zimmer, A., Calkins, E., Hadley, E., et al.: Conducting clinical research in geriatric populations. *Ann Intern Med* 103:276–283, 1985.

2
Neurological Assessment in Aging

5 Neurological Evaluation of the Elderly Patient

David A. Drachman and Joan M. Swearer

Complaints and dysfunction related to the nervous system are frequent among the elderly. The most common disorders involve memory and intellect; strength, coordination, and balance; and sensation. Neurological disorders are the most frequent cause of major disability in the elderly, and account for almost half the incapacitation occurring beyond age 65 and more than 90% of serious dependency (Broe et al. 1976; Cape and Gibson 1994).

Why should the nervous system be more susceptible to deterioration with age than other body systems? In part, it is because the nervous system consists largely of postmitotic neuronal elements. Although neural stem cells are available in two sites (the subventricular zone, and the hippocampal subgranular zone) to replace some neurons throughout adult life, the vast majority of the 100 billion neurons in the brain (20 billion neocortical) are post-mitotic, and have been present from birth. With learning, synaptic modulation takes place, and under certain circumstances axonal growth can repair damaged circuitry ("sprouting") and replace lost synapses (Cotman 1990), but even this capacity declines with advancing age.

Over time, and with increasing "entropy"—disorder—the function of the nervous system inevitably deteriorates (Drachman 2006). Neurons lose the ability to sustain their large dendritic and axonal arbors, which shrink, and eventually the "housekeeping" molecular functions necessary for neuronal survival fall below a threshold of viability. Even in a system with a large safety factor, the ability to compensate for losses declines as its reserve diminishes, the capacity of neural stem cells to replace failing neurons wanes, and sprouting decreases (Cotman 1990).

For these reasons, neurological deterioration in the elderly is due to the cumulative summation of four interacting factors:

1. "Normal" neuronal functional decline and loss over time

2. Previous damage to the nervous system, and losses

3. Decline in neural reserve, or "plasticity"

4. Specific disease(s) of the nervous system at the time of examination

Individuals vary considerably in the rate of involutional change, the burden of previous damage, the amount of neural reserve, and the presence and extent of nervous system disease. Clinical neurological disorders become evident when a combination of these factors reaches the threshold of clinical deficit. In practice, this threshold may depend not only on the initial neural endowment of the individual minus the sum of neural losses, but also on the demands of the particular situation in which a deficit becomes apparent. Thus, a clinically apparent deficit may be the result of rapidly advancing involution alone, specific disease alone (e.g., a major stroke), previous traumatic injury combined with "normal" age-related changes, or a mild new disease process (e.g., a small lacunar stroke) in someone who must perform at an exceptionally high level.

To understand the neurological problems of the elderly, physicians must consider both the variations in individual performance with age, and the multiplicity of factors contributing to deficits. The clinical application of "Ockham's razor"—i.e., the concept that the correct diagnosis is the *single* condition that explains all the clinical problems—often fails beyond the age of 65 (Drachman 2000).

Physicians evaluating elderly patients must first be able to distinguish between normal and abnormal neurological function commensurate with the individual's age. Second, they must determine whether the neurological impairment is the result of a specific current disease state, previous damage, neural attrition, or loss of neural reserve. Finally, they should identify those features of the patient's condition that contribute to the disability, and modify as many of the problems limiting function as possible.

Normal and Abnormal Functions: Health and Disease

"Normal" function, most simply, is regarded as the mean performance on a given test ± 2 standard deviations (SD) for an individual of a given age. As reasonable as this concept of normal may seem—i.e., the age-related average, or "usual aging" function—it presents many problems. Because there is much scatter of function in the aged compared with young adults, performance is less homogeneous (Sprott 1988). A number of changes commonly seen in the aged (e.g., decreased glucose tolerance, diminished ankle jerk reflexes) are considered to be abnormalities, or even diseases, in the young. Indeed, the fact that almost 75% of individuals over age 65 have at least one significant chronic illness (Calkins, Boult and Wagner 1999; Fried, Bandeen-Roche, Kasper, and Guralnik 1999) makes it impossible to equate normal (average) function in the elderly with a state of health, or the absence of disease.

The difficulties arising from this concept of normality have led to two other definitions of normal function. The first defines normal function as the *average performance of healthy aged individuals*—that is, those functioning independently, who are free of known disease. While this is a useful compromise, the difficulty of defining a "healthy person," and the circular, self-fulfilling nature of the definition limit its value. The second defines normal function in the elderly as identical to *ideal function for all healthy adults,* independent of age. Viewed in this way, findings that occur even frequently in an aged population may be considered abnormal if they fail to meet some definable minimum standard.

In order to evaluate the neurological status of an aged individual, and to attempt to distinguish neurological disease from non-disease, each of these three concepts of normality should be considered. In some elderly patients normal age-related changes will masquerade as an apparent disease, whereas in others an actual disease appears to be part of the normal aging process. Because specific diseases are often treatable, while involution usually is not, this distinction is critical in the neurological assessment.

Neurological Evaluation

The neurological evaluation of any adult, young or old, includes a history, the neurological examination, and a series of laboratory tests. These subjects are well-described elsewhere (e.g., Ropper and Brown 2005) and are not given in detail here. In the elderly, however, a different range of problems is likely to be encountered, and the question of the clinical significance of neurological symptoms or findings becomes more difficult to resolve. The implications of a numb hand or of a Babinski sign are therefore different in the 75-year-old from those in the 25-year-old.

Neurological History

In addition to recording each neurological complaint and obtaining the standard historical information related to the present illness, it is important to document carefully the *rate of decline* of function, to assess the pace of age-related processes, or to diagnose a new neurological disease. A prior history of neurological injury (e.g., head trauma, stroke, encephalitis) defines the extent of previous neural loss. Finally, a review of the neurological system should be carried out, covering the use of alcohol or other drugs, episodes of loss of consciousness, and specific inquiries into cranial nerve, motor, and sensory functions (Table 1).

When obtaining the neurological history of an aged patient, the physician must be prepared to deal with a number of special pitfalls, often due to the plethora of neurological symptoms "normally" seen in the elderly. These complaints make it difficult for both the physician and the patient to distinguish between involutional inevitabilities and real disease. Some of the problems in making this distinction are listed in Table 2.

1. *Inaccurate history in patients with memory loss.* Particularly in the dementing disorders, but also in age-associated memory impairment, the patient may be either unaware of intellectual deficits or may deny them, and the history is then obtainable only from the family. Of course, other aspects of the neurological history become unreliable as well, and the physician cannot depend on reported drug usage or the absence of headache, gait disturbance, and so on. Paradoxically, those patients who do complain of memory loss or of intellectual impairment are less likely to be significantly demented; more often they may be depressed.

2. *Varying expectations for the aged.* Because families' expectations of elderly patients' performance may vary widely, their judgment regarding intactness or degree of impairment may be misleading. The patient who is "very sharp" may be considered so because he or she remembers grandchildren's names; the aged person with a "poor memory" may no longer be able to do the Sunday Times crossword puzzle as quickly as he or she once did, though otherwise functioning at a high level. For this reason, it is especially important to ask questions ranging from the ability of the patient to care for his or her personal needs to competence when playing bridge or discussing world events. "Impairment of memory" is the most frequent initial complaint of both patients and their families in most forms of dementia, although impaired executive functions, loss of interests, or decreased verbal or instrumental skills may be the actual problem. If it is determined that a degree of dementia exists, additional questions must be asked to help clarify the nature and extent of the underlying disorder.

3. *Sudden change versus "revealing events."* Ordinarily, a sudden change in neurological function is an appropriate cause for concern and

medical investigation. In the elderly, however, gradual changes may be suddenly brought to the patient's or family's attention when the circumstances change. A slowly dementing patient may abruptly become totally disoriented on vacation in an unfamiliar place; or if his balance has gradually declined he may now begin to fall when, for example, following the death of his wife, he must walk to the store to shop. Close inquiry is needed to determine the true rate of onset of such events.

4. *Denial; or, excessive somatic concerns.* These polar approaches become more confusing as disability and disease increase with age. Perfectionists report every decline as a probable disease requiring medical investigation, whereas those who are "too prepared" for deterioration fail to regard even serious and debilitating disease as worth mentioning.

Table 1 Review of the Neurological System

Head and Mental Function

Headaches

Dizziness

Mental or memory change

Loss of consciousness

Head trauma

Cerebrovascular accidents

Seizures

Alcoholism

Cranial Nerves

Loss of smell

Blurring or loss of vision

Diplopia

Numbness or weakness of the face

Hearing loss, tinnitus

Difficulty swallowing or speaking

Motor and Coordination

Weakness of an arm or a leg

Clumsiness

Difficulty walking

Reflexes

Involuntary spasms of legs

Bladder or bowel dysfunction

Sensation

Numbness or abnormal sensation in limbs

Table 2 Pitfalls in the Neurological History of the Aged

Inaccurate history in patients with memory loss

Varying expectations for the aged

Sudden change, versus "revealing events"

Denial; or, excessive somatic concern

Impact of life style changes

Decreased activity versus depression

Impaired senses—vision, hearing, taste

5. *Impact of lifestyle changes.* The resources of the elderly—personal, professional, social and financial—modify the perception and effect of normal aging and disease. The octogenarian who moves to the "Sunbelt" may suddenly lose all sources of support and knowledge of the environment acquired over a lifetime. Deprived of friends, family, and transportation, and with a diminished capacity to adapt readily, minor disabilities become major obstacles to coping with the environment.

6. *Decreased activity versus depression.* Ordinarily, decreased energy, interests, and activities; disordered sleep, bowel, and sexual function; and feelings of helplessness are regarded as evidence of depression. These complaints may be physiological in some elderly individuals. The line between physiologically decreased activity and psychopathological withdrawal is a fine one, and the distinction requires the physician's careful judgment.

7. *Impaired senses.* Loss of hearing, vision, and other senses are discussed below. The cumulative impact of multi-sensory isolation may have a global effect on the patient's capacity to absorb new information, in addition to the expected impairment of primary sensations. Frequently, the hard of hearing are regarded as cognitively impaired, and those with visual impairments may have problems with balance.

Neurological Examination

During the neurological examination of the elderly patient, the physician assesses the integrity of the central and peripheral nervous systems using a standard series of maneuvers, described elsewhere (Ropper and Brown 2005) (Table 3).

Assessment of the elderly patient requires that standards of performance be adjusted in accordance with the patient's age, and that particular attention be given to certain areas. Areas of special interest are memory function, vision and hearing, gait, frontal release signs, axial and limb tone, diminution of ankle jerks and distal vibratory sensation, and the presence of cervical or cranial arterial bruits. The significance of these findings is discussed below.

Laboratory Studies

Table 4 lists a number of laboratory studies that are useful during the evaluation of aged patients with a variety of complaints. It is by no means complete, yet even a superficial discussion of the techniques and interpretations is beyond the scope of this chapter. The tests listed provide the means of evaluating the anatomical integrity of the aged patient's nervous system, intellectual performance, hearing, visual acuity, cerebral blood flow, and so on. Numerous other studies are often needed to evaluate the effects of the cardiac, renal, respiratory, and other systems on neurological functions.

Neurobiological Changes with Age

Clinically significant neurological changes that occur with age in an un-diseased population can be attributed to neurobiological deterioration. Anatomical, biochemical, physiological, pharmacological, and support system changes occur in the nervous system and underlie the variable, but eventually inevitable and progressive, involution of the nervous system.

Of all the changes, the anatomical changes have been the most extensively studied and are the best understood. The weight of the brain declines on average by about 2–3% per decade after age 50, accelerating in later years (Esiri, Hyman, Beyreuther, and Masters 1997); by age 80 it has normally decreased by about 10% from its maximum weight during early adult life. Brain volume, reliably measured by MRI

Table 3 Examination of the Nervous System

Mental Status

State of consciousness

Orientation

Information

Memory

Calculation

Language function

Special testing for aphasia, apraxia, or agnosia

Cranial Nerves

Sense of smell

Visual acuity, visual fields, optic fundi

Ocular motility, pupillary response

Facial sensation, corneal reflexes, jaw movement, jaw jerk

Facial movement and symmetry, taste

Hearing (whispered speech; finger rub)

Gag reflex, swallowing, phonation

Sternocleidomastoid and trapezius movement

Tongue motion

Motor and Coordination

Gait, station, walking on heels and toes, tandem gait

Direct testing of strength, tone, and coordination of extremities

Reflexes

Deep tendon reflexes, plantar reflexes, abdominal reflexes

Sensation

Primary (touch, pinprick, vibration, position sense)

Cortical (e.g., face-hand, double simultaneous stimulation)

Vascular System

Carotid palpation, auscultation for bruits

during life, undergoes a decrease of frontal lobes of about 12%, and temporal lobes of 9%, while parietal and occipital lobes show relatively little change; the majority of the change occurs after age 50 (DeCarli et al. 2005). The ventricles and sulci enlarge in volume, and both gray and white matter appear to shrink. On MRI studies, white matter hyperintensities increase exponentially with age, and are present to some extent in 90% of normal elderly subjects aged 65–75 (Soderlund, Nyberg, Adolfsson, Nilsson, and Launer 2003). The number of neurons in the cerebral cortex declines, with decreases of about 10% of the 20 billion neocortical neurons by age 90 (Pakkenberg et al. 2003). Neurons are variably lost in different cortical areas, with the hippocampal region showing little change in number of neurons during normal aging (West, Coleman, Flood, and Troncoso 1995) despite a decline of hippocampal volume (Scahill et al. 2003), loss of synapses (Bertoni-Freddari et al. 2003), and neuronal loss in the adjacent entorhinal cortex (Lippa, Hamos, Pulaski-Salo, DeGennaro, and Drachman 1992). Neuronal losses also occur in the cerebellum, locus ceruleus, nucleus basalis, and anterior horn cells of the spinal cord. The losses of myelinated nerve fibers are far more severe than those of neuronal perikarya; 40% are lost by age 90 (Pakkenberg et al. 2003). Thus, much of the capacity of neurons to communicate, and many of the established connections representing memories, may be lost.

Table 4 Neurological Laboratory Tests Useful in the Aged

Neuroimaging Procedures

MRI/MRA scan, CT scan, PET scan

Electrophysiological Tests

Electromyography; nerve conduction velocities

Electroencephalography

Audiometry

Electronystagmography

Psychometric Tests

WAIS-IV

WMS-IV

MMPI-2

MMSE

Vascular Tests

Duplex scan of carotid, vertebral arteries

Neuro-ophthalmological Tests

Visual acuity

Visual fields

Slit lamp

Lumbar puncture

Other microscopic changes that occur in the brain with normal aging include senile plaques, neurofibrillary tangles (NFTs), granulovacuolar degeneration, Hirano bodies, glial proliferation and neuropil threads. Although plaques and tangles are regarded as the hallmarks of Alzheimer's disease (AD), they are found in many normal elderly subjects. Senile plaques consist of dystrophic neurites (axons and dendrites) surrounding an amyloid core; NFTs are intraneuronal silver-staining bodies that are formed by hyperphosphorylated tau protein, and ultrastructurally appear as paired helical filaments. There is considerable overlap between the microscopic findings in normal aged brains and those of patients with AD; Davis and colleagues noted that only 17% of brains from elderly, cognitively normal individuals had few or none of the changes typical of AD (Davis, Schmitt, Wekstein, and Markesbery 1999). In other studies, brains from as few as 18% to as many as 65% of cognitively normal individuals met the CERAD (Consortium to Establish a Registry for Alzheimer's Disease) or the National Institute on Aging—Reagan neuropathologic criteria for AD. It is likely that neuronal, synaptic, and myelinated fiber losses and dysfunction are responsible for the memory and cognitive impairment that occur with normal aging; and that the senile plaques and NFTs do not cause the decline, but serve rather as markers of the processes that are degrading cognitive function.

The total number of motor units (anterior horn cells of the spinal cord and their related muscle fibers (Zhang, Goto, Suzuki, and Ke 1996)) decreases, as does the number of muscle fibers (Faulkner, Larkin, Claflin, and Brooks 2007), with loss of about 50% by age 80. In peripheral nerves, the number of fibers may decline moderately with age (Moriyama, Amano, Itoh, Shimada, and Otsuka 2007).

The *biochemical* basis for neurological deterioration with age is less well understood. Numerous changes have been observed with advancing age, including the accumulation of lipofuscin in neurons, accumulation of oxygen free radicals (Mancuso et al. 2007), impaired mitochondrial function (Barja 2004), damage to neurons due to excitotoxin accumulation with excessive calcium influx into neurons, failure of the normal DNA repair mechanisms (Weissman et al. 2007), disordered processing and accumulation of beta-amyloid, and many other changes. Which of these alterations in the biochemical processes results in, or contributes significantly to, loss of neurons and decline in function of the remaining neurons is uncertain, but the decline in neural function with aging is most likely the result of decreased efficiency of multiple interacting age-related changes (ARCs) (Drachman 2006).

Physiologically, there is evidence that cerebral blood flow (Stoquart-ElSankari et al. 2007) and cerebral metabolic rate of oxygen and glucose diminish, although not dramatically; in aged individuals selected for high levels of cognitive performance ("supernormals"), these metabolic changes are minimized (Cutler 1986). Central synaptic delays in reflex arcs as well as in complex pathways are increased in the elderly; as a result, evoked potential responses, which summate sequences of neural interactions, are prolonged and show a tendency to dyssynchrony. In aged subjects, the overall amount of spontaneous physical activity is reduced (Buchman, Boyle, Wilson, Bienias, and Bennett 2007), a clinical observation that is reflected in studies of the diminished "activity levels" of aged versus young rats.

Pharmacological changes occur with aging. Cortical cholinergic receptors decline with age, and choline acetyltransferase (ChAT)—an important enzyme required for the synthesis of acetylcholine (ACh)—decreases during extreme old age and in the presence of Alzheimer's dementia (Contestabile, Ciani, and Contestabile 2008; Schliebs and Arendt 2006). Basal forebrain cholinergic axons are thickened and their terminals are ballooned with aging (Geula, Nagykery, Nicholas, and Wu 2008), and hippocampal cholinergic neurons undergo degeneration (Ypsilanti, Girao da Cruz, Burgess, and Aubert 2008). The decline in cholinergic neural function has been shown to be closely related to impairment of cognitive function (Drachman and Glosser 1981). Enzymes involved in catecholamine and γ-aminobutyric acid (GABA) synthesis diminish with age (Dreher, Meyer-Lindenberg, Kohn, and Berman 2008), whereas monoamine oxidase (MAO), which is concerned with catecholamine degradation, increases especially in the basal ganglia, adding to decrease of catecholamine levels in the basal ganglia.

Because the nervous system depends on other organs for life support, the decline of a wide variety of other functions, from cardiac output to basal metabolic rate (Masoro 1991), also affects the functional integrity of the central and peripheral nervous systems.

Neurology of the "Normal" Aged in the Absence of Disease

As a result of involutional processes occurring with age, a number of neurological changes occur in the absence of specific disease. Some are noted by elderly individuals, such as diminished memory; others may be detected only by a neurological examination. Not only is the midpoint of the normal distribution curve shifted in the elderly, but the variance seems to increase considerably (Masoro 2001; Sprott 1988). As a result, the distinction between the low end of normal function and a disease-induced abnormality becomes blurred. The neurologist must often decide whether the findings represent a disease or simple involution, based on the context in which the signs appear. For example, Babinski signs may (rarely) be seen in the absence of disease in the elderly, but if they occur asymmetrically and in the presence of weakness they are most likely part of a disease process, rather than merely age-related findings. Neurological changes in the elderly should be interpreted with this variation in mind.

Clinical Changes

Mental Status

The complaint of memory impairment is common among the elderly. Memory complaints may, however, include other disorders of cognitive function, but it is difficult for most elderly people to identify or specify changes in other cognitive domains, ranging from impaired attention to problem-solving. Subjective reports of memory and cognitive function by the elderly are of value for several reasons. Self-report of memory problems has been associated with performance on psychometric tests of memory and cognitive function in some studies (Jessen et al. 2007; Jonker, Launer, Hooijer, and Lindeboom 1996; Miranda et al. 2008), and is consistently found to be related to depression, as well as to some personality traits and to generally poor physical health (Jorm et al. 2004). In addition, self-report of memory impairment may be an early sign of dementing disorders (Jonker, Geerlings, and Schmand 2000).

On formal psychometric assessment, the elderly show, on average, age-related decrements on learning and memory tasks that require active and effortful manipulation of material (Balota, Dolan, and Ducheck 2000). Among memory tests, those concerned with learning and storage of new information—free recall of "declarative" or "episodic" memory (for specific facts and events)—or manipulation of information held in "working memory," show impairments in the elderly compared with young adults. Immediate memory span is relatively unimpaired in the elderly, however (e.g., digit span forward, frequency estimation). Fluid intelligence (the type required for solving novel problems) is impaired more often and earlier in the elderly than is crystallized intelligence (which reflects breadth of prior knowledge) (Craik and Bialystok 2006). Many psychometric tests have been used to measure intellectual function in both young and aged adults; the tests that rely more on fluid intelligence tend to show differences with age. With the Wechsler Adult Intelligence Scale, 4th Edition (WAIS-IV) (Wechsler 2008), standardized norms adjust for the effects of aging on test performance. To illustrate the similarities and the differences, an IQ of 140 in a 64-year-old would translate to an IQ of 130 in a 34-year-old, a modest correction. Yet to obtain an IQ of 100 at age 80, one need obtain only two-thirds as many correct answers as at age 21; with significantly different standards for the subtests of fluid intelligence (one-half as many correct answers), compared with an equal number expected of the young and the elderly on a test of general knowledge base of facts.

The solving of complex novel problems and abstract reasoning also show declines with age, but problem-solving performance on practical, real-life tasks may improve with age. Visual perception and spatial abilities consistently show age decrements; rapid responses under time constraints, especially where complex actions are required, show the most consistent age-related declines of all psychometric tests (Salthouse 1996). Other observations indicate that the aged as a group have diminished energy, tend to be cautious, and show decreased initiative (Kausler 1990).

Despite the many changes in memory and cognitive function that have been shown to decline with advancing age, it is important to understand that these differences are evident between *groups* of young and elderly adults. Even with the most age-sensitive psychometric tests, such as those involving timed responses to complex stimuli, only about one-fourth of the variability in intelligence scores can be accounted for by age (Salthouse 1982). This finding reflects the fact that *individual differences*, regardless of age, account for much more of the variation than age-related differences; an intelligent 70-year-old may well perform better than a less gifted 21-year-old.

It is often valuable when assessing the mental function of the aged to observe performance not only on direct tests of mental status, but also on the ability to function in everyday activities. The normal elderly individual should be able to manage personal, family, and financial affairs, maintain a knowledge of world events, and keep up with contemporaries in conversation, card games, and so on. A significant change in interactions with close family members should be carefully considered; the previously dominant husband who now turns to his wife for answers to questions, no longer trusting his memory or judgment, exemplifies this change. Assessment of functional status may also be of value for identifying elderly individuals in need of social services in order to maintain their personal independence in the least restrictive setting possible. Finally, it is important to recognize that depression, common in the elderly (Blazer 2003), is associated with cognitive and memory deficits (Dotson, Resnick, and Zonderman 2008)—or "pseudodementia." A high index of suspicion should be maintained for this treatable functional disorder.

When it becomes important to document either the extent of mental deterioration or its absence, psychometric instruments available for this purpose are helpful. Few standardized instruments are available for the self-report of memory complaints (see Reid and Maclullich 2006). There are a number of brief screening tests of mental status by an examiner and for the functional assessment of activities of daily living (see (Holsinger, Deveau, Boustani, and Williams 2007). Computerized test batteries have been developed more recently as screening measures of cognitive decline in the elderly (Wild, Howieson, Webbe, Seelye, and Kaye 2008). Formal psychometric testing is useful for objective testing and measurement of cognitive capacity and performance. The WAIS-IV (Wechsler 2008) is among the most frequently used tests of general intelligence; the Wechsler Memory Scale, 4th Edition (WMS-IV) (Wechsler 2009) and the Rey Complex Figure Test (Meyers and Meyers 1995) for various aspects of memory; the Boston Naming Test (Goodglass and Kaplan 2000) and Boston Diagnostic Aphasia Examination, 3rd Edition (Goodglass, Kaplan, and Barresi 2001) for language disorders; and the Stroop Color and Word Test (Golden and Freshwater 2002) and Hooper Visual Organization Test (Hooper 1983) among others, for additional aspects of cognitive function. (For additional references see Lezak, Howieson, Loring, Hannay, and Fischer 2004; Weintraub 2000). For the diagnosis of functional or affective disorders, the Minnesota Multiphasic Personality Inventory-2 (Graham 2000), the Beck Depression Inventory–II (Beck, Steer, and Brown 1996) and the Geriatric Depression Scale (Yesavage et al. 1982) are useful.

Compared with these tests, the clinical impression of a skilled physician may be, paradoxically, both cruder and more subtle. A skillful interview and brief mental status screening may detect minor disorders that affect objective tests minimally if at all; yet it may miss surprisingly gross deficits of isolated cognitive functions in patients whose alertness and energy is retained. Much of the difficulty of determining whether an elderly person is cognitively and emotionally "normal" relates to the physician's lack of information regarding the true baseline. Thus in the absence of the examining physician's prior personal knowledge of the patient, a highly intelligent individual may seem competent despite a considerable degree of intellectual loss, whereas a person of limited initial endowment may appear to be demented in the absence of significant intellectual decline.

Cranial Nerves

Significant alterations in cranial sensory functions are seen in the normal elderly. With age, impairment of visual accommodation for near objects is nearly universal (Charman 2008); distant vision also requires corrective lenses by age 70 in many individuals. Dark adaptation diminishes with age (Jackson, Owsley, and Curcio 2002), and greater illumination is needed for accurate vision. Yellowing of the lens impairs color vision for the blue end of the spectrum (Weale 1986), and alterations of the crystalline protein structure of the lens results in opacities that eventuate in cataract formation (Srivastava, Chaves, Srivastava, and Kirk 2008). Centrally, visual evoked responses are delayed, suggesting slowing in the central visual pathways (Celesia, Kaufman, and Cone 1987). Pupillary responses are diminished or even absent in the elderly, and pupil size decreases on average (Fotiou et al. 2007). Ocular motility tends to be slowed, and upward gaze is often limited. Perception of visual stimuli also diminishes in the elderly: Critical flicker fusion frequency declines with age, and embedded figures are less easily extracted from confusing pictures (Kline and Schieber 1985).

Hearing is similarly diminished in the aged, beginning at about age 50. High frequencies are chiefly affected, and the suggestion has been advanced that it may be due to acoustic trauma suffered over a lifetime (Dobie 2008). Dichotic auditory stimuli are less often correctly identified simultaneously (Drachman, Noffsinger, Sahakian, Kurdziel, and Fleming 1980); this observation suggests that central processing of auditory information becomes limited with advancing age. Diminution of the senses of taste and smell has been noted but is less well documented (Rawson 2006). Impairment of other cranial nerve functions may be seen with specific disease entities but is not commonly associated with the normal aging process. Occasionally, it is difficult to distinguish between neurogenic dysarthria and that due to oral pathology (ill-fitting dentures, for example).

Motor System

Second to impairment of mental function, deterioration of gait and motility are the most frequent neurological changes seen with advancing age (Brach, Studenski, Perera, VanSwearingen, and Newman 2007; Marigold and Patla 2008). The confident stride of youth changes to a hesitant, broad-based, small-stepped gait that has many of the characteristics of early parkinsonism: stooped posture, diminished arm-swing, en bloc turns (Critchley 1956; Mortimer 1988). The difference between this gait change and certain of the clinical disorders described below may appear to be subtle, but from a practical viewpoint, the distinction between a normal gait in an elderly person and one due to dysfunction is the ability of the normal individual to walk without serious limitations or falls. The physiological changes that result in the disordered gait of the elderly are numerous and include a decline in extrapyramidal function, which is associated with significant loss of dopaminergic neurons in the pars compacta of the substantia nigra during normal aging (Mortimer 1988). In addition, however, a wide variety of other central structural changes—cerebellar, prefrontal and parietal cortex, basal ganglia, subcortical white matter—have been correlated with gait impairment. In addition, impaired peripheral nerve function and orthopedic changes may combine to shorten the stride, resulting in a "kinematic profile of walking in an older person… often referred to as a senile gait" (Elble, Hughes, and Higgins 1992). Other clinical characteristics include stooped posture, slowed cadence, reduced arm swing, increased time with both feet on the floor, loss of normal heel-toe sequence, and decreased foot-floor clearance (Elble, Hughes, and Higgins 1992). Peripheral changes in the motor system are limited in extent: There is a slight decrease in nerve conduction velocity (see below), a moderate decrease in muscle mass (Dey, Bosaeus, Lissner, and Steen 2009) and power, and a significant decline in the number of anterior horn cells (Zhang, Goto, Suzuki, and Ke 1996). Tremor is often regarded as a normal occurrence in advanced age, and some degree of tremor is present on detailed testing in about a third of elderly individuals; but fewer than 3% of the elderly consider it to be significant (Louis, Wendt, and Ford 2000). Subjective complaints of tremor should be regarded as a potential neurological dysfunction. Increased muscle tone may be seen (Critchley 1956) in the

form of mild axial rigidity, slight limb rigidity (resistance to passive stretch), or mild paratonic rigidity (gegenhalten), often in association with other evidence of "frontal lobe release" signs. The role of arthritic or orthopedic changes, including mechanical limitation of joint motion, pain on motion, and inelastic tendons or ligaments, is difficult to assess, but it is certain that they contribute to the impaired mobility of the elderly (Critchley 1956).

Reflexes

The reflex change most commonly noted in the aged is diminution or absence of ankle jerks, which may occur in 5% to 10% of patients (Hobson and Pemberton 1955; Impallomeni, Kenny, Flynn, Kraenzlin, and Pallis 1984). Whether it reflects a simple degenerative change or any of a variety of neuropathies (e.g., diabetes) is uncertain. The finding may occur in the absence of a typical peripheral neuropathy. Plantar reflexes are neutral or extensor in about 5% of the aged (Hobson and Pemberton 1955), and superficial abdominal reflexes are often absent. The latter finding is often attributed to obesity, abdominal surgery, or multiparity (Critchley 1956). Suck and grasp reflexes, often regarded as signs of general cerebral or frontal lobe damage, occur in many elderly patients; and the snout reflex, a "corticobulbar" sign, is also frequently present (Damasceno et al. 2005).

Sensation

Vibratory sensation is regularly diminished or lost in the lower extremities, increasing from about one-tenth of individuals at age 60, to one-third to one-half beyond age 75 (Hobson and Pemberton 1955). An increase in the thresholds for touch and pinprick may be found but is not ordinarily present at the level of clinical testing. This diminution may be due to changes in skin and connective tissue (Lin, Hsieh, Chao, Chang, and Hsieh 2005). The face-hand test, a measure of cortical perceptual ability, may show extinction of the hand stimulus in the elderly (Bender, Fink, and Green 1951). Other measures of cortical perception (e.g., stereognosis, graphesthesia, double simultaneous stimulation) ordinarily remain intact.

Laboratory Changes
Clinical Neurophysiology

Clinical neurophysiology has long incorporated the concept of age-specific normal ranges. Computers extract quantitative digitized data from the qualitative analogue signals derived from nervous system electrical activity. As a result, the age-related changes have been well characterized for many quantitative measures of brain and peripheral nerve function. As for the clinical examination, however, the demarcation between normal aging changes and disease is imprecise. The distributions of normal populations not only shift with age, but they usually broaden as variability increases. As a result, there is significant overlap for many electrophysiological measures between normal elderly subjects and aged patients with disease. Thus when data from normal controls are compared with those from age-matched patients with a given disease, the groups differ significantly, but many individuals from each group overlap with the other group. This fact limits the diagnostic utility of physiological measures that change with age; and disease is more reliably identified by serial observations that show accelerated change over time than by data from a single point in time.

Electroencephalographic Changes

During normal aging, the background rhythm in the EEG characteristically may slow, with a shift of the mean alpha frequency from 11 to

12 Hz to as low as 8 Hz. Studies that scrupulously exclude the diseased elderly confirm this finding but indicate that EEG slowing with an alpha frequency below 8 Hz suggests the presence of disease at any age (Katz and Horowitz 1982). Both slow and sharp transients may be observed with increasing frequency in the elderly; this finding may reflect normal aging changes but, alternatively, may indicate disease. Quantitative EEG readings employing spectral analysis of EEG activity and "topographic brain mapping" in color provide additional views of brain electrical activity. Although these techniques have led to many reports of age-related changes (Breslau, Starr, Sicotte, Higa, and Buchsbaum 1989; Williamson et al. 1990), the findings vary from study to study owing to technical differences. Many studies, particularly with quantitative EEG methods, indicate that increased delta (1.5 to 3.5 Hz) or theta (3.5 to 7.7 Hz) power, decreased mean total spectral frequency, or decreased occipital dominant alpha rhythm may be associated with cognitive decline from normal to mild cognitive impairment or dementia (Jackson and Snyder 2008; Prichep 2007).

Evoked Potentials

Short-latency auditory, visual, and somatosensory evoked potentials, used clinically to reveal lesions within sensory pathways, as well as P300 waves, show changes with normal aging (Gaal, Csuhaj, and Molnar 2007; Guillaume et al. 2009; Jackson and Snyder 2008; O'Donnell, Friedman, Swearer, and Drachman 1992; Schiff et al. 2008). These changes may reflect aging effects in the periphery as well as in the central nervous system, however, such as the effects of sensorineural hearing loss on brainstem auditory evoked potentials. The interpretation of evoked potential changes in the elderly may be confounded by these peripheral changes in sensitivity, and their clinical utility must be considered in that light.

Peripheral Electrodiagnosis

The amplitudes of sensory nerve action potentials and, to a lesser degree, compound muscle action potentials decrease with age (Kimura 1989; Lauretani et al. 2006). The median nerve sensory amplitude falls roughly 50% from the second to the eighth decade. Both motor and sensory conductions slow somewhat with age, particularly along distal segments; and H-reflex responses may be absent bilaterally in the normal elderly. On needle electrode studies, electromyographic (EMG) changes are also seen with age. Motor unit potential amplitude, duration, and complexity increase with age—most likely reflecting an ongoing (but largely subclinical) process of denervation and reinnervation (Howard, McGill, and Dorfman 1988; Klass, Baudry, and Duchateau 2008).

Neuroimaging

Computed tomography (CT) and magnetic resonance imaging (MRI) provide direct images of the brain. CT images are produced by converting the local differences in X-ray absorption of brain structures into computer-generated brain slices, while MRI provides considerably higher resolution brain images by converting the differences in the alignment of hydrogen ions (protons) contained in water within brain structures to radiofrequency signals in the presence of magnetic forces some 30,000 times greater than the earth's magnetic field. Both imaging techniques have been used in an effort to determine brain changes that occur normally with aging and to distinguish normal aging changes from those that occur in age-associated pathological conditions, such as dementia.

When groups of elderly subjects are studied, both CT and MRI show mild enlargement of the ventricular system and widening of the sulci due to a decrease in brain volume (Jagust et al. 2008), which may

increase—particularly in the mesial temporal lobes—in Alzheimer's disease, and in frontal and temporal areas in lobar (fronto-temporal) dementia. The technology of MRI also reveals an increase in the frequency of occurrence of subcortical white matter hyperintensities, particularly on T2-weighted scans, in normal elderly subjects, with 90% of those 65 to 75 years of age showing these changes (Soderlund, Nyberg, Adolfsson, Nilsson, and Launer 2003). Neither the presence nor the number of these small hyperintense areas distinguishes the brains of normal aged subjects from those with AD, but findings similar in appearance are associated with vascular disease (Young, Halliday, and Kril 2008). From a clinical standpoint, these imaging techniques are often more valuable for their ability to identify, or rule out, specific disease (e.g., stroke, brain tumor, certain dementias) than for recognition of specific age-related changes.

Although their clinical usefulness has not yet been defined, single photon emission computer tomography (SPECT) and positron emission tomography (PET) add additional metabolic dimensions to brain imaging. Both techniques provide images of injected or inhaled radioisotope tracers that distribute in specific ways in the brain. SPECT uses predominantly technetium 99m (99mTc) radioisotope that distributes with the cerebral blood flow; PET typically uses 18F-fluorodeoxyglucose radioisotope to assess regional glucose metabolism. Only minor decreases in blood flow and cerebral metabolism are seen in normal aged subjects, although most such studies have been done in the resting state. Although these techniques may reveal supportive evidence for cerebrovascular disease and AD, the findings are often neither unique nor diagnostic (Fazekas et al. 1989). The potential for using PET, SPECT, or functional MRI (fMRI) techniques to assess preclinical decreases in specific metabolic capabilities may prove them to be valuable additions to the neuroimaging techniques useful for the study of aging.

Neurological Dysfunction Due to Involution: Disability without Disease

Even in the absence of specific disease states, normal attrition of neural function leads to a significant degree of disability in some individuals. This area is the no-man's land in the neurology of aging: a statistical inevitability situated between normal age-related changes and specific disease. Several conditions are worth noting because of their frequency of occurrence in a nondiseased population: Age-associated memory impairment/mild cognitive impairment, dizziness, gait disorders, and cervical spondylosis.

Age-associated Memory Impairment, Mild Cognitive Impairment, and Dementia

Human memory is not a single, uniform function (Drachman 2008). It includes *immediate memory*, for transient holding of small amounts of information, such as telephone numbers (e.g. with a limited length), or *span*. Memory *storage* relates to the longer-term learning of information, and includes both *declarative* and *procedural* memory. *Declarative* memory involves those remembered items that can be conveyed in oral or written speech, while *procedural* memory refers to learned behaviors, such as driving a car or playing the piano. Declarative memory includes both *episodic* memory—the remembering of events and experiences that one has personally experienced—and *semantic* memory, which is the verbal knowledge of deeply-learned factual material, such as one's birthday or the capital of the United States.

Older adults often have greater difficulty than younger adults primarily with *episodic memory*; immediate memory span, procedural memory, and semantic memory remain largely intact. The decrease of memory is evident on tests of free recall (recall of studied test material without cues), associative learning (creation and recall of novel associative links between items), source memory tests (e.g., recall of where a fact was learned rather than its content), and prospective memory tests (e.g., holding an intention for a future act in mind and executing it without cues) (Luo and Craik 2008). These normal age-related changes in memory, and other cognitive functions as outlined earlier, have been termed "benign senescent forgetfulness," or "age-associated memory impairment" (AAMI).

When cognitive changes exceed this level of age-adjusted decline, but do not reach the extent of dementia, without *significant functional impairment* involving activities of daily living, they have been termed "cognitive impairment–no dementia" (CIND) and "mild cognitive impairment" (MCI) (DeCarli 2003). The construct of MCI refers to an intermediate level of cognitive performance, between normal age-related cognitive functioning and early, clinically identifiable dementia. MCI may involve only memory impairment (MCI-amnestic), or other cognitive domains—either single or multiple. An individual with amnestic-MCI, for example, has memory complaints, greater than age-adjusted memory impairment on exam, but otherwise intact general cognitive functioning and preserved activities of daily living. Individuals with MCI do not meet clinical criteria for dementia, but are at increased risk of developing AD (Petersen 2004).

While MCI indicates that the individual's cognitive function is less than expected for his/her age, it does not necessarily predict further, greater-than-normal decline. About 13% of individuals with MCI progress to dementia annually, and about half over a period of five years; but some have a stable course, while others may return to normal function over time (Fellows, Bergman, Wolfson, and Chertkow 2008). A study group on mild cognitive impairment recommended the following criteria for MCI (Winblad et al. 2004):

"(i) the person is neither normal nor demented; (ii) there is evidence of cognitive deterioration shown by either objectively measured decline over time and/or subjective decline by self and/or informant in conjunction with objective cognitive deficits; and (iii) activities of daily living are preserved and complex instrumental functions are either intact or minimally impaired."

Age-related changes in memory and cognition are not always trivial or "benign," even when occurring in the absence of a specific dementing disease. In part, this confusion relates to our inability to determine clinically where the consequences of normal neuronal attrition end and AD begins. There is considerable evidence that the hallmark pathological changes of AD—senile plaques and neurofibrillary tangles—accumulate in increasing numbers with advancing age in a nondemented population (Davis, Schmitt, Wekstein, and Markesbery 1999), although neuronal and synaptic losses in critical brain areas are moderate (Bertoni-Freddari et al. 2003; Lippa, Hamos, Pulaski-Salo, DeGennaro, and Drachman 1992). With advancing age, an increasing proportion of the "normal" population shows declines on cognitive testing compared to young adults (Drachman 1986); past the age of 75 only a fraction of individuals can compete at an intellectual level permitting continued employment. Although this decline in cognitive ability is not a specific disease state—and by itself does not necessarily progress to significant dementia—the cognitive decline in AAMI, and the cognitive impairment in MCI, may prove limiting in the context of the elderly individual's usual social or occupational requirements.

Dizziness

Dizziness, a frequent complaint in the elderly, is commonly the result of sensory changes involving multiple sensory modalities (Drachman

1998). Normal spatial orientation requires accurate visual, vestibular, proprioceptive, tactile, and auditory perception. Impairment of several of these orienting senses is perceived by patients as "dizziness"—an elusive complaint that results from the patient's uncertainty of position or motion in space. The elderly individual complaining of multisensory dizziness typically walks with a broad-based, unsteady gait, having particular difficulty turning and walking on uneven ground. Carrying a cane or holding someone's arm improves the balance somewhat. This multisensory dizziness results from a combination of two or more diminished sensory modalities. Deficits may be the result of age-related changes, and the patient complaining of dizziness may be unaware of the primary sensory problems.

There are many other causes of dizziness in the aged. Elderly patients often wear "progressive lens" glasses, with gradually decreasing focal lengths from above to below. When looking down—especially when walking downstairs—vision is distorted by the near-vision correction of the lens, which may cause loss of balance. A mild degree of positional vertigo also occurs with increased frequency in the elderly. This is usually caused by small calcium carbonate crystals (otoliths) being dislodged from their normal location in the utricle, and falling into the posterior semicircular canal. This can typically be corrected by an Epley (canalith repositioning) maneuver (Prokopakis et al. 2005), which relocates the otoliths in the utricle. Because postural blood pressure adjustments occur more slowly in the aged, *transient* orthostatic hypotension is common on rapidly arising from a recumbent position. Numerous medications commonly used by the elderly, including antihypertensive agents and antidepressants, may produce dizziness as an unwanted side effect. Finally, pathological causes of dizziness due to specific disease states are also frequent, ranging from Meniere's disorder to brainstem cerebrovascular accidents.

Gait Disorders

When disorders of gait interfere with the elderly patient's independence, the distinction between an age-related process and a specific disease state must be carefully considered. In the absence of specific disease, gait disturbances produce disability in many aged individuals (Kerber, Enrietto, Jacobson, and Baloh 1998). The variable combination of an extrapyramidal syndrome, Bruns' frontal lobe gait apraxia, multisensory dizziness, and/or mechanical impairment due to joint degeneration often leads to significant disability. Other aspects of the "senile gait" have already been mentioned.

Diagnostically, it is important to determine whether any aspect of this combination of conditions is due to a specific disease state. In particular, diseases of the frontal lobes (brain tumor, subdural hematoma), Parkinsonism, peripheral neuropathy, normal pressure hydrocephalus, drug intoxication, and cerebellar disorders should be ruled out with appropriate studies. The course of the gait disturbance should be followed long enough to confirm that no additional disease process is evolving.

Cervical Spondylosis

Degenerative changes of the cervical spine and the resulting symptoms occur with great frequency in the aged. Radiologically, a large proportion of individuals over age 55 show evidence of cervical disk degeneration on MRI, and by age 75 the finding is almost universal. Osteoarthritic changes of the zygapophyseal (facet) joints are almost as common as disk disease. Roughly half of patients with radiological evidence of cervical spondylosis may experience symptoms of local cervical pain or nerve root or spinal cord compression. Signs of cervical spinal cord compression are uncommon; but some degree of bony degeneration of the cervical spine and accompanying pain—either local or referred from nerve root compromise—can be seen as a frequent consequence of aging.

Exaggerated Vulnerability

Drug Sensitivity

The elderly typically take more medications than young adults because of the increased occurrence of medical illnesses (Routledge, O'Mahony, and Woodhouse 2004). This more frequent use of drugs, and the use of multiple drugs, adds to the age differences in pharmacokinetics and pharmacodynamics to explain the two- to threefold greater incidence of adverse drug effects in older patients compared to young adults.

Pharmacokinetics deals with the metabolism, distribution, and elimination of a drug. In the elderly, distribution of a drug may differ, and typically metabolism of the drug in the liver is decreased, as is the renal clearance. Any of these differences may result in drug accumulation and toxicity (Zubenko and Sunderland 2000). For example, the half-life of diazepam is normally 48 hours, but may extend to twice this time in elderly individuals. Because drugs continue to accumulate for approximately four half-lives, the steady-state blood level in elderly patients may be much higher than in younger individuals, even when given the same dose, repeated at the same intervals. With diazepam, the maximum plasma level of drug may not be achieved until 1 to 2 weeks after treatment is begun, and seemingly innocuous individual doses may eventually produce dangerous sedation.

Pharmacodynamics refers to the physiological effects of interaction of a drug with its receptors, and has received less attention in the aged. Age-related change in the sensitivity to a drug at a given plasma level is postulated to result from decreased numbers of receptors or diminished receptor sensitivity (Salzman 1990). For example, the effectiveness of a given level of propranolol diminishes with age and is presumed to reflect a reduction in receptor sensitivity. An enhanced response to certain drugs may be due to age-related losses of particular neural elements in the aged. For example, confusion and hallucinations may be produced in the elderly by even small doses of anticholinergic medications (Tune 2001). It is postulated to be due to loss of central (cortical) cholinergic neurons and receptors as well as decreased receptor function, leaving the remaining cholinergic system highly susceptible to even moderate blockade. Small doses of tricyclic antidepressants, antihistamines, and scopolamine may produce confusional states in the aged by this mechanism.

Head Trauma

Head injuries of moderate or severe degree are much more likely to result in lasting and severe neurological impairment and cognitive deficits in the aged than in young adults (Jennett and Teasdale 1981). Whereas loss of consciousness without focal neurological deficit is usually benign in young adults, it is likely to result in permanent cognitive impairment in those over age 60. The increased susceptibility to permanent injury after head trauma reflects both a diminished "neural reserve" in the elderly and a decrease in "plasticity,"—i.e., the ability for neural structures to recover function following a deficit. Elderly adults are particularly susceptible to tearing of the bridging veins in the subdural space, and may develop subacute subdural hematomas several weeks after the initial trauma. For this reason, a normal brain CT scan immediately following head injury sufficient to cause even very brief loss of consciousness should be followed by a repeat scan two weeks later.

Confusional States

Metabolic alterations of many sorts may impair memory and cognitive function in the elderly. Hyponatremia, uremia, and hepatic encephalopathy are well known systemic disorders that may produce confusional states (Ravin 2008). Aged patients may become disoriented and confused—particularly at night ("sun-downing") or following surgery, during febrile episodes, or with myocardial infarctions—for reasons that are not clear. The relation of the alteration of mental status to the underlying metabolic derangement should be kept in mind; when the underlying condition resolves, the patient's mental status should return to normal, or another cause must be sought (Hayward and Drachman 2008).

Postoperative Cognitive Impairment

Following surgery, many elderly patients experience cognitive dysfunction (Swearer and Nanjundaswamy 2008). The International Study of Post-Operative Cognitive Dysfunction, a multi-center study, evaluated 1218 patients aged 60 or older who had completed neuropsychological testing prior to surgery. The authors found that cognitive performance had declined in about a quarter of the patients at 1 week, and remained lower than baseline in almost 10 percent at 3 months post-operatively. While age and many aspects of anesthesia, surgery, and its complications contributed to the initial (one week) decrease in function, *only age* was significantly related to the later impairment at 3 months (Moller et al. 1998). Cardiac surgery presents a somewhat greater risk of cognitive decline in the elderly than other surgical procedures, although to some degree this is associated with the underlying cardiac disease (Selnes, McKhann, Borowicz, and Grega 2006).

Recognition of Neurological Disease in the Aged

Most often the recognition of real neurological disease in the aged presents little difficulty; paralysis of the limbs, loss of speech, or onset of severe tremor and rigidity are easily recognized by both patient and physician. Yet, with other less obvious complaints, the determination of significant neurological disease becomes far more difficult. Diseases affecting the elderly are discussed in detail elsewhere in this volume; here we point out certain complaints and findings that should be recognized as especially likely to be related to significant neurological disease (Table 5).

Headache

New headaches in aged patients should always be regarded seriously. Although lifelong muscle contraction headaches often persist through old age, neither these headaches nor migraine headaches are likely to appear *de novo* past age 50. The physician must always be alert for intracranial space-occupying lesions, subdural hematomas, cranial arteritis, and cranial neuralgias. A full-scale evaluation is necessary whenever an elderly individual first develops a new headache.

Table 5 Significant Neurological Symptoms in the Aged

New headache
"Blackout" spells
Transient neurological event
Uncorrectable visual impairment
Numb hand / weak hand
Increasing lethargy
Acute mental change
Focal neurological deficits

"Blackouts"

Episodes of loss or alteration of consciousness in the aged require careful evaluation. Even in patients who "fainted in church as children," loss of consciousness may indicate cardiac arrhythmias, seizures, orthostatic hypotension, or posterior circulation ischemia. An especially difficult diagnostic problem is presented by the elderly patient who experiences unwitnessed loss of consciousness in the bathroom during the night. This "bathroom fall syndrome" may be the result of an extensive array of serious or trivial problems and requires an appropriately extensive evaluation to establish the cause. In most states, unexplained loss of consciousness requires suspension of the patient's driver's license for six months, or when appropriate, until the cause is identified and definitively removed (e.g., with a cardiac pacemaker).

Transient Neurological Events

Brief episodes of visual loss, difficulty finding words, weakness of an arm or a leg, and other neurological symptoms clearly require an evaluation for transient ischemic events or focal seizure disorders.

Impaired Vision

Whenever loss in visual acuity is not easily restored by a refractive correction or diagnosable through the ophthalmoscope, a disorder of the visual or ocular motor pathways should be considered. Cataract formation is very common with advancing age, and is easily recognized with ophthalmoscopic examination. Macular degeneration occurs in about 13% of individuals over age 85, and is the most frequent cause of blindness in the elderly (Coleman, Chan, Ferris, and Chew 2008). Diabetic retinopathy and glaucoma are additional common causes of visual impairment that should be carefully evaluated. "Floaters," or "muscae volitantes," are usually benign, but the sudden appearance of large numbers of new floaters may occur following retinal detachment.

Numb Hand or Weak Hand

Numbness or weakness of a hand occurs transiently—lasting for a few minutes—in normal people, particularly after sleeping in an unusual position. In the absence of a precipitating cause, if the duration exceeds one hour or is progressive, neurological disease—from cerebral cortex to peripheral nerves—must be considered. Brain tumors, strokes, cervical spondylosis, thoracic outlet syndrome, amyotrophic lateral sclerosis, and peripheral neuropathies may present this way.

Lethargy

Although the elderly can be expected to nap more frequently than young adults, lethargy—particularly increasing drowsiness or falling asleep at inappropriate times—requires evaluation. Possibilities range from brain tumors or subdural hematomas to sleep apnea, dehydration and drug toxicity.

Acute Mental Changes

Although mild and gradual decline of memory and cognitive function may be "normal" to some extent in the very old, the *sudden* decline of intellectual function requires thorough evaluation. Poorly localized strokes, meningitis, subdural hematomas, and drug intoxication may present in this manner.

Focal Objective Neurological Deficits

Focal, localized, or lateralized neurological deficits are always of significance at any age. With, or without, a history of neurological disease, the finding of a mild hemiparesis with motor, reflex, and sensory changes demands investigation. The allowances made for neurological changes with aging, described above, never imply that the physician should accept focal neurological signs as a consequence of the normal aging process.

Assessment and Management of Neurological Disorders of the Aged

Unlike the situation in the healthy young adult, in whom neurological symptoms and signs generally indicate significant disease, the assessment and management of neurological complaints and findings in the elderly require a careful approach, based on the awareness of normal aging changes, and the different array of disorders that may occur. As already indicated, the neurological status of the aged patient reflects the summation of multiple processes: Some due to specific disease, some the result of age-related physiological changes; some that are curable or treatable, some that are not; some that can be named, some that are nameless. The physician must often attempt to analyze a confusing array of complaints and signs, where the specific combination of findings may relate to the individual's genetic background and life history, as well as to the present disease state. It is also critical to keep in mind the multiplicity of medical comorbidities, and the polypharmacy that often complicate the situation.

The purpose of the neurological assessment must be sharply focused: (1) identification of specific disease processes, particularly those that are treatable or curable; (2) an explanation for the abnormal neurological symptoms or signs; and (3) relief or reduction of disability, whatever the cause.

A few examples may serve to illustrate these points: among the dementing disorders, most disabled patients have a diagnosis of Alzheimer's disease, and a second large group has vascular dementia. Fewer than 25% of dementing disorders are due to treatable disease, and in some populations, fewer than 10% are due to reversible conditions. How far should an investigation be carried out when the probability of identifying a treatable disease, such as a subdural hematoma, normal pressure hydrocephalus, extrapyramidal dementia or depression, is relatively small? Aside from the humanitarian considerations, the cost of caring for a single patient in a nursing home environment for several years far exceeds that of many detailed clinical evaluations. The overall benefits of reasonable investigations of dementia are therefore substantial, even when many patients are found to have disappointingly untreatable conditions. Explanation of the cause of symptoms or signs is often of considerable value as well. For example, the concerned professional who is disabled by fears that his/her memory is declining at age 60 may be restored to normal function by assurance (based on an adequate evaluation) that mental functioning is still superior compared with coevals, and that neither a brain tumor nor a dementing process is present.

The reduction of *disability* due to noncurable disease, age-related changes, or both is also important. With multisensory dizziness, for example, where the underlying neuropathy, cervical spondylosis, and vestibular impairments may not be cured, patients may often be restored to independent function by attention to details: Training in "cane-trailing" to substitute hand sensation for the impaired lower extremity sensation, and the use of a foam collar to eliminate excessive mobility and false cervical proprioceptive sensations.

The ultimate goal of this neurological approach is not an attempt to eliminate the inevitable decline in function that occurs with aging—the "increase of entropy" that affects everything in our universe as a result of the *second law of thermodynamics*. Rather, it is to maintain sufficient neural integrity in aging individuals to enable them to function independently and with satisfaction, until the entire human machine wears down—a human counterpart of the Holmesian "wonderful one horse shay."

References

Balota, D. A., Dolan, P. O., and Ducheck, J. M. (2000). Memory changes in healthy older adults. In E. Tulving & F. I. M. Craik (Eds.), The Oxford handbook of memory (pp. 395–409). New York: Oxford University Press.

Barja, G. (2004). Free radicals and aging. *Trends Neurosci, 27*(10), 595–600.

Beck, A., Steer, R., and Brown, G. (1996). *Beck Depression Inventory-II manual.* San Antonio: Psychological Corporation.

Bender, M. B., Fink, M., and Green, M. (1951). Patterns in perception on simultaneous tests of face and hand. *AMA Arch Neurol Psychiatry, 66,* 355–362.

Bertoni-Freddari, C., Fattoretti, P., Solazzi, M., Giorgetti, B., Di Stefano, G., Casoli, T., et al. (2003). Neuronal death versus synaptic pathology in Alzheimer's disease. *Ann N Y Acad Sci, 1010,* 635–638.

Blazer, D. G. (2003). Depression in late life: review and commentary. *J Gerontol A Biol Sci Med Sci, 58,* 249–265.

Brach, J. S., Studenski, S. A., Perera, S., VanSwearingen, J. M., and Newman, A. B. (2007). Gait variability and the risk of incident mobility disability in community-dwelling older adults. *J Gerontol A Biol Sci Med Sci, 62,* 983–988.

Breslau, J., Starr, A., Sicotte, N., Higa, J., and Buchsbaum, M. S. (1989). Topographic EEG changes with normal aging and SDAT. *Electroencephalogr Clin Neurophysiol, 72,* 281–289.

Broe, G. A., Akhtar, A. J., Andrews, G. R., Caird, F. I., Gilmore, A. J., and McLennan, W. J. (1976). Neurological disorders in the elderly at home. *J Neurol Neurosurg Psychiatry, 39,* 362–366.

Buchman, A. S., Boyle, P. A., Wilson, R. S., Bienias, J. L., and Bennett, D. A. (2007). Physical activity and motor decline in older persons. *Muscle Nerve, 35,* 354–362.

Calkins, E., Boult, C., and Wagner, E., et al. (1999). *New ways to care for older people. Building systems based on evidence.* New York: Springer.

Cape, R. D., and Gibson, S. J. (1994). The influence of clinical problems, age and social support on outcomes for elderly persons referred to regional aged care assessment teams. *Aust N Z J Med, 24,* 378–385.

Celesia, G. G., Kaufman, D., and Cone, S. (1987). Effects of age and sex on pattern electroretinograms and visual evoked potentials. *Electroencephalogr Clin Neurophysiol, 68,* 161–171.

Charman, W. N. (2008). The eye in focus: accommodation and presbyopia. *Clin Exp Optom, 91,* 207–225.

Coleman, H. R., Chan, C. C., Ferris, F. L., 3rd, and Chew, E. Y. (2008). Age-related macular degeneration. *Lancet, 372,* 1835–1845.

Contestabile, A., Ciani, E., and Contestabile, A. (2008). The place of choline acetyltransferase activity measurement in the "cholinergic hypothesis" of neurodegenerative diseases. *Neurochem Res, 33,* 318–327.

Cotman, C. (1990). Synaptic plasticity, neurotrophic factors and transplantation in the aged brain. In E. Schneider & J. Rowe (Eds.), *Handbook of the biology of aging,* Ed 2, (pp. 255–274). San Diego: Academic Press.

Craik, F. I., and Bialystok, E. (2006). Cognition through the lifespan: Mechanisms of change. *Trends Cogn Sci, 10,* 131–138.

Critchley, M. (1956). Neurologic changes in the aged. *J Chronic Dis, 3*(5), 459–477.

Cutler, N. R. (1986). Cerebral metabolism as measured with positron emission tomography (PET) and [18F] 2-deoxy-D-glucose: healthy aging, Alzheimer's disease and Down syndrome. *Prog Neuropsychopharmacol Biol Psychiatry, 10,* 309–321.

Damasceno, A., Delicio, A. M., Mazo, D. F., Zullo, J. F., Scherer, P., Ng, R. T., et al. (2005). Primitive reflexes and cognitive function. *Arq Neuropsiquiatr, 63,* 577–582.

Davis, D. G., Schmitt, F. A., Wekstein, D. R., & Markesbery, W. R. (1999). Alzheimer neuropathologic alterations in aged cognitively normal subjects. *J Neuropathol Exp Neurol, 58,* 376–388.

DeCarli, C. (2003). Mild cognitive impairment: prevalence, prognosis, aetiology, and treatment. *Lancet Neurol, 2,* 15–21.

DeCarli, C., Massaro, J., Harvey, D., Hald, J., Tullberg, M., Au, R., et al. (2005). Measures of brain morphology and infarction in the Framingham heart study: establishing what is normal. *Neurobiol Aging, 26,* 491–510.

Dey, D. K., Bosaeus, I., Lissner, L., and Steen, B. (2009). Changes in body composition and its relation to muscle strength in 75-year-old men and women: A 5-year prospective follow-up study of the NORA cohort in Goteborg, Sweden. *Nutrition Feb 9 e-Pub.*

Dobie, R. A. (2008). The burdens of age-related and occupational noise-induced hearing loss in the United States. *Ear Hear, 29,* 565–577.

Dotson, V. M., Resnick, S. M., and Zonderman, A. B. (2008). Differential association of concurrent, baseline, and average depressive symptoms with cognitive decline in older adults. *Am J Geriatr Psychiatry, 16,* 318–330.

Drachman, D. A. (1986). Memory and cognitive function in normal aging. *Dev. Neuropsychol, 2,* 277–285.

Drachman, D. A. (1998). A 69-year-old man with chronic dizziness. *JAMA, 280,* 2111–2118.

Drachman, D. A. (2000). Occam's razor, geriatric syndromes, and the dizzy patient. *Ann Intern Med, 132,* 403–404.

Drachman, D. A. (2006). Aging of the brain, entropy, and Alzheimer disease. *Neurology, 67,* 1340–1352.

Drachman, D. A. (2008). Memory and the brain: beyond intracranial phrenology. *Curr Neurol Neurosci Rep, 8,* 269–273.

Drachman, D. A., and Glosser, G. (1981). Pharmacologic strategies in aging and dementia: the cholinergic hypothesis. In T. Crook and S. Gershon (Eds.), *Strategies for the development of an effective treatment for senile dementia* (pp. 35–52). Canaan, CT: Mark Powley Associates.

Drachman, D. A., Noffsinger, D., Sahakian, B. J., Kurdziel, S., and Fleming, P. (1980). Aging, memory, and the cholinergic system: A study of dichotic listening. *Neurobiol Aging, 1,* 39–43.

Dreher, J. C., Meyer-Lindenberg, A., Kohn, P., and Berman, K. F. (2008). Age-related changes in midbrain dopaminergic regulation of the human reward system. *Proc Natl Acad Sci U S A, 105,* 15106–15111.

Elble, R. J., Hughes, L., and Higgins, C. (1992). The syndrome of senile gait. *J Neurol, 239,* 71–75.

Esiri, M. M., Hyman, B. T., Beyreuther, K., and Masters, C. L. (1997). Ageing and dementia. In D. I. Graham and P. L. Lantos (Eds.), *Greenfield's neuropathology* (6th ed., pp. 153–234). London: Arnold.

Faulkner, J. A., Larkin, L. M., Claflin, D. R., and Brooks, S. V. (2007). Age-related changes in the structure and function of skeletal muscles. *Clin Exp Pharmacol Physiol, 34,* 1091–1096.

Fazekas, F., Alavi, A., Chawluk, J. B., Zimmerman, R. A., Hackney, D., Bilaniuk, L., et al. (1989). Comparison of CT, MR, and PET in Alzheimer's dementia and normal aging. *J Nucl Med, 30,* 16071615.

Fellows, L., Bergman, H., Wolfson, C., and Chertkow, H. (2008). Can clinical data predict progression to dementia in amnestic mild cognitive impairment? *Can J Neurol Sci, 35,* 314–322.

Fotiou, D. F., Brozou, C. G., Tsiptsios, D. J., Fotiou, A., Kabitsi, A., Nakou, M., et al. (2007). Effect of age on pupillary light reflex: evaluation of pupil mobility for clinical practice and research. *Electromyogr Clin Neurophysiol, 47,* 11–22.

Fried, L. P., Bandeen-Roche, K., Kasper, J. D., & Guralnik, J. M. (1999). Association of comorbidity with disability in older women: The Women's Health and Aging Study. *J Clin Epidemiol, 52,* 27–37.

Gaal, Z. A., Csuhaj, R., and Molnar, M. (2007). Age-dependent changes of auditory evoked potentials—effect of task difficulty. *Biol Psychol, 76,* 196–208.

Geula, C., Nagykery, N., Nicholas, A., and Wu, C. K. (2008). Cholinergic neuronal and axonal abnormalities are present early in aging and in Alzheimer disease. *J Neuropathol Exp Neurol, 67,* 309–318.

Golden, C., and Freshwater, S. (2002). *Stroop Color and Word Test: Revised examiner manual.* Wood Dale, IL: Stoelting Co.

Goodglass, H., and Kaplan, E. (2000). *Boston Naming Test.* Philadelphia: Lippincott Williams & Wilkins.

Goodglass, H., Kaplan, E., and Barresi, B. (2001). *The Boston Diagnostic Aphasia Examination* (3rd ed.). Philadelphia: Lippincott Williams & Wilkins.

Graham, J. (2000). *MMPI-2: Assessing personality and psychopathology* (3rd ed.). New York City, NY: Oxford University Press.

Guillaume, C., Clochon, P., Denise, P., Rauchs, G., Guillery-Girard, B., Eustache, F., et al. (2009). Early age-related changes in episodic memory retrieval as revealed by event-related potentials. *Neuroreport, 20,* 191–196.

Hayward, L., and Drachman, D. (2008). Evaluating the patient with altered consciousness in the intensive care unit. In: R. Irwin and J. Rippe (Eds.), *Irwin and Rippe's intensive care medicine* 6th Ed., (pp. 1959–1966). Philadelphia: Wolters Kluwer / Lippincott Williams & Wilkins.

Hobson, W., and Pemberton, J. (1955). *The health of the elderly at home.* London: Butterworth.

Holsinger, T., Deveau, J., Boustani, M., and Williams, J. W., Jr. (2007). Does this patient have dementia? *JAMA, 297,* 2391–2404.

Hooper, H. (1983). *Hooper Visual Organization Test manual.* Los Angeles, CA: Western Psychological Services.

Howard, J. E., McGill, K. C., and Dorfman, L. J. (1988). Age effects on properties of motor unit action potentials: ADEMG analysis. *Ann Neurol, 24,* 207–213.

Impallomeni, M., Kenny, R. A., Flynn, M. D., Kraenzlin, M., and Pallis, C. A. (1984). The elderly and their ankle jerks. *Lancet, 1,* 670–672.

Jackson, C. E., and Snyder, P. J. (2008). Electroencephalography and event-related potentials as biomarkers of mild cognitive impairment and mild Alzheimer's disease. *Alzheimers Dement, 4*(Suppl 1), S137–143.

Jackson, G. R., Owsley, C., and Curcio, C. A. (2002). Photoreceptor degeneration and dysfunction in aging and age-related maculopathy. *Ageing Res Rev, 1,* 381–396.

Jagust, W. J., Zheng, L., Harvey, D. J., Mack, W. J., Vinters, H. V., Weiner, M. W., et al. (2008). Neuropathological basis of magnetic resonance images in aging and dementia. *Ann Neurol, 63,* 72–80.

Jennett, B., and Teasdale, G. (1981). *Management of head injuries.* Philadelphia: Davis.

Jessen, F., Wiese, B., Cvetanovska, G., Fuchs, A., Kaduszkiewicz, H., Kolsch, H., et al. (2007). Patterns of subjective memory impairment in the elderly: Association with memory performance. *Psychol Med, 37,* 1753–1762.

Jonker, C., Geerlings, M. I., and Schmand, B. (2000). Are memory complaints predictive for dementia? A review of clinical and population-based studies. *Int J Geriatr Psychiatry, 15,* 983–991.

Jonker, C., Launer, L. J., Hooijer, C., and Lindeboom, J. (1996). Memory complaints and memory impairment in older individuals. *J Am Geriatr Soc, 44,* 44–49.

Jorm, A. F., Butterworth, P., Anstey, K. J., Christensen, H., Easteal, S., Maller, J., et al. (2004). Memory complaints in a community sample aged 60-64 years: associations with cognitive functioning, psychiatric symptoms, medical conditions, APOE genotype, hippocampus and amygdala volumes, and white-matter hyperintensities. *Psychol Med, 34,* 1495–1506.

Katz, R. I., and Horowitz, G. R. (1982). Electroencephalogram in the septuagenarian: studies in a normal geriatric population. *J Am Geriatr Soc, 30,* 273–275.

Kausler, D. (1990). Motivation, human aging, and cognitive performance. In J. Birren & K. Schaie (Eds.), *Handbook of the psychology of aging* (3rd ed., pp. 172–183). San Diego: Academic press.

Kerber, K. A., Enrietto, J. A., Jacobson, K. M., and Baloh, R. W. (1998). Disequilibrium in older people: a prospective study. *Neurology, 51,* 574–580.

Kimura, J. (1989). *Electrodiagnosis in diseases of nerve and muscle: Principles and practice.* Philadelphia: FA Davis.

Klass, M., Baudry, S., and Duchateau, J. (2008). Age-related decline in rate of torque development is accompanied by lower maximal motor unit discharge frequency during fast contractions. *J Appl Physiol, 104,* 739–746.

Kline, D., and Schieber, F. (1985). Vision and aging. In J. Birren and K. Schaie (Eds.), *Handbook of the psychology of aging* (2nd ed., pp. 296–331). New York: Van Nostrand Reinhold.

Lauretani, F., Bandinelli, S., Bartali, B., Di Iorio, A., Giacomini, V., Corsi, A. M., et al. (2006). Axonal degeneration affects muscle density in older men and women. *Neurobiol Aging, 27,* 1145–1154.

Lezak, M., Howieson, D., Loring, D., Hannay, H., and Fischer, J. (2004). *Neuropsychological assessment* (4th ed.). New York City, NY: Oxford University Press.

Lin, Y. H., Hsieh, S. C., Chao, C. C., Chang, Y. C., and Hsieh, S. T. (2005). Influence of aging on thermal and vibratory thresholds of quantitative sensory testing. *J Peripher Nerv Syst, 10,* 269–281.

Lippa, C. F., Hamos, J. E., Pulaski-Salo, D., DeGennaro, L. J., and Drachman, D. A. (1992). Alzheimer's disease and aging: effects on perforant pathway perikarya and synapses. *Neurobiol Aging, 13,* 405–411.

Louis, E. D., Wendt, K. J., and Ford, B. (2000). Senile tremor. What is the prevalence and severity of tremor in older adults? *Gerontology, 46,* 12–16.

Luo, L., and Craik, F. I. (2008). Aging and memory: a cognitive approach. *Can J Psychiatry, 53,* 346–353.

Mancuso, C., Scapagini, G., Curro, D., Giuffrida Stella, A. M., De Marco, C., Butterfield, D. A., et al. (2007). Mitochondrial dysfunction, free radical generation and cellular stress response in neurodegenerative disorders. *Front Biosci, 12,* 1107–1123.

Marigold, D. S., and Patla, A. E. (2008). Age-related changes in gait for multi-surface terrain. *Gait Posture, 27,* 689–696.

Masoro, E. J. (1991). Biology of aging: facts, thoughts, and experimental approaches. *Lab Invest, 65,* 500–510.

Masoro, E. J. (2001). Physiology of aging. *Int J Sport Nutr Exerc Metab, 11 Suppl,* S218–222.

Meyers, J. E., and Meyers, K. R. (1995). *Rey Complex Figure Test and Recognition Trial.* Odessa, FL: Psychological Assessment Resources.

Miranda, B., Madureira, S., Verdelho, A., Ferro, J., Pantoni, L., Salvadori, E., et al. (2008). Self-perceived memory impairment and cognitive performance in an elderly independent population with age-related white matter changes. *J Neurol Neurosurg Psychiatry, 79,* 869–873.

Moller, J. T., Cluitmans, P., Rasmussen, L. S., Houx, P., Rasmussen, H., Canet, J., et al. (1998). Long-term postoperative cognitive dysfunction in the elderly ISPOCD1 study. ISPOCD investigators. International Study of Post-Operative Cognitive Dysfunction. *Lancet, 351,* 857–861.

Moriyama, H., Amano, K., Itoh, M., Shimada, K., and Otsuka, N. (2007). Morphometric aspects of peripheral nerves in adults and the elderly. *J Peripher Nerv Syst, 12,* 205–209.

Mortimer, J. A. (1988). Human motor behavior and aging. *Ann N Y Acad Sci, 515,* 54–66.

O'Donnell, B. F., Friedman, S., Swearer, J. M., and Drachman, D. A. (1992). Active and passive P3 latency and psychometric performance: influence of age and individual differences. *Int J Psychophysiol, 12,* 187–195.

Pakkenberg, B., Pelvig, D., Marner, L., Bundgaard, M. J., Gundersen, H. J., Nyengaard, J. R., et al. (2003). Aging and the human neocortex. *Exp Gerontol, 38,* 95–99.

Petersen, R. C. (2004). Mild cognitive impairment as a diagnostic entity. *J Intern Med, 256,* 183–194.

Prichep, L. S. (2007). Quantitative EEG and electromagnetic brain imaging in aging and in the evolution of dementia. *Ann N Y Acad Sci, 1097,* 156–167.

Prokopakis, E. P., Chimona, T., Tsagournisakis, M., Christodoulou, P., Hirsch, B. E., Lachanas, V. A., et al. (2005). Benign paroxysmal positional vertigo: 10-year experience in treating 592 patients with canalith repositioning procedure. *Laryngoscope, 115,* 1667–1671.

Ravin, P. (2008). Metabolic encephalopathy. In: R. Irwin and J. Rippe (Eds.), *Irwin and Rippe's intensive care medicine,* 6th Ed., (pp. 1967–1975). Philadelphia: Wolters Kluwer / Lippincott Williams & Wilkins.

Rawson, N. E. (2006). Olfactory loss in aging. *Sci Aging Knowledge Environ, 2006,* pe6.

Reid, L. M., and Maclullich, A. M. (2006). Subjective memory complaints and cognitive impairment in older people. *Dement Geriatr Cogn Disord, 22,* 471–485.

Ropper, A. H., and Brown, R. H. (2005). *Adams and Victor's principles of neurology* (8th ed.). New York: McGraw-Hill.

Routledge, P. A., O'Mahony, M. S., and Woodhouse, K. W. (2004). Adverse drug reactions in elderly patients. *Br J Clin Pharmacol, 57,* 121–126.

Salthouse, T. A. (1982). *Adult cognition: The experimental psychology of human aging.* New York: Springer-Verlag.

Salthouse, T. A. (1996). The processing-speed theory of adult age differences in cognition. *Psychol Rev, 103,* 403–428.

Salzman, C. (1990). Practical considerations in the pharmacologic treatment of depression and anxiety in the elderly. *J Clin Psychiatry, 51 Suppl,* 40–43.

Scahill, R. I., Frost, C., Jenkins, R., Whitwell, J. L., Rossor, M. N., and Fox, N. C. (2003). A longitudinal study of brain volume changes in normal aging using serial registered magnetic resonance imaging. *Arch Neurol, 60,* 989–994.

Schiff, S., Valenti, P., Andrea, P., Lot, M., Bisiacchi, P., Gatta, A., et al. (2008). The effect of aging on auditory components of event-related brain potentials. *Clin Neurophysiol, 119,* 1795–1802.

Schliebs, R., and Arendt, T. (2006). The significance of the cholinergic system in the brain during aging and in Alzheimer's disease. *J Neural Transm, 113,* 1625–1644.

Selnes, O. A., McKhann, G. M., Borowicz, L. M., Jr., & Grega, M. A. (2006). Cognitive and neurobehavioral dysfunction after cardiac bypass procedures. *Neurol Clin, 24,* 133–145.

Soderlund, H., Nyberg, L., Adolfsson, R., Nilsson, L. G., and Launer, L. J. (2003). High prevalence of white matter hyperintensities in normal aging: Relation to blood pressure and cognition. *Cortex, 39,* 1093–1105.

Sprott, R. L. (1988). Age-related variability. *Ann N Y Acad Sci, 515,* 121–123.

Srivastava, K., Chaves, J. M., Srivastava, O. P., and Kirk, M. (2008). Multi-crystallin complexes exist in the water-soluble high molecular weight protein fractions of aging normal and cataractous human lenses. *Exp Eye Res, 87,* 356–366.

Stoquart-ElSankari, S., Baledent, O., Gondry-Jouet, C., Makki, M., Godefroy, O., and Meyer, M. E. (2007). Aging effects on cerebral blood and cerebrospinal fluid flows. *J Cereb Blood Flow Metab, 27,* 1563–1572.

Swearer, J. M., and Nanjundaswamy, S. (2008). Mental status dysfunction in the intensive care unit: Postoperative cognitive impairment. In: R. Irwin and J. Rippe (Eds.), *Irwin and Rippe's intensive care medicine* (6th ed., pp. 2036–2038). Philadelphia: Wolters Kluwer / Lippincott Williams & Wilkins.

Tune, L. E. (2001). Anticholinergic effects of medication in elderly patients. *J Clin Psychiatry, 62 Suppl 21,* 11–14.

Weale, R. A. (1986). Aging and vision. *Vision Res, 26,* 1507–1512.

Wechsler, D. (2008). *Wechsler Adult Intelligence Scale - IV edition manual* (4th ed.). San Antonio: NCS Pearson, Inc.

Wechsler, D. (2009). *Wechsler Memory Scale - IV edition manual* (4th ed.). San Antonio: NCS Pearson, Inc.

Weintraub, S. (2000). Neuropsychological assessment of mental state. In M. M. Mesulam (Ed.), *Principles of behavioral and cognitive neurology* (pp. 121–173). New York City, NY: Oxford University Press.

Weissman, L., Jo, D. G., Sorensen, M. M., de Souza-Pinto, N. C., Markesbery, W. R., Mattson, M. P., et al. (2007). Defective DNA base excision repair in brain from individuals with Alzheimer's disease and amnestic mild cognitive impairment. *Nucleic Acids Res, 35*(16), 5545–5555.

West, M. J., Coleman, P. D., Flood, D. G., and Troncoso, J. C. (1995). [Differential neuronal loss in the hippocampus in normal aging and in patients with Alzheimer disease]. *Ugeskr Laeger, 157*(22), 3190–3193.

Wild, K., Howieson, D., Webbe, F., Seelye, A., and Kaye, J. (2008). Status of computerized cognitive testing in aging: A systematic review. *Alzheimer's Dement, 4*(6), 428–437.

Williamson, P. C., Merskey, H., Morrison, S., Rabheru, K., Fox, H., Wands, K., et al. (1990). Quantitative electroencephalographic correlates of cognitive decline in normal elderly subjects. *Arch Neurol, 47*(11), 1185–1188.

Winblad, B., Palmer, K., Kivipelto, M., Jelic, V., Fratiglioni, L., Wahlund, L. O., et al. (2004). Mild cognitive impairment—beyond controversies, towards a consensus: report of the International Working Group on Mild Cognitive Impairment. *J Intern Med, 256*(3), 240–246.

Yesavage, J. A., Brink, T. L., Rose, T. L., Lum, O., Huang, V., Adey, M., et al. (1982). Development and validation of a geriatric depression screening scale: A preliminary report. *J Psychiatr Res, 17*(1), 37–49.

Young, V. G., Halliday, G. M., and Kril, J. J. (2008). Neuropathologic correlates of white matter hyperintensities. *Neurology, 71*(11), 804–811.

Ypsilanti, A. R., Girao da Cruz, M. T., Burgess, A., and Aubert, I. (2008). The length of hippocampal cholinergic fibers is reduced in the aging brain. *Neurobiol Aging, 29*(11), 1666–1679.

Zhang, C., Goto, N., Suzuki, M., and Ke, M. (1996). Age-related reductions in number and size of anterior horn cells at C6 level of the human spinal cord. *Okajimas Folia Anat Jpn, 73*(4), 171–177.

Zubenko, G. S., & Sunderland, T. (2000). Geriatric psychopharmacology: Why does age matter? *Harv Rev Psychiatry, 7*(6), 311–333.

6 Mental Status Examination in the Elderly

Alan M. Mandell

"Mental status" and "dementia" are frequent referral issues for practicing neurologists, psychiatrists, and geriatricians. This chapter describes a comprehensive mental status evaluation (MSE) consisting of behavioral observation, data acquisition from an independent historian and previous records if available, and neurological and focused general physical examinations.

Why Do a Routine Geriatric Mental Status Exam?

The response depends on the context of the referral. Not every patient requires a complete MSE (Strub and Black 2000). In the emergency department, where the goal is quick disposition, screening neuroimaging and a "metabolic panel" may already have been completed, or at least are in process, when there is a question of change in mental status (MS). The MSE in this setting is necessarily brief and geared primarily to differentiating among acute confusional state (ACS), aphasia, a dementia syndrome (if not already known), or some combination of these. The foci are obtaining an adequate history, testing of orientation and attention, and brief language assessment.

The inpatient setting is similar. The responsible inpatient team presumably is in tune with the patient's behavior and cognition, and some change or reported change in MS has occurred in the absence of obvious markers (e.g., hemiplegia). The task again is to determine the presence or absence of an ACS or language impairment, to generate a differential diagnosis, and to specify a diagnostic pathway. Sometimes, however, the inpatient team, focusing on acute medical or surgical issues, may not ever have noticed that the patient is unable to sustain a coherent conversation, or that her memory is grossly impaired.

The outpatient clinic is the typical setting in which questions of non-acute cognitive or behavioral changes are addressed. Many clinicians, including neurologists, do not routinely test mental status in older individuals unless they receive complaints either from the patient or the patient's family. Not testing is justifiable in many instances, for example, when the presenting complaint is radiating back pain and the patient can provide a clear, sequential, and logical history. Many elderly cognitively impaired patients do not, however, have a cognitive complaint and in the case of indolent intellectual dissolution, most family members do not seek medical attention for the patient for several years. Most patients, therefore, escape diagnosis when cognitive change is mild, particularly in primary care settings (Cummings 2004).

Dementia, the "Coming Plague of the 21st Century" (Evans et al. 1989; Ferri et al. 2005)

The prime directive in performing an MSE is to identify cognitive decline when available therapies are most likely to be salutary.

"Dementia," as used in this chapter, is a syndrome of *acquired, persistent* intellectual impairments characterized by deterioration in at least three of the following domains: memory, language, visuospatial skills, behavioral comportment, and executive function (Cummings 2004). These domains are the focus of the MSE.

Management and treatment of dementia begin with its recognition (Knopman, Boeve, and Petersen 2003), which is reasonably straightforward either when the patient or an independent historian expressly raises cognitive or behavioral deterioration as an issue, or it becomes obvious in context with other medical issues. Cognition and behavior are not, however, issues for a large proportion of "community dwelling elderly," who nevertheless are already demented and are just one fall, fever, or injury away from health system entry for these issues (Albert et al. 1991). Recognition is further hindered because widespread neuropsychologic, imaging, and laboratory screenings for asymptomatic elderly people are not economically feasible, nor are they always wanted (Guerriero et al. 2006).

Many health professionals as well as the general public persist in believing that substantial cognitive loss is an inevitable and "natural" consequence of aging. There indeed is evidence that general cognition "normally" recedes in later life (Albert 1994; Brayne et al. 1999). Episodic memory, especially as reflected on tests of delayed free recall, clearly deteriorates as we age, beginning perhaps as early as one's 40s (Albert, Heller, and Milberg 1988; Cullum et al. 1990). Nevertheless, longitudinal studies of regularly-evaluated, optimally healthy older adults suggest that overall cognitive function may slow somewhat but does not reflect a significant decline (Schaie 1989). Therefore, in the absence of *disease*, and when account is taken of other aging-related impairments (vision, hearing, joints), older adults can expect reasonably stable overall cognitive function and little or no interference with performance of everyday activities (Rowe and Kahn 1987). Dementia, or even modest cognitive impairment, is NOT an inevitable consequence of aging (Andersen-Ranberg, Vasegaard, and Jeune 2001; Ritchie 1998; Ritchie 1997). Clinicians should not automatically attribute cognitive problems which interfere with everyday activities to "normal aging." What to do about a cognitive disturbance that does NOT interfere with ADLs, so-called mild cognitive impairment (MCI) (Flicker, Ferris, and Reisberg 1991; Mitchell and Shiri-Feshki 2008; Petersen 2007; Petersen et al. 1999; Tuokko et al. 2003; Winblad et al. 2004), a heterogeneous disorder which may or may not worsen (Jicha et al. 2006), is the subject of Chapter 15.

Still debatable is what, in fact, constitutes "usual" or "normal" cognitive aging, an issue discussed in detail in Chapter 14 and elsewhere (Ball et al. 2004). Much of the cognitive decline previously attributed to aging alone probably reflects the effect of unrecognized brain damage, which may or may not correlate with ante-mortem cognitive status (Howieson et al. 2003; Roe et al. 2007; Silver et al. 2002).

Dementia is a differential diagnosis not a diagnostic term. By far the most common cause of the dementia syndrome in persons over the age of about 65 is the pathologic entity of Alzheimer's disease (AD) (Hebert et al. 2003). The most common presentation of AD is pernicious memory loss: The syndrome of progressive amnestic dysfunction (Mesulam 2003) (Dementia of the Alzheimer type [DAT]) (Cummings 2004). Consequently, this is the most common initial symptom of dementia in the elderly. Published diagnostic criteria have therefore routinely included memory impairment and irreversibility as a sine qua non for "dementia" (Association AP 2000). In other words, "dementia" is often used as a synonym for AD. The clinician must realize that, while the association between dementia and memory disorder is relatively robust, amnesia is not a salient feature of every dementing process, and all dementia is not AD (Taing-Wai and Mapstone 2006). Some dementias are heralded by language disturbance, or impaired judgment, or psychiatric symptoms (Alexopoulos et al. 1993), or are otherwise "atypical" (Jagust, Tiller-Borich, and Redd 1990). The point is that any perceived or reported persistent intellectual or behavioral change should trigger an MSE.

The prevalence of truly treatable dementia has been debated (Clarfield 1995; Weytingh, Bossuyt, and van Crevel 1995). The probability of finding a reversible cause for dementia has nevertheless likely declined greatly in the past 20 years (Clarfield 2003; Mok et al. 2004). Prompt recognition of dementia (Boustani et al. 2003) remains important all the same because emerging diagnostic techniques and increasingly effective therapeutic interventions are altering the definition of "treatable" (Fagan et al. 2007; Knopman et al. 2001; Ritchie and Portet 2006). Advantages of an early-as-possible diagnosis of dementia are listed in Table 1.

Nothing described in this chapter, bowing to realities of clinical practice, is fully comprehensive. The ideal evaluation is clinically practical, easily interpretable, sensitive (minimizing false-negative results), specific (minimizing false positives), valid (the test indeed measures the intended cognitive domain), reliable (the test should garner the same results independently of its administrator over a brief time period), culturally independent, acceptable (non-threatening) to the patient, detects change over time, distinguishes between current performance and the optimal capacity of the patient (circumvents both

Table 1 Advantages of Early Diagnosis in Dementing Conditions

For Every Case
- Provide a diagnostic answer and education for the patient and/or family.

For Patients With Reversible or Static Diseases
(e.g., depression, stroke)
- Relieve the fear of an irreversible or progressive disease.
- Treat the underlying disease.
- Initiate prevention and/or rehabilitation strategies.

For Patients With Irreversible and Progressive Diseases
(e.g., Alzheimer's disease)
- Treat cognitive and behavioral symptoms.
- Plan legal and financial future while patient is still competent.
- Initiate management strategies that will postpone dependence and institutionalization.

From Green RC, 2005 Professional Communications, Inc. With Permission.

"ceiling" and "floor" effects), guides clinical decisions, is not influenced by the examiner's specialization bias (Plugge et al. 1991), and accounts for the patient's physical, emotional and social state (Mandell, Knoefel, and Albert 1994). The ideal, "all purpose" MSE is an instrument not likely to be realized within our lifetimes (Weintraub 2000). However, an approach is needed nonetheless.

The goals of the practical geriatric MSE herein presented are several:

- Determine, with high enough accuracy, the presence or absence of behavioral perturbations and cognitive impairment
- Determine whether impairments, if detected, are the result of focal, multi-focal or diffuse brain insult
- Generate a reasonably narrow differential diagnosis
- Guide further testing in the most effective and cost-efficient manner in the service of reaching a diagnosis

One accomplishes this by performing a systematic assessment of cognition and behavior. "Systematic" does not necessarily mean regimented. An adequate MSE consists of both unstructured and structured modules, the content of which is flexible, depending on the clinical setting: ICU, ED, noisy/quiet office or inpatient room, computer availability, lighting, patient positioning (e.g., able or not able to sit upright), presence of family members and/or assistants, etc. Content also depends on the patient's intrinsic "set." The marked attention (state dependent) disturbance of someone in considerable pain, for example, affects the patient's ability to cooperate with testing of "instrumental," or channel-dependent (Weintraub 2000) domains like memory and language.

The geriatric MSE reflects years of clinical and research experience with elderly patients in a variety of settings, and is similar to other published approaches. (Cummings and Mega 2003; Strub and Black 2000; Weintraub 2000) Many items are shared among other brief or more detailed screening instruments. (Milberg, Hebben, and Kaplan 1996; Stern and White 2003) While several of the recommended subtests can be scored, the geriatric MSE by necessity is essentially a *qualitative* instrument. Fully quantitative approaches, which allow relatively unbiased test-re-test and inter-rater comparisons, require much more of a time investment and are the domain of the neuropsychologist.

The tests of individual cognitive functions are in most cases hierarchically arranged, so that good initial performance often obviates the need for more detailed probing. If, for example, the patient's delivery is fluent, organized and he has no conversational word finding problem or difficulty naming objects and body parts, formal testing of auditory comprehension and repetition usually is not indicated. Conversely, poor performance triggers additional testing.

The ultimate goal is, of course, diagnosis and treatment. This may be as simple as recommending discontinuation of narcotics or other sedative agents. Very often, however, none is specifically available and the focus turns to appropriate pharmacologic (disease-modifying and adjunctive) and non-pharmacologic strategies (caregiver/family education, discussion of safety issues, reduction of incontinence and pacing) (Gitlin et al. 2005; Green 2005).

The following tests are often recommended and usually the ones I include in my own clinical MSE:

- Mini-Mental State Examination (MMSE) (Folstein, Folstein, and McHugh 1975)
- Digit Span (Wechsler 1997)

- Controlled Word Association (Lezak et al. 2004) (word list generation)
- Limb and facial praxis (Heilman and Gonzalez Rothi 2003)
- Visual confrontation naming of objects, parts of objects, body parts and colors
- Clock drawing (Cosentino et al. 2004; Freedman et al. 1994)
- Brief dictated writing sample (Chedru and Geschwind 1972)

Why these? Collectively and most importantly, this "battery" requires, in most cases, less than 15 minutes to administer. The MMSE is a brief, standardized, validated instrument which probes multiple cognitive domains. Digit span is a simple test of attention. Word list generation and confrontation naming increase sensitivity in detecting language impairment. Clock drawing harnesses multiple cognitive domains and, when used in conjunction with other tests, also increases sensitivity. Handwriting is affected by even mild inattention, aphasia, or visuospatial perturbation.

If this battery elicits no clear abnormality but the history suggests cognitive or behavioral deterioration, I add a test of episodic memory (Blacker et al. 2007). This combination, comprising a well-known standardized screening instrument plus selected neurobehavioral assays provides, in most cases, useful information. The data so-gathered allow reasonable judgment of language, orientation, attention, memory, executive and non-verbal visuospatial skills. That is, a survey reflecting both state-dependent and channel-dependent domains of bilateral cortical and subcortical structures (Weintraub 2000). This examination, when well-practiced, rarely requires more than one hour.

Screening Instruments

All screening tests are surrogates for more extensive neuropsychologic testing. Some mentioned in this chapter have been the subjects of numerous reviews and analyses (Applegate, Blass, and Williams 1990). A first issue is the purpose of the screen: A rough assessment in a primary care setting, or a more comprehensive instrument to guide further testing and aid in differential diagnosis? Another issue relates to the qualities specific to the instrument. Some screens are highly verbal, thus penalizing patients with relatively greater language impairment or limited education. Some tests are directed to the patient, others are informant-based (generally more sensitive), still others are dual purpose and can be combined with elements from other tests to increase sensitivity and specificity (Galvin, Roe, and Morris 2007), albeit at the expense of additional administration time.

The advantages of screening instruments, other than their brevity, include their standardized—although not necessarily well-validated (Ritchie 1988)—format and content, which allows uniformity of administration and comparisons of data. They work best for detecting moderate to severe dementia and confusional states, and their test-retest reliability is relatively high. They are therefore useful for:

- Community screening for significant, often unreported cognitive or behavioral disturbance
- Supporting a clinical observation of abnormal cognition
- Documenting changes, albeit not fully reliably, resulting from treatment or disease progression

The major criticisms of brief screening instruments are their insensitivity to mild cognitive decline and their low specificity in providing reliable information about precisely which domains are affected (Milberg 1996). This is particularly a problem for patients with high premorbid intelligence (ceiling effect). The highly verbal scheme, non-inclusion of independent information, and reliance on total "score" contribute to the insensitivity of many of these screens.

Significant false positive results from floor effect (i.e., incorrectly identifying a normal but poorly educated person as demented) are another limitation of screening tests. Many have been validated on populations that are too heterogeneous, too poorly defined, or too homogeneous and therefore not representative of the "at large" elderly (Eslinger et al. 1985).

In summary, brief screening instruments can be and often are used as initial guides to mental status function. They are not, however, and never were intended to be, diagnostic examinations. If due regard is given to their limitations and when time is a primary constraint, they are useful for discerning and quantifying moderate to severe cognitive impairment, regardless of whether the impairment has previously been noted. Some screens are described here; other more specific screens are reviewed subsequently.

The most commonly used brief screening instrument is the MMSE (Folstein, Folstein, and McHugh 1975). Originally developed to compare hospitalized psychiatric patients with age-matched "community dwelling elderly," it has since been used as a cognitive screen to quantify severity of dementia and to monitor cognitive worsening.

The MMSE is divided into sections assessing orientation, language, attention, "short-term" and working memory, and visuospatial competence. A score below 24 out of a possible 30 is considered abnormal.

Its advantages are its ease and brevity of administration (5 to 10 minutes), ready availability, and accuracy in detecting moderate dementia in patient populations with an elevated prevalence of cognitive impairment (Grut et al. 1993; Petersen et al. 2001). It is available in several languages. Application does not require extensive training. Test-retest reliability is fairly high within a one to thirty-day interval, and inter-rater reliability also is high. Used sequentially over several years, moreover, scores in general track cognitive decline, at least for dementia of the Alzheimer type, reasonably consistently (Tangalos et al. 1996) (see Figure 1).

Nevertheless, although I use it routinely in a busy outpatient practice, I do so cautiously in view of several criticisms. Like all screening instruments (Milberg 1996), both specificity and sensitivity, depending on the population for which it's utilized, are sacrificed in the service of time savings. The 24 cutoff score is too high for many persons older than 60, especially those with limited education, thus overestimating (lower specificity) cognitive impairment (Fillenbaum et al. 2007). It is insensitive to mild cognitive deterioration, particularly for highly educated persons, i.e., those with large "cognitive reserve," even

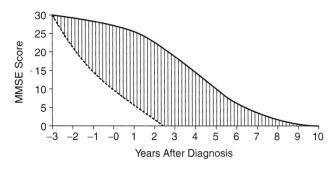

Figure 1 Deterioration in Mini-Mental State scores over time. From: Green RC, 2005. Professional Communications, Inc., by permission.

when history or more extensive testing suggests at least a mild dementia (O'Bryant et al. 2008). As already noted, the MMSE also is culturally biased, i.e., individuals from minority cultures, in general, score lower. Its heavy emphasis on orientation and language, absence of behavioral and mood questions (Riviere et al. 2002), and dependence on total score all temper its ability to detect non-Alzheimer dementia and to provide reliable information about particular cognitive domains. Finally, it has limited value as a method to mark cognitive changes in people with AD during brief clinical trials (Bowie, Branton, and Holmes 1999; Clark et al. 1999).

Examples of screening instruments designed to overcome at least some of its flaws are the Modified Mini-Mental State Exam (3MS) (Teng and Chui 1987), the Saint Louis University Mental Status Examination (SLUMS) for Detecting Mild Cognitive Impairment and Dementia (Tariq et al. 2006) and the CERAD Battery (Welsh et al. 1994). These, too, are not ideal but are more sensitive and specific instruments, albeit with the costs of longer administration time and necessity for at least some training.

A recently published brief informant-based test, the AD8 (Galvin et al. 2005), appears to distinguish dementia from non-dementia reasonably well and may also be useful as a self-assessment tool in the absence of an informant, at least when dementia is mild (Galvin et al. 2007).

The EXIT interview of executive function (Royall, Mahurin, and Gray 1992; Stokholm et al. 2005) is of interest because it appears not only to capture executive cognitive deficits not primarily related to general intellect, but also to predict behavioral disturbance and functional decline. It requires about 15 minutes to administer and correlates well with more standard tests.

Geriatric Mental Status Evaluation (GMSE)

The evaluation begins by noting the patient's level of alertness. Assessment of any cognitive domain will be compromised unless she is fully alert and can respond even to subtle cues. Much of the MSE is verbally-mediated and therefore not very useful if the patient is aphasic. Similarly, the MSE must be edited and pared when the patient has primary visual, hearing, motor (including speech) or other sensory impairments which interfere with test comprehension or execution. The examiner, in brief, must verify language and relevant primary sensory and motor integrity before proceeding with the MSE.

Assessment proceeds before formally engaging the patient, for example by listening or watching for the tell-tale pattern of a shuffling or hemiparetic gait, labored breathing, or agitation as he approaches the exam site. Is the patient in a wheelchair? Some patients become guarded or uncooperative as soon as they are addressed, or may be mute or otherwise incommunicative. During the several seconds necessary for introduction, one notes the patient's gender, race, attire (appropriate, disheveled, incomplete), nutritional status (obese, malnourished), hygiene, eye contact, attitude, and engagement. Equally important is observation of psychomotor activity: bradykinesia or hyperkinesias (tremor, tic, dyskinesia, compulsive rituals or postures), affect (euphoric, grandiose; sad, angry or irritable; apathetic), the manner in which he locates (or not) the chair and how he sits down. These observations are a base from which initial diagnostic theses may be formulated (Cummings and Mega 2003; Othmer and Othmer 2002).

The examiner must be cognizant about anxieties common to the elderly, who may resent or feel threatened by the questions required for assessment. Adoption of a supportive respectful attitude may obviate cautious, evasive, or even hostile responses. Several techniques are appropriate. When others are present, avoid third person references to the patient. When possible, include him in the discussion even if cognitive abnormalities are evident. Reassure him of the routineness of the questions. The pace of the examination should be slow enough for the patient to follow comfortably but not so slow as to appear condescending. Note prolonged response latencies but allow sufficient time, at least initially, for him to respond to questions or problems. Clearly inform him of proposed additional testing. If errors appear to multiply with time, fragment the MSE and, if possible, return to it later. In some cases, an MSE may be impossible if not performed by a health care practitioner already known and trusted by the patient. (Cooper and Bickel 1984)

The History

Formal evaluation begins, as with any diagnostic encounter, by obtaining a history. An adequate history provides information about the patient's personality, behavioral patterns, and judgment which, in general, are poorly if at all testable, even with sophisticated neuropsychological batteries. The history often illuminates obvious functional impairments. Sometimes, however, there has been no significant activities of daily living (ADL) or occupational deterioration. The examiner must therefore discern whether the patient has had any consistent decline from her **usual** level of competence.

History may provide the only evidence of malfunction in previously high-functioning individuals who may "score" within the normal range on all neuropsychological tests (ceiling effect). Highly educated persons with minimal or no cognitive symptoms or signs may nevertheless harbor high plaque and tangle counts, enough to satisfy current pathologic criteria for AD. Their cognitive reserve (Stern 2002) allows them to remain relatively asymptomatic despite extensive pathology, although once (if) symptoms develop, they endure shorter duration of disease before death (Roe et al. 2008; Roe et al. 2007; Scarmeas et al. 2006). Conversely, poor performance on formal tests may not be the result of cognitive decline in a poorly educated person with limited skills. Those with limited education, in less demanding jobs, or who already are significantly impaired, are vulnerable to "floor effect," a similar test insensitivity to change. A *reliable* history of no cognitive or behavioral change may circumvent this type of error.

The patient may offer "poor memory" as a chief complaint. Even without this history, his inability to provide a coherent, logically sequenced record of his problem, vague reportage, frequent "I don't know" or "I'm not sure" responses, not knowing the reason for the encounter, or explicit denial of independent histories should at least trigger suspicion of cognitive impairment. Conversely, if he can fluidly contribute correct dates, sequences, and substantive information (e.g., relating a symptom to a generally-known event), significant cognitive impairment is unlikely. The examiner must, if possible, verify any aspect of a patient's history that does not relate to common knowledge.

The requirement for an *independent, reliable* historian, other than the patient, cannot be over-emphasized. This requirement nevertheless is often not practical because elderly patients often live alone or are otherwise socially isolated. Furthermore, there is no guarantee that family members' or friends' histories are more reliable than that of the patient. For example, the family sometimes attributes cognitive impairment directly to fever, surgery, new stresses, or a disorienting vacation because subtler symptoms have previously been missed or ignored. Some informants, including spouses, may lie or otherwise be less than forthcoming about alcoholism, physical aggression, or sexual indiscretions in the patient's presence; for this reason it's sometimes helpful to interview the informant, particularly a spouse, separately.

Information to be gleaned includes medical history, particularly of stroke, hypertension, diabetes, cancer, alcohol, tobacco, caffeine (Hedges, Woon, and Hoopes 2009) or other substance abuse, HIV risk factors, heart disease, head trauma, sleep disturbance and **all** current medications. The examiner should specifically inquire about the patient's:

♦ Handedness—for writing (if right, has it **always** been right?) **and** for a variety of other activities such as throwing, kicking, threading a needle, using a bottle opener, toothbrush, shovel, or hammer

♦ Memory—repetitive questioning, forgetting important recent events or family member names, greater reliance on written or computerized reminders, frequent wrong turns or needing directions when traveling in or to familiar locales, frequent misplacement of objects, misidentifications of people

♦ Activities of daily living—personal care such as dressing, toileting, cooking, house cleaning, bathing, **driving**, shopping, bookkeeping, problem solving skills

♦ Social functions—preservation (or not) of hobbies and other interests, community affairs, friendships, judgment

♦ Behavior—any consistent change, including apathy and withdrawal, irritability, aggression or resistance, excessive mirth, sexual indiscretions, wandering, delusions, ritualistic or compulsive actions

♦ Language—word finding difficulty, less spontaneity and engagement, invasion of words without clear referents such as "thing/it/ this" into speech; paraphasias

♦ Mood—formal diagnoses of depression or bipolar disorder; expressions of guilt, loss of pleasure, libido or appetite change (up or down); weight loss or significant gain; somatic complaints; anxiety; inappropriate mirth or eutonia

♦ Family History—dementia, "senility," "trouble with memory loss," "hardening of the arteries," depression or bipolar disorder in any 1st degree relative, if known

The Interview

The clinician assumes a dialectical approach by integrating initial observations, history, and the content and the manner of execution of the patient's responses. Her speech, language, ideation, and ability to focus her attention are continuously assessed and diagnostic assumptions altered accordingly. Avoid providing encouraging (or discouraging) feedback and giving assistance for specific tests unless explicitly required (e.g., coin switch test). Occasional general encouragements ("keep plugging; we're almost done") are acceptable although specific response type (correct or incorrect; generated with ease or with difficulty) should not trigger them. "I don't know" or "I give up" responses should be noted but the patient should be encouraged to guess or to try again (Stern and White 2003).

Orientation

Very early during the interview, the examiner should confirm that the patient can state correctly her own name and age and the reason for her appearance in the office. Some persons can recite their birth dates by rote yet cannot come up with their actual age. Failure on any of these items indicates some combination of language, memory, executive (apathy) or attention impairments and reinforces the need for further testing. Also important to establish is whether the patient knows where she is (state, town or city, immediate environment) and the month, day and year.

Arousal and Attention

Arousal

Performance of the MSE depends on the patient's state of arousal. *Arousal* refers to cortical activation from deep brain structures (e.g., brainstem reticular formation) (Strub and Black 2000); impairment results from focal brainstem lesions or from diffuse bilateral hemispheric dysfunction. Neither somnolence nor excessive vigilance can provide a matrix suitable for meaningful assessment. When arousal is an issue, the clinician should ascertain whether the problem is acute, chronic, or periodic. While terms such as obtundation, stupor, lethargy, and coma are useful, the type and intensity of the stimuli required to evoke a response, and the nature (including verbatim transcription) and duration of that response should be documented.

Attention

"Attention" is a difficult-to-describe construct (Lezak et al. 2004). Assessment depends on multimodality inputs and outputs and therefore on the integrity of neuroanatomical networks that subserve other domains (Flicker et al. 1985). A large body of research documents age-related decrements in attention (McDowd and Birren 1990), although many other studies indicate that normal aging does not substantially alter important attentional mechanisms (Nissen and Corkin 1985).

Attention has been described by several models. One posits separate components: selective (phasic), sustained (tonic), and divided attention (Perry and Hodges 1999). "Inattention" is characterized to variable degrees by easy distractibility, perseveration and inappropriate focusing on and response to irrelevant environmental stimuli. It may be sufficiently subtle to be revealed only by specific tests (Chedru and Geschwind 1972).

Inattention is the essential element of the confusional state (CS). Patients in a CS may be quiet (and therefore difficult to diagnose). Agitated CS (delirium) features affective and thought disorders (fear, paranoia, delusions), hallucinations, motor disorders (tremor, myoclonus, asterixis), repetitive, purposeless behavior (picking at bedclothes, dressing/undressing, standing up/sitting down), and autonomic disturbances (tachycardia, diaphoresis).

Inattention also underlies uncommon linguistic disorders such as isolated misnaming of illness-related objects (non-aphasic misnaming) (Weinstein and Kahn 1952). Confusional states typically wax and wane in severity. The same patient may derail the examination either by perseverating actions or verbal responses and then, seconds later, by responding transiently to any sound, sight, or tactile sensation within his environment.

The confusional state is not a particularly localizing malfunction. Focal lesions of many brain areas, particularly fronto-limbic, may be responsible, although the most common substrate of the CS is widespread cortical dysfunction by a variety of metabolic, post-operative, post-ictal, systemic infectious, and intoxicating perturbations (Rummans et al. 1995).

Attention disturbance may also be unilateral: the phenomenon of hemispatial/body **neglect**. Neglect is the

> "failure to report, respond, or orient to novel or meaningful stimuli presented to the side opposite a brain lesion, when this failure cannot be attributed to either sensory or motor deficits"
> (Heilman, Watson, and Valenstein 2003).

Behaviors associated with unilateral neglect include directing responses to questions contralateral to their source, sitting consistently rotated (usually to the patient's left) on the body's axis, extinction of one of two simultaneously delivered right and left stimuli (auditory, visual, tactile), denying ownership of a limb or a tendency not to use it, and denial of illness altogether.

The bedside geriatric MSE is not designed to assess all aspects of attention. We emphasize selective (directed) attention (Mesulam 2000) and vigilance. The ability to filter and ignore extraneous, irrelevant stimuli is basic to goal-oriented behavior and is most clinically relevant. In response to criticism that evaluation of the CS often is too subjective, multiple delirium assessment scales have been published (Broshek and Marcopulos 1999).

Tests of Attention

Series counting is perfomed by asking the patient to count from 1 to 20 and then in reverse, from 20 to 1. Non-aphasic patients who cannot perform this test flawlessly likely are significantly inattentive and will probably perform poorly on subsequent tests.

The digit span test provides basic quantitative assessment of data apprehension. Although education level influences virtually all tests, even poorly-schooled people should succeed in repeating five numbers (Baddeley 1992). Normal span is 7 ± 2 (Miller 1956; Strub and Black 2000).

Using digits 1–9, tell the patient: "Listen carefully. I will say some numbers. When I am all finished, please repeat the numbers in exactly the same order." Prime the patient to make sure she understands the test: "If I say 'one two three,' what do you say?" Speak aloud each digit with equal emphasis (loudly for the hearing impaired) in random order at a rate of about one per second. Begin with a two digit span ("2-7") and continue increasing span ("3-8-4") until reproduction is inaccurate. Terminate the test, noting the patient's optimum span, when she fails *two* sequences of a given length.

Backward digit span, in which the task is recall of digits in their exact reverse order, requires mental manipulation and is more challenging. It taps executive (working memory) as well as attentional mechanisms (Weintraub 2000).

Vigilance (sustained attention) can be assessed simply with any of several **continuous response tasks**. For the 'A' test, the examiner reads aloud, again at a rate of about one per second, a long random series of letters in which a target letter occurs with more than random frequency (Strub and Black 2000). Instruct the patient to tap the bed/table, or raise a hand each and every time she hears the target letter ("A"). Errors include those of omission (failure to indicate the target), commission (signaling to a non-target letter), and perseveration (repetitive signaling in response to any of the stimuli). Non-brain-damaged elderly should perform at least with 90% accuracy.

A somewhat more challenging variant may be useful when previous tests have been normal but subtle inattention is still suspected. Instruct the patient to signal only when he hears two odd numbers in succession. One again primes the patient to ensure understanding of the task, and specifically not to signal when he hears only one odd number. Record the number of errors, if any. Persons from ages 50 through at least 90 should err no more than twice from a series of about 50 numbers.

Another useful test is timed (one minute) recitation of overlearned series (months, days of week). This test is not specific for attention, but is a reasonably good marker for it in the absence of language impairment.

Score correction for age is not necessary for most of these tests. An 80 year old should perform as well as a 40 year old. Because inattention may wax and wane, be prepared to accept variable results and to re-test as needed. For any aspect of the geriatric MSE, flexibility in test administration is necessary. Normal or superior performance by a patient who, by history, is suspected of having a dementia should lead the examiner to apply more rigorous tests, or to generate appropriate subspecialty referral.

Dysgraphia may be the only manifestation of an otherwise inapparent confusional state (Chedru and Geschwind 1972). A brief writing sample may therefore yield useful information if the patient has done well with previous testing. Handwriting is a complicated skill dependent on multiple factors, not the least of which are educational level, mechanical factors (arthritis, neuropathy, tremor), and language competency. Handwriting analysis can be as obsessive as one has time for, measuring, for example, legibility, spacing, size of words and letters, generation speed, presence or absence of paragraphias, word crowding, line slant and other misalignments, margin size, etc. If non-cognitive causes (e.g., tremor, arthritis, hemisensory defect) are not operative, dysgraphia, in short, is a sensitive albeit nonspecific indicator of brain malfunction.

I generally limit testing to a brief dictated sentence, such as, "Big dogs like to chase small cats." Ask the patient to transcribe this verbatim. The writing sample can be expanded (or contracted) during language testing (see following). Copying (cursive or print) letters, numbers, words, sentences of variable complexity, writing these to dictation, and asking for a free narrative sample are all appropriate but time-consuming tasks.

Neglect is the subject of an extensive literature and entire batteries have been designed for its evaluation (Heilman, Watson, and Valenstein 2003). Suspect neglect if the patient fails to attend to stimuli on one side of extra-personal space during the interview, or if he fails consistently to move a non-plegic limb. Other portions of the MSE may elicit neglectful behavior: ignoring half of written words or sentences when reading aloud, or of vertically arranged arithmetic problems ("neglect paralexia"), or copying or drawing only one-half of an object (e.g., a flower or clock face). During the neurological examination, note persistent unilateral *extinction* to double simultaneous visual, tactile, or auditory stimulation. Sometimes extinction is elicited only after repetitive stimulations.

The examiner must ensure that the patient acknowledges unilateral stimuli from or on either side of his body (absence of primary sensory deficit). Hemianopic patients, however, may or may not also have contra-lesional neglect. Those without neglect often will deliberately compensate during tests by turning their eyes or head toward the blind field. Those with neglect tend to rotate away from the blind field.

Time allowing, neglect may also be discerned by simple line bisection or cancellation tests. For the latter, draw several approximately two inch straight lines in various orientations in all four quadrants of an otherwise blank sheet of paper (Figure 2). Place this sheet in front of the patient in her saggital midline. Ask her to cross every line in its middle. Lines in the neglected field will be uncrossed more often than those in the good field, and the executed crosses may be biased toward the good field (Albert 1973). For the former (bisection), simply draw a single long horizontal line and ask the patient to bisect it. Look for a consistent crossing bias well to either side of the midline.

Neglect occurs contralateral to the offending lesion. It generally is more severe and chronic when brain damage is right-sided because, as one example of hemispheric specialization, the right hemisphere is *dominant* for mechanisms underlying attention.

Language and Speech

Language refers to the communication of meaningful symbols. A language is a symbolic system used by persons of the same cultural background (Benson and Ardila 1996). *Speech* refers to the mechanical execution of language through the vocal apparatus. Language is clearly associated with speech; there is considerable overlap among their organizational networks but they often are dissociated by afflictions common to the elderly, such as stroke, parkinsonism, and myasthenia gravis.

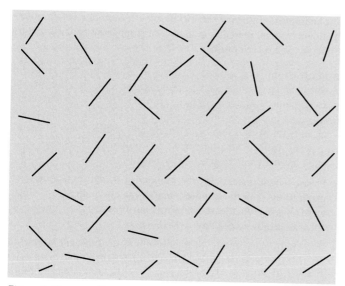

Figure 2 Line cancellation test. From Albert, 1973. Used with permission from A Simple Test of Visual Neglect. *Neurology* 23: 658–664.

For this reason, a few words are in order regarding speech disorders although detailed speech evaluation is beyond the scope of this MSE.

Ill-fitting dentures, edentulism, and laryngectomy, all usually obvious, are common non-neurogenic causes of speech impairment. Lesions at any level of the nervous system, from muscle to cerebrum, may also disrupt speech. When neurally mediated, brief speech analysis may aid the diagnostic process. Several speech impairments deserve mention, all of which, when severe, may eliminate effective spoken communication:

◆ Dysarthia: A disorder of articulation. When responsible lesions are above brainstem level, they are usually bilateral and subcortical and may or may not be associated with cognitive impairment (Benson and Ardila 1996).

◆ Dysphonia (hoarseness): A result of brainstem, neuromuscular, or laryngeal disease.

◆ Hypophonia: Reduction in voice volume, most often caused by bilateral subcortical/basal ganglionic malfunction. Common causes in the elderly are stroke and parkinsonism. Hypophonia often is associated with cognitive impairment.

◆ Mutism: Usually refers to complete inability by alert patients to produce sounds with their vocal apparatus. Laryngeal infections, neoplasms, neuromuscular disorders, and laryngectomy are causes. Mutism in this sense is equivalent to *aphonia*. It is also is caused by multiple psychiatric and CNS disorders through a variety of pathologies, in multiple locations, via a variety of mechanisms (Cummings and Mega 2003) including those responsible for aphasia. A writing sample should therefore always be obtained, if possible, from a mute patient. Patients who are both mute and (acutely) aphasic will generate aphasic dysgraphia. Handwriting should be normal from mute patients who are not also aphasic. Centrally-mediated mutism in an alert person without aphasia indicates damage to unilateral (relatively brief-duration) or bilateral (longer duration) medial frontal cortex.

◆ Stuttering: When acquired beyond childhood, may be a residuum of otherwise recovered aphasia, a product of bilateral, right hemispheric (Ardila and Lopez 1986) or multi-focal brain damage, a feature of basal ganglionic degenerative diseases, and may associate with cognitive deterioration. It is itself a poorly-localizing disorder (Benson and Ardila 1996).

Finally, dialects and accents are important speech parameters and may affect interpretation. Proper assessment clearly is not possible within context of a practical MSE, but the interested reader can consult the website http://web.ku.edu/~idea/readings/rainbow.htm for introduction to the "rainbow passage," which allows clinicians and researchers to compare the sounds of different dialects applied to a standard text.

If by listening to the patient's speech you suspect a subtle impairment, testing of non-verbal and verbal agility sometimes can augment it. For the former, ask the patient to repeat rapidly a series of phonemes, such as "la-la-la" "ma-ma-ma," "puh-ta-kuh puh-ta-kuh." For the latter, direct her to repeat tongue twisters like:

◆ full riding artillery brigade

◆ which wristwatches are Swiss wristwatches?

◆ the myth of Miss Muffet.

Language embodies propositional (linguistic), prosodic (Ross 2000), and gestural elements which may be distorted together or separately. The geriatric MSE is designed primarily for qualitative identification of *aphasia*. Aphasia is the loss or impairment of *language* function caused by brain damage (Benson and Ardila 1996). The differential diagnosis of aphasia, as well as relevant neuroanatomic correlations, are discussed in detail in Chapter 49. Related disorders are *alexia, agraphia, acalculia,* and *apraxia.* Aphasia usually incorporates all of these, but all can be independent of aphasia and of each other. Recognition of aphasia is critical because any but the mildest language disturbance renders much of the remainder of the MSE difficult or impossible.

Language evaluation is home to the relevance of handedness. *Handedness* is a complex attribute and does not refer simply to the limb favored for writing, which itself may be culturally dependent. Many persons older than about 60, products of parochial schools and social backgrounds in which left-handedness was actively disfavored, were trained to write right-handed ("switched" left-handers).

Few people are 100% right or left-handed; preference depends, among other variables, on the specific task "at hand" (Annett 1970). Although the right hemisphere mediates some aspects of language in just about everyone (Landis, Graves, and Goodglass 1982), the left hemisphere is usually dominant for language for both right and left-handers; aphasia thus requires at least some left hemisphere damage in about 90% of us.

Handedness becomes an issue when aphasia can be associated reliably with unilateral right hemisphere damage. "Crossed" aphasia among true right-handers is rare, but aphasia is relatively common (40%) in non-right-handers, in whom language competence often is shared significantly between the hemispheres. The practical consequence is that non-right-handers acquire aphasia more easily but less severely than right-handers from brain damage.

Keep in mind that, as with any other cognitive domain, "language" is not an isolated function. Aphasics often have additional, non-language impairments, particularly in the context of traumatic brain injury or neoplasm. Besides inattention or drowsiness, other privations which can influence language testing or performance include slowed information processing, perseveration (Sandson J, and Albert 1987), loss of "abstract attitude" (ability to think symbolically) (Goldstein and Scheerer 1941), and stimulus boundness (the tendency to respond to a stimulus in terms of its immediate sensory attributes) (Albert 1991).

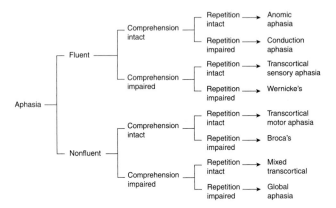

Figure 3 Systematic approach to aphasia diagnosis. Adapted from Cummings and Mega 2003, by permission of Oxford University Press, Inc.

The approach to language evaluation for this MSE follows closely that of the so-called "Boston School" (Benson and Ardila 1996). This "localizationist," or syndromic, approach is inadequate for exact anatomic correlation (Alexander, Naeser, and Palumbo 1987; Dronkers et al. 2007), the aphasia of many patients does not "fit" well into this schema, there is much clinical variability among aphasics sharing the same diagnostic label (Alexander, Benson, and Stuss 1989), and it does not account for curious phenomena such as category-specific anomia (Hart, Berndt, and Caramazza 1985). "Classic" aphasia correlative anatomy is nevertheless accurate enough for the MSE (Kreisler et al. 2000). The beauty of classical taxonomy is that it facilitates clinical communication. Colleagues instantly understand that when I refer to a "conduction aphasia," I mean someone with fluent, paraphasic speech, virtually normal auditory comprehension, but poor repetition. This is a starting point for more detailed language analysis (Figure 3).

Language Testing

Responsive and conversational language, referred to as **spontaneous speech** is appraised simultaneously with analysis of speech. The examiner notes the patient's response (or lack thereof) to introductory and salutary remarks ("How can I help you; why are you in the hospital?"). "Response" means any sign that the patient is aware of the examiner's attempt to engage him. If the patient is known in advance to be aphasic, begin with small talk designed to elicit everyday phrases such as "yes," "no," "I don't know," "I hope so," then proceed to more open-ended conversation. Useful topics include details of her illness, her work, hobbies, and family (Albert 1991). Alternatively, provide an image from a magazine, the Internet, etc. and ask the patient to describe it.

Fluency of speech is assessed next. If she is not mute, the first step is to note whether language output is fluent or nonfluent. Decreased output, less than about 50 words per minute, is the cardinal feature of nonfluent aphasia. Output may be limited to verbal stereotypies such as "boy," "ba-ba," "Jesus Christ," "shit," or other expletives. Word production for fluent aphasics is normal (roughly 150 words per minute) or even supernormal, approaching 200 words per minute.

Note that even severe nonfluent language **may** improve markedly when the patient is asked to count (in standard order) or recite over-learned "serial speech" such as the alphabet, days of the week, or months of the year. Nonfluency often also is improved by singing familiar songs.

The important fluency parameters are effort, phrase length, informational content, presence or absence of paraphasias and articulatory difficulty, and speech prosody.

- Effort. Nonfluent aphasics struggle to initiate speech, grope for words, and pause often and for prolonged epochs. The effort may be accompanied by gestures or facial grimaces. Fluent aphasic speech is effortless but also is subject to brief pauses when a semantically meaningful word is required (Benson and Ardila 1996). The pause may end with *circumlocutions*, a series of descriptive phrases in an often failed attempt to generate the target word.

- Phrase length. Essentially, the number of words spoken between inspirations. Nonfluent phrase length may be limited to a single word. Normal is at least 5–6 words per breath unit. Some fluent aphasics greatly exceed this.

- Informational content. Markedly reduced nonfluent output is often information-plentiful because of reliance on semantically rich words ("hate...nurse...glasses") to the exclusion of "functors": syntactical articles, prepositions, pronouns, etc. (*agrammatism*). Fluent aphasics, on the other hand, generate long phrases and sentences with few substantive nouns and verbs, but full of syntactical constructions which often are misused (*paragrammatism*), thus conveying little or no information to the listener (*empty speech*).

- Paraphasias. A *paraphasia* is a substitution within language; an incorrect word or an incorrectly produced word (Benson and Ardila 1996), that is, "production of unintended syllables, words, or phrases during the effort to speak" (Goodglass and Kaplan 1983). Paraphasia analysis occupies its own linguistic sub-universe. For the purpose of the geriatric MSE, paraphasias are classified as *literal (phonemic)*, *verbal (semantic)*, and *neologistic*. Literal paraphasia refers to omission, displacement, substitution, or addition of phonemes to words (tree branches have *breaves*; my friend gets *larried*) and are characteristic of nonfluent aphasia. Verbal paraphasias are erroneous substitutions of real words for the proper words. The substitutions may or may not be semantically or phonologically related to the proper target (Don't *dress* the coffee; the *cat* barks all day). Neologistic (new word) paraphasias do not belong to the language lexicon (Don't *groget* the floor); in some cases they represent multiple superimposed phonemic substitutions (Benson and Ardila 1996). Verbal and neologistic paraphasias typify fluent aphasia, are more prominent when aphasia is acute, and may be so plentiful that output is incomprehensible. Fluent aphasics in general are not aware of their paraphasias and, when aphasia is acute, may be unaware of any language disturbance at all. Nonfluent aphasics, on the other hand, frequently attempt to correct their own paraphasic errors, resulting in more paraphasias (Albert 1991).

- Prosody. Prosody refers to rhythmic, melodic, and inflectional elements of speech, which, accompanied by learned movements such as forehead furrowing, head tilt, smirking, and other body postures convey meaning independently of, and sometimes contrary to, the words themselves. A listener, for example, comprehends "he's really funny" differently when proclaimed sarcastically, as an interrogative, or by a laughing person. *Dysprosody* alludes to monotonous and affectless production and to impaired comprehension of others' inflected speech and usually reflects right hemisphere damage in **non**-aphasics (Ross 2000). Melodic line is as well, however, invariably disrupted in the agrammatic and labored speech of nonfluent aphasics. Dysprosody indeed is a major differentiating feature of nonfluent vs. fluent aphasia, (Albert 1991; Benson and Ardila 1996) although it may be so mild as to be mistaken merely for a foreign accent (Monrad-Krohn 1947).

- Articulatory difficulty. Nonfluent aphasics are typically, but not always, dysarthric. Fluent aphasics typically, but not always, have normal *speech*.

With adequate exposure, one gains adequate qualitative appreciation and technique of reporting language fluency. Some texts (Strub and Black 2000) recommend controlled word association tests (animal naming, "FAS") as a measure of fluency. Virtually every aphasic, fluent or nonfluent, is impaired on this test, and poor performance may be the only indication of subtle language dysfunction. Normal generation is at least 20 words per minute and anything less than 15 is probably abnormal. Be aware, however, that this test is not specific for language, and can reflect motivational, attentional and psychiatric disorders.

The next step is assessment of auditory **comprehension**, which in aphasics virtually is never either fully normal or absent (Benson and Ardila 1996). Be aware of several pitfalls. In addition to the obvious importance of hearing, intact output pathways are necessary. Apraxia and perseveration may invalidate responses in spite of good comprehension, as can inattention, hemispatial neglect, and hemianopia and visual scanning impairment (Helm-Estabrooks and Albert 2004). One should nevertheless attempt to isolate comprehension by limiting as much as possible the required motor response.

As with any task, there is a hierarchy of difficulty. Length and grammatical complexity of the stimulus are obvious factors. Stimuli with high affective content ("Is this a gun; are you married?") evoke correct responses more often than neutral stimuli ("Is this a spoon?"). Naturally occurring, functional commands ("Pull up your chair") are followed more accurately than low frequency commands ("Twirl the pencil"). Similarly, lower usage words (flotilla) may not register as well as words used frequently (family). Actions involving axial or midline muscles (bowing, walking, eyelid opening or closure) often are performed correctly by even the severest aphasics, who may fail tasks requiring use of one limb. Prepositions, word tenses, word order, passive constructions, and possessives complicate comprehension ("touch *your* knee" vs. "touch *my* knee;" "my uncle's brother" vs. "my brother's uncle;" "touch the keys with the pen" vs. "with the pen, touch the keys;" "Joe slapped Carl" vs. "Joe was slapped by Carl"), which may fluctuate in any given patient. Fluent aphasics especially tend to "fatigue" (i.e., auditory comprehension worsens), particularly when the subject is changed, whereas understanding might improve, usually briefly, if a topic is maintained. Finally, examiners may overestimate the patient's ability if they are not careful to avoid cues such as changes in their own vocal prosody, facial expression, or gestures which accompany questions or commands (e.g., looking at the ceiling when you command the patient to point to it).

Begin by asking the patient to locate several of his own body parts ("Point to/show me your_____"), followed by several easily visible room objects, one at a time. Gradually increase the number of actions to be performed per command sequence until she fails. Normal pointing span is at least four. If he succeeds with all commands, proceed with several single-step "natural context" commands ("Close the door; Take off your shoes.") Time permitting, challenge the patient with more complex constructions ("Show me the source of illumination in this room; point to where I wash my hands; point to an object which marks the passage of time.")

If the patient has difficulty, signal a brief delay to the patient, then switch to a "yes-no" response mode. Ask several questions so that correct responses alternate between "yes" and "no" randomly ("Is this a car? Are these brown? Do you put your shoes on before your socks?").

If possible, challenge him with more complex linguistic structures ("Is my father's sister a man; do football players use bats?"). Responses may be verbal or via gesture (head nodding or shaking). Other nonverbal means may be useful. The examiner may, for example, designate a red object as "yes" and a black object as "no" and then instruct the patient to point to or otherwise indicate the appropriate color following each question.

Repetition should be tested in the language-impaired elderly for two reasons. First, presence or absence of repetition difficulty narrows aphasia differential diagnosis (Figure 3). Second, if DAT is suspected, repetition disturbance not attributable to deafness, inattention, or dysarthria renders unlikely Alzheimer's disease as the sole pathological entity.

The same variables that affect performance on other language tasks, word frequency and length, phrase length, emotional relevance, semantic category, and syntactic content, also influence repetition. Severe comprehension impairment may prevent the patient even from getting into proper testing set (Helm-Estabrooks and Albert 2004). Listen for paraphasias, altered word order, span limitation, and omissions of words, particularly articles.

Tell the patient, "I want you to repeat everything I say, exactly as I say it." Speak in an even, deliberate manner; try not to alter prosodic intonation among your offerings. Begin with single words and numbers, one-syllable words at first then gradually increase syllabic content. Include some fractions. Proceed with short and then longer phrases and sentences, some with a preponderance of substantive nouns and verbs, some loaded with functors. For example:

One

Five

Thirty-eight

Seven-eighths

Seventy-five

Four hundred twenty-three

Boy

Donut

Committee

He is here

If he comes, I will go

She is also there now

We went home at supper time

The bear bit the wolf on his cold nose

Basketball players are usually very tall

When the man returned he found the house filled with his son's friends

Naming refers to the ability to produce a correct word label for objects, concepts, actions and colors and is a basic language function. Naming disturbance in a responsive, attentive patient with intelligible speech implies either a psychiatric disorder or aphasia although, as always, there are uncommon causes. Non-aphasic patients with callosal disconnection, for example, may be unable to name any stimulus presented ipsilateral to their language-dominant (usually left) hemisphere.

All aphasics are *anomic* to some degree. Anomia (dysnomia) is manifest by word-finding difficulty in spontaneous discourse, by inability to produce the correct word when asked to do so, or by both. Tests are described below, but the examiner must be flexible in his/her approach for several reasons. First, naming ability on any task is related to educational level and socio-economic status in the context of the given language. Second, and again worth emphasizing, what constitutes "normal" aging remains largely an unresolved issue. Mild word-finding difficulties in everyday discourse are virtually universal from about the sixth decade, and slight verb and noun confrontation naming difficulty also may be "normal" (Ramsay et al. 1999), Third, naming disorders may be dependent on the input channel. Visually impaired elders may not *perceive* a wristwatch but may correctly identify it instantly by description ("a timepiece worn on your arm") or if it is placed in her hand. In addition, aphasic misnaming may be modality (e.g., color anomia) or category specific. Some patients name room objects better than body parts, others the reverse. They may not be able to name any mammal but have no difficulty with other animals or other word categories.

Begin by listening for word-finding pauses (obvious for nonfluent aphasics) during conversation. Be attentive for *circumlocution*: a description of the target word or of its use instead of the word itself, which in turn may require other inaccessible words, thus generating fairly meaningless, "empty" speech. Another phenomenon is word substitution by an "all-purpose paraphasia," that is, generalizations and demonstrative pronouns and adjectives like "thing," "them," "it," "these," "that," etc.

The simplest test is confrontation naming. Targets can be presented in any modality (tactile, auditory), and multi-modality testing is routine for comprehensive language assessment. Visual confrontation naming is sufficient unless sight is significantly impaired. Provide photographs, computer images, or line drawings of objects if available, and ask the patient to name ("Tell me what this is") body parts and room objects. Once again, grade the targets for word frequency. Start with common body parts and objects (shoulder, foot, nose, hand, elbow; floor, table, door, sink, glasses, pants), then parts of objects (knuckles, nails, crease, cuff, [ear]lobe; [watch] crystal, hinge, lens, faucet, knob) then actions (throw, kick, hit, mash, stomp, chop, etc.). Some patients may name common objects and actions flawlessly, yet may hesitate, circumlocute, or generate a paraphasia with low frequency words. In response to naming failures, provide a semantic cue (pencil: "you write with it"). If this is ineffective, try successive (if necessary) phonemic cues ("it's a p/peh/pen/penc," etc.).

Show the patient a few highly saturated colors, on special testing plates, cards, room objects or clothes. Ask him to name them. *Color anomia* in isolation, i.e., without aphasia, strongly suggests a lesion of the posterior (splenium) corpus callosum.

Aphasic anomia is diagnostically non-specific. If, however, a patient displays no evidence of naming disorder with testing, and his conversational language is unremarkable, clinically significant language disorder is unlikely. The examiner may then pare the language examination with the exception of reading. Conversely, if naming ability is only mildly diminished, the response to cuing may be critical. Failure of cuing to elicit a correct word in more than one or two instances is probably abnormal.

Determine the patient's literacy and, as always, his level of education and primary visual competency. If he is literate and can see, **reading** evaluation is important because alexia, impairment of the ability to comprehend written language, may occur in the absence of any other language disorder. Aphasics are always, at least to some extent, alexic.

Full analysis of alexia is beyond the scope of the geriatric MSE. Time permitting, however, reading aloud and reading comprehension should both be tested, as either may be disrupted in isolation.

Conduction aphasics, for example, comprehend written material very well, but may become more paraphasic when reading aloud even than when engaged in conversation. Reading for nonfluent aphasics is struggle enough so that most don't, although comprehension of written material, while not normal, often is adequate (Benson and Ardila 1996). Nevertheless, they may be completely unable to read aloud a single word. Some fluent (Wernicke-type) aphasics are relatively word blind (auditory comprehension better than reading comprehension), others relatively word deaf (reading comprehension better than auditory comprehension).

In addition to education, variables that influence reading comprehension include passage length, semantic/functor word ratio, emotional valence, and whether the word is imageable (Helm-Estabrooks and Albert 2004).

Lesions in either hemisphere can produce alexia. Hemispatial (neglect) alexics, for example, ignore either the initial (right hemisphere lesions) or the end (left hemisphere) morphemes of words and of halves of sentences (Basketball >>> "ball"). In general, alexia is a left hemisphere issue and can occur with anterior or posterior lesions. The purpose of testing is to determine whether a reading disorder represents a language disturbance or a visuospatial perturbation, and whether it is isolated, with or without accompanying agraphia, or embedded within a more pervasive aphasia.

Bedside/office testing for alexia is graded in complexity:

- Ask the patient to read several education level-appropriate sentences, or a paragraph from a magazine, computer screen, or newspaper. Then ask her to relate to you what she has just read, or ask specific questions regarding the content of the passage. If there is a problem:
- Present single large-print words of objects and body parts and ask the patient to read them aloud, then to identify the appropriate targets; alternatively, point to the target and instruct the patient to indicate, "yes" or "no," whether there is a match
- Present a few printed short sentences ("We pound a nail with a _____") as well as several alternative endings (car, weather, hammer) and ask the patient to select the correct word
- Proffer sentences of varying complexity then ask about the content (The tiger was killed by the lion. "Which animal is dead?")
- Reading aloud is assessed simultaneously with comprehension. The examiner attends to phonemic and semantic *paralexias*, evidence of hemialexia, and the rate and prosody of speech while he is reading. Note particularly whether prosody differs significantly from his conversational speech

See Chapter 8 and other sources (Benson and Ardila 1996) for discussions of various types of alexia.

Memory

The importance of memory impairment in the elderly need hardly be emphasized. It is by far the most common cognitive complaint and usually the earliest symptom of the dementia syndrome in older persons. Poor memory is probably the best prognostic indicator for detecting incipient dementia (Eias et al. 2000).

That which we call *memory* by any other name, however, may or may not be "memory." In other words, memory is not a unitary phenomenon. Impairments in a variety of mechanisms may produce a range of memory disorders of variable severity. Examples include relatively non-disabling "gist memory" impairment characteristic of early DAT (Budson, Todman, and Schacter 2006), seizure-induced loss of autobiographical memory (Butler and Zeman 2008), and forgetfulness which in fact may be consequent to an attention or language disturbance. The complexity of the cognitive functions we refer to collectively as "memory" can in part be appreciated by considering the still-evolving nomenclature of both normal memory and memory disorders. Some familiarity with this terminology (e.g., "semantic memory", "encoding", "storage"), discussed in Chapter 7 and elsewhere (Petersen R, and Weingartner 1991), is necessary to assess that which we call memory.

Longevity allows people with memory disturbance to acquire numerous pathologic substrates as its basis. Thus an elder with mild AD may also have endured years of alcohol abuse and/or suffered traumatic brain injury. This can scramble the patterns of memory loss which are more or less typical of single pathologic entities. As with language impairment, memory loss can be modality (auditory, visual) (Ross 1980), material (verbal, non-verbal), or category specific, and testing results are education level-dependent. Anterograde amnesia may or may not accompany significant retrograde memory loss, and may change over time (Blass 1985).

The goals of memory assessment by the MSE are relatively limited: to determine whether-or-not impairment in fact is present and if so, its severity and relationship to other cognitive and behavioral disorders. Bedside screening of memory in many cases is insufficient to achieve these goals. The MMSE, for example and as already noted, simply is too insensitive and subject to ceiling and floor effects (O'Bryant et al. 2008) unless the history is suggestive of a dementia. The Memory Impairment Screen (Buschke et al. 1999) and its expanded (therefore more time-consuming) version (Ivanoiu et al. 2005) are useful and relatively brief instruments, but detailed neuropsychological testing usually is necessary to distinguish between "normal" age-associated memory from that associated with a variety of dementias.

Another popular screening test is the Hopkins Verbal Learning Test, (Brandt 1991) published in several forms, all of which are essentially equivalent. It is composed of 12 items, organized into three semantic categories, and presented over three consecutive learning trials. Its relative brevity and ease of administration makes it an attractive memory screen and it likely is useful for many elderly people. However, it lacks a delayed recall component (which adds to testing time) and thus is insensitive to ceiling effects (Lacritz and Cullum 1998).

Ivnik (Ivnik 1991) has summarized the advantages and limitations of standardized, structured memory tests.

Memory Testing

Assessment initially can be relatively informal. **Orientation** has already been emphasized. Assuming verifiability of responses, obtain personal data such as the patient's hometown, current and previous residences, phone number, children's/grandchildren's and parent's names, names and types of pets, model and color of current and previous cars, current and past medical problems, surgeries and current prescriptions, location and name of current church/synagogue/mosque and of previous schools, previous jobs, year and location of marriage or military service, current and past hobbies, and activities of the previous few days.

Ask the patient if he reads the paper or watches TV news. If yes, inquire about current news/weather/sports events, then locations (e.g., north, west) of major cities and states, widely known historical events (JFK's assassination, Viet Nam, 9-11, Obama election) and recognition of famous political, entertainment, and sports figures, always keeping in mind the possibility that the patient may never have acquired some of this information in the first place. Flawless performance indicates unlikelihood of an ADL-disrupting memory problem. In addition, integrity (or no) of memory for remote events might help

differentiate an alcoholic Korsakoff-type amnesia, in which information learned decades previously is usually retrievable, from that typical of Alzheimer's disease, in which remote (episodic and semantic) memory is impaired.

I always include a restricted test of **prospective memory** (remembering to remember) (McDaniel and Einstein 2007). Instruct the patient, verifying that she understands the task, to interrupt proceedings 15 minutes hence and to perform then a task such as pointing to one or two pre-determined room objects, or standing up and raising one arm. As with virtually any other assessment, this task taps an array of cognitive processes besides "memory," particularly motivation. Its value in the MSE is that, in the absence of inattention, failure may be one of the earliest signs of DAT (Huppert and Beardsal l993).

A very useful, easy-to-administer instrument in the clinic and usually at the bedside is the **Three Words-Three Shapes Test** (3W3ST) (Weintraub 2000) (Figure 3), which incorporates several important features of more detailed memory tasks: acquisition, free recall, and recognition of both verbal and non-verbal material. The leaning phase comprises several trials which tend to neutralize mild attention deficit, differentiate between incidental and rote acquisition, and blunt the effect of different learning capacities among individuals. It is useful not only as a screen for mild memory problem, but also for more advanced impairments when more difficult tests are susceptible to floor effect (Weintraub et al. 2000). As with many other instruments, performance may be affected by low education (Armantano and Quayle 2007).

Provide the patient with the six stimuli (Figure 4). Ask him to copy all six items but do not inform that this is a memory test. Note problems with copying either words or shapes. Remove the stimuli and ask (urge, if necessary) him to reproduce all on a blank page. If successful (at least five items), test for delayed recall at 5, 15 and (if possible) 30 minutes with intervening interference tasks. If unsuccessful, allow the patient to study the items for 30 seconds (first study period), remove, again instruct him to reproduce them. For recall of less than five items, allow a maximum four additional study periods. Once he reaches successful criterion, or after five study periods, perform the delayed recall trials. If criterion is never reached, assess recognition by showing him other words and shapes in which are embedded the original stimuli. His task is to identify which items were seen previously. Note both commission and omission errors.

Immediate reproduction of the stimuli is a measure of incidental learning, which is impaired early in DAT, even when most other tests are preformed normally (Weintraub et al. 2000). Normal persons less

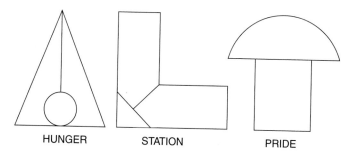

HUNGER   STATION   PRIDE

Figure 4 "Three Words–Three Shapes test" From Weintraub and Mesulam, 1985 "Mental state assessment of young and elderly adults in behavioral neurology," in M-M Mesulam (editor): *Principles of behavioral neurology.* Philadelphia, PA: Davis (ISBN 803661517 - OUP Inc acquisition), and from Mandell, Knoefel and Albert, 1994 "Mental status examination in the elderly," in *"Clinical neurology of aging, 2nd edition"* Albert, M and Knoefel, J, (Eds.). By permission of Oxford University Press, Inc.

than 65 years old require no or only one study period to reach criterion; over age 65, two study periods may be required (Petersen 1991; Weintraub 2000). The delayed recall portion allows assessment of retention and retrieval of novel verbal and nonverbal information over time. Deterioration of reproduction over time and recognition failure indicate retention deficit. Free recall impairment with accurate recognition suggests retrieval deficit.

To correct for ceiling effect (i.e., for persons known to have high cognitive reserve), the number of test items can be increased. I suggest execution of this test early in the MSE. This ensures an abundance of interference tasks for the delayed portion.

The 3W3ST consumes more time than other bedside memory tests and it may be impractical for the slow, apathetic patient with prolonged response latencies, or for those with prominent visuoperceptual impairment, disabling perseveration, or disruptive movement disorder. For most such cases, however, the question usually is "how much" and not whether brain damage is present. If administration is practical, the 3W3ST provides significantly more information than simpler tasks.

When time is very short, or if additional testing is impractical, a brief **Hidden Objects Test** (Strub and Black 2000) is a simple if crude measure of verbal and non-verbal memory, and is useful for at least some aphasic patients. Hide four or five easily recognizable objects (glasses, shoe, cell phone, paper currency), including a few of the patient's personal items as she watches, naming each item in the process. To minimize inattention, tell the (non-aphasic) patient to repeat object names and locations as you hide them. Then immediately ask what was hidden and where, repeating the procedure if she can indicate the location of only one or two items. If she eventually can locate (and preferably also name) all the items, administer other MSE tests as interference, then re-test after 10–20 minutes. Specifically ask her search the room and then to point to or actually locate the hidden objects. If she can't recall the locations, ask her to name the hidden items. Non-recall of at least three items likely indicates a significant memory impairment.

Another useful if crude test for non-aphasic patients is brief paragraph recall. Have the patient read or, if necessary, read to him a news item in which are embedded four or five substantive details. Administer an interference task, such as reciting the months in reverse order, then tell the patient to recall as much as he recalls from the stimulus paragraph. There are many possible reasons for a poor response. In the absence of aphasia, inattention, or primary hearing/visual impairment, your job is to notice whether at least three details are successfully recalled.

Praxis

Praxis refers to the ability to produce purposive movements (Helm-Estabrooks and Albert 2004). Evaluation of praxis is important because performance on virtually all other tests involving the limbs requires a reliable output pathway. *Apraxia* can interfere with assessment of many other cognitive skills.

Apraxia ("loss of the idea of movement") is a family of *cognitive* motor disorders that entail the loss or impairment of the ability to program motor systems to perform purposeful skilled movements (Heilman and Gonzalez Rothi 2003). More simply put, and for the purposes of this MSE, apraxia is an inability to perform purposeful gestures correctly—in response to command or imitation—as a consequence of brain damage. It thus represents a high level disorder of stimulus-response processing, and apraxic patients often perform actions spontaneously which they fail to perform on command. Muscle weakness, ataxia, involuntary movement disorders, uncooperation,

sensory impairment, inattention, and inability to comprehend the command must be ruled out as primary causes of failure.

Apraxia is more severe with pantomime than with use of actual tools or objects. Since most people rarely pantomime and because most patients are unaware of their own apraxia, it is rarely elicited as a problem in the history. Praxis must therefore be tested (Heilman and Gonzalez Rothi 2003). The definition does not include entities such as constructional, dressing, eye opening, and gait "apraxias" because these primarily are non-cognitive motor or sensory disorders.

Unilateral limb apraxia from a callosal lesion (Geschwind and Kaplan 1962; Heilman et al. 1973; Liepmann and Maas 1907) is a dramatic example. Apraxia nevertheless usually is bilateral and referable to left hemisphere pathology. Assessment is consequently often hampered by right hemiparesis and concomitant aphasia, although severities of apraxia and aphasia are not strongly correlated. If there is any doubt about language competency, auditory comprehension must be tested as thoroughly as possible; if it is normal or nearly so, the examiner may then avoid missing apraxia as a cause of performance failure (Alexander et al. 1992; Heilman and Gonzalez Rothi 2003).

There are a variety of "apraxias." (Heilman and Gonzalez Rothi 2003) Full evaluation of praxis can thus be quite time-consuming. The following abbreviated method of praxis testing should nonetheless effectively screen for apraxia likely to complicate other aspects of the MSE. Detection may then require referral for more elaborate, formal testing and interpretation.

Apraxia Testing

The examiner should ask the patient to perform, without speaking, actions involving buccal and lingual musculature, proximal and distal limbs, and whole body (axial) movements. The order of difficulty of praxis testing from hardest to easiest is 1. pantomime to command, 2. imitation of the examiner's pantomime, 3. use of actual tool or object (Albert et al. 1981).

Transitive (miming use of an object or tool), distal, toward-the-body gestures (e.g., brushing teeth) are more difficult and therefore more sensitive tests of limb praxis than are intransitive, proximal, away-from-body actions (wave good-bye). Likewise, intransitive, non-respiratory buccofacial actions (blow a kiss) are easier than transitive, respiratory gestures (blow out a match). The patient should attempt to execute all of the commands with limbs on one side then repeat the actions with the contralateral limbs (i.e., do not alternate from side to side during the testing). Table 2 contains examples of praxis tests.

Apraxic errors vary in severity. Relatively mild errors include inaccurate representation of an object (holding the phantom toothbrush too close to the mouth), and body part as tool substitutions (using the fingers instead of a mimed comb). More severe errors include perseverations and content errors (miming sawing when asked to hammer a nail, or executing an indecipherable action).

A normal response is flawless execution of the command. If performance is imperfect, it may improve with imitation and then again with actual tool use (for transitive actions). Continued impairment may indicate some combination of inattention, aphasia, neglect, or visual object agnosia in addition to, or instead of, apraxia. Suspect an anterior callosal lesion if apraxia is unilateral.

Visuospatial and Manipulospatial Skills

The raison d'être of visuospatial (constructional) tasks is assessment of integrity of brain structures, primarily parietal association cortex, responsible for non-verbal competence. The usual caveats apply. First, as with other aspects of the MSE, few tests are entirely "non-verbal." The examiner's directions are in most cases verbally mediated even

Table 2 Tests of Praxis

Limb praxis, proximal actions	Buccofacial praxis
Throw a ball	Blow a kiss
Wave good-bye	Sniff a flower
Use a saw	Blow out a match
Kick a ball	Lick your lips
Salute	Cough
Limb praxis, distal actions	Whole body (axial) praxis
Thumb a ride	Take a bow
Flip a coin	Stand like a boxer
Snap your fingers	Pretend you're in the batter's box
Brush your teeth	Lean forward
Crush out a cigarette	March in place
Comb/brush your hair	Look up
Use a screwdriver	Look Down
Hammer a nail	Turn around

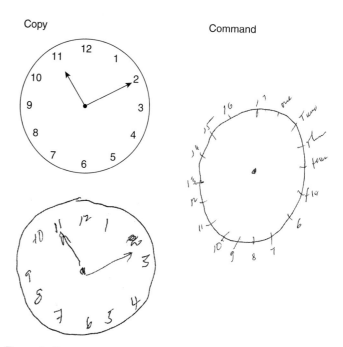

Copy Command

Figure 5 Command and copy clocks by an eighty year-old with probable Alzheimer's disease. Note the regular contour and spacing of the time segments (outside the contour border), initial stimulus boundess (words instead of numerals), lack of hands despite origin mark at center, stuck-in-set ("hyperkinetic") graphomotor perseveration in the command condition, marked improvement with copy.

though the responses may not be. Some "constructional" tasks (e.g., clock drawing) rely on the integration of multiple domains: language (writing numbers), praxis, memory, executive skills (motivation, planning, sequencing, etc.), and visuomotor coordination. In other words, since multiple brain areas and their connections are necessary for successful performance on most of these tasks, they are fairly sensitive in detecting even subtle brain damage. The goal nevertheless is to isolate visuospatial skills to the extent possible. Testing is particularly important because patients rarely complain of this type of impairment.

Visuospatial Testing

Numerous tests are available (Lezak et al. 2004; Strub and Black 2000; Weintraub 2000), reflecting the many mechanisms underlying visuospatial and visuoconstructional impairment. The choice and number of tests one employs influence the power of interpretation. One may, for example, infer hemispheric localization by analyzing both the patient's errors and the strategies used to derive them (Kaplan 1990). The examiner can increase or decrease the complexity and number of stimuli to control for floor and ceiling effects among individual patients. Recall and recognition measures can assist with assessment of non-verbal memory, although adding a memory component may complicate interpretation. Most clinicians lack the time and neuropsychological sophistication for proper interpretation of the many possible errors associated with these tests.

This portion of the MSE requires copying and reproduction of drawings. Pre-drawn standardized designs are preferable, but the examiner who generates her own stimuli should do so as precisely as possible (e.g., drawing a circle as a circle, not as an oval) so that deciding whether the patient's copy is distorted versus a slavish reproduction of the original is unnecessary (Lezak et al. 2004). Poor performance, particularly gross distortion of the figure, particularly in the copy condition, particularly when the general neurologic examination is unremarkable, strongly suggests parietal pathology. Following are examples of tests I routinely employ.

The **clock drawing test** (CDT) is a prime example of an instrument which taps multiple cognitive domains (Powlishta et al. 2000; Tuokko et al. 1992), including auditory comprehension, verbal and

visuospatial memory, visuomotor skills, and executive function (Cosentino et al. 2004; Shah 2001). The CDT is widely used as a screening test for dementia. It has little educational bias, is suitable for non-English speaking populations, may be superior to the MMSE in differentiating demented from normal persons (Borson et al. 2006; Juby, Tench, and Baker 2002; Tuokko et al. 1992), has reasonably good inter-rater reliability, and is often said to be easy to administer and score. Basically, one commands the patient to draw the face of a clock with all of its numbers and to set the clock (draw the hands) to a specified time. The examiner then compares the product with the patient's copy of an already drawn and set clock face. By employing both test conditions, it may be possible, for example, to differentiate between frontal or temporal pathology (poor command) from parietal (poor copy).

In fact, there are many variants of the CDT and interpretation depends greatly on exactly what directions are given. Multiple quantitative scoring systems of varying complexity have been established in an attempt to improve sensitivity and specificity (Royall, Cordes, and Polk 1998). For the command condition, some clinicians advocate using a pre-drawn circle to reduce the effects of a poorly-executed contour (Wolf-Klein et al. 1989), others argue that an irregular or micrographic circle is precisely one of the failings we are to detect. Some prefer segregating the directions for the command condition, asking the patient first to draw the clock face and numerals then, if completed reasonably accurately, to set the time. If higher specificity is desired, this is appropriate. If higher sensitivity (for general cognitive impairment) is the goal, issuing both directions simultaneously is better.

Another variable is the time to which the clock is to be set. The recommended setting ("10 after 11") requires using both halves of the clock face (to uncover neglect), abets the patient to recode number meaning (e.g., converting "10 after" to a hand pointing to the

Copy   Command

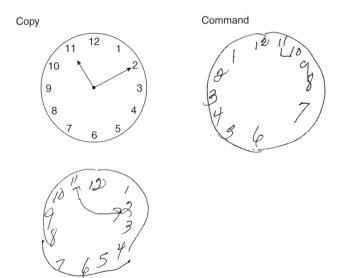

Figure 6 Command and copy clocks by a sixty-eight year old with multiple small bilateral subcortical infarcts. This patient has no functional/ADL impairments. Note irregular spacing, border encroachment of numerals, reversal of numeral order and stimulus boundness with small, markedly off-center hands, again with significant copy improvement. The command clock suggests mostly right hemisphere pathology (Kumral E and Evyapan 2000; Wolf-Klein et al. 1989).

numeral 2) and may unmask stimulus boundness (e.g., pulling the patient into concretely drawing one hand toward the numeral 10 instead of to the 2) (Shah 2001).

An emerging variable is the visual "engram" of clock time. Younger individuals are at least as likely to envision "10 after 11" as digital time, 11:10, rather than its analog representation on a clock face. Interpretation of the CDT will require adjustment as these individuals move into their at-risk ages for dementia (Chan et al. 2008).

Procedure: Say to the patient: "Please draw a face of a clock, writing in all the numbers, then set the hands to read ten after eleven." A square border is permissible and I credit clocks without a border as long as all numerals are present, in proper sequence and evenly spaced.

As noted, the literature pertaining to interpretation of the CDT is voluminous. Interpretation can be qualitative or quantitative. The former approach is appropriate for this MSE. The important variables for the command clock are (Figures 5–7):

♦ Size and shape of clock face—too small for all the numerals? Distorted shape? Incomplete circle?

♦ Both hands present, intersecting at or near center, clearly of different lengths?

♦ All numerals present, reasonably evenly spaced, within the contour of the face, perseverations?

♦ Time correctly set? Stimulus bound response?

I use the CDT routinely. Nevertheless, as with most other cognitive screens, it's stand-alone value is questionable. Its sensitivity in discriminating MCI/very mild dementia from normal controls, and specificity in differentiating MCI from otherwise detectable AD is unacceptably low (Nair et al. 2009; Nishiwaki et al. 2004; Powlishta et al. 2002). The CDT should always be used in the context of additional testing and independent, reliable sources of history.

Many published copying tests, such as the Rey Complex Figure, (Lezak et al. 2004) are well-suited both for qualitative and quantitative analysis, and may be necessary to unmask mild hemispatial neglect

and to overcome ceiling effects in persons who have high pre-morbid capacity. The drawings we suggest (**Line Drawings**) though relatively simple, are in most cases sufficiently sensitive and are commonly used by neurologists.

Present several large line drawings one at a time, each covering the top half of white unlined paper, equidistant from the vertical margins. Place each sheet directly in front of the patient and ask him to copy each drawing exactly as he sees it, directly underneath the original. If possible, provide the patient with a pen/pencil of different color than yours in case the patient "closes in" on the stimulus. Label each drawing as "examiner" or "patient" as appropriate and record the date and time of the test. Simple two dimensional figures go first, followed by relatively more complex 3-D drawings (Figure 7). Note qualitatively the following deviations:

♦ Rotation and fragmentation of the drawing

♦ Neglect: non-reproduction of one side of the figure or consistent copying on one side of the sheet

♦ Perseveration of details (single lines, figure fragments) either within that drawing or carrying over parts of one drawing into another

♦ Closing in: overlapping of the patient's copy directly onto the examiner's figure

♦ Omissions and elaborations of details

♦ Angulation errors, including inaccurate line intersections

♦ Gross aberration of copy size, particularly smallness

Drawing without a model (**Drawing to Command**) requires visual memory, visuomotor coordination, and imaging ability (Farah 1989), related processes that nevertheless are partially dependent on the integrity of different brain regions. It is thus a more challenging task for most people.

The examiner may begin by asking the patient to reproduce any of the figures recently copied as a test of nonverbal memory. Otherwise, ask her to draw such common objects as a daisy, a light bulb, a tree, or a house showing at least two sides.

Higher Cognitive Functions

The focus of this portion of the MSE is a group of skills generally referred to as "higher cognitive functions" (HCF). These skills, virtually all of which are learned over many years, include concept and goal formulation, reasoning, judgment, manipulation of information, motor regulation (initiation and termination or inhibition of behavioral responses), sequencing, insight, abstracting ability, analysis of relationships, and mental flexibility. All are required for maintenance of

Copy   Command

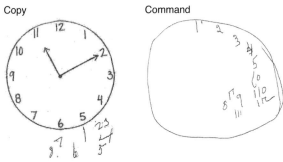

Figure 7 Command and copy clocks by a 72-year-old patient with Alzheimer's disease. Note distortion of circle contour, neglect of left half of circle, improper spacing, perseverations, virtual loss of "clock" concept, no improvement with copy.

socially responsible activities of daily living and job performance, stability of interpersonal relationships, and social independence. HCF integrity is of course dependent on the complex interactions among language, attention, and memory, but insight and judgment, for example, may be grossly disrupted in the absence of these "instrumental" functions.

Exceptionally important in the analysis of HCF is a cluster of skills collectively termed "executive," or "frontal-executive," which encompass volition, planning, purposive action, and effective performance (Lezak et al. 2004). The goal of some of the following tests is to uncover a "dysexecutive syndrome" which, while often attributed to frontal cortical damage, is often the result of extra-frontal lesions as well as subcortical and diffuse brain lesions, regardless of etiology (Perry and Hodges 1991).

Testing of Higher Cognitive Functions

Assessment of HCF is not easy. The examiner typically determines the goals, directions, materials, and timing of any given test. Lezak (Lezak et al. 2004) in particular attends to "the paradoxical need to structure a situation in which patients can show whether and how well they can make structure for themselves." Executive function testing especially requires transferring "goal setting, structuring, and decision making from the clinician to the subject within the structured examination" (pp. 611–612) (Lezak et al. 2004). Structured tests, for example, present little or no difficulty to some brain-damaged patients with major behavioral aberrations.

Assessment of "judgment" is necessarily arbitrary. What, for example, is the "correct" procedure were one to find an addressed, stamped envelope on the sidewalk? The person who reports that she would discretely inform the theater manager of smelling smoke may act impulsively in the real situation (Strub and Black 2000).

Adequate assessment sometimes is possible only by directly observing the patient in his usual environment (Lhermitte 1983; Shallice and Burgess 1991). This obviously is impractical, as is the administration of long "executive" batteries when encounter times rarely exceed one hour. The following tests tap adequately into clinical HCF and can be supplemented by tests detailed elsewhere. (Lezak et al. 2004; Strub and Black 2000; Weintraub 2000)

The purpose of the **Coin Switch Test**, which essentially is a simplified version of the Wisconsin Card Sorting Test (Grant and Berg 1993), is to estimate, albeit crudely, the patient's ability to guide her behavior on the basis of abstract, unspoken rules rather than by reflex. Poor performance has multiple, non-mutually exclusive attributions, including hypomotivation to form and test hypotheses on the basis of experience, inability to inhibit previous responses (perseveration) (Sandson and Albert 1987), defect in working memory, and, less securely (Drewe 1975), a pathologic dissociation between action and the governing influence of language for failure even when the rule is explicitly stated (Luria 1980).

The patient's task is to guess the hand in which you have hidden a coin. The test has two sections, Switching and Holding, each comprising multiple trials. Show the patient a coin in your palm. Say to him: "I am going to hide this coin in one of my hands. I want you to guess in which hand the coin is hidden." Before each trial, switch the coin from one hand to the other out of his view (behind your back or under a table). Extend your pronated fists and say, "point to the hand you think the coin is in." Be sure not to cue the patient via subtle differences in fist shape. For each trial, consistently alternate the coin (e.g., trial 1 in left hand, trial 2 in right hand) until he responds correctly five times consecutively (criterion) or until ten trials are administered. After each guess, open your hands and say either "you're right" or "you're wrong." Meeting criterion within ten trials indicates adequate

conceptualization of unspoken, implicit rules. If he fails within the ten trials, prompt by saying, "I'm not trying to trick you. If you pay close attention, you should be able to guess where the coin is every time," then repeat. If he still fails, say, "watch carefully. All I'm doing is switching the coin each time from hand to hand. Let's try again." Further failure engenders this prompt: "Each time I place my hands behind my back, I am switching the coin to the other hand. Now see if you can guess which hand the coin is in." Note the response to whichever cue is necessary to elicit criterion.

When and if the patient succeeds, proceed to the Holding section. Without warning, change the pattern by retaining the coin in the same hand for each trial until he again guesses correctly five times in succession. In the event of failure (patient remains "stuck in set" of switching in spite of negative feedback), provide the same sequence of progressively more explicit prompts until he either succeeds or fails altogether.

The Coin Switch Test has not been statistically validated on a large patient population. Clinical observations nevertheless suggest that elderly intact persons should establish criterion within 20 trials on both switching and holding portions.

Many distinct cognitive operations are necessary for performing **calculations**, whether written or verbal ("in one's head"). Calculating is a learned skill, so results are highly correlated with education and to a lesser extent with occupation. The patient must be able to read and write numbers and to comprehend arithmetic signs. Differential disability is possible between written and verbal proficiency. Calculation is in general a sensitive measure of cognitive ability but, as with all tasks, ceiling and floor effects are possible. Specificity depends on the examiner's competence to segregate the various causes of acalculia (Benson and Ardila 1996):

- Anarithmetria (virtually never an isolated impairment)—loss of mathematical concepts including "carrying over," inability to understand quantities

- Aphasic, alexic, and agraphic acalculias

- Frontal acalculia—inattention, difficulty handling multiple step problems, perseverations

- Spatial acalculia—related most often to right hemisphere damage, frequently associated with neglect; reiteration of numbers, writing over a previously used paper segment, difficulty using multiplication tables, misalignment of columns; verbal ability better than written ability

Establish, if possible, the previous level of calculating competence. Was the patient always "bad at numbers," independently of his education?

1. Rote arithmetic. The ability to utilize overlearned arithmetic tables is not a reliable measure of calculating ability. Inability to perform these operations suggests, in the absence of aphasia, limited education or inattention. It is not uncommon for patients to respond "14" when given the verbal problem, "what is 7 plus 2?" When this occurs, it may be useful to alter the wording of the question. For example:

- What is 7 *and* 2?

- What is 7 *add* 2?

- What is 7 *multiplied by* 2?

- What is 16 *take away* (instead of "minus") 5

- What is 16 *subtract* 5?

If he cannot respond correctly to rote problems, more difficult problems are unlikely to be solved correctly.

2. More demanding verbal calculations. Carrying and borrowing add to calculating complexity. Adjust problem difficulty as a function of the patient's education and occupational background. Some otherwise "normal" persons fail tests of pure arithmetic but perform adequately if the problem is presented in a "real life" format, e.g., handling money, "making change." Mental calculation should be untimed, but note prolonged response latencies: patients with "subcortical" dementias (Benson 1983) may generate consistently correct responses if given sufficient time.

3. Written calculations. Written problems tend to mute attentional disturbance and even educational discrepancies, but open for inspection errors secondary to spatial misalignment, neglect, alexia, agraphia, and perseveration (including change of sign between problems). If possible, each problem should be presented on its own sheet of unlined paper, or the examiner can cover previous problems once completed.

Abstraction, Reasoning, Concept Formation are related but not identical constructs. Interpreting or scoring responses is problematic and may even be arbitrary, reflecting the examiner's experience, biases, cultural background and, obviously, her choice of instruments. The previously discussed CDT is one such device. Multiple standardized tests have been designed to evaluate what essentially is the ability to solve problems by applying one's fund of general information to novel situations (Lezak et al. 2004). With the geriatric MSE, we are concerned with whether or not the patient's responses are "concrete" or "abstract," reflecting his adroitness in generalizing and converting ideas and concepts while avoiding a "pull" to superficial meanings and solutions. Two tests from the many available are proverb interpretation and similarities. Both are influenced by education and even subtle aphasia can significantly impair performance.

Probably all neurology residents are taught to use **Proverb Interpretation** as a measure of abstracting ability. Many proverbs are understood by people with high school-equivalent education. Failure to *interpret* proverbs by a well-educated person likely is a signal of cognitive impairment. Be aware, however, that familiar proverbs (e.g., a rolling stone gathers no moss) are more a feature of older individuals' everyday conversation than they are for younger people. Elderly patients may thus be able to convey "abstract" meaning in the absence of abstracting ability. Be also aware, for this and other tests, of possible practice effect: some people eventually learn, after repeated experience with the same material, the "correct" response. At least a few proverbs which are not common currency should be used (Van Lancker 1990). Proverb interpretation can also be useful in eliciting idiosyncratic and depressive responses from psychiatrically ill patients (Cummings and Mega 2003).

Begin with familiar or easy proverbs and idioms, such as:

- He's feeling blue
- She's level headed
- He gave her the cold shoulder
- She's got a chip on her shoulder
- He's wearing a loud necktie
- Strike while the iron is hot
- Rome wasn't built in a day

Patients unable to handle these are unlikely to be successful with more complicated proverbs, examples of which follow. Say to the patient: "I'm going to say some proverbs to you. I want you to tell me their meanings." If she can provide an abstract generalization, proceed to the next proverb. If not, say, "but what if..." then repeat the proverb by prefacing it with the prompt specified. If she still fails, provide her with multiple choice responses and judge them as correctly abstract

(CA), incorrect and unrelated (IU), correct but concrete (CC) or incorrect/phonemic (IP). Other scoring schemata and proverbs are equally useful (Lezak et al. 2004; Strub and Black 2000).

1. You can't judge a book by its cover.
Prompt: "But what if I just finished talking to someone and I tell you, 'you know something'..."

- One should read a novel before judging it (CC)
- You can't buy any book that covers one topic (IP)
- Initial appearances can be misleading (CA)
- One can catch more flies with honey than with vinegar (IU)

2. Shallow brooks are noisy.
Prompt: "But what if a parent gives advice to a child about how to act and says, 'remember'..."

- When the water is low, the rapids are louder (CC)
- Shallow brooks are not necessarily safe (IP)
- People with little wisdom often talk too much (CA)
- There is an exception to every rule (IU)

3. Don't keep a dog and bark yourself.
Prompt: "But what if someone believes you are working too hard and says..."

- The two of you would make a lot of noise (CC)
- Keeping a dog is expensive (IP)
- Don't pay someone to do a task and then do it regardless (CA)

Similarities is another popular test for probing verbal concept formation, including categorization and understanding of relationships. The task is to explain what a pair of superficially dissimilar words has in common. Although reasonably sensitive to brain damage almost regardless of location, poor performance is more likely a consequence of left temporal and/or bilateral frontal pathology (Lezak et al. 2004). Impaired performance in middle age may also presage later-onset dementia (La Rue and Jarvik 1987).

Say to the patient, "I'm going to say some pairs of words. I'd like you to tell me how they are alike. What do a _____ and a _____ have in common?" Begin with some easy pairs and, if responses are appropriate, proceed to more difficult pairs. The judgment is whether he can successfully provide an abstract generalization, or only specific attributes shared by both. Be attentive to the tendency for subjects to be pulled to the *differences* between the words or to a property of only one of them. See Table 3 for examples.

Manual Position Sequencing otherwise known as the "Luria 3-step" (fist-edge-palm) test and serial hand sequencing, it can be administered during the MSE or as part of the general neurologic examination. This test is useful for determining, in Luria's (translated) words,

"preservation of (a) flow of kinesthetic afferent impulses adequate to direct the motor efferent impulse to its proper destination and to maintain constant control over the movements" (Luria 1980).

Table 3 Some Word Pairs for Similarities Test

Easy	Moderate	Difficult
Coat/Shirt	Poem/Novel	Praise/Punishment
Apple/Banana	Desk/Bookcase	Fly/Tree
Fish/Turtle	Fish/Carrot	Fish/Boat

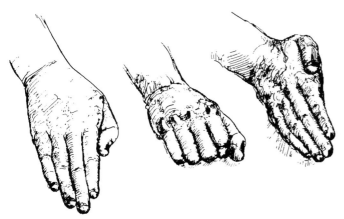

Figure 8 Luria's Alternating Sequences (3-step) Test From: Neuropsychiatry and Behavioral Neuroscience by Cummings, Jeffery and Mega, Michael (2003). By permission of Oxford University Press, Inc.

Failure indicates some combination of inability to establish/initiate, maintain, or to change set in response both to verbal and non-verbal cues. Non-impaired older patients may require several tries but eventually learn to execute the sequence flawlessly. Response to the patient's own verbal mediation, if necessary, allows gradation of imperfect performance.

Say to the patient, "I'm going to demonstrate something with my hand. First, just watch what I do, then you'll do it a few times with me, then you'll do it on your own until I tell you to stop." Demonstrate the sequence (Figure 8) on your lap or the table top several times, then say, "now follow along with me" (time permitting, both limbs should be tested, in succession). When (if) she can perform the sequence, say, "now try it on your own, keep doing it until I tell you to stop." At first, do not allow her to verbalize the task.

Many persons who cannot perform this correctly by example can do so, or at least can improve significantly, via their own verbal mediation. If it's too difficult, assist her by saying, "it might be easier if you talk while you do it, by saying 'fist-slap-side' with each movement, like this."

Summary

Performance on the MSE depends not only on the structural and physical integrity of the patient's nervous system, but also on the presence or absence of systemic perturbations, medications, primary sensory integrity (e.g., vision, hearing), examination setting, and the rapport between examiner and the patient. The patient's educational, occupational, and cultural backgrounds are of paramount importance and, when not obvious, should be determined. In the absence of a gross confusional state or dementia syndrome, the bedside examiner may have difficulty deciding whether poor performance is a function of disadvantaged upbringing or brain disease. Conversely, persons of high intelligence or who previously successfully held demanding jobs may perform standard MSEs flawlessly or with minimal error despite an unequivocal history of personality or behavioral deterioration.

Mental status testing and the clinician's judgment may have far-reaching implications for patients and their families. Hence, their execution and interpretation deserve the meticulous attention described in this chapter.

References

Albert M. A simple test of visual neglect. *Neurology* 23: 658–664, 1973.

Albert M, Goodglass H, Helm N, Rubens A, and Alexander M. *Clinical aspects of dysphasia.* New York, NY: Springer-Verlag, 1981.

Albert M, Goodglass H, Helm N, Rubens A, and Alexander M. *Clinical aspects of dysphasia.* New York, NY: Springer-Verlag, 1981.

Albert M, Smith LA, Scherr PA, Taylor JO, Evans DA, and Funkenstein HH. Use of brief cognitive tests to identify individuals in the community with clinically diagnosed Alzheimer's disease. *Int J Neurosci* 57: 167–178, 1991.

Albert MS. Age-related changes in cognitive function. In: *Clinical neurology of aging,* edited by Albert ML, and Knoefel JE. New York: Oxford University Press, 1994, p. 314–346.

Albert MS, Heller HS, and Milberg W. Changes in naming ability with age. *Psychology and aging* 3: 173–178, 1988.

Alexander M, Baker E, Naeser M, Kaplan E, and Palumbo C. Neuropsychological and neuroanatomical dimensions of ideomotor apraxia. *Brain* 115: 87–107, 1992.

Alexander MP, Benson DF, and Stuss DT. Frontal lobes and language. *Brain and language* 37: 656–691, 1989.

Alexander MP, Naeser MA, and Palumbo CL. Correlations of subcortical CT lesion sites and aphasia profiles. *Brain* 110 (Pt 4): 961–991, 1987.

Alexopoulos GS, Meyers BS, Young RC, Mattis S, and Kakuma T. The course of geriatric depression with "reversible dementia": A controlled study. *Am J Psychiatry* 150: 1693–1699, 1993.

Andersen-Ranberg K, Vasegaard L, and Jeune B. Dementia is not inevitable: A population based study of Danish centenarians. *J Gerontol B Psychol Sci Soc Sci* 56: P152–P159, 2001.

Annett M. A classification of hand preference by association analysis. *Br J Psychol* 61: 303–321, 1970.

Applegate WB, Blass JP, and Williams TF. Instruments for the functional assessment of older patients. *N Engl J Med* 322: 1207–1214, 1990.

Ardila A and Lopez MV. Severe stuttering associated with right hemisphere lesion. *Brain and language* 27: 239–246, 1986.

Armantano C and Quayle J. Performance of elderly on the three words-three shapes test. A Brazilian study. *Dement Neuropsychol* 1: 396–401, 2007.

Association AP. *Diagnostic and statistical manual of mental disorders.* Washington, DC: American Psychiatric Association, 2000.

Baddeley A. Working memory. *Science* 255: 556–559, 1992.

Ball KK, Vance DE, Edwards JD, and Wadley VG. Aging and the brain. In: *Principles and practice of behavioral neurology and neuropsychology,* edited by Rizzo M, Eslinger, PJ. Philadelphia: WB Saunders, 2004, p. 795–809.

Benson D and Ardila A. *Aphasia A clinical perspective.* New York: Oxford University Press, 1996.

Benson DF. Subcortical dementia: A clinical approach. In: *Advances in neurology,* edited by Mayeux R, and Rosen WG. New York: Raven Press, 1983, p. 185–194.

Blacker D, Lee H, Muzikansky A, et al. Neuropsychological measures in normal individuals that predict subsequent cognitive decline. *Arch Neurol* 64: 862–871, 2007.

Blass JP. Mental status tests in geriatrics. *Journal of the American Geriatrics Society* 33: 461–462, 1985.

Borson S, Scanlan JM, Watanabe J, Tu SP, and Lessig M. Improving identification of cognitive impairment in primary care. *International Journal of Geriatric Psychiatry* 21: 349–355, 2006.

Boustani M, Peterson B, Hanson L, Harris R, and Lohr KN. Screening for dementia in primary care: A summary of the evidence for the U.S. Preventive Services Task Force. *Annals of Internal Medicine* 138: 927–937, 2003.

Bowie P, Branton T, and Holmes J. Should the Mini Mental State Examination be used to monitor dementia treatments? *Lancet* 354: 1527–1528, 1999.

Brandt J. The Hopkins Verbal Learning Test: Development of a new memory test with six equivalent forms. *The Clinical Neuropsychologist* 5: 125–142, 1991.

Brayne C, Spiegelhalter DJ, Dufouil C, et al. Estimating the true extent of cognitive decline in the old old. *Journal of the American Geriatrics Society* 47: 1283–1288, 1999.

Broshek DK, and Marcopulos BA. Delirium assessment in older adults. In: *Handbook of assessment in clinical gerontology*, edited by Lichtenberg PA. New York, NY: John Wiley & Sons, 1999, pp. 167–204.

Budson AE, Todman RW, and Schacter DL. Gist memory in Alzheimer's disease: Evidence from categorized pictures. *Neuropsychology* 20: 113–122, 2006.

Buschke H, Kuslansky G, Katz M, Stewart WF, Sliwinski MJ, Eckholdt HM, and Lipton RB. Screening for dementia with the memory impairment screen. *Neurology* 52: 231–238, 1999.

Butler CR and Zeman AZ. Recent insights into the impairment of memory in epilepsy: Transient epileptic amnesia, accelerated long-term forgetting and remote memory impairment. *Brain* 131: 2243–2263, 2008.

Chan A, Remington R, Paskavitz J, and Shea TB. The clock-drawing test: Time for a change? *American journal of Alzheimer's Disease and Other Dementias* 23: 377–381, 2008.

Chedru F and Geschwind N. Writing disturbances in acute confusional states. *Neuropsycholocia* 10: 343–353, 1972.

Clarfield AM. Reversible dementia. *Neurology* 45: 601, 1995.

Clarfield AM. The decreasing prevalence of reversible dementias: An updated meta-analysis. *Archives of Internal Medicine* 163: 2219–2229, 2003.

Clark CM, Sheppard L, Fillenbaum GG, et al. Variability in annual Mini-Mental State Examination score in patients with probable Alzheimer disease: A clinical perspective of data from the Consortium to Establish a Registry for Alzheimer's Disease. *Archives of Neurology* 56: 857–862, 1999.

Cooper B and Bickel H. Population screening and the early detection of dementing disorders in old age: A review. *Psychological Medicine* 14: 81–95, 1984.

Cosentino S, Jefferson A, Chute DL, Kaplan E, and Libon DJ. Clock drawing errors in dementia: Neuropsychological and neuroanatomical considerations. *Cogn Behav Neurol* 17: 74–84, 2004.

Cullum C, Butters N, Troster AI, and Salmon DP. Normal aging and forgetting rates on the Wechsler Memory Scale-Revised. *Arch Clin Neuropsychol* 5: 23–30, 1990.

Cummings JL. Alzheimer's disease. *New Engl J Med* 351: 56–67, 2004.

Cummings JL and Mega MS. Disorders of speech and language. In: *Neuropsychiatry and behavioral neuroscience*, edited by Cummings JL, and Mega MS. New York: Oxford University Press, 2003, p. 70–96.

Cummings JL and Mega MS. Neuropsychiatric assessment. In: *Neuropsychiatry and behavioral neuroscience*. New York: Oxford University press, 2003, pp. 24–42.

Cummings JL and Mega MS. *Neuropsychiatry and behavioral neuroscience*. New York, NY: Oxford University Press, 2003.

Drewe EA. An experimental investigation of Luria's theory on the effects of frontal lobe lesions in man. *Neuropsychologia* 13: 421–429, 1975.

Dronkers NF, Plaisant O, Iba-Zizen MT, and Cabanis EA. Paul Broca's historic cases: High resolution MR imaging of the brains of Leborgne and Lelong. *Brain* 130: 1432–1441, 2007.

Elias MF, Beiser A, Wolf PA, Au R, White RF, and D'Agostino RB. The preclinical phase of Alzheimer's disease: A 22-year prospective study of the Framingham Cohort. *Archives of Neurology* 57: 808–813, 2000.

Eslinger PJ, Damasio AR, Benton AL, and Van Allen M. Neuropsychologic detection of abnormal mental decline in older persons. *JAMA* 253: 670–674, 1985.

Evans DA, Funkenstein HH, Albert MS, et al. Prevalence of Alzheimer's disease in a community population of older persons. Higher than previously reported. *JAMA* 262: 2551–2556, 1989.

Fagan AM, Roe CM, Xiong C, Mintun MA, Morris JC, and Holtzman DM. Cerebrospinal fluid tau/beta-amyloid42 ratio as a prediction of cognitive decline in nondemented older adults. *Archives of Neurology* 64: 2007.

Farah M. The neuropsychology of mental imagery. In: *Handbook of neuropsychology*, edited by Boller F, and Grafman J. New York: Elsevier Science Publ., 1989, pp. 395–413.

Ferri CP, Prince M, Brayne C, et al. Global prevalence of dementia: a Delphi consensus study. *Lancet* 366: 2112–2117, 2005.

Fillenbaum G, Hughes D, Heyman A, George L, and Blazer D. Relationship of health and demographic characteristics to Mini-Mental State Examination score among community residents. *Psychological medicine* 18: 719–726, 1988.

Flicker C, Ferris SH, and Reisberg B. Mild cognitive impairment in the elderly: Predictors of dementia. *Neurology* 41: 1006–1009, 1991.

Flicker C, Ferris SH, Crook T, Bartus RT, and Reisberg B. Cognitive function in normal aging and early dementia. In: *Senile dementia of the Alzheimer type*, edited by Traber J, Gispen, WH. Berlin: Springer-Verlag, 1985.

Folstein MF, Folstein SE, and McHugh PR. "Mini-Mental State": A practical method for grading the cognitive state of patients for the clinician. *J Psychiatr Res* 12: 189–198, 1975.

Freedman M, Leach L, Kaplan E, Winocur G, Shulman K, and Delis D. *Clock drawing. A neuropsychological analysis.* New York: Oxford University Press, 1994.

Galvin JE, Roe CM, Coats MA, and Morris JC. Patient's rating of cognitive ability: Using the AD8, a brief informant interview, as a self-rating tool to detect dementia. *Archives of Neurology* 64: 725–730, 2007.

Galvin JE, Roe CM, and Morris JC. Evaluation of cognitive impairment in older adults: Combining brief informant and performance measures. *Archives of Neurology* 64: 718–724, 2007.

Galvin JE, Roe CM, Powlishta KK, et al. The AD8: A brief informant interview to detect dementia. *Neurology* 65: 559–564, 2005.

Geschwind N, and Kaplan E. A human cerebral deconnection syndrome-A preliminary report. *Neurology* 12: 675–685, 1962.

Gitlin LN, Hauck WW, Dennis MP, and Winter L. Maintenance of effects of the home environmental skill-building program for family caregivers and individuals with Alzheimer's disease and related disorders. *J Gerontol A Biol Sci Med Sci* 60: 368–374, 2005.

Goldstein K, and Scheerer M. Abstract and concrete behavior: An experimental study with special tests. *Psychological Monographs* 53: 1–151, 1941.

Goodglass H, and Kaplan E. *The assessment of aphasia and related disorders.* Philadelphia: Lea and Febiger, 1983.

Graff MJ, Vernooij-Dassen MJ, Thijssen M, Dekker J, Hoefnagels WH, and Rikkert MG. Community based occupational therapy for patients with dementia and their care givers: Randomised controlled trial. *BMJ* 333: 1196, 2006.

Grant D, and Berg E. *Wisconsin Card Sorting Test.* Odessa, Fl.: Psychological Assessment Resources, 1993.

Green RC. *Diagnosis and management of Alzheimer's disease and other dementias.* Caddo, OK: Professional Communications, Inc., 2005, p. 224.

Grut M, Fratiglioni L, Viitanen M, and Winblad B. Accuracy of the Mini-Mental Status Examination as a screening test for dementia in a Swedish elderly population. *Acta Neurologica Scandinavica* 87: 312–317, 1993.

Guerriero Austrom M, Hartwell C, Patricia Moore P, et al. An integrated model of comprehensive care for people with Alzheimer's disease and their caregivers in a primary care setting. *Dementia* 5: 339–352, 2006.

Hart J, Jr., Berndt RS, and Caramazza A. Category-specific naming deficit following cerebral infarction. *Nature* 316: 439–440, 1985.

Hebert LE, Scherr PA, Bienias JL, Bennett DA, and Evans DA. Alzheimer disease in the US population: Prevalence estimates using the 2000 Census. *Archives of Neurology* 60: 1119–1122, 2003.

Hedges DW, Woon FL, and Hoopes SP. Caffeine-induced psychosis. *CNS Spectrums* 14: 127–129, 2009.

Heilman K, and Gonzalez Rothi L. Apraxia. In: *Clinical neuropsychology*, edited by Heilman K, and Valenstein E. New York, NY: Oxford University Press, 2003, pp. 215–235.

Heilman K, Watson R, and Valenstein E. Neglect and related disorders. In: *Clinical neuropsychology*, edited by Heilman K, and Valenstein E. New York: Oxford University Press, 2003, pp. 296–346.

Heilman KM, Coyle JM, Gonyea EF, and Geschwind N. Apraxia and agraphia in a left-hander. *Brain* 96: 21–28, 1973.

Helm-Estabrooks N, and Albert M. *Manual of aphasia therapy.* Austin, Texas: Pro-Ed, 2004.

Henderson AS and Huppert FA. The problem of mild dementia. *Psychological medicine* 14: 5–11, 1984.

Howieson DB, Camicioli R, Quinn J, et al. Natural history of cognitive decline in the old old. *Neurology* 60: 1489–1494, 2003.

Huppert FA, and Beardsall L. Prospective memory impairment as an early indicator of dementia. *Journal of Clinical and Experimental Neuropsychology* 15: 805–821, 1993.

Ivanoiu A, Adam S, Van der Linden M, Salmon E, Juillerat AC, Mulligan R, and Seron X. Memory evaluation with a new cued recall test in patients with mild cognitive impairment and Alzheimer's disease. *Journal of Neurology* 252: 47–55, 2005.

Ivnik R. Memory testing. In: *Memory disorders research and clinical practice*, edited by Yanagihara T, and Petersen R. New York, NY: Marcel Dekker, 1991.

Jagust J, Davies P, Tiller-Borich JK, and Redd B. Focal Alzheimer's disease. *Neurology* 40: 14–19, 1990.

Jicha GA, Parisi JE, Dickson DW, et al. Neuropathologic outcome of mild cognitive impairment following progression to clinical dementia. *Archives of Neurology* 63: 674–681, 2006.

Juby A, Tench S, and Baker V. The value of clock drawing in identifying executive cognitive dysfunction in people with a normal Mini-Mental State Examination score. *CMAJ* 167: 859–864, 2002.

Kaplan E. The process approach to neuropsychological assessment of psychiatric patients. *The Journal of Neuropsychiatry and Clinical Neurosciences* 2: 72–87, 1990.

Knopman DS, Boeve BF, and Petersen RC. Essentials of the proper diagnoses of mild cognitive impairment, dementia, and major subtypes of dementia. *Mayo Clinic Proceedings* 78: 1290–1308, 2003.

Knopman DS, DeKosky ST, Cummings JL, et al. Practice parameter: Diagnosis of dementia (an evidence-based review). Report of the Quality Standards Subcommittee of the American Academy of Neurology. *Neurology* 56: 1143–1153, 2001.

Kreisler A, Godefroy O, Delmaire C, Debachy B, Leclercq M, Pruvo JP, and Leys D. The anatomy of aphasia revisited. *Neurology* 54: 1117–1123, 2000.

Kumral E and Evyapan D. Reversed clock phenomenon: A right-hemisphere syndrome. *Neurology* 55: 151–152, 2000.

La Rue A and Jarvik LF. Cognitive function and prediction of dementia in old age. *Int J Aging Hum Dev* 25: 79–89, 1987.

Lacritz LH, and Cullum CM. The Hopkins Verbal Learning Test and CVLT: A preliminary comparison. *Arch Clin Neuropsychol* 13: 623–628, 1998.

Landis T, Graves R, and Goodglass H. Aphasic reading and writing: Possible evidence for right hemisphere participation. *Cortex: A Journal Devoted to the Study of the Nervous System and Behavior* 18: 105–112, 1982.

Lezak M, Howieson D, Loring D, Hannay H, and Fischer J. *Neuropsychological Assessment.* New York, NY: Oxford University Press, 2004.

Lhermitte F. 'Utilization behaviour' and its relation to lesions of the frontal lobes. *Brain* 106 (Pt 2): 237–255, 1983.

Liepmann H, and Maas O. Fall von linksseitiger Agraphie und Apraxie bei rechtsseitiger Lähmung. *Journal für Psychology und Neurologie* 10: 214–227, 1907.

Luria AR. *Higher cortical functions in man.* New York: Basic Books, Inc., 1980.

Mandell A, Knoefel J, and Albert M. Mental status examination in the elderly. In: *Clinical neurology of aging.* New York, NY: Oxford University Press, 1994, pp. 277–313.

McDaniel M, and Einstein G. *Prospective memory: An overview and synthesis of an emerging field.* Thousand Oaks, Ca: Sage Publications, Inc., 2007.

McDowd JM, and Birren JE. Aging and attentional processes. In: *Handbook of the psychology of aging*, edited by Birren JE, and Schare KW Academic Press, Inc., 1990.

Mesulam M-M. Attentional networks, confusional states, and neglect syndromes. In: *Principles of behavioral and cognitive neurology*, edited by Mesulam M-M. New York, NY: Oxford University Press, 2000, pp. 174–256.

Mesulam MM. Primary progressive aphasia—A language-based dementia. *New Engl J Med* 349: 1535–1542, 2003.

Milberg W. Issues in the assessment of cognitive function in dementia. *Brain and Cognition* 31: 114–132, 1996.

Milberg WP, Hebben N, and Kaplan E. The Boston process approach to neuropsychological assessment. In: *Neuropsychologic Assessment of Neuropsychiatric Disorders*, edited by Grant I, and Adams KM. New York: Oxford University Press, 1996.

Miller GA. The magical number seven plus or minus two: Some limits on our capacity for processing information. *Psychological Review* 63: 81–97, 1956.

Mitchell AJ, and Shiri-Feshki M. Temporal trends in the long term risk of progression of mild cognitive impairment: A pooled analysis. *Journal of Neurology, Neurosurgery, and Psychiatry* 79: 1386–1391, 2008.

Mok W, Chow TW, Zheng L, Mack WJ, and Miller C. Clinicopathological concordance of dementia diagnoses by community versus tertiary care clinicians. *American Journal of Alzheimer's Disease and Other Dementias* 19: 161–165, 2004.

Monrad-Krohn GH. Dysprosody or altered melody of language. *Brain* 70: 405–415, 1947.

Nair AK, Gavett BE, and Damman M, et al. Clock Drawing Test ratings by dementia specialists—inter-rater reliability and diagnostic accuracy. *J Neuropsychiat Clin Neurosci* 2009.

Nishiwaki Y, Breeze E, Smeeth L, Bulpitt CJ, Peters R, and Fletcher AE. Validity of the Clock-Drawing Test as a screening tool for cognitive impairment in the elderly. *American Journal of Epidemiology* 160: 797–807, 2004.

Nissen MJ, and Corkin S. Effectiveness of attentional cueing in older and younger adults. *Journal of Gerontology* 40: 185–191, 1985.

O'Bryant SE, Humphreys JD, Smith GE, et al. Detecting dementia with the mini-mental state examination in highly educated individuals. *Archives of Neurology* 65: 963–967, 2008.

Othmer E, and Othmer S. *The clinical interview using DSM-IV-TR* Washington, D.C.: American Psychiatric Publishing, Inc., 2002, pp. 104–111.

Perry RJ, and Hodges JR. Attention and executive deficits in Alzheimer's disease. A critical review. *Brain* 122 (Pt 3): 383–404, 1999.

Petersen R and Weingartner H. Memory nomenclature. In: *Memory disorders research and clinical practice*, edited by Yanagihara T, and Petersen R. New York, NY: Marcel Dekker, 1991, pp. 9–22.

Petersen RC. Memory assessment at the bedside. In: *Memory disorders research and clinical practice*, edited by Yanagihara T, and Petersen R. New York, NY: Marcel Dekker, 1991, pp. 137–152.

Petersen RC. Mild cognitive impairment: Current research and clinical implications. *Semin Neurol* 27: 22–31, 2007.

Petersen RC, Smith GE, Waring SC, Ivnik RJ, Tangalos EG, and Kokmen E. Mild cognitive impairment. Clinical characterization and outcome. *Archives of Neurology* 56: 303–308, 1999.

Petersen RC, Stevens JC, Ganguli M, Tangalos EG, Cummings JL, and Dekosky ST. Practice parameter: Early detection of dementia: Mild cognitive impairment (an evidence-based review). *Neurology* 56: 1133–1142, 2001.

Plugge LA, Verhey FR, van Everdingen JJ, and Jolles J. Differential diagnosis of dementia: Intra- and interdiscipline agreement. *Journal of Geriatric Psychiatry and Neurology* 4: 90–97, 1991.

Powlishta KK, Von Dras DD, Stanford A, Carr DB, Tsering C, Miller JP, and Morris JC. The clock drawing test is a poor screen for very mild dementia. *Neurology* 59: 898–903, 2002.

Ramsay CB, Nicholas M, Au R, Obler LK, and Albert ML. Verb naming in normal aging. *Applied Neuropsychology* 6: 57–67, 1999.

Ritchie K. Establishing the limits of normal cerebral ageing and senile dementias. *Br J Psychiatry* 173: 97–101, 1998.

Ritchie K. Eugeria, longevity, and normal ageing. *British Journal of Psychiatry* 171: 501, 1997.

Ritchie K. The screening of cognitive impairment in the elderly: A critical review of current methods. *Journal of Clinical Epidemiology* 41: 635–643, 1988.

Ritchie K, Allard M, Huppert FA, Nargeot C, Ledersert BP, and Ledersert B. Computerized cognitive examination of the elderly (ECO): The development of a neuropsychological examination for clinic and population use. *Int J Geriatr Psychiatry* 8: 899–914, 1993.

Ritchie K, and Portet F. 'I think therefore I am': Improving cognition. *Current Opinion in Psychiatry* 19: 570–574, 2006.

Riviere S, Gillette-Guyonnet S, Andrieu S, et al. Cognitive function and caregiver burden: Predictive factors for eating behaviour disorders in Alzheimer's disease. *International Journal of Geriatric Psychiatry* 17: 950–955, 2002.

Roe CM, Mintun MA, D'Angelo G, Xiong C, Grant EA, and Morris JC. Alzheimer disease and cognitive reserve: Variation of education effect with carbon 11-labeled Pittsburgh Compound B uptake. *Archives of Neurology* 65: 1467–1471, 2008.

Roe CM, Xiong C, Miller JP, and Morris JC. Education and Alzheimer disease without dementia: Support for the cognitive reserve hypothesis. *Neurology* 68: 223–228, 2007.

Ross ED. Affective prosody and the aprosodias. In: *Principles of behavioral and cognitive neurology*, edited by Mesulam M-M. New York, NY: Oxford University Press, 2000.

Ross ED. Sensory-specific and fractional disorders of recent memory in man. I. Isolated loss of visual recent memory. *Archives of Neurology* 37: 193–200, 1980.

Rowe J, and Kahn R. Human aging: Usual and successful. *Science* 237: 143–149, 1987.

Royall DR, Cordes JA, and Polk M. CLOX: An executive clock drawing task. *Journal of Neurology, Neurosurgery, and Psychiatry* 64: 588–594, 1998.

Royall DR, Mahurin RK, and Gray KF. Bedside assessment of executive cognitive impairment: The executive interview. *JAGS* 40: cc, 1992.

Rummans TA, Evans JM, Krahn LE, and Fleming KC. Delirium in elderly patients: Evaluation and management. *Mayo Clinic Proceedings* 70: 989–998, 1995.

Sandson J and Albert M. Perseveration in behavioral neurology. *Neurology* 37: 1736–1741, 1987.

Scarmeas N, Albert SM, Manly JJ, and Stern Y. Education and rates of cognitive decline in incident Alzheimer's disease. *Journal of Neurology, Neurosurgery, and Psychiatry* 77: 308–316, 2006.

Schaie KW. The hazards of cognitive aging. *Gerontologist* 29: 484–493, 1989.

Shah J. Only time will tell: Clock drawing as an early indicator of neurologic dysfunction. *P & S Medical Review* 7: 30–34, 2001.

Shakespeare W. King Richard III. 1594.

Shallice T, and Burgess P. Deficits in strategy application following frontal lobe damage in man. *Brain* 114: 727–741, 1991.

Silver MH, Newell K, Brady C, Hedley-Whyte ET, and Perls TT. Distinguishing between neurodegenerative disease and disease-free aging: Correlating neuropsychological evaluations and neuropathological studies in centenarians. *Psychosom Med* 64: 54–69, 2002.

Stern R, and White T. *Neuropsychological Assessment Battery (NAB)*. Lutz, FL: Psychological Assessment Resources (PAR), 2003.

Stern Y. What is cognitive reserve? Theory and research application of the reserve concept. *Journal of the International Neuropsychological Society* 8: 448–460, 2002.

Stokholm J, Vogel A, Gade A, and Waldemar G. The executive interview as a screening test for executive dysfunction in patients with mild dementia. *Journal of the American Geriatrics Society* 53: 1577–1581, 2005.

Strub RL, and Black FW. *The mental status examination in neurology*. Philadelphia, PA: FA Davis Company, 2000.

Tang-Wai D, and Mapstone M. What are we seeing? Is posterior cortical atrophy just Alzheimer disease? *Neurology* 66: 300–301, 2006.

Tangalos EG, Smith GE, Ivnik RJ, et al. The Mini-Mental State Examination in general medical practice: Clinical utility and acceptance. *Mayo Clinic Proceedings* 71: 829–837, 1996.

Tariq SH, Tumosa N, Chibnall JT, Perry MH, 3rd, and Morley JE. Comparison of the Saint Louis University mental status examination and the mini-mental state examination for detecting dementia and mild neurocognitive disorder—a pilot study. *Am J Geriatr Psychiatry* 14: 900–910, 2006.

Teng EL, and Chui HC. The Modified Mini-Mental State (3MS) Examination. *J Clin Psychiatry* 48: 314–318, 1987.

Trachtenberg DI, and Trojanowski JQ. Dementia: A word to be forgotten. *Archives of Neurology* 65: 593–595, 2008.

Tuokko H, Frerichs R, Graham J, et al. Five-year follow-up of cognitive impairment with no dementia. *Archives of Neurology* 60: 577–582, 2003.

Tuokko H, Hadjistavropoulos T, Miller JA, and Beattie BL. The clock test: A sensitive measure to differentiate normal elderly from those with Alzheimer disease. *Journal of the American Geriatrics Society* 40: 579–584, 1992.

Valcour VG, Masaki KH, Curb JD, and Blanchette PL. The detection of dementia in the primary care setting. *Arch Intern Med* 160: 2964–2968, 2000.

Van Lancker D. The neurology of proverbs. *Behavioural Neurology* 3: 169–187, 1990.

Wechsler D. *Wechsler Memory Scale, 3rd edition (WMS-III) Manual*. San Antonio, TX: Psychological Corporation, 1997.

Weinstein EA, and Kahn RL. Non-aphasic misnaming (paraphasia) in organic brain disease. *Arch Neurol Psychiatry* 67: 72–79, 1952.

Weintraub S. Neuropsychological assessment of mental state. In: *Principles of behavioral and cognitive neurology*, edited by Mesulam M-M. New York, NY: Oxford University Press, 2000, pp. 121–173.

Weintraub S, Peavy GM, O'Connor M, Johnson NA, Acar D, Sweeney J, and Janssen I. Three words three shapes: A clinical test of memory.

Journal of Clinical and Experimental Neuropsychology 22: 267–278, 2000.

Welsh KA, Butters N, Mohs RC, et al. The Consortium to Establish a Registry for Alzheimer's Disease (CERAD). Part V. A normative study of the neuropsychological battery. *Neurology* 44: 609–614, 1994.

Weytingh MD, Bossuyt PM, and van Crevel H. Reversible dementia: More than 10% or less than 1%? A quantitative review. *Journal of Neurology* 242: 466–471, 1995.

Winblad B, Palmer K, and Kivipelto M, et al. Mild cognitive impairment: Beyond controversies, toward a consensus: Report of the international working group on mild cognitive impairment. *Journal of Internal Medicine* 256: 240–246, 2004.

Wolf-Klein GP, Silverstone FA, Levy AP, and Brod MS. Screening for Alzheimer's disease by clock drawing. *Journal of the American Geriatrics Society* 37: 730–734, 1989.

7 The Process of Geriatric Neuropsychological Assessment

Melissa M. Amick, Laura J. Grande, and William P. Milberg

Introduction

The segment of the population aged 65 and older has continued to steadily increase from 29.6 million in 1990 to 36 million in 2007 (US Bureau 2006) and is expected to reach 70 million by 2030 (Plassman et al. 2007). The prevalence of dementia and related disorders of cognition increases with age and as the number of elderly rises, particularly in the oldest-old range (85+), so will the incidence of dementia. While roughly 5% of those aged 71–79 have the diagnosis, 37% of those aged 90 and older meet criteria for dementia (Plassman et al. 2007). Concerns related to cognitive function are commonly expressed by older individuals, with many elderly patients and their families worried specifically about memory changes and the possibility of a progressive dementing illness such as Alzheimer's disease (O'Connor, Pollitt, Roth, Brook, and Reiss 1990). These concerns are not unwarranted, as studies have revealed a relationship between cognitive decline and mortality in community-dwelling, non-demented elderly individuals (Lavery, Dodge, Snitz, and Ganguli 2009). In addition, a challenge for health care providers working with older patients is the increasing need to differentiate normal, age-related cognitive changes from those associated with an underlying disease process.

In this chapter, we will focus on the neuropsychological evaluation of older patients (i.e., age 65 and older) and discuss salient assessment issues. The first part of the chapter focuses on age-related factors (sensation and perception, mood, medical issues, and normative data development and selection) that must be considered when interpreting the neuropsychological performance of older adults. The second part of the chapter focuses on a discussion of the basic components of the geriatric neuropsychological report.

Covering all aspects of geriatric neuropsychological assessment is well beyond the scope of this short chapter, as entire books have been written on this topic (e.g., Attix and Welsh-Bohmer 2006). To narrow our scope, we review our process of neuropsychological assessment with older adults rather than focus on diagnosis of specific age-related neuropsychological syndromes. There already exists a number of comprehensive articles and book chapters on the topic of diagnostic criteria for neurodegenerative disease processes (e.g., Bondi et al. 2008; Tröster 2008; Welsh-Bohmer and Warren 2006). In this chapter, we attempt to explain the neuropsychological process by explicitly stating the steps taken, considerations made, and techniques used when performing this type of evaluation. By creating this condensed guide, we hope to fill the perceived gap in the current geriatric assessment literature.

Age-related Factors Affecting Assessment and Interpretation

Geriatric neuropsychological assessment should not be a simple extension of the assessment procedures implemented with the general population. Compared to young and middle aged adults, consideration of the potential impact of factors that could artificially depress cognitive performance is even more critical in geriatric patients. Consider that aging is associated with declines in sensation and perception and increased prevalence of medical illnesses, all of which may effect performance on cognitive measures. For example, during the neuropsychological assessment, a geriatric patient with uncorrected hearing loss might struggle to recall a word list. In this case, failure to consider that poor hearing may have caused the deficient word recall could lead to overestimation of cognitive impairment and worse yet, an inaccurate diagnosis of dementia. Inaccurate labeling of cognitive impairment and dementia can have significant consequences both psychologically and financially.

The potential for underestimating cognitive impairment in older adults is also a concern when interpreting neuropsychological performance of geriatric patients. For instance, the inclusion of individuals with an emerging dementia in normative data samples could make it even more difficult to detect abnormal performance in this population. The consequence of failing to diagnosis the presence of cognitive impairment in older adults is also worrisome since functional decline related to cognitive change may go undetected, creating an unsafe environment (e.g., poor medication compliance or driving impairments). Below we detail the most common age-related issues that must be considered when interpreting neuropsychological performance by older adults.

Vision

Visual disease becomes more prevalent with age. According to the results from the National Health Interview Survey, in the 75 or older age group, 53% had cataracts, 10% had glaucoma, and 9% had macular degeneration, which is markedly more frequent than reports from the 18–44 age group (0.5%, 0.4%, and 0.2%, respectively, Ryskulova et al. 2008). It is predicted that the number of Americans aged 65 years or older with diabetic retinopathy will increase from 2.5 million in 2005 to 9.9 million in 2050, and vision-threatening diabetic retinopathy will increase from 0.5 million to 1.9 million in this age group (Saaddine et al. 2008). Age-related structural changes occur within the visual system (Chapter 29). The pupils become smaller and the cornea and lens thicken and yellow with age (reviewed in Matjucha and Katz 1994). The aging retina experiences a loss of cones (important for acuity and color vision) and rods (important for vision under low lighting), and a decline in retinal ganglion cell axons occurs (decreasing the size of the optic nerve) (reviewed in Kline and Scialfa 1996).

Structural aging of the eye impacts visual perception, which can, in turn, affect performance on visually mediated cognitive tasks. The most common age-related visual change is presbyopia, the decline in near vision attributed to the loss of accommodative power of the aging lens (reviewed in Jackson and Owsley 2003). Compared to younger adults, older adults require greater differences in luminance to discriminate an object from its background (contrast sensitivity), higher levels of coherent dot movement to perceive motion, color vision along the blue-yellow axis declines, smooth pursuit eye movements slow with age, and older adults are more susceptible to glare (reviewed in Kline and Scialfa 1996; Matjucha and Katz 1994). Age-related neurological diagnoses appear to be associated with even greater declines in visual abilities. Individuals with Parkinson's disease (PD) or Alzheimer's disease (AD) have been found to demonstrate poorer contrast sensitivity, color vision, and motion perception compared to healthy age-matched control groups (Jackson and Owsley 2003; Mendola, Cronin-Golomb, Corkin, and Growdon 1995).

Demonstrating the association between visual abilities and neuropsychological performance, Valentinijn and colleagues (2005) found that age-related decline in far acuity predicted decline on cognitive measures of memory and executive functions. Despite the presence of significant cognitive impairment, visual abilities were found to be the best predictors of visually mediated cognitive performance in AD patients (Cronin-Golomb, Corkin, and Growdon 1995). Illustrating the potential negative impact of visual changes upon neuropsychological performance, it was found that color vision errors significantly predicted AD patients' Stroop performance, which requires discrimination of green and blue stimuli (Cronin-Golomb et al. 1995). In sum, consideration of the potential contribution of visual deficits is critical when interpreting neuropsychological performance, and failure to do so could result in the inaccurate characterization of a patient's cognitive abilities.

A brief visual acuity screening measure can ensure that the patient has adequate corrected binocular acuity to view visual stimuli. Given the dramatic effects of aging upon visual perception in low lighting environments (see Matjucha and Katz 1994), a well lit testing environment and reduction of shadow or glare are essential. Use of visual test materials that are of high contrast is also crucial. Cronin-Golomb and colleagues (2007) found that when AD patients viewed enhanced contrast visual stimuli, their ability to recognize faces or pictures became comparable to a healthy control group. Despite attempts to mitigate the effects of age-related visual changes, visual deficits may continue to impact neuropsychological performance. In the neuropsychological report, recognition of these factors and their impact on visually-mediated tests should be acknowledged.

Hearing

The auditory system is also affected by the aging process. The tympanic ring and the ossicles of the middle ear calcify, hair cell loss occurs, and the lateral wall of the inner ear (cochlea) and spiral ganglion cells degenerate (For review, see chapter 30, as well as Gates and Mills 2005; Kline and Scialfa 1996; Martin and Jerger 2005). Genetic factors, noise exposure, ototoxic agents, and other disease processes also impact auditory functioning of older adults (reviewed in Fozard and Gordon-Salant 2001). Age-associated functional declines in hearing (presbycusis) are characterized by reduced hearing sensitivity, speech comprehension, and sound localization. While 10% of the general population has hearing loss sufficient to interfere with communication, 40% of adults over age 65 have hearing loss of this severity (Ries 1994).

Declines in auditory acuity predict changes on verbal memory measures (Valentijn et al. 2005). One study has found that a 10dB reduction in hearing was equivalent to aging six years in terms of negative impact on verbal memory performance (van Boxtel et al. 2000). This finding is even more striking when considering that the verbal memory measure was administered through a sound system set to an optimal hearing level for each participant. In older adults with hearing loss, there is

the potential that verbal memory performance may be underestimated. Clinically, verbal memory performance is heavily weighted in dementia evaluations, given its strong predictive utility for detecting AD (Devanand et al. 2008; Tabert et al. 2006). Without proper consideration, hearing impaired older adult patients could be inaccurately labeled as cognitively impaired.

For patients with significant hearing impairment, use of a portable sound amplifier may be helpful, particularly because many patients arrive to their appointments without their hearing aids. To be noted, attempts to correct age-related hearing loss have not resulted in improved cognitive functioning. An intervention study assessing verbally mediated cognitive abilities found no difference in patients' performance before or after they were fitted with hearing aids (van Hooren et al. 2005), and hearing ability remained associated with verbal memory performance even though auditory stimuli were presented at individual-specific optimal levels (van Boxtel et al. 2000). Though issues with non-standard administration occur, for tasks with lengthy aurally presented information, provision of written material should be considered when assessing hearing-impaired older adults. The testing environment should be free of distracting background noises and in some cases sound machines may be necessary to mask extraneous sounds in the clinic.

Motor

Motoric functioning declines with age. Structural changes in the primary motor cortex (Ziegler et al. 2008), basal ganglia (Cherubini, Péran, Caltagirone, Sabatini, and Spalletta 2009; Walhovd et al. 2005), and cerebellum (Raz, Rodrigue, Kennedy, et al. 2003) have been documented when comparing structural images of older to younger adult brains. With increased age there is a loss of muscle mass that results in decreased strength and the skeleton becomes less movable and able to sustain stress (Erber 2005). Behaviorally, older adults perform more poorly on a range of motor functions compared to a younger comparison group, including reaction times for simple and complex tasks, proprioception, and sensorimotor integration (reviewed in Ketcham and Stelmach 2001). Additionally, osteoarthritis, rheumatoid arthritis, osteoporosis, stroke, and peripheral neuropathy are common age-related diseases that can impact neuropsychological tasks requiring motoric output. In instances when the patient presents with significant motor dysfunction not accounted for in their medical history, referral to a neurologist or a movement disorders specialist is recommended.

Mood

A significant literature exists regarding the relationship between depression and cognitive functioning, and studies involving older participants have implicated depression, as a risk factor for dementia (Devanand, et al. 1996; Geerlings, et al. 2000; Green, et al. 2003; Steffens, et al. 2004). The temporal relationship between depression and dementia is not well-understood, and whether they are concomitant unrelated clinical syndromes or two aspects of the same clinical entity is currently debated (Fioravanti 1998; Han, McCusker, Abrahamowicz, Cole, and Capek 2006). Memory complaints are common in elderly patients experiencing depression and these complaints may reflect depressed affect and poor self-efficacy rather than actual cognitive performance (Zimprich, Martin, and Kliegel 2003). However, a number of studies have noted impaired executive functions in depressed elderly patients (e.g., Kioses, Klimstra, Murphy, and Alexopoulos 2009). There is evidence that the reported memory impairments in this patient population may, in fact, reflect the lack of a learning strategy or organized approach to encoding (i.e., executive functioning; Balardin, et al. 2009; King, Cox, Lyness, Conwell, and Caine 1998). Fisher and colleagues (2008) reported negative findings when comparing depressed and non-depressed older adults. These inconsistent findings emphasize the importance of including screening measures of mood when performing geriatric neuropsychological assessments.

Medical Conditions

Health status should be considered for any patient in whom cognitive impairment is suspected; however, the likelihood of compromised health is greater in the elderly as the percentage of individuals living with chronic medical illnesses is considerably larger in the aged population. Brain and cognitive functioning can be impacted both directly and indirectly by medical status. Common neurological diseases such as Parkinson's disease, Alzheimer's disease, and cerebrovascular diseases are well-known to impact cognitive abilities and, as a result, patients with these diagnoses are often referred for evaluation. In contrast, many providers may not be as familiar with the potential cognitive changes associated with common illnesses and diseases. Here we focus on some of the prevalent medical illnesses of the elderly that have been associated with altered cognitive functioning.

Cardiovascular Disease and Cardiovascular Risk Factors

Cardiovascular disease, in some form, has been diagnosed in an estimated 80 million Americans and represents a major public health issue (AHA 2008). Significant gains have been made in the screening and diagnosing of cardiovascular disease, and considerable efforts have been made to educate the public regarding the implications of cardiovascular disease and the need for "heart-healthy" living. By contrast, considerably less effort has been spent on understanding the relationship between cardiovascular health and cognitive functioning. The term vascular cognitive impairment (VCI) was proposed in 2003 (O'Brien, Erkinjuntti, and Reisberg 2003) to identify the pattern of cognitive dysfunction commonly observed in patients with vascular illness. The idea of VCI developed as the term multi-infarct dementia fell out of favor due to the growing realization that a considerable number of vascular patients with significant cognitive deficits did not have infarct-related brain changes and consequently did not meet diagnostic criteria for vascular dementia (Moorhouse and Rockwood 2008). Rather than focusing on specific diagnostic labels, below we highlight the complex relationship between common cardiovascular illnesses and cognitive impairment.

Two of the most common diseases impacting cardiovascular function are hypertension and diabetes mellitus, affecting 73 million and 21 million Americans, respectively (AHA, 2008) and both have been linked to changes in cognitive function. The relationship between blood pressure and cognitive dysfunction in older adults is not as straightforward as initially conceptualized. Several studies have implicated an inverse relationship between elevated blood pressure and cognitive function (Birns and Kalra 2009; Hannesdottir, et al. 2008; Kuo, et al. 2005; Kuo, et al. 2004) even for patients in which systolic blood pressure is in the high-normal range (i.e., 140 mm Hg (Dahle, Jacobs, and Raz 2009; Knecht, et al. 2008)). An increasing number of studies have revealed inconsistent findings, with some studies reporting a non-linear relationship (Waldstein, Giggey, Thayer, and Zonderman 2005), better cognitive performance associated with variability of BP (Keary, et al. 2007), or better cognitive functioning with elevated BP (Birns and Kalra 2009; Paran, Anson, and Reuveni 2003). Interestingly, the potential negative effects of blood pressure on cognition in later life may commence several years earlier, with cognitive decline more strongly associated with hypertension in younger (70 years or younger) relative to older (70 years or older) patients (Freitage, et al. 2006; J. Kivipelto, et al. 2001; Koenig, et al. 2008; Paran, et al. 2003; Qui, Winblad, and Fratiglioni 2005; Skoog, et al. 1996). A similar pattern of

midlife medical diagnoses impacting later life cognitive functioning has also been noted for elevated total cholesterol (M. Kivipelto, et al. 2001; van Vliet, van de Water, de Craen, and Westendorp 2009).

In general, studies evaluating the relationship between blood pressure and cognitive functioning in older participants have reported deficits of executive functioning (Dahle, et al. 2009; Hannesdottir, et al. 2008; Knecht, et al. 2008; Kuo, et al. 2005; Kuo, et al. 2004; Oosterman, deVries, and Scherder 2007; Paran, et al. 2003; Pugh, Kiely, Milberg, and Lipsitz 2003; Raz, Rodrigue, and Acker 2003; Verfelho, et al. 2009; Waldstein, et al. 2005). Executive dysfunction is most often detected with measures involving verbal fluency, switching attention, and working memory. Deficits in memory functions have also been reported, though less frequently than executive dysfunction (Hannesdottir, et al. 2009; Llwewllyn, et al. 2008; Sims, et al. 2008). The majority of studies evaluating memory functions with this patient population have employed measures of verbal learning and memory (e.g., word lists, narratives), and published reports have almost entirely noted deficits on measures of free or spontaneous recollection, though some evidence exists for impaired non-verbal memory (Waldstein, et al. 2005). Frequently, measures assessing recognition of the to-be-remembered information are not administered, making it hard to determine if the observed difficulties are associated with learning and memory issues (i.e., information was not encoded or consolidated) or a retrieval-based deficit (i.e., information has been encoded, but cannot be retrieved). If related to the latter, the difficulties may be viewed less as an amnestic disorder and more as evidence of executive dysfunction. These executive function and memory deficits persist even when possible confounding factors such as age, education, and mood have been controlled (Kuo, et al. 2005; Kuo, et al. 2004; Pugh, et al. 2003; Waldstein, et al. 2005).

Investigations of cognitive function in patients with more serious cardiovascular disease, such as heart failure and congestive heart failure, have also implicated deficits of memory and executive functioning (Hoth, Popas, Moser, Paul, and Cohen 2008; Trojano, et al. 2003; Vogels, et al. 2007). In general, the few studies examining language and visuospatial abilities have reported intact performance (Vogels, et al. 2007). Interestingly, Stanek and colleagues (2009) reported improved performance over one year in a group of heart failure patients on the attention, initiation/perseveration, and conceptualization tasks of the Dementia Rating Scale (Jurica, Leitten, and Mattis 2001). This was in contrast to a non-heart failure cardiovascular disease control group who evidenced no performance improvement. This study again highlights the complicated relationship between medical burden and cognitive functioning, as it is possible that the heart failure group, because of their fragile medical status, received more aggressive medical care relative to the control group. As with the studies summarized above for blood pressure and hypertension, these investigations did not include specific measures of recognition memory. Consequently, it is unclear if severe cardiovascular disease is associated with amnestic and executive-type deficits.

Pulmonary Disease

The majority of studies investigating pulmonary function and cognitive performance have included patients with chronic obstructive pulmonary disease (COPD). Given the essential role of oxygen in brain function, the notion of cognitive deficits linked with respiratory disease seems intuitive. The most consistent deficits noted in COPD are in the domain of executive functions (Fioravanti, Nacca, Amati, Buckley, and Bisetti 1995; Incalzi, et al. 2003; Liesker, et al. 2004; Stuss, Peterkin, Guzman, Guzman, and Troyer 1997), with specific impairment noted on measures requiring speeded responding (e.g., Trail Making). A number of studies have also implicated memory difficulties

(Fioravanti, et al. 1995; Incalzi, et al. 2003; Stuss, et al. 1997), and there is some indication that learning and memory dysfunction is linked to more advanced or severe COPD (Incalzi, et al. 2003). Impaired memory functions may reflect more significant interruption of hippocampal and limbic functions (Stuss, et al. 1997), brain regions well known to be sensitive to oxygen depletion. Similar to cardiovascular disease described above, however, it is difficult to know if the impairment reported in these studies on measures of memory reflects a primary encoding deficit or retrieval difficulty since recognition memory is almost never assessed. In general, performance in other domains of cognition remains relatively intact (e.g., visuospatial abilities, Incalzi, et al. 2003; language, Stuss, et al. 1997).

Other Medical Illnesses and Symptoms

Cognitive impairment has also been noted in illnesses affecting other systems including the kidney (Chiu, Markowitz, Cook, and Jassal 2008; Slinin, et al. 2008; Thornton, Shapiro, Deria, Gelb, and Hill 2007) and lungs (Crews, et al. 2003; Fioravanti, et al. 1995; Incalzi, et al. 2003). Additionally, cognitive deficits have also been linked with peripheral artery disease (Thornton, et al. 2007). In many of these medical conditions, interrupted executive functions are the most frequently documented cognitive issue and may have a more profound impact on functional independence (Schillerstrom, Horton, and Royall 2005).

Pain

Symptoms of pain are commonly experienced by elderly adults, with reported estimates of 31% to 76% in community-dwelling elderly (Blay, Andreoli, and Gastal, 2007; Blyth, March, and Brnabic 2002; Mobily, Herr, Clark, and Wallace 1994). The experience of post-surgical pain in elderly patients has been shown to be predictive of post-surgical cognitive decline and delirium (Duggleby and Lander 1994; Heyer, Sharma, and Winfree 2000). Chronic and persistent pain has been reported to affect attention, memory, and executive abilities in older adults (Buckalew, Haut, Morrow, and Weiner, 2008; Karp, et al. 2006; Kewman, Vaishampayan, Zald, and Han 1991; Weiner, Rudy, Morrow, Slaboda, and Lieber 2006). Additionally, there is evidence of structural brain differences (i.e., volume loss) in older adults with chronic pain, although the exact mechanism or etiology of these neuroanatomical differences remains unknown (Buckalew, et al. 2008).

Sleep Disorders

Sleep disturbance is also common in older adults, including frequent interruption of sleep by long periods of wakefulness, decreased total sleep time, reduced sleep efficiency (percent time sleeping while in bed), and disruption of the physiological stages of sleep (reviewed in Bloom et al. 2009). Increased excessive daytime sleepiness and/or napping accompany age-related disruption of the nocturnal sleep cycle (Foley, et al. 2007, Martin, et al. 2006). Medical problems common in the elderly, such as hypertension, cardiovascular disease, cerebrovascular disease, depression, nocturia, pain, respiratory disorders, and restless leg syndrome can account for or contribute to sleep disturbance (Bloom, et al. 2009). Cognitive performance declines with increased age-related sleep complaints (e.g., Jelicic et al. 2002), and this association persists despite controlling for the potential confounding factors of age, education, stroke risk, anticholinergic use, depression scores, medical comorbidity, use of hypnotic medication, and body mass index (Nebes, Buysse, Halligan, Houck, and Monk 2009; Schmutte, Harris, Levin, Zweig, Katz and Lipton 2007). Elderly patients are more susceptible to fatigue, which may negatively impact the validity of lengthy neuropsychological assessments.

Normative Data

Evaluation of cognitive functioning relies on understanding how a particular individual compares to the population of individuals of similar age and background. Raw scores on an objective test may be meaningless until placed in appropriate context. There are a few central issues in normative data development and selection of available normative data, highlighted below, that uniquely threaten the validity of neuropsychological assessment in older adults.

Cohort Effects

A major challenge to developing appropriate normative data for older adults stems from the lack of a clear distinction between normal and abnormal cognitive aging. Methodological design can strongly influence the characterization of age-related cognitive change. Studies employing a cross-sectional design compare older and younger participant performance on tests collected at a single point in time. Cross-sectional studies tend to inflate cognitive changes associated with aging, due to cohort effects (historical era-related experiences) and differences in disease burden (see Hebben and Milberg 2002). A factor to consider in the serial assessment of older adults is the Flynn effect (Hiscock 2007). This is the generational inflation of performance on tests of intellectual abilities, which may reflect another consequence of cohort effects. This highlights the importance of utilizing recently updated, age-appropriate normative data.

Longitudinal studies that measure cognitive functioning at several time points can parse out cohort effects, but these studies are susceptible to attrition bias (death or withdrawal). Older adults who do not return for reassessment have been found to perform more poorly on cognitive tests and differ demographically (older age and less education) from those who remain in longitudinal studies (Holtzer, et al. 2008). Consequently, it is possible that data derived from longitudinal studies may represent an exceptional subset of the general older adult population and underestimate the cognitive decline associated with normal aging (Ritchie and Tuokko 2007).

Impact of Emerging Dementia

Presently, most neuropsychological tests have normative data that were derived from cross-sectional studies of specific age ranges. The inclusion of patients with subtle cognitive impairments who later develop dementia is an important issue for normative studies that employ a cross-sectional design. Inclusion of people who may have an emerging dementia could artificially increase variability in normative data (Holtzer, et al. 2008) and possibly depress averaged performance (Rentz, et al. 2007), which will impact a test's ability to detect or rule out cognitive impairment. To address this issue, some studies have included follow-up assessment and removed incident cases of dementia from the normative sample (Holtzer, et al. 2008; Marcopulos and McLain 2003; Rentz, et al. 2006; Sliwinski, Lipton, Buschke, and Stewart 1996). Underscoring the importance of eliminating this subset, Holtzer and colleagues found that baseline cognitive performance differed between their healthy and incident dementia groups. Repeat assessment may be too difficult for large normative studies, but methods for excluding emerging dementia cases will need to be considered in future normative studies involving older adults.

Premorbid Functioning

In most instances, referral for neuropsychological testing will be made because of concerns related to a change or loss in cognitive functioning. When evaluating for acquired cognitive deficits, consideration of baseline level of cognitive functioning is essential so that current performance can be considered in relation to the individual's prior level of functioning. Most patients referred for testing, however, rarely have been assessed prior to symptom onset so baseline data are not typically available to the clinician. We encourage examiners to make use of interview and objective data to assist in estimating an individual's premorbid functioning.

Since low levels of education may be associated with poorer performance on some cognitive measures, older adults with limited education might be at increased risk for a misdiagnosis of dementia (false positive error). For example, in a group of older adults with intact cognitive functioning but limited education (0–10 years), approximately 50% were incorrectly classified as having cognitive impairment when their scores on neuropsychological measures were interpreted using normative data based on individuals with higher levels of education (Marcopulos and McLain 2003). Normative data are available for assessing older adults with limited education, which may improve diagnostic accuracy (Heaton, Miller, Taylor, and Grant 2004; Marcopulos and McLain 2003).

By contrast, highly educated/very bright older adults are at risk for being misclassified as cognitively intact (false negative error). For instance, average range performance in very intelligent patients was associated with the emergence of MCI and signs of AD pathology on functional neuroimaging (Rentz, et al. 2007). Intelligence based normative data sets for very bright older adults are available (Rentz, et al. 2007; Steinberg, Bieliauskas, Smith, Langellotti, and Ivnik 2005). In sum, fair assessment of older adults whose premorbid functioning is quite different from the general population may require use of education or intelligence-based normative data sets.

Ethnicity

When assessing individuals from varying ethnic groups, it is necessary to evaluate the similarities and differences between the individual and the reference group. Manly (2006) recommends that acculturation, literacy, quality of education, and racial socialization are critical factors to consider when interpreting neuropsychological performance of people from all ethnicities and races. Inattention to these background variables can lead to reduced diagnostic accuracy (e.g., Campbell, et al. 2002; Manly 2006). Literacy, rather than years of education, has been found to be a better proxy of academic training, and accounting for literacy significantly reduced or eliminated racial or ethnic group differences on most neuropsychological measures (Manly, Jacobs, Touradji, Small, and Stern 2002; Manly, Touradji, Tang, and Stern 2003). Of note, racial differences have been found to persist even after accounting for literacy, emphasizing the complex factors that may affect performance on neuropsychological measures (Jefferson, et al. 2007). Normative data for specific ethnic groups have been developed (Cherner, et al. 2007; Dotson, Kitner-Triolo, Evans, and Zonderman 2008; Heaton, et al. 2004; La Rue, Romero, Ortiz, Liang, and RD. 1999; Lucas, et al. 2005), which might offer a more appropriate reference group if the patient and normative group share similar cultural and educational experiences. However, creating normative data for specific ethnic groups will not be feasible given the growing diversity of the U.S. population. Rather, the development of normative data that includes variables known to predict neuropsychological performance across ethnic groups may be the most useful method for accurately assessing this expanding portion of the aging population (Manly 2006).

Use of Co-normed Tests

As discussed above, there are a number of common age-related changes (sensory, perceptual, and medical) that can affect older adults'

performance in normative studies. Therefore, a normative study's inclusion and exclusion criteria for participant selection can greatly impact the applicability of the data. This becomes critical when trying to parse out a patient's cognitive strengths and weaknesses on a battery of tests from differences between the various tests normative samples. Use of a battery of neuropsychological measures that have normative data derived from the same population can resolve this issue. The Mayo's Older Americans Normative Studies (MOANS) (Ivnik, et al. 1990; Ivnik, et al. 1991; Machulda, et al. 2007) or The Revised Comprehensive Norms for an Expanded Halstead-Reitan Battery (Heaton, et al. 2004) offer normative data for a range of neuropsychological measures derived from the same group of older adults. A critique of the MOANS normative data is on the uniqueness of the sample participants, who tend to be Caucasian, possess above average intelligence, and have high levels of education and stable socio-economic backgrounds (see Machulda, et al. 2007). Consequently, similarity between the test-taker and the normative sample is critical when using the MOANS normative data.

The Neuropsychological Assessment

The neuropsychological assessment can be thought of as containing four parts: behavioral observation/clinical interview, administration of objective and self-report measures, report preparation/case formulation and interpretive feedback.

Clinical Interview

A thorough and thoughtful clinical interview is critical in geriatric neuropsychological assessments. While objective measures of neuropsychological performance are necessary for diagnosis, information derived from the clinical interview provides the necessary context to substantiate clinical impressions. The most basic elements of the clinical interview include the patient's subjective description of their current cognitive difficulties; medical, educational and occupational history; and the patient's current social and living situations.

Subjective memory complaints are predictive of cognitive impairment (Clement, Belleville, and Gauthier 2008; Jorm, et al. 2004; Saykin, et al. 2006) and should be thoroughly reviewed in the clinical interview. Questions about forgetting appointments, repetitiveness, becoming lost or disoriented while driving, difficulty retrieving names, and impaired recognition of familiar people can be useful opening questions, which should be followed-up by asking the patient to describe specific episodes when these difficulties occurred. Clinically, this informal assessment of memory functioning can provide a wealth of information. Interestingly, we often find that patients who can provide examples of their memory lapses in exquisite detail often perform within the normal range on objective memory testing. In these cases, we find that the subjective memory complaints frequently reflect either an underlying depression or other psychosocial factors. Consistent with our clinical experience, Metternich and colleagues (Metternich, Schmidtke, and Hüll 2009) report that persisting subjective memory impairments in older adults with normal objective memory performance is associated with higher levels of depressive symptoms and perceived stress. (See Learning and Memory section for further discussion). It is noted that people with true memory impairments may not be able to provide detailed examples of their cognitive difficulties. Sometimes this reflects memory loss and other times anosognosia, impaired self-awareness of cognitive impairments (Cosentino and Stern 2005). For this reason, the presence of an informant (someone who sees the patient regularly) can provide invaluable information about observed cognitive decline and current daily functioning.

In addition to inquiring about the specifics of cognitive difficulties and seeking additional sources of information, we utilize the interview to assess for incidental learning and memory. In an effort to reduce test anxiety, we employ an informal, conversational approach, and ask the patient to discuss and describe current events. It is important to find a topic that is meaningful and relevant to the patient such as the recent status of his/her favorite sports team, news stories, or the obituary section of the local newspaper. Vague or fragmented recall can raise suspicion of memory impairment, whereas accurate and detailed reporting may indicate preserved learning and memory abilities. When the patient is unable to spontaneously generate any current event or recent news item, the clinician may wish to provide a series of multiple-choice items to examine the patient's recognition memory of these recent events.

As discussed above, there are a number of age-related sensory, motor, and medical conditions that can affect performance on the assessment. Knowledge regarding medical history may assist the clinician in developing hypotheses regarding domains of cognition likely to be impaired, as well as intact, and serve to focus the clinical assessment. A thorough review of these conditions and their treatments will inform the duration of the assessment (in cases of pain and fatigue), test selection (to compensate for sensory or physical disabilities), as well as interpretation of the findings (limitations of measures to detect cognitive impairments).

A detailed discussion of educational history is important to gauge an estimate of the patient's premorbid level of functioning. For many older adults who lived through the Great Depression, pressure to earn a wage and support their family often outweighed the need for schooling. Therefore, bright individuals who grew up during this time might have limited educational experience as well as lower levels of professional achievement. In these instances, education history is unlikely to provide useful information related to the individual's level of functioning. However, critical questioning about employment and specific job duties can provide a wealth of information and reveal that these individuals typically managed complex tasks often associated with a higher-level position or greater educational experience. When inquiring about work history for this purpose, it is essential that information related to responsibilities and duties be queried, as job titles often are ambiguous (e.g., manager).

Finally, the current social and living environment should be reviewed. This includes the number of residents in the home, type of housing, services received within the home, and quality and quantity of social contact. At times, it can be difficult for family members to recognize the early signs of cognitive decline (Ala, Berck, and Popovich 2005; Maust, et al. 2006). The caregiver may be experiencing his/her own cognitive deficits or anxiety related to the deficits of his/her loved-one, which impairs their ability to fully appreciate the difficulties of the patient. In some cases, cognitive decline may proceed so gradually that the caregiver does not recognize the steps they have taken to compensate for the patient's cognitive loss (e.g., spouse fills pillbox, son pays monthly utilities). Sensitive questioning about the patient's responsibilities within the home and changes in the division of labor between the patient and caregiver can reveal evidence of cognitive impairment. Further, this discussion can provide critical information to ensure that the patient and their caregiver are receiving adequate support and services within the home.

Behavioral Observations

Our clinical assessment begins upon observing and greeting the patient in the waiting room; that is, incidental behavior should be noted from the beginning of the assessment to the moment the patient leaves the clinic. Informal interactions even at the initial introduction and arrival at the clinic testing room can alert the examiner to a variety of difficulties (e.g., language, gait/motor, anxiety). In some cases, patient behavior is noted even before the assessment, such as missing the appointment or calling the office multiple times (without awareness) to confirm the same appointment. Behavioral signs of memory loss/executive dysfunction can also include forgetting to bring requested forms, eyeglasses and hearing aids to the evaluation. Memory-impaired older adults may often repeat the same information multiple times, without awareness, throughout the assessment. Incidental signs of executive dysfunction can include disinhibited language and behavior (e.g., using foul language or stimulus-bound behavior), poor initiation (absence of verbal responses without prompt), and disorganized behavior. Additionally, observation of the patient's attire and cleanliness can often provide insight into his/her functional abilities.

Level of cooperation and effort must also be considered to determine the validity of the assessment. Some patients may not spontaneously report pain or fatigue, so careful monitoring throughout the assessment is necessary to determine if these factors are interfering with the patient's ability to comply with the testing situation. Behavioral signs of fatigue may manifest as increased slowing as the assessment progresses, whereas pain can present as irritability or as frequent fidgeting to achieve a comfortable sitting position. The patient's emotional response to the assessment (particularly in the context of very impaired performance) may also impact compliance and motivation.

Activities of Daily Living

The evaluation of activities of daily living (ADLs) is critical in geriatric neuropsychological assessment. According to the DSM-IV-TR (APA 2000), a dementia diagnosis requires a decline in performance of everyday functions due to cognitive impairment. ADLs have generally been separated into two categories: Basic self-care behaviors such as dressing and grooming and the more cognitively challenging instrumental tasks including driving, bill paying, and medication management. Informant-based questionnaires such as the Lawton and Brody ADL Questionnaire (Lawton and Brody 1996) or the Measurement of Everyday Cognition scale (Farias, et al. 2008) are efficient ways to quantify functional declines in older adults. Performance based measures involving completion of functional tasks rated by a trained observer such as the ALFA: Assessment of Language-Related Functional Activities (pro-Ed 1999) or Direct Assessment of Functional Status (Loewenstein, et al. 1989) allow direct assessment of these skills. Performance-based ADL measures have been critiqued for their expense, length of administration, and artificial conditions (Cahn-Weiner, et al. 2007; Farias, et al. 2008), whereas questionnaires can be influenced by informant characteristics such as perceived burden (Razani, et al. 2007; Zanetti, Geroldi, Frisoni, Bianchetti, and Trabucchi 1999).

Declines in ADLs are associated with increased distress and decreased quality of life for patients and their caregivers (Andersen, Wittrup-Jensen, Lolk, Andersen, and Kragh-Sørensen 2004; Clyburn, Stones, Hadjistavropoulos, and Tuokko 2000). ADL assessment is critical for dementia diagnosis, and by assessing functional independence, neuropsychologists have the opportunity to address patient and caregiver quality of life. Measuring functional independence provides critical information for the interpretation of objective test findings; consistencies and inconsistencies across both should be carefully considered when formulating a diagnosis and generating recommendations. Obtaining this information becomes critical when formulating recommendations. Integration of the ADL and cognitive assessments can form the basis for developing compensatory strategies to help patients maintain their highest level of functional independence.

Standardized Test Measures

The use of abbreviated assessment is strongly recommended when assessing older adults. Reviewed above, there are a number of age-related factors that may limit an older adults' stamina during the testing session and artificially depress their performance on cognitive testing. A review of all the neuropsychological measures appropriate for use with geriatric patients is beyond the scope of this article. Below, we discuss some of the neuropsychological measures that are commonly utilized in the assessment of older adults. We focus primarily on measures of learning and memory and executive functioning, as these domains represent the most common impairments in our elderly patients. We have grouped the measures according to cognitive areas but caution the reader from assuming these tests to be process pure. Performance on any measure will reflect the contribution of a number of cognitive actions, and impairment on any single measure should not be taken to indicate domain-specific deficits.

Global Measures

A number of measures of global cognitive functioning have been developed and normed for use with the geriatric population. These relatively brief (less than sixty minutes) instruments assess cognitive performance across many domains and provide specific index scores as well as an overall rating of general level of cognitive functioning. The Repeatable Battery for the Assessment of Neuropsychological Status (RBANS) assesses attention, visual spatial skills, language, and memory (Randolph, Tierney, Mohr, and Chase 1998) and normative data are available for older adults through age 89. Unfortunately, it does not sample executive functions, which can make it less useful when assessing patients with suspected subcortical or frontal lobe dysfunction. By contrast, the Dementia Rating Scale-2 (Jurica, et al. 2001) more thoroughly measures executive functions in addition to other aspects of cognition and is broadly used as an assessment tool for patients with disease involving the basal ganglia or the frontal lobes (Gunning-Dixon, Murphy, Alexopoulos, and Young 2008; Stanek, et al. 2009; Witt, et al. 2008). Overall, these measures are not sufficient for diagnosing neuropsychological syndromes but are helpful to determine a patient's current level of functioning and inform further test selection.

Attention

Basic attention, such as repeating a string of numbers (Digit Span, WAIS-IV, Pearson, New York, NY), can be used to assess level of alertness as well as the presence of confusion. Considering that older adults are vulnerable to delirium and acute confusional states given the underlying medical conditions and the potential for polypharmacy, it is critical to assess the ability to attend to basic information. Given the broad involvement of attention in all aspects of cognition, disrupted attention can have a blunting effect across all cognitive domains.

Learning and Memory

Memory problems are the most common cognitive difficulties reported by geriatric patients. Oftentimes, these self-reports are incorrect and reflect the subjective experience of difficulties in other cognitive domains such as word finding or executive dysfunction. When patients do present with memory impairment, it is typically related to declarative (explicit) and episodic material, in which information is consciously recalled and context specific. This is in contrast to non-declarative (implicit) memory in which performance does not rely on the conscious retrieval of information (e.g., procedural memory or priming). Additionally, impairment is most likely to be related to difficulty learning new information.

Most clinical evaluations of memory focus on episodic memory and include either verbal or non-verbal (e.g., geometric designs) stimuli. The most useful measures provide information related to learning/encoding, retrieval, retention, and recognition. The evaluation of encoding ideally occurs over a number of trials and provides information related to the patient's ability to learn information over repeated presentations. The evaluation of retrieval typically occurs ~ 30 minutes after the learning trials, in which the patient is asked to spontaneously generate the to-be-remembered information. Comparison across the learning and spontaneous recall trials provides an index of savings, or amount of information retained. The final task includes a measure of recognition in which the patient is asked to discriminate novel from previously presented material. To reiterate, the recognition trial, while frequently overlooked by many research studies, provides essential clinical information regarding the distinction of a retrieval, rather than a storage-based memory deficit.

A number of published tests are available to assess learning and memory across the verbal and non-verbal domains. The Hopkins Verbal Learning Test-Revised (HVLT-R) (Brandt and Benedict 2001) is a memory measure with normative data for adults through age 80. The 12-item list-learning test includes three learning trials, delayed recall, recognition trials, and includes an index of retention. Additionally, the HVLT-R includes six alternate forms, making it very useful for serial assessment. The Rey Auditory Verbal Learning Test (Schmidt 1996) and the short-form of the California Verbal Learning Test-Second Edition (Delis, Kramer, Kaplan, and Ober 2000) are also well suited for elderly patients.

The Logical Memory Subtest of the Wechsler Memory Scale-IV (Pearson, New York, NY) provides information related to an individual's ability to encode and retrieve verbal information presented within a contextually meaningful format. Performance is based on the recollection of both the story details as well as the overarching theme. Information presented in this organized and meaningful format provides an inherent structure (i.e., reduced execute demands), providing a foil for the unstructured list-learning tasks (i.e., greater executive demands). Clinicians typically administer both list and narrative memory tasks to compare performance across measures in order to infer the impact of executive dysfunction upon memory performance.

The Brief Visuospatial Memory Test- Revised (BVMT-R) was developed as a non-verbal analog to the HVLT-R and includes three learning trials of six simple geometric designs, delayed recall, recognition, and a copy trial (Benedict 1997). It also provides normative data for individuals aged 18–79 and includes an index of retention and three alternate forms. The Rey Complex Figure (Meyers and Meyers 1996) also provides age-appropriate norms for adults through age 90, though it has been critiqued as being too difficult for many elderly patients.

Executive Functions

Executive function refers to a wide range of skills that are necessary for goal-directed behavior. There are a number of abilities that fall under executive functioning including: planning, organization, problem solving, initiation, inhibition and cognitive flexibility. Many excellent measures are commercially available (e.g., Wisconsin Card Sorting Test, Paced Auditory Serial Addition Test, Continuous Performance Test), though many are too difficult or lengthy for use with elderly patients. The Delis-Kaplan Executive Function Scale (D-KEFS, Delis, Kaplan, and Kramer 2001) was designed to assess executive functions across the verbal and non-verbal modalities and includes a number of subtest items that can be administered in isolation. Normative data are available for ages 8–89.

A few measures of executive functioning that are brief and well-tolerated by older patients include verbal fluency, Trail Making Test part B (TMTB, Army Individual Test Battery 1946), and the Frontal Systems Behavior Scale (FrSBe, Grace and Malloy 1996). Verbal fluency involves the generation of as many words as possible within a limited time to a provided phonemic or semantic cue. This test provides information related to speed of processing, working memory, and initiation of behavior, and normative data are available for children through age 97. Performance is generally based on the number of generated items, although errors and clustering and switching (Troyer 2000) can also provide useful information. Another commonly administered test of executive function is TMTB (Army Individual Test Battery 1946). This test requires the individual to connect circles containing letters and numbers in alternating sequence and provides information about speed of information processing, set shifting, and planning. Performance is based on time to completion. Normative data are available for children through age 80.

In some instances, objective measures of executive dysfunction do not capture problematic behaviors of patients with impaired functioning of the frontal lobes (either by direct insult to the frontal lobes, or via subcortical structures) (Grace, Malloy, and Stout 1997). The Frontal Systems Behavior Scale (FrSBe) is a questionnaire that measures behavioral symptoms of frontal lobe dysfunction across three domains (apathy, executive dysfunction, and disinhibition) and can be completed in less than 15 minutes by the patient or an informant (Grace and Malloy 1996). When issues of insight are suspected in a patient, which is common in individuals with executive deficits, an informant's report can prove invaluable.

Language

Language includes the system of symbolic expression that may include verbal symbols, hand gestures, or other modalities (e.g., braile). Most evaluations of language functioning in the clinical setting are focused on verbal communication, both receptive and generative. Much qualitative language assessment, such as the evaluation of tone, rate, prosody, word finding, paraphasias, and comprehension can be done informally during the interview and test administration. For patients who exhibit language deficits during the interview, a more thorough evaluation of language functioning should be completed. For those individuals whose language appears intact, a screening measure may prove useful for documentation. The Boston Naming Test (Kaplan, Goodglass, and Weintraub 2000) is a commonly used test of confrontation naming that includes normative data through age 79 and is quickly and easily administered. The Test of Adolescent and Adult Word Finding (TAWF), specifically the Brief subtest, provides a more comprehensive evaluation of language functioning including: subtests of verb and noun picture naming, sentence completion, and naming to description. Normative data are available through age 80 (German 1990).

Visuospatial Abilities

The visual perception and construction of objects and features, and the spatial relationships among them, are evaluated in measures of visuospatial functioning. A number of simple measures of target cancellation and line bisection can provide qualitative information, but intact performance is typically observed in all but the most impaired patients (e.g., hemi-spatial neglect). The Judgment of Line Orientation (JLO) (Benton, Sivan, Hamsher, Varney, and Spreen 1994) requires patients to match angles, which requires perception of orientation and spatial relations. Two alternate test forms have been published and normative data are available for ages 7–96. The clock drawing test provides useful information related to visuospatial, constructional, and executive

functioning. A number of different versions exist, with both subtle and not-so subtle differences between versions, although excellent psychometric properties have been demonstrated across versions (Shulman 2000). This commonly administered test involves asking the patient to draw an analog clock, write in all of the numbers within the clock face, and set the hands to a specified time. Normative data are available for the elderly (Hubbard, et al. 2008). The copy conditions of non-verbal memory measures such as the Rey Complex Figure and the BVMT-R can also provide useful information related to visuospatial abilities.

Mood

The relationship between mood disorders and cognitive functioning is a complicated one, with impaired mood impacting cognitive abilities (Airaksinen, Larsson, Lundberg, and Forsell 2004; Ganguli, Snitz, Bilt, and Chang 2009; Hammar and Ardal 2009) and changes in cognitive functioning impacting mood (Ferro, Caeiro, and Santos 2009; Nazem, et al. 2008; Stella, Banzato, Quagliato, and Viana 2008). Given the prevalence of depression in the elderly (Kok, Heeren, Hooijer, Dinkgreve, and Rooijmans 1995; Newman, Sheldon, and Bland 1998), it is suggested that neuropsychological evaluation also include an assessment of mood. The Beck Depression Inventory-II (BDI, (Beck 1996) is a common brief screening tool that has normative data for ages 13–86, although there is some suggestion that this measure includes a number of somatic items that may be endorsed by the elderly not because of mood, but related to health and aging. The Geriatric Depression Scale (GDS) is also a brief screening tool that eliminates the somatic items that may be less sensitive to depression. Performance on the GDS does not appear to differ across age as the recommended cutoff score for depression is consistent across all ages (Yesavage, et al. 1983).

Recommendations

The goal of the recommendations section is to offer useful and explicit suggestions to assist the patient and caregiver in improving the patient's functioning. Our approach incorporates recommendations written in a detailed and simple language outlining all the steps necessary for easy implementation by the patient, caregiver, and health care providers. We view the recommendations as the most important portion of the neuropsychological report. Within this part of the report, the neuropsychologist explains how the findings and diagnosis translates into everyday behavior and outlines steps to enhance functioning.

Typically, recommendations focus on strategies to compensate for observed cognitive weaknesses. For example, a patient with poor free recall on a list learning task (and general mild memory loss), would be encouraged to start using a small notepad to record important information such as grocery lists and tasks that need to be completed. For patients with mild memory loss, regular use of external mnemonic devices is emphasized. Through the use of external memory aids, we attempt to train the patient to use procedural memory skills (regular writing and checking of the notepad) rather than their failing episodic memory functions. Consequently, the patient's cognitive strengths become the mechanism for compensation of their cognitive deficits. In the case of most memory disordered patients, use of routines and behavior patterns (relying upon implicit memory) is recommended, as these abilities tend to be better preserved for a longer period of time relative to episodic memory skills (Harrison, Son, Kim, and Whall 2007; Koenig, et al. 2008; van Halteren-van Tilborg, Scherder, and Hulstijn 2007).

A second major area often addressed in this part of the report is referrals for supportive services within the home or community.

In patients with early diagnosis of Alzheimer's disease, telephone numbers for the local Alzheimer's Association and a list of educational and support groups are provided (see http://www.alz.org). This can be helpful to both the patient and his/her caregiver. In addition, we frequently generate recommendations stressing the importance of self-care and support for caregivers. This may include suggestions of outside assistance and respite care. In the cases of patients with insufficient home support, referral to a local community center, adult day-care, or meal programs (meals on wheels, http://www.mowaa.org) may be suggested.

In the aging population with cognitive impairment, driving safety is an important topic addressed in the recommendations section. The neuropsychologist may offer referrals for driving evaluations and remediation. In cases where cessation of driving is recommended, it is necessary to discuss alternative sources for transportation. Often the state's Department of Elder Affairs will have a list of transportation services available to the elderly portion of the population.

Issues with mental health may also be addressed. Referrals to psychiatry and psychology are frequently offered. We keep a regularly updated list of treatment providers and their specialty areas to facilitate care. Recommendations for healthy cognitive and emotional functioning may also be offered when appropriate, such as increasing pleasant events or engaging in cognitive exercises. For the latter, it is often framed that just like working out the body is necessary for good physical health, a mental workout can be beneficial for cognitive health.

Feedback Session

There is no standard format for the follow-up, feedback session. In fact, considering the importance of clear communication of the assessment findings, our approach is tailored to the strengths and needs of each patient. A few overarching themes persist across all feedback styles including explaining the purpose of the different components of the assessment, reviewing the findings, providing psychoeducation about the diagnosis, and reviewing of the recommendations.

The feedback session starts by reviewing the referral question with the patient. This leads to an explanation about the purpose of the clinical interview and choice of cognitive domains assessed. Next, the findings are reviewed. Frequently, visual aids are employed to help patients understand how their performance on the assessment was interpreted. Since cognitive performance is measured along a normative curve, we often draw this out for the patient. This provides an opportunity to visually demonstrate normal and abnormal performance. For patients with premorbid intellectual functioning at the extreme ranges, using the normative curve as a visual aid is very important. To illustrate cognitive strengths and weaknesses, drawing bar graphs to reflect the differing levels of performance can also be useful.

Discussion of dementia diagnoses can be challenging, especially when the family and patient appear to be very anxious about the label. Regardless of the prognosis, it is often a relief for patients to have a diagnosis and explanation for their experiences. Furthermore, the diagnosis is often not a surprise, as the patient's or family's concerns frequently prompt the referral. When discussing the diagnostic impressions, education about the disease and possible progression are reviewed. When appropriate, possible treatments can be discussed.

During the feedback session, it is recommended that all patients receive a written copy of the recommendations and an easy-to-understand summary of the diagnostic impressions. In many cases, there is too much information conveyed in the feedback session for the patient to retain. By providing a written copy of these suggestions, the patient has ample time to listen (and not take notes) during the feedback session and can review the material in his/her own home. In some cases, a follow up phone call to assess the usefulness and implementation of recommendations can be helpful. A second feedback session sometimes occurs to answer new questions about the findings or to refine implementation of recommendations.

Summary

The process of neuropsychological assessment is complicated by the aging process. Increasing age is accompanied by a number of physical changes that can artificially depress performance on cognitive testing. Similarly, development of normative data samples is laden with potential issues that can weaken the clinician's ability to detect true cognitive impairment. The geriatric neuropsychological assessment, more so than other age groups, requires careful consideration of these factors. The detailed review of our approach to geriatric neuropsychological evaluation provides a concrete way to model clinical thinking during this type of assessment and highlights future issues in assessment that will need to be addressed as this section of the population continues to expand.

References

Airaksinen, E., Larsson, M., Lundberg, I., and Forsell, Y. (2004). Cognitive functions in depressive disorders: Evidence from a population-based study. *Psychological Medicine*, 31(1), 83–91.

Ala, T., Berck, L., and Popovich, A. (2005). Using the telephone to call for help and caregiver awareness in Alzheimer disease. *Alzheimer Dis Assoc Disord*, 19(2), 79–84.

American Heart Association. (2008). *Heart disease and stroke statistics*. Dallas, TX.

Andersen, C., Wittrup-Jensen, K., Lolk, A., Andersen, K., and Kragh-Sørensen, P. (2004). Ability to perform activities of daily living is the main factor affecting quality of life in patients with dementia. *Health Qual Life Outcomes*, Sep 21(2), 52.

Army Individual Test Battery. (1944). *Manual of directions and scoring*. Washington, DC: War Department, Adjutant General's Office.

Association, A. P. (2000). *Diagnostic and statistical manual of mental disorders (4th ed.)*. Washington, DC: American Psychiatric Association.

Attix, D. and Welsh-Bohmer, K. (2006). *Geriatric neuropsychology*. In D. K. Attix & K. A. Welsh-Bohmer (Eds.), (pp. 467). New York: Guilford Press.

Balardin, J., Vedana, G., Ludwig, A., deLima, D., Argimon, I., Schneider, R., et al. (2009). Contextual memory and encoding strategies in young and older adults with and without depressive symptoms. *Aging and Mental Health*, 13(3), 313–318.

Beck, A. (1996). *Beck Depression Inventory*. San Antonio, TX: The Psychological Corporation.

Benedict, R. (1997). *Brief Visuospatial Memory Test—Revised*. Odessa, FL Psychological Assessment Resources, Inc.

Benton, A., Sivan, A., Hamsher, K., Varney, S., and Spreen, O. (1994). *Contributions to neuropsychological assessment. A clinical manual* (2nd ed). New York: Oxford University Press.

Birns, J., and Kalra, L. (2009). Cognitive function and hypertension. *Journal of Human Hypertension*, 23, 86–96.

Blay, S., Andreoli, S., and Gastal, F. (2007). Chronic painful physical conditions, disturbed sleep and psychiatric morbidity: Results from an elderly survey. *Annals of Clinical Psychiatry*, 19(3), 169–174.

Bloom, H., Ahmed, I., Alessi, C., Ancoli-Israel, S., Buysse, D., Kryger, M., et al. (2009). Evidence-based recommendations for the assessment and management of sleep disorders in older persons. *J Am Geriatr Soc*, 57(5), 761–789.

Blyth, F., March, L., and Brnabic, A. (2002). Chronic pain in Austraila: A prevalence study. *Pain*, 89(2–3).

Bondi, M., Jak, A., Delano-Wood, L., Jacobson, M., Delis, D., and Salmon, D. (2008). Neuropsychological contributions to the early identification of Alzheimer's disease. *Neuropsychol Rev*, 18(1), 73–90.

Brandt, J. and Benedict, R. (2001). *Hopkins Verbal Learning Test—Revised professional manual*. Lutz, FL: Psychological Assessment Resources, Inc.

Buckalew, N., Haut, M., Morrow, L., and Weiner, D. (2008). Chronic pain is associated with brain volume loss in older adults: Preliminary evidence. *Pain Medicine*, 9(20), 240–248.

Cahn-Weiner, D., Farias, S., Julian, L., Harvey, D., Kramer, J., Reed, B., et al. (2007). Cognitive and neuroimaging predictors of instrumental activities of daily living. *J Int Neuropsychol Soc*, 13(5), 747–757.

Campbell, A., Ocampo, C., DeShawn Rorie, K., Lewis, S., Combs, S., Ford-Booker, P., et al. (2002). Caveats in the neuropsychological assessment of African Americans. *J Natl Med Assoc*, 94(7), 591–601.

Cherner, M., Suarez, P., Lazzaretto, D., Fortuny, L., Mindt, M., Dawes, S., et al. (2007). Demographically corrected norms for the Brief Visuospatial Memory Test-revised and Hopkins Verbal Learning Test-revised in monolingual Spanish speakers from the U.S.-Mexico border region. *Arch Clin Neuropsychol*, 22(3), 343–353.

Cherubini, A., Péran, P., Caltagirone, C., Sabatini, U., and Spalletta, G. (2009). Aging of subcortical nuclei: Microstructural, mineralization and atrophy modifications measured in vivo using MRI. *Neuroimage*.

Chiu, E., Markowitz, S., Cook, W., and Jassal, S. (2008). Visual impairment in elderly patient receiving long-term hemodialysis. *American Journal of Kidney Diseases*, 52(6), 1131–1138.

Clement, F., Belleville, S., and Gauthier, S. (2008). Cognitive complaint in mild cognitive impairment and Alzheimer's disease. *J Intl Neuropsychol Soc*, 14(2), 222–232.

Clyburn, L., Stones, M., Hadjistavropoulos, T., and Tuokko, H. (2000). Predicting caregiver burden and depression in Alzheimer's disease. *J Gerontol B Psychol Sci Soc Sci*, 55(1), S2–S13.

Cosentino, S., and Stern, Y. (2005). Metacognitive theory and assessment in dementia: Do we recognoize our areas of weakness? *J Intl Neuropsychol Soc*, 11(7), 910–919.

Crews, W., Jefferson, A., Broshek, D., Rhodes, R., Williamson, J., Brazil, A., et al. (2003). Neuropsychological dysfunction in patients with end-stage pulmonary disease: lung transplant evaluation. *Archives of Clinical Neuropsychology*, 18(4), 353–362.

Cronin-Golomb, A., Corkin, S., and Growdon, H. (1995). Visual dysfunction predicts cognitive deficits in Alzheimer's disease. *Optometry and Vision Science*, 72(3), 168–176.

Cronin-Golomb, A., Gilmore, G., Neargarder, S., Morrison, S., & Laudate, T. (2007). Enhanced stimulus strength improves visual cognition in aging and Alzheimer's disease. *Cortex*, 43(7), 952–966.

Dahle, C., Jacobs, B., and Raz, N. (2009). Aging, vascular risk and cognition: Blood glucose, pulse pressure, and cognitive performance in healthy adults. *Psychology and Aging*, 24(1), 154–162.

Delis, D., Kramer, J., Kaplan, E., and Ober, B. (2000). *California Verbal Learning Test- Second edition*. San Antonio, Texas: Pearson.

Delis, D. C., Kaplan, E., and Kramer, J. (2001). *Delis Kaplan Executive Function System. San* Antonio, Texas: Pearson.

Devanand, D., Liu, X., Taber, t. M., Pradhaban, G., Cuasay, K., Bell, K., et al. (2008). Combining early markers strongly predicts conversion from mild cognitive impairment to Alzheimer's disease. *Biological Psychiatry*, 15(64), 871–879.

Devanand, D., Sano, M., Tan, M., Taylor, S., Gurland, B., Wilder, D., et al. (1996). Depressed mood and the incidence of Alzheimer's disease in the elderly living in the community. *Arch Gen Psychiatry*, 53(2), 175–182.

Dotson, V., Kitner-Triolo, M., Evans, M., and Zonderman, A. (2008). Literacy-based normative data for low socioeconomic status African Americans. *Clinical Neuropsychology*, 22(6), 989–1017.

Duggleby, W., and Lander, J. (1994). Cognitive status and postoperative pain: Older adults. *J Pain Symptom Management*, 9, 19–27.

Erber, J. (2005). *Aging and Older Adulthood*. Toronto Canada: Wadsworth.

Farias, S., Mungas, D., Reed, B., Cahn-Weiner, D., Jagust, W., Baynes, K., et al. (2008). The measurement of everyday cognition (ECog): Scale development and psychometric properties. *Neuropsychology*, 22(4), 531–544.

Ferro, J., Caeiro, L., and Santos, C. (2009). Poststroke emotional and behavior impairment: A narrative review. *Cerebrovascular Diseases*, 27, 197–203.

Fioravanti, M. (1998). The quest for distinction between old-age depression and dementia. *Arch of Gerontol and Geriatrics*, 29(Suppl1), 201–206.

Fioravanti, M., Nacca, D., Amati, S., Buckley, A. E., and Bisetti, A. (1995). Chronic obstructive pulmonary-disease and associated patterns of memory decline. *Dementia*, 6(1), 39–48.

Fischer, C., Schweizer, T., Atkins, J., Bozanovic, R., Norris, M., Herrmann, N., et al. (2008). Neurocognitive profiles in older adults with and without major depression. *Intl J Geri Psychiatry* (23), 851–856.

Fozard, J., and Gordon-Salant, S. (2001). Changes in vision and hearing with aging. In B. J.E. and K. W. Scaie (Eds.), *Handbook of the psychology of aging*. Fifth Edition (pp. 181–203). San Diego: Academic Press.

Freitage, H., Peila, R., Masaki, K., Petrovitch, H., Ross, G., White, L., et al. (2006). Midlife pulse pressure and incidence of dementia: the Honolulu-Asia Aging Study. *Stroke*, 37, 33–37.

Ganguli, M., Snitz, B., Bilt, J., and Chang, C. (2009). How much do depressive symptoms affect cognition at the population level? The Monongahela-Youghiogheny Healthy Aging Team (MYHAT) study. *International Journal of Geriatric Psychiatry*, 24(11), 1277–1284.

Gates, G., and Mills, J. (2005). Presbycusis. *Lancet*, 366(9491), 1111–1120.

Geerlings, M., Schoevers, R., Beekman, A., Jonker, C., Deeg, D., Schmand, B., et al. (2000). Depression and risk of cognitive decline and Alzheimer's disease: Results of two prospective community-based studies in The Netherlands. *British Journal of Psychiatry*, 176, 568–175.

German, D. (1990). National College of Education Test of Adolescent/ Adult Word Finding. Austin, TX: PRO-ED.

Grace, J., and Malloy, P. (1996). *Frontal Systems Behavior Scale*. Lutz, FL: Psychological Assessment Resources.

Grace, J., Malloy, P., and Stout, J. (1997). Assessing frontal behavioral syndromes: Reliability and validity of the frontal lobe personality scale. *Archives of Clinical Neuropsychology*, 12(4), 327.

Green, R., Cupples, A., Kurz, A., Auerbach, S., Go, R., Sadovnick, D., et al. (2003). Depression as a risk factor for Alzheimer's disease. *Arch Neurol*, 60, 753–759.

Gunning-Dixon, F., Murphy, C., Alexopoulos, G., M., M.-T., and Young, R. (2008). Executive dysfunction in elderly bipolar manic patients. *Am J Geriatr Psychiatry*, 16(6), 506–512.

Hammar, A., and Ardal, G. (2009). Cognitive function in major depression - a summary. *Frontiers in Human Neuroscience*, 3(26).

Han, L., McCusker, J., Abrahamowicz, M., Cole, M., and Capek, R. (2006). The temporal relationship between depression symptoms and cognitive functioning in older medical patients – Prospective or concurrent? *J of Gerontology Series A-Biological Sciences and Medical Sciences*, 61(12), 1319–1323.

Hannesdottir, K., Nitkunan, A., Charlton, R., Barrick, T., MacGregor, G., and Markus, H. (2008). Cognitive impairment and white matter damage in hypertension: A pilot study. *Acta Neurol Scan*, 119, 261–268.

Hannesdottir, K., Nitkunan, A., Charlton, R., Barrick, T., MacGregor, G., and Markus, H. (2009). Cognitive impairment and white matter damage in hypertension: A pilot study. *Acta Neurological Scandinavica*, 119(4), 261–268.

Harrison, B., Son, G., Kim, J., and Whall, A. (2007). Preserved implicit memory in dementia: A potential model for care. *Am J Alzheimer's Dis Other Demen*, 22(4), 286–293.

Heaton, R., Miller, S., Taylor, M., and Grant, I. (2004). *Revised comprehensive norms for an expanded Halstead-Reitan Battery: Demographically adjusted neuropsychological norms for African American and Caucasian adults. Professional Manual.* Lutz, FL: Psychological Assessment Resources, Inc.

Hebben, N., and Milberg, W. (2002). *Essentials of neuropsychological assessment.* New York, NY: John Wiley and Sons.

Heyer, E., Sharma, R., and Winfree, C. (2000). Severe pain confounds neuropsychological test performance. *J Clin Exp Neuropsychol*, 22(5), 663–639.

Hiscock, M. (2007). The Flynn effect and its relevance to neuropsychology. *J Clin Exp Neuropsychol*, 29(5), 514–529.

Holtzer, R., Goldin, Y., Zimmerman, M., Katz, M., Buschke, H., and Lipton, R. (2008). Robust norms for selected neuropsychological tests in older adults. *Arch Clin Neuropsychol*, 23(5), 531–541.

Hoth, K., Popas, A., Moser, D., Paul, R. F., and Cohen, R. (2008). Cardiac dysfunction and cognition in older adults with heart failure. *Cognitive and Behavioral Neurology*, 21(2), 65–72.

Hubbard, E., Santini, V., Blankevoort, C., Volkers, K., Barrup, M., Byerly, L., et al. (2008). Clock drawing performance in cognitively normal elderly. *Arch Clin Neuropsychol*, 23(3), 295–327.

Incalzi, R., Marra, C., Girodano, A., Calcagni, M., Capa, A., Basso, S., et al. (2003). Cognitive impairment in chronic obstructive pulmonary disease – A neuropsychological and spect study. *Journal of Neurology*, 250(3), 325–332.

Ivnik, R., Malec, J., Tangalos, E., Petersen, R., Kokmen, R., and Kurland, L. (1990). The Auditory-Verbal Learning Test (AVLT): Norms for ages 55 years and older. *Psychological Assessment*, 2, 304–312.

Ivnik, R., Smith, G., Tangalos, E., Petersen, R., Kokmen, R., and Kurland, L. (1991). Wechsler Memory Scale (WMS): IQ dependent normas for persons age 65–97. *Psychological Assessment*, 3, 156–161.

Jackson, G., and Owsley, C. (2003). Visual dysfunction, neurodegenerative diseases, and aging. *Neurol Clin*, 21(3), 709–729.

Jefferson, A., Wong, S., Gracer, T., Ozonoff, A., Green, R., and Stern, R. (2007). Geriatric performance on an abbreviated version of the Boston Naming Test. *Appl Neuropsychol*, 14(3), 215–223.

Jorm, A., Masaki, K., Davis, D., Hardman, J., Nelson, J., Markesbery, W., et al. (2004). Memory complaints in nondemented men predict future pathologic diagnosis of Alzheimer disease. *Neurology*, 63(10), 1960–1961.

Jurica, P., Leitten, C., and Mattis, S. (2001). *Dementia Rating Scale-2 (DRS-2).* Lutz, FL: Psychological Assessment Resources Inc.

Kaplan, E., Goodglass, H., and Weintraub, S. (2000). *Boston Naming Test (2nd ed.).* Philadelphia: Lippincott, Williams & Wilkins.

Karp, J., Reynolds, C., Butters, M., Dew, M., Maxumdar, S., Begley, A., et al. (2006). The relationship between pain and mental flexibility in older adult pain clinic patients. *Pain Medicine*, 7, 444–452.

Keary, T., Gunstad, J., Poppas, A., Paul, R., Jefferson, A., Hoth, K., et al. (2007). Blood pressure variability predicts Dementia Rating Scale performance in older adults with cardiovascular disease. *Cognitive and Behavioral Neurology*, 20, 73–77.

Ketcham, C., and Stelmach, G. (2001). Age-related declines in motor control. In B. J.E. and K. W. Scaie (Eds.), *Handbook of the pychology of aging.* Fifth edition. (pp. 313–348). San Diego: Academic Press.

Kewman, D., Vaishampayan, N., Zald, D., and Han, B. (1991). Cognitive impairment in musculoskeletal pain patients. *Intl J Psychiatry Med*, (21), 3.

King, D., Cox, C., Lyness, J., Conwell, Y., and Caine, E. (1998). Quantitative and qualitative differences in verbal learning performance of elderly depressives and healthy controls. *JINS*, 4, 115–126.

Kioses, D., Klimstra, S., Murphy, C., and Alexopoulos, G. (2009). Executive dysfunction and disability in elderly patients with major depression. *Am J Geri Psychiatry*, 9(3), 269–274.

Kivipelto, J., Helkala, E., Hanninen, T., Laakso, M., Hallikainen, M., Alhainen, K., et al. (2001). Midlife vascular risk factors and late-life mild cognitive impairment: A population-based study. *Neurology*, 56(12), 1683–1689.

Kivipelto, M., Helkala, E., Hanninen, T., Laakso, M., Hallikainen, M., Alhzinen, K., et al. (2001). Midlife vascular risk factors and late-life mild cognitive impairment: A population based study. *Neurology*, 56, 1683–1689.

Kline, D., and Scialfa, C. (1996). Visual and auditory aging. In B. J.E. and K. W. Scaie (Eds.), *Handbook of the psychology of aging* (pp. 181–203). San Diego: Academic Press.

Knecht, S., Wersching, H., Lohmann, H., Bruchmann, M., Duning, T., Dziewas, R., et al. (2008). High-normal blood pressure is associated with poor cognitive performance. Hypertension, 51, 663–668.

Koenig, P., Smith, E., Troiani, V., Anderson, C., Moore, P., and Grossman, M. (2008). Medial temporal lobe involvement in an implicit memory task: evidence of collaborating implicit and explicit memory systems from FMRI and Alzheimer's disease. *Cereb Cortex*, 18(12), 2831–2843.

Kok, R., Heeren, T., Hooijer, C., Dinkgreve, M., and Rooijmans, H. (1995). The prevalence of depression in elderly medical inpatients. *Journal of Affective Disorders*, 33(2), 77–82.

Kuo, H., Jones, R., Milberg, W., Tennstedt, S., Talbot, L., Morris, J., et al. (2005). Effect of blood pressure and diabetes mellitus on cognitive and physical functions in older adults: A longitudinal analysis of the advanced cognitive training for independent and vital elderly cohort. *JAGS*, 53, 1154–1161.

Kuo, H., Sorond, F., Iloputaife, I., Gagnon, M., Milberg, W., and Lipsitz, L. (2004). Effect of blood pressure on cognitive functions in elderly persons. *Journals of Gerontology Series A – Biological Sciences and Medicine*, 59(11), 1191–1194.

La Rue, A., Romero, L., Ortiz, I., Liang, H., and RD., L. (1999). Neuropsychological performance of Hispanic and non-Hispanic older adults: An epidemiologic survey. *Clin Neuropsychol*, 13(4), 474–486.

Lavery, L., Dodge, H., Snitz, B., and Ganguli, M. (2009). Cognitive decline and mortality in a community-based cohort: The Monongahela Valley Independent Elders Survey. *JAGS*, 57, 94-100.

Lawton, M., and Brody, E. (1996). Assessment of older people: Self-maintaining and instrumental activities of daily living. *Gerontologist*, 9(3), 179–186.

Liesker, J., Postma, D. F., Beukema, R., ten Hacken, N., van der Molen, T., Riemersma, R., et al. (2004). Cognitive performance in patients with COPD. *Respiratory Medicine*, 98, 351–356.

Llwewllyn, D., Lang, I., Xie, J., Huppert, F., Melzer, D., and Langa, K. (2008). Framingham stroke risk profile and poor cognitive function: A population-based study. *BMC Neurology*, 8(12).

Loewenstein, D., Amigo, E., Duara, R., Guterman, A., Hurwitz, D., Berkowitz, N., et al. (1989). A new scale for the assessment of functional status in Alzheimer's disease and related disorders. *J Gerontol*, 44(4), 114–121.

Lucas, J., Ivnik, R., Smith, G., Ferman, T., Willis, F., Petersen, R., et al. (2005). Mayo's Older African Americans Normative Studies: Norms for Boston Naming Test, Controlled Oral Word Association, Category Fluency, Animal Naming, Token Test, Wrat-3 Reading, Trail Making Test, Stroop Test, and Judgment of Line Orientation. *Clin Neuropsychol*, 19(2), 243–269.

Machulda, M., Ivnik, R., Smith, G., Ferman, T., Boeve, B., Knopman, D., et al. (2007). Mayo's Older Americans Normative Studies: Visual form discrimination and copy trial of the Rey-Osterrieth Complex Figure. *J Clin Exp Neuropsych*, 29(4), 377–384.

Manly, J. (2006). Cultural issues. In Attix and Welsch-Bohmer (Eds.), *Geriatric neuropsychology* (pp. 198–222). New York: Guilford.

Manly, J., Jacobs, D., Touradji, P., Small, S., and Stern, Y. (2002). Reading level attenuates differences in neuropsychological test performance between African American and White elders. *J Int Neuropsychol Soc*, 8(3), 341–348.

Manly, J., Touradji, P., Tang, M., and Stern, Y. (2003). Literacy and memory decline among ethnically diverse elders. *J Clin Exp Neuropsychol*, 25(5), 680–690.

Marcopulos, B., and McLain, C. (2003). Are our norms "normal"? A 4-year follow-up study of a biracial sample of rural elders with low education. *Clin Neuropsychol*, 17(1), 19–33.

Martin, J., and Jerger, J. (2005). Some effects of aging on central auditory processing. *J Rehabil Res Dev*, 42(4 (suppl)), 25–44.

Matjucha, I., and Katz, B. (1994). Neuro-ophthalmology of aging. In M. L. Albert and J. E. Knoefel (Eds.), *Clinical neurology of aging* (2nd ed., Vol., pp. 427–447). Oxford: Oxford University Press.

Maust, D., Onyike, C., Sheppard, J., Mayer, L., Samus, Q., Brandt, J., et al. (2006). Predictors of caregiver unawareness and nontreatment of dementia among residents of assisted living facilities: The Maryland Assisted Living Study. *Am J Geriatr Psychiatry*, 14(8), 668–675.

Mendola, J., Cronin-Golomb, A., Corkin, S., and Growdon, J. (1995). Prevalence of visual deficits in Alzheimer's disease. *Optom Vis Sci*, 72(3), 155–167.

Metternich, B., Schmidtke, K., and Hüll, M. (2009). How are memory complaints in functional memory disorder related to measures of affect, metamemory and cognition? *J Psychosom Res*, 66(5), 435–444.

Meyers, and Meyers, K. (1996). *The Rey Complex Figure Memory and Recognition Trial Manual.* Lutz, FL: Psychological Assessment Resources, Inc.

Mobily, P., Herr, K., Clark, M., and Wallace, R. (1994). An epidemiologic analysis of pain in the elderly: The Iowa 65+ Rural Health Study. *J Aging Health*, 6, 139–154.

Moorhouse, P., and Rockwood, K. (2008). Vascular cognitive impairment: Current concepts and clinical developments. *Lancet Neurol*, 7, 246–255.

Nazem, S., Siderowf, A., Duda, J., Brown, G., Ten Have, T., Stern, M., et al. (2008). Suicidal and death ideation in Parkinson's disease. *Movement Disorders*, 23(11), 1573–1579.

Newman, S., Sheldon, C., and Bland, R. (1998). Prevalence of depression in an elderly community sample: A comparison of GMS-AGECAT and DSM-IV diagnostic criteria. *Psychological Medicine*, 28, 1339–1345.

O'Connor, D., Pollitt, P., Roth, M., Brook, C., and Reiss, B. (1990). Problems reported by relatives in a community study of dementia. *Br J Psychiatry*, 156, 835–841.

O'Brien, J., Erkinjuntti, T., and Reisberg, B. (2003). Vascular cognitive impairment. *Lancet Neurol*, 2, 89–98.

Oosterman, J., deVries, K., and Scherder, E. (2007). Executive ability in relation to blood pressure in residents of homes for the elderly. *Archives of Clinical Neuropsychology*, 22, 731–738.

Paran, E., Anson, O., and Reuveni, H. (2003). Blood pressure and cognitive functioning among independent elderly. *American Journal of Hypertension*, 16, 818–826.

Plassman, B., Langa, K., Fisher, G., Heeringa, S., Weir, D., Ofstedal, M., et al. (2007). Prevalence of dementia in the United States: The aging, demographics, and memory study. *Neuroepidemiology*, 29(1-2), 125–132.

Pugh, K., Kiely, D., Milberg, W., and Lipsitz, L. (2003). Selective impairment of frontal-executive cognitive function in African Americans with cardiovascular risk factors. *JAGS*, 51, 1439–1444.

Qui, C., Winblad, B., and Fratiglioni, L. (2005). The age-dependent relation of blood pressure to cognitive function and dementia. *Lancet Neurol*, 4(8), 487–499.

Randolph, C., Tierney, M., Mohr, E., and Chase, T. (1998). The Repeatable Battery for the Assessment of Neuropsychological Status (RBANS): Preliminary clinical validity. *J Clin Exp Neuropsychol*, 20(3), 310–319.

Raz, N., Rodrigue, K., and Acker, J. (2003). Hypertension and the brain: Vulnerability of the prefrontal regions and executive functions. *Behavioral Neuroscience*, 117(6), 1169–1180.

Raz, N., Rodrigue, K., Kennedy, K., Dahle, C., Head, D., and Acker, J. (2003). Differential age-related changes in the regional metencephalic volumes in humans: A 5-year follow-up. *Neurosci Lett*, 349(3), 163–166.

Razani, J., Kakos, B., Orieta-Barbalace, C., Wong, J., Casas, R., Lu, P., et al. (2007). Predicting caregiver burden from daily functional abilities of patients with mild dementia. *J Am Geriatr Soc*, 55(9), 1415–1420.

Rentz, D., Huh, T., Sardinha, L., Moran, E., Becker, J., Daffner, K., et al. (2007). Intelligence quotient-adjusted memory impairment is associated with abnormal single photon emission computed tomography perfusion. *J Int Neuropsychol Soc*, 13(5), 821–831.

Rentz, D., Sardinha, L., Huh, T., Searl, M., Daffner, K., and Sperling, R. (2006). IQ-based norms for highly intelligent adults. *Clin Neuropsychol*, 20(4), 637–648.

Ries, P. (1994). Prevalence and characteristics of persons with hearing trouble: United States, 1990-91. *Vital Health Stat 10*, 10(188), 1–75.

Ritchie, L., and Tuokko, H. (2007). Neuropsychological prediction of attrition due to death. *J Clin Exp Neuropsychol*, 29(4), 385–394.

Ryskulova, A., Turczyn, K., Makuc, D., Cotch, M., Klein, R., and Janiszewski, R. (2008). Self-reported age-related eye diseases and visual impairment in the United States: Results of the 2002 National Health Interview Survey. *Am J Public Health*, 93(3), 454–461.

Saaddine, J., Honeycutt, A., Narayan, K., Zhang, X., Klein, R., and Boyle, J. (2008). Projection of diabetic retinopathy and other major eye diseases among people with diabetes mellitus: United States, 2005–2050. *Arch Ophthalmol*, 126(12), 1740–1777.

Saykin, A., Wishart, H., Rabin, L., Santulli, R., Flashman, L., West, J., et al. (2006). Older adults with cognitive complaints show brain atrophy similar to that of amnestic MCI. *Neurology*, 12(67), 834–842.

Schillerstrom, J., Horton, M., and Royall, D. (2005). The impact of medical illness of executive function. *Psychosomatics*, 46(6), 508–516.

Schmidt, M. (1996). *Rey Auditory and Verbal Learning Test. A handbook.* Los Angeles: Western Psychological Services.

Shulman, K. (2000). Clock-drawing: Is it the ideal cognitive screening test? *International Journal of Geriatric Psychiatry*, 15(6), 548–561.

Sims, R., Madhere, S., Gordon, S., Clark, E., Abayomi, K., Callender, C., et al. (2008). Relationships among blood pressure, triglycerides and verbal learning in African Americans. *Journal of the National Medical Association*, 100(10), 1193–1198.

Skoog, I., Lernfelt, B., Landahl, S., Plamertz, B., Andreasson, L., Nilsson, L., et al. (1996). A 15-year longitudinal study of blood pressure and dementia. *Lancet*, 374, 1141–1145.

Slinin, Y., Paudel, M., Ishani, A., Taylor, B., Yaffe, K., Murray, A., et al. (2008). Kidney function and cognitive performance and decline in older men. *JAGS*, 56(11), 2082–2088.

Sliwinski, M., Lipton, R., Buschke, H., and Stewart, W. (1996). The effects of preclinical dementia on estimates of normal cognitive functioning in aging. *J Gerontol B Psychol Sci Soc Sci*, 51(4), 217–225.

Stanek, K., Gunstad, J., Paul, R., Poppas, A., Jefferson, A., Sweet, H., et al. (2009). Longitudinal cognitive performance in older adults with cardiovascular disease evidence for improvement in hear failure. *J of Cardiovascular Nursing*, 24(3), 192–197.

Stanek, K., Gunstad, J., Paul, R., Poppas, A., Jefferson, A., Sweet, L., et al. (2009). Longitudinal cognitive performance in older adults with cardiovascular disease: evidence for improvement in heart failure. *J Cardiovasc Nurs*, 24(3), 192–197.

Steffens, D., Welsh-Bohmer, K., Burke, J., Plassman, B., Beyer, J., Gersing, K., et al. (2004). Methodology and preliminary results from the Neurocognitive Outcomes of Depression in the Elderly Study. *J Geriatric Psychiat and Neurol*, 17, 202–211.

Steinberg, B., Bieliauskas, L., Smith, G., Langellotti, C., and Ivnik, R. (2005). Mayo's Older Americans Normative Studies: Age- and IQ-Adjusted Norms for the Boston Naming Test, the MAE Token Test, and the Judgment of Line Orientation Test. *Clin Neuropsychol*, 19(3–4), 280–328.

Stella, F., Banzato, C., Quagliato, E., and Viana, M. (2008). Depression in patients with Parkinson's disease: Impact on functioning. 272, 1–2(158–163).

Stuss, D., Peterkin, I., Guzman, D., Guzman, C., and Troyer, A. (1997). Chronic obstructive pulmonary disease: Effects of hypoxia on neurological and neuropsychological measures. *J Clin Exp Neuropsychology*, 19(4), 515–524.

Tabert, M., Manly, J., Liu, X., Pelton, G., Rosenblum, S., Jacobs, M., et al. (2006). Neuropsychological prediction of conversion to Alzheimer disease in patients with mild cognitive impairment. *Arch Gen Psychiatry*, 63(8), 916–924.

Thornton, W., Shapiro, R., Deria, S., Gelb, S., and Hill, A. (2007). Differential impact of age on verbal memory and executive functioning in chronic kidney disease. *JINS*, 13, 334–353.

Trojano, L., Incalzi, R., Acanfora, D., Picone, C., Mecocci, P., Rengo, F., et al. (2003). Cognitive impairment: A key feature of congestive heart failure in the elderly. *J Neurol*, 250, 1456–1463.

Tröster, A. (2008). Neuropsychological characteristics of dementia with Lewy bodies and Parkinson's disease with dementia: Differentiation, early detection, and implications for "mild cognitive impairment" and biomarkers. *Neuropsychol Rev*, 18(1), 103–119.

U.S. Census Bureau. (2006). Current Population Survey.

Valentijn, S., van Boxtel, M., van Hooren, S., Bosma, H., Beckers, H., Ponds, R., et al. (2005). Change in sensory functioning predicts change in cognitive functioning: Results from a 6-year follow-up in the Maastricht aging study. *Am Geriatr Soc*, 53(3), 374–380.

van Boxtel, M., van Beijsterveldt, C., Houx, P., Anteunis, L., Metsemakers, J., and Jolles, J. (2000). Mild hearing impairment can reduce verbal memory performance in a healthy adult population. *J Clin Exp Neuropsychol*, 22(1), 147–154.

van Halteren-van Tilborg, I., Scherder, E., and Hulstijn, W. (2007). Motor-skill learning in Alzheimer's disease: A review with an eye to the clinical practice. *Neuropsychol Rev*, 17(3), 203–212.

van Hooren, S., Anteunis, L., Valentijn, S., Bosma, H., Ponds, R., Jolles, J., et al. (2005). Does cognitive function in older adults with hearing impairment improve by hearing aid use? *Int J Audiol*, 44(5), 265–271.

van Vliet, P., van de Water, W., de Craen, A., and Westendorp, R. (2009). The influence of age on the association between cholestoral and cognitive function. *Experimental Gerontology*, 44, 112–122.

Verfelho, A., Madureira, S., Ferro, J., Basile, A., Chabriat, H., Erkinjuntti, T., et al. (2009). Differential impact of cerebral white matter changes, diabetes, hypertension and stroke on cognitive performance among non-disabled elderly. The LADIS study. *J Neurol Neurosurg Psychiatry*, 78, 1325–1330.

Vogels, R., Oosterman, J., van Harten, B., Scheltens, P., van der Flier, W., Schroeder-Tanka, J., et al. (2007). Profile of cognitive impairment in chronic heart failure. *JAGS*, 55, 1764–1770.

Waldstein, S., Giggey, P., Thayer, J., and Zonderman, A. (2005). Nonlinear relations of blood pressure to cognitive function. The Baltimore Longitudinal Study of Aging. *Hypertension*, 45, 374–379.

Walhovd, K., Fjell, A., Reinvang, I., Lundervold, A., Dale, A., Eilertsen, D., et al. (2005). Effects of age on volumes of cortex, white matter and subcortical structures. *Neurobiol Aging*, 26(9), 1261–1270.

Weiner, D., Rudy, T., Morrow, L., Slaboda, J., and Lieber, S. (2006). The relationship between pain, neuropsychological performance, and physical function in community-dwelling older adults with chronic low back pain. *Pain Med*, 7(1), 60–70.

Welsh-Bohmer, K., and Warren, L. (2006). Neurodegenerative dementias. In Attix and Welsch-Bohmer (Eds.), *Geriatric neuropsychology* (pp. 89–102). New York: Guilford.

Witt, K., Daniels, C., Reiff, J., Krack, P., Volkmann, J., Pinsker, M., et al. (2008). Neuropsychological and psychiatric changes after deep brain stimulation for Parkinson's disease: A randomised, multicentre study. 7, 7(605–614).

Yesavage, J., Brink, T., Rose, T., Lum, O., Huang, V., Adey, M., et al. (1983). Development and validation of a geriatric depression screening scale—A preliminary report. *Journal of Psychiatric Research*, 17(1), 37–49.

Zanetti, O., Geroldi, C., Frisoni, G., Bianchetti, A., and Trabucchi, M. (1999). Contrasting results between caregiver's report and direct assessment of activities of daily living in patients affected by mild and very mild dementia: The contribution of the caregiver's personal characteristics. *Journal of the American Geriatrics Society*, 47(2), 196–202.

Ziegler, D., Piguet, O., Salat, D., Prince, K., Connally, E., and Corkin, S. (in press). Cognition in healthy aging is related to regional white matter integrity, but not cortical thickness. *Neurobiol Aging*.

Zimprich, D., Martin, M., and Kliegel, M. (2003). Subjective cognitive complaints, memory performance, and depressive affect in old age: A change-oriented approach. *Intl J Aging and Human Development*, 57(4), 339–366.

8 Anatomical Neuroimaging in Aging

Joseph C. Masdeu

In aging, anatomical or structural imaging helps in the diagnosis of a variety of nervous system syndromes that may also affect younger people and therefore are not characteristic of aging. However, there are two conditions that are characteristic of the older population and that require the use of anatomical imaging: dementia and gait disorders. In this chapter, imaging in both conditions will be reviewed in detail, after a brief introduction to anatomical neuroimaging in older people.

Anatomical neuroimaging is performed with computed tomography (CT) and magnetic resonance imaging (MRI). The physical principles of these two modalities are outside of the scope of this chapter. However, something should be said about their application to the study of older patients. CT uses ionizing radiation, which can cause tissue injury by interfering with DNA repair mechanisms (Sanders 2000). In the older person the concern is with the addition of radiation doses by the combination of radiological procedures that use X-rays. MRI does not present this problem. But it is not devoid of side effects that may be more common in aging. For instance, the occasional complaint of dizziness or frank vertigo while in the scanner could be due to the deposition of iron in structures of the vestibular system in the inner ear, which could be more frequent in older people. Vestibular effects are more pronounced with higher field magnets (Patel 2008).

The methodology of structural imaging in aging is currently undergoing a major transformation. Traditional visual evaluation of images by experts to rule-out obvious pathology is being increasingly complemented by quantitative image-analysis methods (Colliot 2008; Duchesne 2008; Kloppel 2008; Brewer 2009). These methods are based on the determination of the subtle but reliably present regional atrophy characteristic of many neurodegenerative disorders. For instance, atrophy of medial temporal structures occurs at the onset of Alzheimer's disease. In contrast, the frontal pole is more affected in some varieties of fronto-temporal dementia. Sophisticated imaging methods are able to measure reliably the volume or thickness of the cortex on a T1-weighted MRI, better than the human eye is able to do. Machine learning techniques have shown in some studies greater accuracy than trained physicians in classifying the MRIs of patients with autopsy-proven Alzheimer's disease as compared to normal controls or patients with fronto-temporal dementia (Kloppel 2008). Some software packages to perform quantitative cortical measurements in commercial MRI units have already been approved by the United States Federal Drug Administration (FDA) (Brewer 2009).

Imaging in Dementia

A practice guideline on the management of dementia states: *Neuroimaging is now the most important ancillary investigation in the work-up of dementia to aid in differential diagnosis and management decisions* (Waldemar 2007). Currently around 24 million people in the world have dementia, with the number being projected to double every 20 years (Qiu 2007). Moreover, therapeutic intervention is likely to be most effective in the preclinical stages of the dementing process, or at least in the early stages of cognitive impairment, when the halting of progressive neuronal loss seems most feasible. At these early stages of the process, neuroimaging provides key information to determine whether the patient has a degenerative dementing disease and which type, particularly when neuroimaging is combined with genetics (Masdeu 2005).

Non-degenerative Dementias

Potentially reversible neurological or psychiatric conditions leading to cognitive impairment may be diagnosed with the help of neuroimaging (Figure 1). For this reason, the 1994 American Academy of Neurology (AAN) guideline on the management of dementia, which did not require the use of imaging to diagnose a degenerative dementia in a patient with progressive memory loss and no motor or sensory findings or epilepsy, was changed to require structural imaging (CT or MRI) in the 2001 guideline (Knopman 2001). A clinical picture of progressive memory loss or psychomotor slowing may be caused by *tumors or subdural hematomas* (Figures 2 and 3) (Chui 1997). Unless a tumor infiltrates the cortex, for instance in the case of very rare lymphomas or metastases from malignant melanoma, a CT without contrast is enough to rule out potentially reversible structural brain lesions (Knopman 2001). The European guidelines for the work up of dementia suggest that, if possible, an MRI be performed to increase specificity, given that MRI provides additional information on vascular causes of dementia and to distinguish the various degenerative dementias (Waldemar 2007).

The role of *vascular disease* as a cause of dementia continues to need further definition. Small vessel infarction, of the subcortical type, seems more likely to contribute to dementia than large cortical infarctions (Esiri 1997). The effect of vascular and degenerative changes is cumulative (Chui 2006; Schneider 2007). When vascular disease is the primary cause of dementia, multiple infarctions are generally present on CT or MRI (Figure 4), particularly involving the thalamic nuclei bilaterally (Liem 2007; Viswanathan 2007). By contrast, the extent of white matter involvement on T2-weighted images does not correlate with cognitive impairment in many studies (Liem 2007; Viswanathan 2007) but does in some (Grau-Olivares 2007). Medial temporal atrophy, a feature of Alzheimer's disease (AD), also correlates with cognitive impairment in vascular dementia (Chui 2006; O'Sullivan 2007). Cognitive impairment is a prominent feature of cerebral amyloid angiopathy (CAA), which presents with white matter hyperintensity on T2 MRI and cortical microhemorrhages, best seen on gradient echo MRI sequences (Figure 5). In rare cases, CAA can be worsened by regional inflammation, susceptible to immunosuppresive treatment (Figure 6) (Eng 2004). Involvement of the white matter of the frontal

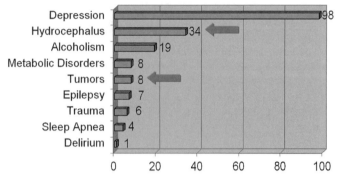

Figure 1 Potentially reversible primary etiologies for cognitive symptoms in 1000 patients referred to a memory disorders clinic (Hejl, 2002). A potentially reversible primary etiology for cognitive symptoms was identified in 19% and a potentially reversible concomitant condition in 23% of all patients. As this was a referral sample, it may not represent the proportion of these disorders among the population with dementia at large. Note that vascular dementia is not included here. Arrows indicate the main etiologies ruled out by structural brain imaging.

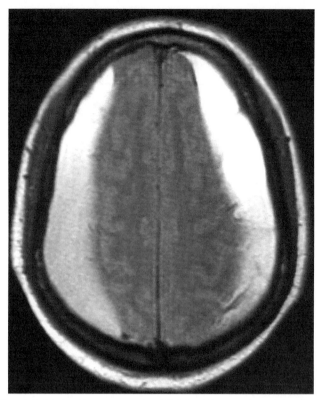

Figure 3 Subdural hematomas. Axial FLAIR MRI image showing bilateral convexity subdural hematomas in an 82-year-old man with gait freezing and an attentional disorder.

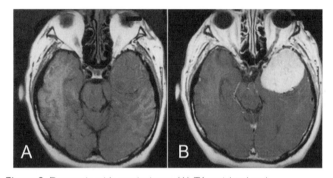

Figure 2 Dementia with meningioma. (A) T1-weighted and (B) gadolinium-enhanced T1-weighted MRI of the brain of a 65-year-old woman, showing a large contrast-enhancing mass lesion in the right temporal lobe that compresses the left hippocampus and displaces the midbrain. Modified from Chui H and Zhang Q (Chui, 1997), with permission.

and temporal poles on MRI may help differentiate cerebral autosomal-dominant arteriopathy with subcortical infarcts and leukoencephalopathy (CADASIL) from sporadic subcortical arteriosclerotic encephalopathy (Figure 7) (Auer, 2001).

Prion diseases may present as a rather rapidly progressive dementing process, often accompanied by clinical manifestations of basal ganglia or cerebellar involvement (Knopman 2001). Imaging is very helpful and tends to be abnormal before the onset of any characteristic EEG pattern. Bilateral caudate or thalamic areas of high signal intensity on diffusion-weighted or FLAIR MR imaging are characteristic (Figure 8). The cortical ribbon is often affected, particularly in the paramedial regions of the frontal lobes (Kallenberg 2006).

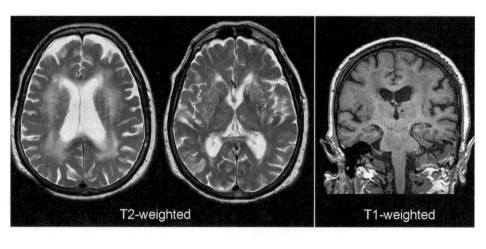

Figure 4 Vascular dementia. Shown are axial T2-weighted and coronal T1-weighted images from an 80-year-old woman with impairment of cognition and gait. Note the thalamic infarctions and the large areas of altered signal (increased on T2 and decreased on T1) in the centrum semiovale. The thalamic lacunes are bright on T2 and dark on T1-weighted images.

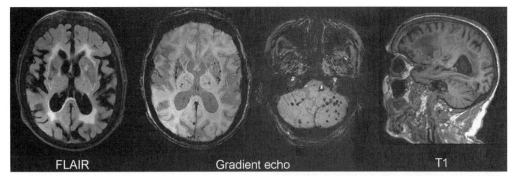

Figure 5 Cerebral amyloid angiopathy (CAA). Shown are MR images from a 72-year-old woman with dementia and CAA. The white matter contains many abnormal areas, which appear hyperintense on the transverse FLAIR image and hypointense on the sagittal T1-weighted image. Multiple lacunar infarcts are present in the lenticular nuclei and few in the thalami. Microbleeds, best seen on the gradient echo images, dot the lenticular nuclei, thalami and the cerebellum. Scattered microbleeds can also be seen in the cortex or subcortical white matter.

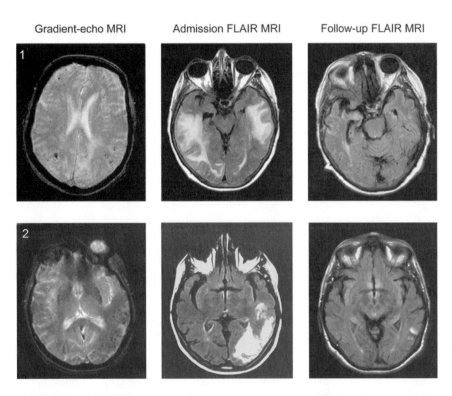

Figure 6 Amyloid-angiopathy-related inflammation. Magnetic resonance imaging (MRI) appearance in patients with cerebral amyloid angiopathy (CAA)-related inflammation, managed with immunosuppressive treatment. The gradient-echo images from Patients 1 and 2 show multiple small hypointense lesions characteristic of CAA-related microhemorrhages. The fluid-attenuated inversion recovery (FLAIR) images performed at presentation and after follow-up intervals of 2 months (Patient 1) or 22 months (Patient 2) demonstrate confluent regions of white matter hyperintensity that largely resolve at follow-up. Modified from (Eng, 2004) with permission.

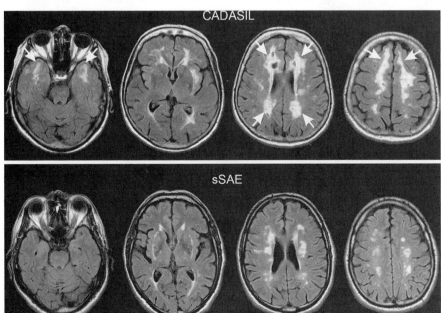

Figure 7 CADASIL. Images obtained in representative patients with biopsy-proved cerebral autosomal-dominant arteriopathy with subcortical infarcts and leukoencephalopathy (CADASIL, top row) and sporadic subcortical arteriosclerotic encephalopathy (sSAE, bottom row) display the differentially involved temporopolar and superior frontal white matter. Note the marked symmetry of lesions and the extension of lesions into the superficial white matter in CADASIL (arrows). Modified from Auer (Auer, 2001) with permission.

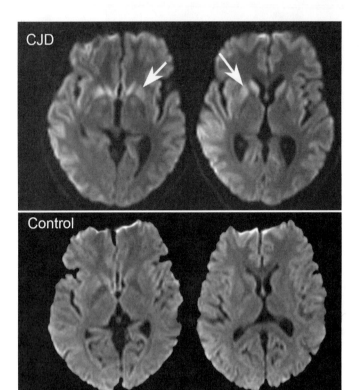

Figure 8 Creutzfeldt-Jakob disease. Images shown (FLAIR MRI) are from a 39-year-old woman who developed chorea, followed by anxiety and progressive cognitive and motor impairment, leading to inability to walk and marked dysarthria and dementia by the time this imaging study was obtained, five months after symptom onset. Note the high intensity of the caudate and of the anterior portion of the lenticular nuclei (arrows). For comparison purposes, the lower image row was obtained with a similar technique, but from a control individual.

Most cognitive impairment from *depression or mania* can be readily diagnosed from the clinical findings and response to therapy. However, in some older patients, making these diagnoses may not be straightforward. In a patient with impairment in various areas of cognition, likely to be attributable to an attentional deficit, and who has a structural imaging study that appears to be normal, a quantitative MRI may help to reduce the probability of diagnosing a neurodegenerative disorder (Colliot 2008; Kloppel 2008; Brewer 2009). Even a semiquantitative visual estimation of medial temporal atrophy, using atrophy templates,

can be useful (Scheltens 2002; Urs 2009). The absence of medial temporal atrophy will lessen the probability of the patient being at a preclinical stage of AD and therefore will encourage a more aggressive approach to the treatment of a potential psychiatric disorder. It must be remembered, however, that at this point the sensitivity and specificity of quantitative imaging ranges between 80–88% (Colliot 2008; Kloppel 2008; Brewer 2009) and therefore is only a helpful ancillary method. As discussed in Chapter 10 on functional neuroimaging, positron emission tomography with fluorodeoxyglucose, and, particularly, with [11]C Pittsburgh Compound B (PiB) can be very helpful to improve the probability of the diagnoses of AD or dementia with Lewy bodies.

Degenerative Dementias

In this section I will review the most characteristic imaging findings in the most frequent types of neurodegenerative dementia. Many of the disorders that we now consider unitary diseases, such as Alzheimer's, may turn out to be caused by a variety of genetic and environmental conditions. As an example, the genetic heterogeneity of the frontotemporal dementias has become apparent in the past few years (Baker 2006). Thus, the classification I follow is mostly syndromic, based on the clinical presentation and some associated imaging or neuropathological changes.

Alzheimer's disease (AD). Most cases of AD start with mesial temporal atrophy, which can be appreciated by a dilation of the temporal horn of the lateral ventricle on CT (Masdeu 1985) or by atrophy of the entorhinal and hippocampal cortex on MRI (Figure 9) (Masdeu 2005). The same is true of MCI leading to AD (Whitwell 2007). Scheltens (2002) has developed a visual rating scale to gauge medial temporal atrophy (Scheltens 2002) (Table 1). The sensitivity and specificity of this scale for the detection of mild to moderate Alzheimer's disease compared with controls has been estimated as 85% and 88%, respectively. In practical terms, if before temporal atrophy is taken into account, the probability of Alzheimer's disease were of 60% (in line with the sensitivity values for the NINCDS-ADRDA criteria; McKhann 1984), the presence of temporal atrophy raises the probability to 91% and its absence lowers the probability to 20%. As the disease progresses, atrophy extends from the limbic cortex to the neocortex, particularly in regions posterior to the rolandic sulcus. Medial temporal atrophy is not specific for AD and happens in frontotemporal dementia (FTD) and vascular dementia as well (Likeman 2005). Greater bilateral symmetry and predominantly posterior atrophy tend to suggest AD over FTD (Likeman 2005). In some patients, early atrophy of areas in the parietal, occipital, or posterior temporal

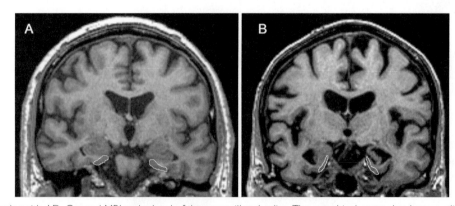

Figure 9 Temporal atrophy with AD. Coronal MRI at the level of the mammillary bodies. The entorhinal cortex has been outlined in a normal control (A) and a person with mild cognitive impairment of the amnesic type (B).

Table 1 Scheltens' Scale for the Visual Assessment of Medial-Temporal-Lobe Atrophy

Score	Width of Choroid Fissure	Width of Temporal Horn	Height of Hippocampus
0	Normal	Normal	Normal
1	↑	Normal	Normal
2	↑↑	↑	↓↓
3	↑↑↑	↑↑	↓↓
4	↑↑↑	↑↑↑	↓↓↓

↑ = increased, ↓ = decreased.
Reproduced from (Scheltens, 2002) with permission.

lobe can be prominent, giving rise to presentations such as Balint's syndrome (Figure 10). In such cases, regional atrophy may be determined by automated methods, such as *voxel-based morphometry*, now available in some clinical units (Good 2002; Karas 2003). By facilitating the comparison of two or more studies, automated methods greatly simplify the determination of the annual rate of volume change in temporal cortex, which distinguishes AD from controls with greater sensitivity and specificity than one-time measurements (Du 2003). Whereas the annual volume loss in normal aging is less than 1%, annual rates as high as 4% occur in early AD (Thompson 2003).

Lewy-body Dementia (LBD). There are very few neuropathologically-confirmed imaging studies of LBD. More occipital atrophy in LBD than in AD has been reported by a group with a good diagnostic record (Beyer 2007). In agreement is the finding of decreased metabolism in occipital association cortex (Okamura 2001).

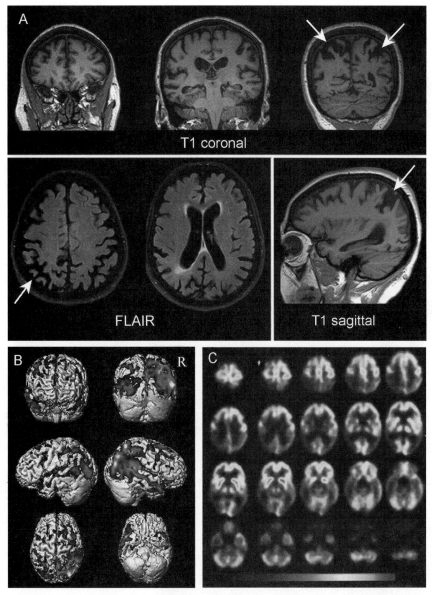

Figure 10 Balint's syndrome with AD. Shown are the MRI and PET studies from a 61-year-old woman with a 3-year history of progressive reading difficulties, agraphia, and dressing apraxia. On examination, she had Balint's syndrome, with simultanagnosia, apraxia of eye movements, optic ataxia and "tunnel vision." Note the marked atrophy in the lateral parietal lobe with dilation of the intraparietal sulcus (arrows). There is also less prominent hippocampal atrophy. See Figure 8.10 on the color insert.

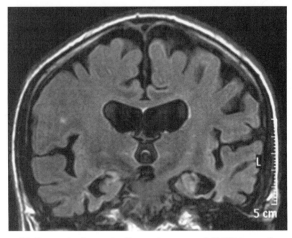

Figure 11 Semantic dementia. Shown is a coronal FLAIR image from a 72-year-old man with a progressive anomic aphasia. Although the patient's spontaneous language was almost normal, he could not name by confrontation objects as common as a table. Note the marked atrophy in the anterior portion of the temporal lobes, more pronounced on the left.

Frontotemporal Dementias (FTD), *Corticobasal Degeneration* (CBD). Clinically, neuropathologically, and genetically, FTD comprises a heterogeneous group of disorders (Josephs 2006). It can present with a *frontal-lobe syndrome*, characterized by impulsivity and disinhibition (Liscic 2007), or as a *progressive aphasia*, either semantic (Figure 11) or non-fluent (Figure 12). Atrophy on MRI or decreased metabolism on FDG-PET tends to be regional and corresponds well to the area preferentially affected by the pathology. Except for rare cases with motor neuron involvement, these disorders tend to affect association cortex, rather than primary motor or sensory cortices. Clinical, imaging, and neuropathological findings are summarized in Table 2. The most common clinical variety, frontotemporal dementia, is also the most neuropathologically and genetically heterogeneous (Josephs 2006; Liscic 2007), as is the more recently characterized hippocampal sclerosis dementia (Probst 2007). Fronto-temporal abnormalities on FDG-PET / SPECT may antedate the atrophy that eventually becomes obvious on MRI (Figure 13) (Foster 2007; Mendez 2007).

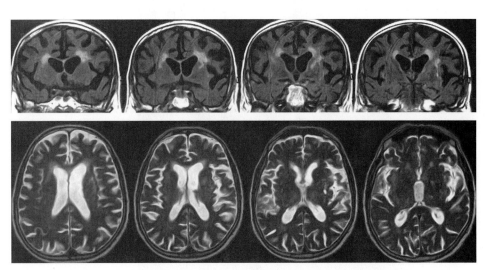

Figure 12.a Primary progressive aphasia. MRI from an 80-year-old right-handed man who had a progressive non-fluent aphasia with a stuttering course. Coronal FLAIR (top row) and axial T2-weighted (bottom row) MRI images showing mild to moderate leukoaraiosis of the frontal periventricular white matter and lacunar infarctions in the left putamen, globus pallidus, pulvinar, and internal and extreme capsules. The MRI findings could be interpreted as showing evidence of vascular disease.

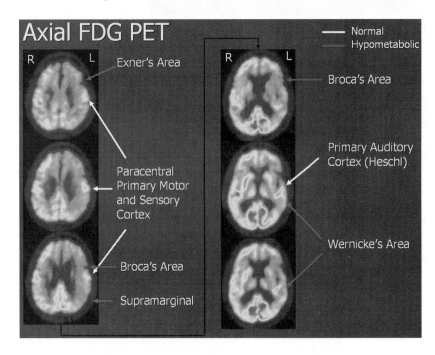

Figure 12.b Axial FDG PET showing hypometabolism in the perisylvian association cortex of the frontal, parietal, and temporal lobes of the left hemisphere. The primary auditory and motor-sensory cortices are spared. The findings on PET are highly characteristic of a degenerative disorder. See Figure 8.12b on the color insert.

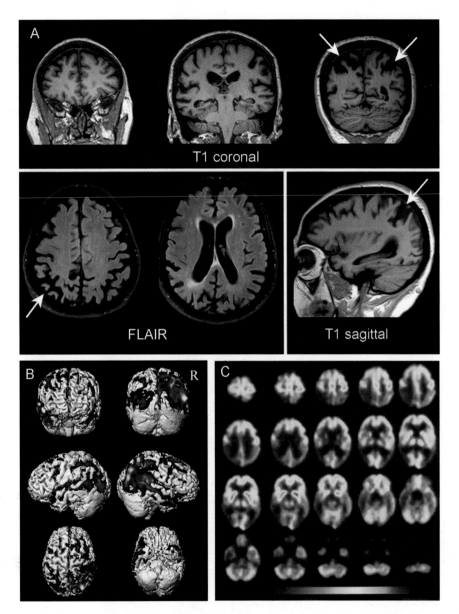

Figure 8.10 Balint's syndrome with AD. Shown are the MRI and PET studies from a 61-year-old woman with a 3-year history of progressive reading difficulties, agraphia, and dressing apraxia. On examination, she had Balint's syndrome, with simultanagnosia, apraxia of eye movements, optic ataxia and "tunnel vision." Note the marked atrophy in the lateral parietal lobe with dilation of the intraparietal sulcus (arrows). There is also less prominent hippocampal atrophy.

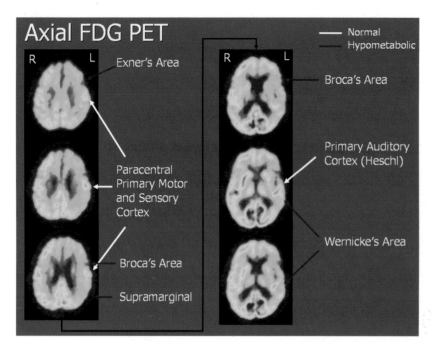

Figure 8.12b Axial FDG PET showing hypometabolism in the perisylvian association cortex of the frontal, parietal, and temporal lobes of the left hemisphere. The primary auditory and motor-sensory cortices are spared. The findings on PET are highly characteristic of a degenerative disorder.

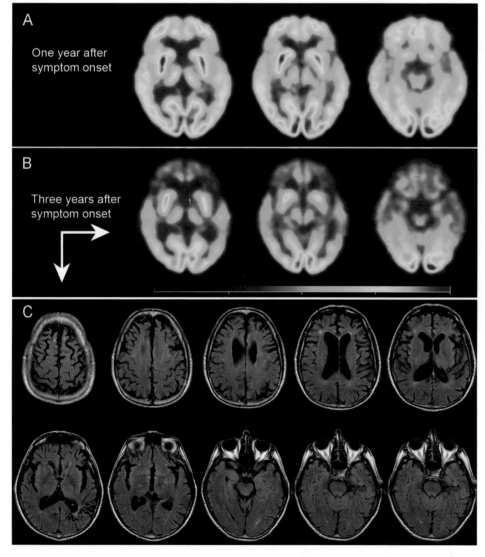

Figure 8.13 Frontotemporal dementia. Shown are FDG-PET (A, B) and FLAIR MRI (C) studies from a 51-year-old man with progressive speech apraxia and impaired planning, to the point of mutism and complete dependency for activities of daily living when studies B and C were obtained, on the same day. Metabolism was already decreased on the initial PET study, particularly on the frontal opercula and temporal tips, but it is much more obvious on the follow up study, showing extensive fronto-temporal hypometabolism. Note that the fronto-temporal abnormality is much more obvious on the PET study (A, B) than on the MRI study (C), which shows frontal atrophy.

Table 2 Non-Alzheimer Neurodegenerative Dementias

Dementia Type	Clinical Findings	Atrophy (MRI)	Motor Neuron Disease	Ubiquitinated Bodies (TDP-43)	Tau	Known Genetics
Behavioral variant frontotemporal dementia (bvFTD)	Behavioral and personality changes & executive dysfunction	Bilateral frontotemporal	20%	50%	50%	Progranulin (PGRN) and microtubule associated protein tau (MAPT)
Frontotemporal dementia with motor neuron disease (FTD-MND)	Similar to bvFTD	Frontal > temporal lobe atrophy	100%	100%	0%	Possible Chromosome 9
Semantic dementia (SD)	Anomic aphasia, loss of comprehension, surface dyslexia	Bilateral (L>R) anterior temporal, atrophy	<5%	80%	20%	None determined
Progressive non-fluent aphasia (PNFA)	Non-fluent speech with agrammatism	Left perisylvian association cortex atrophy	<5%	20%	80%	PGRN & MAPT
Corticobasal syndrome (CBS)	Apraxia, rigidity	Asymmetric frontoparietal, lenticular & thalamic atrophy	<5%	5%	95%	MAPT H1 haplotype and PGRN (4 families)
Progressive supranuclear palsy syndrome (PSPS)	Vertical supranuclear palsy, apathy, symmetric parkinsonism	Midbrain atrophy. Mild frontal lobe atrophy	<1%	1%	99%	MAPT H1 haplotype

(Baker, 2006; Josephs, 2006; Neumann, 2006; Liscic, 2007). Courtesy of Dr. Keith Josephs

Imaging in Gait Disorders of Aging

Imaging plays an important role in the work-up of the characteristic gait disordes of aging. The clinical appearance of this disorder was masterfully described by Critchley in 1948 (Critchley 1948):

> There exists a large group of cases where the gait in old people becomes considerably disordered, although the motor power of the legs is comparatively well preserved. A paradoxical state of affairs is the result: testing of the individual movements of the legs while the patient reclines upon the couch shows little, if any, reduction in the strength. The tonus may not be grossly altered and the reflexes may betray only minor deviations. Sensory tests show no unusual features. But when the patient is instructed to get out of bed and to walk, remarkable defects may be witnessed. The patient, first of all, appears most reluctant to make the attempt. His stance is bowed and uncertain. He props himself against the end of the bed and seeks the aid of the bystanders. Encouraged to take a few steps, he advances warily and hesitatingly. Clutching the arms of two supporters, he takes short, shuffling steps. The legs tend to crumble by giving way suddenly at the knee joints. Progression, as far as it is possible, is slow and tottery. The patient veers to one side or the other. Frequently the legs cross, so that one foot gets in the way of the other.

The clinical picture described by Critchley is one of an advanced gait disorder. Earlier stages present only with impaired balance and a propensity to tripping and falling. At this point, the patients or, more often, their families, may consult a physician. The responsible lesion could be at a number of places in the neuraxis. Often, several lesions combine to produce the gait disorder (Rubenstein 1997). Most frequent lesions detectable by anatomical neuroimaging are cervical myelopathy from spondylosis, vascular brain disease, and hydrocephalus. They will be reviewed in succession.

Cervical Myelopathy from Cervical Spondylosis

Cervical myelopathy from cervical spondylosis has been reported as the second most-common cause of gait impairment in the older adult (Fuh 1994; Sudarsky 1997). Because it is potentially treatable, cervical myelopathy should be considered in any older adult presenting with gait impairment (Holly 2008). Some patients present with the characteristic clinical picture of cervical radicular pain and spastic paraparesis, but most do not have radicular pain. Initially, at the time when surgery is most likely to be successful and prevent further deterioration, the gait impairment may be very subtle, noticeable to the patient but yielding minimal findings on neurological examination (Sadasivan 1993). The paucity of findings may delay the diagnosis. In the Yale series, the investigators felt that the diagnosis had been delayed in the average by 6.3 years. The earliest consistent symptom in all of their 22 patients was a gait abnormality. These patients may become unsteady when closing their eyes and standing with feet together. They are unable to walk in tandem. The brachioradialis reflex may be depressed and instead, a brisk finger flexor response is elicited when percussing the brachioradialis tendon (inverted radial reflex). Careful testing of vibratory sense may reveal a sensory level in the cervical region. Sometimes the patient perceives the stimulus better in the thumb than in the small finger. Early diagnosis is important, because the myelopathy of cervical spondylosis is often progressive if untreated (Sadasivan 1993).

MRI of the cervical spine is helpful in the diagnosis of cervical myelopathy from cervical spondylosis, but, in the absence of the clinical findings, the presence of spondylitic changes by themselves does not make the diagnosis. Rather severe changes can be seen in asymptomatic older adults (Weis 1991; Reul 1995; Healy 1996). Baseline plain x-rays are useful when surgery is being considered for

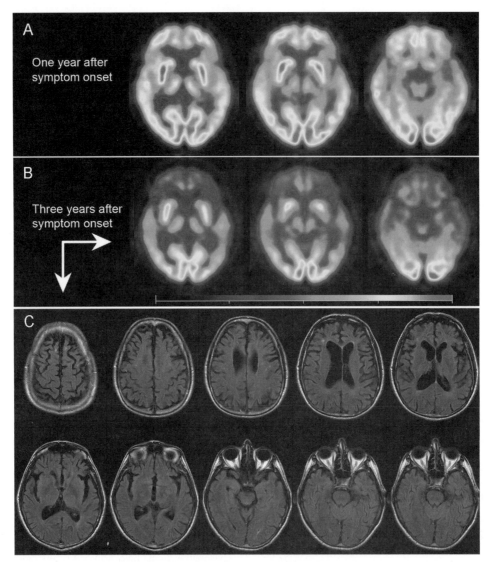

Figure 13 Frontotemporal dementia. Shown are FDG-PET (A, B) and FLAIR MRI (C) studies from a 51-year-old man with progressive speech apraxia and impaired planning, to the point of mutism and complete dependency for activities of daily living when studies B and C were obtained, on the same day. Metabolism was already decreased on the initial PET study, particularly on the frontal opercula and temporal tips, but it is much more obvious on the follow up study, showing extensive fronto-temporal hypometabolism. Note that the fronto-temporal abnormality is much more obvious on the PET study (A, B) than on the MRI study (C), which shows frontal atrophy. See Figure 8.13 on the color insert.

comparison with postoperative x-rays or when the patient cannot undergo MRI, for instance in the case of someone bearing a pacemaker. However, MRI is the screening test of choice in most instances (Sadasivan 1993). Boney osteophytes can be seen as black ridges compressing the canal and, if the compression is severe, causing high-intensity changes in the spinal cord on T2-weighted images (Figure 14). The patient whose MRI is shown in Figure 14 had a quadriparesis with a spastic-ataxic gait.

In addition to the narrowing of the spinal canal by spondylitic hypertrophy of bones and ligaments, two changes are frequently observed in the cord itself: decreased diameter and a hyperintense signal on T2-weighted images. How often a hyperintense area is observed depends on the stage of progression, with gliosis and microcavitation of the gray matter and other poorly understood factors. In some series, as many as 40% of the patients have this finding (Yone 1992). Whereas some have found the presence of this finding and its irreversibility after surgery to predict a poor outcome, others have not (Matsuda 1991;

Yone 1992). MRI may show other changes within the spinal cord itself due to chronic compression such as syrinx formation. MRI is also of great value in the differential diagnosis of myelopathy, as conditions such as tumor and infection can be easily ruled out. MRI scan is not as good as CT in showing osteophytes or ossification of the posterior longitudinal ligament (Rao 2007; Matsunaga 2008). If surgical treatment is contemplated, thin-slice CT of the cervical spine after intrathecal introduction of a non-ionic water soluble contrast material is of great help (Figure 15). MRI scan, CT scan, and CT myelography are all complementary tests and not mutually exclusive. CT myelography is most valuable when deciding on the surgical approach, either anterior or posterior. CT myelography also allows for accurate measurement of the spinal canal in the axial, sagittal, and coronal planes. A canal diameter of less than 12 mm in the antero-posterior plane is considered stenotic. Ossification of the posterior longitudinal ligament (OPLL) is sometimes found in patients with cervical spondylotic myelopathy. OPLL may be segmental or continuous in the cervical spine.

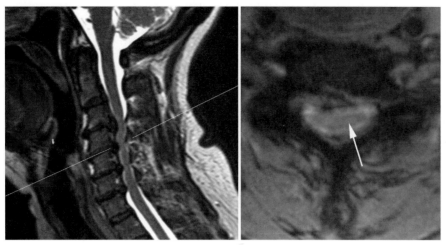

Figure 14 Cervical myelopathy from spondylosis. Sagittal MRI images showing spinal cord compression by a horizontal osteophyte at the C5–C6 (arrow) and C6–C7 levels. At those levels the spinal cord is abnormally hyperintense in these T2-weighted images.

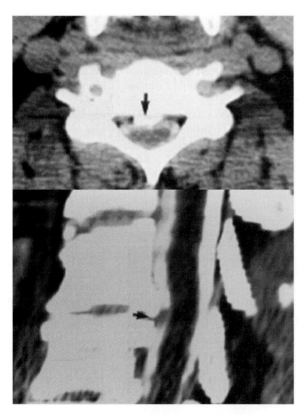

Figure 15 Posterior longitudinal ligament calcification. Axial (top) and sagittal (bottom) CT images of the cervical spine, obtained after the infusion of metrizamide in the subarachnoid space through a lumbar puncture. Note that the bony details are better visualized than with MRI (Figure 14). But changes in the spinal cord itself are better seen with MRI (Figure 14).

CT myelography is particularly useful for diagnosing this entity which has significant bearing on the type of surgical procedure to be performed (Figure 15).

Vascular Brain Disease

Vascular disease of the brain ranks among the three top causes of gait impairment in the older adult (Fuh 1994; Sudarsky 1997). These are patients referred for progressive gait impairment; they are not those with a clear-cut stroke that causes hemiparesis and gait difficulty. Ischemic brain disease tends to follow one of three patterns, discernible by clinical evaluation and with the help of neuroimaging procedures: (1) cortical infarcts, most often related to embolic disease; (2) subcortical disease, often in the form of widespread lacunes and white matter changes, most often related to arteriolar disease; and (3) a mixture of the two patterns, often related to atheromatous disease of the major vessels (Masdeu 2004). Subcortical infarcts strategically located may impair equilibrium and gait with little or no limb weakness on isometric testing (Masdeu 2004). Although acute stroke tends to be associated with overt neurological findings, gait impairment may be neglected as a neurological finding and yet be the result of small, "silent" lacunar strokes (Franch 2009). Vascular disease causing this syndrome most often affects the supratentorial compartment in the form of lacunar disease or ischemic disease of the white matter. Less often, it involves the posterior circulation, involving vestibular or cerebellar structures, and very rarely, other brainstem structures important for gait, such as the mesencephalic locomotor center (Figure 16).

Lacunar disease of gait-critical structures. CT and MRI are the diagnostic tests most useful for the study of these syndromes. Whereas hemorrhagic lesions can be readily detected by either modality (Figure 16), acute lacunar lesions may pass unnoticed unless MR diffusion imaging is used (Figure 17). Very small older lacunes may also be missed, because the infarcted tissue retracts and healthy tissue takes up its place. The resulting atrophy can be quantified using region of interest (ROI) methods or voxel-based morphometry. Larger lacunes can be easily appreciated on MRI as elongated lesions, following the trajectory of the arteriolar perforators, bright on T2-weighted images, including fluid-attenuated inversion recovery (FLAIR) images, and dark on T1-weighted images (Figure 4). Although in the supratentorial compartment small lacunes are easier to spot on FLAIR images, conventional T2-weighted images are superior for lesions in the brainstem

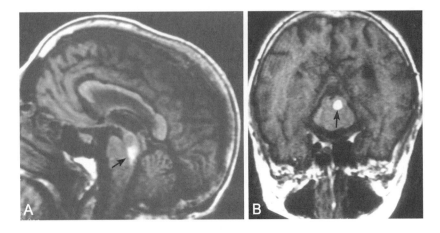

Figure 16 Mesencephalic gait failure. MRI of an 83-year-old woman with gait failure after a hemorrhage in the locomotor mesencephalic region. Lesion is shown in the sagittal (A) and coronal (B) planes, arrow. Reprinted with permission from Masdeu et al. (Masdeu, 1994).

(Brant-Zawadzki 1996). Supratentorial lacunes most likely to affect gait and balance affect the ventrolateral nucleus of the thalamus, suprathalamic white matter, basal ganglia, and the paracentral white matter. In order to cause persistent impairment, the lesions have to be bilateral and reach a volume threshold. The correlation of the imaging data with the clinical findings is often difficult because the gait impairment caused by these lesions affects the unconscious control of gait and posture (the "automatic pilot") (Masdeu 1988; Masdeu 1994). Often, patients with a shuffling, unsteady gait at home perform normally at a physician's office: they are successfully engaging the cortical mechanisms of gait to compensate for the impaired subcortical mechanisms (Masdeu 2001; Masdeu 2004). Here, the history, coupled with the neuroimaging findings, can be most helpful (Srikanth 2009).

White matter disease. White matter changes on CT or MRI are very frequent in older people (Figure 4). On MRI, some degree of white matter change is present in about 95% of subjects over the age of 60 and increases with age (de Leeuw 2001; Qiu 2009). Areas in the hemispheric white matter hypodense on CT appear markedly hyperintense on T-2 weighted images, and hypointense on T-1 weighted images (Figure 4). However, high intensity areas on T-2 MRI are often undetected on CT. On T-2 MR images, it may be difficult to differentiate tissue damage from increased water content due to dilation of perivascular spaces with normal aging because both have increased intensity

values (Kirkpatrick 1987). For this reason, in older persons it seems preferable to make the diagnosis of significant white matter changes only when the abnormalities are visible on T-1 weighted images or CT. However, there are no data available in this age group exploring the functional significance of white matter changes on only T2 images versus changes on both T-2 and T-1 weighted images. In multiple sclerosis, and therefore in a younger age group, it is known that T1 lesion volume correlates better than T2 volume with hemispheric dysfunction (Comi 2000).

A number of techniques are available to evaluate the extent of white matter changes. Initial methods were semiquantitative and involved the visual inspection of images. Changes could be compared among individuals on a cross-sectional basis or longitudinally in the same individual. Cross-sectional comparisons have been made by grouping the scans from 1 (least amount of white matter changes) to 8 (largest amount) (Masdeu 1989). Most often used are scales describing the amount of white matter changes. The Fazekas Scale (Fazekas 1987) has a range of 1–6. In the periventricular regions scores 0–3 can be given, and in the subcortical region scores 1–3 can be given for mild, moderate, or severe lesions, respectively. The ARWMC scale (Wahlund 2001) has a range from 0 to 30, where scores 0–3 can be given in 5 regions, each left and right. The Scheltens Rating Scale (Scheltens 1993) ranges from 0 to 84 (scores 0–6 can be given in 13 subcortical regions and

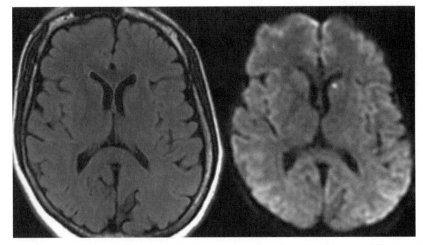

Figure 17 Acute lacunar stroke. MRI from a 60-year-old man with a left caudate nucleus infarct, visible on the diffusion-weighted image (right), but not on the acute FLAIR image (left).

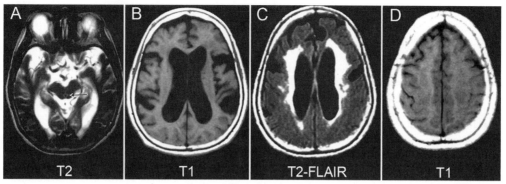

Figure 18 Hydrocephalus. (A–D) are axial sections of the MRI from a 71-year-old woman with progressive gait and cognitive impairment, as well as urinary incontinence. Notice the low signal in the Sylvian aqueduct, due to a flow void from a vigorous CSF flow in this structure (A, arrow). Although the basal cisterns (A) and the interhemispheric and sylvian fissures (B–C) are dilated, the sulci in the high convexity (D) are compressed. Transependymal reabsorption of CSF, suggested by the homogeneous high signal in the periventricular white matter (C), need not occur in all cases of symptomatic hydrocephalus.

scores 0–2 for 3 periventricular regions). An example of longitudinal scale is the Rotterdam Progression Scale (Prins 2004) (range –7 to 7), which measures decrease, no change, or increase (–1, 0, 1, respectively) of white matter changes for three periventricular regions and four subcortical regions. These visual methods are giving way to semiautomatic (Gouw 2008) or even completely automatic methods, which use the matrix output from the scanner to select voxels likely to correspond to abnormal white matter (Tiehuis 2008). Ideally, images to be processed automatically should be obtained with good magnetic field homogeneity, small voxel size (1–2 cubic mm), and with 3D acquisitions, where the entire brain is imaged with voxels having the same size in all three planes. In good quality scans, automatic or semiautomatic segmentation methods can measure the extent of white matter changes accurately and with a minimum of operator effort (de Boer 2009).

Because the histology underlying white matter changes in older people remains elusive in many cases, Hachinski (1987) coined the descriptive term "leukoaraiosis" for the CT findings and this term was later applied to the MRI findings as well. In many papers, other purely descriptive terms, such as white matter hyperintensities, are used (Srikanth 2009). Several authors have reported normal histology, but ischemic changes similar to the findings in subcortical arteriosclerotic encephalopathy (SAE) have been present in cases with pronounced changes on T1-weighted MRI or CT (Yamanouchi 1991; Gold 2009). Cerebrovascular disease and hypertension are frequent correlates of subcortical arteriosclerotic encephalopathy (Awad 1986; van Swieten 1991). Amyloid angiopathy can also cause white matter disease in the elderly (Dubas 1985; Gray 1985). In addition to white matter changes, amyloid angiopathy results in subcortical hemorrhages (Figure 5). Other characteristics of this disorder were reviewed in the section on dementia.

Disorders of gait and equilibrium are the most prominent correlate of white matter CT or MRI changes in older people (Masdeu 2001; Masdeu 2004; Franch 2009). In controlled studies of elderly prone to falling, impaired gait and balance correlated with the presence of white matter disease on CT or MRI (Masdeu 1989; Srikanth 2009).

Hydrocephalus

Although not a frequent cause of gait disorders in older people, patients with symptomatic hydrocephalus initially present with a gait disorder and it should be recognized because it is potentially treatable (Marmarou 2005; Graff-Radford 2007). Particularly after CT became

available, several authors found enlarged ventricles to be frequently present in patients with gait disorders (Fisher 1982). From this finding they concluded that symptomatic hydrocephalus was common and thus shunting procedures multiplied. However, even in series with carefully selected patients, some failed to improve after shunting, suggesting that hydrocephalus was not the cause of their gait disorder (Graff-Radford 1989). For this reason, it is important to apply more sensitive diagnostic criteria in the work up of these patients (Graff-Radford 2007). On CT or MRI, the ventricles are enlarged (Figure 18). Often, the cortical sulci are compressed. However, in many patients they may be enlarged, sometimes greatly so (Holodny 1998; Kitagaki 1998). Sulcal enlargement involves particularly the basal cisterns, sylvian fissures, and other major sulci on the convexity of the hemispheres. Typically, the sulci in the high parietal convexity and medial aspect of the parietal lobe are compressed, unlike the situation in hydrocephalus ex-vacuo produced by atrophy (Figure 14). Another finding that helps distinguish sulcal dilation due to hydrocephalus is that the sulci are ballooned out, with the depth of the sulcus in the shape of a U. By contrast, sulci dilated from atrophy have the shape of a V (compare Figures 9 and 18).

Cerebrovascular disease, in the form of lacunar strokes or abnormal white matter on CT or MRI, is more frequent in patients with hydrocephalus than in controls (Krauss 1997) and is an important confounder in the diagnosis of treatable hydrocephalus (Caplan 2002). It has predicted a poorer outcome after shunting in some large studies (Boon 1999), but not in smaller ones (Tullberg 2001). When the clinical or CT-MR diagnosis is dubious, a pattern of decreased perfusion or metabolism in the association cortex of the parietal lobes on SPECT or PET may predict a poor outcome (Graff-Radford 1989). This pattern is usually seen in Alzheimer's disease and Parkinson's with dementia.

Structural neuroimaging aids in the diagnosis of a variety of nervous system syndromes that may affect older people. In two of these complex conditions, dementia and gait disorders, imaging adds important information to assist in diagnosis and treatement.

References

Auer, D. P., Putz, B., Gossl, C., et al. Differential lesion patterns in CADASIL and sporadic subcortical arteriosclerotic encephalopathy: MR imaging study with statistical parametric group comparison. *Radiology* 218(2): 443–451, 2001.

Awad, I., Johnson, P., Spetzler, R., et al. Incidental subcortical lesions identified on magnetic resonance imaging in the elderly. II. Postmortem pathological correlations. *Stroke* 17: 1090–1097, 1986.

Baker, M., Mackenzie, I. R., Pickering-Brown, S. M., et al. Mutations in progranulin cause tau-negative frontotemporal dementia linked to chromosome 17. *Nature* 442(7105): 916–919, 2006.

Beyer, M. K., Larsen, J. P. and Aarsland, D. Gray matter atrophy in Parkinson disease with dementia and dementia with Lewy bodies. *Neurology* 69(8): 747–754, 2007.

Boon, A. J., Tans, J. T., Delwel, E. J., et al. Dutch Normal-Pressure Hydrocephalus Study: The role of cerebrovascular disease. *J Neurosurg* 90(2): 221–226, 1999.

Brant-Zawadzki, M., Atkinson, D., Detrick, M., et al. Fluid-attenuated inversion recovery (FLAIR) for assessment of cerebral infarction. Initial clinical experience in 50 patients. *Stroke* 27(7): 1187–1191, 1996.

Brewer, J. B., Magda, S., Airriess, C., et al. Fully-automated quantification of regional brain volumes for improved detection of focal atrophy in Alzheimer disease. *AJNR Am J Neuroradiol* 30(3): 578–580, 2009.

Caplan, L. R. White-matter hyperintensities and subcortical infarcts as predictors of shunt surgery outcome. *AJNR Am J Neuroradiol* 23(5): 894; author reply 894–895, 2002.

Chui, H. and Zhang, Q. Evaluation of dementia: A systematic study of the usefulness of the American Academy of Neurology's practice parameters. *Neurology* 49(4): 925–935, 1997.

Chui, H. C., Zarow, C., Mack, W. J., et al. Cognitive impact of subcortical vascular and Alzheimer's disease pathology. *Ann Neurol* 60(6): 677–687, 2006.

Colliot, O., Chetelat, G., Chupin, M., et al. Discrimination between Alzheimer disease, mild cognitive impairment, and normal aging by using automated segmentation of the hippocampus. *Radiology* 248(1): 194–201, 2008.

Comi, G., Rovaris, M., Leocani, L., et al. Assessment of the damage of the cerebral hemispheres in MS using neuroimaging techniques. *J Neurol Sci* 172(Suppl 1): S63–66, 2000.

Critchley, M. On senile disorders of gait, including the so-called "senile paraplegia." *Geriatrics* 3: 364–370, 1948.

de Boer, R., Vrooman, H. A., van der Lijn, F., et al. White matter lesion extension to automatic brain tissue segmentation on MRI. *Neuroimage* 45(4): 1151–1161, 2009.

de Leeuw, F. E., de Groot, J. C., Achten, E., et al. Prevalence of cerebral white matter lesions in elderly people: A population based magnetic resonance imaging study. The Rotterdam Scan Study. *J Neurol Neurosurg Psychiatry* 70(1): 9–14, 2001.

Du, A. T., Schuff, N., Zhu, X. P., et al. Atrophy rates of entorhinal cortex in AD and normal aging. *Neurology* 60(3): 481–486, 2003.

Dubas, F., Gray, F., Roullet, E., et al. Leucoencéphalopathies artériopathiques (17 cas anatomo-cliniques). *Rev Neurol (Paris)* 141: 93–l08, 1985.

Duchesne, S., Caroli, A., Geroldi, C., et al. MRI-based automated computer classification of probable AD versus normal controls. *IEEE Trans Med Imaging* 27(4): 509–520, 2008.

Eng, J. A., Frosch, M. P., Choi, K., et al. Clinical manifestations of cerebral amyloid angiopathy-related inflammation. *Ann Neurol* 55(2): 250–256, 2004.

Esiri, M. M., Wilcock, G. K. and Morris, J. H. Neuropathological assessment of the lesions of significance in vascular dementia. *J Neurol Neurosurg Psychiatry* 63(6): 749–753, 1997.

Fazekas, F., Chawluk, J. B., Alavi, A., et al. MR signal abnormalities at 1.5 T in Alzheimer's dementia and normal aging. *AJR Am J Roentgenol* 149(2): 351–356, 1987.

Fisher, C. Hydrocephalus as a cause of disturbances of gait in the elderly. *Neurology* 32: 1358–1363, 1982.

Foster, N. L., Heidebrink, J. L., Clark, C. M., et al. FDG-PET improves accuracy in distinguishing frontotemporal dementia and Alzheimer's disease. *Brain* 130(Pt 10): 2616–2635, 2007.

Franch, O., Calandre, L., Alvarez-Linera, J., et al. Gait disorders of unknown cause in the elderly: Clinical and MRI findings. *J Neurol Sci* 280(1–2): 84–86, 2009.

Fuh, J. L., Lin, K. N., Wang, S. J., et al. Neurologic diseases presenting with gait impairment in the elderly. *J Geriatr Psychiatry Neurol* 7(2): 89–92, 1994.

Gold, G. Defining the neuropathological background of vascular and mixed dementia and comparison with magnetic resonance imaging findings. *Front Neurol Neurosci* 24: 86–94, 2009.

Good, C. D., Scahill, R. I., Fox, N. C., et al. Automatic differentiation of anatomical patterns in the human brain: validation with studies of degenerative dementias. *Neuroimage* 17(1): 29–46, 2002.

Gouw, A. A., van der Flier, W. M., van Straaten, E. C., et al. Reliability and sensitivity of visual scales versus volumetry for evaluating white matter hyperintensity progression. *Cerebrovasc Dis* 25(3): 247–253, 2008.

Graff-Radford, N., Godersky, J. and Jones, M. Variables predicting outcome in symptomatic hydrocephalus in the elderly. *Neurology* 39: 1601–1604, 1989.

Graff-Radford, N. R. Normal pressure hydrocephalus. *Neurol Clin* 25(3): 809–832, vii-viii, 2007.

Grau-Olivares, M., Bartres-Faz, D., Arboix, A., et al. Mild cognitive impairment after lacunar infarction: Voxel-based morphometry and neuropsychological assessment. *Cerebrovasc Dis* 23(5–6): 353–361, 2007.

Gray, F., Dubas, F., Roullet, E., et al. Leukoencephalopathy in diffuse hemorrhagic cerebral amyloid angiopathy. *Ann Neurol* l8: 54–59, 1985.

Hachinski, V., Potter, P. and Merskey, H. Leuko-araiosis. *Arch Neurol* 44: 21–23, 1987.

Healy, J. F., Healy, B. B., Wong, W. H., et al. Cervical and lumbar MRI in asymptomatic older male lifelong athletes: Frequency of degenerative findings. *J Comput Assist Tomogr* 20(1): 107–112, 1996.

Hejl, A., Hogh, P. and Waldemar, G. Potentially reversible conditions in 1000 consecutive memory clinic patients. *J Neurol Neurosurg Psychiatry* 73(4): 390–394, 2002.

Holly, L. T., Moftakhar, P., Khoo, L. T., et al. Surgical outcomes of elderly patients with cervical spondylotic myelopathy. *Surg Neurol* 69(3): 233–240, 2008.

Holodny, A. I., George, A. E., de Leon, M. J., et al. Focal dilation and paradoxical collapse of cortical fissures and sulci in patients with normal-pressure hydrocephalus. *J Neurosurg* 89(5): 742–747, 1998.

Josephs, K. A., Petersen, R. C., Knopman, D. S., et al. Clinicopathologic analysis of frontotemporal and corticobasal degenerations and PSP. *Neurology* 66(1): 41–48, 2006.

Kallenberg, K., Schulz-Schaeffer, W. J., Jastrow, U., et al. Creutzfeldt-Jakob disease: Comparative analysis of MR imaging sequences. *AJNR Am J Neuroradiol* 27(7): 1459–1462, 2006.

Karas, G. B., Burton, E. J., Rombouts, S. A., et al. A comprehensive study of gray matter loss in patients with Alzheimer's disease using optimized voxel-based morphometry. *Neuroimage* 18(4): 895–907, 2003.

Kirkpatrick, J. and Hayman, L. White-matter lesions on MR imaging of clinically healthy brains of elderly subjects: Possible pathologic basis. *Radiology* 162: 509–511, 1987.

Kitagaki, H., Mori, E., Ishii, K., et al. CSF spaces in idiopathic normal pressure hydrocephalus: Morphology and volumetry. *AJNR Am J Neuroradiol* 19(7): 1277–1284, 1998.

Kloppel, S., Stonnington, C. M., Barnes, J., et al. Accuracy of dementia diagnosis: A direct comparison between radiologists and a computerized method. *Brain* 131: 2969–2974, 2008.

Knopman, D. S., DeKosky, S. T., Cummings, J. L., et al. Practice parameter: Diagnosis of dementia (an evidence-based review).

Report of the Quality Standards Subcommittee of the American Academy of Neurology. *Neurology* 56(9): 1143–1153., 2001.

Krauss, J. K., Regel, J. P., Vach, W., et al. White matter lesions in patients with idiopathic normal pressure hydrocephalus and in an age-matched control group: A comparative study. *Neurosurgery* 40(3): 491–495; discussion 495–496., 1997.

Liem, M. K., van der Grond, J., Haan, J., et al. Lacunar infarcts are the main correlate with cognitive dysfunction in CADASIL. *Stroke* 38(3): 923–928, 2007.

Likeman, M., Anderson, V. M., Stevens, J. M., et al. Visual assessment of atrophy on magnetic resonance imaging in the diagnosis of pathologically confirmed young-onset dementias. *Arch Neurol* 62(9): 1410–1415, 2005.

Liscic, R. M., Storandt, M., Cairns, N. J., et al. Clinical and psychometric distinction of frontotemporal and Alzheimer dementias. *Arch Neurol* 64(4): 535–540, 2007.

Marmarou, A., Young, H. F., Aygok, G. A., et al. Diagnosis and management of idiopathic normal-pressure hydrocephalus: A prospective study in 151 patients. *J Neurosurg* 102(6): 987–997, 2005.

Masdeu, J. Cerebrovascular disease and hydrocephalus. In *Clinical disorders of balance, posture and gait*. (A. Bronstein, T. Brandt, M. Woollacott and J. Nutt, Eds). Arnold, London, 2004: 222–244.

Masdeu, J., Alampur, U., Cavaliere, R., et al. Astasia and gait failure with damage of the pontomesencephalic locomotor region. *Ann Neurol* 35: 619–621, 1994.

Masdeu, J. and Aronson, M. CT findings in early dementia. *The Gerontologist* 25(special issue): 82, 1985.

Masdeu, J. and Gorelick, P. Thalamic astasia: Inability to stand after unilateral thalamic lesions. *Ann Neurol* 23: 596–603, 1988.

Masdeu, J. C. Dysequilibrium syndromes. *In Gait disorders*. (E. Ruzicka, M. Hallet and J. Jankovic, Eds). Lippincott Williams and Wilkins, Philadelphia, 2001.

Masdeu, J. C., Wolfson, L., Lantos, G., et al. Brain white-matter changes in the elderly prone to falling. *Arch Neurol* 46(12): 1292–1296, 1989.

Masdeu, J. C., Zubieta, J. L. and Arbizu, J. Neuroimaging as a marker of the onset and progression of Alzheimer's disease. *J Neurol Sci* 236(1–2): 55–64, 2005.

Matsuda, Y., Miyazaki, K., Tada, K., et al. Increased MR signal intensity due to cervical myelopathy. Analysis of 29 surgical cases. *J Neurosurg* 74(6): 887–892, 1991.

Matsunaga, S., Nakamura, K., Seichi, A., et al. Radiographic predictors for the development of myelopathy in patients with ossification of the posterior longitudinal ligament: A multicenter cohort study. *Spine* 33(24): 2648–2650, 2008.

McKhann, G., Drachman, D., Folstein, M., et al. Clinical diagnosis of Alzheimer's disease: Report of the NINCDS-ADRDA Work Group under the auspices of Department of Health and Human Services Task Force on Alzheimer's Disease. *Neurology* 34(7): 939–944., 1984.

Mendez, M. F., Shapira, J. S., McMurtray, A., et al. Accuracy of the clinical evaluation for frontotemporal dementia. *Arch Neurol* 64(6): 830–835, 2007.

Neumann, M., Sampathu, D. M., Kwong, L. K., et al. Ubiquitinated TDP-43 in frontotemporal lobar degeneration and amyotrophic lateral sclerosis. *Science* 314(5796): 130–133, 2006.

O'Sullivan, M., Ngo, E., Viswanathan, A., et al. Hippocampal volume is an independent predictor of cognitive performance in CADASIL. *Neurobiol Aging* 2007.

Okamura, N., Arai, H., Higuchi, M., et al. [18F]FDG-PET study in dementia with Lewy bodies and Alzheimer's disease. *Prog Neuropsychopharmacol Biol Psychiatry* 25(2): 447–456, 2001.

Patel, M., Williamsom, R. A., Dorevitch, S., et al. Pilot study investigating the effect of the static magnetic field from a 9.4-T MRI on the vestibular system. *J Occup Environ Med* 50(5): 576–583, 2008.

Prins, N. D., van Straaten, E. C., van Dijk, E. J., et al. Measuring progression of cerebral white matter lesions on MRI: Visual rating and volumetrics. *Neurology* 62(9): 1533–1539, 2004.

Probst, A., Taylor, K. I. and Tolnay, M. Hippocampal sclerosis dementia: A reappraisal. *Acta Neuropathol* 114(4): 335–345, 2007.

Qiu, C., Cotch, M. F., Sigurdsson, S., et al. Microvascular lesions in the brain and retina: The age, gene/environment susceptibility-Reykjavik study. *Ann Neurol* 65(5): 569–576, 2009.

Qiu, C., De Ronchi, D. and Fratiglioni, L. The epidemiology of the dementias: An update. *Curr Opin Psychiatry* 20(4): 380–385, 2007.

Rao, R. D., Currier, B. L., Albert, T. J., et al. Degenerative cervical spondylosis: Clinical syndromes, pathogenesis, and management. *J Bone Joint Surg Am* 89(6): 1360–1378, 2007.

Reul, J., Gievers, B., Weis, J., et al. Assessment of the narrow cervical spinal canal: A prospective comparison of MRI, myelography and CT-myelography. *Neuroradiology* 37(3): 187–191, 1995.

Rubenstein, L. and Josephson, K. Interventions to reduce the multifactorial risks for falling. In *Gait disorders of aging. Falls and therapeutic strategies*. (J. Masdeu, L. Sudarsky and L. Wolfson, Eds). Lippincott & Raven, Philadelphia, 1997: 309–326.

Sadasivan, K. K., Reddy, R. P. and Albright, J. A. The natural history of cervical spondylotic myelopathy. *Yale J Biol Med* 66(3): 235–242, 1993.

Sanders, J. A. Computed tomography and magnetic resonance imaging. In *Neuroimaging*. (W. W. Orrison, Eds). W. B. Saunders, Philadelphia, 2000, 1: 12–36.

Scheltens, P., Barkhof, F., Leys, D., et al. A semiquantitative rating scale for the assessment of signal hyperintensities on magnetic resonance imaging. *J Neurol Sci* 114(1): 7–12, 1993.

Scheltens, P., Fox, N., Barkhof, F., et al. Structural magnetic resonance imaging in the practical assessment of dementia: Beyond exclusion. *Lancet Neurol* 1(1): 13–21, 2002.

Schneider, J. A., Arvanitakis, Z., Bang, W., et al. Mixed brain pathologies account for most dementia cases in community-dwelling older persons. *Neurology*, 2007.

Srikanth, V., Beare, R., Blizzard, L., et al. Cerebral white matter lesions, gait, and the risk of incident falls: A prospective population-based study. *Stroke* 40(1): 175–180, 2009.

Sudarsky, L. Clinical approach to gait disorders of aging: An overview. In *Gait disorders of aging. Falls and therapeutic strategies*. (J. Masdeu, L. Sudarsky and L. Wolfson, Eds). Lippincott & Raven, Philadelphia, 1997: 147–157.

Thompson, P. M., Hayashi, K. M., de Zubicaray, G., et al. Dynamics of gray matter loss in alzheimer's disease. *J. Neurosci.* 23(3): 994–1005, 2003.

Tiehuis, A. M., Vincken, K. L., Mali, W. P., et al. Automated and visual scoring methods of cerebral white matter hyperintensities: Relation with age and cognitive function. *Cerebrovasc Dis* 25(1–2): 59–66, 2008.

Tullberg, M., Jensen, C., Ekholm, S., et al. Normal pressure hydrocephalus: Vascular white matter changes on MR images must not exclude patients from shunt surgery. *AJNR Am J Neuroradiol* 22(9): 1665–1673, 2001.

Urs, R., Potter, E., Barker, W., et al. Visual rating system for assessing magnetic resonance images: a tool in the diagnosis of mild cognitive impairment and Alzheimer disease. *J Comput Assist Tomogr* 33(1): 73–78, 2009.

van Swieten, J. C., Geyskes, G. G., Derix, M. M., et al. Hypertension in the elderly is associated with white matter lesions and cognitive decline. *Ann Neurol* 30(6): 825–830, 1991.

Viswanathan, A., Gschwendtner, A., Guichard, J. P., et al. Lacunar lesions are independently associated with disability and cognitive impairment in CADASIL. *Neurology* 69(2): 172–179, 2007.

Wahlund, L. O., Barkhof, F., Fazekas, F., et al. A new rating scale for age-related white matter changes applicable to MRI and CT. *Stroke* 32(6): 1318–1322, 2001.

Waldemar, G., Dubois, B., Emre, M., et al. Recommendations for the diagnosis and management of Alzheimer's disease and other disorders associated with dementia: EFNS guideline. *Eur J Neurol* 14(1): e1–26, 2007.

Weis, E., Jr. Abnormal magnetic-resonance scans of the cervical spine in asymptomatic subjects. *J Bone Joint Surg [Am]* 73(7): 1113, 1991.

Whitwell, J. L., Przybelski, S. A., Weigand, S. D., et al. 3D maps from multiple MRI illustrate changing atrophy patterns as subjects progress from mild cognitive impairment to Alzheimer's disease. *Brain* 130(Pt 7): 1777–1786, 2007.

Yamanouchi, H. Loss of white matter oligodendrocytes and astrocytes in progressive subcortical vascular encephalopathy of Binswanger type. *Acta Neurol Scand* 83(5): 301–305, 1991.

Yone, K., Sakou, T., Yanase, M., et al. Preoperative and postoperative magnetic resonance image evaluations of the spinal cord in cervical myelopathy. *Spine* 17(10 Suppl): S388–392, 1992.

9 Functional Neuroimaging in Aging

Gary R. Turner and Mark D'Esposito

Introduction

Functional neuroimaging methods have been used to study cognitive aging for almost two decades. Much of the work over this period has utilized these methods to identify the neural correlates of behavior-based theories of age-related cognitive decline across a myriad of domains (e.g. sensory functioning, processing speed, working memory, dual task coordination, inhibitory function). More recently, functional neuroimaging has moved beyond this supporting role to advance hypotheses with respect to the neural basis of age-related cognitive decline and these are now leading to novel diagnostic markers of cognitive aging (Gazzaley, Cooney, Rissman, and D'Esposito 2005).

In the first section of the chapter, we provide a brief review of the leading behavioral theories of cognitive aging and how these have informed our clinical understanding of non-pathological, age-related cognitive change. Next we examine brain-based theories emerging from cognitive neuroscience studies of aging, their key assumptions, strengths and weaknesses, and utility in mapping the neural correlates of cognitive decline in non-pathological aging. We argue that these neural theories represent the first step towards developing functional neural markers for assessing cognitive decline in older adults. In the final sections we review work ongoing in our laboratory to establish reliable markers that can aid in the assessment of age-related cognitive decline and identify brain-based targets for remediative interventions.

Behavior-based Theories of Cognitive Aging

The dual nature of cognitive decline in aging has been well characterized in the literature and is only briefly reviewed here (for a comprehensive review see: Park, Polk, Mikels, Taylor, and Marshuetz 2001). Performance on tasks dependent upon consistent (i.e., non-contingent) application of well learned cognitive schemas or tapping 'crystallized' knowledge structures (e.g. declarative memory, vocabulary, antonym or synonym knowledge) is generally well preserved even into advanced age. In contrast, performance on tasks requiring controlled or speeded processing involving novel behavior or contingent responding based on variable temporal, social, or environmental contexts (e.g. strategic encoding into and retrieval from memory; selective attention, complex working memory) show steady declines into advanced age.

Behavioral theories typically point to either common-cause or domain-specific hypotheses to explain this duality. For example, Salthouse (1996) has argued that deficits in controlled processing are secondary to a generalized reduction in processing speed in older adults. Building upon a large body of empirical data, Salthouse argues that reduced speed of processing limits both the rate of cognitive operations and their fluency as operations become temporally decoupled. This loss of simultaneity and fluency degrades controlled processing

capacity that is essential to higher cognition, and indeed, the author has reported that most age-related variance in memory and cognitive performance can be explained by performance on speeded tasks (Salthouse 1996). A second common cause hypothesis has been proposed by Baltes and Lindenberger (1997). They argue that age-related loss of sensory functioning results in degraded mental representations and, in turn, the quality of controlled processing operations that depend upon the integrity of these representations. Similar to claims put forth by Salthouse, they report that simple sensory task performance is able to explain a significant portion of age-related variance in cognitive performance.

Two of the most prominent domain-specific hypotheses of age-related cognitive decline emphasize the susceptibility of memory and inhibitory processing to normal aging. Moscovitch and Winocur (1992) argue that healthy aging is associated with reductions in the capacity to encode into, maintain, and retrieve mnemonic representations from medial temporal memory systems—a series of control processes they collectively refer to as 'working with memory.' In their account, the mnemonic representations themselves remain relatively intact. This is in contrast to pathological aging, including Alzheimer's disease, where medial temporal lobe memory structures are typically compromised, impacting the formation, consolidation, and reconstitution of the memory representations themselves while generally sparing controlled encoding and retrieval capacity. This distinction between preserved memory and degraded control (i.e. executive) processing in healthy aging was also emphasized in a recent review of healthy and pathological age-related cognitive decline by Buckner (2004) who argued that degraded executive control was indicative of normal age-related decline whereas degraded mnemonic representations suggested the presence of more pathological aging processes. He attributed these declines to perturbations in frontal and medial temporal brain structures respectively, thus suggesting a brain basis for this control versus content distinction in cognitive aging.

A second domain-specific cognitive theory of healthy aging argues that a selective deficit in the capacity to suppress distracting stimuli is a central feature of cognitive aging. The inhibitory deficit hypothesis (Hasher and Zacks 1988) posits that reduced inhibitory processing capacity enables non-goal path related information to compete for limited cognitive processing resources with goal-relevant mental representations. This competition results in greater distractibility, slowed and error-prone retrieval, and greater forgetting rates as both goal and non-goal relevant representations vie for processing capacity. While hypothesizing a specific deficit in inhibitory processing, this theory is consistent with other domain-specific accounts of cognitive aging that implicate controlled processing over representational integrity as a central mechanism of age-related cognitive decline.

Each of these leading behavioral theories, irrespective of whether they argue for a common cause or a domain-specific explanation of cognitive aging, draws a sharp distinction between control operations and mental representations that serves as the fulcrum upon which the vast majority of cognitive aging research has come to rest. In a recent review of cognitive changes across the lifespan, Craik and Bialystok (2006) summarized this pattern simply as preserved 'representation' in the context of declining 'control.' In this formulation, mental representations that include highly practiced or learned behaviors ("Always take the third freeway exit to get to work" or "Do not step on that squeaky third step when coming in late"), general semantic knowledge ("Paris is the capital of France"; Christmas is in December"), or personal semantics ("my childhood address was…") are considered to be robust to decline over the lifespan, and serve as foundational knowledge structures that we use to guide behavior in the absence of, or perhaps in spite of, bottom-up contextual or environmental influences. Control processes are considered to be a set of fluid operations that enable intentional processing and adaptive cognitive performance in cases where novel responses are required or where learned behaviors and knowledge structures must be overridden to meet shifting contexts or contingencies ("Always take the third freeway exit to get work—but not on Tuesday when I have a dentist appointment just off the fourth exit"). As described above, these control processes, whether considered in the context of speeded operations, sensory perception, working with memory, or inhibition, are considered to be vulnerable to age-related decline and thus have received the greatest attention with respect to the behavioral correlates of cognitive aging.

While the distinction between control and content has become the de facto explanation of the duality observed in age-related cognitive decline, it remains unclear whether this dichotomy is a true reflection of disparate cognitive phenomenon or simply an artifact of existing behavioral assessment methods. Control processes and the quality of the representations upon which they operate are difficult to disentangle in a single behavioral measure. Put another way, demands for controlled processing may increase with advanced age in response to degraded or unstable mental representations and thus these demands approach capacity limits earlier in older than younger adults. In this case, the robustness of these mental representations themselves or the quality of the interactions between representations and control processes may more accurately reflect age-related cognitive decline. If, as has been hypothesized by Buckner (2004) and others, control processes and mental representations are subserved by distinct neural architectures, functional neuroimaging methods which are able to measure activity across the whole brain at a high temporal and spatial resolution, open the possibility of charting the trajectories of age-related changes in representational integrity and controlled processing independently as well as mapping functional interactions between underlying brain regions. Thus, using functional neuroimaging methods, it is possible to discern age-related changes in control processes and representational integrity, a distinction heretofore inaccessible to behavioral assessment methods. This will allow development of more mechanistic, brain-based theories of cognitive aging. In the next section we review several of the leading cognitive neuroscience theories and how these may lead to more sensitive and specific markers of age-related cognitive decline.

Brain-based Theories of Cognitive Aging

Early functional neuroimaging studies of cognitive aging typically adopted a domain-centric approach, with investigators enumerating age-related changes in the neural implementation of cognitive task performance using cross-sectional study designs (for reviews see: Grady 2008; Greenwood 2007; Hedden and Gabrieli 2004; Park, Polk, Mikels, Taylor, and Marshuetz 2001; Park and Reuter-Lorenz 2009;

Reuter-Lorenz and Lustig 2005). Emerging from these early studies there was also evidence for domain-general patterns of functional brain changes in aging, suggesting that the behavioral deficits associated with age-related cognitive decline may share a common neural mechanism. In this section we review two brain-based theories of cognitive aging—dedifferentiation and neuromodulation—that have emerged from cognitive neuroscience research and consider how these may facilitate the development of neural markers of age-related cognitive decline, thus opening new avenues for assessment and treatment protocols.

Dedifferentiation

In one of the earliest functional neuroimaging investigations of cognitive aging, Grady et al. (1994) utilized positron emission tomography (PET) scanning methods to measure changes in metabolism across brain regions while younger and older subjects performed perceptual tasks. They reported that older subjects displayed greater functional activation during cognitive task performance than younger subjects. Moreover, unlike the lateralized pattern of functional activity within the prefrontal cortex (PFC) observed in the young, older subjects demonstrated greater bilateral activation of PFC regions. Since this seminal work, this pattern of decreased lateralization in functional brain response in aging has been replicated in numerous reports using PET and functional MRI (fMRI) methods and spanning a range of cognitive domains including memory encoding and retrieval (Cabeza et al. 2004; Grady 1996; McIntosh et al. 1999; Velanova, Lustig, Jacoby, and Buckner 2007), visual attention (Madden et al. 2007); working memory (Mattay et al. 2006; Reuter-Lorenz et al. 2000; Rypma and D'Esposito 2000), selective attention and inhibition (Colcombe, Kramer, Erickson, and Scalf 2005).

The finding that cortical representations of cognitive activities become more diffuse and distributed with advancing age has been referred to as dedifferentiation and has become a leading account of functional brain changes in older adults. Dedifferentiation has been operationalized in a number of ways in the neurocognitive aging literature. Zarahn and colleagues (2007) describe it simply as non-identical brain activity patterns between younger and elder populations. Craik and Bialystok (2006) characterize dedifferentiation as more diffuse and distributed cortical representations of cognitive activities while Cabeza et al. (2002) argue that it reflects a failure to engage specialized neural mechanisms during cognitive performance. Park and colleagues (2001) describe three forms of dedifferentiation which they label as contralateral, unique, or substitutive functional recruitment. In this schema, contralateral recruitment refers to the age-related recruitment of brain regions homologous to those recruited in younger subjects first reported by Grady and colleagues (1994). Unique recruitment describes the engagement of additional (non-homologous) brain regions (e.g. Davis, Dennis, Daselaar, Fleck, and Cabeza 2008; Madden et al. 2007; McIntosh et al. 1999) while substitution reflects activation of entirely novel neural networks in older relative to younger adults, perhaps signaling strategy differences or functional reorganization, potentially in response to more pathological age-related brain changes (e.g. Hazlett et al. 1998).

Accumulating evidence for dedifferentiation in older versus younger adults suggests that reduced neural specialization may provide a neural marker of age-related cognitive decline. Unfortunately, as a theory of cognitive aging, it is ambivalent with respect to whether these brain changes are compensatory or deleterious. In other words, does dedifferentiated neural response reflect compensatory functional responses or inefficient processing in older adults? Several studies have addressed this question directly and these are reviewed briefly below.

Dedifferentiation as compensation. Decreased lateralization has been positively correlated with cognitive performance. In an early report, Cabeza et al. (2002) examined the behavioral performance of healthy older subjects who had undergone fMRI scanning while performing a recognition memory task. The investigators observed that older subjects who performed better on the task showed greater bilateral PFC activation than those who performed more poorly. They considered these results to be provisional evidence that this dedifferentiated neural pattern was indeed a compensatory functional response to degraded neural circuitry in healthy aging. Similar studies have also observed compensatory bilateral PFC recruitment (e.g. Cabeza et al. 2004; Madden et al. 2007; Reuter-Lorenz et al. 2000; Rosen et al. 2002). Dedifferentiation through substitution has also been positively associated with behavior. In a recent report, Gutchess et al. (2005) investigated patterns of functional brain responses while young and older subjects incidentally encoded scene images, a task known to engage medial temporal lobe structures. Older adults recruited medial temporal lobe (MTL) regions less and lateral PFC regions more than their younger counterparts. Moreover, recruitment of lateral PFC and MTL structures were inversely correlated in older but not younger subjects. The investigators concluded that since the analysis was only conducted on 'remembered' stimuli, dedifferentiation was compensatory for recognition performance in the older adults. This pattern of compensatory dedifferentiation through substitution has since been replicated in other functional domains (e.g. selective working memory, Payer et al. 2006) and in a longitudinal study of structural and functional brain changes in aging (Persson et al. 2006). Perhaps the most compelling evidence that dedifferentiation is compensatory comes from a report by Rossi et al. (2004) who applied repetitive transcranial magnetic stimulation (rTMS) to older and younger subjects during an episodic memory task. While memory retrieval was disrupted by rTMS to a right PFC region in younger subjects, older subject performance was disrupted by rTMS applied to both right and left PFC, suggesting that dedifferentiation was compensatory in these subjects.

Dedifferentiation as neural inefficiency. Several functional neuroimaging studies have now reported that dedifferentiated neural response is associated with poorer, not improved, cognitive performance. This has been demonstrated in individual difference studies of healthy young adults (e.g. Rypma and D'Esposito 1999) as well as in brain disease and dysfunction (e.g. Callicott et al. 2000; Turner and Levine 2008). In a recent study of visual attention in healthy aging, Colcombe et al. (2005) observed that greater bilateral recruitment in older subjects was associated with poorer performance on the task. In the only study that we are aware of to directly contrast these competing behavioral accounts of neural dedifferentiation, Zarahn et al. (2007), tested the functional compensation and neural inefficiency hypotheses in a sample of healthy older and younger adults during performance of a delayed recognition task. The authors observed evidence of inefficient neural responding (i.e., greater activity for equivalent performance) in older relative to younger subjects across a large area of cortex during encoding and maintenance epochs of the task. Moreover, the spatial patterns of response in younger subjects were more similar to the pattern observed in higher performing than lower performing older adults; a finding clearly inconsistent with a compensatory account.

From the earliest report of Grady and colleagues (1994), dedifferentiation of neural response in older relative to younger adults has been one of the most ubiquitous findings in the cognitive neuroscience of aging. The robustness of this finding suggests that neural dedifferentiation and its various manifestations (e.g. contralateral, unique, or substitutive recruitment) may serve as reliable neural markers of cognitive aging. Moreover, this account is consistent with the proposal of Baltes and Lindenberger (1997), who have argued that cognitive

performance becomes increasingly dedifferentiated across the lifespan as representational schemas become increasingly degraded. Unfortunately, the neural dedifferentiation account is ambivalent with respect to the behavioral correlates of these functional brain changes. Thus its potential clinical utility as an assessment marker or an intervention target is limited. While neural dedifferentiation is an influential brain-based theory, it remains a descriptive rather than a predictive account of cognitive aging. In the next section we review evidence for an alternative neural mechanism of age-related cognitive decline, reduced neuromodulatory capacity, and suggest that, unlike dedifferentiation, this account leads to robust, reliable, and behaviorally relevant neural markers for assessing cognitive changes in aging.

Neuromodulation

As reviewed briefly above, cognitive theorists have posited a duality of behavioral decline in cognitive aging with relatively preserved representations and degraded control processing. While neural dedifferentiation is consistent with this behavioral profile, we have argued for its utility as a descriptive rather than a mechanistic account of cognitive aging. An alternate account argues that age-related reduction in the top-down modulation of neural representations serves as a central mechanism of cognitive aging. Consistent with this theory, Payer et al. (2006) reported reduced selectivity in neural responses in category-selective regions of visual association cortex in older relative to younger subjects during a working memory task. This reduced selectivity of neural response was accompanied by enhanced activity in PFC, which the authors interpreted as compensatory modulation of VAC regions in response to degraded representations. Gazzaley et al. (2005) reported a similar pattern of age-related deficits in the modulation of neural responses within the VAC. The authors observed age-related reductions in goal-directed modulation of posterior cortices that resulted in poor filtering of goal-irrelevant stimuli and subsequent impairments on a recognition memory paradigm. Using computational modeling techniques, Li and colleagues (2001, 2002) demonstrated that impaired modulatory capacity attenuates neural responsiveness to afferent signaling in posterior brain regions, producing poorly regulated (i.e. noisy) information processing. Resultant reductions in signal-to-noise ratios effectively degrade the integrity of mental representations, thus reducing the quality of information throughput to higher cognitive processes. Thus, reduced modulatory capacity should preferentially impact those domains dependent upon the highest levels of representational integrity, including episodic memory encoding and retrieval, selective attention, and working memory, and these are indeed considered to be amongst the most vulnerable to age-related decline.

Mechanistically, Li et al. (2001, 2002) emphasize the role of dopamine in modulating the integrity of neural representations through top down biasing of goal-relevant versus irrelevant representations. This biasing mechanism serves to allocate limited cognitive resources to goal-relevant information processing. The importance of dopaminergic modulation has recently been demonstrated by Erixon-Lindroth and colleagues (2005) who measured the extent of dopamine transport mechanisms in the striatum and observed a strong positive correlation with episodic memory and executive functioning in young, healthy subjects. Recently, we observed increased functional connectivity between lateral PFC and VAC regions during goal-directed responding on a selective working memory task (Gazzaley et al. 2007), suggesting that top down modulation may be implemented through multiple neural mechanisms, each of which may be implicated in cognitive aging.

In contrast to dedifferentiation, neuromodulation theory extends beyond descriptions of functional brain changes to propose a more mechanistic account of cognitive aging in which dynamic functional interactions between control operations and representational integrity is a central feature. Thus alterations in the efficiency of control processes, the integrity of the neural representations upon which they operate, or the strength of the functional and structural connections supporting these interactions may each serve as neural markers of age-related cognitive decline. Moreover, unlike dedifferentiation theory, neuromodulation is not concerned with overall differences in the quantity of task-related neural activity, but rather the relative responses to goal-relevant versus irrelevant representations between young and old. Thus, it is equally plausible that poor modulation of neural representations will result in increases (e.g. poor suppression) or decreases (e.g. poor enhancement) in neural activity. It is this emphasis on relative versus absolute differences in functional brain response that facilitates the development of behaviorally meaningful neural markers which can, in turn, serve as brain-based metrics for assessing age-related cognitive decline. In the next section we review work ongoing in our laboratory to develop three of these neural markers based upon the neuromodulation theory of cognitive aging.

Measuring Age-related Cognitive Decline—A Functional Neural Marker Approach

There is now compelling evidence for functional brain changes in healthy aging. In the previous section we reviewed the two prominent brain-based theories of age-related cognitive decline, dedifferentiation, and neuromodulation, and argued that only the latter provides a sufficiently mechanistic account of functional brain changes in aging to serve as the basis for the development of clinically relevant neural markers. In this section we describe a functional-imaging based approach to defining specific markers of cognitive aging that emerge from a neuromodulation account of age-related cognitive decline. These functional markers can be used to complement behavioral and structural brain measures, thus informing clinical assessments and setting the stage for the design of targeted treatment protocols. Here we describe the central features of this approach.

Theory and Mechanisms

Developing functional neural markers of age-related cognitive decline requires a coherent theoretical account of how cognitive processes most susceptible to aging are implemented in the brain. Building upon the behavioral theories of cognitive aging which posit a relative decline in controlled processing and the functional neuroimaging findings of poor PFC modulation of neural responses within posterior cortices, we theorize that impaired neuromodulation is a central feature of the functional brain changes observed in healthy aging. As described above, top down modulation enhances the integrity of mental representations providing a critical mechanism for biasing limited capacity resources towards goal-relevant representations while filtering irrelevant information. Poor modulation would thus lead to distractibility, behavioral inflexibility, and loss of strategic control over mnemonic processing, each of which is a common behavioral consequence of cognitive aging (Park et al. 2001).

Neuromodulation is likely an emergent property of functional interactions between frontal and posterior brain regions. In this account, control processes associated with lateral PFC function influence representational architectures within domain-specific posterior cortical regions, in a top-down or goal-directed manner. It is now well established that prefrontal cortex, and specifically its lateral aspect, is extensively and reciprocally connected to posterior and subcortical cortices in humans (Petrides and Pandya 1999), providing the structural

architecture necessary for this region to implement top-down modulation. Yet, evidence of functional interaction between PFC and posterior brain regions has been slow to emerge. In one of the earliest reports, Fuster et al. (1985) cooled lateral PFC in non-human primates and recorded from sites in a higher visual processing region in inferior temporal cortex (ITC) while the animals performed a color working memory task. Cooling at either site resulted in both increased and decreased firing rates amongst cells in the other location, providing evidence that these regions are functionally connected. Moreover, cooling of lateral PFC diminished the task-related selectivity of neural responses within ITC to distinct color stimuli, consistent with a functional modulation account. Thus, perturbation of PFC altered the selectivity of neural response to bottom-up inputs in ITC, providing the first direct evidence that top-down modulation can influence the integrity of mental representations in posterior brain regions.

Chao and Knight (1995) tested this modulation hypothesis in a neuropsychological study of patients with lateral PFC lesions. Patients were asked to perform an auditory discrimination task with and without distractions, thus testing their capacity to effectively resolve goal-relevant from irrelevant stimuli. As predicted, frontal lesion patients were impaired on the task, but only during the distractor condition. This result is consistent with a role for the PFC in selectively modulating representations in a goal-directed manner. In a follow-up study, the authors obtained electrophysiological recordings from a sample of healthy older adults while they performed the same auditory discrimination task. As with the PFC lesion patients, performance of the older subjects was attenuated by the presence of distractions. Importantly, this decline was associated with reduced frontal but enhanced auditory functional brain response (Chao and Knight 1997). The authors argued that age-related reductions in PFC activity was associated with poor goal-directed modulation of responses to goal relevant versus irrelevant stimuli, resulting in poorer behavioral performance during the distractor condition and increased neural response in auditory processing regions.

In a recent functional MRI investigation, Park et al. (2004) compared the pattern of neural responses within visual association cortex to discrete categories of visual stimuli between younger and older adults. They observed a more diffuse pattern of response to the stimulus categories in older relative to younger adults, suggesting a loss in selectivity of neural responses to visual stimuli in visual association cortex. Consistent with the previous report by Fuster (1985), the researchers interpreted these findings as evidence for dedifferentiation of neural responses in older adults and hypothesized that these functional changes were secondary to structural changes occurring within frontal cortices and/or their connections to visual association cortex. These findings were recently replicated using a more attentionally demanding working memory task (Payer 2006).

Converging evidence from animal, human lesion, and functional neuroimaging investigations is consistent with a role for frontal cortex and frontally-mediated neural networks in modulating the integrity of neural representations within posterior brain regions in a top-down, goal-directed manner. This neuromodulatory account of goal-directed or top-down control processing has enabled us to develop specific neural markers that may be used to assess the neural basis of age-related cognitive decline. We describe three of these markers below.

Neural Markers of Cognitive Aging

Electrophysiological, neuropsychological and functional neuroimaging investigations have now highlighted the importance of frontally-mediated functional brain networks in cognitive control and suggest that age-related changes to these networks may serve as a marker of age-related cognitive decline. To this end we have been working to identify specific functional brain measures to measure top-down modulation and goal directed neural activity in young and older adults. Once validated, these neural markers may be used to characterize successful or, as importantly, unsuccessful aging.

Neural Marker 1: Goal-directed modulation of neural responses. Using an experimental protocol developed in our laboratory, we have demonstrated top-down modulation of posterior representational areas during encoding into working memory (Fiebach, Rissman, and D'Esposito 2006; Gazzaley, Cooney, Rissman, and D'Esposito 2005, Ranganath, DeGutis, and D'Esposito 2004, see Figure 1, marker 1). We asked younger adults to view four stimuli in random order, two faces and two scenes, while undergoing fMRI scanning. In different blocks of trials, they were instructed to remember the scenes and ignore the faces, remember the faces and ignore the scenes, or passively view both with no attempt to remember. Relative to passive viewing of the stimuli, activity in the parahippocampal place area (PPA) was greater in the remember scenes condition and less in the ignore scenes condition. Thus, activity within this region of visual association cortex was modulated by the goal of the task. Moreover, the extent of this modulation predicted subject performance on a subsequent recognition memory task such that attended stimuli were better recognized than those passively viewed, which were in turn recognized better than those stimuli which were ignored (Gazzaley, Cooney, McEvoy, Knight, and D'Esposito 2005).

In a subsequent study using this protocol (Gazzaley et al. 2005), older adults failed to show suppression of response within the PPA during the ignore scenes condition. Moreover, they rated the ignored scenes as significantly more familiar than the younger adults rated them on the post-experiment recognition test. This result revealed increased incidental long-term memory for distracting information, suggesting that poor modulation of neural responses to goal irrelevant stimuli had a measurable negative impact on mnemonic functioning in the older adults. Thus goal-directed modulation, or more specifically, goal-directed suppression, of neural response within visual association cortex provides a reliable neural marker of cognitive decline in healthy aging (see Figure 1).

Neural Marker 2: Goal-directed modulation of anterior to posterior functional connectivity. The extensive and reciprocal connectivity between frontal and posterior brain regions and its functional significance has been well established (Fuster et al. 1985). As described above, functional connectivity between frontal and posterior brain regions serves as a neural mechanism for goal-directed, or top-down modulation. Thus, alterations in the strength of these connections in response

to shifting goal states may represent a second candidate neural marker of top-down modulation. The inherently multivariate nature of fMRI data is ideally suited to investigate this functional connectivity and how anatomically disparate brain areas interact during cognitive tasks. Such interactions have typically been characterized by identifying regions that show correlated fluctuations in their fMRI time series data, with the assumption that temporal correlations in the BOLD signal reflect synchronous neural firing in the communicating, or "functionally connected," regions. We recently assessed functional connectivity during the face/scene memory task described above and observed that the PFC demonstrated greater functional connectivity with the posterior scene-selective area in the remember scenes condition (task-relevant) as compared to the ignore scenes (task-irrelevant) condition, providing evidence that functional connectivity is enhanced in a goal-directed manner (Gazzaley et al. 2007). Thus the strength of these functional connections in response to goal-directed processing provides a second neural marker of goal-directed processing that may be used to identify neurofunctional changes associated with age- or injury-related brain damage. We have obtained some support for the utility of this marker in a recent pilot study of an intervention protocol to enhance goal-directed processing in a sample of healthy older adults (see below and Figure 1, marker 2).

Neural Marker 3: Goal-directed sharpening of distributed neural representations. While these first two markers are consistent with a neuromodulatory account of cognitive aging, a more specific claim emerging out of the theoretical framework hypothesizes that reduced goal-directed modulation impairs the integrity of neural representations in posterior cortices, contributing to noisy processing and ultimately poor goal direction (e.g. Li and Lindenberger 2001; Fuster 1985). Thus, a more direct measure of the representational integrity of neural responses to goal relevant versus irrelevant stimuli may provide a more sensitive marker of neuromodulatory deficits in aging (see Figure 1, marker 3).

Recently, we identified a novel multivariate metric for assessing the integrity of goal relevant representations in the visual association cortex that capitalizes on the rich spatial and temporal information in fMRI data. We have applied multi-voxel pattern analysis (Norman, Polyn, Detre, and Haxby 2006) to fMRI data acquired during the face/scene working memory task we described earlier (see Norman et al. 2006 for a detailed review of MVPA analysis methods). In brief, MVPA uses a multi-layer, feed forward, back-propagation algorithm (i.e., a multi-level perceptron) to learn the pattern of neural responses within visual association cortex for faces and scene stimuli which are viewed during the four memory conditions of our task (i.e., remember faces,

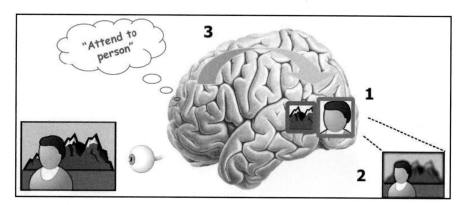

Figure 1 Schematic representation of functional markers of goal-directed neuromodulation. (1) Modulation of neural representations in visual association cortex (VAC) in response to top-down goal direction (enhancement of goal-relevant and suppression of goal-irrelevant stimulus features) (2) Functional connectivity between lateral prefrontal cortex and VAC is enhanced by goal-direction (3) Integrity of neural representations is enhanced for goal-relevant versus goal irrelevant stimuli.

remember scenes, remember both faces and scenes, and categorize the images as faces or scenes). The pattern classifier algorithm is trained on the patterns of neural responses associated with faces and scenes over multiple scan runs and experimental conditions and is then required to interpret the activation patterns (i.e., guess whether the person was viewing a scene or a face) in a novel set of data that was not included in the training set.

Based on the evidence that goal-directed neuromodulation enhances the representational integrity of goal-relevant versus irrelevant stimuli, we predicted that the integrity of neural representations for goal-relevant stimuli within category-selective regions of VAC would be enhanced relative to those stimuli that were goal-irrelevant (i.e., distractors). Thus classification accuracy, or the ability of the classification algorithm to learn and correctly guess the category of stimulus being viewed, would be higher for goal-relevant versus irrelevant stimuli. Our preliminary data in a sample of healthy young subjects is consistent with this account. In a pilot study of healthy older subjects, we failed to observe this pattern of an enhanced classification accuracy for goal-relevant stimuli, suggesting that the representational integrity for goal-relevant stimuli was not enhanced relative to the distractor stimuli in this sample. These data, while preliminary, suggest that pattern classification methods may be sensitive to age-related changes in the integrity of neural representations in posterior cortices, providing a potentially robust and sensitive marker of neurofunctional change associated with healthy aging.

In this section we have described three potential neural markers that may be used to assess neurofunctional changes in healthy aging. While validation of these markers is continuing, we argue that functional neuroimaging can be used to establish reliable functional neural markers of cognitive aging that will complement existing behavioral and structural measures, thereby leading to more comprehensive assessments of age-related cognitive decline. In the final section of the chapter we briefly describe how we have begun to utilize these functional neural markers in the design, implementation, and evaluation of a brain-based intervention to enhance goal-directed control processing in a cohort of healthy older subjects.

A Brain-based Approach to Remediate Age-related Cognitive Change

A theory-driven, brain-based approach to assessing age-related cognitive decline is crucial both for designing cognitive intervention therapies and measuring the efficacy of such therapies. Inappropriate outcome measures are as likely to result in 'negative' treatment trials as inappropriate treatments, and these failures are difficult to distinguish post hoc. To date, there has been little evidence that interventions to remediate age-related changes in cognition generalize to untrained domains or to real-world functional improvements (Salthouse 2007). We argue that strong prospective planning that includes clear delineation of the target cognitive and neural processes can lead to specific prescriptions, and matched measurements to gauge the expected cognitive and neural effects of those prescriptions. By isolating a core cognitive process (i.e., goal-directed modulation) and identifying the specific neural mechanisms and functional neural markers that characterize the implementation of this behavior in the brain using fMRI methods, we have designed a targeted cognitive intervention protocol to remediate age-related declines in this domain.

As outlined above, we have developed a theoretical framework to describe the implementation of goal directed processing in the brain (and see D'Esposito and Chen 2006; Gazzaley and D'Esposito 2007), We have used this framework to design and implement a comprehensive training protocol based on the Goal Management Training program (Levine et al. 2000). This protocol specifically targets top-down neuromodulation through an active process of re-direction of attention to goal-relevant processes, in effect, training participants to selectively filter "noise" (non-relevant information) via mindfulness-based attention regulation training. Thus the intervention is expressly targeted at the mechanism (neuromodulation) and the markers (enhancement/suppression, functional connectivity and representational integrity) we previously identified as central to goal-directed modulation. Unpublished data from our first pilot study implementing this protocol in a sample of healthy aging subjects is encouraging. We observed significant change from pre-post-intervention on each of our functional neural markers including greater suppression of neural response to distractor stimuli, greater goal-directed functional connectivity between PFC and visual association cortex, and enhanced representational integrity for goal-relevant stimuli from pre- to post-training. While preliminary, these results suggest that brain-based intervention protocols aimed at specific neural mechanisms may be an effective strategy for remediating age-related cognitive decline.

This brain-based approach to cognitive interventions represents the next step in the translation of functional neuroimaging methods into clinical practice. Consideration of both neural and behavioral outcome measures may provide a more comprehensive account of intervention efficacy. This strategy may allow us to push beyond behavioral measures of intervention success or failure to more rigorously assess the neural basis of treatment efficacy and thus continuously tune our interventions to maximize both neural and behavioral outcomes.

Conclusion

The functional neural marker approach described here represents a new frontier in characterizing, measuring, and ultimately treating deficits associated with cognitive aging. We contend that advances in functional neuroimaging methods and analyses have provided a unique *in vivo* window into the neural mechanisms of cognitive aging that will lead to an expanding array of diagnostic markers and treatment targets. While cognitive psychology has laid the groundwork for understanding age-related cognitive decline through an emphasis on theory and measurement, cognitive neuroscience is now well placed to build on this foundation through its focus on neural mechanisms and functional neural markers of cognitive aging. The importance of such an integrated approach to the assessment of age-related cognitive decline is perhaps most salient in efforts to design efficacious treatments to slow or remediate cognitive changes associated with healthy or pathological aging.

References

Baltes, P. B., and Lindenberger, U. (1997). Emergence of a powerful connection between sensory and cognitive functions across the adult life span: A new window to the study of cognitive aging? *Psychol Aging, 12*(1), 12–21.

Buckner, R. L. (2004). Memory and executive function in aging and AD: Multiple factors that cause decline and reserve factors that compensate. *Neuron, 44*(1), 195–208.

Cabeza, R., Anderson, N. D., Locantore, J. K., and McIntosh, A. R. (2002). Aging gracefully: compensatory brain activity in high-performing older adults. *Neuroimage, 17*(3), 1394–1402.

Cabeza, R., Daselaar, S. M., Dolcos, F., Prince, S. E., Budde, M., and Nyberg, L. (2004). Task-independent and task-specific age effects on brain activity during working memory, visual attention and episodic retrieval. *Cereb Cortex, 14*(4), 364–375.

Callicott, J. H., Bertolino, A., Mattay, V. S., Langheim, F. J., Duyn, J., Coppola, R., et al. (2000). Physiological dysfunction of the dorsolateral prefrontal cortex in schizophrenia revisited. *Cereb Cortex, 10*(11), 1078–1092.

Chao, L. L., and Knight, R. T. (1995). Human prefrontal lesions increase distractibility to irrelevant sensory inputs. *Neuroreport, 6*(12), 1605–1610.

Chao, L. L., and Knight, R. T. (1997). Prefrontal deficits in attention and inhibitory control with aging. *Cereb Cortex, 7*(1), 63–69.

Colcombe, S. J., Kramer, A. F., Erickson, K. I., and Scalf, P. (2005). The implications of cortical recruitment and brain morphology for individual differences in inhibitory function in aging humans. *Psychol Aging, 20*(3), 363–375.

Craik, F. I., and Bialystok, E. (2006). Cognition through the lifespan: Mechanisms of change. *Trends Cogn Sci, 10*(3), 131–138.

D'Esposito, M., and Chen, A. J. (2006). Neural mechanisms of prefrontal cortical function: Implications for cognitive rehabilitation. *Prog Brain Res, 157*, 123–139.

Davis, S. W., Dennis, N. A., Daselaar, S. M., Fleck, M. S., and Cabeza, R. (2008). Que PASA? The posterior-anterior shift in aging. *Cereb Cortex, 18*(5), 1201–1209.

Erixon-Lindroth, N., Farde, L., Wahlin, T. B., Sovago, J., Halldin, C., and Backman, L. (2005). The role of the striatal dopamine transporter in cognitive aging. *Psychiatry Res, 138*(1), 1–12.

Fiebach, C. J., Rissman, J., and D'Esposito, M. (2006). Modulation of inferotemporal cortex activation during verbal working memory maintenance. *Neuron, 51*(2), 251–261.

Fuster, J. M., Bauer, R. H., and Jervey, J. P. (1985). Functional interactions between inferotemporal and prefrontal cortex in a cognitive task. *Brain Res, 330*(2), 299–307.

Gazzaley, A., Cooney, J. W., McEvoy, K., Knight, R. T., and D'Esposito, M. (2005). Top-down enhancement and suppression of the magnitude and speed of neural activity. *J Cogn Neurosci, 17*(3), 507–517.

Gazzaley, A., Cooney, J. W., Rissman, J., and D'Esposito, M. (2005). Top-down suppression deficit underlies working memory impairment in normal aging. *Nat Neurosci, 8*(10), 1298–1300.

Gazzaley, A., and D'Esposito, M. (2007). Top-down modulation and normal aging. *Ann N Y Acad Sci, 1097*, 67–83.

Gazzaley, A., Rissman J., Cooney, J. Rutman, A., Seibert, T., Clapp, W., and D'Esposito, M. (2007). Functional interactions between prefrontal and visual association cortex contribute to top-down modulation of visual processing. *Cerebral Cortex, 17*:i125–135.

Grady, C. L. (1996). Age-related changes in cortical blood flow activation during perception and memory. *Ann N Y Acad Sci, 777*, 14–21.

Grady, C. L. (2008). Cognitive neuroscience of aging. *Ann N Y Acad Sci, 1124*, 127–144.

Grady, C. L., Maisog, L. M., Horwitz, B., Ungerleider, L. G., Mentis, M. J., Salerno, J. A., et al. (1994). Age-related changes in cortical blood flow activation during visual processing of faces and location. *Journal of Neuroscience, 14*, 1450–1462.

Greenwood, P. M. (2007). Functional plasticity in cognitive aging: Review and hypothesis. *Neuropsychology, 21*(6), 657–673.

Gutchess, A. H., Welsh, R. C., Hedden, T., Bangert, A., Minear, M., Liu, L. L., et al. (2005). Aging and the neural correlates of successful picture encoding: Frontal activations compensate for decreased medial-temporal activity. *J Cogn Neurosci, 17*(1), 84–96.

Hasher, L. and Zacks, R. T. (1988). Working memory, comprehension, and aging: A review and a new view. In G. H. Brower (Ed.), *The psychology of learning and motivation* (pp. 193–225). San Diego, CA: Academic Press.

Hazlett, E. A., Buchsbaum, M. S., Mohs, R. C., Spiegel-Cohen, J., Wei, T. C., Azueta, R., et al. (1998). Age-related shift in brain region activity during successful memory performance. *Neurobiol Aging, 19*(5), 437–445.

Hedden, T. and Gabrieli, J. D. (2004). Insights into the ageing mind: A view from cognitive neuroscience. *Nat Rev Neurosci, 5*(2), 87–96.

Levine, B., Robertson, I. H., Clare, L., Carter, G., Hong, J., Wilson, B. A., et al. (2000). Rehabilitation of executive functioning: an experimental-clinical validation of goal management training. *J Int Neuropsychol Soc, 6*(3), 299–312.

Li, S. C., Lindenberger, U., and Sikstrom, S. (2001). Aging cognition: From neuromodulation to representation. *Trends Cogn Sci, 5*(11), 479–486.

Li, S. C. and Sikstrom, S. (2002). Integrative neurocomputational perspectives on cognitive aging, neuromodulation, and representation. *Neurosci Biobehav Rev, 26*(7), 795–808.

Madden, D. J., Spaniol, J., Whiting, W. L., Bucur, B., Provenzale, J. M., Cabeza, R., et al. (2007). Adult age differences in the functional neuroanatomy of visual attention: a combined fMRI and DTI study. *Neurobiol Aging, 28*(3), 459–476.

Mattay, V. S., Fera, F., Tessitore, A., Hariri, A. R., Berman, K. F., Das, S., et al. (2006). Neurophysiological correlates of age-related changes in working memory capacity. *Neurosci Lett, 392*(1–2), 32–37.

McDowell, S., Whyte, J., and D'Esposito, M. (1998). Differential effect of a dopaminergic agonist on prefrontal function in traumatic brain injury patients. *Brain, 121* (Pt 6), 1155–1164.

McIntosh, A. R., Sekuler, A. B., Penpeci, C., Rajah, M. N., Grady, C. L., Sekuler, R., et al. (1999). Recruitment of unique neural systems to support visual memory in normal aging. *Current Biology, 9*(21), 1275–1278.

Moscovitch, M., and Winocur, G. (1992). The neuropsychology of memory and aging. In T. A. Salthouse & F. I. M. Craik (Eds.), *The handbook of aging and cognition* (pp. 315–372). Hillsdale, NJ: Erlbaum.

Norman, K. A., Polyn, S. M., Detre, G. J., and Haxby, J. V. (2006). Beyond mind-reading: Multi-voxel pattern analysis of fMRI data. *Trends Cogn Sci, 10*(9), 424–430.

Park, D. C., Polk, T. A., Mikels, J. A., Taylor, S. F., and Marshuetz, C. (2001). Cerebral aging: Integration of brain and behavioral models of cognitive function. *Dialogues in Clinical Neuroscience, 3*(3).

Park, D. C., Polk, T. A., Park, R., Minear, M., Savage, A., and Smith, M. R. (2004). Aging reduces neural specialization in ventral visual cortex. *Proc Natl Acad Sci U S A, 101*(35), 13091–13095.

Park, D. C., and Reuter-Lorenz, P. (2009). The adaptive brain: Aging and neurocognitive scaffolding. *Annu Rev Psychol, 60*, 173–196.

Payer, D., Marshuetz, C., Sutton, B., Hebrank, A., Welsh, R. C., and Park, D. C. (2006). Decreased neural specialization in old adults on a working memory task. *Neuroreport, 17*(5), 487–491.

Persson, J., Nyberg, L., Lind, J., Larsson, A., Nilsson, L. G., Ingvar, M., et al. (2006). Structure-function correlates of cognitive decline in aging. *Cereb Cortex, 16*(7), 907–915.

Petrides, M., and Pandya, D. N. (1999). Dorsolateral prefrontal cortex: Comparative cytoarchitectonic analysis in the human and the macaque brain and corticocortical connection patterns. *Eur J Neurosci, 11*(3), 1011–1036.

Ranganath, C., DeGutis, J., and D'Esposito, M. (2004). Category-specific modulation of inferior temporal activity during working memory encoding and maintenance. *Brain Res Cogn Brain Res, 20*(1), 37–45.

Reuter-Lorenz, P. A., Jonides, J., Smith, E. E., Hartley, A., Miller, A., Marshuetz, C., et al. (2000). Age differences in the frontal lateralization of verbal and spatial working memory revealed by PET. *J Cogn Neurosci, 12*(1), 174–187.

Reuter-Lorenz, P. A., and Lustig, C. (2005). Brain aging: Reorganizing discoveries about the aging mind. *Curr Opin Neurobiol, 15*(2), 245–251.

Rosen, A. C., Prull, M. W., O'Hara, R., Race, E. A., Desmond, J. E., Glover, G. H., et al. (2002). Variable effects of aging on frontal lobe contributions to memory. *Neuroreport, 13*(18), 2425–2428.

Rossi, S., Miniussi, C., Pasqualetti, P., Babiloni, C., Rossini, P. M., and Cappa, S. F. (2004). Age-related functional changes of prefrontal cortex in long-term memory: A repetitive transcranial magnetic stimulation study. *J Neurosci, 24*(36), 7939–7944.

Rypma, B., and D'Esposito, M. (1999). The roles of prefrontal brain regions in components of working memory: Effects of memory load and individual differences. *Proc Natl Acad Sci U S A, 96*(11), 6558–6563.

Rypma, B., and D'Esposito, M. (2000). Isolating the neural mechanisms of age-related changes in human working memory. *Nat Neurosci, 3*(5), 509–515.

Salthouse, T. A. (1996). The processing-speed theory of adult age differences in cognition. *Psychol Rev, 103*(3), 403–428.

Salthouse, T. A. (2007). Comment on Greenwood (2007): Functional plasticity in cognitive aging. *Neuropsychology, 21*(6), 678–679; discussion 680–673.

Turner, G. R., and Levine, B. (2008). Augmented neural activity during executive control processing following diffuse axonal injury. *Neurology, 71*(11), 812–818.

Velanova, K., Lustig, C., Jacoby, L. L., and Buckner, R. L. (2007). Evidence for frontally mediated controlled processing differences in older adults. *Cereb Cortex, 17*(5), 1033–1046.

Zarahn, E., Rakitin, B., Abela, D., Flynn, J., and Stern, Y. (2007). Age-related changes in brain activation during a delayed item recognition task. *Neurobiol Aging, 28*(5), 784–798.

10 Electroencephalography and Evoked Potentials in Geriatrics

Barry S. Oken and Alexandra Amen

Electroencephalography (EEG) consists of dynamic voltage fluctuations that represent field potentials generated by cortical neurons. The most common EEG application evaluates free running cerebral activity as a measure of cerebral physiology. The EEG can be evaluated visually as the standard clinical approach, or more quantitatively based on digital signal processing. Field potentials that represent a time-locked response to a stimulus are referred to as evoked potentials and are a more focused measure of subcortical and peripheral as well as cortical physiology. For clinical purposes, the stimuli used to elicit EPs are usually exogenous, e.g. a click in the ear or an electrical stimulation of a peripheral nerve. Higher levels of attentional processing may also serve as endogenous stimuli. For example, if several auditory stimuli are presented, the stimuli that are different based on task demands may elicit different potentials. The two physiologic techniques, EEG and evoked potentials, will be reviewed separately in this chapter.

EEG

The EEG is a reflection of cerebral cortical activity that is heavily dependent on the state of arousal, which reflects the state of the thalamocortical projections as well as the other relatively non-specific cortical projection systems (Oken et al. 2006; Steriade, McCormick, and Sejnowski 1993). For example, people with a strong sleep tendency of any cause have different frequencies in their EEG. The EEG has two aspects that will be discussed separately. The background EEG activity consists of dynamically fluctuating waveforms of various frequencies and amplitudes over the different head regions. The EEG also may contain episodic paroxysmal discharges, referred to as epileptiform activity, which may be related to the presence of epilepsy but may also be seen in other disorders.

The EEG is generally recorded by placing electrodes on the scalp, although in special circumstances invasive electrodes (subdural and intracortical) or magnetoencephalography, a technique measuring the magnetic rather than electrical fields produced in the brain, may be performed (Papanicolaou et al. 2005). Magnetoencephalography has not gained wide clinical use in the geriatric population and will not be discussed further. For the same reason, we will not review very low frequency EEG (near direct current signals less than 1.0 Hz), or high frequency—above 32 Hz (gamma frequency). The EEG recording for clinical purposes has the best quality when performed by trained and registered EEG technologists. Interpretation of EEG is more subjective than other clinical lab tests in part because the interpretation is based primarily on visualization of the EEG, a practice not dissimilar to that in radiology. However, there is reasonably good inter-rater reliability between neurologists who are fellowship trained and certified in EEG or clinical neurophysiology. Quantitative EEG (QEEG) assigns numbers to components of the EEG based on various signal processing algorithms such as frequency analysis. QEEG is better suited as a measure of cerebral physiology for many research purposes but still has not gained wide use in clinical EEG (Nuwer 1997). There are textbooks on the physiology, performance, and clinical interpretation of EEG (Niedermeyer and da Silva 2004).

Most adults in the awake state have posteriorly dominant rhythmic EEG activity that increases in amplitude with eyes closed, referred to as the posterior rhythm. The posterior rhythm has a peak frequency in the alpha (8–13 Hz) range. Slow frequencies are grouped as theta (4–8 Hz) and delta (1–4 Hz), and such activity is not common in normal awake adult EEGs. Delta frequency activity is considered an abnormality in awake adults but some low amplitude fronto-central delta may be seen during drowsy transitions in elders (Santamaria and Chiappa 1987).

Other activity generated by sources near to the brain may confound EEG interpretations. Significant head movement or facial muscle contraction may obscure the EEG signal, though eye blinks and other eye movements are common artifacts that only rarely impede interpretation. While patients with Parkinson's disease may have decreased blinks, tremors may produce rhythmic artifact on the EEG at the same frequency as the tremor. EEG recordings in intensive care units are sensitive to 60 Hz line frequency, movement and vibration artifacts caused by ventilators, infusions pumps, and electrical beds, and thus the expertise of a trained EEG technologist is especially required to minimize such artifacts.

The EEG portion of this chapter will be divided into sections reflecting the most common changes: Both focal and generalized frequency changes (usually slowing), and epileptiform patterns.

Focal Slowing

Temporal Slowing

Focal slowing in younger adults is generally suggestive of a focal brain lesion interrupting normal EEG activity. While focal slowing in older adults may have a similar etiology, episodic temporal slowing in the elderly is not necessarily associated with a specific lesion or pathology, and has repeatedly been shown to be present in overtly healthy subjects (Holschneider and Leuchter 1999; Oken and Kaye 1992; Shigeta et al. 1995; see Figure 1). Episodic slow activity in temporal regions, more frequent on the left side of the brain although with a shifting laterality, is common in the aging population. Beginning in approximately the sixth decade of life, elderly populations have episodic temporal slowing with a prevalence of 17–59% (Holschneider and Leuchter 1999; Arenas 1986; Oken and Kaye 1992), demonstrated through the use of both visual EEG (Shigeta et al. 1995) and QEEG (Prichep 2007) analysis. The slow waves are intermittent, sporadic, and are attenuated during active mental states. In contrast, they may increase in prevalence during drowsiness (Klass and Brenner 1995).

Temporal slowing in the elderly may be positively correlated with MRI white matter hyperintensities (Oken and Kaye 1992) although

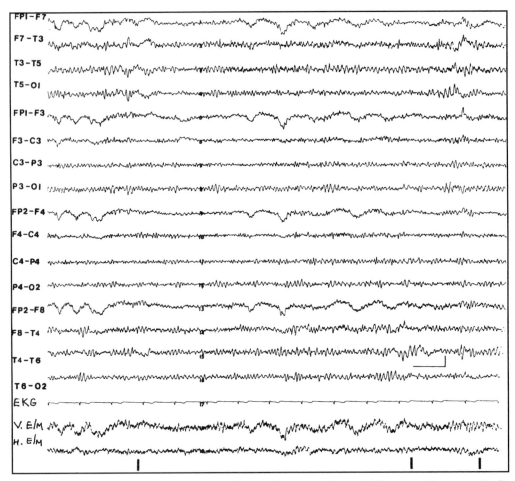

Figure 1 Temporal slowing. Temporal slowing as demonstrated via a 15-second segment of bipolar EEG recorded from a healthy 91-year-old woman. ECG, vertical and horizontal eye movement channels, and a 1-second 50 μV calibration mark are shown. Vertical marks at the bottom denote three episodes of temporal slowing, the first and the third being primarily left-sided and the second being right-sided. Note that the subject is awake, evidenced by the presence of vertical eye movements, the absence of slow lateral eye movements, and the persistence of the subject's 8 Hz posterior rhythm.

this is not a consistent finding (Shigeta et al. 1995). Evidence is controversial as to whether it is associated with age-related anatomical brain changes such as increased ventricle size (Solomon 1998; Shigeta et al. 1995). Increased hypertension has been hypothesized to play a role in the occurrence of focal slowing (Visser 1991). However, the presence of hypertension is not necessary to observe temporal slowing in the elderly (Holschneider and Leuchter 1999; Oken and Kaye 1992).

Most commonly, performance on neuropsychological measures has been shown to have no correlation with the degree of focal temporal slowing present (Holschneider and Leuchter 1999; Shigeta et al. 1995; Oken and Kaye 1992). Such research suggests that temporal slow activity in the elderly is not clinically relevant in terms of cognitive decline. However, a small number of studies have indicated that the presence of temporal slowing may correlate with lower cognitive performance in elderly persons characterized as otherwise "healthy." In one example, Visser et al. (1987) were able to divide a cohort of healthy elderly subjects (65–83 years of age) who had been pre-screened to exclude psychiatric, neurological, metabolic, and cardiovascular diseases into one group that exhibited left temporal focal slowing, and another group that did not. The group with temporal slow activity performed significantly less well on a verbal fluency task than did the group without these focal abnormalities. Such findings suggest that temporal slowing in the aged population is not benign, but instead an indication of potential early pathology.

Temporal Slowing and Dementia

Though temporal slow activity is observed in healthy elderly subjects, it can be seen to an even greater extent in patients diagnosed with Alzheimer's disease (AD). Subjects with both AD and mild cognitive impairment (MCI) exhibit a significantly greater degree of focal temporal slowing than healthy age-matched controls (Prichep 2007; Rice et al. 1990). Temporal abnormalities (specifically left hypometabolism) have been observed using PET in patients with AD, and have been correlated with EEG measures of temporal slowing. Therefore, such EEG changes could be a result of temporal hypometabolism in AD (Buchan et al. 1997; Miller et al. 1987). Significant increases in transient temporal slowing have also been demonstrated in patients with Lewy body dementia (Briel et al. 1999) and in Parkinson's disease with dementia (Korczyn 2001). Focal abnormalities (though not specific) are common as well in cases of vascular dementia (Jeong 2004). Such research again supports the idea that perhaps temporal slowing in the elderly may be a sign of early pathologic changes associated with dementia. It is reasonable that abnormal temporal activity would be associated with temporal lobe deficits. However, because delta and theta waves in low levels are present in most EEGs, it is difficult to know when the presence of temporal slowing may be normal (or a result of normal aging) and when temporal slowing may be a sign of early pathology (Holschneider and Leuchter 1999). The next step in research related to these issues will be to perform longitudinal studies following clinically normal, healthy elderly subjects who exhibit

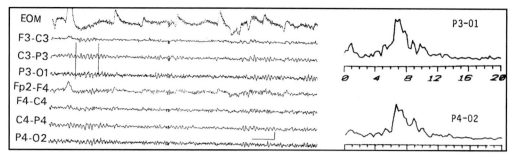

Figure 2 Posterior alpha slowing. *Left* Evidence of posterior rhythm slowing in an 8-channel EEG segment from a healthy 80-year-old subject with an MMSE score of 30. The subject is awake, which can be determined by the presence of eye blinks. Lower right calibration mark is 1 second and 50 μV. A 7 Hz posterior rhythm is demonstrated through the 1 second segment marked on the left side of the figure. *Right* Average spectra from the same subject across 1.5 to 20 Hz with a 0.25 Hz resolution from the P3-O1 and P4-O2 channels. The peak-power frequency was 7 Hz in the average spectra and using visual analysis, and 7.6 Hz using QEEG techniques.

temporal slowing, and to observe at what levels focal slowing may tend to precede more severe dementia.

Generalized Frequency Changes

Slow Activity

By around the fifth decade of life, generalized changes are apparent in the EEG (Dustman et al. 1993). Early studies described generalized EEG slowing in the elderly, as evidenced by an increase in delta and theta activity and a decrease in overall EEG frequency, to be a result of normal aging. However, many such findings stemmed from the failure to control for cognitive state and use of medications. Current research shows that "healthy" aging actually does not involve a pathologic increase in background EEG slow activity through age 80. Traditional visual EEG analysis in a population of pre-screened very healthy elderly up to the eighth and ninth decades of life has indicated no overall increase in slow wave occurrence or decrease in dominant frequency below 8 Hz (Shigeta et al. 1995). Based on such evidence, a significant increase in slow activity is considered to be indicative of encephalopathies, both in younger adults and the elderly population—in fact, generalized EEG slowing has been called the primary sign of pathology in the geriatric population without overt brain disease (Kaszniak et al. 1979).

Using QEEG, several observations involving slow waves and aging have been made. Frequency analysis has indicated an increase in posterior relative theta power in the very healthy elderly over 85 years of age (Oken and Kaye 1992). In terms of more general activity, the elderly population (71–90 years old) exhibited an increase in relative delta activity but a less clear change in relative theta activity (Dustman, Shearer, and Emmerson 1999). The results of these studies on very healthy elders imply that background EEG slowing in the elderly, at least until around 85 years of age, should be seen as potentially clinically significant, and not merely a by-product of aging.

Alpha and Beta Activity

Alpha (8–13 Hz) and beta (13–32 Hz) activity are affected by the aging process. Overall, alpha wave amplitude tends to decrease with age (Obrist 1954) and the mean frequency of posterior alpha rhythm and the alpha amplitude appears to decrease starting in the fifth decade of life (Holschneider and Leuchter 1999; Roubicek 1977; Dustman, Shearer, and Emmerson 1999; Oken and Kaye 1992) (see Figure 2). Some QEEG research suggests that healthy elders maintain their posterior alpha rhythm frequency at or above 8 Hz through the aging process up to the oldest old (Dustman, Shearer, and Emmerson 1999; Smith 1989). "Alpha blocking" refers to the fact that in response to sensory (particularly visual) and cognitive stimulation, alpha activity and amplitude are dramatically decreased. Healthy elderly subjects do not show this reaction to the same extent as younger controls (Duffy et al. 1984).

In contrast, beta amplitude is thought to increase with normal aging over a wide age spectrum (Holschneider and Leuchter 1999; Holschneider and Leuchter 1995). Original studies noted that an increase in beta wave amplitude was correlated with cognitive decline when looking at a range of aging subjects (Duffy et al. 1984). However, most current research suggests that such an increase (particularly in the frontocentral regions of the brain) is associated with stable or even increased cognitive performance in the elderly. Use of QEEG has demonstrated a significant positive correlation between beta activity and cognitive performance during laboratory tasks (Williamson et al. 1990). In fact, cognitive impairment in the elderly has been shown to be related to reduced beta amplitude as compared to healthy age-matched controls. Williamson et al. (1990) observed a significant positive correlation between beta activity and cognitive performance using QEEG in 53 healthy elderly subjects, and a significant decrease in beta activity in 5 elderly subjects showing signs of early cognitive decline as determined by neuropsychological testing.

Generalized Changes in Dementia

AD is one of the most common pathologic dementias studied with EEG. It is clear that patients suffering from AD exhibit a significantly higher rate of EEG abnormalities than healthy controls, unaffected by the presence of possible concurrent psychological disorders such as depression (Brenner, Reynolds, and Ulrich 1989). Using traditional visual EEG analysis, patients with AD tend to show an overall slowing of EEG frequencies with an increase in theta and delta activity and a decrease in alpha and beta activity. QEEG analysis demonstrates a similar trend, with theta and delta power increases and alpha and beta power decreases in cases of AD (Jeong 2004; Holschneider and Leuchter 1999; Claus et al. 1998). Alpha power specifically tends to decrease to a significantly greater degree in AD patients carrying the ApoE epsilon4 allele (Ponomareva, Korovaitseva, and Rogaev 2008). The slowing is observed in both early and late-onset AD, but they may have different spatial distributions (Duffy et al. 1984). In response to photic stimulation, patients with AD tend to show smaller changes in EEG power between rest and stimulus conditions, and lower alpha and beta powers during stimulus conditions (Wada et al. 1997). In terms of the effects of AD drug therapies, responsiveness to acetylcholinesterase inhibitors has been positively correlated with short-term memory increase, alpha power increase, theta power decrease, and alpha-theta power ratio (Adler et al. 2004; Lanctot, Herrmann, and LouLou 2003).

EEG and QEEG changes associated with AD are directly related to the severity of the disease. The Mini-Mental State Examination (MMSE) and other neuropsychological test scores are significantly correlated with EEG abnormality in AD even in situations of minimal impairment (van der Hiele 2007a; van der Hiele 2007b; Babiloni et al.

2006; Kowalski et al. 2001; Robinson, Merskey, and Blume 1994; Brenner et al. 1988; Reynolds, and Ulrich 1988). Additionally, the clinical decline of patients with mild to severe cases of AD is mirrored by changes in the EEG. The earliest EEG changes associated with AD tend to include an increase in theta and decrease in beta activity. This is followed by a decrease in alpha activity, and finally, in the most severe stages of the disease, an increase in delta activity (Jeong 2004). Longitudinal studies have demonstrated this relationship between disease progression (as measured via cognitive testing) and EEG. In a 2.5 year follow-up study of patients with AD, specific changes in the various frequency wave activities of the EEG were shown to be predictive of the patient's cognitive decline as assessed by neuropsychological measures, as well as particular stage and severity of the disease (Coben et al. 1985). It has also been shown to be possible to distinguish between patients suffering from MCI, patients with AD, and control subjects, using QEEG. Specifically, an increase in theta and a decrease in alpha powers are suggested as the best distinguishing features between AD as compared to MCI and control groups (van der Hiele 2007; Huang et al. 2000). Despite these group observations, the conventional clinical EEG is often normal in early AD. Thus normal EEG background frequencies on conventional EEG, and even QEEG, do not rule out a diagnosis of AD. Despite the poor sensitivity of the EEG, the specificity of abnormal background EEG slowing may be helpful. For example, background EEG slowing may help rule out depression as a primary cause of cognitive decline.

Previous studies have evaluated the idea of using EEG as a predictor of future dementia and AD. It has been suggested that not only the severity of the disease but the probability of decline itself can be predicted using EEG technology. Longitudinal studies have been performed using patients suffering from dementia, all of whom are initially assessed to be near the same levels of impairment using cognitive measures. Those patients who initially show greater EEG changes from the norm also experience greater cognitive decline between baseline and follow-up laboratory visits (Rossini et al. 2006; Helkala et al. 1991). In fact, using QEEG in a longitudinal study, Clause et al. (1998) demonstrated a correlation between increased theta and decreased alpha and beta powers and the probability of mortality in subjects with AD. Even more intriguing research has suggested EEG as a predictor of future cognitive decline for those without clinically diagnosed pathologies (Brickman et al. 2005; Prichep et al. 2006; van der Hiele et al. 2008). Prichep et al. (2006) evaluated 44 elderly subjects with no objective signs of dementia, but subjective complaints of cognitive deficits. Those subjects initially showing increased theta power and an overall decrease in dominant frequency underwent significantly greater cognitive decline as assessed at a 7–9 year follow-up.

Other EEG measures that are observed to be affected by AD include EEG complexity, coherence, and cordance (Jeong 2004). Coherence is a measure of the relationship in EEG recorded from different locations, with synchrony and cordance being measures related to coherence. Complexity is a systems science measure that tries to capture the number of interacting subcomponents necessary to produce an unpredictable signal. In AD patients, coherence (as studied using QEEG technology) is affected presumably because of a reduction in neuronal signaling related to AD, leading to less functional connectivity and decreased interaction between certain regions of the brain. Specifically, AD results in decreased coherence of alpha and beta powers across the cortex (Jelles et al. 2008; Locatelli et al. 1998; Dunkin et al. 1994; Leuchter 1992). It is potentially interesting to note that theta and delta power coherence do not significantly change in varying levels of dementia in AD, suggesting that AD affects brain connectivity differently across the various physiological processes giving rise to separate frequencies (Jelles et al. 2008). Coherence has been demonstrated to

decrease in vascular dementia as well as AD. Interestingly, coherence evaluated via long corticocortical fibers is significantly decreased in AD but not vascular dementia, while coherence evaluated via broad connective networks shows a larger decrease in patients with vascular dementia. These finding have clinical implications in terms of differential nervous system changes in AD and vascular dementia, and in terms of accurate diagnosis of pathologies (Leuchter et al. 1992).

Though here we have focused primarily on dementia related to AD, pathologic conditions such as vascular dementia (Signorino 1995) and Parkinson's disease (Korczyn 2001) are also associated with generalized slowing of the EEG. Soikkeli et al. (1991) demonstrated a significant overall increase in theta activity and a decrease in dominant overall frequency in Parkinson's patients (with and without dementia) as compared to control subjects. Parkinson's patients with dementia also exhibited a significant increase in delta activity as compared to both controls and Parkinson's patients without dementia. Patients with transient global amnesia (TGA), in both the acute and later stages, tend to show an increase in beta activity, and a decrease in beta frequency (Tikhonova et al. 2003). Metabolic encephalopathies also produce an increase in slowing. Overall, given the various etiologies of cognitive dysfunction, it is not surprising that they each would lead to multiple and overlapping changes in overall EEG patterns. However, because each condition presumably gives rise to slightly different physiologic changes, one future aim will be the use of EEG in clearly differentiating between various pathologic conditions. For example, QEEG has demonstrated a significantly greater loss of beta power in AD than in vascular dementia (Holschneider et al. 1997) as well as a greater preservation of alpha power in occipital areas in vascular dementia than AD (Rosen et al. 1993). In addition, fronto-temporal dementia has been associated with smaller increases in slow wave activity but larger decreases in fast wave activity than is typically observed in AD (Lindau et al. 2003). Such findings may have clinical significance in terms of the use of EEG as an ancillary diagnostic tool in neurologic conditions associated with the geriatric population.

Pharmacology and the EEG

Background EEG frequencies may be affected by widely used and prescribed drugs. Certain central nervous system drugs, barbiturates, and benzodiazepines, tend to cause an increase in beta activity when administered in therapeutic doses. Generalized slowing may also be a result of the use of most central nervous system depressants. For example, neuroleptics and narcotic analgesics cause a decrease in alpha frequency and an increase in delta and theta slow wave activity. While tricyclic antidepressants are associated with an increase in slower frequencies, serotonin reuptake inhibitor antidepressants have little effect on the EEG. Lithium is the antidepressant with the most marked and consistent changes on the EEG, resulting in frontally maximal slowing and even epileptiform activity at therapeutic doses. Antiepileptic drugs may also cause slowing on the EEG, especially using QEEG (Meador et al. 2007; Salinsky et al. 2003). The changes caused by all these substances clearly necessitate that interpretation of an EEG on a patient or subject incorporates the knowledge of drug use.

Paroxysmal Activity

EEGs are often performed to assess the likelihood that a patient's intermittent symptoms may be related to seizures. The EEG changes that are most specific for epilepsy are epileptiform discharges. These waves are visually characterized as rapid voltage change that is more linear than the average EEG waveform and the waveform has a pointed peak. The common types of epileptiform discharges are spikes and sharp waves, the distinction between the two being whether the waveform duration is 20–70 msec (spikes) or 70–200 msec (sharp waves). While some sharp activity is pathologic, there is some sharp activity on the EEG that is not abnormal. The most common normal sharp activity consists of vertex waves and K complexes, which are centrally and frontally maximal, symmetric discharges seen during normal sleep. There are also some epileptiform-appearing discharges that are not associated with epilepsy, referred to as benign variants (Klass and Westmoreland 1985). Perhaps the least understood pattern is referred to as 'subclinical rhythmic electrographic discharge of adults' (SREDA) (Westmoreland and Klass 1981). This pattern generally includes rhythmic sharp waves, which later converge into a non-evolving theta rhythm and its resemblance to frank seizures have resulted in reference to both normal and abnormal SREDA patterns (Westmoreland and Klass 1997). While epileptiform activity that is not a benign variant may be related to the presence of epilepsy, it is not specific and there are other neurological disorders that may produce epileptiform activity as well.

Epilepsy

Patients with epilepsy may or may not have epileptiform discharges on their routine EEG. The sensitivity of a single, 30-minute EEG, i.e., the likelihood the EEG contains epileptiform discharges, is only 30–60%, although the sensitivity increases with repeated studies (Salinsky, Kanter, and Dasheiff 1987; Marsan and Zivin 1970). There are also some people who have epileptiform discharges on their EEG but have no history of seizures. This is seen in a very low percent of people (in younger adults, only 1–2%), and may even be occasionally associated with a family risk of epilepsy. The sensitivity of EEG for epilepsy can increase with activation techniques that increase the likelihood of the EEG containing epileptiform activity. Both sleep deprivation as well as recording transitions in and out of stage 1 sleep may increase the sensitivity. Photic stimulation and hyperventilation are other activating techniques that increase the likelihood of recording epileptiform discharges. These latter two techniques are best at activating primary generalized epilepsies, so are most critical for children and younger adults, but can also activate focal or secondary generalized epilepsies as well. The other method to increase the yield of an EEG for epileptiform activity or for frank seizure activity is to increase the EEG recording period. Patients who are having occasional clinical events may be monitored with 24-hour video EEG to capture the event visually as well by EEG. This is the most definitive way to determine whether a clinical event is a seizure or some non-epileptic event. Non-convulsive seizures in the intensive care unit may also be hard to diagnose and require long-term EEG monitoring (Jordan 1999). In general, seizures have characteristics in the EEG consisting of abrupt onset of a change, rhythmicity, evolution, abrupt offset, and post-ictal changes. Counterintuitively, these characteristic changes may be harder to detect in cases of status epilepticus because of the absence of non-seizure EEG.

While interictal epileptiform discharges are the most common, relatively specific abnormality for epilepsy, there are other patterns that may be seen as well. Paroxysmal slowing is the abrupt onset of higher amplitude slower frequency activity than is otherwise seen in the background EEG. Paroxysmal slowing may be related to epilepsy, but most paroxysmal slowing, including frontal intermittent rhythmic delta activity, is more likely secondary to non-epileptic encephalopathies such as metabolic encephalopathies. Generalized slowing may be seen post-ictally so this finding may occasionally be clinically relevant to seizures. Similarly, focal slowing is a marker for focal cerebral dysfunction. As such it may be related to cerebral infarcts or ischemia, tumor, or other lesions, but may also be seen following a focal seizure. However, EEG during episodes of TGA have indicated that while TGA patients exhibit a non-significant increase in sharp waves and bilaterally synchronized spikes, TGA is not believed to be epileptic in origin (Tikhonova et al. 2003). EEG is still used to evaluate some patients with transient cognitive dysfunction because such symptoms are occasionally secondary to complex partial seizures.

Dementia

Individuals at high risk for AD as assessed by ApoE epsilon4 allele presence tend to show greater synchronous high-voltage delta and theta activity and sharp wave occurrence in response to hyperventilation, as well a decrease in alpha and increase in slow wave relative powers (Ponomareva, Korovaitseva, and Rogaev 2008). However, AD and most of the neurodegenerative dementia syndromes only infrequently produce epileptiform activity on the EEG. In contrast, Creutzfeldt-Jakob disease often produces epileptiform discharges on the EEG, which are usually periodic. While most of the dementias may produce slowing on the EEG, the sensitivity of the EEG for Creutzfeldt-Jakob, i.e., the presence of periodic sharp waves on the EEG, is likely greater than 90% if several EEGs are obtained two months or more after symptom onset (Levy et al. 1986). These discharges are not indicative of ongoing epilepsy and have no obvious correlation to the myoclonus associated with CJD.

Acute Brain Lesions

Any acute brain lesion, most commonly strokes, may produce periodic lateralized epileptiform discharges (PLEDs) at a rate varying across etiologies but most often at about one per sec (Walsh and Brenner 1987). While the periodic discharges of CJD may be lateralized, there are many more common acute lesions that may produce PLEDS. Acute strokes, especially hemorrhagic may produce PLEDS. Herpes simplex encephalitis commonly produces either generalized slowing or focal temporal slowing but can produce periodic epileptiform discharges, with a repetition rate slower than the usual PLEDs, being only one per 2 to 4 seconds rather than about 1 per second.

Metabolic Encephalopathies

Patients with severe metabolic encephalopathies, especially hepatic and uremic, may have anteriorly predominant sharp waves with a triphasic morphology. While such patients may have increased likelihood of seizures because of their encephalopathy, these triphasic sharp waves do not necessarily imply the presence of seizures. While the specificity varies by exact morphology, triphasic sharp waves are not specific to metabolic encephalopathy.

Hypoxic-ischemic Encephalopathy

EEG is often used to assess patients with hypoxic-ischemic encephalopathy, most often due to cardiac arrest. The EEG is used to assess for possible seizures, especially in the presence of abnormal motor movements, and to help prognosticate. Two EEG patterns are helpful in negative prognostication: severe generalized attenuation of all EEG activity and the presence of a burst-suppression pattern. For prognostication purposes, the EEG needs to be obtained more than 24 hours after the causative event. The burst-suppression pattern consists of moderate to high amplitude EEG activity often with intermixed epileptiform activity alternating with episodes of generalized attenuation of all EEG activity. While burst-suppression pattern may be seen without an irreversible brain injury in patients on extremely high doses of sedatives, e.g., barbiturate infusions or high dose of general anesthetics, the presence of this pattern following a cardiac arrest has a grim prognosis (Synek 1988). Generalized attenuation of all EEG activity has a similar grim prognosis. Other types of epileptiform patterns or generalized slowing have limited prognostic significance. Sometimes, there may be motor activity during the burst of a burst suppression pattern.

Most commonly this is some myoclonic movement, but there may be more rhythmic epileptiform activity during the bursts associated with more rhythmic motor movements. Independent of the rhythmicity of the bursts, this pattern of myoclonus status has a grim prognosis (Wijdicks, Parisi, and Sharbrough 1994). Treating it with conventional antiepileptic drugs may decrease the motor symptoms, but given the refractory nature and grim prognosis, most would not treat it more aggressively with, for example, propofol infusions. The other electrophysiologic study that may be helpful at prognostication of coma is median nerve somatosensory evoked potentials (see below).

Evoked Potentials (EPs)

EPs are obtained by averaging the neural response to a stimulus. It requires many stimuli to elicit the EP potential that is time-locked to the stimulus, by averaging out the background EEG activity that is not time-locked to the stimulus. For example, brainstem auditory evoked potentials, which are about 1% the amplitude of the background EEG activity, may require averaging as many as 1000 post-stimulus epochs to eliminate the EEG not time-locked to the stimulus. Higher amplitude EPs, such as visual EPs and long-latency EPs, require averaging many fewer stimuli. Interpretation of EPs is more quantitative than EEG since the primary interpretation is simply based on latency and amplitude of the EP waveforms specific to the modality being tested. Nomenclature for EP waveforms is not completely standardized but often the waves are named by polarity (P for positive and N for negative) and latency (either the mean latency in controls, e.g., P100 for a positive wave at about 100 msec, or its position in a sequence of waves, e.g., P3 being the 3^z positive wave). There are textbooks and chapters on the physiology of EPs, performing EPs, and interpreting EPs that discuss these issues in more detail (Oken and Phillips 2008; Chiappa 1997).

Visual Evoked Potentials

The functionality of visual conduction pathways may be assessed through the study of visual evoked potentials (VEPs). VEPs are EPs useful in evaluating patients with possible visual dysfunction, since they depend on neural conduction from the eye to the visual cortex. In order to examine each conduction pathway separately, the left and right eyes are tested individually. The most reliable VEPs tend to be produced using pattern-reversal stimuli (e.g. a "checkerboard" pattern with alternating black and white squares), most commonly with checks at angles of 10 min to 1 degree, with a screen size of 15–20 degrees. VEPs may be elicited through other visual stimuli such as light flashes, but these waveforms tend to be more variable across individuals and thus have less clinical utility (Tobimatsu and Celesia 2006). Contrast sensitivity gratings are likely better than checkerboard patterns from a visual physiology perspective but have not gained wide use clinically.

Pattern-reversal VEPs occur as a negative-positive-negative waveform pattern maximal in amplitude midline and posteriorly, involving N75, P100, and N145 components. The P100 waveform (occurring about 100ms post stimulus onset) is the most consistent, and therefore is considered to be the most clinically useful of the peaks (Gilmore 1995; Tobimatsu 1994). The generator of the P100 has been located in the occipital cortex (Lesevre and Joseph 1979; Michael and Halliday 1971). Pattern-reversal VEPs are sensitive to inattention and drowsiness that lead to an attenuation of the expected waveforms. The characteristics of the waveforms are also affected by spatial and temporal frequency of the checkerboard pattern, as well as luminance and contrast (Oken and Phillips 2008; Tobimatsu and Celesia 2006).

Ocular pathologies, such as severe macular degeneration and cataracts, may result in a decrease of light transferred to the retina and may contribute to VEP changes associated with age. However, the age-related VEP changes seem to exceed what would be expected from purely ocular disease (Tobimatsu 1995). Overall, VEP component latencies increase in elderly populations (Tobimatsu 1995; Celesia 1987; Allison et al. 1984). Allison et al. (1984) evaluated age-related changes in pattern-reversal VEP waveforms using a population of subjects ranging from 4–95 years of age. While N75 latency showed a constant gradual increase with age, the P100 and N145 component latencies increased more noticeably after the age of 60. Given that the generator of the N75 is in the striate cortex, before the extrastriate generation of the P100 and N145, this suggests that age-related degeneration of the visual system occurs primarily in extrastriatal regions. Looking specifically at the P100 component, there is a generally observed 1–3ms increase in latency per decade, in part dependent on check size (Gilmore 1995; Sokol, Moskowitz, and Towle 1981). This could be the result of multiple age-related degenerative processes located anywhere from the retina to visual cortex. It is also important to take into account previously-mentioned pattern characteristics such as frequency, luminance, and contrast, particularly when testing elderly subjects. For example, it has been observed that a decrease in both luminance and contrast of checks in pattern-reversal stimuli leads to a significant increase in P100 latency in the elderly (Gilmore 1995).

In patients with dementia, both pattern-reversal and flash VEPs appear to be delayed (Visser et al. 1985; Wright, Harding, and Orwin 1984). A meta-analysis of VEPs in an elderly demented population showed significantly greater P100 latencies as compared to controls, particularly in response to pattern-reversal stimuli (Pollock et al. 1989). In terms of specific dementias, P100 latency appears to be delayed in both AD and vascular dementia as compared to controls (Sloan and Fenton 1992). In addition, overall prolonged VEP latencies are commonly observed in Parkinson's disease. Treatment with levodopa tends to reverse this effect, suggesting that visual cortex impairment in Parkinson's disease is a result of dopamine deficiency (Rodnitzky 1998; Onofrj et al. 1986; Bodis-Wollner and Yahr 1978). However, though P100 latencies are prolonged in Parkinsonian patients as a group, there is still enough individual overlap with control populations to limit its clinical utility in this group. Other diseases affecting the visual pathway, especially locations anterior to the optic chiasm, can also produce abnormal VEPs. While optic neuritis secondary to multiple sclerosis is more common in younger patients, ischemic optic neuropathy also produces abnormal VEPs.

Somatosensory Evoked Potentials

Somatosensory evoked potentials (SEPs) allow for the noninvasive evaluation of peripheral and central somatosensory system integrity. SEPs are neurally generated waveforms in response to peripheral nerve stimulation. The median, ulnar, radial, posterior tibial, and peroneal nerves have been used in the study of SEPs, though median and posterior tibial nerve stimulation are the most well studied (Gilmore 1995). The short-latency SEP components arising from peripheral or central nervous system somatosensory pathways up to the primary sensory cortex are the most commonly clinical used SEPs. Generally speaking, mixed-nerve electrical stimulation of peripheral nerves is used to evaluate the function of the large 1A afferent-posterior column-medial lemniscus-thalamus-sensory cortex pathway (Oken and Phillips 2008). Typically, electromyography and nerve conduction studies are better than SEPs to evaluate the peripheral component of this pathway. SEP responses following upper limb stimulation show a greater signal to noise ratio, resulting in clearer waveform peaks. SEP responses following lower limb stimulation are more sensitive to possible demyelination of conduction pathways because of the longer spinal cord segment being tested. The choice of which stimulation site to use depends on the specific problem being studied.

A range of short-latency waveforms occur following peripheral site stimulation (Figure 3a). In response to upper limb (e.g. median nerve) stimulation, the N9 (Erb's point, recorded from the brachial plexus) occurs 9ms post stimulus. The N13 and P14 occur 12–13ms post stimulus, recorded from the dorsal column nucleus and medial lemniscus. The N18, thought to be generated in the thalamus, occurs 18ms post stimulus, and the N20 and P22/P25 occur around 20–25ms post stimulus and are generated in the sensory cortex (Oken and Phillips 2008; Gilmore 1995). SEP middle-latency potentials have been studied but do not have significant clinical applications (Zumsteg and Weiser 2002). In response to lower limb (e.g. tibial nerve) stimulation, the N29 arises from the cervicomedullary region, the N34 from the thalamus, and the P37 from the sensory cortex (Oken and Phillips 2008). SEPs have been demonstrated to be affected by height, and therefore must be normalized in order to be of clinical utility (Tanosaki et al. 1999; Allison et al. 1984; Hume et al. 1982; Desmedt and Cheron 1980).

Currently published literature shows a clear correlation between SEP latency and amplitude changes and aging. Latencies of all SEP components tend to increase in elders (Zumsteg and Weiser 2002; Allison et al. 1984; Ito 1994; Hume et al. 1982; Desmedt and Cheron 1980). Age-related effects on SEP amplitudes may depend on whether it is short or middle latency components that are being studied (Hume

1982; Desmedt and Cheron 1981). In most subjects, peripheral conduction time is increased with age (Allison et al. 1984; Desmedt and Cheron 1980). Therefore, in order to assess central function and exclude peripheral pathologies, it is necessary to study changes in central conduction time (CCT) by subtracting the latency of the peripheral component. Using medial nerve stimulation, Hume et al. (1982) found that CCT was stable up until the 5th decade of life, at which point it increased. In addition, the N20 to P14 peak ratio was significantly increased in elderly subjects. An increase in CCT with age has been demonstrated in additional studies as well (Tanosaki et al. 1999; Allison et al. 1984) though others have found that SEP latency changes with age are entirely due to alterations in peripheral pathways (Desmedt and Cheron 1980). The differences in these study results may be in part due to variations in the calculation of CCT, i.e., which waveform latency is subtracted from the sensory cortex latency (Desmedt and Cheron 1980; Tanosaki et al. 1999; Hume 1982; Allison et al. 1984).

Clinically, SEP latencies and interpeak latencies increase in conditions such as multiple sclerosis and myelopathy although anatomical imaging studies are generally performed first. SEPs may be useful to evaluate central somatosensory pathways when there is a known peripheral pathology or when it is uncertain if there is a significant neurologic process affecting central pathways and producing sensory symptoms. Following cardiac arrest and hypoxic-ischemic encephalopathy, bilateral absence of the thalamo-cortical waveforms in the median SEPs has been shown to be highly predictive of a poor outcome (Figure 3b).

A clear correlation does not exist between SEP components and dementia. A pilot study of patients with senile dementia suggested a delay in middle-latency SEPs (Huisman et al. 1985), though short-latency SEPs and CCT have been observed to remain unaffected in AD, Parkinsonian dementia, and dementia with Lewy bodies (Caviness 2000; Ito 1994; Tachibana, Takeda, and Sugita 1989; Abbruzzese et al. 1984). On the other hand, patients with vascular dementia have been shown to exhibit prolonged CCTs, as well as increased N13 and N20 latencies in vascular dementia (Ito 1994; Abbruzzese et al. 1984). If future research confirms this is the case, the use of SEPs may be helpful in differentiating between pathologic dementias (Abbruzzese et al. 1984).

Auditory Evoked Potentials

Auditory evoked potentials (AEPs) are typically divided into brainstem auditory evoked potentials (called the auditory brainstem response), and the middle and long-latency components. The brainstem auditory evoked potentials are the most widely used clinical AEPs (Golob, Johnson, and Starr 2002).

Brainstem Auditory Evoked Potentials

The auditory brainstem response (ABR) allows, among other things, for the evaluation of brainstem integrity. The ABR occurs as a series of seven waves generated in brainstem auditory areas within around 10ms of an auditory stimulus (Boettcher 2002). Various acoustic signals may be used to elicit this response—pure tones, for example—but generally the best waveforms are produced in using broadband click stimuli 60–70 dB above hearing threshold. Of the waveforms, termed I–VII, the most clinically useful are waves I, III, and V, thought to arise from the auditory nerve, the superior olive, and the inferior colliculus, respectively (Boettcher 2002).

When using the ABR to study brainstem function in an elderly population, it is important to control for age-related hearing loss (Boettcher 2002). Typically, as individuals age, an increase in latency of all ABR waveforms is observed (Costa et al. 1990; Allison et al. 1984; Don and Eggermont 1978) as well as a decrease in various wave amplitudes (Psatta and Matei 1988; Don and Eggermont 1978). Peripheral pathologies associated with hearing loss, as in the case of presbycusis, result in

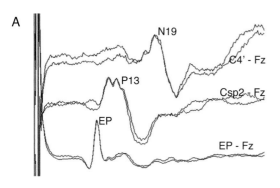

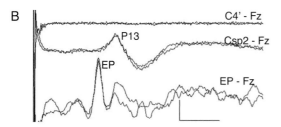

Figure 3 SEPs for prognosis post cardiac arrest. (Top, A): Normal median nerve SEPs. Three channels each with two averages, each of 500 stimuli. Calibration mark is 1 micv amplitude and 5 msec duration. Note brachial plexus potential recorded from Erb's point (EP), cervicomedullary junction potential, P13, recorded from 2nd cervical spinous process (Csp2), and sensory cortex potential (N19). (Bottom, B): Median SEPs two weeks following in-hospital cardiac arrest. Patient had eye blinking, head movement, and intact cranial nerve function but no response to commands and no purposeful movements. Same recording as above. Note the normal Erb's point (EP) and cervico-medullary junction potential (P13) but no cortical potentials. These changes were bilateral. Calibration mark is 1 micv amplitude and 5 msec duration.

alterations of ABR waveforms (Gilmore 1995). Therefore, in order to assess central changes or abnormalities it is necessary to study interpeak as opposed to absolute latencies, and potentially peak amplitude ratios. Because of this, multiple studies have attempted to observe ABR inter-peak latencies (IPLs) in relation to age, with varying results. Allison et al. (1984) observed a positive correlation between increasing age and greater I–V latencies in all subjects. In addition, the use of nonlinear temporal interactions (a quasi-random sequence of clicks and silences) demon-strated a significant change in the I–V interval. The authors suggest that this is indicative of an alteration in temporal processing of auditory information within the auditory brainstem in the elderly (Lavoie, Mehta, and Thornton 2008). In contrast, other studies have found no changes in IPLs with aging in healthy subjects (Costa et al. 1990; Ottaviani et al. 1990). Ottaviani et al. (1990) compared elderly subjects diagnosed with presbycusis to elderly subjects with normal hearing and young controls. It appeared that changes seen in the ABR of elderly subjects with presby-cusis was related to hearing loss and not to age per se.

Several studies have attempted to study the ABR in relation to cen-tral pathologies such as dementia. Some results have indicated that there is no change in ABR waveforms between controls and patients diagnosed with AD (Grimes, Grady, and Pikus 1987). However, in one study, there was an increase in I–III and III–V IPLs in patients with vascular dementia and an increase in III–V IPLs in patients with AD as compared to controls (Tachibana, Masanaka, and Sugita 1989). Differences between the vascular dementia and AD groups IPLs were not significant, and therefore the use of ABR was not effective in distinguishing the two types of dementia. However, these results may suggest the presence of brainstem lesions in the auditory pathways in patients with vascular dementia and AD (Tachibana, Taketa, and Sugita 1989).

While ABRs are sensitive to some focal brainstem pathologies, e.g. acoustic neurinoma, demyelination, or brainstem infarcts, MRI pro-vides much more useful information. Thus, its clinical use in the geri-atric population is limited to rare cases where the MRI is ambiguous and information about brainstem auditory physiology might be help-ful. In cases of coma, including following closed head injury, ABRs may be used to help with prognosis and to evaluate hearing.

Middle Latency Potentials—P50

The majority of research relating AEPs to dementia has focused on middle and long-latency components in response to auditory stimuli. Relevant components include middle-latency AEPs P30 and P50, and earlier long-latency AEPs such as the N100 and P200. It has been sug-gested that all of these components arise from the temporal lobe pri-mary cortex and nearby areas (Scherg and Picton 1991). As is the case with previously discussed evoked potentials, latencies and amplitudes of each waveform are sensitive to stimulus parameters, though the N100 and P200 components also depend on arousal and attention (Naatanen and Picton 1987). Overall, it appears that the normal aging process does not have a major effect on the middle latency and the earlier long-latency AEP components (Chambers and Griffiths 1991; Goodin et al. 1978).

Dementia affects the middle-latency AEPs, specifically the P50. It appears that in patients with probable AD, P50 latency may increase and amplitude may decrease. However, other AEP components remain unchanged (Buchwald et al. 1989; Golob, Johnson, and Starr 2001). Using a subject population of probable AD patients, Parkinson's patients with and without dementia, and control subjects, Green et al. (1992) demonstrated that patients with dementia (as a result of either AD or Parkinson's disease) were significantly more likely to lack the P50 component than those without dementia. Existing P50 latency and amplitude, however, appeared to be unchanged in dementia.

P50 generation has been hypothesized to be a reflection of brainstem cholinergic pathway activity (Buchwald et al. 1991; Erwin and Buchwald 1986).

In contrast to those with moderate dementia and probable AD, P50 amplitude has been demonstrated to increase in patients with MCI and early AD, especially using a paired-pulse paradigm which is sensi-tive to the usual loss of inhibition of response to the second stimulus (Golob, Johnson, and Starr 2001; Golob and Starr 2000; Jessen et al. 2001; Cancelli et al. 2006). This loss of inhibition of response has been observed in cortical SEP response to simultaneous median and ulnar nerve stimulation (Haavik, Taylor, and Murphy 2007). It has been suggested that abnormalities in the P50 component are a result of pathologic effects on the prefrontal cortex and its interactions with the auditory cortex. Clinically speaking, this could imply that P50 latency and amplitude changes are associated with an increased risk for AD, although in later, more severe cases of AD, that the P50 waveform is reduced or absent.

Long-latency Evoked Potentials

Long-latency evoked potentials are generated above the brainstem and occur later than 100ms post stimulus. These EPs requiring cognitive processing of the stimulus are commonly referred to as endogenous event-related potentials. An example of a long-latency EP could be a waveform that occurs when a subject recognizes a stimulus to which they are supposed to be attending. Thus, recording of long-latency EPs requires the patient to be alert and awake and this type of EP may be useful to evaluate abnormalities in cognitive function.

P300

The P300, also referred to as the P3, is the only long-latency EP that may be of clinical use. Other long-latency potentials, e.g., mismatch negativity and N400, will not be discussed. The P300 is a symmetrical positive waveform that occurs maximally over the midline central and parietal regions in response to stimuli of any modality, including vis-ual, auditory, and somatosensory tasks (Oken 1997). The P300 has been recorded over multiple different brain areas, including the infe-rior parietal lobe, frontal lobe, hippocampus, and medial temporal lobe. Thus, there is a brain network rather than a specific brain region that serves as the generator of the P300. Cognitive states such as attention and alertness, as well as response accuracy, affect the P300. Inattention or drowsiness will decrease P300 amplitude, and may extinguish it altogether (Oken 1997).

The P300 is most commonly elicited using an 'oddball' paradigm, which involves the random inclusion of an infrequent or unexpected stimulus among a group of frequent, expected stimuli. The P300 com-ponent is observed at approximately 300ms following the infrequent stimulus in such a paradigm. If a subject is asked to attend to target stimuli and ignore non-relevant stimuli, the P300 amplitude (observed following target stimulus presentation) is observed to increase. Therefore, the P300 is related to both stimulus infrequency and task-relevance. The effects of infrequency and task-relevance appear to function independently, resulting in two different P300 waveform components, termed P300a and P300b. The P300a occurs earlier and with a more frontal distribution in response to infrequent stimuli. The P300b occurs in response to task-relevance, and is maximal over pari-etal areas of the brain. In most cases of clinical P300 analysis, these two components are assessed as one waveform (Oken and Phillips 2008). In contrast to the P300 amplitude, the P300 latency increases with task difficulty.

There is a very well documented positive correlation between P300 latency and age. In general, it appears that P300 peak latency increases by around 1–2ms per year (Schiff et al. 2008; Oken 1997; Polich 1996) while P300 amplitude has been shown to decrease with advancing age (Schiff et al. 2008). In addition, one study suggested that latency increases exponentially with advancing age (Brown, Marsh, and LaRue 1983) though other studies have indicated a general linear increase in latency with age (Schiff et al. 2008). Advanced age has also been associated with less well-defined P300 waveforms (Oken and Kaye 1992) (see Figure 4). In middle-aged adults the P300 amplitude usually increases from fronto-central to parietal regions, while in the elderly population the P300 may be more evenly distributed across the scalp (Gilmore 1995). Polich (1997) demonstrated a correlation between P300 amplitude decrease and decreasing delta, theta, and particularly alpha power with age, leading to the hypothesis that P300 changes are associated with age-related changes in background EEG frequencies.

P300 latency may be clinically useful in terms of its ability to assess cognitive aging, since it reflects the time required for the brain to process information (Polich 1996), but is potentially independent of a motor response which is often affected by aging or age-related pathologies. The P300 has been suggested to be related to overall cognitive function (Polich 1997) and indeed, Verleger et al. (1991) demonstrated a significant positive correlation between P300 latency, age, and decreased auditory verbal learning test scores. However, the strength of the relationship between P300 and factors of aging tend to vary widely among studies. A meta analysis of 34 P300 research studies suggested that variance in subject demographics as well as factors such as task design, stimulus modality, and stimulus intensity led to altered effect size (Polich 1996). Still, despite sources of variability in P300 study data, P300 latency clearly increases with age. It is suggested that

for the P300 to be useful clinically, it first needs to be made reliable through normalization of study parameters (Polich 1996).

P300 and Dementia

In many cases, cognitive dysfunction in neurologic disorders is seen in conjunction with increased P300 latencies (Polich 1996). P300 latency may be delayed in demented but not non-demented Parkinson's patients (Matsui et al. 2007), AD (Juckel et al. 2008), vascular dementia (Muscoso et al. 2006), and even Down's syndrome (Vieregge et al. 1992), which is of note given that nearly all patients with Down's syndrome develop AD later in life (Wisniewski, Wisniewski, and Wen 1985). In fact, subjective general age-associated memory impairment has been shown to correlate with increased P300 latency and decreased amplitude as compared to controls (Anderer et al. 2003). These P300 changes may reflect reduced attentional capacity in all types of dementia and memory deficits (Anderer et al. 2003). In line with such an idea, P300 latency has been observed to increase with growing cognitive dysfunction (Muscoco et al. 2006; Polich et al. 1986), and longitudinal studies have linked disease progression to increasing P300 latency as well (Ball et al. 1989). It is important, however, to be aware of paradigm design when analyzing such data since (as previously discussed) differing paradigm stimuli may produce differing results in studies of dementia as well as normative aging (Polich 1996). In one example, P300 latency and amplitude differences between subjects with AD and controls were diminished when the infrequent 'oddball' stimulus was made more frequent, which may have interesting implications in terms of the pathophysiology of AD (Polich, Ladish,

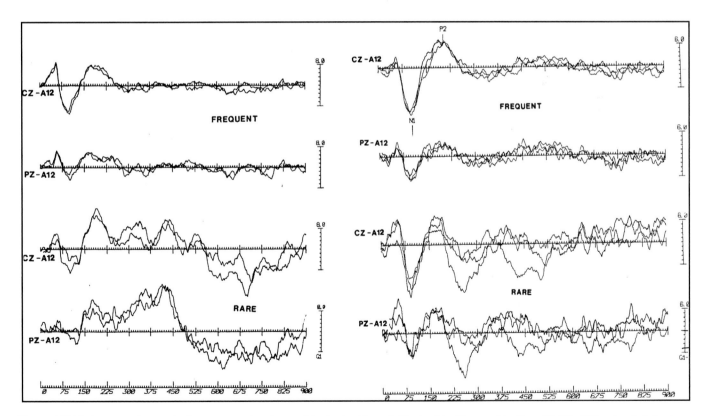

Figure 4 P300 changes with age.   Auditory event-related potentials obtained from (left) a healthy 90-year-old with an MMSE of 27 and well-defined, although broad, P3, with a latency more than 2 standard deviations above the mean for 20–50 year olds, and (right) a healthy 86-year-old with an MMSE of 30 and a poorly reproducible P3. Two channels, Cz and Pz referenced to linked ares, are shown for the frequent and the rare (attended) tones. There is a 900-msec sweep, calibration voltages are on the right, and negativity from the scalp channels is displayed down.

and Bloom 1990). Additionally, TGA has been shown to be associated with unstable P300 peaks and decreased P300 amplitude, though peak latency remained stable (Tikhonova et al. 2003).

Despite clear evidence of group differences in P300 latencies, the sensitivity of P300 latency prolongation has varied greatly, with 10% to 80% of demented patients diagnosed with AD having been reported in various studies to have latencies outside of normal limits (usually two standard deviations) (Oken 1997). Duffy et al. (1984a) demonstrated that EEG frequency analysis was a better discriminator between patients with AD and controls than was the P300. Therefore, though overall group differences in the P300 between demented and non-demented subjects are observed, the P300 has had limited clinical utility in terms of classifying an individual subject. Still, more recent research has demonstrated advancement in these issues. It has been suggested that though the P300 as a general waveform is not always a clear indicator of pathologic dementia, individual components P300a and P300b may be useful in differentiating between patients with and without dementia (Juckel et al. 2008).

Movement-related Potentials

Premotor Potentials

Premotor potentials refer to evoked potentials that occur before the initiation of a movement. The most well studied of these is the readiness potential, or Bereitschaftspotential (BP), which is observed prior to a voluntary movement (Shibasaki and Hallett 2006). It tends to be maximal over the contralateral central scalp in response to upper limb movements, and the midline central scalp in response to lower limb movements. The waveform can be divided into two components, typically termed the early BP and late BP (or NS'). The early BP waveform appears initially as a very low frequency negative slope, with the late BP leading to an increase in negative slope. The early BP begins around 2.0 s before movement initiation, and is thought to be generated in the pre-supplementary motor area, supplementary motor area, and lateral premotor cortex (Shibasaki and Hallett 2006). It appears to be influenced in amplitude and duration by factors such as movement speed and precision, muscle force, and movement selection, to name a few (Oken and Phillips 2008). The late BP occurs around 500 ms before movement initiation, and originates in the contralateral primary motor cortex and lateral premotor cortex (Shibasaki and Hallett 2006). This component may be influenced by factors such as discreteness and complexity of movement. Thus, for the BP to be of any practical use, a clearly standardized motor task and instructions must be provided. Still, significant variability in the waveform severely limits its clinical utility. For a complete overview of the BP, see Shibasaki and Hallet (2006).

Currently, very little research has attempted to directly observe the correlation between premotor potentials and aging. However, several pathologies common with aging have been linked to abnormal premotor potentials. Patients with Parkinson's disease tend to exhibit abnormal BPs, particularly the early BP component. Commonly, PD patients show a smaller early BP waveform amplitude than controls, which is then increased in response to L-dopa drug administration (Dick et al. 1987; Fattapposta et al. 2002). Unfortunately, in terms of clinical significance, the size of BP components is so variable among individuals and movement types that these potentials are not useful in terms of disease severity (Shibasaki and Hallett 2006).

Potentials Prior to Abnormal Movements

In addition to the longer duration, slow frequency premotor potentials prior to voluntary movement, there may be different potentials prior to myoclonus. Most particularly, the use of jerk-locked backaveraging

from the onset of activity in myoclonus may help to determine etiologies of the condition (Shibasaki and Hallett 2005). Myoclonus occurs in conjunction with many neurologic disorders and it is often important to determine whether its cause is cortical or subcortical (Alvarez and Caviness 2008). In cortical myoclonus, a premotor potential is observed via jerk-locked backaveraging at 50 ms prior to involuntary movement in the sensorimotor cortex. Subcortical myoclonus will not show this wave. Interestingly, myoclonus arising from psychogenic causes will result in BP waveforms prior to the movement, which are not seen in myoclonus due to nervous system damage (Oken and Phillips 2008).

Motor Evoked Potentials

Motor evoked potentials (MEPs) are useful in terms of assessing the functionality of the descending corticospinal tract. They are measured by recording EMG of a muscle twitch from surface electrodes in response to an electrical current in the motor cortex, usually occurring 20–45 ms following stimulation. Transcranial electrical stimulation (TES) was originally used to induce this current, but because of the coincidental stimulation of scalp nociceptors, TES is painful for the subject and is now used only when a patient is under general anesthesia. Transcranial magnetic stimulation (TMS) utilizes the magnetic field caused by current flow in a stimulation coil to painlessly induce a cortical current and produce MEP waveforms (Rossini et al. 2007; Sohn and Hallett 2004).

MEP amplitudes vary widely between and within individuals, so the latency (either absolute or central conduction times) is the more clinically useful variable (Oken and Phillips 2008). Peripheral and central conduction times are also variables of interest. Peripheral conduction time is assessed by measuring MEP latency in response to stimulation over the spinal roots. Central conduction time is then computed by subtracting peripheral conduction time from the latency following cortical stimulation. MEP latency and central conduction time increased with age, while maximum MEP amplitude decreased (Eisen and Shtybel 1990), likely reflecting age-related changes in the functionality of large, fast-conducting upper motor neurons.

Increased MEP latencies may also be observed in pathologies affecting motor system such as ischemic stroke, multiple sclerosis, and amyotrophic lateral sclerosis (Oken and Phillips 2008; Mitsumoto et al. 2007; Homberg, Steph, and Netz 1991; Mitsumoto 2007). Parkinson's disease has been associated with increases in MEP amplitudes, though not latency, and there are changes related to on-off state (Lou et al. 2003; Eisen and Shtybel 1990).

Transcranial magnetic MEPs may be used for research to explore the motor system beyond amplitudes and latencies of single pulse evoked muscle response. Resting motor threshold evaluates the baseline excitability of motor cortex. TMS paired-pulse protocols can be used to assess intracortical inhibition (ICI) and intracortical facilitation (ICF). The cortical silent period, a period of EMG silence following TMS motor cortex stimulation of a contracting muscle, can also be assessed. Excitability threshold for TMS does not appear to change in the elderly (Rossini et al. 2007). Still, ventricular volume and white matter hyperintensity volumes in the otherwise healthy elderly have both been shown to be positively correlated with resting motor threshold via TMS studies (Silbert et al. 2006). Both ICI and the cortical silent period decrease in amyotrophic lateral sclerosis, with ICI decrease specifically correlating with disease severity and duration (Zanette al. 2002). Parkinson's disease is associated with lower resting threshold and shorter silent period (Cantello et al. 2007; Lefaucheur 2005). The ICI has been observed to decrease in patients with Parkinson's disease and AD, though not fronto-temporal dementia (Pierantozzi et al. 2004; Cantello, Tarletti, and Civardi 2002).

MEP motor thresholds are decreased and MEP amplitudes are increased in patients with AD, in correlation with the severity of the disease (Alagona et al. 2001). In general, TMS results indicate a hyperexcitability of the motor cortex in AD (Rossini et al. 2007). In a recent study, Julkunen et al. (2008) used TMS to show significant differences between patients with AD (via a decrease in P30), patients with MCI (via a decrease in N100), and controls. These differences are hypothesized to be a result of changes in frontal connectivity during progressive dementia (Julkunen et al. 2008). Additionally, transcranial magnetic stimulation may be used to interfere with ongoing cortical information processing. For example, it has been used to measure subjects' ability to encode simple motor-related memories, anability believed to decrease with advancing age (Sawaki et al. 2003).

Repetitive TMS (rTMS) involves repeated electrical signals to a specific area of the brain, and has been considered as a possible treatment for some neurologic conditions and for depression. Theoretically, it may improve cognitive performance by stimulating the brain (Rossini et al. 2007). Administration of rTMS on the dorsolateral prefrontal cortex in patients with AD significantly improved action naming performance (Cotelli et al. 2006). Associative memory task performance in subjects diagnosed with MCI has been shown to improve in response to rTMS (Sole-Padulle et al. 2006). Based on these findings, rTMS may be a useful rehabilitation strategy (Rossi and Rossini. 2004). However, further research will be necessary in order to determine the duration of improvement, and whether these results are consistent.

Intraoperative Neurophysiologic Monitoring (IONM)

IONM consists of performing EPs and other electrophysiologic tests during surgery and is used to give information in real-time to surgeons operating in or near relevant neural structures (Nuwer, 2008). IONM is not ordered by the primary care provider but IONM must be accessible to any surgeon performing a procedure where neural tissue is at risk. IONM is used for several general purposes. The information may consist of ongoing assessment of signal conduction integrity. For example, changes in cortical SEP components following posterior tibial nerve stimulation during cervical spine surgery suggest a posterior column dysfunction. While under general anesthesia, acute changes in EPs secondary to central nervous system perfusion perhaps related to physical maneuver, e.g., retraction or distraction, indicates the surgical team has about 10–20 minutes to reverse the underlying etiology until the pathology is more likely to become irreversible. EPs may also be used for localization purposes, for example localizing motor cortex by recording SEP field potentials from subdural electrode or from direct neural stimulation and recording EMG.

The EP modalities used for IONM include SEP (upper and lower limb), ABR, and MEP. Due to the marked attenuation of magnetically evoked MEPs by general anesthesia, intraoperative MEPs are performed using transcranial electrical stimulation. VEPs using goggles have not been reliable intraoperatively. In addition to EPs, EMG from relevant muscles is often recorded if cranial nerves or nerve roots are at risk. Nerve conductions from pedicle screw stimulation or direct nerve stimulation may also be used. EEG may be used to help determine and guide the depth of anesthesia (e.g., until suppression-burst pattern is observed) or determine focal or global cerebral dysfunction during cerebrovascular or cardiovascular surgery.

EEG and EPs during surgery are sensitive to level of anesthesia. Intravenous anesthetics such as propofol and narcotics have less of an effect on EPs than inhalants. ABRs are relatively insensitive to anesthesia with SEPs having a sensitivity to anesthesia in between MEPs and ABRs. This is important in the geriatric population because the same percent of inhalant anesthetics might produce a much greater depth of anesthesia (and greater attenuation of EPs) in older compared to younger adults. EPs are also sensitive to changes in other physiologic parameters during surgery including blood pressure and temperature. EP recording within the operating room requires much expertise in managing the numerous causes of artifacts potentially obliterating the signals (e.g., electrocautery) as well as knowledge of the surgical procedures and anesthesiology.

While IONM has become standard for many neurosurgical, orthopedic, vascular, and otolaryngology surgeries, there are no prospective randomized trials demonstrating IONM utility at improving outcomes. There have been several studies using historical or non-monitored controls that strongly suggest IONM utility for preventing paraparesis (scoliosis surgery) or preserving hearing (resection of small acoustic neuromas and microvascular decompression for trigeminal neuralgia). Currently, IONM is commonly performed in surgeries where there is significant risk to neural structures (e.g., multilevel spine surgery with myelopathy, posterior fossa surgery, and aneurysm surgery).

Summary

EEGs and EPs demonstrate consistent changes related to relatively healthy aging, but show greater and clinically significant changes when associated with certain pathologies. EEGs and EPs are most helpful clinically when there is a specific clinical question that can be facilitated by the presence of a normal or abnormal result. In healthy elders, intermittent temporal slowing is present in some who are over 65 years of age, though the posterior alpha rhythm does not drop below 8 Hz at least through 85 years of age. Encephalopathies of any etiology produce increased amounts of focal and generalized slowing. Abnormal epileptiform activity is not seen in healthy aging, but is associated with epilepsy, acute cerebral lesions, some metabolic encephalopathies, and some neurodegenerative diseases. EP latencies generally increase in latency with age, independent of any clear disease etiology, with longer latency waves showing greater age-related increases. This suggests that intracerebral conduction times may decline more than peripheral, spinal cord, and brainstem conduction times through the aging process. Newer recording and analysis techniques have aided our understanding of more fine-grained physiologic function in aging and age-related diseases and may provide future research directions.

Acknowledgments

This work was funded in part from grants from NIH (AG008017 and AT002656).

References

Abbruzzese, G., Reni, L., Cocito, L., Ratto, S., Abbruzzese, M., and Favale, E. (1984). Short-latency somatosensory evoked potentials in degenerative and vascular dementia. *J Neurol Neurosurg Psychiatry*, 47(9), 1034–1037.

Adler, G., Brassen, S., Chwalek, K., Dieter, B., and Teufel, M. (2004). Prediction of treatment response to rivastigmine in Alzheimer's dementia. *J Neurol Neurosurg Psychiatry*, 75(2), 292–294.

Alagona, G., Bella, R., Ferri, R., Carnemolla, A., Pappalardo, A., Costanzo, E., et al. (2001). Transcranial magnetic stimulation in Alzheimer disease: Motor cortex excitability and cognitive severity. *Neurosci Lett*, 314(1–2), 57–60.

Allison, T., Hume, A. L., Wood, C. C., and Goff, W. R. (1984). Developmental and aging changes in somatosensory, auditory and visual evoked potentials. *Electroencephalogr Clin Neurophysiol, 58*(1), 14–24.

Alvarez, M. and Caviness, J. N. (2008). Primary progressive myoclonus of aging. *Mov Disord, 23*(12), 1658–1664.

Anderer, P., Saletu, B., Semlitsch, H. V., and Pascual-Marqui, R. D. (2003). Non-invasive localization of P300 sources in normal aging and age-associated memory impairment. *Neurobiol Aging, 24*(3), 463–479.

Arenas, A. M., Brenner, R. P., and Reynolds III, C. F. (1986). Temporal slowing in the elderly revisited. *American Journal of EEG Technology, 26*, 105–114.

Babiloni, C., Binetti, G., Cassetta, E., Dal Forno, G., Del Percio, C., Ferreri, F., et al. (2006). Sources of cortical rhythms change as a function of cognitive impairment in pathological aging: A multicenter study. *Clin Neurophysiol, 117*(2), 252–268.

Ball, S. S., Marsh, J. T., Schubarth, G., Brown, W. S., and Strandburg, R. (1989). Longitudinal P300 latency changes in Alzheimer's disease. *Journal of Gerontology, 44*, M195–200.

Bodis-Wollner, I. and Yahr, M. D. (1978). Measurements of visual evoked potentials in Parkinson's disease. *Brain, 101*(4), 661–671.

Boettcher, F. A. (2002). Presbyacusis and the auditory brainstem response. *J Speech Lang Hear Res, 45*(6), 1249–1261.

Brenner, R. P., Reynolds, C. F., and Ulrich, R. F. (1988). Diagnostic efficacy of computerized spectral versus visual EEG analysis in elderly normal, demented and depressed subjects. *Electroencephalography and Clinical Neurophysiology, 69*, 110–117.

Brenner, R. P., Reynolds, C. F., and Ulrich, R. F. (1989). EEG findings in depressive pseudodementia and dementia with secondary depression. *Electroencephalography and Clinical Neurophysiology, 72*, 298–304.

Brickman, A. M., Paul, R. H., Cohen, R. A., Williams, L. M., MacGregor, K. L., Jefferson, A. L., et al. (2005). Category and letter verbal fluency across the adult lifespan: relationship to EEG theta power. *Arch Clin Neuropsychol, 20*(5), 561–573.

Briel, R. C., McKeith, I. G., Barker, W. A., Hewitt, Y., Perry, R. H., Ince, P. G., et al. (1999). EEG findings in dementia with Lewy bodies and Alzheimer's disease. *J Neurol Neurosurg Psychiatry, 66*(3), 401–403.

Brown, W. S., Marsh, J. T., and LaRue, A. (1983). Exponential electrophysiological aging: P3 latency. *Electroencephalogr Clin Neurophysiol, 55*(3), 277–285.

Buchan, R. J., Nagata, K., Yokoyama, E., Langman, P., Yuya, H., Hirata, Y., et al. (1997). Regional correlations between the EEG and oxygen metabolism in dementia of Alzheimer's type. *Electroencephalogr Clin Neurophysiol, 103*(3), 409–417.

Buchwald, J. S., Erwin, R. J., Read, S., and Van Lancker, D. (1989). Midlatency auditory evoked responses: Differential abnormality of P1 in Alzheimer's disease. *Electroencephalography and Clinical Neurophysiology, 74*, 378–384.

Buchwald, J. S., Rubinstein, E. H., Schwafel, J., and Strandburg, R. J. (1991). Midlatency auditory evoked responses: Differential effects of a cholinergic agonist and antagonist. *Electroencephalogr Clin Neurophysiol, 80*(4), 303–309.

Cancelli, I., Cadore, I. P., Merlino, G., Valentinis, L., Moratti, U., Bergonzi, P., et al. (2006). Sensory gating deficit assessed by P50/Pb middle latency event related potential in Alzheimer's disease. *J Clin Neurophysiol, 23*(5), 421–425.

Cantello, R., Tarletti, R., and Civardi, C. (2002). Transcranial magnetic stimulation and Parkinson's disease. *Brain Res Brain Res Rev, 38*(3), 309–327.

Cantello, R., Tarletti, R., Varrasi, C., Cecchin, M., and Monaco, F. (2007). Cortical inhibition in Parkinson's disease: New insights from early, untreated patients. *Neuroscience, 150*(1), 64–71.

Caviness, J. N., Gwinn-Hardy, K., Adler, C. H., and Muenter, M. D. (2000). Electrophysiological observations in hereditary parkinsonism-dementia with Lewy body pathology. *Mov Disord, 15*(1), 140–145.

Celesia, G. G., Kaufman, D., and Cone, S. (1987). Effects of age and sex on pattern electroretinograms and visual evoked potentials. *Electroencephalogr Clin Neurophysiol, 68*(3), 161–171.

Chambers, R. D., and Griffiths, S. K. (1991). Effects of age on the adult auditory middle latency response. *Hear Res, 51*(1), 1–10.

Claus, J. J., Ongerboer de Visser, B. W., Walstra, G. J., Hijdra, A., Verbeeten, B., Jr., and van Gool, W. A. (1998). Quantitative spectral electroencephalography in predicting survival in patients with early Alzheimer disease. *Arch Neurol, 55*(8), 1105–1111.

Coben, L. A., Danziger, W., and Storandt, M. (1985). A longitudinal EEG study of mild senile dementia of Alzheimer type: Changes at 1 year and 2.5 years. *Electroencephalography and Clinical Neurophysiology, 61*, 101–112.

Costa, P., Benna, P., Bianco, C., Ferrero, P., and Bergamasco, B. (1990). Aging effects on brainstem auditory evoked potentials. *Electromyogr Clin Neurophysiol, 30*(8), 495–500.

Cotelli, M., Manenti, R., Cappa, S. F., Geroldi, C., Zanetti, O., Rossini, P. M., et al. (2006). Effect of transcranial magnetic stimulation on action naming in patients with Alzheimer disease. *Arch Neurol, 63*(11), 1602–1604.

Desmedt, J. E., and Cheron, G. (1980). Somatosensory evoked potentials to finger stimulation in healthy octogenarians and in young adults: Wave forms, scalp topography and transit times of parietal and frontal components. *Electroencephalogr Clin Neurophysiol, 50*(5–6), 404–425.

Desmedt, J. E., and Cheron, G. (1981). Non-cephalic reference recording of early somatosensory potentials to finger stimulation in adult or aging normal man: Differentiation of widespread N18 and contralateral N20 from the prerolandic P22 and N30 components. *Electroencephalogr Clin Neurophysiol, 52*(6), 553–570.

Dick, J. P. R., Cantello, R., Buruma, O., Gioux, M., Benecke, R., Day, B. L., et al. (1987). The Bereitschaftspotential, L-DOPA, and Parkinson's disease. *Electroencephalography and Clinical Neurophysiology, 66*, 263–274.

Don, M., and Eggermont, J. J. (1978). Analysis of the click-evoked brainstem potentials in man using high-pass noise masking. *J Acoust Soc Am, 63*(4), 1084–1092.

Duffy, F. H., Albert, M. S., and McAnulty, G. (1984a). Brain electrical activity in patients with presenile and senile dementia of the Alzheimer type. *Annals of Neurology, 16*, 439–448.

Duffy, F. H., Albert, M. S., McAnulty, G., and Garvey, A. J. (1984b). Age-related differences in brain electrical activity of healthy subjects. *Annals of Neurology, 16*, 430–438.

Dunkin, J. J., Leuchter, A. F., Newton, T. F., and Cook, I. A. (1994). Reduced EEG coherence in dementia: State or trait marker? *Biol Psychiatry, 35*(11), 870–879.

Dustman, R. E., Shearer, D. E., and Emmerson, R. Y. (1993). EEG and event-related potentials in normal aging. *Prog Neurobiol, 41*(3), 369–401.

Dustman, R. E., Shearer, D. E., and Emmerson, R. Y. (1999). Life-span changes in EEG spectral amplitude, amplitude variability and mean frequency. *Clin Neurophysiol, 110*(8), 1399–1409.

Eisen, A. A., and Shtybel, W. (1990). AAEM minimonograph #35: Clinical experience with transcranial magnetic stimulation. *Muscle Nerve, 13*(11), 995–1011.

Erwin, R. J., and Buchwald, J. S. (1986). Midlatency auditory evoked responses: Differential recovery cycle characteristics. Electroencephalogr Clin Neurophysiol, 64(5), 417–423.

Fattaposta, F., Pierelli, F., My, F., Mostarda, M., Del Monte, S., Parisi, L., et al. (2002). L-dopa effects on preprogramming and control activity in a skilled motor act in Parkinson's disease. *Clin Neurophysiol, 113*(2), 243–253.

Gilmore, R. (1995). Evoked potentials in the elderly. *J Clin Neurophysiol, 12*(2), 132–138.

Golob, E. J., Johnson, J. K., and Starr, A. (2002). Auditory event-related potentials during target detection are abnormal in mild cognitive impairment. *Clin Neurophysiol, 113*(1), 151–161.

Golob, E. J., and Starr, A. (2000). Effects of stimulus sequence on event-related potentials and reaction time during target detection in Alzheimer's disease. *Clin Neurophysiol, 111*(8), 1438–1449.

Goodin, D. S., Squires, K. C., Henderson, B. H., and Starr, A. (1978). Age-related variations in evoked potentials to auditory stimuli in normal human subjects. *Electroencephalography and Clinical Neurophysiology, 44*, 447–458.

Green, J. B., Flagg, L., Freed, D. M., and Schwankhaus, J. D. (1992). The middle latency auditory evoked potential may be abnormal in dementia. *Neurology, 42*(5), 1034–1036.

Grimes, A. M., Grady, C. L., and Pikus, A. (1987). Auditory evoked potentials in patients with dementia of the Alzheimer type. *Ear Hear, 8*(3), 157–161.

Haavik Taylor, H., and Murphy, B. A. (2007). Altered cortical integration of dual somatosensory input following the cessation of a 20 min period of repetitive muscle activity. *Exp Brain Res, 178*(4), 488–498.

Helkala, E. L., Laulumaa, V., Soininen, H., Partanen, J., and Riekkinen, P. J. (1991). Different patterns of cognitive decline related to normal or deteriorating EEG in a 3-year follow-up study of patients with Alzheimer's disease. *Neurology, 41*(4), 528–532.

Holschneider, D. P., and Leuchter, A. F. (1995). Beta activity in aging and dementia. *Brain Topogr, 8*(2), 169–180.

Holschneider, D. P., and Leuchter, A. F. (1999). Clinical neurophysiology using electroencephalography in geriatric psychiatry: Neurobiologic implications and clinical utility. *J Geriatr Psychiatry Neurol, 12*(3), 150–164.

Holschneider, D. P., Leuchter, A. F., Uijtdehaage, S. H., Abrams, M., and Rosenberg-Thompson, S. (1997). Loss of high-frequency brain electrical response to thiopental administration in Alzheimer's-type dementia. *Neuropsychopharmacology, 16*(4), 269–275.

Homberg, V., Stephan, K. M., and Netz, J. (1991). Transcranial stimulation of motor cortex in upper motor neurone syndrome: Its relation to the motor deficit. *Electroencephalogr Clin Neurophysiol, 81*(5), 377–388.

Huang, C., Wahlund, L., Dierks, T., Julin, P., Winblad, B., and Jelic, V. (2000). Discrimination of Alzheimer's disease and mild cognitive impairment by equivalent EEG sources: A cross-sectional and longitudinal study. *Clin Neurophysiol, 111*(11), 1961–1967.

Huisman, U. W., Posthuma, J., Hooijer, C., Visser, S. L., and de Rijke, W. (1985). Somatosensory evoked potentials in healthy volunteers and in patients with dementia. *Clin Neurol Neurosurg, 87*(1), 11–16.

Hume, A. L., Cant, B. R., Shaw, N. A., and Cowan, J. C. (1982). Central somatosensory conduction time from 10 to 79 years. *Electroencephalogr Clin Neurophysiol, 54*(1), 49–54.

Ito, J. (1994). Somatosensory event-related potentials (ERPs) in patients with different types of dementia. *Journal of the Neurological Sciences, 12*, 139–146.

Jelles, B., Scheltens, P., van der Flier, W. M., Jonkman, E. J., da Silva, F. H., and Stam, C. J. (2008). Global dynamical analysis of the EEG in Alzheimer's disease: Frequency-specific changes of functional interactions. *Clin Neurophysiol, 119*(4), 837–841.

Jeong, J. (2004). EEG dynamics in patients with Alzheimer's disease. *Clin Neurophysiol, 115*(7), 1490–1505.

Jessen, F., Kucharski, C., Fries, T., Papassotiropoulos, A., Hoenig, K., Maier, W., et al. (2001). Sensory gating deficit expressed by a disturbed suppression of the P50 event-related potential in patients with Alzheimer's disease. *Am J Psychiatry, 158*(8), 1319–1321.

John, E. R., Prichep, L. S., Fridman, J., and Easton, P. (1988). Neurometrics: Computer-assisted differential diagnosis of brain dysfunctions. *Science, 239*(4836), 162–169.

Jordan, K. G. (1999). Continuous EEG monitoring in the neuroscience intensive care unit and emergency department. *J Clin Neurophysiol, 16*(1), 14–39.

Juckel, G., Clotz, F., Frodl, T., Kawohl, W., Hampel, H., Pogarell, O., et al. (2008). Diagnostic usefulness of cognitive auditory event-related p300 subcomponents in patients with Alzheimers disease? *J Clin Neurophysiol, 25*(3), 147–152.

Julkunen, P., Jauhiainen, A. M., Westeren-Punnonen, S., Pirinen, E., Soininen, H., Kononen, M., et al. (2008). Navigated TMS combined with EEG in mild cognitive impairment and Alzheimer's disease: A pilot study. *J Neurosci Methods, 172*(2), 270–276.

Kaszniak, A. W., Garron, D. C., Fox, J. H., Bergen, D., and Huckman, M. (1979). Cerebral atrophy, EEG slowing age, education, and cognitive functioning in suspected dementia. *Neurology, 29*(9 Pt 1), 1273–1279.

Klass, D. W., and Brenner, R. P. (1995). Electroencephalography of the elderly. *J Clin Neurophysiol, 12*(2), 116–131.

Klass, D. W., and Westmoreland, B. F. (1985). Nonepileptogenic epileptiform electroencephalographic activity. *Ann Neurol, 18*(6), 627–635.

Korczyn, A. D. (2001). Dementia in Parkinson's disease. *J Neurol, 248 Suppl 3*, III1–4.

Kowalski, J. W., Gawel, M., Pfeffer, A., and Barcikowska, M. (2001). The diagnostic value of EEG in Alzheimer disease: Correlation with the severity of mental impairment. *J Clin Neurophysiol, 18*(6), 570–575.

Lanctot, K. L., Herrmann, N., and LouLou, M. M. (2003). Correlates of response to acetylcholinesterase inhibitor therapy in Alzheimer's disease. *J Psychiatry Neurosci, 28*(1), 13–26.

Lavoie, B. A., Mehta, R., and Thornton, A. R. (2008). Linear and nonlinear changes in the auditory brainstem response of aging humans. *Clin Neurophysiol, 119*(4), 772–785.

Lefaucheur, J. P. (2005). Motor cortex dysfunction revealed by cortical excitability studies in Parkinson's disease: Influence of antiparkinsonian treatment and cortical stimulation. *Clin Neurophysiol, 116*(2), 244–253.

Lesevre, N., and Joseph, J. P. (1979). Modifications of the pattern-evoked potential (PEP) in relation to the stimulated part of the visual field (clues for the most probable origin of each component). *Electroencephalogr Clin Neurophysiol, 47*(2), 183–203.

Leuchter, A. F., Newton, T. F., Cook, I. A., Walter, D. O., Rosenberg-Thompson, S., and Lachenbruch, P. A. (1992). Changes in brain functional connectivity in Alzheimer-type and multi-infarct dementia. *Brain, 115 (Pt 5)*, 1543–1561.

Levy, S. R., Chiappa, K. H., Burke, C. J., and Young, R. R. (1986). Early evolution and incidence of electroencephalographic abnormalities in Creutzfeldt-Jakob disease. *J Clin Neurophysiol, 3*(1), 1–21.

Lindau, M., Jelic, V., Johansson, S. E., Andersen, C., Wahlund, L. O., and Almkvist, O. (2003). Quantitative EEG abnormalities and cognitive dysfunctions in frontotemporal dementia and Alzheimer's disease. *Dement Geriatr Cogn Disord, 15*(2), 106–114.

Locatelli, T., Cursi, M., Liberati, D., Franceschi, M., and Comi, G. (1998). EEG coherence in Alzheimer's disease. *Electroencephalogr Clin Neurophysiol, 106*(3), 229–237.

Lou, J. S., Benice, T., Kearns, G., Sexton, G., and Nutt, J. (2003). Levodopa normalizes exercise related cortico-motoneuron excitability abnormalities in Parkinson's disease. *Clin Neurophysiol, 114*(5), 930–937.

Marsan, C. A., and Zivin, L. S. (1970). Factors related to the occurrence of typical paroxysmal abnormalities in the EEG records of epileptic patients. *Epilepsia, 11*(4), 361–381.

Matsui, H., Nishinaka, K., Oda, M., Kubori, T., and Udaka, F. (2007). Auditory event-related potentials in Parkinson's disease: prominent correlation with attention. *Parkinsonism Relat Disord, 13*(7), 394–398.

Meador, K. J., Gevins, A., Loring, D. W., McEvoy, L. K., Ray, P. G., Smith, M. E., et al. (2007). Neuropsychological and neurophysiologic effects of carbamazepine and levetiracetam. *Neurology, 69*(22), 2076–2084.

Michael, W. F., and Halliday, A. M. (1971). The topography of occipital responses evoked by pattern-reversal in different areas of the visual field. *Vision Res, 11*(10), 1202–1203.

Miller, J. D., de Leon, M. J., Ferris, S. H., Kluger, A., George, A. E., Reisberg, B., et al. (1987). Abnormal temporal lobe response in Alzheimer's disease during cognitive processing as measured by 11C-2-deoxy-D-glucose and PET. *J Cereb Blood Flow Metab, 7*(2), 248–251.

Mitsumoto, H., Ulug, A. M., Pullman, S. L., Gooch, C. L., Chan, S., Tang, M. X., et al. (2007). Quantitative objective markers for upper and lower motor neuron dysfunction in ALS. *Neurology, 68*(17), 1402–1410.

Muscoso, E. G., Costanzo, E., Daniele, O., Maugeri, D., Natale, E., and Caravaglios, G. (2006). Auditory event-related potentials in subcortical vascular cognitive impairment and in Alzheimer's disease. *J Neural Transm, 113*(11), 1779–1786.

Naatanen, R., and Picton, T. (1987). The N1 wave of the human electric and magnetic response to sound: A review and an analysis of the component structure. *Psychophysiology, 24*(4), 375–425.

Niedermeyer, E. and da Silva, F. L. (Eds.). (2004). *Electroencephalography: Basic principles, clinicalapplications, and related fields.* Baltimore: Lippincott Williams & Wilkins.

Nuwer, M. (1997). Assessment of digital EEG, quantitative EEG, and EEG brain mapping: Report of theAmerican Academy of Neurology and the American Clinical Neurophysiology Society. *Neurology, 49*(1), 277–292.

Nuwer, M.R. (Ed). (2008). *Intraoperative monitoring of neural function.* Amsterdam: Elsevier.

Obrist, W. D. (1954). The electroencephalogram of normal aged adults. *Electroencephalogr Clin Neurophysiol, 6*(2), 235–244.

Oken, B., and Phillips, T. (2008). Evoked potentials—Clinical. In S. LB (Ed.), *New Encyclopedia of Neuroscience.* Elsevier Press.

Oken, B. S. (1997). Endogenous event-related potentials. In K. H. Chiappa (Ed.), *Evoked potentials in clinical medicine* (3rd ed., pp. 529–564). Philadelphia: Lipplincott-Raven.

Oken, B. S., and Kaye, J. A. (1992). Electrophysiologic function in the healthy, extremely old. *Neurology, 42,* 519–526.

Oken, B. S., Salinsky, M. C., and Elsas, S. M. (2006). Vigilance, alertness, or sustained attention: Physiological basis and measurement. *Clinical Neurophysiology, 117,* 1885–1901.

Onofrj, M., Ghilardi, M. F., Basciani, M., and Gambi, D. (1986). Visual evoked potentials in parkinsonism and dopamine blockade reveal a stimulus-dependent dopamine function in humans. *J Neurol Neurosurg Psychiatry, 49*(10), 1150–1159.

Ottaviani, F., Maurizi, M., D'Alatri, L., and Almadori, G. (1990). Auditory brainstem responses in the aged. *Acta Otolaryngol Suppl, 476,* 110–112; discussion 113.

Papanicolaou, A. C., Castillo, E. M., Billingsley-Marshall, R., Pataraia, E., and Simos, P. G. (2005). A review of clinical applications of magnetoencephalography. *Int Rev Neurobiol, 68,* 223–247.

Pierantozzi, M., Panella, M., Palmieri, M. G., Koch, G., Giordano, A., Marciani, M. G., et al. (2004). Different TMS patterns of intracortical inhibition in early onset Alzheimer dementia and frontotemporal dementia. *Clin Neurophysiol, 115*(10), 2410–2418.

Polich, J. (1996). Meta-analysis of P300 normative aging studies. *Psychophysiology, 33*(4), 334–353.

Polich, J. (1997). On the relationship between EEG and P300: Individual differences, aging, and ultradian rhythms. *Int J Psychophysiol, 26*(1–3), 299–317.

Polich, J., Ehlers, C. L., Otis, S., Mandell, A. J., and Bloom, F. E. (1986). P300 latency reflects the degree of cognitive decline in dementing illness. *Electroencephalography and Clinical Neurophysiology, 63,* 138–144.

Polich, J., Ladish, C., and Bloom, F. E. (1990). P300 assessment of early Alzheimer's disease. *Electroencephalography and Clinical Neurophysiology, 77,* 179–189.

Pollock, V. E., Schneider, L. S., Chui, H. C., Henderson, V., Zemansky, M., and Sloane, R. B. (1989). Visual evoked potentials in dementia: a meta-analysis and empirical study of Alzheimer's disease patients. *Biol Psychiatry, 25*(8), 1003–1013.

Ponomareva, N. V., Korovaitseva, G. I., and Rogaev, E. I. (2008). EEG alterations in non-demented individuals related to apolipoprotein E genotype and to risk of Alzheimer disease. *Neurobiol Aging, 29*(6), 819–827.

Prichep, L. S. (2007). Quantitative EEG and electromagnetic brain imaging in aging and in the evolution of dementia. *Ann N Y Acad Sci, 1097,* 156–167.

Prichep, L. S., John, E. R., Ferris, S. H., Rausch, L., Fang, Z., Cancro, R., et al. (2006). Prediction of longitudinal cognitive decline in normal elderly with subjective complaints using electrophysiological imaging. *Neurobiol Aging, 27*(3), 471–481.

Psatta, D. M., and Matei, M. (1988). Age-dependent amplitude variation of brain-stem auditory evoked potentials. *Electroencephalogr Clin Neurophysiol, 71*(1), 27–32.

Rice, D. M., Buchsbaum, M. S., Starr, A., Auslander, L., Hagman, J., and Evans, W. J. (1990). Abnormal EEG slow activity in left temporal areas in senile dementia of the Alzheimer type. *J Gerontol, 45*(4), M145–151.

Robinson, D. J., Merskey, H., Blume, W. T., Fry, R., Williamson, P. C., and Hachinski, V. C. (1994). Electroencephalography as an aid in the exclusion of Alzheimer's disease. *Arch Neurol, 51*(3), 280–284.

Rodnitzky, R. L. (1998). Visual dysfunction in Parkinson's disease. *Clin Neurosci, 5*(2), 102–106.

Rosen, I., Gustafson, L., and Risberg, J. (1993). Multichannel EEG frequency analysis and somatosensory-evoked potentials in patients with different types of organic dementia. *Dementia, 4*(1), 43–49.

Rossi, S., and Rossini, P. M. (2004). TMS in cognitive plasticity and the potential for rehabilitation. *Trends Cogn Sci, 8*(6), 273–279.

Rossini, P. M., Del Percio, C., Pasqualetti, P., Cassetta, E., Binetti, G., Dal Forno, G., et al. (2006). Conversion from mild cognitive impairment to Alzheimer's disease is predicted by sources and coherence of brain electroencephalography rhythms. *Neuroscience, 143*(3), 793–803.

Rossini, P. M., Rossi, S., Babiloni, C., and Polich, J. (2007). Clinical neurophysiology of aging brain: From normal aging to neurodegeneration. *Prog Neurobiol, 83*(6), 375–400.

Salinsky, M., Kanter, R., and Dasheiff, R. M. (1987). Effectiveness of multiple EEGs in supporting the diagnosis of epilepsy: An operational curve. *Epilepsia, 28*(4), 331–334.

Salinsky, M. C., Oken, B. S., Storzbach, D., and Dodrill, C. B. (2003). Assessment of CNS effects of antiepileptic drugs using quantitative EEG measures. *Epilepsia, 44,* 1042–1050.

Santamaria, J., and Chiappa, K. H. (1987). The EEG of drowsiness in normal adults. *J Clin Neurophysiol, 4*(4), 327–382.

Sawaki, L., Yaseen, Z., Kopylev, L., and Cohen, L. G. (2003). Age-dependent changes in the ability to encode a novel elementary motor memory. *Ann Neurol, 53*(4), 521–524.

Scherg, M., and Picton, T. W. (1991). Separation and identification of event-related potential components by brain electric source analysis. *Electroencephalogr Clin Neurophysiol Suppl, 42,* 24–37.

Schiff, S., Valenti, P., Andrea, P., Lot, M., Bisiacchi, P., Gatta, A., et al. (2008). The effect of aging on auditory components of event-related brain potentials. *Clin Neurophysiol, 119*(8), 1795–1802.

Shibasaki, H., and Hallett, M. (2005). Electrophysiological studies of myoclonus. *Muscle Nerve, 31*(2), 157–174.

Shibasaki, H., and Hallett, M. (2006). What is the Bereitschaftspotential? *Clin Neurophysiol, 117*(11), 2341–2356.

Shigeta, M., Julin, P., Almkvist, O., Basun, H., Rudberg, U., and Wahlund, L. O. (1995). EEG in successful aging: A 5 year follow-up study from the eighth to ninth decade of life. *Electroencephalogr Clin Neurophysiol, 95*(2), 77–83.

Signorino, M., Pucci, E., Belardinelli, N., Nolfe, G., and Angeleri, F. (1995). EEG spectral analysis in vascular and Alzheimer dementia. *Electroencephalogr Clin Neurophysiol, 94*(5), 313–325.

Silbert, L. C., Nelson, K., Holman, S., Eaton, R., Oken, B. S., Lou, J. S., et al. (2006). Cortical excitability and age-related volumetric MRI changes. *Clinical Neurophysiology, 117*, 1029–1036.

Sloan, E. P., and Fenton, G. W. (1992). Serial visual evoked potential recordings in geriatric psychiatry. *Electroencephalogr Clin Neurophysiol, 84*(4), 325–331.

Smith, M. C. (1989). Neurophysiology of aging. *Semin Neurol, 9*(1), 68–81.

Sohn, Y. H. and Hallett, M. (2004). Motor evoked potentials. *Phys Med Rehabil Clin N Am, 15*(1), 117–131, vii.

Soikkeli, R., Partanen, J., Soininen, H., Paakkonen, A., and Riekkinen, P., Sr. (1991). Slowing of EEG in Parkinson's disease. *Electroencephalogr Clin Neurophysiol, 79*(3), 159–165.

Sokol, S., Moskowitz, A., and Towle, V. L. (1981). Age-related changes in the latency of the visual evoked potential: Influence of check size. *Electroencephalogr Clin Neurophysiol, 51*(5), 559–562.

Sole-Padulles, C., Bartres-Faz, D., Junque, C., Clemente, I. C., Molinuevo, J. L., Bargallo, N., et al. (2006). Repetitive transcranial magnetic stimulation effects on brain function and cognition among elders with memory dysfunction. A randomized sham-controlled study. *Cereb Cortex, 16*(10), 1487–1493.

Solomon, P. R., Hirschoff, A., Kelly, B., Relin, M., Brush, M., DeVeaux, R. D., et al. (1998). A 7 minute neurocognitive screening battery highly sensitive to Alzheimer's disease. *Arch Neurol, 55*(3), 349–355.

Steriade, M., McCormick, D. A., and Sejnowski, T. J. (1993). Thalamocortical oscillations in the sleeping and aroused brain. *Science, 262*, 679–685.

Synek, V. M. (1988). Prognostically important EEG coma patterns in diffuse anoxic and traumatic encephalopathies in adults. *J Clin Neurophysiol, 5*(2), 161–174.

Tachibana, H., Takeda, M., and Sugita, M. (1989). Short-latency somatosensory and brainstem auditory evoked potentials in patients with Parkinson's disease. *Int J Neurosci, 44*(3–4), 321–326.

Tanosaki, M., Ozaki, I., Shimamura, H., Baba, M., and Matsunaga, M. (1999). Effects of aging on central conduction in somatosensory evoked potentials: Evaluation of onset versus peak methods. *Clin Neurophysiol, 110*(12), 2094–2103.

Tikhonova, I. V., Gnezditskii, V. V., Stakhovskaya, L. V., and Skvortsova, V. I. (2003). Neurophysiological characterization of transitory global amnesia syndrome. *Neurosci Behav Physiol, 33*(2), 171–175.

Tobimatsu, S. (1994). [Visual information processing in humans]. *Rinsho Shinkeigaku, 34*(12), 1250–1252.

Tobimatsu, S. (1995). Aging and pattern visual evoked potentials. *Optom Vis Sci, 72*(3), 192–197.

Tobimatsu, S., and Celesia, G. G. (2006). Studies of human visual pathophysiology with visual evoked potentials. *Clin Neurophysiol, 117*(7), 1414–1433.

van der Hiele, K., Bollen, E. L., Vein, A. A., Reijntjes, R. H., Westendorp, R. G., van Buchem, M. A., et al. (2008). EEG markers of future cognitive performance in the elderly. *J Clin Neurophysiol, 25*(2), 83–89.

van der Hiele, K., Vein, A. A., Reijntjes, R. H., Westendorp, R. G., Bollen, E. L., van Buchem, M. A., et al. (2007). EEG correlates in the spectrum of cognitive decline. *Clin Neurophysiol, 118*(9), 1931–1939.

van der Hiele, K., Vein, A. A., van der Welle, A., van der Grond, J., Westendorp, R. G., Bollen, E. L., et al. (2007). EEG and MRI correlates of mild cognitive impairment and Alzheimer's disease. *Neurobiol Aging, 28*(9), 1322–1329.

Verleger, R., Neukater, W., Kompf, D., and Vieregge, P. (1991). On the reasons for the delay of P3 latency in healthy elderly subjects. *Electroencephalography and Clinical Neurophysiology, 79*, 488–502.

Vieregge, P., Verleger, R., Schulze-Rava, H., and Kompf, D. (1992). Late cognitive event-related potentials in adult Down's syndrome. *Biol Psychiatry, 32*(12), 1118–1134.

Visser, S. L. (1991). The electroencephalogram and evoked potentials in normal aging and dementia. *Electroencephalogr Clin Neurophysiol Suppl, 42*, 289–303.

Visser, S. L., Hooijer, C., Jonker, C., Van Tilburg, W., and De Rijke, W. (1987). Anterior temporal focal abnormalities in EEG in normal aged subjects: Correlations with psychopathological and CT brain scan findings. *Electroencephalography and Clinical Neurophysiology, 66*, 1–7.

Visser, S. L., Van Tilburg, W., Hooijer, C., Jonker, C., and De Rijke, W. (1985). Visual evoked potentials (VEPs) in senile dementia (Alzheimer type) and in non-organic behavioral disorders in the elderly: Comparison with EEG parameters. *Electroencephalography and Clinical Neurophysiology, 60*, 115–121.

Wada, Y., Nanbu, Y., Jiang, Z. Y., Koshino, Y., Yamaguchi, N., and Hashimoto, T. (1997). Electroencephalographic abnormalities in patients with presenile dementia of the Alzheimer type: Quantitative analysis at rest and during photic stimulation. *Biol Psychiatry, 41*(2), 217–225.

Walsh, J. M., and Brenner, R. P. (1987). Periodic lateralized epileptiform discharges—long-term outcome in adults. *Epilepsia, 28*(5), 533–536.

Westmoreland, B. F., and Klass, D. W. (1997). Unusual variants of subclinical rhythmic electrographic discharge of adults (SREDA). *Electroencephalogr Clin Neurophysiol, 102*(1), 1–4.

Wijdicks, E. F., Parisi, J. E., and Sharbrough, F. W. (1994). Prognostic value of myoclonus status in comatose survivors of cardiac arrest. *Ann Neurol, 35*(2), 239–243.

Williamson, P. C., Merskey, H., Morrison, S., Rabheru, K., Fox, H., Wands, K., et al. (1990). Quantitative electroencephalographic correlates of cognitive decline in normal elderly subjects. *Archives of Neurology, 47*, 1185–1188.

Wisniewski, K. E., Wisniewski, H. M., and Wen, G. Y. (1985). Occurrence of neuropathological changes and dementia of Alzheimer's disease in Down's syndrome. *Ann Neurol, 17*(3), 278–282.

Wright, C. E., Harding, G. F., and Orwin, A. (1984). Presenile dementia—the use of the flash and pattern VEP in diagnosis. *Electroencephalogr Clin Neurophysiol, 57*(5), 405–415.

Zanette, G., Tamburin, S., Manganotti, P., Refatti, N., Forgione, A., and Rizzuto, N. (2002). Changes in motor cortex inhibition over time in patients with amyotrophic lateral sclerosis. *J Neurol, 249*(12), 1723–1728.

Zumsteg, D., and Wieser, H. G. (2002). Effects of aging and sex on middle-latency somatosensory evoked potentials: Normative data. *Clin Neurophysiol, 113*(5), 681–685.

11 Nerve Conduction Studies and Electromyography

Jau-Shin Lou

Introduction

Electromyographic (EMG) or electrodiagnostic (EDX) studies consist of nerve conduction studies (NCV) and needle examination. EDX studies are an extension of the neurological examination. Electromyographers perform a brief history and focused neurological examination and use the information to design the EMG studies. Electromyographers design each study specifically based on history and initial neurological findings to modify the study as information is obtained. A well-designed and executed EDX study should obtain necessary information needed for the diagnosis, provide guidance for treatment, and minimize patient discomfort.

Peripheral and Central EMG

Traditionally, electromyography (EMG) is used to diagnose disorders of the peripheral nervous system. The term EMG is used to refer to both nerve conduction studies and needle examination of the muscles. The nerve conduction studies include examination of both motor and sensory nerves. The commonly studied motor nerves include the median, radial, ulnar, tibial, peroneal, femoral, and facial nerves. The commonly studied sensory nerves studies include median, radial, ulnar, tibial, superficial peroneal, and sural nerves. Because this traditional EMG is used to study peripheral nerve systems, it is also called peripheral EMG.

Over the last twenty years, the technique of transcranial magnetic stimulation (TMS) has been used to study motor conduction from the motor cortex to the spinal cord. TMS is useful in studying spinal cord lesions. Because it studies part of the central nervous system, TMS can be called central EMG.

Peripheral EMG is useful in diagnosing disorders in the peripheral nervous system such as lower motor neuron diseases, sensory neuronopathy, radiculopathy, plexopathy, neuropathy, neuromuscular junction transmission disorders, and myopathy.

The goals of the peripheral EMG include the following:

1. To localize a lesion.
   EMG is useful in localizing a lesion to peripheral nerve, neuromuscular junction, or muscles. The disorders that involve the peripheral nerve include mononeuropathy, mononeuritis multiplex, polyneuropathy, plexopathy, radiculopathy, polyradiculopathy, and neuronopathy. The neuromuscular junction disorders include presynaptic disorders such as the myasthenic syndrome and post synaptic disorders such as myasthenia gravis. Muscle disorders include inflammatory or metabolic myopathy and muscular dystrophy.

2. To reveal underlying pathophysiology.
   EMG is useful in characterizing neuropathy as a predominant motor, predominant sensory, or mixed motor and sensory neuropathy. It also plays an important role in differentiating demyelinating neuropathy such as acute or chronic inflammatory demyelinating polyneuropathy (AIDP or CIDP) from primary axonal neuropathy.

3. To evaluate the temporal course of the condition.
   EMG is helpful in deciding if the disease is hyperacute (less than a week), acute (a couple of weeks), subacute (weeks to a few months), or chronic (more than a few months).

4. To assess the severity of nerve damage.
   The findings from an EMG can be useful in assessing the severity of the nerve damage.

The above information is helpful for both diagnosis and for making treatment decisions. For example, a 21-year-old man presented with 3 weeks' history of acute onset weakness of the right hand and numbness of the right 4th and 5th digits. The differential diagnosis includes the following:

1. Right C8-T1 cervical radiculopathy.

2. Right brachial plexopathy involving the lower trunk.

3. Mononeuropathy of the ulnar nerve not caused by entrapment, such as vasculitis.

4. Right ulnar nerve entrapment at elbow.

5. Right ulnar nerve entrapment at the wrist.

The EMG will be very helpful in arriving at the diagnosis.

Each EMG should be customized to answer the relevant clinical questions for each patient. At the beginning of an EMG, an electromyographer explains to patients what is about to take place. For example, electrical shocks will be used to perform the nerve conduction studies and a needle, which serves as a small microphone, will be used to "listen" to the muscle. Although these tests can cause some discomfort, they are not unbearable. Most importantly, the patients should be informed that they can ask the tests be stopped at any time if they cannot tolerate it any longer. Patients usually tolerate the procedure well. The electromyographer will take a brief history, perform a focused physical examination, and formulate the differential diagnosis. This information is crucial in designing an EMG. The electromyographer needs to decide which nerve conduction studies need to be performed. Based on the findings in the nerve conduction studies, the electromyographer will decide which muscles need to be tested with needle examination. As more data is collected during the test, the design of the study may need to be modified to collect appropriate data for the diagnosis. A good EMG should be designed in such a way that it answers the clinical questions and yet minimizes patients' discomfort.

Classification of Nerve Injury

Nerve injury is classified in relation to the location of the damage to a nerve. In the normal nerve, the axons which are surrounded by myelin sheaths are grouped into a funiculus. The connective tissue that surrounds each axon and myelin sheath is called endoneurium. The connective tissue that surrounds each funiculus is called perineurium. A peripheral nerve such as median or ulnar nerve typically contains several funiculii which are surrounded by epineurium. Depending on whether the injury is to the axon, myelin sheath, or surrounding connective tissue (see Figure 1), there are three classes of nerve injury:

1. Neuropraxia.

    This type of injury is characterized by a segmental block of the conduction of the nerve action potential caused by structural damage to the myelin sheath. The axon and connective tissues including endoneurium, perineurium, and epineurium are not affected. In neuropraxia, a nerve can conduct above and below a certain area, but not across the region of injury. This phenomenon is due to a focal demyelination of the nerve. Conduction block correlates extremely well with demyelination. Neuropraxia is most commonly seen in nerve entrapment such as in carpal tunnel syndrome and in demyelinating neuropathies such as AIDP or CIDP.

2. Axonotmesis.

    In this type of injury, there is a loss of continuity of nerve axons but the continuity of the connective tissue is intact. The myelin sheath and the surrounding connective tissue are not affected. Axonotmesis leads to Wallerian degeneration of the distal part of the nerve characterized by breakdown of the axon in ovoids with secondary degeneration of the myelin sheath. Typically, Wallerian degeneration takes at least 3 to 5 days to occur and, for at least several days, the distal part of the axon may retain relatively normal excitability. For example, after a complete transection of the median nerve in the upper arm, the compound muscle action potential obtained by stimulating at the wrist may remain normal for up to a week.

    Following Wallerian degeneration, the proximal part of the nerve attempts to re-grow. Schwann cells along the course of the degenerated distal nerve proliferate and form tubes. The distal ends of the intact nerve fibers become specialized for growth and attempt to grow down through the tubes of Schwann cells to their original destination. Under the optimal conditions, this growth occurs at the rate of approximately 1mm per day, 1 cm per week, or 1 inch per month.

3. Neurotmesis.

    In this type of nerve injury, all components of the nerve including axon, myelin sheath, and connective tissues are affected. This process leads to Wallerian degeneration of the axons, but there is less chance for re-growth in the appropriate direction due to loss of continuity in the supporting connective tissue surrounding the nerve. In this condition the nerve may not grow much beyond the site of the injury and may ball up and develop into a neuroma.

Motor Nerve Conduction Studies

In the motor nerve conduction study a pair of recording electrodes (referred to as active electrode and reference electrode) are placed on a muscle and the corresponding motor nerve is stimulated along its path. For example, in the ulnar motor nerve conduction study, the active electrode is placed on the muscle belly of the abductor digiti minimi and the reference electrode is placed on the tendon. The ulnar nerve can be stimulated at the wrist, below and above the elbow, and at the axilla.

When motor nerves are stimulated, the action potential generated travels distally and proximally. The distal-traveling action potentials cause the release of acetylcholine. The acetylcholine molecules that are released diffuse across the neuromuscular junction and bind with the acetylcholine receptors and this generates muscle fiber action potentials. The summation of all the muscle fiber action potentials constitutes the compound muscle action potential (Figure 2).

The key parameters in the motor nerve conduction study include the following:

1. Distal latency (DL, measured in ms). The DL measures the time from stimulation to the onset of a compound muscle action potential. DL is most commonly prolonged in entrapment neuropathies such as median nerve entrapment at the wrist or demyelinating neuropathy such as AIDP or CIDP. DL is usually normal in axonal neuropathies.

2. Compound muscle action potential (CMAP, measured in mV). The CMAP represents the summation of all muscle action potentials generated by intact motor axons. A reduction in the amplitude of CMAP, therefore, represents motor axonal loss. This is most commonly seen in axonal neuropathy or axonal damage due to entrapment or demyelinating lesions.

3. Conduction velocity (CV, measured in m/s). The CV is calculated by dividing the distance between two stimulation sites and the difference in latency. Moderate to severe slowed CV is seen in demyelinating polyneuropathies. However, a mild reduction in CV can be seen in severe axonal neuropathies or entrapment neuropathies.

Sensory Nerve Conduction Studies

In the sensory nerve conduction study, a pair of recording electrodes (referred to as active electrode and reference electrode) are placed along a nerve path and the corresponding sensory nerve is stimulated at a site proximal or distal to the recording electrode. When the sensory nerve axons are stimulated, the action potential activated travels in both directions and the recording electrode records the

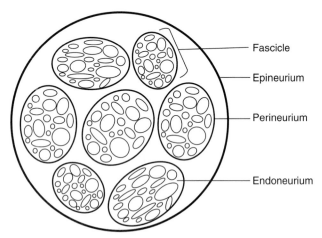

Figure 1 Anatomy of a Nerve. Each nerve fascicle is surrounded by the perineurium and the connective tissue around each fiber within a fascicle is the endoneurium. Multiple fascicles are surrounded by the epineurium. The degree to which endoneurium, perineurium, and epineurium are damaged will affect the recovery of the nerve.

Fascicle

Epineurium

Perineurium

Endoneurium

Ulnar

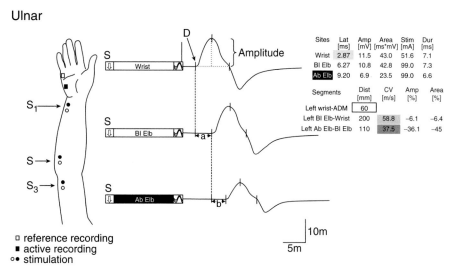

Sites	Lat [ms]	Amp [mV]	Area [ms*mV]	Stim [mA]	Dur [ms]
Wrist	2.87	11.5	43.0	51.6	7.1
Bl Elb	6.27	10.8	42.8	99.0	7.3
Ab Elb	9.20	6.9	23.5	99.0	6.6

Segments	Dist [mm]	CV [m/s]	Amp [%]	Area [%]
Left wrist-ADM	60			
Left Bl Elb-Wrist	200	58.8	−6.1	−6.4
Left Ab Elb-Bl Elb	110	37.5	−36.1	−45

□ reference recording
■ active recording
○● stimulation

Figure 2 Motor nerve conduction study of an ulnar nerve. The stimulation is applied at the wrist, below the elbow, and above the elbow with the CMAP recorded from the abductor digiti minimi. In this case the CMAP was measured from the negative peak to the baseline with an amplitude of 11.5 mV. The DL (distal latency) represents the time from the stimulation to the deflection of the CMAP. In this case the DL is 2.87 ms. The conduction velocity from below the elbow to the wrist is calculated by dividing the distance (in this case 200 mm) by the difference in the latency at the wrist and below the elbow (a, which is 6.27−2.87). The CV from below elbow to wrist in this case is 200 mm/3.4 ms = 58.8 m/s. Likewise, the CV from above elbow to below elbow is calculated by dividing the distance (in this case110 mm) by the difference in latency (b, which is 9.20−6.27), the CV from above to below elbow = 37.5 m/s, which is reduced. This nerve conduction study shows evidence of ulnar nerve entrapment at the elbow. There is also a reduced CMAP from 10.8 mV at below elbow to 6.9 mV at above elbow. This phenomenon is called conduction block.

summation of the traveling action potentials from either a proximal site (orthodromic) or from a distal site (antidromic) (see Figure 3). In an orthodromic sensory nerve conduction study, the sensory nerve action potential (SNAP) is recorded from a site proximal to the stimulation site because the nerve action potential travels in the physiological direction. In an antidromic sensory nerve conduction study, the sensory nerve action potential (SNAP) is recorded from a site distal to the stimulation site because the nerve action potential travels opposite the physiological direction. For example, for the orthodromic sensory conduction study of the median nerve the stimulation is applied at the palm with the SNAP recorded at the wrist, and for the antidromic sensory conduction study of the median nerve the stimulation is applied at the wrist with the SNAP recorded from the thumb or second digit.

The key parameters of the sensory nerve conduction study include:

1. Distal latency (DL, measured in ms). The DL represents the time from the stimulation to the onset of the SNAP. DL is prolonged in entrapment lesions between the stimulation and recording sites such as ulnar nerve entrapment at the wrist or demyelinating neuropathy. DL is usually normal in axonal neuropathies.

2. Sensory nerve action potential (SNAP, measured in μV). The amplitude of SNAP reflects the summation of all the action potentials from all intact sensory nerve axons. A reduction in the amplitude of SNAP, therefore, represents sensory axonal loss. This is most commonly seen in axonal neuropathy or axonal damage due to entrapment or demyelinating lesions.

3. Sensory nerve conduction velocity (CV, measured in m/s). The CV is calculated by dividing the distance between the stimulation site and the recording site by the latency. Moderately to severely slowed CV is seen in demyelinating polyneuropathies. However, a mild reduction in CV can be seen in severe axonal neuropathies or entrapment neuropathies.

Radial

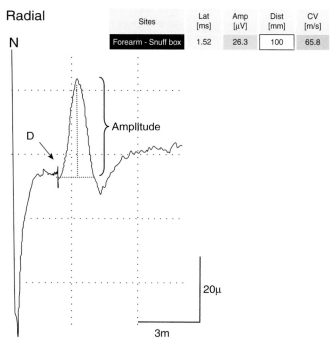

Sites	Lat [ms]	Amp [μV]	Dist [mm]	CV [m/s]
Forearm - Snuff box	1.52	26.3	100	65.8

Figure 3 Sensory nerve conduction study of a radial nerve. The stimulation is applied at the forearm with the sensory nerve action potential (SNAP) recorded from the first interdigital space (the snuff box). The DL represents the time from stimulation to the deflection of the SNAP. In this case the DL is 1.52 ms. The NCV from the forearm to the first interdigital space is calculated by dividing the distance between the stimulation and recording sites. In this case it is 100mm/1.52 ms = 65.8 m/s. The amplitude of the SNAP is measured from the peak to the baseline. In this case it is 29.3 μV.

Needle Examination

In a needle examination, a specially designed needle is inserted into the muscle.

The key observations in a needle examination include:

1. Insertion activity.

   During this examination, the examiner advances the needle with fine abrupt movements to irritate the muscle membrane. In normal innervated muscles, the needle movement evokes normal insertion activity that lasts for 40–60ms. The duration of the insertion activity may increase in denervated muscles or muscle disorders with increased muscle membrane excitability such as myotonic disorders. In denervated muscles, a local muscle action potential, called a positive-wave or fibrillation potential, will be generated in addition to prolonged duration of insertion activity.

2. Spontaneous activity.

   (a) *Normal spontaneous activity.* Normal muscle has no spontaneous activity at rest other than end plate noise or end plate spike in the motor end plate region.

   (b) *Abnormal spontaneous activity.*

   (i) Positive waves and fibrillation potentials. These two potentials are generated by denervated muscle fibers. They can be observed in neurogenic disorders that cause motor axonal damage such as lower motor neuron disease, radiculopathy, or neuropathy. In addition, positive waves and fibrillation potentials can be observed in myopathic disorders where the destruction of muscle fiber occur such as inflammatory myopathy, muscular dystrophy, or severe neuromuscular transmission disorders such as myasthenia or botulism. Therefore, positive waves and fibrillation potentials are not specific for neurogenic disorders.

   (ii) Myotonic discharges. Myotonic discharges are spontaneous discharges of muscle fibers triggered by needle movements. Myotonic discharges are characterized by their waxing and waning, both in amplitude and frequency. Myotonic discharges are typically observed in myotonic disorders such as myotonic dystrophies, myotonia congenita and paramyotonia congenita.

   (iii) Complex repetitive discharges (CRDs). CRDs are generated by rapid, repetitive discharges of a group of muscle fibers following the depolarization of a single muscle fiber. CRDs are observed in chronic neurogenic or myopathic disorders.

   (iv) Myokymic discharges. Myokymic discharges are spontaneous, rhythmic discharges of the same motor neurons. They are commonly observed in radiation brachial plexopathy, AIDP or CIDP, multiple sclerosis (facial muscles), brainstem tumors, radiculopathies, hypocalcemia, or timber rattlesnake poisoning.

   (v) Fasciculation potentials. Fasciculation potentials are random, irregular spontaneous discharges of single motor units. It is generated at the cell body or axon level. The most commonly observed fasciculation potentials are benign fasciculation that are not associated with weakness or neuromuscular disorders. Benign fasciculation potentials have the normal waveforms (including amplitude and duration) of normal motor units. Pathologic fasciculation potentials are associated with disease process affecting the lower motor neurons such as motor neuron diseases, radiculopathies, plexopathies, neuropathies, and nerve entrapment.

   (vi) Cramp potentials. Cramp potentials are muscle potentials recorded during painful muscle cramps. Cramp potentials are similar to EMG activities of maximally contracted muscles with full interference patterns. Cramp potentials can be seen in normal individuals, neuropathies, or myopathies.

   (vii) Neuromyotonic discharges. Neuromyotonic discharges are spontaneous high-frequency (100 to 200 Hz), decremental discharges of a single motor unit. It is observed in chronic neuropathic disorders or in Issac's syndrome (syndrome of spontaneous muscle activity).

3. Motor unit potential (MUP).

   A motor unit constitutes a motor neuron and all of the muscle fibers it innervates. During the needle examination, after evaluating the insertion activity, the examiner will ask the patient to minimally activate the muscle so that only a few motor units (low-threshold motor units) are activated. The duration and amplitude of these motor units will be evaluated. At least ten low-threshold motor units will be evaluated from two or three different insertion sites. The duration and amplitude of the MUP depend on the muscle fiber size, the number of muscle fibers innervated by the same motor axons, and the size of the motor axon territory. In a neurogenic disorder, the denervated muscle fibers will be re-innervated by the sprouting of the remaining functioning motor axons. Therefore, these healthy motor axons will have a larger territory and an MUP of longer duration and larger amplitude than normal. On the contrary, in a myopathic disorder the muscle fibers are smaller in size and some of the muscle fibers are damaged; therefore, the MUP is of shorter duration and smaller amplitude.

4. Recruitment pattern.

   Recruitment pattern refers to the order in which motor units are activated with voluntary effort. As a patient increases the effort in muscle contraction, more motor units will be activated. Physiologically, motor units with small MUPs are activated with lower effort and larger motor units are activated with increasing effort (Heinemann Principle). Physiologically, only a few motor units are recruited with lower force generation. However, in a myopathic disorder, because of loss of normal muscle fibers, the force generated by each motor unit is much smaller than normal. Therefore, more motor units (compared to normal) need to be activated to generate a desired force. This phenomenon is called "early recruitment."

5. Interference pattern.

   Interference pattern refers to the degree of overlap of MUPs on a computer screen. In normal muscles, it is impossible to delineate each individual MUP with maximum voluntary effort because they overlap with each other; however, in a moderate to severe neurogenic disorder the MUP can still be somewhat delineated due to loss of motor units—a phenomenon called reduced interference pattern. The interference pattern is normal in a myopathic disorder because there is no loss of motor axons.

Late Responses

Two late responses, F-waves and the H-reflex, are commonly studied in clinical EMG laboratories (see Figure 4).

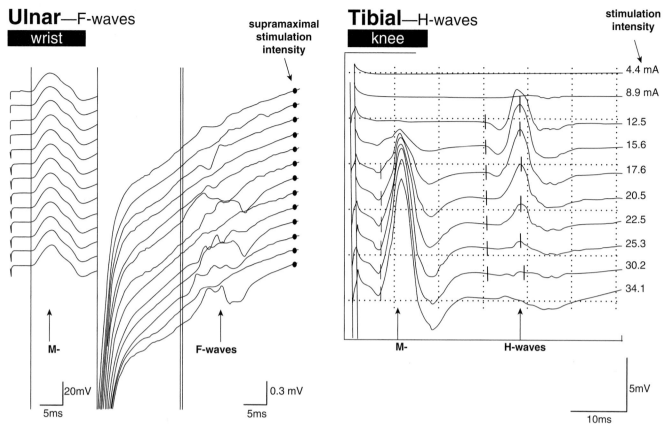

Figure 4 F-wave vs. H-wave. The left panel displays F-waves recorded from an ulnar nerve and the right panel H-waves from a tibial nerve. In an F-wave study, the nerve is stimulated at a supramaximal intensity. Usually a total of more than ten trials are performed. Each F-wave represents the combined MUPs of a few motor units. Usually different motor units contribute to different F-waves; therefore, each F-wave may have a different wave form and a different latency. In an H-wave study, the nerve is stimulated with a very small stimulation intensity. The stimulation intensity is then increased gradually. In this illustration, the stimulation intensity was increased from 4.4 mA for the first trial to 34.1 mA for the 10th trial. Please note that the H-wave appears before the M-response (the 3rd trace). As the stimulation intensity increases, an increase in the size of the M-response is accompanied by a decrease in the size of the H waves.

1. F-waves.
   F-waves are so named because this response was first observed in the abductor hallucis muscle in the "foot" with the stimulation of the tibial nerve. When a motor nerve is stimulated, the action potential evoked travels both distally and proximally. The distal-traveling action potential evokes the CMAP response from the muscle (M-response) while the proximally-traveling action potential reaches the cell bodies of the anterior horn cells. This causes the cells to back-fire and generate distally traveling action potentials. These action potentials in turn activate muscles and are recorded as F-waves. There is no synapse involved in the generation of F-waves. Due to the fluctuation of the excitability of anterior horn cells, usually only about 5% of the motor neuron pool (usually less than ten motor neurons) generates F-waves. Each supramaximal stimulation may activate different anterior horn cells to generate distinct F-waves with each stimulation. Therefore, the F-wave latency may vary from stimulation to stimulation. Clinically, we measure the shortest F-wave latencies from 10–20 supramaximal stimulations.

   In a normal motor nerve, F-waves are characterized by a large variety of each wave forms. Lack of variability in F-waves may be indicative of a proximal nerve lesion such as AIDP or CIDP. The absence of F-waves is very useful in the diagnosis of early AIDP. F-waves are not useful in diagnosing radiculopathy because each commonly tested motor nerve contains motor axons from two or more roots.

2. The H-reflex.
   The H-reflex is named after a German physiologist Johann Hoffmann who first described it. The H-reflex is the physiological equivalent of the ankle reflex clinically. The H-reflex is recorded from the soleus muscle with the stimulation of the tibial nerve at the popliteal fossa. The H-reflex, like the ankle reflex, is a monosynaptic reflex. The H-reflex is optimally evoked with an electrical stimulation of long duration (such as 1 ms), and it is generated at a lower stimulation intensity than is required to evoke any M-response. As the stimulation intensity increases, the M-response amplitude increases and the H amplitude is reduced. At the maximal stimulation for the M-response, the H-response disappears (see Figure 4). In S1 radiculopathy, the H latency is prolonged. It should be noted that H latency is also prolonged in a variety of disorders such as axonal or demyelinating polyneuropathy involving the tibial nerve.

Blink Reflex

Blink reflex is the physiological equivalent of the corneal reflex. The blink reflex is recorded from bilateral orbicularis muscles with the stimulation applied to the supraorbital nerve on one side. The afferent limb of the blink reflex is the supraorbital branch of the 5th cranial nerve. The efferent limb is the facial nerve. There are two components in the blink reflex: an R1 component and an R2 component. The R1 component is a unilateral response (ipsilateral to the stimulation side) with a latency of about 10 ms. It is a monosynaptic response. The R2 component can be observed bilaterally with a latency of about 30 ms. It is an oligosynaptic response involving several synapses in the brainstem. The blink reflex is useful in studying lesions involving the 5th nerve, 7th nerve, and brainstem lesions.

Repetitive Nerve Stimulation (RNS)

The examiner performs RNS when a neuromuscular transmission disorder, such as myasthenia gravis (MG) or Lambert-Eaton myasthenic syndrome (LEMS), is suspected.

Physiology of the Neuromuscular Junction Transmission

A neuromuscular junction consists of the pre-synaptic axonal terminals of a motor neuron and the post-synaptic end-plate of muscle fibers with a synaptic cleft separating these two structures. When a nerve action potential arrives at the pre-synaptic terminal, it triggers a release of ACh vesicles into the synaptic cleft. The ACh then diffuses across the cleft and binds with the ACh receptors in the end-plate zone of the muscle fiber. There are three different ACh vesicle pools in the pre-synaptic terminals: the immediately available pool (~1000 vesicles), intermediately available pool (~10,000 vesicles), and the mobilization pool (~300,000 vesicles). Each vesicle contains about 1000 ACh molecules (called a quantum). When the action potential arrives at the presynaptic terminal, it triggers the release of vesicles from the immediately available pool which is then replenished by the vesicles from the intermediately available pool.

Even when the presynaptic terminal is not activated by an action potential (at rest), there is random spontaneous release of quanta of ACh into the synaptic cleft. Each quantum of ACh induces a miniature excitatory postsynaptic potential (MEPP) in the muscle. Simultaneous release of several quanta of ACh induces several MEPPs that are summated into an end-plate potential (EPP). The arrival of an action potential in the presynaptic motor neuron triggers a synchronous release of about 100 quanta of ACh which induces an EPP above the threshold to generate a muscle action potential.

The release of ACh from a presynaptic terminal is calcium (Ca) dependent. The extracellular Ca enters the presynaptic terminal when the presynaptic voltage gated Ca channels open upon the arrival of the action potential. Increasing the intracellular Ca in the presynaptic terminal facilitates the release of ACh vesicles into the synaptic cleft. It takes about 100–200ms for this intracellular Ca to be pumped back out to the extracellular space.

Physiology of RNS

Two RNS techniques are commonly used: low-rate (2–5 Hz) and high rate (>20 Hz). There is a net accumulation of Ca in the presynaptic terminal at high rate stimulation, but not at low rate stimulation, because it takes about 100–200ms for Ca to be pumped out to the extracellular space.

When a nerve is stimulated at 2–5 Hz, the number of available ACh quanta from the presynaptic terminal reduces with each successive stimulus; however, there is a large "safety margin" in a healthy neuromuscular junction. Because of this safety margin, there is no reduction in the amplitude of the M response in both high rate and low rate stimulation.

Pathophysiology of MG

In myasthenia gravis, the ACh receptor antibodies destroy the ACh receptors at the postsynaptic end-plate; therefore, there are fewerACh receptors available.

In a diseased state, such as myasthenia gravis, the safety margin is greatly reduced due to the loss of ACh receptors in the postsynaptic end plate zone. The amplitude of the M response will be reduced with each successive stimulus and reach its nadir at the 4th stimulus. This phenomenon is referred to as abnormal decrement. Abnormal decrement is also observed in high rate stimulation in patients with MG.

Pathophysiology of LEMS

In LEMS there are reduced numbers of voltage-gated Ca channels in the presynaptic terminal. Therefore, less Ca enters the presynaptic terminal upon the arrival of an action potential, which results in the release of fewer quanta of ACh. This ultimately leads to a reduction in the CMAP amplitude in a postsynaptic muscle. A commonly observed abnormality in LEMS is a severe reduction in CMAP amplitude.

At low rate stimulation there will be abnormal decrement observed in LEMS. However, at high rate stimulation, a marked increment in CMAP amplitude (as high as 1000%) is observed due to the accumulation of Ca in the presynaptic terminal which facilitates the release of ACh vesicles.

The Effect of Exercise on Neuromuscular Transmission

Contracting a muscle maximally requires the rapid activation of motor neurons similar to that of high rate stimulation; therefore, contracting the muscle maximally will cause the accumulation of calcium in the presynaptic terminal.

Repetitive nerve stimulation can be performed before and 0, 1, 2, and 3 minutes after brief (30–60 s) exercise. In patients with MG, the abnormal decrement observed before exercise is often partially or completely abolished (known as post-exercise facilitation). Post exercise facilitation is most likely due to the higher concentration of Ca in the presynaptic terminal. However, the abnormal decrement observed before exercise is often exacerbated at 2 to 3 minutes after exercise, probably due to the depletion of the immediately available ACh vesicles.

Transcranial Magnetic Stimulation (TMS)

TMS is a technique developed in the 1980s that allows a painless stimulation of the motor cortex which evokes a recordable response in a muscle. These recordings are useful in evaluating the corticospinal tract. During TMS a magnetic coil is placed on the scalp of a patient. A large current is released from a capacitor in a short burst (<1ms). The current flows through the coil and induces a magnetic field. This magnetic field can penetrate the skull painlessly and induce current in the motor cortex. The current activates interneurons which in turn activate pyramidal cells (Figure 5). The action potential induced in the cortical pyramidal cells travels down the spinal cord, activates a lower motor neuron, which in turn activates a muscle. The most important clinical application of TMS is to measure the central motor conduction time (CMCT).

CMCT, which is the conduction time in the cortico-spinal tract, can be calculated as follows:

$$CMCT = latency\ (MEP) - \tfrac{1}{2}\ (M\ latency + F\ latency - 1)$$

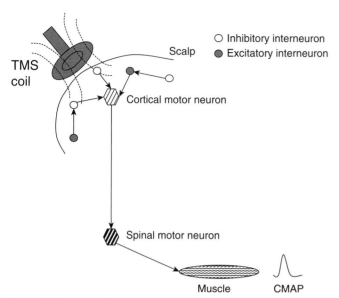

Figure 5 Transcranial magnetic stimulation (TMS). During TMS, a TMS coil is placed in the appropriate position on the scalp. A very high intensity current is passed through the coil which induces a magnetic field. The magnetic field in turn induces current in the cerebral cortex. The induced current then activates inhibitory and excitatory interneurons which in turn activate cortical motor neurons. The cortical motor neurons in turn activate spinal motor neurons which in turn activate the muscles. The output of TMS is recorded as the CMAP from the target muscle.

Latency (MEP): the latency of the motor response evoked by TMS (in ms).

M latency: the latency of the M response evoked by stimulation of the peripheral nerve (in ms).

F latency: the minimum latency of the F-waves (in ms).

−1: is to account for the turn-around time of the F-waves at the motor neuron cell body.

M latency + F latency −1: is twice the time required for the action potential to travel from the lower motor neuron cell body to the muscle. This value is multiplied by ½ to represent the time for a one-way conduction.

For example, when TMS is applied to the cortical motor area with the motor response recorded from the abductor pollicis muscles, the latency (MEP) = 20.6 ms. With the stimulation of the median nerve at the wrist, the M latency = 3.4 ms and the minimum F-wave latency = 28.6 ms. In this example, the CMCT is calculated as follows:

$$CMCT = 20.6 - \tfrac{1}{2}\,(3.4 + 28.6 - 1) = 5.1\ ms$$

CMCT is usually prolonged in patients with compression myelopathy or central demyelinating disorder such as multiple sclerosis (MS).

Factors Affecting Nerve Conduction Studies and Needle Examination

Several factors may influence the findings in EDX studies and lead to misinterpretations of the results.

Temperatures

Temperature affects almost every parameter measured in the nerve conduction study and needle examination.

In nerve conduction studies, low limb temperature can result in increased distal latency, reduced nerve conduction velocities, increased CMAP amplitudes, and increased SNAP amplitudes.

In needle examination, low limb temperature can result in MUPs of larger amplitude, longer duration, and increase in the number of phases. Cold temperature also may reduce spontaneous activity such as positive waves and fibrillation potentials.

The EMG laboratories should be kept warm (room temperature at 75°F). Limb temperatures should be routinely monitored in every patient. The ideal temperature for the EMG is at least 33°C measured at the forearm and at least 32°C measured at anterior tibialis muscles. Immersing the limbs in a warm water bath or warming packs are the best ways to warm up a cold limb. Surface heating with a heating lamp is not recommended.

Age

Age affects nerve conduction velocity (NCV). NCV in newborns is about 50% of normal adult values. It increases to 75% of adult values by 12 months of age and reaches normal adult value by 24 months of age. NCVs reach their peak at about 20 years of age and start to decline at about 40 years of age at a rate of about 1–4 meter per second per decade. A motor NCV of 35 m/s (lower limit of normal 40 m/s) in the tibial nerve of an 80-year-old man should not be considered as abnormal.

Age affects the amplitude of CMAP and SNAP. Both CMAP and SNAP increase their amplitude during first two years of life and decline slowly after 50 years of age. Low SNAP amplitude or absent SNAP in the lower extremities are not necessarily abnormal in the elderly.

Older people also tend to have MUP of longer duration and larger amplitude due to gradual, physiological drop-out of motor neurons.

Height

Taller individuals tend to have slower NCV than shorter individuals due to the difference in nerve length. The longer the nerve length, the slower the NCV. It is not uncommon to see a NCV of 37 m/s in the lower extremities of a 6.5 feet tall basketball player.

Summary

EMG and NCV studies are useful in the evaluation of peripheral sensorimotor disturbances in individuals of any age. The changes seen with aging are well documented and are of a modest degree of difference when compared to younger individuals.

Examples of Common EDX Cases

CASE #1. A 71-Year-old Woman with Foot Drop

This 71-year old woman presented with a two-week history of right foot drop and numbness of the lateral aspect of her right lower extremity below knee. She enjoyed gardening and knelt on the ground preparing her flower bed for spring planting for a few days three weeks ago.

Physical examination showed 2/5 weakness of the right anterior tibialis, peroneal longus, and extensor hallucis longus muscles on the right. Sensory examination showed reduced sensation to light touch and pin prink in the lateral aspect of the calf. The EDX study showed (**abnormal values in bold text**):

Case 1 Motor Nerve Conduction Studies

Nerve	DL (ms)	Amp (mV)	CV (m/s)
R. Peroneal—EDB	5.1	2.1	49 (below knee—ankle) **28 (above—below knee)**
Tibial—AH	5.3	6.5	43 (knee—ankle)

EDB: extensor digitorum brevis; AH: abductor hallucis

Case 1 Sensory Nerve Conduction Studies

Nerve	DL (ms)	Amp (μV)	CV (m/s)
L. Sural		2.5	40

Case 1 EMG Findings

Muscle	IA	Fib	POS	AMP	Dur	IP
R Lower E						
VL	N	N	N	N	N	N
TA	Inc	2+	2+	N	N	−2
Posterior Tibialis	N	N	N	N	N	N
Gastro	N	N	N	N	N	N
FDI(foot)	N	N	N	N	N	N
AH	N	N	N	N	N	N

VL: vastus lateralis; TA: tibialis anterior; FDI: first dorsal interosseus

Summary

The clinical history and physical examination suggested that the patient may suffer from right peroneal entrapment at the fibular head. A right L5 radiculopathy also needs to be considered. The EDX showed that the conduction velocity of the peroneal nerve was normal from below the knee to the ankle. However, the NCV was reduced from above to below knee, which confirms the clinical impression. Needle examination showed there was denervation observed in the anterior tibialis muscle.

CASE #2. A 75-Year-old Man with Dementia and Weakness

A 75-year-old man who had been seen at the dementia clinic for frontotemporal dementia was referred to the EMG laboratory because of progressive weakness of the right side of his body and diffuse fasciculation. His wife stated that he developed weakness of his right hand about six months ago and now he is having trouble with his left hand as well. She also noted that he is not walking as well as he did before. On physical examination, you noted that the patient has 4/5 weakness of proximal right upper extremity and 3/5 weakness in the distal right upper extremity. The left upper extremity was 4/5 distally and 4+/5 proximally. You also noted 4/5 weakness in both lower extremities. The reflexes were 3/4 diffusely with bilateral upgoing toes. You performed the EDX study (**abnormal values in bold text**).

Case 2 Motor Nerve Conduction Studies

Nerve	DL (ms)	Amp (mV)	CV (m/s)	Minimal F-latency (ms)
R. Median—APB	3.4	**3.5**	51	27.3
R. Ulnar—ADM	2.6	**2.8**	47	28.8
R. Peroneal—EDB	5.6	2	49 (below knee–ankle) 43 (above–below knee)	58
R. Tibial—AH	4.7	6	45	56

APB: abductor pollicis brevis; ADM: abductor digiti minimi

Case 2 Sensory Nerve Conduction Studies

Nerve	DL (ms)	Amp (μV)	CV (m/s)
R. Median—2nd		15	54
R. Ulnar—5th		13	51
R. Radial—Thumb		10	52
R. Sural		4	38

Case 2 EMG Findings

Muscle	IA	Fib	POS	AMP	Dur	IP
R Upper E						
Deltoid	Inc	2+	2+	Inc	Inc	−2
Triceps	Inc	3+	3+	Inc	Inc	−2
EDC	Inc	2+	2+	Inc	Inc	−2
APB	Inc	4+	4+			−4
FDI	Inc	4+	4+			−4
L Lower E						
VL	Inc	2+	2+	Inc	Inc	−2
TA	Inc	1+	1+	Inc	Inc	−1
Gastro	Inc	1+	1+	Inc	Inc	−1
R Upper E						
Deltoid	Inc	2+	2+	Inc	Inc	−2
Triceps	Inc	1+	1+	Inc	Inc	−1
EDC	Inc	1+	1+	Inc	Inc	−1
Thoracic paraspinal	Inc	1+	1+			

EDC: extensor digitorum communis

Summary

The clinical history and physical examination suggested that the patient most likely has amyotrophic lateral sclerosis associated with frontotemporal lobe dementia. Motor nerve conduction studies showed reduced CMAP amplitude in the right APB and FDI, suggesting axonal loss. Sensory nerve conduction studies were normal. Needle examination showed he has diffuse acute and chronic denervation in three extremities and thoracic paraspinal muscle.

The findings are diagnostic for a widespread lower motor neuron disease such as ALS.

CASE #3. An 88-Year-old Woman with Gait Disturbance

This 88-year-old woman presented with progressive difficulty walking over the last five years. She had a history of arthritis, osteoporosis, and diabetes controlled by diet alone. She complained of numbness and tingling in her feet starting about five years ago and the symptoms had been creeping up to her knees. She felt that her legs were always cold.

Physical examination showed distal weakness of both lower extremities and reduced sensation to light touch, pinprick, and vibration up to the knee. The bilateral knee jerk was trace and bilateral ankle jerk was absent (**abnormal values in bold text**).

Case 3 Motor Nerve Conduction Studies

Nerve	DL (ms)	Amp (mV)	CV (m/s)	Minimal F-latency (ms)
R. Median—APB	3.4	5.5	51	27.3
R. Ulnar—ADM	2.6	6.7	53 (wrist—below elbow)60 (below—above elbow)	28.8
R. Peroneal—EDB	5.6	**0.1**	49 (below knee—ankle)43 (above—below knee)	58
R. Tibial—AH	4.7	**0.9**	45	56

Case 3 Sensory Nerve Conduction Studies

Nerve	DL (ms)	Amp (µV)	CV (m/s)
R. Median—2nd		12	52
R. Ulnar—5th		11	54
R. Radial—Thumb		15	58
R. Sural		**Abs**	

Case 3 EMG Findings

Muscle	IA	Fib	POS	AMP	Dur	IP
R Upper E						
Deltoid	N	N	N	N	N	N
Triceps	N	N	N	N	N	N
EDC	N	N	N	N	N	N
APB	N	N	N	N	N	N
FDI	N	N	N	N	N	N
R Lower E						
VL	N	N	N	N	N	N
TA	**Inc**	**1+**	**1+**	**Inc**	**Inc**	**-1**
Gastro	**Inc**	**1+**	**1+**	**Inc**	**Inc**	**-1**
FDI (foot)	**Inc**	**3+**	**3+**	**Inc**	**Inc**	**-3**

Summary

The clinical examination was suggestive of a length-dependent polyneuropathy. The NCS showed that the CMAP amplitudes were markedly reduced in the abductor hallucis and extensor digitorium brevis. The sural sensory nerve action potential was absent. Needle examination showed mild acute and chronic denervation in the anterior tibialis and gastronemius muscles and very severe acute and chronic denervation in the first dorsal interrosseus muscles. These findings confirmed the clinical impression of a length-dependent axonal polyneuropathy.

CASE #4. A 93-Year-old Man in ICU with Failure to Wean Off Ventilator

He was admitted to ICU a month prior to the neurological consultation for acute respiratory failure secondary to a bout of pneumonia. His ICU course was complicated by pneumothorax. As the patient gradually recovered, the ICU doctors found that they could not wean him off the ventilator.

Physical examination of the patient showed 3/5 weakness of proximal muscles and 4/5 weakness of distal muscles in both upper and lower extremities. Sensory examination showed only minimal reduction in all modalities in distal lower extremities. The reflexes were 1/4 throughout (**abnormal values in bold text**).

Case 4 Motor Nerve Conduction Studies

Nerve	DL (ms)	Amp (mV)	CV (m/s)	Minimal F-latency (ms)
L. Median—APB	3.7	6.5	55	29.3
R. Ulnar—ADM	2.9	7.7	54 (wrist—below elbow) 55 (below—above elbow)	28.4
R. Peroneal—EDB	5.6	1.9	47 (below knee—ankle) 45 (above—below knee)	58
R. Tibial—AH	4.7	6.7	43	59

Case 4 Sensory Nerve Conduction Studies

Nerve	DL (ms)	Amp (µV)	CV (m/s)
L. Median—2nd		10	54
L. Ulnar—5th		11	51
L Radial—Thumb		15	53

Case 4 EMG Findings

Muscle	IA	Fib	POS	AMP	Dur	Recruitment	IP
R Upper E							
Deltoid	**Inc**	2+	2+	**Reduced**	**Reduced**	**Early**	N
Biceps	**Inc**	1+	1+	**Reduced**	**Reduced**	**Early**	N
EDC	N	N	N	N	N	N	N
APB	N	N	N	N	N	N	N
FDI	N	N	N	N	N	N	N
R Lower E							
VL	**Inc**	2+	2+	**Reduced**	**Reduced**	**Early**	N
TA	N	N	N	N	N		N
Gastro	N	N	N	N	N		N
FDI (foot)	N	N	N	N	N		N

Summary

The clinical examination suggested a myopathic process. The needle examination showed acute denervation as well as motor units of small amplitudes and short duration in the proximal muscles of upper and lower extremities. The findings support the diagnosis of a myopathy.

CASE #5. A 68-Year-old Man with Intermittent Double Vision and Slurred Speech

This gentleman, who was previously healthy, started to experience double vision and droopy eyelids toward the end of the day six months ago. These symptoms would improve after a brief nap. He started to notice that he had slurred speech when he was tired starting about three months ago. Over the last two weeks he would get tired easily with physical activity. This fatigue would improve with rest.

Physical examination showed drooping of the eyelid after five seconds of upward gaze. The deltoid muscle developed fatigability with repeat contraction. Sensory examination and reflexes were normal. An MRI of the brain including the brainstem was also normal.

An EMG/NCV study was performed. The motor nerve conduction studies of the left median and tibial nerves and the sensory nerve conduction studies of the left radial and sural nerves were normal. The needle examination of left deltoid, biceps, EDC, FDI, vastus lateralis, tibialis anterior, and gastronemius muscles were normal.

The repetitive nerve conduction study of the left facial nerve at 3 Hz, recording from the orbicularis oris was performed. The decrement was measured by the difference between the 1st and the 4th CMAP amplitude.

Case 5

	Baseline	0 min after exercise	1 min after exercise	2 min after exercise	3 min after exercise
Decrement	12%	6%	9%	15%	12%

Summary

The repetitive nerve stimulation study of the right facial nerve at 3Hz, recorded from the obicularis oculi, showed that there was abnormal decrement of 12% at rest and with 30 seconds of exercise the decrement was 6% at 0 minutes, 9% at 1 minute, 15% at 2 minutes, and 12% at 3 minutes. The laboratory test showed that he also had elevated ACh receptor antibodies. These findings supported the diagnosis of a neuromuscular junction transmission disorder such as myasthenia gravis.

References

Amassian VE, Cracco RQ, and Maccabee PJ. Focal stimulation of human cerebral cortex with the magnetic coil: A comparison with electrical stimulation. *Electroencephalogr Clin Neurophysiol* 1989;74:401–416.

American Association of Electromyography and Electrodiagnosis Nomenclature Committee. Glossary of terms in clinical electromyography. *Muscle Nerve* 1987;10(8 Suppl):G1–G60.

Aminoff MJ: *Electrodiagnosis in clinical neurology*, 5th ed. New York, Churchill Livingstone, 2005.

Brown WE and Bolton CF: *Clinical electromyography*, 2nd ed. Boston, Butterworth-Heinemann, 1993.

Buchthal F. Electromyography in the evaluation of muscle diseases. *Neurological Clinics* 1985;3:573–598.

Cornblath DR, Sumner AJ, Daube J, et al. Conduction block in clinical practice. *Muscle Nerve* 1991;14:869–871.

Dumitru D, Amato AA, and Zwarts M. *Electrodiagnostic medicine.* 2001, Elsevier Science.

Daube JR. Needle examination in clinical electromyography. *Muscle Nerve* 1991;14(8):685–700.

Daube J. *Clinical neurophysiology*, 2nd Edition, 2002, Oxford University Press.

Drachman DB. Myasthenia gravis. *N Engl J Med* 1994;330:1797–1810.

Falck B and Alaranta H: Fibrillation potentials, positive sharp waves and fasciculations in the intrinsic muscles of the foot in healthy subjects. *J Neurol Neurosurg Psychiatry* 46:681, 1983

Falck B and Stalberg E. Motor nerve conduction studies: measurement principles and interpretation of findings. *J Clin Neurophysiol* 1995;12:254–279.

Gutmann L. Pearls and pitfalls in the use of electromyography and nerve conduction studies. *Semin Neurol* 2003; 23:77–82.

Howard JF, Sanders DB, and Massey JM. The electrodiagnosis of myasthenia gravis and the Lambert-Eaton myasthenic syndrome. *Neurologic Clin N Amer* 1994;12:305–329.

Kimura, J. *Electrodiagnosis in diseases of nerve and muscle: Principles and practice.* 2001, Oxford University Press.

Kobayashi M and Pascual-Leone A. Transcranial magnetic stimulation in neurology. *Lancet Neurol* 2003;2:145–156.

Nielsen VK, Friis ML, and Johnsen T. Electromyographic distinction between paramyotonia congenita and myotonia congenita: Effect of cold. *Neurology* 32:827, 1982.

Oh J, ed. *Clinical electromyography, nerve conduction studies,* 3rd Edition, 2003, Lippincott Williams & Wilkins, Philadelphia.

Preston DC and Shapiro B. *Electromyography and neuromuscular disorders: Clinical-electrophysiologic correlations.* 2005, Butterworth-Heinmann.

Rothwell JC, Hallett M, Berardelli A, et al. Magnetic stimulation: Motor evoked potentials. The International Federation of Clinical Neurophysiology. *Electroencephalogr Clin Neruophysiol Suppl* 1999;52:97–103.

Tim RW and Sanders DB. Repetitive nerve stimulation studies in the Lambert-Eaton myasthenic syndrome. *Muscle Nerve* 1994;17:995–1001.

Vincent A, Lang B, and Newsom-Davis J. Autoimmunity to the voltage-gated calcium channel underlies the Lambert-Eaton myasthenic syndrome, a paraneoplastic disorder. *Trends in Neruoscience* 1989;12:496–502.

Wilbourn AJ: The value and limitations of electromyographic examination in the diagnosis of lumbosacral radiculopathy, in Hardy RW (ed): *Lumbar disc disease.* New York, Raven Press, 1982, pp 65–109.

Wilbourn AJ. Sensory nerve conduction studies. *J Clin Neurophysiol* 1994;11:584–601.

Wilbourn AJ, Aminoff MJ: AAEE Minimonograph 32: The electrophysiologic examination in patients with radiculopathies. *Muscle Nerve* 11:1099, 1988.

12 Competency, Capacity, and Self-determination in Aging

Scott Y. H. Kim

Neurological illnesses can often compromise patients' decision-making capacity (DMC). Acute confusional states, neurodegenerative conditions, immune disorders of the brain, CVAs, and traumatic and anoxic brain injuries, among others, can impair a patient's cognition, which can, in various degrees, affect the capacity to make decisions. When the impairment is severe enough and a major decision must be made, the usual presumption of capacity may need to be put aside and the physician must determine whether the patient retains sufficient abilities to make his or her own decision. The decisions may be of various types, such as providing informed consent to treatment, diagnostic procedures, or participation in research. At other times, the task may involve choosing a place to live or even voting in elections. Although each of these capacities must be evaluated on its own (rather than a generic "global" decision-making capacity), the basic conceptual approach to the variety of 'competencies' (Grisso 2003) is quite similar. In this chapter, we will examine the DMC necessary for providing informed consent to treatment; the approach outlined can then be used for assessing other types of DMC.

Informed Consent and Decision-making Capacity

Informed consent to a treatment or a diagnostic procedure requires three conditions: Sufficient decision-making *capacity* of the patient; disclosure of adequate *information* by the health care provider; and the patient's voluntary choice without coercion or undue influence (Berg, Appelbaum, Lidz, and Parker 2001). Although the requirement of informed consent is pervasive in modern medicine, from a historical perspective it is a relatively new doctrine. The key court cases underlying the current doctrine date back only to the 1950s to 1970s (Berg et al. 2001; Faden and Beauchamp 1986). The concept of decision-making capacity, which arises out of the informed consent doctrine, is therefore a relatively new concept as well.

Although the criteria for DMC for treatment consent are generally enumerated in various state statutes (Berg, Appelbaum, and Grisso 1996), the practice of assessing it has tended to remain within the clinical realm, mainly because it is impractical to adjudicate every case of questionable DMC and our society tends to give clinicians considerable responsibility in the determination of patients' DMC (Appelbaum 2007). Thus, the boundary between the legal and the clinical in capacity assessments is not always distinct. In general, "decision-making capacity" (DMC) can be used interchangeably with "competence" because laws do not prefer one term over the other. In fact, most modern laws tend to use the term decision-making capacity to refer to the concept. The important distinction between adjudicated competence and clinical judgments of competence can be noted as needed.

Prevalence of Incapacity in Various Treatment Settings

With the aging of the population and the attendant rise in the prevalence of cognitive problems among hospital inpatients (Inouye 2006), the lack of treatment consent capacity is quite common in general hospitals. Recent estimates are that 37% to 48% of general hospital patients lack the capacity to consent to treatment (Etchells et al. 1999; Raymont et al. 2004). In a variety of studies on consent capacity conducted in nursing homes, high proportions of decisional impairment were found, ranging from 44% to as high as 69% (Kim, Karlawish, and Caine 2002a). The most common condition associated with incapacity in these settings is cognitive impairment associated with delirium and/or dementia.

It is informative to compare these numbers with the rates of incapacity in other clinical contexts, such as among psychiatric inpatients. Recent studies found that approximately 30% to 60% of patients lack the capacity to consent to medication treatment or to be admitted to the hospital (Okai et al. 2007; Owen et al. 2008). The main conditions associated with incapacity in these settings are psychotic illnesses and mood disorders (especially mania).

Conditions Likely to Affect Capacity
Delirium

Despite its high prevalence, there have been relatively few studies that have specifically studied the relationship between delirium and capacity (Adamis, Martin, Treloar, and Macdonald 2005; Auerswald, Charpentier, and Inouye 1997). However, in a sense, because delirium is the major cause of incapacity in general hospitals and other institutional settings, studies that examine decision-making capacity in hospital inpatients can generally be interpreted to reflect the impact of delirium on treatment consent capacity.

Although delirium is generally defined as a dysfunction of cognitive abilities (such as attention, memory, visual-spatial and other functions—thus the term 'global' impairment), there are instances where some psychotic symptoms are present without a similar degree of cognitive impairment (Meagher et al., 2007). In a recent study of 100 consecutive patients on a palliative care service who exhibited delirium, 49 had evidence of psychosis. They tended to be younger patients with more severe affect lability, and hallucinations and delusions tended not to be associated with cognitive disturbance (although another psychotic symptom—thought process disturbance—was closely correlated with attention, memory, orientation, and comprehension) (Meagher et al. 2007). For these patients, brief cognitive screens (such as the Mini Mental State Folstein, Folstein, and McHugh 1975) may be misleading. A highly educated, delirious patient, for instance, could have a score that is in the normal range and yet have an underlying delusion that prevents the person from making a competent medical decision.

Dementia

A recent population-based study found that nearly 14% of adults over the age of 70 suffer from dementia in the U.S. Of these, 74% have Alzheimer's disease and another 16% suffer from vascular dementia (Plassman et al. 2007). Another 22% suffer from pre-dementia states of cognitive impairment (Plassman et al. 2008). Not unexpectedly, persons with dementia or cognitive impairment are more likely to be incompetent or have impaired decisional abilities than their elderly counterparts without these diagnoses of dementia or cognitive impairment (Kim, Caine, Currier, Leibovici, and Ryan 2001; Marson, Ingram, Cody, and Harrell 1995; Marson, Annis, McInturff, Bartolucci, and Harrell 1999).

However, it is worth noting that even among those with known diagnoses of dementia (such as Alzheimer's disease) there is sufficient heterogeneity that one cannot simply equate a diagnosis of dementia with incapacity. For example, in one study (Marson et al. 1995), all mild to moderate AD (mean MMSE=19.4) patients were decisionally impaired (defined psychometrically as performing 2 SDs below the mean score) on the understanding legal standard, yet 28% to 83% had adequate decisional abilities on the other relevant legal standards of appreciation, reasoning, or choice (see below for a discussion of these criteria). Others have found that the quality of AD patients' reasoning, and comprehension of risks and benefits, was similar to those of elderly controls'(Stanley, Stanley, Guido, and Garvin 1988). Two other studies reported that 34% of the mild to mild-moderate AD patients (mean MMSE=22.9) performed above a clinician panel validated threshold on all four standards of decision-making ability (Kim et al. 2001), and 50% of AD patients performed above the threshold for adequate ability on a measure of comprehension for advance directives (Bassett 1999).

Nevertheless, the dementing illnesses in general do have a major impact on treatment consent capacity, even when the disease is in the early stages. In a recent study of 60 patients with mild cognitive impairment with a mean MMSE score of 28.4 (0–30 scale), 33% were marginal or below on a test of appreciation, 27% were marginal or below on reasoning, and 53% were marginal or below on the understanding standard. In this study, "marginal or below" was defined psychometrically as persons falling 1.5 standard deviations below the control group mean (Okonkwo et al. 2007).

Other neurodegenerative disorders such as Parkinson's disease, when accompanied by cognitive dysfunction, also lead to impairment in decision-making capacity. Depending on the legal standard used, 25% to 80% of PD patients with 'mild' level of cognitive impairment (Mattis Dementia Rating Scale mean score of 117.3 SD 14.5) were marginally incapable or incapable (Dymek, Atchison, Harrell, and Marson 2001).

Multiple cognitive functions seem to account for impaired decision-making abilities in Alzheimer's disease, but one consistent theme is the importance of executive functions. Bedside assessments (Royall, Mahurin, and Gray 1992) and neuropsychological tests such as Trails A (Bassett 1999), word fluency (Marson, Cody, Ingram, and Harrell, 1995) and tests of conceptualization (Marson, Chatterjee, Ingram, and Harrell 1996) that measure aspects of executive function predict impairments in decisional abilities. A qualitative analysis of error behaviors of Alzheimer disease patients also supports the link between executive function and decisional abilities (Marson et al. 1999). A factor analysis revealed that decision-making capacity seems to involve two broad domains: Verbal reasoning/conceptualization and verbal memory (Dymek, Marson, and Harrell 1999). Neuropsychological measures of conceptualization, executive function, language/semantic memory, and attention appear correlated with the reasoning/conceptualization factor, while measures of immediate and delayed verbal recall are closely related to the verbal memory factor (Dymek et al. 1999).

Psychiatric Disorders

The influence of psychotic disorders on treatment consent capacity has been extensively studied over the past three decades. The research to date can be summarized as follows. First, chronic psychotic disorders are a risk factor for impaired consent capacity but there is considerable heterogeneity. A multi-center study involving 498 subjects found that about 25% of the persons with schizophrenia failed a psychometric threshold for overall capacity, with 52% failing on at least one capacity standard (Grisso and Appelbaum 1995). But among stable outpatients in assisted living, the performance is much better. In a recent study comparing 59 relatively older (mean age 50.2) patients with schizophrenia with control subjects, only the measure of understanding showed a significant difference between controls and patients, and on average the patient group performed quite well on that ability (Palmer, Dunn, Appelbaum, and Jeste, 2004). Second, performance on abilities related to consent capacity are more a function of cognitive symptoms (and negative symptoms) than of classic positive psychotic symptoms (Palmer and Savla 2007; Carpenter, Jr. et al. 2000; Moser et al. 2002; Palmer et al. 2004). Third, several studies have suggested that understanding of factual information can be improved through interventions in persons with chronic psychotic disorders (Dunn et al. 2002; Carpenter, Jr. et al. 2000; Moser et al. 2002).

A manic episode, a hallmark of bipolar disorder (sometimes referred to as manic depressive illness), is accompanied by several of the following symptoms: Impulsivity, grandiose thinking, distractibility, rapid speech and "racing thoughts," increased activity, and lack of need for sleep. It is often accompanied by frank psychotic beliefs and poor judgment in personal interactions, spending money, and engaging in risky activities. In a recent study, manic patients' ability to provide consent for research was worse than non-manic bipolar patients, but repeated disclosures erased any differences between the groups (Misra, Socherman, Park, Hauser, and Ganzini 2008). But recent British studies found that most (62–97%) patients admitted to a psychiatric unit in a manic state were deemed to be incapable of making a treatment decision (either for medications or for psychiatric admissions) (Owen et al. 2008; Beckett and Chaplin 2006). The more severe the manic state, the more likely the patient was incapacitated.

Mild to moderate depression has little effect on the abilities relevant for consent capacity (Appelbaum, Grisso, Frank, O'Donnell, and Kupfer 1999). However, some persons with severe depression, especially if accompanied by psychotic symptoms, may evidence significant loss of decision-making abilities (Lapid et al. 2003).

Traumatic Brain Injury

An estimated 5.3 million Americans (just over 2% of the population) live with disabilities resulting from traumatic brain injury (TBI) (as of 1999). The annual societal cost of traumatic brain injury is estimated to be $48.3 billion (National Center for Injury Prevention and Control 2008). The issue of decision-making capacity looms large in the brain injury rehabilitation setting (Mukherjee and McDonough 2006; Marson et al. 2005). In a study of 24 moderate to severe TBI patients 6 months after their acute hospitalization, 25% still were marginally capable or incapable in terms of their appreciation ability, and 34%

were marginally capable or incapable in their understanding (Marson et al. 2005).

Other Disorders

Medical conditions that do not directly impair cognitive functions generally have not been shown to affect abilities relevant to treatment consent, including cardiac illness (Appelbaum and Grisso 1997), diabetes mellitus (Palmer et al. 2005), and HIV infection (as long as there is no additional cognitive impairment) (Moser et al. 2002). One study of ambulatory cancer patients showed that significant impairment in understanding for research consent may occur in this population, but most of this seems to be explained by cognitive dysfunction, age, and education (the study sample contained a relative high proportion of persons without a high school diploma, 40%) (Casarett, Karlawish, and Hirschman, 2003).

Criteria for Capacity: The Four Abilities Model

Informed consent for a treatment assumes that a patient will competently use the information disclosed by the health care provider. The concept of capacity therefore focuses on the patient's capacity to use the disclosed information to arrive at a free choice, rather than on some feature of the person like diagnosis, age, legal status, or a quasi-psychological concept that functions as a proxy for "normal" (e.g., "of sound mind"). A comprehensive review of state laws, court cases, commission reports, and other ethico-legal literature reveals that the most widely used set of criteria for capacity, with slight variations, can be reduced to four standards or abilities: Communicating a choice, understanding, appreciation, and reasoning (Berg et al. 1996).

Communicating a Choice

The ability to communicate a choice simply requires the patient communicate a decision regarding a treatment or procedure. It is a necessary but insufficient basis for competence in most instances. The choice, however, must be stable to some degree. If the choice flip flops such that the choice cannot be carried out, it is unclear that the patient is making a meaningful choice at all and thus would fail to meet this criterion.

Understanding

The ability to understand the information relevant to decision-making is perhaps the most intuitive standard, and indeed some version of it is present in all discussions of competency standards and in all legal definitions of capacity (Berg et al. 1996). The ability to understand, however, is broader than a mere retention and regurgitation of what the doctor tells the patient. The patient must be able to "grasp the fundamental meaning" (Appelbaum 2007) of the disclosed information. One can get at this by asking, "Can you tell me in your own words what the doctors have told you so far?" and asking the patient to explain the relevant concepts in his answer ("What's involved in the surgery?" "What do you mean by 'the treatment will work'?"), if necessary to confirm that the patient truly comprehends the meaning of the information.

Appreciation

The ability to appreciate refers to patients' ability to apply the facts that are disclosed to them to their own situation. Thus, appreciation can be truly assessed only if understanding is intact. Indeed, often in the clinical setting, doctors use the term "understand" in a broader, more colloquial sense to include both factual understanding of facts and an application of those facts to one's own situation.

The ability to appreciate encompasses two broad domains:

"Whether patients (1) acknowledge, or appreciate, that they are suffering from the disorder with which they have been diagnosed, and (2) acknowledge the consequences of the disorder and of potential treatment options for their own situation" (Grisso and Appelbaum 1998).

One can assess this ability by first confirming the patient's understanding ("What have the doctors told you about your condition and what are they recommending?") and then probing for the patient's ability to apply those facts to his or her situation. This typically involves probing for patient's beliefs regarding the facts conveyed to him or her. A delusional patient, for example, may be able to convey a perfect factual understanding of what the doctors said, but deny that those facts apply to him or her.

Reasoning

Even if patients understand and appreciate the facts of their clinical situation, some process must connect the factual understanding, the beliefs surrounding that understanding, and the outcome of expressing a preference. Court decisions may refer to "rational thought processes" or statutes refer to the "ability to reach a decision" in order to capture this "process" that is involved in "manipulating the information" that is presented to the patients (Berg et al. 1996). This ability to reason refers to a constellation of abilities that are involved in processing information that leads to a decision. This involves being able to compare options, make cogent inferences, weigh evidence, etc. which are formal features of *processes* leading to a choice, rather than the rationality of the *content* of the choice. That is, the standard does *not* refer to the reasonableness of the decision made by the patient. Although a very unconventional decision (say, refusing a high-benefit-but-no-burden intervention) may trigger an evaluation, the "reasonableness" of the content of a choice cannot be the sole basis for judging someone incompetent.

In general, the reasoning standard should not be used alone. It is not as commonly delineated by the courts or statutes and is never used alone by the courts, but rather always in conjunction with other standards (Berg et al. 1996).

Variations in Terminology

Despite its broad acceptance within the medical community in the U.S., most statutes, published ethico-legal analyses, and various policies do not always use the same terminology in referring to the four abilities. Generally, however, the descriptions of these different terms, upon reflection, show that similar abilities are at issue. However, there are jurisdictions that may not use all four standards, and the clinician needs to be aware of the specific requirements in his or her jurisdiction (Grisso et al. 1998).

Principles in Applying the Criteria for Capacity: Function in Context

Although courts and state laws have delineated the various criteria for capacity, how they are applied in practice depends on a set of additional principles that have evolved over the years that reflect not only a functional approach to capacity assessment but also the trend toward increased emphasis on patient autonomy in modern medical practice. These principles will not be found in the law (Grisso et al. 1998), but they are widely endorsed by various reports and guidelines nationally (President's Commission for the Study of Ethical Problems in Medicine and Biomedical and Behavioral Research 1982; National Bioethics

Advisory Commission 1998) and internationally (WHO, 2005). In general, these principles rest on the fact that the determination of capacity must take into account both the patient's abilities and the context in which he or she is expected to exercise those abilities (Buchanan & Brock 1989).

Function and Task-specific Assessment of Capacity

The requirement for capacity assessment flows out of the doctrine of informed consent, which is in turn an expansion of the role of the patient in medical decision-making. This emphasis on patient self-determination implies that the assessment of capacity tends to be geared toward preserving and maximizing patient autonomy. Thus, capacity assessments are task specific: Just because a person is deemed incapable of consenting to research participation, it does not mean that the person is also incapable of other decisions, such as making treatment decisions. In fact, if at all possible, the capacity evaluator must attempt to evaluate the patient's capacity for the specific decision at hand rather than rely on diagnostic categories or broad pronouncements (e.g., "sound mind"). Also, the assessment cannot rely on generic cognitive tests. Of course, this hardly means that diagnostic and cognitive dysfunction do not matter. But they are better conceived as risk factors of incapacity, rather than defining incapacity.

Risk-benefit Considerations and Thresholds for Categorical Determinations of Capacity

It is a widely accepted practice to vary the thresholds for capacity according to the risk-benefit profile of the patient's choice (National Bioethics Advisory Commission 1998; President's Commission for the Study of Ethical Problems in Medicine and Biomedical and Behavioral Research 1982; Buchanan et al. 1989; Grisso et al. 1998) Thus, other things being equal, the lower the risk and greater the potential for benefit, the lower the level of abilities needed to be deemed competent. The capacity evaluator therefore needs to ask the following questions: Are the reasonably anticipated risks and burdens high or low (or, high, moderate, or low)? Are the reasonably anticipated benefits high or low (or, high, moderate, or low)? Finally, how do the risks and benefits of the patient's chosen course compare with the risk-benefit profile of other alternatives (including no treatment at all)? By systematically asking these questions and making these risk-benefit assessments explicit, and, when needed, consulting with other colleagues, the capacity evaluator should be able to reach a medically sound assessment of the risks and benefits.

Use of Capacity Instruments

There are a number of interview instruments that have been used to evaluate DMC. Two recent reviews examine 15 instruments for the assessment of either research or treatment consent capacity (Moye 2003; Dunn, Nowrangi, Palmer, Jeste, and Saks 2006). Using an established instrument—an instrument that has been well conceptualized and operationalized in relation to the accepted legal standards—does have significant advantages. It helps the interviewer to be comprehensive, to use questions and probes that are conceptually on target and have been validated, and allows the interviewer to document the interview in systematic and domain-specific ways. Also, if the instrument has been used in a variety of research studies, the body of evidence gathered using that instrument lends further support for using it. One instrument that meets these criteria, and probably the most widely used and tested, is the MacArthur Competence Assessment Tool-Treatment (MacCAT-T) (Grisso et al., 1998). It can be administered in about 20 minutes, and a manual and training video are available (http://www.prpress.com/books/mact-setfr.html).

In using such instruments, the evaluator should be aware that although a capacity instrument can contribute valuable information to the evaluation process, it is not possible to impose a decision-making rule to its outcome solely based on the outcome of the structured evaluation. Instruments at best measure degrees and types of impairment. Additional clinical judgment (especially a risk-benefit assessment) is necessary to arrive at a categorical judgment.

Uses of Cognitive Screens

Although capacity assessments must be task-specific, routinely obtained brief cognitive screens can often be used to provide a sense of the prior probability of incapacity. The Mini-Mental State examination (MMSE) (Folstein et al. 1975) is perhaps the most widely used bedside cognitive screen.

The preponderance of evidence supports the view that MMSE can be helpful, if used with realistic expectations (Kim et al. 2002a). Specifically, the use of a single cutoff score on the MMSE to aid one's assessment of a cognitively impaired subject is not recommended. Instead, it is most useful to divide the results into three domains with two cutoff scores: The lower cutoff (probably somewhere around 16 to 18) score and an upper cutoff score (24 to 26) (Kim and Caine 2002b). One study of general hospital patients noted that the most useful range of scores was 16 or below for predicting incapacity, and 24 or above for predicting capacity (Etchells et al. 1999). A study of nursing home residents suggests MMSE scores of 18 and 26, along with scores from an understanding assessment instrument as the first screening step: Only persons falling in between those two scores would need further, intensive capacity assessment (Pruchno, Smyer, Rose, Hartman-Stein, and Henderson-Laribee, 1995). We found in a study of Alzheimer's disease patients that a fairly wide range MMSE scores of 21–25 were uninformative in predicting the capacity status of these patients; however, scores below and above were quite predictive of these patients' capacity to provide consent for research (Kim et al. 2002b). Thus, the utility of the MMSE depends on the context and the use to which it is put. Because the test is so routinely obtained, the utility gained comes at virtually no extra cost or effort. In dementia specialty clinics and research centers where other simple neuropsychological tests are widely used, those other tests may be of use as well (Marson et al. 1995a; Marson et al. 1996, Bassett 1999).

Enhancement of Capacity when Possible

As noted above, at least for some patient groups, there is a strong body of evidence that educational interventions can improve comprehension abilities. As long as the neuropsychiatric impairment does not severely impair the ability to learn itself, there is the hope of improving the patient's treatment consent capacity. But it is unlikely, for example, that educational interventions would reduce delusional beliefs that impair one's ability to appreciate. However, there is a duty to conduct the informed consent conversation in such a way that it maximizes the chance that even a mildly impaired patient may be able to exercise his or her capacity to the fullest.

Averting a Capacity Evaluation May Sometimes Be the Best Course

Sometimes it is better to avert a capacity evaluation altogether by changing the contextual factors in the patient's favor. An example of this is an elderly patient, perhaps mildly demented, who is at risk if she goes home by herself. However, it may well be true that if sufficient resources were available and provided, she may still be able to live in her own apartment for a longer time if the safety risks are reduced. Since the threshold for capacity must be adjusted to the potential consequences of the choices at hand, if the choice of the patient can be made safe enough, it may prove to be a better solution than forcing a capacity evaluation.

After the Assessment: Issues in Surrogate Decision-making

Decision-making for an incapacitated patient can be divided into two broad types of situations: When some type of formal advance care planning has taken place versus when there has not. Advance care planning in turn falls into two types of mechanisms: The instructional health care directive (also often called the living will) and proxy advance directive (as health care proxies or as durable power of attorney for health care). All states have some type of advance directive statutes, and most have provisions for both types (American Bar Association Commission on Law and Aging 2008a).

Instructional Directives

Instructional health care directives, sometimes called the living will, record the explicit treatment preferences of the patients. They can vary in complexity and specificity. Usually the directives address end of life decision-making. Those who complete instructional directives anticipate potential future situations of incapacity, and express the individual's preference. There are some limitations to the living will (Fagerlin and Schneider 2004). Most people do not complete living wills. Even if people do fill out a living will, they may not know what they want, given the complexity of medical decisions. Also, even if they do know what they want, describing and anticipating the unknown future can be a daunting task, whether it be about what might happen to them or in regard to changes in their preferences over time. Further, an instructional directive must still be interpreted by the medical team and by the patient's surrogates.

All of this is not to deny that living wills can sometimes be helpful, especially when a patient already has a terminal illness with a predictable course and has anticipated key decision points and has been able to discuss and document his or her treatment preferences. However, in most cases, most of the decision-making for an incapacitated person must still rest on a third-party who has to exercise some degree of judgment.

Proxy Directives

Another form of advance directive involves appointing a proxy who can take on the role of a substitute decision-maker when the patient becomes incapacitated. The obvious advantage of a proxy over an instructional directive is that the details of the future need not be anticipated in detail. The proxy can take in the relevant information at the time that the decision needs to be made, and does his or her best to represent the patient's preferences (see below). However, even with an instructional directive determining what the patient would have wanted is not always straightforward (Shalowitz, Garrett-Mayer, and Wendler 2006).

When There Are No Advance Directives

Most people still do not complete an advance directive, so that the surrogate decision-maker is not a previously designated person. The de facto surrogate decision-maker (traditionally 'next of kin' decision-makers) has a long and respected tradition in medicine and this tradition has been formalized in specific laws in most states. As of January 2008, 43 states and Washington, D.C. had at least *some* form of de facto surrogate treatment decision-making law that explicitly gives decision-making authority to family members (and, rarely, to other close associates) (American Bar Association Commission on Law and Aging 2008b).

These laws are useful because they provide legal clarity to what has been de facto practice based on custom. Further, they usually spell out the hierarchy of authority that can be useful when there is a disagreement among available surrogates. The order is almost always spouse, adult child, sibling, then usually next nearest relative, but sometimes a close friend. Some states explicitly mention life partners or "long-term spouse-like relationships" as taking precedence over even an adult child, taking the place of 'spouse' in the traditional hierarchy of surrogates (e.g., New Mexico). It is a reasonable presumption that even when specific surrogate treatment laws do not exist, family surrogates generally will play the role of decision-makers for their incapacitated relatives. But physicians should familiarize themselves with the limitations and exceptions for such a presumption in his or her own jurisdiction by consulting with the hospital's counsel or an ethics committee.

Decision-making Standards for Substitute Decision-makers

When an appropriate surrogate decision-maker is present (either a previously appointed proxy, or a de facto surrogate specified in statute, or a next of kin in states without surrogate treatment laws), what is the standard that such a surrogate should use to make his or her decision about the patient's treatment? Given the priority given to patient autonomy, there is a natural hierarchy, at least in theory, regarding how a treatment decision should be made for an incapacitated patient: (a) previously stated specific preferences (as expressed in a living will, for example), (b) substituted judgment ("If this incompetent patient were in fact competent, what would he choose to do in this situation?"), and (c) best interests. In reality, some mixture of the three approaches is commonly used. Most terminally ill patients prefer some combination of their own preferences (in the form of substituted judgment) and the views of their loved ones or physicians (Nolan et al. 2005). Another recent longitudinal study of patients with cancer, heart failure, or amyotrophic lateral sclerosis found that such a preference for shared decision-making was fairly stable (Sulmasy et al. 2007).

Cases that Need Judicial Review

Although the majority of treatment consent capacity evaluations are directly incorporated into medical decision-making for the patient, some cases do need to go to court.

Inability to Care for Oneself Independently

Perhaps the most common reason for going to court is when an elderly patient with dementia who had been living alone but no longer can do so safely needs to be placed in a living facility. When a decisionally incapable patient insists on going back home to an unsafe environment, there may be no choice but to go to court. Ideally, a caring family member would petition to become the patient's guardian. But if the patient has no family members, or lacks the financial means to hire an attorney, sometimes a hospital may need to petition the courts for a guardian.

Special Medical Treatments or Procedures

Some medical interventions are controversial because there is the specter of exposing the patient to some risk, burden, harm, or indignity, not for the sake of the patient's welfare or preference, but because it may or could serve someone else's purpose. Such interventions with incompetent patients who decline those interventions must be reviewed by the courts. For psychiatric interventions—such as antipsychotics, electroconvulsive therapy, and psychosurgery—a primary concern has been the issue of using medical procedures for social control. In the case of psychosurgery, for example, thousands of patients, primarily housed in long term facilities, were exposed to what amounted to unregulated neurosurgical experimentation (Valenstein 1986). Another example of "extraordinary" intervention that requires judicial review is sterilization (Committee on Bioethics 1999; Dubler and White 1995; Reilly 1991).

Patient Disagrees with Proxy Decision-maker

Sometimes a person with an advance proxy directive who is deemed incompetent by a clinician then disagrees with the recommendation of the proxy and the team, or disagrees with the determination of incompetence made by the evaluator. Most health care proxy laws do not authorize a proxy to override the active objection of a patient, even if that patient has been deemed incapacitated by a physician who has conducted a formal capacity evaluation. Such a case needs judicial review.

Surrogate Decision-maker(s) Not Available, Unqualified, or in Conflict

When a surrogate is not present and the situation is urgent, a judgment call is necessary regarding whether an emergency court hearing is required. Sometimes there is no bright line between an emergency (in which one would proceed with an exception to informed consent justification) and a situation in which an urgent court hearing is the best option. Factors that favor proceeding to court include (a) availability of urgent court hearing in the jurisdiction, (b) the relative invasiveness of the procedure, and (c) a benefit to risk ratio becomes less clear cut in favor of intervention.

When the surrogate decision-maker is not able (due to incapacity) or unwilling (due, for example, to conflicts of interest) to carry out his or her duties, the courts may need to appoint an alternative decision-maker.

When there are intractable conflicts among potential surrogates, courts may have to decide who will have the final decision-making authority for the patient, especially if the state does not have a surrogate treatment law or the application of the law is not clear.

Guardianship should be sought when other mechanisms for surrogate decision-making are not available for an incapacitated patient who is likely to face a series of major medical decisions. For example, a long time resident of a residential facility for mentally handicapped adults is admitted to a general hospital with a newly diagnosed cancer. The patient may have no family and is without a guardian. Suppose the patient's prognosis is quite good but the treatment may be burdensome and lengthy. The best scenario for a patient like this is to have an experienced guardian who can work closely with the treatment team across time, as well as with others such as the hospital's ethics committee or ethics consultants.

A slight variation on the above case is more common, namely, the very ill ICU patient (for example, after a CVA) who is incapacitated and without a surrogate decision-maker (White et al. 2007). In a recent study of seven medical centers (East and West coast centers), 5.5% (range: 0–27%) of all ICU deaths occurred in persons without capacity and without surrogates. Most major medical societies recommend judicial review of decisions to limit life-sustaining treatment but data show that such decisions are currently made without judicial review (White et al. 2007). No doubt this will remain an area of continuing legal and clinical controversy.

Other Competencies of Interest
Capacity to Consent to Research

By 2050, the number of persons in the US diagnosed with AD is projected to be 12.5 million if no effective interventions are found to alter the current trend (Hebert, Scherr, Bienias, Bennett, and Evans 2003). Also, current treatments are of only modest benefit. Research, even with its attendant risks (Orgogozo et al. 2003; Tuszynski et al. 2005), is necessary in order to develop effective treatments. Because the disease usually leads to early decisional incapacity (Kim et al. 2001; Okonkwo et al. 2007), surrogate consent is necessary for research (Kim, Appelbaum, Jeste, and Olin 2004).

Because research involving persons with dementia is becoming more common, a neurologist may need to evaluate the DMC of such patients to give informed consent to research. It may be useful to review what remains the same and what is different about DMC for research when compared to DMC for treatment consent. The overall framework remains the same. The assessment of DMC for research consent should be assessed in a task specific way, rather than using a generic cognitive test or inferring from a diagnosis. The four abilities model discussed is widely used in the research context, and considerable amount of data are available using the framework (Kim et al. 2001; Kim et al. 2002b). But there is one notable difference.

The risk-benefit analysis is different than the treatment context. It is not the individual subjects' welfare that is the primary goal of the research enterprise. Indeed, in most situations of research, the subject forgoes some advantage in order to enhance the goals of science (Lidz and Appelbaum 2002). This is why there is such an elaborate system of regulatory oversight of human subject research. The implication for capacity assessment is that the threshold for competence must take into account this different risk-benefit context. This will not be an algorithm-based decision, but a clinical judgment.

Capacity to Vote

Given that the elderly are both most likely to vote and most likely to develop dementia, important social questions arise regarding what constitutes the capacity to vote and how to assess it. Researchers are beginning to put this question to both policy analysis (Karlawish et al. 2004) and empirical study. According to the Doe standard, the capacity to vote requires an understanding of the nature and effect of voting and the ability to choose among the candidates (or questions) on a ballot (Karlawish et al. 2004). A recent study of persons with Alzheimer's disease using this federal standard found that most persons with very mild or mild cases of AD appeared capable of voting, whereas persons with severe dementia were not, and persons with moderate dementia were unpredictable in terms of their voting capacity (Appelbaum, Bonnie, and Karlawish 2005).

Summary

Neurological conditions of old age that compromise the patient's capacity to make important decisions are common. This fact in combination with the rise of the doctrine of informed consent—which requires a function-based assessment of DMC—have made competency assessments a common issue in clinics and hospitals. The current practice is guided by fairly broad legal guidelines relying on considerable clinical judgment by clinicians. There are now widely accepted practice principles which interpret the general legal guidelines, and an increasing amount of research on the DMC of patients is beginning to provide an important evidence base for the clinician.

References

Adamis, D., Martin, F. C., Treloar, A., and Macdonald, A. J. (2005). Capacity, consent, and selection bias in a study of delirium. *Journal of Medical Ethics, 31,* 137–143.

American Bar Association Commission on Law and Aging (2008a). *Health care power of attorney and combined advance directive legislation - January 2008.*

American Bar Association Commission on Law and Aging (2008b). *Surrogate consent in the absence of an advance directive - January 2008.*

Appelbaum, P. S. (2007). Assessment of patients' competence to consent to treatment. *New England Journal of Medicine, 357,* 1834–1840.

Appelbaum, P. S. and Grisso, T. (1997). Capacities of hospitalized, medically ill patients to consent to treatment. *Psychosomatics, 38,* 119–125.

Appelbaum, P. S., Grisso, T., Frank, E., O'Donnell, S., and Kupfer, D. (1999). Competence of depressed patients for consent to research. *American Journal of Psychiatry, 156,* 1380–1384.

Appelbaum, P. S., Bonnie, R. J., and Karlawish, J. H. (2005). The capacity to vote of persons with Alzheimer's disease. *American Journal of Psychiatry, 162,* 2094–2100.

Auerswald, K. B., Charpentier, P. A., and Inouye, S. K. (1997). The informed consent process in older patients who developed delirium: A clinical epidemiologic study. *American Journal of Medicine, 103,* 410–418.

Bassett, S. S. (1999). Attention: Neuropsychological predictor of competency in Alzheimer's disease. *Journal of Geriatric Psychiatry & Neurology, 12,* 200–205.

Beckett, J. and Chaplin, R. (2006). Capacity to consent to treatment in patients with acute mania. *Psychiatric Bulletin, 30,* 419–422.

Berg, J. W., Appelbaum, P. S., Lidz, C. W., and Parker, L. S. (2001). *Informed consent: Legal theory and clinical practice.* (Second ed.) New York: Oxford University Press.

Berg, J. W., Appelbaum, P. S., and Grisso, T. (1996). Constructing competence: Formulating standards of legal competence to make medical decisions. *Rutgers Law Review, 48,* 345–396.

Buchanan, A. E. and Brock, D. W. (1989). *Deciding for others: The ethics of surrogate decision making.* New York: Cambridge University Press.

Carpenter, W. T., Jr., Gold, J., Lahti, A., Queern, C., Conley, R., Bartko, J. et al. (2000). Decisional capacity for informed consent in schizophrenia research. *Archives of General Psychiatry, 57,* 533–538.

Casarett, D. J., Karlawish, J. H. T., and Hirschman, K. B. (2003). Identifying ambulatory cancer patients at risk of impaired capacity to consent to research. *Journal of Pain and Symptom Management, 26,* 615–624.

Committee on Bioethics (1999). Sterilization of minors with developmental disabilities. *Pediatrics, 104,* 337–340.

Dubler, N. and White, A. (1995). Fertility control: Legal and regulatory issues. In W.T.Reich (Ed.), *Encyclopedia of bioethics* (pp. 839–847). New York: Simon & Shuster Macmillan.

Dunn, L. B., Nowrangi, M. A., Palmer, B. W., Jeste, D. V., and Saks, E. R. (2006). Assessing decisional capacity for clinical research or treatment: A review of instruments. *American Journal of Psychiatry, 163,* 1323–1334.

Dunn, L., Lindamer, L., Palmer, B. W., Golshan, S., Schneiderman, L., and Jeste, D. V. (2002). Improving understanding of research consent in middle-aged and elderly patients with psychotic disorders. *American Journal of Geriatric Psychiatry, 10,* 142–150.

Dymek, M., Atchison, P., Harrell, L., and Marson, D. C. (2001). Competency to consent to medical treatment in cognitively impaired patients with Parkinson's disease. *Neurology, 56,* 17–24.

Dymek, M., Marson, D., and Harrell, L. (1999). Factor structure of capacity to consent to medical treatment in patients with Alzheimer's disease: An exploratory study. *Journal of Forensic Neuropsychology, 1,* 27–48.

Etchells, E., Darzins, P., Silberfeld, M., Singer, P. A., McKenny, J., Naglie, G. et al. (1999). Assessment of patient capacity to consent to treatment. *Journal of General Internal Medicine, 14,* 27–34.

Faden, R. and Beauchamp, T. (1986). *A history and theory of informed consent.* New York: Oxford University Press.

Fagerlin, A. and Schneider, C. E. (2004). Enough: The failure of the living will. *Hastings Center Report, 34,* 30–42.

Folstein, M. F., Folstein, S. E., and McHugh, P. (1975). Mini-Mental State. A practical guide for grading the cognitive state of patients for the clinician. *Journal of Psychiatric Research, 12,* 189–198.

Grisso, T. and Appelbaum, P. S. (1998). *Assessing competence to consent to treatment: A guide for physicians and other health professionals.* New York: Oxford University Press.

Grisso, T. and Appelbaum, P. S. (1995). The MacArthur Treatment Competence Study III: Abilities of patients to consent to psychiatric and medical treatments. *Law & Human Behavior, 19,* 149–174.

Grisso, T. (2003). *Evaluating competencies.* (Second ed.) New York: Kluwer/Plenum.

Hebert, L. E., Scherr, P. A., Bienias, J. L., Bennett, D. A., and Evans, D. A. (2003). Alzheimer disease in the US population: Prevalence estimates using the 2000 Census. *Archives of Neurology, 60,* 1119–1122.

Inouye, S. K. (2006). Delirium in older persons. *New England Journal of Medicine, 354,* 1157–1165.

Karlawish, J. H., Bonnie, R. J., Appelbaum, P. S., Lyketsos, C., James, B., Knopman, D. et al. (2004). Addressing the ethical, legal, and social issues raised by voting by persons with dementia. *JAMA: The Journal of the American Medical Association, 292,* 1345–1350.

Kim, S. Y. H., Caine, E. D., Currier, G. W., Leibovici, A., and Ryan, J. M. (2001). Assessing the competence of persons with Alzheimer's disease in providing informed consent for participation in research. *American Journal of Psychiatry, 158,* 712–717.

Kim, S. Y. H., Karlawish, J. H. T., and Caine, E. D. (2002a). Current state of research on decision-making competence of cognitively impaired elderly persons. *American Journal of Geriatric Psychiatry, 10,* 151–165.

Kim, S. Y. H., Appelbaum, P. S., Jeste, D. V., and Olin, J. T. (2004). Proxy and surrogate consent in geriatric neuropsychiatric research: Update and recommendations. *American Journal of Psychiatry, 161,* 797–806.

Kim, S. & Caine, E. D. (2002b). Utility and limits of the Mini Mental State examination in evaluating consent capacity in Alzheimer's disease. *Psychiatric Services, 53,* 1322–1324.

Lapid, M., Rummans, T., Poole, K., Pankratz, S., Maurer, M., Rasmussen, K. et al. (2003). Decisional capacity of severely depressed patients requiring electroconvulsive therapy. *Journal of ECT, 19,* 67–72.

Lidz, C. W. and Appelbaum, P. S. (2002). The therapeutic misconception: Problems and solutions. *Medical Care, 49,* V55–V63.

Marson, D. C., Annis, S. M., McInturff, B., Bartolucci, A., and Harrell, L. E. (1999). Error behaviors associated with loss of competency in Alzheimer's disease. *Neurology, 53,* 1983–1992.

Marson, D. C., Chatterjee, A., Ingram, K. K., and Harrell, L. E. (1996). Toward a neurologic model of competency: Cognitive predictors of capacity to consent in Alzheimer's disease using three different legal standards. *Neurology, 46,* 666–672.

Marson, D. C., Cody, H. A., Ingram, K. K., and Harrell, L. E. (1995). Neuropsychological predictors of competency in Alzheimer's disease using a rational reasons legal standard [comment]. *Archives of Neurology, 52,* 955–959.

Marson, D. C., Dreer, L. E., Krzywanski, S., Huthwaite, J. S., Devivo, M. J., and Novack, T. A. (2005). Impairment and partial recovery of medical decision-making capacity in traumatic brain injury: A 6-month longitudinal study. *Arch Phys Med Rehabil, 86,* 889–895.

Marson, D. C., Ingram, K. K., Cody, H. A., and Harrell, L. E. (1995). Assessing the competency of patients with Alzheimer's disease under different legal standards. A prototype instrument. *Archives of Neurology, 52,* 949–954.

Meagher, D.J., Moran, M., Raju, B., Gibbons, D., Donnelly, S., Saunders, J. et al. (2007). Phenomenology of delirium: Assessment of 100 adult cases using standardised measures. *The British Journal of Psychiatry, 190,* 135–141.

Misra, S., Socherman, R., Park, B. S., Hauser, P., and Ganzini, L. (2008). Influence of mood state on capacity to consent to research in patients with bipolar disorder. *Bipolar Disord, 10,* 303–309.

Moser, D. J., Schultz, S. K., Arndt, S., Benjamin, M. L., Fleming, F. W., Brems, C. S. et al. (2002). Capacity to provide informed consent for participation in schizophrenia and HIV research. *American Journal of Psychiatry, 159,* 1201–1207.

Moye, J. (2003). Competence to consent to treatment. In T. Grisso (Ed.), *Evaluating competencies: Forensic assessments and instruments* (Second ed., pp. 391–458). New York: Kluwer Academic/Plenum Publishers.

Mukherjee, D. and McDonough, C. (2006). Clinician perspectives on decision-making capacity after acquired brain injury. (Ethics in Practice). *Topics in Stroke Rehabilitation, 13,* 75.

National Bioethics Advisory Commission (1998). *Research involving persons with mental disorders that may affect decision-making capacity.* (Volume 1 ed.) Rockville, MD: NBAC.

National Center for Injury Prevention and Control (2008). *Traumatic brain injury.* Centers for Disease Control and Prevention.

Nolan, M. T., Hughes, M., Narendra, D. P., Sood, J. R., Terry, P. B., Astrow, A. B. et al. (2005). When patients lack capacity: The roles that patients with terminal diagnoses would choose for their physicians and loved ones in making medical decisions. *J Pain Symptom Manage, 30,* 342–353.

Okai, D., Owen, G., McGuire, H., Singh, S., Churchill, R., and Hotopf, M. (2007). Mental capacity in psychiatric patients: Systematic review. *The British Journal of Psychiatry, 191,* 291–297.

Okonkwo, O., Griffith, H. R., Belue, K., Lanza, S., Zamrini, E. Y., Harrell, L. E. et al. (2007). Medical decision-making capacity in patients with mild cognitive impairment. *Neurology, 69,* 1528–1535.

Orgogozo, J. M., Gilman, S., Dartigues, J. F., Laurent, B., Puel, M., Kirby, L. C. et al. (2003). Subacute meningoencephalitis in a subset of patients with AD after A 42 immunization. *Neurology, 61,* 46–54.

Owen, G., Richardson, G., David, AS., Szmukler, G., Hayward, P., and Hotopf, M. (2008). Mental capacity to make decisions on treatment in people admitted to psychiatric hospitals: Cross sectional study. *BMJ, 337,* a448.

Palmer, B. W. and Savla, G. N. (2007). The association of specific neuropsychological deficits with capacity to consent to research or treatment. *J Int Neuropsychol Soc, 13,* 1047–1059.

Palmer, B. W., Dunn, L. B., Appelbaum, P. S., and Jeste, D. V. (2004). Correlates of treatment-related decision-making capacity among middle-aged and older patients with schizophrenia. *Archives of General Psychiatry, 61,* 230–236.

Palmer, B. W., Dunn, L. B., Appelbaum, P. S., Mudaliar, S., Thal, L., Henry, R. et al. (2005). Assessment of capacity to consent to research among older persons with schizophrenia, Alzheimer disease, or diabetes mellitus: Comparison of a 3-item questionnaiwwwre with a comprehensive standardized capacity instrument. *Archives of General Psychiatry, 62,* 726–733.

Plassman, B. L., Langa, K. M., Fisher, G. G., Heeringa, S. G., Weir, D. R., Ofstedal, M. B. et al. (2008). Prevalence of cognitive impairment without dementia in the United States. *Annals of Internal Medicine, 148,* 427–434.

Plassman, B. L., Langa, K. M., Fisher, G. G., Heeringa, S. G., Weir, D. R., Ofstedal, M. B. et al. (2007). Prevalence of dementia in the United States: The aging, demographics, and memory study. *Neuroepidemiology, 29,* 125–132.

President's Commission for the Study of Ethical Problems in Medicine and Biomedical and Behavioral Research (1982). *Making health care decisions: The ethical and legal implications of informed consent in the patient-practitioner relationship* (Rep. No. One).

Pruchno, R. A., Smyer, M. A., Rose, M. S., Hartman-Stein, P. E., and Henderson-Laribee, D. L. (1995). Competence of long-term care residents to participate in decisions about their medical care: A brief, objective assessment. *Gerontologist, 35,* 622–629.

Raymont, V., Bingley, W., Buchanan, A., David, A. S., Hayward, P., Wessely, S. et al. (2004). Prevalence of mental incapacity in medical inpatients and associated risk factors: Cross-sectional study. *The Lancet, 364,* 1421–1427.

Reilly, P. (1991). *The surgical solution: A history of involuntary sterilization in the United States.* Baltimore, MD: Johns Hopkins University Press.

Royall, D. R., Mahurin, R. K., and Gray, K. F. (1992). Bedside assessment of executive cognitive impairment: The executive interview. *Journal of the American Geriatrics Society, 40,* 1221–1226.

Shalowitz, D. I., Garrett-Mayer, E., and Wendler, D. (2006). The accuracy of surrogate decision makers: A systematic review. *Archives of Internal Medicine, 166,* 493–497.

Stanley, B., Stanley, M., Guido, J., and Garvin, L. (1988). The functional competency of elderly at risk. *Gerontologist, 28,* 53–58.

Sulmasy, D. P., Hughes, M. T., Thompson, R. E., Astrow, A. B., Terry, P. B., Kub, J. et al. (2007). How would terminally ill patients have others make decisions for them in the event of decisional incapacity? A longitudinal study. *J Am Geriatr Soc, 55,* 1981–1988.

Tuszynski, M. H., Thal, L., Pay, M., Salmon, D. P., Hoi, S., Bakay, R. et al. (2005). A phase 1 clinical trial of nerve growth factor gene therapy for Alzheimer disease. *Nature Medicine, 11,* 551–555.

Valenstein, E. S. (1986). *Great and desperate cures: The rise and decline of psychosurgery and other radical treatments for mental illness.* New York: Basic Books.

White, D. B., Curtis, J. R., Wolf, L. E., Prendergast, T. J., Taichman, D. B., Kuniyoshi, G. et al. (2007). Life support for patients without a surrogate decision maker: Who decides? *Annals of Internal Medicine, 147,* 34–40.

WHO. *Resource book on mental health, human rights and legislation* (2005). Geneva: World Health Organization.

13 Functional Assessment in Geriatric Neurology

Germaine L. Odenheimer and Linda Hunt

Physicians are frequently asked to determine their patients' capacities for functioning safely and adequately in common situations. Such situations involve everyday tasks but may also include demanding, perhaps dangerous, occupations, such as driving a police car or handling firearms. This issue focuses on patient-relevant activities and contributes to the patient-centered model of health care.

Neurologists are trained to localize, diagnose, prognosticate, and treat neurological disorders but are often ill-prepared to assess and help older patients adapt to the nearly inevitable erosion of independent living skills. Despite the availability of practical instruments, functional assessment continues to be underutilized in current clinical neurological practice. Thus, functional deficits are under recognized (Fleming et al.1995). This chapter will discuss multiple aspects of functional decline with a focus on cognitive changes affecting function. It will present an overview of terminology, common neurological causes of functional decline, methods for measuring function, and the impact on management. Since occupational therapy (OT) is the discipline most likely to perform detailed functional assessments, an OT perspective is also included.

Although cognitive, physical, and functional skills are related (Heaton and Pendleton 1981), they are distinct concepts that should be measured independently (Skurla et al. 1988; Applegate et al. 1990) Measures of cognitive, motor, and sensory function do not adequately predict how people will perform tasks of daily living. This discrepancy is particularly evident in patients with mild degrees of dementia (Reed et al. 1989) and has given standardized functional assessment great importance in our evaluations. In most busy practices, if functional status is addressed at all, it is typically based on self or caregiver reports. The value of collateral input cannot be over emphasized in obtaining valid information. When collateral sources are used to describe functional capacity, dementing disorders may be identified much earlier and more accurately than by traditional clinical assessments (Morris et al. 1991).

Functional assessment tools were developed because traditional medically based clinical measures did not adequately predict function. It is an approach specifically intended to capture the ability of a person to perform common self-care skills deemed relevant for living independently. Such skills are classically divided into basic and complex activities of daily living. Activities of daily living (ADLs) traditionally include the most fundamental of self-care skills such as toileting and bathing (Table 1a) (Katz et al. 1963, Mahoney and Barthel 1965). More complex skills have been referred to as instrumental activities of daily living (IADLs). They require greater planning and experience and include such tasks as managing money or taking medications appropriately (Table 1b) (Lawton and Brody 1969). Advanced skills that might be considered more individualized IADLs [Ind-IADLs] (Table 1c) would include those required for functioning in a particular job, signing legal documents or using heavy equipment. The first presumption in measuring IADLs and Ind-IADLs is that the individual had been capable of and performed these functions previously.

Domains of Daily Living Skills

The detection and documentation of impaired ADLs is relatively straightforward. ADLs are fundamental for self-sufficient existence and are largely independent of gender, culture, education, or socio economic status. Impairments in these functions often, though not inevitably, lead to placement in nursing homes or similar institutions.

On the other hand, measurements of IADLs and Ind-IADLs have been much more difficult to standardize because the tasks are variably influenced by gender, culture, education, or socio economic status. Although telephone use is comparatively free of these biases, women more typically have done the cooking and laundering, whereas men, especially in the current elderly cohort, have more often performed home maintenance and driving. This is likely to change as the baby boomers enter the aged playing field.

Decline in IADLs tends to require increased supervision as well as restrictions in paying the bills or picking up the grandkids from school. A strong social support system can dramatically prolong the ability of an individual to live safely in the community. But when social support systems fail, patients with decline in IADLs tend to land in long-term care facilities.

Ind-IADLs tend to be the first skills to deteriorate in dementing disorders. They are often overlooked because the person is often still working and socializing with apparent competence. But these situations can have disastrous results: For example the attorney who makes significant errors in defense of a client, the surgeon who forgets the sequence of a surgical procedure, the architect whose building collapses. These scenarios end up in court before anyone is aware that a disease is behind these failures [personal observation].

Table 1a Activities of Daily Living (ADLs)

Communicating
Walking on level surfaces and on stairs
Transferring from and to toilet, bed, chair
Dressing
Grooming
Bathing
Controlling bowels and bladder
Feeding

Table 1b Instrumental Activities of Daily Living (IADLs)

Managing money

Taking medications

Meeting transportation needs

Cooking

Cleaning

Shopping

Laundering

Maintaining house

Using the telephone

Thoughtful functional assessment can help us advise our patients and their caregivers in making reasonable decisions regarding major alterations in lifestyles and changing roles. In light of time constraints and lack of experience by physicians, occupational therapists (OTs) are our strongest allies in performing structured functional assessments. Their role is described in more detail later in the chapter.

Neurological Changes of Functional Relevance in the Elderly

Functional decline can result from both common age-associated neurological diseases as well as so called "normal" aging processes. Physical decline has been associated with aging for almost every aspect of the nervous system [i.e., reaction time (Birren et al. 1980), complex cognitive skills (Albert and Heaton 1988), vision (Kline and Scheiber 1985), and hearing (Olsho and Harkins 1985)]. Pupillary size and pupillary response to light are reduced (Prakash and Stern 1973; Kokmen et al. 1977; Carter 1979). Decline in proximal muscle strength is often described (Kokmen et al. 1977; Jacobs and Gossman 1980; Jenkyn et al. 1985).

Although many neurological changes have been described with aging, the studies rarely excluded individuals with diseases known to cause neurological signs. When studies of neurologic changes with advancing age exclude diseases with known neurological consequences (such as diabetes, stroke or Parkinson's disease), most changes in the neurological examination commonly attributed to age became the exception, not the rule. (Odenheimer et al. 1994). From here forward, "normal" will refer to those populations without known neurologic

Table 1c Examples of Individualized IADLs (Ind-IADLs)

Working the microwave or the computer

Playing bridge or performing magic tricks

Planning a party or a trip

Signing a will or voting in an election

Running heavy machinery

Supervising a medical laboratory

Directing a research team or an army

Flying an airplane or driving a school bus

Designing a tower or a bridge

disease and "typical" will refer to the common or average findings in an aging population.

Of the neurological changes described in apparently normal elderly, only a few have significant impact on function. Those changes that do affect function relate primarily to motor slowness, difficulty with cognitive complexity, and visual and auditory decline.

Normal functional decline is evident only under circumstances with high demand. For example, slowness is generally not a major problem except for professional athletes. Pupillary changes make driving at night difficult (Graca 1986). Hearing loss has been independently associated with decreased mobility, although the reasons for this relationship remain undetermined (Bess et al. 1989).

Neurological Diseases that Impair Function

Although the majority of those over age 85 remain independent, rates of disability clearly increase with "typical" advancing age. Many age-associated neurological conditions can dramatically impair function, particularly Alzheimer's disease, Parkinson's disease, and stroke. Neurological diseases appear to account for the majority of disabilities in the elderly. In one study, 25% of community-dwelling elderly were fully dependent in their ADLs. Of those, 93% were functionally impaired by neurological disorders (Akhtar et al. 1973).

Rapid decline in function often signals disease or even imminent death. The elderly often present with non-specific neurological signs and symptoms of common non neurological medical diseases. For example, a person with a urinary tract infection may present with a fall. Delirium may be the presenting sign of a myocardial infarction. These non-specific patterns of disease presentation are referred to as *geriatric syndromes* (Fleming et al.1995). These appear to be a consequence of co-morbid diseases and multiple medications superimposed on age-related changes. The precise mechanisms of the geriatric syndromes are under investigation. The geriatric syndromes typically include urinary incontinence, dizziness, instability of gait and falls, and/or delirium (AMA 1990). The risk factors for causing any of the geriatric syndromes are largely the same for all (Tinetti 1995).

Neurological disorders that predispose to incontinence include neuropathies, myelopathies, normal-pressure hydrocephalus, and multiple cerebral infarcts (Resnick 1988). But non-neurologic medical diseases are just as likely. Regardless of the etiology, this common geriatric syndrome usually leads to medical attention when it is acute or severe but is often dismissed by the patient, caregivers, or doctors if it develops gradually or occurs sporadically.

Dizziness is an extremely common complaint in the elderly that has been associated with sensory dysfunction, depression, and cardiovascular diseases as well as a "geriatric syndrome." It is independently associated with increase in institutionalization (Sloane et al. 1989). This symptom is often accompanied by gait instability and falls.

Disorders of gait have a profound impact on the lives of the elderly with increased risk of falls, hip fractures, and death (Tinetti and Speechley 1989). Even fear of falling can lead to severely restricted activity. It is a common geriatric syndrome, although the more recognized culprits for gait instability are medications; visual, musculoskeletal, and neurological disorders such as myelopathy, Parkinson's disease, frontal lobe disorders; and sensory and cerebellar dysfunction (Sudarsky 1990; Lipsitz et al. 1991).

Risk factors for delirium include advanced age, vision and hearing impairments, polypharmacy, psychosocial stress, and intracranial disease (Lipowski 1989). Delirium is associated with high morbidity and mortality and presents major management challenges. Patients with delirium are particularly at risk for additional iatrogenic complications from medications and physical restraints. More than any of the other geriatric syndromes, delirium significantly increases lengths of stay in the hospital, resulting in higher medical care costs (Inouye et al. 1998).

Despite the classic description of delirium as an acute confusional state, the onset of delirium may be insidious in the elderly [personal observation]. This is most often seen in the outpatient setting where new medications and increased dosages accumulate gradually. With aging changes in metabolism and fat/lean muscle mass ratios, serum drug levels and sensitivity to even low levels can increase despite stability in medications or dosing for years. Abrupt decompensation of cognition or function in the face of otherwise relatively trivial illness such as upper respiratory tract infection or cataract surgery may be an indication of incipient dementia.

Purposes of Functional Assessment

Functional assessment can facilitate important clinical decisions. Functional status measures can serve as powerful predictors of morbidity and mortality (Milan-Calenti, et al, 2010). They are useful for assessing the combined impact of aging and neurological disorders. Different clinical settings have developed specialized assessment tools, as goals vary with type and stage of disease and the living arrangements. At home the agenda usually involves maximizing independence without compromising safety. In acute care facilities, prognosis, response to treatment, and discharge planning are major objectives. In rehabilitation settings the emphasis tends to be on functional improvement and appropriate placement. Nursing homes often concentrate on determining levels of care and staffing needs.

Tools have also been designed to follow patients with specific diagnoses, such as Alzheimer's disease (Blessed 1968), Parkinson's disease (Richards et al. 2004), and stroke (American Stroke Association 2009; Hajek 1997). Depending on the setting, the assessment tools may include measures of gait, tremor, or spasticity, or track symptoms such as pain or depression (Table 2).

Functional concepts are commonly used to describe degrees or stages of dementia (Wilson et al. 1973; Shader et al. 1974; Berger 1980; Hughes et al. 1982; Pfeffer et al. 1982; Reisberg et al. 1982; Galasko et al. 1991). Most definitions of dementia require that the symptoms are severe enough to impact function: "significantly interfere with work or usual social activities" (APA 2000).

When impairments are obvious, it is relatively straight forward to make recommendations that restrict activities. However, most of our patients consult us when their function is marginal. Unfortunately, health care providers tend to miss all but the most severe functional impairment (Pinholt et al. 1987). A standardized functional assessment tool can help to objectify and guide our clinical decision making (Wasson et al. 1990). There are a number of valuable reviews available on functional assessment instruments (Kane and Kane 1981; Applegate et al. 1990, Burns et al. 2001).

Methods of Functional Assessment

Treatment teams with skills in functional assessment and knowledge about available social services are invaluable when caring for the elderly patient with functional decline. Functional information can be obtained by having the family fill out a form while the clinician examines the patient. The functional information should then be supplemented by an observational assessment of the patient, ideally by a trained specialist such as a nurse practitioner or occupational therapist. In the event that such specialists are unavailable, it behooves the practitioner to observe at least those functions that are of concern to

Table 2 Some Goals of Functional Assessment

Predict outcomes, including morbidity, mortality

Estimate length of stay in acute care

Maximize balance between independence & safety

Establish & measure Quality of Life goals

Establish baseline function

Stage severity of illness

Follow progression

Adjust medication

Monitor change after treatment

Measure impact of co-morbidity

Document results of study interventions

Determine eligibility for services or admission

Determine key environmental, emotional & social supports

Guide rehabilitation

Select assistive devices

Plan for discharge

Select appropriate placement and level of care

Determine staffing needs

the patient or family. The patient may also be referred for outpatient or home care therapies as well as for a driving assessment, available at rehabilitation facilities or by the state's Department of Motor Vehicles (AAAM 1991; AMA 2003)

Functional status can be determined by report and or direct observation. Clinicians usually rely on reports from the patient and the family about the patient's abilities to perform designated skills (Lawton and Brody 1969). Although accepting such reports may seem efficient, the information is often of limited value. In general, families tend to underestimate and patients tend to overestimate their capabilities when compared with direct observation by trained staff (Rubenstein et al. 1984). This is especially evident for highly emotionally charged tasks like driving a car (Odenheimer 1994).

Direct observation of the patient in his or her own setting at home, at work, or in the car, has been shown to be the most valid approach. This method allows evaluation of the interaction of the medical, environmental, and psychosocial factors that impact functional status. In one study, office-based assessments were compared with in-home evaluations. The home evaluations revealed a significant increase in recognition of serious problems and led to improvement in management (Ramsdell et al. 1989).

Structured tasks can be incorporated into the home setting to add reliability to the evaluation, including asking the patient to find the house key, give the examiner a tour of the house, prepare a cup of tea, dial a phone number, or demonstrate the strategy for handling emergencies (Kapust and Weintraub 1988).

Methods of direct observation have also been developed for the office setting (Kuriansky and Gurland 1976). The patient may be provided with the necessary props to make a purchase, make a cup of instant coffee, telephone a designated place, and select and dress from an array of clothing (Skurla et al. 1988).

Standardized equipment also exists for measuring and timing task performance. We can reliably quantify tasks such as manipulating a button and a zipper, putting on a shirt, tying a bow, cutting with a knife, and threading a needle. Scoring is dependent on the time it takes to complete each task (Potvin and Tourtellotte 1985). Slowness in task performance has been shown to be a useful predictor of long-term care needs (Williams 1987).

Relationship between ADLs, IADLs, and Cognition

Some studies suggest that cognitive skills can predict functional capacity (Kahn et al. 1960; Wilson et al. 1973; Vitaliano et al. 1984). Other investigators have shown cognitive testing to be insufficient to adequately predict functional competence (Winograd 1984; Weintraub 1986; Teri et al. 1989; Akki et al. 1991). The discrepancies in these findings may be explained largely by differences in types of illnesses (psychiatric, medical, and neurological diseases), settings (rehabilitation, nursing home, acute care facility, community dwelling), and the measures used to determine cognitive and functional status (Heaton and Pendleton 1981). Performance on the Blessed Dementia Scale (which includes a large component of functional assessment) has been correlated with the neuropathological changes seen in Alzheimer's disease (Blessed 1968). The Clinical Dementia Rating scale which is widely used in research settings to stage dementia also relies heavily on functional status (Morris 1993).

The relationship between measures of cognitive status and measures of ADLs and IADLs is illustrated by the following description of patients referred to a dementia specialty clinic (Odenheimer and Minaker 1998). Of 190 consecutive patients, the duration of dementia symptoms averaged 5 years, largely due to subtle decline in function. The Mini-Mental State Examination (MMSE) scores (Folstein et al. 1975) ranged from 0 to 30 (mean 18), with 30 as the best possible score. Functional assessment was determined by interviewing the patients and families. The patients' functional status in ADLs and IADLs were categorized as fully independent, fully dependent, or mixed for each category. On initial evaluation 13% of the patients were fully independent in their IADLs and 68% were fully dependent. For ADLs, 48% of the patients were independent and 21% totally dependent. The rest were mixed or unknown. Significant correlations were found between IADLs and ADLs ($r = 0.52$), IADLs and MMSE ($r = -0.51$), and ADLs and MMSE ($r = -0.52$). Although there was a significant relation between ADLs and IADLs and between each functional assessment scale and mental status, cognitive function alone did not adequately account for the functional decline observed. Certainly there are more sensitive measures of cognitive function, but these are rarely used in a typical practice.

Use of Functional Assessment in Management

In general, the ultimate goal of management is to maximize the balance between independence and safety of the patient. However, the goals of assessment should be defined explicitly, e.g., baseline measures, establish therapeutic goals, emphasize patient preferences, or monitor the clinical course of a patient (Applegate et al. 1990). When concerns arise for the safety of the patient or others, determination of capacity and competency issues must be addressed.

All reasonable and acceptable alternatives should be explored if we are to effectively help patients and families make choices that may lead to loss of autonomy. Rarely do current transportation options suit the frail or confused older person. Share-a-ride programs or church groups may provide fragmented transportation. Special transportation programs, such as the Independent Transportation Network, that offer 24/7 service is prepaid and will provide assistance to the older

passenger can greatly enhance the ability of frail elderly to age in place (ITN 2009).

Daycare and assisted living arrangements can be transitional options to nursing homes. Visiting nurses, home health aides, senior companions and food delivery programs may provide enough support to maintain a frail senior at home for an extended period. There are a number of community-based comprehensive services that facilitate living at home despite high care needs that would ordinarily lead to a nursing home. These include the Program of All-Inclusive Care for the Elderly (PACE) (www.medicare.gov/nursing/Alternatives/Pace.asp) and the Home Based Primary Care (HBPC) program offered to veterans (Department of Veterans Affairs 2007).

PACE is a capitated managed care program offered through Medicare and Medicaid for frail elderly who have been certified as eligible for nursing home care. An interdisciplinary team assesses participants' needs, develops care plans, and delivers all services (including acute care services and when necessary, nursing facility services), which are integrated for a seamless provision of total care. PACE programs provide social and medical services primarily in an adult day health center, supplemented by in-home and referral services in accordance with the participant's needs. As of 2009 there were 72 programs in 30 states.

The Department of Veteran Affairs HBPC program provides comprehensive, interdisciplinary, primary care in the homes of veterans with complex medical, social, and behavioral conditions for whom routine clinic-based care is not effective. The primary focus of HBPC is longitudinal care for complex chronic disabling disease. HBPC consists of a multidisciplinary team that travels to veterans' homes to provide services for veterans whose medical or physical problems limit their ability to come to the hospital or clinics for medical care. HBPC primarily targets the following three types of patients in need of home care:

(1) Longitudinal care patients with chronic complex medical, social, and behavioral conditions, particularly those at high risk of hospital, nursing home, or recurrent emergency care.

(2) Longitudinal care patients who require palliative care approach for an advanced disease that is life limiting and refractory to disease-modifying treatment.

(3) Patients whose home care needs are expected to be of short duration or for a focused problem, when such services best help the facility meet the needs of this population.

Increasingly some of the services are being offered through telehealth set ups.

The services include:

1. Functional and cognitive screening

2. Assessment, diagnosis, and treatment

3. Education of the veteran and caregivers to improve outcomes

4. Interventions for pain, disability, sleep problems, smoking cessation, and medical compliance.

5. Psychotherapy to support veterans coping with grief and loss associated with disability and other life transitions.

The Role of Occupational Therapists (OTs)

Occupational therapists facilitate engagement in activities that are meaningful and important to the patient. Skilled OTs also determine the patient's readiness for assessment and intervention. For example, if an assessment/intervention requires reading, the OT would make sure that the patient can properly see the material and that visual acuity is appropriate for the task. In addition, the OT would screen for pain and depression, since both may impact the results of cognitive and functional performance. Finally, OTs would check for overall comfort of the patient regarding fatigue level, positioning, and posture for the task to be performed, and other factors that may compromise optimal performance.

Researchers in occupational therapy have developed tools to measure patients' perceptions, goals, and function in performance of their everyday activities or occupations.

Two assessment tools are the *Canadian Occupational Therapy Measure* (COPM) and the *Activity Card Sort* (ACS). These are powerful measures that provide a rich portrait of patients' lives and allow patients' concerns to emerge.

In the 1980s, the Department of National Health and Welfare Canada and the Canadian Association of Occupational Therapists developed quality assurance guidelines for the practice of occupational therapy (Department of National Health and Welfare 1983, 1986, 1987). This task force recommended that tools be developed for occupational therapy practitioners to determine the effectiveness of their work. In response to the recommendations, the COPM was developed to be compatible with the Canadian Guidelines for client-centered practice (Law et al. 2005).

The COPM is a semi-structured interview aimed at identifying problems in occupational performance with an additional emphasis on what is important to the patient, how an activity is performed, and the patient's satisfaction with that performance (Table 3). The occupational performance problems are weighted in terms of the importance of those activities. This serves to establish the client's priorities and leads very naturally into goal setting and treatment planning.

The COPM requires interviewing skills to administer and costs around $52 for the materials. Administration takes 40–60 minutes and involves reviewing issues of self-care (ADLs and IADLs), productivity (education and work), and leisure (play and social participation) with the patient, then having the patient identify those activities that he or she needs to do, wants to do, or is expected to do but that are presenting challenges. After the issues are identified, the patient rates each issue's importance and current satisfaction and performance for each issue (Law et al. 2005). The COPM provides two scores: performance and satisfaction with performance, both of which are self-rated by the patient; although this may be a limitation in patients with poor insight and cognitive impairment.

The measurement properties (reliability, validity, responsiveness) of the COPM have been satisfactory to excellent (Carswell et al. 2004). The COPM has been used successfully with a wide variety of patients, including older adults with hip fractures (Edwards et al. 2007), in a wide variety of settings and has been translated into 22 languages used in over 35 countries. It is ideal for evaluation of older adults and their family members. It has also been shown to be highly responsive to change.

Studies using this approach have addressed consumer and expert ratings on an ADL scale for predicting functional outcomes after acute care (Chen and Kane 2001). It has been demonstrated to measure changes in performance and satisfaction that are comparable to changes in overall function as perceived by caregivers, occupational therapists, and patients. A review article summarizes the results of approximately 85 research articles involving the COPM (Carswell et al. 2004).

Activity Card Sort (ACS)

The ACS is a tool that identifies: 1) types of activities in which patients participate, 2) deficits in participation of activities, and 3) how these influence quality of life (Baum and Edwards 2008). The ACS captures differences in activity patterns that have clinical usefulness and gives the OT an immediate impression of the activities to use in individual treatment planning. It provides clinicians with an activity history that can be used in intervention planning, allows the therapist and client to consider the impact of a disability or condition on occupations and participation, and fosters the use of activities meaningful to the client in treatment (Letts et al. 2002). Benefits of using this instrument include:

- Identify the impact of a disability on an individual's activity pattern

- Foster the use of treatment activities that are meaningful to the client

- Guide family members and friends to enable activity and social participation

The ACS was developed with a population of older adults in the United States. Through a series of 80 photographs, the ACS offers a full scope of activities that engage the time and interests of older adults, including instrumental, leisure (high and low physical demand), and social activities. It can be used with clients in institutional and community settings and also when people are recovering from a specific health issue. It requires approximately 20 minutes to administer. The materials cost about $150.

Although not as commonly used as the COPM, the ACS has been taught in all OT schools over the last six plus years, so that most OTs are familiar with it. Some OTs use the ACS prior to the COPM, which helps older adults better identify the ADLs and IADLs that are most important to them. The ACS also functions as an instrument to develop rapport with patients, discuss a variety of issues that impact the care of patients, and better understand patients' environment including family and friends' roles in patients' quality of life.

Summary and Policy Implications

Incorporating functional approaches to assessment and management should lead to greater gratification in the treatment of chronic diseases that in the past have discouraged clinicians, patients, and their families.

Aging changes, diseases, and drugs that affect the nervous system can impair skills required for independent living. Geriatric neurology focuses on assisting the aging patient in maintaining autonomy in the face of declining health and psychosocial status. It relies on a close alliance between neurologists, nurses, occupational therapists, psychologists, social workers, and others to understand and manage the functional aspects and complex interactions between aging, disease, and social support systems. An interdisciplinary team can maximize independence of the frail older patient by assisting in the determination of the presence and impact of disease, prioritizing and coordinating desired outcomes, and resolving conflicting interventions (Besdine 1988).

When we cannot adequately gauge the critical skills required for a complex task, we tend to capitulate with age-based criteria. This method is unsatisfactory for judging the individual. Age and diagnosis are inadequate predictors of outcome in our patients. The integration of functional abilities into our routine clinical evaluation and management will greatly enhance quality of care.

Table 3 Outcomes from the COPM

- Provide a rating of a patient's priorities in occupational performance
- Evaluate performance & satisfaction relative to those problem areas
- Measure change in a patient's perception of performance over time

A defensible solution will be found only through a dedicated interchange between experts on aging, health, policy, ethics, law, engineering, and others. Should we intervene as health care providers? Can we use our clinical repertoire to impeach the incompetent judge or school bus driver, surgeon, pilot, or captain of an oil tanker (Odenheimer 1999)? Unfortunately, it is often through tragedy that we begin to realize our deficiencies in addressing functional decline.

There is some agreement regarding the general skills needed to live independently despite lack of consensus regarding specific tools to measure these skills (Katz et al. 1963; Lawton and Brody 1969; Kane and Kane 1981). There is a need to improve communication between those who approach the patient from a disease or systems perspective and those who take the functional approach. There is great advantage in combining approaches, using reporting and observational techniques for determining functional abilities.

Clinicians need information and guidance when making rational decisions about maximizing or limiting the independence of their patients. Similar levels of impairment may lead to dramatically different degrees of disability in different individuals. Although physical impairments contribute to functional decline, "disability … appears to be a complex phenomenon influenced by … preexisting factors such as age, gender, socioeconomic status and living situation" (Jette and Branch 1985).

Psychological, social, cultural, and economic conditions contribute significantly to the ability to live independently in the face of physical and cognitive decline (Besdine 1988). In contrast, the number and types of diagnoses or medications for a patient do not accurately predict functional dependence. A comprehensive functional assessment is useful not only for identifying early signs of disease; it is invaluable for determining long-term care needs and appropriate placement. The understanding of disease must broaden to incorporate the effect of that disease on one's lifestyle, preferences, and quality of life.

Finally, concerns have been raised about the danger of inappropriate policies based on findings from the studies, particularly when those policies are used to restrict services, establish overly narrow service guidelines, or discharge a client to an institution such as a skilled nursing facility. For example, if a study concludes that after 90 days following a stroke little further recovery is seen, then we must be clear how recovery was defined and whether the measure used was sensitive to small amounts of functional change. And if a study purports to examine participation, then we should make sure that the content of the outcome measure examines more than basic ADLs or whether the person can walk a mile but also asks about social relationships and engagement in family and community life, work, play, and leisure. A life of quality is about so much more than buttoning a shirt or tying shoes. Costner advocates that we make sure that measures capture life's richness and complexity (Costner 2009).

Acknowledgment

This work was made possible by support from Veterans Administration Medical Center in Oklahoma City, OK & the University of Oklahoma, College of Medicine.

References

Association for the Advancement of Automotive Medicine (AAAM) (1991). Screening and licensing criteria for the older drivers. *Assoc Advancement Automotive Med Bull* 4:6.

Akhtar AJ, Broe GA, Cromble A, McLean WMR, Andrews GR, and Caird FI (1973). Disability and dependence in the elderly at home. *Age Aging* 2:102–111.

Akki S, Lemsky C, and Winograd C (1991). The relationship between mental status scores and ADL status. *J Am Geriatr Soc* 39:A22.

Albert M and Heaton R (1988). *Intelligence testing in geriatric neuropsychology*. New York: Gilford Press, pp. 13–32.

American Medical Association American Medical Association (AMA) (1990). American Medical Association white paper on elderly health: Report of the council on scientific affairs. *Arch Intern Med* 150:2459–2472.

American Medical Association (AMA) (2003). *Physician's guide to assessing and counseling older drivers*. Chicago: AMA, USDOT, NHTSA.

American Stroke Association, National Institute for Neurological disorders and Stroke, Washington University School of Medicine in St Louis (2009). *Stroke scales and clinical assessment tools*. http://www.strokecenter.org/trials/scales/scales-overview.htm

APA (2000). *Diagnostic and statistical manual of mental disorders-Fourth edition-Revised*. Washington, DC: American Psychiatric Association.

Applegate WB, Blass JP, and Williams TF (1990). Instruments for the functional assessment of older patients. *N Engl J Med* 322: 1207–1214.

Baum CM and Edwards D. (2008). *Activity Card Sort* (2nd ed.) Bethesda, MD: AOTA Press.

Beales JL and Edes T. (2009) Veteran's Affairs home-based primary care in clinics. *Geriatric Medicine* 25:149–154.

Berger EY (1980). A system for rating the severity of senility. *J Am Geriatr Soc* 28:234–236.

Besdine RW (1988). Functional assessment as a model for clinical evaluation of geriatric patients. *J US Public Health Service* 103:530–536.

Bess FH, Lichtenstein MJ, Logan SA, Burger MC, and Nelson E (1989). Hearing impairment as a determinant of function in the elderly. *J Am Geriatr Soc* 37:123–128.

Birren J, Woods AW, and Williams MV (1980). Behavioral slowing with age: Causes, organization and consequences. In *Aging in the 1980s: Selected contemporary issues*. Washington, DC: American Psychological Association, pp. 559–612.

Blessed G, Tomlinson BE, and Roth M. (1968). The association between quantitative measures of dementia and of senile change in the cerebral grey matter of elderly subjects. *British Journal of Psychiatry* 114: 797–811.

Carswell A, McColl MA, Baptiste S, Law M, Polatajko H, and Pollock N. (2004). The Canadian Occupational Performance Measure: A research and clinical literature review. *Canadian Journal of Occupational Therapy*, 71(4), 210–222.

Carter AB (1979). The neurologic aspects of aging. In *Clinical geriatrics*. Philadelphia: Lippincott, pp. 292–316.

Chen Q, and Kane, RL (2001). Effects of using consumer and expert ratings of an activities of daily living scale on predicting functional outcomes of post acute care. *Journal of Clinical Epidemiology*, 54:334–342.

Coster WJ. (2008). Embracing ambiguity: Facing the challenge of measurement. *American Journal of Occupational Therapy*, 62, 743–752.

Department of National Health and Welfare. (1983). *Guidelines for the client-centred practice of occupational therapy*. (H39–33/1983E). Ottawa, Ontario.

Department of National Health and Welfare. (1986). *Intervention guidelines for the client-centred practice of occupational therapy*. (H39–100/1986E). Ottawa, Ontario.

Department of National Health and Welfare. (1987). *Towards outcome measures in occupational therapy* (H39–1141/1987E). Ottawa, Ontario.

Edwards M, Baptiste S, Stratford PW, and Law M. (2007). Recovery after hip fracture: What can we learn from the Canadian Occupational Performance Measure? *American Journal of Occupational Therapy* 61:335–344.

Fleming KC, Evans JM, Weber DC, and Chutka DS. (1995) Practical functional Assessment of Elderly Persons: A primary-care approach. *Mayo Clin Proc* 70:890–910.

Folstein MF, Folstein SE, and McHugh PR (1975). Mini-mental state: A practical method for grading the cognitive state of patients for the clinician. *J Psychiatr Res* 12:189–198.

Galasko D, Corey-Bloom J, and Thal LJ (1991). Monitoring progression in Alzheimer's disease. *J Am Geriatr Soc* 39:932–941.

Graca JL (1986). Driving and aging. *Clin Geriatr Med* 2:577–589.

Hajek VE, Gagnon S, and Ruderman JE. (1997) Cognitive and functional assessments of stroke patients: An analysis of their relation *Archives of Physical Medicine and Rehabilitation* 78: 1331–1337.

Heaton RK and Pendleton MG (1981). Use of neuropsychological tests to predict adult patients' everyday functioning. *J Consult Clin Psychol* 49: 807–821.

Hughes CP, Berg L, Danziger WL, Cohen LA, and Martin RL (1982). A new clinical scale for the staging of dementia. *Br J Psychiatry* 140:566–572.

Imms FJ and Edholm OG (1981). Studies of gait and mobility in the elderly. *Age Ageing* 10:147–156.

Independent Transportation Network (2009). http://www.itnamerica.org/

Inouye SK, Rushing JT, Foreman MD, Palmer RM, and Pompei P (1998). Does delirium contribute to poor hospital outcomes? A three-site epidemiologic study. *J Gen Intern Med* 13:234–242.

Jacobs L and Gossman MD (1980). Three primitive reflexes in normal adults. *Neurology* 30:184–188.

Jenkyn LR, Reeves AG, Warren T, Whiting RK, Clayton RJ, Moore WW, et al. (1985). Neurological signs in senescence. *Arch Neurol* 42:1154–1157.

Jette AM and Branch LG (1985). Impairment and disability in the aged. *J Chronic Dis* 38:59–65.

Kahn RL, Goldfarb AI, Pollack M and Gerber IE (1960). The relationship of mental and physical status in institutionalized aged persons. *Am J Psychiatry* 117:120–124.

Kane RA and Kane RL (1981). *Assessing the elderly. A practical guide to measurement.* Lexington, MA: D.C. Health.

Kapust LR and Weintraub S (1988). The home visit: Field assessment of mental status impairment in the elderly. *Gerontologist* 28:112–115.

Katz S, Ford AB, Moskowitz RW, Jackson BA, and Jaffe MW (1963). Studies of illness in the aged. The index of ADL. *JAMA* 185: 914–919.

Kline DW and Scheiber F (1985). *Vision and aging. Handbook of the psychology of aging.* New York: Van Nostrand Reinhold, pp. 296–331.

Kokmen E, Bossemeyer RW, Barney J, and Williams WJ (1977). Neurological manifestations of aging. *J Gerontol* 32:411–419.

Kuriansky J and Gurland B (1976). The performance test of activities of daily living. *Int J Aging Hum Dev* 7:343–352.

Law M, Baptiste S, Carswell A, McColl MA, Polatajko H, and Pollock N (2005). *The Canadian Occupational Performance Measure, manual to the 4th edition.* Ottawa, Ontario: CAOT Publications.

Lawton MP and Brody EM (1969). Assessment of older people: Self-maintaining and instrumental activities of daily living. *Gerontologist* 9:179–186.

Letts L, Baum C, and Perlmutter M (2003). Person-environment-occupation assessment with older adults. *OT Practice* 06/02/03.

Lipowski JZ (1989). Delirium in the elderly patient. *N Engl J Med* 320:578–582.

Lipsitz LA, Jonsson PV, Kelley MM, and Koestner JS (1991). Causes and correlates of recurrent falls in ambulatory frail elderly. *J Gerontol* 46:M114–122.

Mahoney FI and Barthel DW (1965). Functional evaluation: The Barthel Index. *Maryland State Medical Journal* 14:61–65.

Milan-Calenti JC, Tubio J, Pita-Fernandez S, Gonzalez-Abraldes I, Lorenzo T, Fernandez-Arruty T, and Maseda A (2010). Prevalence of functional disability in activities of daily living, (ADL), instrumental activities of daily living (IADL) and associated factors, as predictors of morbidity and mortality. *Archives of Gerontology and Geriatrics*, 50;306-310.

Morris JC, McKeel DW, Storandt M, Rubin EH, Price JL, Grant EA, et al. (1991). Very mild Alzheimer's disease: Informant-based clinical,

psychometric, and pathologic distinction from normal aging. *Neurology* 41:469–478.

Morris JC (1993). The Clinical Dementia Rating (CDR): Current version and scoring rules. *Neurology* 43:2412–2414.

Program of All-Inclusive Care for the Elderly http://www.medicare.gov/nursing/Alternatives/Pace.asp

Odenheimer G, Funkenstein HH, Beckett L, Chown M, Pilgrim D, Evans D, and Albert M (1994). Comparison of neurologic changes in 'successfully aging' persons vs. the total aging population. *Arch Neurol* 51:573–580.

Odenheimer G (1999). Function, flying and the Age-60 Rule. *JAGS* 47:910–911.

Odenheimer GL, Beaudet M, Jette AM, and Albert MS (1994). Driver: Safety, reliability, and validity. *J Gerontol: Med Sci* 49:M153–M159.

Odenheimer GL and Minaker KL. Functional assessment in geriatric neurology. In *Clinical neurology of aging* (2nd ed) 1994 New York, Oxford Press p181–189.

Olsho LW, Harkins SW, and Lenhardt ML (1985). Aging and the auditory system. In *Handbook of the psychology of aging.* New York: Van Nostrand Reinhold, pp. 332–377.

Pfeffer RI, Kurosaki TT, Harrah CH, Chance JM, and Filos S (1982). Measurement of functional activities in older adults in the community. *J Gerontol* 37:323–329.

Pinholt EM, Kroenke K, Hanley JF, Kussman MJ, Twyman PL, and Carpenter JL (1987). Functional assessment of the elderly: A comparison of standard instruments with clinical judgment. *Arch Intern Med* 147:484–488.

Potvin AR and Tourtellotte WW (1985). The instrumented examination of activities of daily living. In *Quantitative examination of neurologic functions.* Boca Raton, FL: CRC Press, pp. 167–180.

Prakash G and Stern C (1973). Neurological signs in the elderly. *Age Ageing* 3:24–27.

Ramsdell JW, Swart JA, Jackson JE, and Renvall M (1989). The yield of a home visit in the assessment of geriatric patients. *J Am Geriatr Soc* 37: 17–24.

Reed BR, Jagust WJ, and Seab JP (1989). Mental status as a predictor of daily function in progressive dementia. *Gerontologist* 29:804–807.

Reisberg B (1988). Functional assessment staging (FAST). *Psychopharmacology Bulletin* 24:653–659.

Reisberg B, Ferris SH, de Leon MJ, and Crook T (1982). The Global Deterioration Scale (GDS) for assessment of primary degenerative dementia. *American J of Psychiatry* 139:1136–1139.

Resnick NM (1988). Urinary incontinence-a treatable disorder. In *Geriatric medicine* (2nd ed.). Boston: Little, Brown, pp. 246–265.

Richards M, Marder K, Cote L, and Mayeux R (2004). Inter-rater reliability of the unified Parkinson's disease rating scale motor examination. *Movement Disorders* 9: 89–91.

Rubenstein LZ, Schairer C, Wieland GD, and Kane R (1984). Systematic biases in functional status assessment of elderly adults: Effects of different data sources. *J Gerontol* 39:686–691.

Shader RI, Harmatz JS, and Salzman C (1974). A new scale for clinical assessment in geriatric populations: Sandoz clinical assessment-geriatric (SCAG). *J Am Geriatr Soc* 22:107–113.

Skurla E, Rogers JC, and Sunderland T (1988). Direct assessment of activities of daily living in Alzheimer's disease. *J Am Geriatr Soc* 36:97–103.

Sloane P, Blazer D, and George LK (1989). Dizziness in a community elderly population. *J Am Geriatr Soc* 37:101–108.

Sudarsky L (1990). Geriatrics: Gait disorders ill the elderly. *N Engl J Med* 322:1441–1446.

Teri L, Borson S, Kiyak HA, and Yamagishi M (1989). Behavioral disturbance, cognitive dysfunction and functional skill: Prevalence and relationship in Alzheimer's disease. *J Am Geriatr Soc* 37: 109–116.

Tinetti ME and Speechley M (1989). Prevention of falls among the elderly. *N Engl J Med* 320: 1055–1059.

Tinetti ME, Inouye SK, Gill TM, and Doucette JT. Shared risk factors for falls, incontinence, and functional dependence. (1995) *JAMA* 273:1348–1353.

Department of Veterans Affairs (2007). Home-Based Primary Care Program, VHA Handbook 1141.01, Veterans Health Administration, Washington DC.

Vitaliano PP, Breen AR, Albert MS, Russo J, and Prinz PN (1984). Memory, attention, and functional status in community-residing Alzheimer type dementia patients and optimally healthy aged individuals. *J Gerontol* 39:58–64.

Wasson JH, Gall V, McDonald R, and Liang MH (1990). The prescription of assistive devices for the elderly: Practical considerations. *J Gen Intern Med* 5:46–54.

Weintraub S (1986). The record of independent living: an informant-completed measure of activities of daily living and behavior in elderly patients with cognitive impairment. *Am J Alzheimers Care Relat Disord Spring*: 35–39.

Williams ME (1987). Identifying the older person likely to require long-term care services. *J Am Geriatr Soc* 35:761–766.

Wilson LA, Grant K, Witney PM, and Kerridge DF (1973). Mental status of elderly hospital patients related to occupational therapist's assessment of activities of daily living. *Gerontol Clin* 15:197–202.

Winograd CH (1984). Mental status tests and the capacity for self-care. *J Am Geriatr Soc* 32:49–55.

3
Cognitive Disorders in Aging

14 Cognitive Function in Healthy Aging

Janet L. Jankowiak

As the baby-boomers creep into their 60s, there is increased interest in forestalling the onset of cognitive decline and especially dementia. Cognitive changes occur over the lifespan, with variable maturation of certain functions and then variable decline of these functions. There is considerable debate over the delineation of where "healthy aging" ends, minimal cognitive impairment (MCI) begins, and where MCI may enter the early stages of dementia. In healthy aging, changes in cognition are very gradual and subtle and do not seriously impact functioning until late in life, often when other organ systems begin to fail. The spectrum of cognitive decline is extremely wide and strongly influenced by multiple factors, including genetics, education, personal habits, socioeconomic status, medical comorbidities, gender, and possibly race. Clearly some of these factors cannot be altered, but many involve lifestyle behaviors that are modifiable. This chapter reviews what is known about various aspects of cognition in terms of expected changes over time, including executive function, memory, language, arithmetic and visuospatial skills, insight, judgment, and emotions, along with their anatomical correlates. It then presents the cognitive reserve hypothesis and data on modifiable risk factors of cognitive decline, providing a strategy for dealing with the inevitable cognitive changes that accompany the privilege of aging.

Measuring Cognitive Changes

One of the difficulties with defining cognitive changes in healthy aging is that many studies are relatively small and generally have few participants in the older old category (over the mid 70s). This is particularly problematic since the mid 70s is when changes become more apparent (Schaie 2005). In addition, samples tend to cluster participants of comparable educational background, particularly those who are highly educated (>15 years of formal education). Comparison between studies is difficult and it is unclear whether findings can be generalized more widely. Cross-sectional studies may overestimate cognitive decline due to cohort effect, based on sensitivity to demographic differences (Small 2001). On the other hand, longitudinal studies may underestimate decline due to the learning effect of repeated testing and attrition of possibly more impaired individuals (Small 2001). Further, it is probable that laboratory tests, e.g. neuropsychological batteries, favor individuals with experience taking tests and it is unclear how results will translate to real-life situations.

In addition, testing can be laborious and time-consuming, creating reluctance for participants to continue. The fatigue effect may also affect performance when tests are too long, generally occurring earlier for older adults than for young adults. Perhaps the biggest hurdle in assessing change in cognition is that true baseline information is not available, especially for older participants. Consequently, selection of tests is variable, depending on resources and cognitive domain targeted. While the Mini-Mental State Examination (MMSE) (Folstein et al. 1975) is commonly used as a gold standard for global cognitive function, it has a well-known ceiling effect and cannot identify slight declines in high levels of cognition, particularly among highly educated people (Tombaugh and MacIntyre 1992). Other tests are more useful to study specific cognitive domains, e.g. memory, language, executive function, but trying to isolate a particular domain for study is challenging and probably artificial due to the interdependence of these functions.

Executive Function

One of the chief complaints of adults as they age is that their memory is not as good. What may not be immediately recognized is that this perception of memory loss may more correctly be attributed to executive dysfunction, and particularly a problem with working memory and processing speed. Executive function does not fare well with aging, being the latest function to develop but among the first to show signs of decline (Craik and Bialystok 2008; Estranges 2008), and may precede memory deficits by three years (Carlson et al. 2009). It appears to impact virtually all other cognitive domains and may be responsible for apparent age-related deficits in these functions as well.

While there is little consensus on a precise definition of executive function (Salthouse 2005), it is generally thought of as higher-order cognitive abilities that allow for problem solving, initiation, execution, and modification of complex goal-directed behavior. Goal selection, planning, set maintenance, self-monitoring, and flexibility are mechanisms hypothesized to be used in executive function (Brennan 1997). Major subcomponents are: focusing attention on relevant information and inhibiting irrelevant information; task management, including switching attention between tasks; planning a sequence of subtasks; updating working memory contents to determine the next step in a sequential task, and coding the context/source of the information in working memory (Smith and Jonides 1999).

It is well established that at least aspects of executive function decline with age and particularly with increasing task complexity (Brennan et al. 1997; Holtzer et al. 2004; Velanova et al. 2007). Healthy older adults show consistently slower processing and response time than younger adults but with similar accuracy, at least for simpler tasks. On more complex tasks with increased demands on control processes (Velanova et al. 2007), older adults make more errors due to failure to maintain problem set, having more difficulty abiding by rules on a novel task (Brennan et al. 1997), although applying logical rules in their responses (Andres and Van de Linden 2000). However, there is considerable inter-individual variability, accentuated with increasing age (Treitz et al. 2007), with some older adults performing as well as younger adults (Rodrigue et al. 2005; Treitz et al. 2007). Within executive processing, Treitz et al. (2007) noted accelerated decline in both task management (i.e., ability to efficiently divide attention) and inhibition of irrelevant information after age 60. Although the oldest group (age 61–75) had the most difficulty, the group of adults 46–60 years also had difficulty with more challenging divided attention tasks if two sensory modalities had to be processed in parallel (Treitz et al. 2007), consistent with earlier decline in executive function. Bopp and Verhaeghen (2007) also concluded that age-related differences in cognitive manipulation are both process specific and domain specific, after studying transformation, supervision, and coordination processes in verbal and visuospatial tasks. Strategic memory processing, cognitive flexibility, reasoning, and self-evaluation of executive abilities did not show age-dependent differences in this young old group (Treitz et al. 2007), while deficits in reasoning (Salthouse 2005; Bowles 2008), flexibility (Velanova et al. 2007), and decreased self-awareness (Gerstorf et al. 2008) have been reported when more participants are older.

However, the major difficulty in assessing executive function is that laboratory tests are based largely on speed measures, and global slowing is part of aging (Salthouse 2005; Treitz et al. 2007). Salthouse (2005) takes this view further and suggests that neuropsychological tests for executive function do not support the notion of executive function as a unique and distinct cognitive dimension because most tests are strongly related to reasoning and perceptual speed abilities, which vary most with age. To assess executive function in more real-life circumstances, performance of activities of daily living (ADLs) and instrumental ADLs (IADLs) are useful in determining functional status (Grigsby et al. 1998; Royall et al. 2004; Royall et al. 2005; Peres et al. 2008; Allaire et al. 2009). Specifically, Peres et al. (2008) found that the ability to handle finances, a complex IADL, is the earliest marker of cognitive decline, observed ten years prior to incident dementia. The autonomous regulation of behavior, which involves executive components of initiation, performance, and monitoring of purposeful tasks, is a stronger predictor of functional status than is the MMSE score (Grigsby et al. 1998). Royall et al. (2004) concluded that executive control function deteriorates over time, even in the absence of abnormal MMSE scores, and is independently associated with longitudinal declines in functional status.

The impact of executive control on measurements of other cognitive domains suggests that age-related declines are domain specific (Jenkins et al. 2000; Bopp and Verhaeghen 2007; Carlson et al. 2009). In addition, age-related cognitive decline appears to be nonlinear (Zimprich and Martin 2002) with an accelerating decline, being most pronounced for spatial and processing speed factors, less for the memory factor and only modest accelerating decline in the verbal factor in late adulthood (Finkel et al. 2007). Quantitatively, Thorvaldsson et al. (2009) found onset of accelerating decline in perceptual speed to occur 14.8 years before death, while terminal decline in spatial ability began 7.8 years and verbal ability 6.6 years before death in older adults without dementia.

Theories regarding the basis of age-related decline of executive function include global slowing of processing speed, interference based on reduced inhibition of distractors, and impaired working memory. While decreased processing speed is accepted as part of normal aging (associated with decreases in white matter integrity, dopamine receptors, and axonal demyelination) (Park and Gutchess 2005), there is debate whether this single factor can explain all changes in cognitive aging (Salthouse 1996; Andres and Van der Linden 2000; Zimprich and Martin 2002; Holtzer et al. 2004; Rodrigue et al. 2005; Finkel et al. 2007; Gazzaley et al. 2008). A dynamic interaction between deficits in neural processing speed and impaired suppression of irrelevant information may act together to explain cognitive deficits in aging (Gazzaley et al. 2008). While older adults are able to suppress irrelevant information, filtering occurs at a later time in processing (Gazzaley et al. 2008),

consistent with a "load shift" model of compensation in executive processing strategy (Velanova et al. 2007). During a simple visual sequential activity—a nonstrategic process—responses were slowed by a factor of 1.6 in older compared to younger adults while a coordinative activity—a strategic process—was slowed by a factor of 13 (Gorman and Fisher 1998). Slowing of the nonstrategic process in the older adults was attributed to generalized slowing while slowing in the strategic process was hypothesized to be due to decreased working memory, strategy difference, and/or increased cautiousness with age (Gorman and Fisher 1998). From a practical standpoint, older adults are involved in many more traffic accidents at left turn intersections than younger adults, possibly because in the prolonged time it takes the older driver to determine that the path is clear, a fast approaching car that was not a threat becomes one (Gorman and Fisher 1998).

Working memory may begin to decline in the thirties (Craik and Bialystok 2008) and is posited to be a pivotal determinant of more general age-related declines in cognitive function. While working memory could be discussed under the heading of memory it is also key in executive processing. By definition, working memory includes a short-term (3–30 seconds) storage of information, which is kept active for processing (Reuter-Lorenz and Sylvester 2005). Verbal information is kept active by a rehearsal process of inner speech (the phonological loop) while visuospatial material is rehearsed by mental images (the visuospatial sketchpad) (Baddeley 1996, 2003). A proposed "central executive" controls the selection, sequencing, and flow of mental operations performed on this stored information (Baddeley 1996). This executive function may not be an undifferentiated supervisory system but a collection of anatomically and functionally independent but interrelated attentional control processes (Stuss and Alexander 2007). The storage component of working memory is relatively preserved in older adults as noted in rote maintenance tasks, e.g. forward and backward digit span (Reuter-Lorenz and Sylvester 2005). On the other hand, age-related deficits in working memory are accentuated by tasks that place greater demand on the executive components of working memory, e.g. selective or executive attention and task management (Braver and West 2008). Selective attention is particularly vulnerable to the effect of competing stimuli due to faulty inhibition and filtering processes associated with aging (West 1999). The clinical manifestation in older adults is increased difficulty with *multitasking*.

Working memory and executive function are localized primarily to the frontal lobes and especially prefrontal cortex (PFC) (Rodrigue 2005; Pardo 2007; Craik and Bialystok 2008). The frontal-striatal systems are particularly vulnerable to white matter change, atrophy, and certain forms of neurotransmitter depletion and may contribute to age-related cognitive impairment on tasks requiring high levels of attention and executive processing (Buckner 2004). Age-associated atrophy occurs earliest in the frontal regions with a 4.9% decrease per decade in the volume of the prefrontal grey matter on MRI (Raz et al. 1997). While a detailed review of the extensive work that is being done with positive emission tomography (PET) and functional magnetic resonance imaging (fMRI) on working memory and aging is beyond the scope of this chapter, a few key observations are important. Older and younger adults tend to activate different brain regions to perform the same task, suggesting that different neural circuitry is engaged. Specifically, older adults may show underactivation in regions activated in younger adults (with associated decline of specific executive processes) and concurrent overactivation in other regions, especially the PFC (Craik and Bialystok 2008), which is activated at lower levels of task demand (Reuter-Lorenz and Sylvester 2005). According to the "selective compensation" hypothesis, this overactivation, and often bilateral activation, of the PFC allows older adults to compensate and perform at comparable levels to younger adults on simpler (e.g. storage/maintenance) tasks, treating the task as a "maintenance-plus-processing task" (Reuter-Lorenz and Sylvester 2005). Therefore, when the task demand level is increased, older adults have already used available resources and performance declines, especially on tasks that explicitly require executive processing. However, when the demand for controlled processing is reduced through practice, the age-related increase in frontal recruitment reverses, showing the plasticity of the older brain (Velanova et al. 2007). Others have argued that overactivation of the PFC in older adults may not be compensatory but dysfunctional, due to nonselective activation (Logan et al. 2002). Recruitment of contralateral regions may be beneficial only when the recruited area mediates a complementary function (Colcombe et al. 2005). Clearly there is considerable variability in the ability of older adults to recruit executive processes for various task demands, with effective compensation in those who age most successfully.

Memory

Memory is multifaceted and has been categorized in numerous ways: fluid/crystallized, short-term/long-term, explicit/implicit, declarative/nondeclarative, primary/secondary/tertiary, episodic/semantic memory, and working memory (discussed above), as well as a host of other terms (Ayd 2000). The abundant research concerning categorization and localization of memory functions is beyond the scope of this chapter (Basar 2004; Cabeza et al. 2005; Eichenbaum 2002; Craik and Salthouse 2008; Desgranges et al. 2008), but an overview is important for understanding functional changes with aging. Memory may be broken down into declarative/explicit memory, which occurs at a conscious level, and nondeclarative/implicit memory, which is nonconscious (performed without awareness of any memory content). *Explicit memory* includes knowledge of facts, independent of specific episodes (i.e., semantic memory) and knowledge of personal events (i.e., episodic memory), both associated with the medial temporal lobe/diencephalon (Squire and Zola 1996). *Implicit memory* includes *procedural memory* (skills and habits, associated with the striatum), priming (recall facilitated by recent exposure, associated with the neocortex), emotional responses (associated with the amygdala), simple classical conditioning of skeletal musculature (associated with the cerebellum) and nonassociative learning (associated with reflex pathways) (Squire and Zola 1996). The various stages of forming memories (acquisition, consolidation, and storage) (Tranel and Damasio 2002) may be dynamic processes and not separable on a time axis (Basar 2004). In a simplified schema of the memory circuit, Small (2001) attributes the medial temporal lobe/ hippocampus with encoding (Park and Gutchess 2005) and consolidation, the posterior association neocortex with storage, and the prefrontal cortex with facilitation of memory retrieval. Arguing against precise localization, Basar (2004) supports the view of overlapping memory networks, such that one neuron or groups of neurons anywhere in the cortex may belong to many networks and thus many memories.

From a functional standpoint, age-related decline in memory is not a diffuse process but appears to have a differential effect on stages of processing as well as domain. Aspects of memory that show only slight changes with aging include implicit /nondeclarative memory (habits, skills, and priming), short term memory (e.g. repetition of a string of words, letters, or numbers that does not require manipulation of information), recognition (as opposed to free recall), and familiarity (i.e., sense of recognition but can not place the source or context of where/how the information was acquired) (Grady and Craik 2000). *Procedural* knowledge, which is acquired earliest, develops through consistent and extensive practice (i.e., becomes automatic), and is most resistant to

age-related decline (Craik and Bialystok 2008). On the other hand, tasks that require effortful, higher-level control processes, e.g. self-initiated activities, show much larger age-related losses. These include free or cued recall, recollection of the original context in which the information was acquired (source memory), prospective memory (i.e., remembering to carry out an action in the future), and working memory (Grady and Craik 2000). *Encoding* of information is particularly vulnerable to the effects of aging, in part due to attentional difficulties. As discussed under working memory, older adults are more sensitive to irrelevant environmental stimuli due to impaired inhibition and filtering, resulting in memory failure (Stevens et al. 2008). Age-related sensory deficits, e.g. hearing, may compete for central processing resources and compromise acquisition of information (McDaniel et al. 2008). Similarly, negative stereotypes regarding aging, e.g. "can't teach an old dog new tricks," may influence effort in attempts to learn (McDaniel et al. 2008). Encoding strategies used to facilitate the memory process include organization of the material by categorization, mental imagery, or attaching significance through association with previous knowledge. Studies in older adults show deficiencies in these strategies, consistent with decline in executive control function, and associated with poorer performance on memory tasks (Isingrini and Taconnat 2008). *Retrieval* of information (Dennis and Cabeza 2008) also shows age-related declines (context>recall>recognition) but less severe than for encoding and is less disadvantaged by interference than is encoding (Park and Gutchess 2005).

Changes in long-term memory that accompany aging may be mediated largely by declines in speed of processing and working memory (Park and Gutchess 2005). Declarative/explicit long-term memory, also called personal memory, includes semantic memory (i.e., general knowledge about the world) and episodic memory (i.e., recollection of personal events and incidents) (Basar, 2004). *Semantic memory*, (knowledge "that") is independent of identifying specific episodes or where the information was learned and tends to be better preserved with aging, although ability to access that information declines (Craik and Bialystok 2008). Acquisition of semantic knowledge increases until about age 60 then slowly declines; knowledge that is initially learned well is much more likely to be retained (Ackerman 2008; Craik and Bialystok 2008). Older adults tend to have larger prior domain knowledge than younger adults, which facilitates acquisition of new information, but only if allowed longer time for processing (Ackerman 2008). In addition, the more often memories are used the better they are retained. *Episodic memory* is particularly vulnerable to the effects of age; it is stable until 50–60 years (longitudinal study), then shows a steeper decline than semantic memory (Ackerman 2008). Age-related deficits are noted when episodic memory tasks involve free recall, context, association, or increased processing demands on retrieval, while tasks that involve recognition and more automatic aspects, e.g. familiarity, show little change with age (Braver and West 2008). Consequently, deficits in episodic memory may not represent deficits in memory storage per se but rather impaired executive control, which again explains marked individual differences noted in older adults (Braver and West 2008). While episodic memory is classically viewed as being subserved by the mediotemporal cortex and hippocampus, there is close linkage to frontal cortex function (Wheeler et al. 1997; Cabeza 2002a). In older adults, larger areas of right frontal regions are activated during encoding and left frontal region during retrieval of episodic memory, leading to more bilateral PFC activation and a reduction of hemispheric asymmetry, i.e., the HAROLD model (Hemispheric Asymmetry Reduction in Older Adults) (Cabeza 2002b). This increased PFC activity may compensate for observed decreases in medial temporal lobe (MTL) activity in older adults (Dennis and Cabeza 2008).

In addition, low-performing older adults recruit a similar network of brain regions as young adults but in an inefficient manner while high-performing adults overcome this age-related neural decline with bilateral PFC activation during a demanding memory task, suggesting plastic reorganization of neurocognitive networks (Cabeza et al 2002). Other studies discuss functional reorganization in the older brain as a reallocation of resources, as well as other possible mechanisms to explain changes in brain function with aging (Rajah and D'Esposito 2005; Restom et al. 2007; Zarahn et al. 2007; Beason-Held 2008).

Memory for recent events is known to decline with age, especially recollection of specific contextual details of events, while familiarity-based recognition of the event is better retained (Yonelinas 2002). Paradoxically, older adults exhibit more *false memory* of events that never occurred, compared with young adults, especially when features of the false event overlap with actual events they have experienced. One hypothesis is that over-reliance on familiarity contributes to elevated false recognition in older adults (Grady and Craik 2000). Against this theory, Duarte et al. (2008) found (using event-related fMRI) that both recollection and familiarity-related activity were diminished in older adults, and posited that the reduced differentiation between neural activity associated with true and false memories may contribute to elevated false recognition in older adults. Individual differences are significant and older adults with high frontal functioning show comparable performance to younger adults, independent of medial temporal lobe function (McDaniel et al. 2008).

Another aspect of memory distortion noted in older adults is the tendency to recall positive events more than negative ones, both for autobiographical information and more general knowledge (Mather and Carstensen 2005). This has been termed the "positivity effect" and has been linked to improved emotion regulation skills found in older adults (Mather and Carstensen 2005). *Emotional memory* is selective, such that attentional biases influence what information is encoded. As for young adults, older adults show enhanced memory for emotionally arousing stimuli, associated with amygdala function. However, older adults also seem to use top-down control processes supported by prefrontal systems to filter out more negative than positive information and reconstruct future memories in a more positive light. In addition, older adults show increased (bilateral) hippocampal activation for autobiographical event retrieval while young adults show only left-lateralized activation, suggesting that personal or emotional information may be less fragile than purely experimental/episodic information (Park and Gutchess 2005). The long-term benefit of the positivity effect may be associated with "successful aging." For example, bereaved spouses who experience some positive emotions while grieving immediately after the death fare better in the following years than those who show more dramatic distress (Bonanno 2004).

Prospective memory (remembering to carry out an intention in the future) is more impaired in older versus younger adults in the laboratory but not on field tasks (Henry et al. 2004; Cuttler and Graf 2007). In real life situations old adults could make use of personal compensatory strategies (Cuttler and Graf 2007) and may have had greater motivation to succeed, e.g., to carry out a promise (Grady and Craik 2000). While a large meta-analysis of studies showed pronounced age-related deficits in prospective memory (Henry et al. 2004), individual differences in working memory capacity and executive functions impact successful prospective memory (Braver and West 2008). Focusing on the contribution of personality and lifestyle variables, Cuttler and Graf (2007) found that conscientiousness and neuroticism correlated positively with performance, reasoning that neurotic adults are more vigilant about monitoring or ruminate more about the need to perform upcoming tasks. A negative correlation was found with perfectionism, predicted by the association of this trait with procrastination, anxiety, and depression. Cuttler and Graf (2007) posited that current theories of episodic prospective memory task performance may overestimate the impact of cognitive factors while underestimating the "potentially equally powerful influence due to personality and lifestyle variables" (p 228).

Source memory, the context in which a memory is acquired (i.e., when, where, how of an event), generally shows age-related decline (McDaniel et al. 2008). However, there is considerable variability among older adults, and those with high frontal function perform as well as young adults on source memory tasks (Glisky et al. 2001). Neuroimaging studies of these high performing older adults show bilateral activity in the PFC, again suggesting compensatory activation (Cabeza et al. 2002).

Strategies to facilitate memory include distinctive processing, e.g. it is easier to learn and recall elements that are inconsistent with expectation (bizarreness effect), unusual, or incongruent in a series (isolation effect) (McDaniel et al. 2008). These strategies work as well for older adults as younger adults as long as there is not too much information and processing is not too fast. Repetition helps to make behavior automatic (habit), which reduces the need for cognitive control of recollection and thus facilitates performance, e.g. routinely putting keys in the same place (McDaniel et al. 2008).

In summary, age-related declines in memory are noted for source memory, free recall, prospective memory, and episodic memory which all require higher-level control processes, while procedural memory, recognition, and familiarity are relatively well preserved. However, there are marked individual differences, i.e., older adults with good frontal function perform at a level comparable to younger adults. Thus, memory changes in normal aging are more like frontal deficits than the temporal lobe deficits that characterize memory deficits of Alzheimer disease (Isingrini and Taconnat 2008).

Language

Language is a cognitive domain that is generally well-preserved in healthy aging in terms of function, although specific aspects of language may be variably affected. Areas of language that show decline with age are word-finding, comprehension, and syntactic complexity. However, at least some of the decline may actually be attributable to nonlinguistic functions. The most-preserved aspects of language appear to be vocabulary, articulation, and story-telling.

Vocabulary is generally noted to increase with age until middle age (40–60 years), when it plateaus and then declines gradually in late adulthood (past 70 years) (Bowles and Salthouse 2008). However, vocabulary tests vary in format and show a differential change in relation to age (Bowles and Salthouse 2008). Different test formats produce different trends with aging, due to association with other cognitive domains and, while a single test of vocabulary is not ideal, the multiple-choice test of synonyms may be closest to an average test (Bowles and Salthouse 2008).

Word-finding: A common complaint as people age is that they have increasing difficulty finding specific words and experience a tip-of-the-tongue (TOT) phenomenon. TOT is a problem in phonological retrieval, characterized by a temporary inability to recall a known word and especially proper names (Burke and Shafto 2004). Semantic knowledge of the word is retained but phonological representation of the word is more vulnerable. Compared to young adults, older adults (over age 73) experience more frequent TOT episodes, have more difficulty finding alternate words, and have less phonological information about the target word (i.e., are not aided by first syllable primes)

(White and Abrams 2002). In keeping with a "use it or lose it" theory, words that are not activated frequently are more susceptible to TOTs (White and Abrams 2002). Young adults are less certain of infrequently used target words than older adults and have more difficulty with pronunciation of low-frequency, irregularly spelled words (Shafto et al. 2007). White and Abrams (2002) reason that older adults have had a lifetime to accumulate a large vocabulary and therefore know more words. TOT rates do not correlate significantly with measures of vocabulary knowledge or articulation, the latter of which does not decline with normal aging (Shafto et al. 2007).

In further support that problems with word retrieval occur slowly over time, Connor et al. (2004) found that object naming on the Boston Naming Test (BNT) declined two percentage points per decade, on average. Individuals with higher initial BNT scores had less decline over 20 years of study (Connor et al. 2004), consistent with a "cognitive reserve" hypothesis (see below) (Stern 2002).

Using fMRI, Wierenga et al. (2008) found that for equivalent naming accuracy, older adults activate a larger frontal network during word retrieval than younger adults. Increased activation in the left basal ganglia is associated with faster response time while increased activity in Broca's area homologue improves accuracy in "high" performing older adults (Wierenga 2008). Since the older adults showed comparable or better performance than younger adults on naming and semantic associations tests, the semantic memory of the words appears to be preserved. However, the older adults were much slower in word retrieval and had much more difficulty manipulating verbal information (Wierenga 2008). Wierenga (2008) concluded that these frontally-mediated problems with executive language function (i.e., selecting, retrieving, and manipulating lexical-semantic information) underlie age-related word-finding difficulty.

Grammatical complexity: Speech production is simplified in older age, characterized by a reduction in the mean number of clauses per utterance, a measure of the complexity of adult language (Kemper et al. 2001). Kemper et al. (2001) found that grammatical complexity and propositional content of older adults' spontaneous speech was relatively stable until around 74 years of age when it showed a period of rapid decline (age 74 to 78) and then a period of more gradual decline (although there were few samples for adults older than 80 years). This decline is attributed to working memory limitations, reductions in processing speed, and decreased resistance to interference (Craik and Bialystok 2008).

Sentence comprehension shows variable decline in healthy older adults. Functional MRI reveals that a core network of left hemisphere regions is recruited to process written sentences, seemingly independent of age, while additional areas are recruited in older adults during the same reading test (Grossman et al. 2002). Grossman et al. (2002) hypothesized that these additional regions, which support verbal working memory, are up-regulated in older adults to achieve comprehension that is equivalent to young adults. Although responses are slower with age, the core aspects of sentence comprehension are unchanged.

Verbal fluency is another aspect of language often measured to assess cognitive change with aging. Phonemic fluency tests require a subject to generate as many words as possible beginning with a specific letter (e.g. F, A, and S) within one minute for each letter. Semantic fluency tests require generation of words in a specific category (e.g. animals, fruits, colors) within one minute per category. Verbal fluency tests are complex tasks, requiring lexical storage and retrieval, articulation and/or graphomotor ability for the written version, and psychomotor speed (Rodriguez-Aranda 2003). Older adults perform comparably to young adults on oral phonemic fluency tests but have significantly lower scores on oral semantic tests as well as written phonemic and semantic tests (Rodriguez-Aranda 2003). These age-related differences are partly attributable to decreased psychomotor speed, especially in written more than oral fluency tests, and do not necessarily reflect a decline in linguistic or cognitive functions (Rodriguez-Aranda 2003).

Narratives: Functional language is characterized by narrative speech and how effectively ideas are communicated. Narratives become less efficient with age; i.e., there is an increase in quantity of speech (number of words and sentences) but a reduction of informational content and cohesive reference (Juncos-Rabadan et al. 2005). However, higher vocabulary scores were correlated with improved density of content and cohesion of ideas and less irrelevant content. Juncos-Rabadan et al. (2005) questioned whether the increased verbosity of the older adults is due to an age-related inhibitory deficit, cognitive decline of executive functions affecting the control and coordination of complex information in working memory, or possibly social context, where isolated older adults seize the opportunity to converse. In any case, the increased quantity of speech is considered an asset in story-telling. Obler (1980) studied narratives told by Palestinian villagers (aged 18 to 83) and noted that older adults were judged to be the most skilled story-tellers. Their narratives contained more detail, more modifiers, and more frequent repetition of elements.

On the other hand, narratives with low idea density written at age 22 from the Nun Study (Riley et al. 2005) were associated with worse cognitive function in old age and increased neuropathological findings associated with Alzheimer disease. This study demonstrates a strong inverse relationship between early life linguistic function and late life memory dysfunction, from MCI to Alzheimer disease. However, Riley left in question: Were the neuropathological changes already operating in early life, resulting in low idea density scores, or did the linguistic measure simply mark those at risk for developing Alzheimer pathology later in life?

Emotional/Behavioral Changes

Communication requires much more than language skills; nonverbal communication may be even more important to social interactions, but has not been studied as extensively as linguistic functions. How an individual relates emotionally plays a key role in social competence and behavior. *Emotional recognition* is a major component of nonverbal communication and relies on facial expression and eye contact, as well as body postures and gestures. Studies suggest that older adults have more difficulty than younger adults in recognizing facial expressions of anger, fear, and sadness, independent of general face processing, fluid intelligence, processing speed, or changes in perceptual abilities (Sullivan and Ruffman 2004). Matching emotional sounds to certain facial expressions is also impaired, while the ability to match non-emotion (e.g. machine) sounds to corresponding objects is preserved (Sullivan and Ruffman 2004). Explanatory hypotheses for this age-related change in emotional recognition include: "right hemi-aging" hypothesis, based on association of negative emotions with the right hemisphere which ages faster than the left (Dolcos 2002); age-related regional brain changes, e.g. orbitofrontal cortex (OFC) and amygdala that correlate with individual emotions, e.g. anger and fear (Sullivan and Ruffman 2004); "positivity bias" of older adults such that they attend and remember more emotionally positive than negative information as an adaptive strategy to maintain emotional regulation (Mather and Carstensen 2005); high load of emotional identification placed on working memory, which declines with age (Phillips et al. 2008); age-related reduction of neurotransmitters, e.g. dopamine and noradrenaline in the amygdala, OFC, and ventral striatum which might be directly related to decrease in physiological responding and self-reports of less negative emotion (Ruffman et al. 2008).

Similar to modality-specific age-related declines in other cognitive domains, emotional recognition deficits are modality-specific. There is a greater age-related differential in recognition on a lexical task describing emotional situations than on photographs of facial expressions (Isaacowitz et al. 2007). How these age-related differences translate into everyday functioning is less clear since older adults may be able to compensate through multiple stimuli, e.g. intonation, gestures, facial expression, and situational context (Isaacowitz et al. 2007).

The question arises whether these age-related differences actually represent a decline in function or perhaps generational differences. Compared to younger adults, older adults spend less time looking at eyes, which provide more information, when examining photographs of facial expression and more time focusing on mouths (Ruffman et al. 2008). One could question whether this may be due to societal changes, as younger generations tend to be much "bolder" in their interactions with authority figures, e.g. teachers, and may be more accustomed to looking at eyes. Another possibility is that older adults with slight hearing impairment may focus on mouths to better comprehend a conversation. In addition, many tests of emotion use people who are instructed to move facial muscles to convey a prototypical emotional expression, but this may not reflect real-life situations where facial expressions are elicited in response to an identifiable stimulus. Some question whether people are better at judging emotions of same-aged individuals (Malatesta et al. 1987). Ruffman et al. (2008) also point out that all 28 studies reviewed were cross-sectional, which raises the possibility of cohort effects.

Emotional responses of younger and older adults are also different. Older adults report fewer arguments and interpersonal tensions (Birditt and Fingerman 2005), fewer conflicts with spouses (Levenson et al. 1993), and are better at resolving interpersonal conflicts (Charles and Carstensen 2008). Age-related differences in response to negative interactions occur immediately at the time of the event, with older adults being adept at using cognitive appraisal strategies, e.g. being less judgmental toward someone directing negative comments and disengaging earlier from the situation (Charles and Carstensen 2008). Following an unpleasant interaction, younger adults more often report higher levels of anger, an emotion associated with action-oriented strategies, while older adults more often note higher levels of sadness, a more passive response. However, according to the "socioemotional selectivity" theory, older adults do not react passively in these situations but seek strategies to enhance emotional regulation and minimize time and energy on negative experiences (Carstensen et al. 2000). Specifically, this theory posits age-related shifts in goals based on increasing awareness of time horizons. As older adults perceive the end of life, goals associated with emotional meaning and well-being take priority over goals associated with acquiring knowledge for future use (Mather and Carstensen 2005).

This increased attention to emotion regulation in older adults is believed to be due to top-down cognitive control by anterior cingulate and other prefrontal brain circuits. While these same areas tend to show decline with age, it is postulated that older adults with best-preserved prefrontal cognitive function, i.e. "successful aging," are more likely to show positivity effects that help regulate emotion (Mather and Carstensen 2005). On the other hand, older adults who have sustained strokes or microvascular lesions in frontal brain regions with impaired executive function are prone to medication-resistant depression (Mast et al. 2004).

While goal-directed emotional attention is associated with prefrontal function, more automatic emotional attention, such as arousal to threat, is associated with amygdala function. Unlike the earlier changes noted in prefrontal brain regions, the amygdala shows relatively little decline with age (Grieve et al. 2005), which supports the observation that older adults show similar threat/arousal detection to young adults, (Mather and Carstensen 2005). Mather and Carstensen (2005) further speculate that older adults may use top-down control processes supported by the anterior cingulate to down-regulate amygdala responses to negative emotions, thus contributing to older adults' improved emotional regulation.

Arithmetic Cognition

Mathematical problem solving and arithmetic processing are skills needed on a daily basis. Arithmetic skills are part of semantic memory (Julien et al. 2008) and are well preserved with age. However, even though older adults may reach the same correct answer as younger adults, the process is slower and strategies may be different (Duverne and Lemaire 2005; Zamarian et al. 2007). Duverne and Lemaire (2005) found that older participants did not switch between strategies or choose the fastest strategies as consistently as younger adults. Rather, they tended to use calculation processes, based on preserved arithmetic skills, regardless of the difficulty of the problem. Older adults with high arithmetic skills preserved these skills while older adults with poor arithmetic skills used more laborious calculation strategies (e.g. counting, decomposition). While older adults did not use faster estimation strategies as often as younger adults, they made fewer errors. This speed-accuracy trade-off effect suggests that older adults may retrieve all arithmetic knowledge before making a decision while younger adults short-circuit this process and make a decision without complete information (Duverne and Lemaire 2005).

The comparable accuracy of older and younger adults on arithmetic problems lead Zamarian et al. (2007) to propose that semantic retrieval of multiplication knowledge is a central process that is preserved with age. The slower processing speed is a peripheral process that declines with age due to decline in executive function (encoding, decision-making, and responding), which worsen with increasing task complexity when more demand is placed on working memory (Zamarian et al. 2007).

Parietal cortico-subcortical networks associated with arithmetic fact retrieval are preserved in normal aging (Zamarian et al. 2007). The temporal lobes may also play an important role in arithmetic understanding (Julien et al. 2008) as well as prefrontal areas for monitoring or strategy selection when complex mental calculation is effortful.

Visuospatial Ability

While verbal skills remain functionally intact well into old age, visuospatial skills tend to show earlier decline. For example, processing speed, memory span, and paired-associate learning, i.e., speeded and unspeeded tasks, are more impaired for visuospatial tasks than for verbal tasks in older adults (Jenkins et al. 2000). Age-related differences in cognitive manipulation (storage and transformation, supervision, and coordination) are also domain specific, with visuospatial tasks more compromised than equivalent verbal tasks (Bopp and Verhaeghen 2007). Increased load on working memory has a more detrimental impact on visuospatial tasks than verbal tasks (Verhaeghen et al. 2006). These age-related deficits in visuospatial processing are associated with reduced activity in the posterior parietal and visual regions on functional neuroimaging with increased, possibly compensatory, PFC activity (Dennis and Cabeza 2008).

Spatial attention shows age-related changes, with older adults maintaining a narrower focus of attention, possibly to compensate for reduced sensory input (Atchley and Hoffman 2004). In addition, older adults are slower in switching focus of attention and are able to visually track fewer objects (Kramer and Madden 2008), which may be important in tasks such as driving. Visual attention, which involves search, selection, and switching, was associated with 25 of 36 driving behaviors including distance judgments, scanning the environment, yielding right of way, and negotiating safe turns and merges (Richardson and Marottoli 2003). Some of these behaviors are associated with the types of crashes most common in elderly drivers, who have the highest rate of crashes per mile driven other than the youngest drivers (Richardson and Marottoli 2003).

While visuospatial testing has traditionally used tests of production and recognition of figures, navigational tests are probably more useful for real-world functioning. Cushman et al. (2008) found a close correlation between real-world and virtual (VR) navigational skills, which decrease with normal aging and early dementia. The greatest difficulties were in associating visual scenes and location, but VR technology may help train older adults in navigational skills (Cushman et al. 2008).

Insight and Judgment

Insight is an area of higher cognition that is sometimes lumped with executive function but is perhaps one of the most difficult to assess. This becomes apparent when one attempts to assess the impact of executive processing deficits on daily functioning. Using a self-report questionnaire, the Dysexecutive Functioning Questionnaire (DEX), Gerstorf et al. (2008) noted that everyday executive dysfunctions occurred frequently throughout adulthood. These were defined as subjective impressions of poor decision-making, distractibility, or planning problems. Interestingly, younger adults report more problems than older adults, suggesting that they may have better insight into their errors compared with older adults whose executive function is known to decline (Gerstorf et al. 2008). In support of this view, Salthouse and Siedlecki (2005) noted a lack of correlation between performance on divided attention tasks in the lab and self-reports of divided attention ability in a group of older adults. However, Gerstorf (2008) noted that reports of executive problems on the DEX also correlated with endorsement of more negative symptoms, e.g. depression, anxiety, neuroticism, more subjective health concerns and negative affect. One theory is that older adults report fewer executive function problems because they may regulate their emotions better, i.e., handle emotionally challenging situations better or manage to avoid such situations (Carstensen et al. 2000).

Stories of older adults falling victim to fraudulent advertising and scams are abundant. Denburg et al. (2007) found that a large subgroup of otherwise cognitively normal older adults (35–40%) showed decision-making impairment on a "gambling task" (the Iowa Gambling Task (IGT)), that factors in risk, reward, punishment, and ambiguity, approximating everyday life. They found a correlation between decision-making ability and psychophysiological responses. Because decision-making is often associated with emotional processes, the "somatic marker" hypothesis suggests a linkage between several large-scale cortical and subcortical brain networks, including the ventromedial PFC, amygdala, insular and somatosensory cortices, and the peripheral nervous system. Skin conductance response (SCR) has been used as a measure of somatic "signaling" activity in response to emotional activation. Specifically, healthy older adults generate anticipatory SCRs during the IGT, as do young adults. On the other hand, older adults who showed impaired decision-making on the IGT lacked discriminatory SCRs to advantageous versus disadvantageous choices. In another experiment, Denburg et al. (2007) noted that the older adults who were poor decision makers on the IGT also were more likely to believe and act on deceptive advertising. From a real-world perspective, the fact that a large subgroup of otherwise cognitively normal older adults has decision-making deficits has profound consequences. Not only does that make them vulnerable to fraudulent advertising, but also other critical life decisions (e.g. driving, housing decisions, allocation of personal finances, and end-of-life medical decisions) may be severely compromised (Denburg et al. 2005). Denburg et al. (2007) postulate that the results of their studies are consistent with the "frontal lobe" hypothesis of aging, with particular implications for ventromedial prefrontal dysfunction (West 2000).

Cognitive Reserve and Brain Plasticity

With all the known declines in cognitive functioning, what hope is there for the aging baby boomers? The theory of *cognitive reserve* is possibly the most promising for some. This hypothesis was proposed to account for repeated observations of a seeming lack of correlation between the severity of brain changes, e.g. amyloid plaques and neurofibrillary tangles or metabolic function (Garibotto et al. 2008) observed in Alzheimer disease and its clinical manifestations (Katzman 1993; Stern 2002; Roe et al. 2007; Erten-Lyons et al. 2009). Specifically, why do some individuals maintain good cognitive function with advancing years while others with apparently similar health status show cognitive decline?

According to a passive model of reserve, the "threshold effect" (Satz 1993), cognitive impairment becomes apparent only after cognitive or neurological resources, defined in terms of synapse count or brain volume, are depleted beyond a certain threshold. Therefore, individuals with higher initial reserve can function longer without showing signs of impairment because they start with or acquire more resources. Larger cortical volume has the strongest association with intelligence, but does not protect against age-related atrophy (Christensen et al. 2008). Mental activity in the form of education (Roe et al. 2007), occupational demands, and mental leisure-time activities, as well as premorbid IQ, are thought to contribute to cognitive reserve (Fritsch et al. 2007).

A more active model of reserve posits compensatory strategies at work (Stern 2002). According to this model, cognitive reserve is viewed as the ability to optimize performance by more efficient utilization of brain networks or "recruiting" alternative brain networks. For example, studies using positron-emission tomography (PET) demonstrate increased activation of specific brain regions in response to increasing task demands in high functioning older adults (Scarmeas et al. 2003; Corral 2006).

However, to explain the paradox of age-related prefrontal/parietal cortex (PC) atrophy with associated increases in task-related activation in these same regions, Greenwood (2007) proposes the concept of *functional plasticity of aging*. Specifically, she argues that brain plasticity allows for adaptation to loss (e.g. age-related decline in brain volume) by driving functional reorganization. Throughout the lifespan there is considerable change in brain structure with 11–12% loss of grey matter and 22–25% loss of white matter from age 22 to 88 years (Allen et al. 2005). Loss of gray matter density before age 40 is believed to be due to remodeling (synapse pruning), while after age 40 reflects processes of degeneration (Sowell et al. 2003). Greenwood (2007) proposes that brain plasticity is manifested by a shift toward greater activity in regions mediating executive function (i.e., PFC and PC), supporting a posterior-anterior shift in activity with age (PASA) (Grady et al. 1994; Dennis and Cabeza 2008). Recruitment of adjacent and contralateral regions is also noted, consistent with the HAROLD (hemispheric asymmetry reduction in older adults) model (Cabeza 2002b). In addition, cortical thickening (seen in response to environmental enrichment in animals) is also noted in posterior cingulate and gyrus cuneus prior to old age in high functioning adults, based on tests of fluid ability (Fjell et al. 2006; Greenwood 2007). Fjell et al. (2006) further suggests that it is the *changes* in cortical thickness that are more important than either thickening or thinning alone and represent plasticity (Greenwood 2007). Another example of plasticity is the increase in hippocampal volume noted in relation to navigation experience in London taxi drivers (Maguire et al. 2006).

Greenwood (2007) summarizes her theory of functional plasticity of aging as follows: regional volume shrinkage, caused by dendritic regression and synaptic loss starting in young adults and white matter degeneration in older adults, causes deficits in processes dependent on that region. Adaptation to these age-related deficits leads to changed processing strategies, which in turn lead to altered cortical innervation and recruitment of adjacent regions, manifested as increased activation in these regions on functional imaging. In addition, training and/or instructions to improve performance induce recruitment of prefrontal and parietal cortices, with associated neuroimaging increases. Individual variability in successful aging may depend on effective adaptation and brain plasticity, i.e., changes in the neuronal circuitry in response to environmental demands. Greenwood (2007) suggests that older adults could be trained to alter strategies to potentially improve age-related cognitive deficits.

Education has been proposed as a proxy for cognitive reserve. Older adults with more education outperform those with less education across most neuropsychological tests, and especially on tasks associated with high-attention demand and frontal lobe function, e.g. fluency, working memory, shifting attention, abstract reasoning, and conceptualization (Corral et al. 2006; Proust-Lima et al. 2008). However, an argument against using education as a proxy for cognitive reserve is that increased education selects individuals who do well taking standardized tests (Proust-Lima et al. 2008). The usual battery of neuropsychological tests most likely tap this same ability and therefore may not fully assess the potential of individuals who have not had as much experience or facility taking tests. In addition, years of education may not be equivalent, depending on regional standards, cohort effect, and international differences in educational systems. There may be a big difference both in terms of IQ and motivation between a student who barely passes and one who is a high academic achiever, yet they may both have a high school diploma (Ackerman 2008). For this reason, others have used premorbid IQ, based on Wechsler Adult Intelligence Scale (WAIS) Vocabulary subtest, as a proxy for cognitive reserve (Corral et al. 2006; Stern et al. 2005).

The question also arises whether cognitive reserve is fixed or able to increase over the lifespan. In a unique longitudinal study, Fritsch et al. (2007) demonstrate that reserve is dynamic but that most changes are relatively small and best acquired before early adulthood. Specifically, higher adolescent IQ, participation in mental extracurricular activities in high school, pursuing further education, and continued mental activities through early adulthood seem to provide a greater protective effect against cognitive decline in late life, with possible smaller benefit from continued activities in midlife and even later (Fritsch et al. 2007).

Others have questioned the impact of education on late life cognition (Van Dijk et al. 2008; Wilson et al. 2009). Also, education may only be protective for selective cognitive domains such as crystallized abilities, and less predictive for fluid abilities and processing speed (Van Dijk et al. 2008). There may be differential decline of function, with a lifelong gradual decline of mental speed, episodic memory, and working memory; a late-life decline of vocabulary, semantic knowledge, and short-term memory; and lifelong stability of implicit and autobiographical memory (Hedden and Gabrieli 2004). Tests involving mental speed show a faster decline when physical health is poorer, while long-term memory and set-shifting are more impaired when depressive symptoms are greater, leading Van Dijk et al. (2008) to suggest that health factors have more effect on cognitive change over time than do effects of education. While Wilson et al. (2009) found a robust association of education with cognitive function at baseline in 6,000 community dwelling older adults, they found no association with rate of cognitive decline but noted considerable individual variability.

Factors other than education alone may contribute to preservation of late-life cognitive function, particularly social, physical, and intellectual activities (Bielak et al. 2007). Consistent with the "use it or lose it" hypothesis, older adults who engage in more activities performed faster and had more consistent responding (i.e., less inconsistency) on all tasks (Bielak et al. 2007). However, the strongest correlation involved novel information processing (e.g. completing income tax forms or playing bridge), which lead Bielak et al. (2007) to posit that the most cognitively challenging activities may have the most long-term benefit.

Measures to Maintain Cognitive Health

"Successful aging" is a hot topic for baby boomers, particularly with regards to cognitive vitality. Studies of the growing population of centenarians, nono-, and octogenarians show common patterns of behavior in those who remain autonomous in late life: regular exercise, nonsmoking, no/moderate alcohol consumption, and better ability coping with stress (Perls and Terry 2003; Barnes et al. 2007; Ozaki et al. 2007; Barondess 2008).

Lifestyle choices are clearly a significant contributor to successful cognitive aging. *Regular physical activity* (three or more times per week) is associated with reduced risk for incident dementia (Larson et al. 2006) and cognitive decline (Yaffe et al. 2001; Weuve et al. 2004; Kramer et al. 2006; Middleton et al. 2008). Exercise may extend longevity without prolonging time in a cognitively impaired state and may even improve cognition in those with cognitive impairment (Lautenschlager et al. 2008; Middleton et al. 2008). Fitness training (aerobic exercise) has the largest positive effect on executive-control processes, functions that show substantial age-related decline (Colombe and Kramer 2003; McDaniel et al. 2008).

Diet, optimal weight, and use of nutritional supplements are areas of considerable controversy. Recent studies suggest a Mediterranean diet, possibly by reducing vascular risk factors, may reduce the risk of Alzheimer disease (Scarmeas et al. 2009). A Mediterranean diet is characterized by high intake of fish, vegetables, legumes, fruits, cereals, and unsaturated fatty acids, e.g. olive oil, and reduced intake of meat, dairy products, and saturated fatty acids, with a regular but moderate intake of alcohol. Low to moderate *alcohol consumption* may delay age-related cognitive decline in older women (less clear for men), including global cognition, speed of information processing, and verbal memory (Stampfer et al. 2005; Stott et al. 2008). Other studies more consistently find a negative association between high alcohol consumption and cognition (Thomas and Rockwood 2001; Stott et al. 2008). While patients with MCI who consumed up to one drink/day of wine or alcohol had a decrease in rate of progression to dementia, Solfrizzi et al. (2007)

cautioned that the effect may not be the alcohol but the moderate life-style with its complex set of favorable social and behavioral factors.

While octogenarians and older who maintain optimal cognitive function are less likely to have *comorbid medical conditions* (Barnes et al. 2007), optimal management of chronic illnesses is key. Kramer et al. (2007) caution that MRI markers of cerebrovascular disease, e.g. white matter hyperintensities, should not be considered benign, even in apparently healthy older adults, because of their association with a decrease in executive function. Thus, good vascular health through control of high blood pressure, diabetes, high cholesterol, excessive weight, stress reduction, and not smoking contribute to health of cerebral blood vessels and may help preserve cognition in later life (Alagiakrishnan et al. 2006). Knopman et al. (2001), suggest that interventions should begin before age 60 based on their observation of decline in cognitive function in participants with diabetes and/or hypertension, aged 47 to 57 years.

Polypharmacy in older adults is a recognized risk factor for adverse drugs reactions, which can affect cognitive function. Combined use of CNS medications (e.g. benzodiazepines, opioids, antipsychotics, and antidepressants), especially at higher doses, is associated with cognitive decline in older adults (Wright et al. 2009). Herbal remedies and other complimentary/alternative compounds are consumed by a large number of older adults (Nahin et al. 2006), use is often underreported, and contribute to potentially harmful drug-drug interactions, especially in combination with prescription medications (Qato et al. 2008). Recognition of medications as a potentially reversible component of cognitive decline in older adults is critical, as well as using the lowest effective dose possible. In 1997, the Beers Criteria for medications considered generally inappropriate in the elderly was published, based on unfavorable risk/benefit ratios and availability of safer, effective alternatives (Beers 1997). Despite widespread dissemination of the criteria, older patients seen in emergency departments (Caterino et al. 2004), as well as health maintenance organization members (Simon et al. 2005) are frequently administered inappropriate medications. Medications with anticholinergic effects are particularly problematic due to age-related changes in pharmacokinetics, greater permeability of the blood-brain barrier, slower metabolism and drug elimination, and diminished function of cholinergic brain receptors (Chew et al. 2008; Han et al. 2008).

Lifelong learning and leisure activity that involves *active cognitive engagement*, e.g. playing board games and reading (Verghese et al. 2003), is associated with a reduced risk of cognitive impairment while more passive activities, e.g. watching television, is associated with an increased risk of cognitive impairment in older adults (Wang et al. 2006; Rundek and Bennett 2006). This large study of older Chinese adults noted that those who played mahjong, a board game that demands attention, memory, calculation, initiative capacity, and planning, also had the benefit of social contact. A longitudinal Swedish study (Wang et al. 2002) as well as American studies (Wilson et al. 2002; Verghese et al. 2003) of older adults came to a similar conclusion that activities that are intellectually stimulating and socially engaging are associated with a decreased risk of incident dementia. "Brain excise" is proposed to help maintain mental alertness, but just doing crossword puzzles, bridge, and reading may not be enough, especially if they become routine. *Novelty* appears to be the key to neuroplasticity, so tasks that require concentrated focus seem to provide the most benefit (Bielak et al. 2007).

Social engagement challenges older adults to communicate and interact emotionally, avoiding isolation, and thus promoting cognitive vitality in later life (Fillit et al. 2002). Positive affect or *emotional well-being* is different from the absence of depression and may protect older adults from functional decline possibly by promoting a healthy lifestyle and increasing social interaction (Ostir et al. 2000). Chronic stress (e.g. the perception of being overwhelmed) may alter the hippocampus and contribute to memory impairment (McDaniel et al. 2008), but may be amenable to *stress reduction* techniques (Fillit et al. 2002), e.g. meditation, muscle relaxation training, and yoga.

While sleep efficiency declines with age (Espiritu 2008), especially after 75 years, the relation of health and sleep is bidirectional. Sleep disorders are common in older adults, including sleep fractionation, sleep-disordered breathing (e.g. sleep apnea and hypopnea), insomnia, and daytime sleepiness, all having negative impact on cognition, especially attention and memory (Cricco et al. 2001; Spira et al. 2008). Sedatives and hypnotics used to treat symptoms often exacerbate cognitive problems (Fillit et al. 2002). Many of these conditions are treatable or can be significantly improved with good sleep hygiene.

Memory training is gaining popularity but research results are mixed. While mnemonic training of older adults can improve performance of word list recognition, there is minimal carryover to untrained tasks. Training of executive processes, e.g. dual-task performance with progressively increasing interference, does show carryover to untrained tasks and offers promise (McDaniel et al. 2008). Practicing a skill until it becomes automatic—a habit—facilitates performance, e.g. routinely putting keys in the same place (Craik and Bailystok 2008).

Even though a number of large observational studies find associations between various preventive strategies and risk for dementia, there are few randomized controlled trials to prove the protective effects of these interventions (Coley et al. 2008). However, because age-related changes in cognition are multifactorial, interventions that target a wide variety of domains seem to be a reasonable preventive strategy (Butler et al. 2004; Hendrie et al. 2006; Karp et al. 2006; Albert 2008; Coley et al. 2008). In the final analysis: hope for good genes, observe moderation in lifestyle choices, stay socially engaged and mentally stimulated, seek novelty, be creative, and preserve a positive outlook.

References

Ackerman, P.L.: Knowledge and cognitive aging. In *The handbook of aging and cognition*, Ed. 3 (Craik, F.I.M. and Salthouse, T.A., Eds.). New York: Psychology Press 2008, pp 445–489.

Alagiakrishnan, K., McCracken, P., and Feldman, H.: Treating vascular risk factors and maintaining vascular health: Is this the way towards successful cognitive ageing and preventing cognitive decline? *Postgrad Med J* 82 (964): 101–105, 2006.

Albert, M.S.: The neuropsychology of the development of Alzheimer's disease. In *The handbook of aging and cognition,* Ed. 3 (Craik, F.I.M. and Salthouse, T.A., Eds.). New York: Psychology Press 2008, pp 97–132.

Allaire, J.C., Gamaldo, A., Ayotte, B.J., et al.: Mild cognitive impairment and objective instrumental everyday functioning: the everyday cognition battery memory test. *J Am Geriatr Soc* 57: 120–125, 2009.

Allen, J.S., Bruss, J., Brown, C.K., and Damasio, H.: Normal neuroanatomical variation due to age: The major lobes and a parcellation of the temporal region. *Neurobiol Aging* 26(9): 1245–1260; discussion 1279–1282, 2005.

Andres, P. and Van der Linden, M.: Age-related differences in supervisory attentional system functions. *J Gerontol B Psychol Sci Soc Sci* 55B (6): 373–380, 2000.

Atchley, P. and Hoffman, L.: Aging and visual masking: Sensory and attentional factors. *Psychol Aging* 19(1): 57–67, 2004.

Ayd, FJ. Jr.: *Lexicon of psychiatry, neurology, and the neurosciences,* Ed 2. Philadelphia: Lippincott Williams & Wilkins, 2000, pp 603–604.

Baddeley, A.: The fractionation of working memory. *Proc Natl Acad Sci USA* 93 (24): 13468–13472, 1996.

Baddeley, A.: Working memory: Looking back and looking forward. *Nature Rev Neurosci*, 4(10): 829–839, 2003.

Barnes, D.E., Cauley, J.E., Lui, L.-Y., Fink, et al.: Women who maintain optimal cognitive function into old age. *J Am Geriatr Soc* 55: 259–264, 2007.

Barondess, J.A.: Toward healthy aging: The preservation of health. *J Am Geriatr Soc* 56: 145–148, 2008.

Basar, E.: Memory and brain dynamics: Oscillations integrating attention, perception, learning, and memory. New York: CRC Press, 2004.

Beason-Held, L.L., Kraut, M.A., and Resnick, S.M.: Longitudinal changes in aging brain function. *Neurobiol Aging* 29: 483–496, 2008.

Beers, M.H.: Explicit criteria for determining potentially inappropriate medication use by the elderly: An update. *Arch Intern Med* 157(14): 1531–1536, 1997.

Bielak, A.A.M., Hughes, T.F., Small, B.J., and Dixon, Roger A.: It's never too late to engage in lifestyle activities: Significant concurrent but not change relationships between lifestyle activities and cognitive speed. *J Gerontol B Psychol Sci Soc Sci* 62B (6): 331–339, 2007.

Birditt, K.S. and Fingerman, K.L.: Do we get better at picking our battles? Age group differences in descriptions of behavioral reactions to interpersonal tensions. *J Gerontol B Psychol Sci Soc Sci* 60(3): 121–128, 2005.

Bonanno, G.A. Loss, trauma, and human resilience: Have we underestimated the human capacity to thrive after extremely aversive events? *Am Psychol* 59(1): 20–28, 2004.

Bopp, K.L. and Verhaeghen, P.: Age-related differences in control processes in verbal and visuospatial working memory: Storage, transformation, supervision, and coordination. *J Gerontol B Psychol Sci Soc Sci* 62B (5): 239–246, 2007.

Bowles, R.P. and Salthouse, T.A.: Vocabulary test format and differential relations to age. *Psychol Aging* 23 (2): 366–376, 2008.

Braver, T.S. and West, R.: Working memory, executive control, and aging. In *The handbook of aging and cognition*, Ed. 3 (Craik, F.I.M. and Salthouse, T.A., Eds.). New York: Psychology Press, 2008, pp 311–372.

Brennan, M., Welsh, M.C., and Fisher, C.B.: Aging and executive function skills: An examination of a community-dwelling older adult population. *Percept Mot Skills* 84: 1187–1197, 1997.

Buckner, R.L.: Memory and executive function in aging and AD: Multiple factors that cause decline and reserve factors that compensate. *Neuron* 44(1): 195–208, 2004.

Burke, D.M. and Shafto, M.A.: Aging and language production. *Curr Dir Psychol Sci*, 13: 21–24, 2004.

Butler, R.N., Forette, F., and Greengross, Baroness S.: Maintaining cognitive health in an ageing society. *Perspect Public Health* 124(3): 119–121, 2004.

Cabeza, R.: Functional neuroimaging of cognitive aging. In *Handbook of functional neuroimaging of cognition* (Cabeza R. and Kingstone, A., Eds.). Cambridge: MIT Press, 2002, pp 331–378.

Cabeza, R.: Hemispheric asymmetry reduction in older adults: The HAROLD model. *Psychol Aging* 17(1): 85–100, 2002.

Cabeza, R., Anderson, N.D., Locantore, J.K., and McIntosh, A.R.: Aging gracefully: Compensatory brain activity in high-performing older adults. *Neuroimage* 17: 1394–1402, 2002.

Cabeza, R., Nyberg L., and Park, D.: *Cognitive neuroscience of aging: Linking cognitive and cerebral aging.* New York: Oxford University Press, 2005.

Carlson, M.C., Xue, Q.-L., Zhou, J., and Fried, L.P.: Executive decline and dysfunction precedes declines in memory: The women's health and aging study II. *J Gerontol A Biol Sci Med Sci* 64 (1): 110–117, 2009.

Carstensen, L.L., Pasupathi M., Mayr, U., and Nesselroade, J.R.: Emotional experience in everyday life across the adult life span. *J Pers Soc Psychol* 79(4): 644–655, 2000.

Caterino, J.M., Emond, J.A., and Camargo, C.A. Jr.: Inappropriate medication administration to the acutely ill elderly: A nationwide emergency department study, 1992-2000. *J Am Geriatr Soc* 52: 1847–1855, 2004.

Charles, S.T. and Carstensen, L.L.: Unpleasant situations elicit different emotional responses in younger and older adults. *Psychol Aging* 23(3): 495–504, 2008.

Chew, M.L., Mulsant, B.H., Pollock, B.G., et al.: Anticholinergic activity of 107 medications commonly used by older adults. *J Am Geriatr Soc* 56: 1333–1341, 2008.

Christensen, H., Anstey, K.J., Leach, L.S., and Mackinnon, A.J.: Intelligence, education, and the brain reserve hypothesis. In *The handbook of aging and cognition*, Ed. 3 (Craik, F.I.M. and Salthouse, T.A., Eds.). New York: Psychology Press, 2008, pp 133–188.

Colcombe, S., and Kramer, A.F.: Fitness effects on the cognitive function of older adults: A meta-analytic study. *Psychol Sci.* 14(2): 125–130, 2003.

Colcombe, S.J., Kramer, A.F., Erickson, K.I., and Scalf, P.: The implications of cortical recruitment and brain morphology for individual differences in inhibitory function in aging humans. *Psychol Aging* 20(3): 363–375, 2005.

Coley, N., Andrieu, S., Gardette, V., et al.: Dementia prevention: Methodological explanations for inconsistent results. *Epidemiol Rev* 30: 35–66, 2008.

Connor, L.T., Sprio, A.III, Obler, L.K., and Albert, M.L.: Change in object naming ability during adulthood. *J Gerontol B Psychol Sci Soc Sci* 59 (5): 203–209, 2004.

Corral, M., Rodriguez, M., Amenedo, E., et al.: Cognitive reserve, age, and neuropsychological performance in healthy participants. *Dev Neuropsychol* 29(3): 479–491, 2006.

Craik, F.I.M. and Bialystok, E.: Lifespan cognitive development: The roles of representation and control. In *The handbook of aging and cognition*, Ed. 3 (Craik, F.I.M. and Salthouse, T.A., Eds.). New York: Psychology Press, 2008, pp 557–601.

Craik, F.I.M. and Salthouse, T.A.: *The handbook of aging and cognition*, Ed. 3. New York: Psychology Press, 2008.

Cricco, M., Simonsick, E.M., and Foley, D.J.: The impact of insomnia on cognitive functioning in older adults. *J Am Geriatr Soc* 49: 1185–1189, 2001.

Cushman, L.A., Stein, K. and Duffy, C.J.: Detecting navigational deficits in cognitive aging and Alzheimer disease using virtual reality. *Neurology* 71: 888–895, 2008.

Cuttler, C. and Graf, P.: Personality predicts prospective memory task performance: An adult lifespan study. *Scand J Psychol*, 48: 215–231, 2007.

Denburg, N.L., Cole, C.A., Hernandez, M., et al.: The orbitofrontal cortex, real-world decision making, and normal aging. *Ann NY Acad Sci.* 1121: 480–498, 2007.

Denburg, N.L., Tranel, D., and Bechara, A.: The ability to decide advantageously declines prematurely in some normal older persons. *Neuropsychologia* 43: 1099–1106, 2005.

Dennis, N.A. and Cabeza, R.: Neuroimaging of healthy cognitive aging. In *The handbook of aging and cognition*, Ed. 3 (Craik, F.I.M. and Salthouse, T.A., Eds.). New York: Psychology Press, 2008, pp 10–54.

Desgranges, B., Kalpouzos, G., and Eustache, F.: Cerebral imaging in healthy aging: contrast with Alzheimer disease. *Rev Neurol* 164: S102–S107, 2008.

Dolcos, F., Rice, H.J., and Cabeza, R.: Hemispheric asymmetry and aging: Right hemisphere decline or asymmetry reduction. *Neurosci Biobehav Rev* 26: 819–825, 2002.

Duarte, A., Graham, K.S., and Henson, R.N.: Age-related changes in neural activity associated with familiarity, recollection and false recognition. *Neurobiol Aging*, doi: 10.1016/j.neurobioloaging.2008.09.014.

Duverne, S. and Lemaire, P.: Arithmetic split effects reflect strategy selection: An adult age comparative study in addition comparison and verification tasks. *Can J Exp Psychol*, 59-4: 262–278, 2005.

Eichenbaum, H.: *The cognitive neuroscience of memory: An introduction.* New York: Oxford University Press, 2002.

Erten-Lyons, D., Woltjer, R.L., Dodge, H., et al.: Factors associated with resistance to dementia despite high Alzheimer disease pathology. *Neurology* 72: 354–360, 2009.

Espiritu, J.R.: Aging-related sleep changes. *Clin Geriatr Med* 24 (1): 1–14, 2008.

Fillit, H.M., Butler, R.N., O'Connell, A.W., et al.: Achieving and maintaining cognitive vitality with aging. *Mayo Clin Proc*, 77: 681–696, 2002.

Finkel, D., Reynolds, C.A., McArdle, J.J., and Pedersen, N.L.: Age changes in processing speed as a leading indicator of cognitive aging. *Psychol Aging* 22 (3): 558–568, 2007.

Fjell, A.M., Walhovd, K.B., Reinvang, I., et al.: Selective increase of cortical thickness in high-performing elderly—structural indices of optimal cognitive aging. *Neuroimage* 29(3): 984–994, 2006.

Folstein, M.F., Folstein, S.E., and McHugh, P.R.: "Mini-mental state": A practical method for grading the cognitive state of patients for the clinician. *J Psychiatr Res* 12: 189–198, 1975.

Fritsch, T., McClendon, M.J., Smyth, K.A., et al.: Cognitive functioning in healthy aging: The role of reserve and lifestyle factors early in life. *Gerontologist* 47 (3): 307–322, 2007.

Garibotto, V., Borroni, B., Kalbe, E., et al.: Education and occupation as proxies for reserve in aMCI converters and AD: FDG-PET evidence. *Neurology* 71 (17): 1342–1349, 2008.

Gazzaley, A., Clapp, W., Kelley, J., et al.: Age-related top-down suppression deficit in the early stages of cortical visual memory processing. *Proc Natl Acad Sci USA* 105 (35): 13122–13126, 2008.

Gerstorf, D., Siedlecki, K.L., Tucker-Drob, E.M., and Salthouse, T.A.: Executive dysfunctions across adulthood: Measurement properties and correlates of the DEX self-report questionnaire. *Neuropsychol Dev Cogn B Aging Neuropsychol Cogn* 15: 424–445, 2008.

Glisky, E.L., Rubin, S.R., and Davidson, P.S.: Source memory in older adults: An encoding or retrieval problem? *J Exp Psychol Learn Mem Cogn* 27(5): 1131–1146, 2001.

Gorman, M.F. and Fisher, D.L.: Visual search tasks: Slowing of strategic and nonstrategic processes in the nonlexical domain. *J Gerontol Psychol Sci* 53B (3): 189–200, 1998.

Grady, C.L. and Craik, F.I.M.: Changes in memory processing with age. *Curr Opin Neurobiol* 10: 224–231, 2000.

Grady, C.L., Maisog, J.M., Horwitz, B., et al.: Age-related changes in cortical blood flow activation during visual processing of faces and location. *J Neurosci* 14: 1450–1462, 1994.

Greenwood, P.M.: Functional plasticity in cognitive aging: Review and hypothesis. *Neuropsychology* 21(6): 657–673, 2007.

Grieve, S.M., Clark, C.R., Williams, L.M., et al.: Preservation of limbic and paralimbic structures in aging. *Hum Brain Mapp* 25(4): 391–401, 2005.

Grigsby, J., Kaye, K., Baxter, J., et al.: Executive cognitive abilities and functional status among community-dwelling older persons in the San Luis Valley Health and Aging Study. *J Am Geriatr Soc* 46: 590–596, 1998.

Grossman, M., Cooke, A., DeVita, C., et al.: Age-related changes in working memory during sentence comprehension: An fMRI study. *Neuroimage* 15: 302–317, 2002.

Han, L., Agostini, J.V., and Allore, H.G.: Cumulative anticholinergic exposure is associated with poor memory and executive function in older men. *J Am Geriatr Soc* 56: 2203–2210, 2008.

Hedden, T. and Gabrieli, J.D.: Insights into the ageing mind: A view from cognitive neuroscience. *Nature Rev Neurosci* 5(2): 87–96, 2004.

Hendrie, H.C., Albert, M.S., Butters, M.A., et al.: The NIH cognitive and emotional healthy project: Report of the critical evaluation study committee. *Alzheimers Dement* 2(1): 12–32, 2006.

Henry, J.D., MacLeod, M.S., Phillips, L.H., and Crawford, J.R.: A meta-analytic review of prospective memory and aging. *Psychol Aging* 19(1): 27–39, 2004.

Holtzer, R., Stern, Y., and Rakitin, B.C.: Age-related differences in executive control of working memory. *Mem Cognit* 32 (8): 1333–1345, 2004.

Isaacowitz, D.M., Lockenhoff, C.E., Lane, R.D., et al.: Age differences in recognition of emotion in lexical stimuli and facial expressions. *Psychol Aging* 22 (1): 147–159, 2007.

Isingrini, M. and Taconnat, L.: Episodic memory, frontal functioning and aging. *Rev Neurol* 164: 591–595, 2008.

Jenkins, L., Myerson, J., Joerding, J.A., and Hale, S.: Converging evidence that visuospatial cognition is more age-sensitive than verbal cognition. *Psychol Aging* 15 (1): 157–175, 2000.

Julien, C.L., Thompson, J.C., Neary, D., and Snowden, J.S.: Arithmetic knowledge in semantic dementia: is it invariably preserved? *Neuropsycholgia* 46(11): 2732–2744, 2008.

Juncos-Rabadan, O., Pereiro, A.X., and Rodriguez, M.S.: Narrative speech in aging: Quantity, information content, and cohesion. *Brain Lang* 95: 423–434, 2005.

Karp, A., Paillard-Borg, S., Wang, H.X., et al.: Mental, physical and social components in leisure activities equally contribute to decrease dementia risk. *Dement Geriatr Cogn Disord* 21(2): 65–73, 2006.

Katzman, R.: Education and the prevalence of dementia and Alzheimer's disease. *Neurology* 43(1): 13–20, 1993.

Kemper, S., Marquis, J., and Thompson, M.: Longitudinal change in language production: Effects of aging and dementia on grammatical complexity and propositional content. *Psychol Aging* 16 (4): 600–614, 2001.

Knopman, D., Boland, L.L., Mosley, T., et al.: Cardiovascular risk factors and cognitive decline in middle-aged adults. *Neurology* 56: 42–48, 2001.

Kramer, A.F., Erickson, K.I., and Colcombe, S.J.: Exercise, cognition and the aging brain. *J Appl Physiol* 101: 1237–1242, 2006.

Kramer, A.F. and Madden, D.J.: Attention. In *The handbook of aging and cognition*, Ed. 3 (Craik, F.I.M. and Salthouse, T.A., Eds.). New York: Psychology Press, 2008, pp 189–249, 2008.

Kramer, J.H., Mungas, D., Reed, B.R., et al.: Longitudinal MRI and cognitive change in healthy elderly. *Neuropsychology* 21 (4): 412–418, 2007.

Larson E.B., Wang, L., Bowen, J.D., et al.: Exercise is associated with reduced risk for incident dementia among persons 65 years of age and older. *Ann Intern Med* 144(2): 73–81, 2006.

Lautenschlager, N.T., Cox, K.L., Flicker, L., et al.: Effect of physical activity on cognitive function in older adults at risk for Alzheimer disease. *J Am Med Assoc* 300 (9): 1027–1037, 2008.

Levenson, R.W., Carstensen, L.L. and Gottman, J.M.: Long-term marriage: Age, gender and satisfaction. *Psychol Aging* 8(2): 301–313, 1993.

Logan, J.M., Sanders, A.L., Snyder, A.Z., et al.: Under-recruitment and nonselective recruitment: Dissociable neural mechanisms associated with aging. *Neuron* 33 (5): 827–840, 2002.

Maguire, E.A., Woollett, K., and Spiers, H.J.: London taxi drivers and bus drivers: A structural MRI and neuropsychological analysis. *Hippocampus* 16: 1091–1101, 2006.

Malatesta, C.Z., Izard, C.E., Culver, C., and Nicolich, M.: Emotion communication skills in young, middle-aged, and older women. *Psychol Aging* 2(2): 193–203, 1987.

Mast, B.T., Yochim, B., MacNeill, S.E. and Lichtenberg, P.A.: Risk factors for geriatric depression: The importance of executive functioning within the vascular depression hypothesis. *J Gerontol A Biol Sci Med Sci* 59 (12): 1290–1294, 2004.

Mather, M. and Carstensen, L.L.: Aging and motivated cognition: The positivity effect in attention and memory. *Trends Cogn Sci* 9 (10): 496–502, 2005.

McDaniel, M.A., Einstein, G.O., and Jacoby, L.L.: New considerations in aging and memory: The glass may be half full. In *The handbook of aging and cognition*, Ed. 3 (Craik, F.I.M. and Salthouse, T.A., Eds.). New York: Psychology Press, 2008, pp 251–310.

Middleton, L.E., Mitnitski, A., Fallah, N., et al.: Changes in cognition and mortality in relation to exercise in late life: A population based study. *PLoS ONE* 3(9): e3124, 2008.

Nahin, R.L., Fitzpatrick, A.L., Williamson, J.D., et al.: Use of herbal medicine and other dietary supplements in community-dwelling older people: Baseline data from the ginkgo evaluation of memory study. *J Am Geriatr Soc* 54: 1725–1735, 2006.

Obler, L.K.: Narrative discourse style in the elderly. In *Language and communication in the elderly: Clinical, therapeutic, and experimental aspects* (L.K. Obler, and M. Albert, Eds.). Lexington, MA: D.C. Heath and Co., 1980, pp 75–90.

Ostir, G.V., Markides, K.S., Black, S.A., and Goodwin, J.S.: Emotional well-being predicts subsequent functional independence and survival. *J Am Geriatr Soc* 48: 473–478, 2000.

Ozaki, A., Uchiyama, M., Tagaya, H., et al.: The Japanese centenarian study: Autonomy was associated with health practices as well as physical status. *J Am Geriatr Soc* 55: 95–101, 2007.

Pardo, J.V., Lee, J.T., Sheikh, S.A., et al.: Where the brain grows old: Decline in anterior cingulate and medial prefrontal function with normal aging. *Neuroimage* 35: 1231–1237, 2007.

Park, D.C. and Gutchess, A.H.: Long-term memory and aging: A cognitive neuroscience perspective. In *Cognitive neuroscience of aging: Linking cognitive and cerebral aging* (Cabeza, R, Nyberg, L., and Park, Denise Eds.). New York: Oxford University Press, 2005, pp 218–245.

Peres, K., Helmer, C., Amieva, H., et al.: Natural history of decline in instrumental activities of daily living performance over the 10 years preceding the clinical diagnosis of dementia: A prospective population-based study. *J Am Geriatr Soc* 56: 37–44, 2008.

Perls, T. and Terry, D.: Understanding the determinants of exceptional longevity. *Ann Intern Med* 139 (5 Pt 2): 445–449, 2003.

Phillips, L.H., Channon, S., Tunstall, M., et al.: The role of working memory in decoding emotions. *Emotion* 8(2): 184–191, 2008.

Proust-Lima, C., Amieva, H., Letenneur, L., et al.: Gender and education impact on brain aging: A general cognitive factor approach. *Psychol Aging* 23 (3): 608–620, 2008.

Qato, D.M., Alexander, G.C., Conti, R.M., et al.: Use of prescription and over-the-counter medications and dietary supplements among older adults in the United States. *J Am Med Assoc* 300 (24): 2867–2878, 2008.

Rajah, M.N. and D'Esposito, M.: Region-specific changes in prefrontal function with age: A review of PET and fMRI studies on working and episodic memory. *Brain* 128: 1964–1983, 2005.

Raz, N., Gunning, F.M., Head, D., et al.: Selective aging of the human cerebral cortex observed in vivo: Differential vulnerability of the prefrontal gray matter. *Cereb Cortex* 7(3): 268–282, 1997.

Restom, K., Bangen, K.J., Bondi, M.W., et al.: Cerebral blood flow and BOLD responses to a memory encoding task: A comparison between healthy young and elderly adults. *Neuroimage*, 37: 430–439, 2007.

Reuter-Lorenz, P.A. and Sylvester, C.-Y.C.: The cognitive neuroscience of working memory and aging. In *Cognitive neuroscience of aging: Linking cognitive and cerebral aging* (Cabeza, R, Nyberg, L., and Park, Denise Eds.). New York: Oxford University Press, 2005, pp 186–217.

Richardson, E.D. and Marottoli, R.A.: Visual attention and driving behaviors among community-living older persons. *J Gerontol A Bio Sci Med Sci* 58 (9): 832–836, 2003.

Riley, K.P., Snowdon, D.A., Desrosiers, M.F., and Markesbery, W.R.: Early life linguistic ability, late life cognitive function, and neuropathology: Findings from the Nun Study. *Neurobiol Aging* 25: 341–347, 2005.

Rodrigue, K.M., Kennedy, K.M., and Raz, N.: Aging and longitudinal change in perceptual-motor skill acquisition in healthy adults. *J Gerontol B Psychol Sci Soc Sci* 60B (4): 174–181, 2005.

Rodriguez-Aranada, C.: Reduced writing and reading speed and age-related changes in verbal fluency tasks. *Clin Neuropsychol* 17 (2): 203–215, 2003.

Roe, C.M., Xiong, C., Miller, J.P., and Morris, J.C.: Education and Alzheimer disease without dementia: Support for the cognitive reserve hypothesis. *Neurology* 68: 223–228, 2007.

Royall, D.R., Palmer, R., Chiodo, L.K, and Polk, M.J.: Declining executive control in normal aging predicts change in functional status: The freedom house study. *J Am Geriatr Soc* 52: 346–352, 2004.

Royall, D.R., Palmer, R., Chiodo, L.K., and Polk, M.J.: Normal rates of cognitive change in successful aging: The freedom house study. *J Int Neuropsychol Soc* 11(7): 899–909, 2005.

Ruffman, T., Henry, J.D., Livingstone, V., and Phillips, L.H.: A meta-analytic review of emotion recognition and aging: Implications for neuropsychological models of aging. *Neurosci Biobeh Rev* 32: 863–881, 2008.

Rundek, T. and Bennett, D.A.: Cognitive leisure activities, but not watching TV, for future brain benefits. *Neurology* 66: 794–795, 2006.

Salthouse, T.A.: The processing-speed theory of adult age differences in cognition. *Psychol Rev* 103 (3): 403–428, 1996.

Salthouse, T.A.: Relations between cognitive abilities and measures of executive functioning. *Neuropsychology* 19 (4): 532–545, 2005.

Salthouse, T.A. and Siedlecki, K.L.: Reliability and validity of the divided attention questionnaire. *Neuropsychol Dev Cogn B Aging Neuropsychol Cogn* 12: 89–98, 2005.

Satz, P.: Brain reserve capacity on symptom onset after brain injury: A formulation and review of evidence for threshold theory. *Neuropsychology* 7(3): 273–295, 1993.

Scarmeas, N., Stern, Y., Mayeux, R., et al.: Mediterranean diet and mild cognitive impairment. *Arch Neurol* 66 (2): 216–225, 2009.

Scarmeas, N, Zarahn, E., Anderson, K.E., et al.: Cognitive reserve modulates functional brain responses during memory tasks: A PET study in healthy young and elderly subjects. *Neuroimage* 19(3): 1215–1227, 2003.

Schaie, K.W.: Developmental influences on adult intelligence: The Seattle longitudinal study. New York: Oxford University Press, 2005.

Shafto, M.A., Burke, D.M., Stamatakis, E.A., et al.: On the tip-of-the-tongue: Neural correlates of increased word-finding failures in normal aging. *J Cogn Neurosci* 19 (12): 2060–2070, 2007.

Simon, S.R., Chan, K.A., Soumerai, S.B., et al.: Potentially inappropriate medication use by elderly persons in U.S. health maintenance organizations, 2000–2001. *J Am Geriatr Soc* 53: 227–232, 2005.

Small, S.A.: Age-related memory decline: Current concepts and future directions. *Arch Neurol* 58: 360–364, 2001.

Smith, E.E. and Jonides, J.: Storage and executive processes in the frontal lobes. *Science*, 283: 1657–1661, 1999.

Solfrizzi, V., D'Introno, A., Colacicco, A.M., et al.: Alcohol consumption, mild cognitive impairment and progression to dementia. *Neurology* 68: 1790–1799, 2007.

Sowell, E.R., Peterson, B.S., Thompson, P.M., et al.: Mapping cortical change across the human life span. *Nat Neurosci* 6(3): 309–315, 2003.

Spira, A.P., Blackwell, T., Stone, K.L., et al.: Sleep-disordered breathing and cognition in older women. *J Am Geriatr Soc* 56: 45–50, 2008.

Squire, L.R. and Zola, S.M.: Structure and function of declarative and nondeclarative memory systems. *Proc Natl Acad Sci USA* 93: 13515–13522, 1996.

Stampfer, M.J., Kang, J.H., Chen, J., et al.: Effects of moderate alcohol consumption on cognitive function in women. *New Engl J Med* 352: 245–53, 2005.

Stern, Y.: What is cognitive reserve? Theory and research application of the reserve concept. *J Int Neuropsychol Soc* 8: 448–460, 2002.

Stern, Y., Habeck, C., Moeller, J., et al.: Brain networks associated with cognitive reserve in healthy young and old adults. *Cereb Cortex* 15 (4): 394–402, 2005.

Stevens, W.D., Hasher, L., Chiews, K.S., and Grady, C.L.: A neural mechanism underlying memory failure in older adults. *J Neurosci* 28(48): 12820–12824, 2008.

Stott, D.J., Falconer, A., Kerr, G.D., et al.: Does low to moderate alcohol intake protect against cognitive decline in older people? *J Am Geriatr Soc* 56: 2217–2224, 2008.

Stuss, D.T. and Alexander, M.P.: Is there a dysexecutive syndrome? *Philos Trans R Soc Lond B Biol Sci* 362 (1481): 901–915, 2007.

Sullivan, S. and Ruffman, T.: Emotion recognition deficits in the elderly. *Int J Neurosci* 114: 403–432, 2004.

Thomas, V.S. and Rockwood, K.J.: Alcohol abuse, cognitive impairment, and mortality among older people. *J Am Geriatr Soc* 49: 415–420, 2001.

Thorvaldsson, V., Hofer, S.M., Berg, S., et al.: Onset of terminal decline in cognitive abilities in individuals without dementia. *Neurology* 71: 882–887, 2009.

Tombaugh, T.N. and McIntyre, N.J.: The mini-mental state examination: A comprehensive review. *J Am Geriatr Soc* 40 (9): 922–935, 1992.

Tranel, D. and Damasio, A.R.: Neurobiological foundations of human memory. In *Handbook of memory disorders*, Ed 2. (Baddeley, A.D., Kopelman, M.D., and Wilson, B.A., Eds). Chichester, UK: J. Wiley, 2002, pp 17–57.

Treitz, F.H., Heyder, K., and Daum, I.: Differential course of executive control changes during normal aging. *Neuropsychol Dev Cogn B Aging Neuropsychol Cogn* 14: 370–393, 2007.

Van Dijk, K.R.A., Van Gerven, P.W.M., Van Boxtel, M.P.J., et al.: No protective effects of education during normal cognitive aging: Results from the 6-year follow-up of the Masstricht aging study. *Psychol Aging* 23(1): 119–130, 2008.

Velanova K., Lustig, C., Jacoby, L.L, and Buckner, R.L.: Evidence for frontally mediated controlled processing differences in older adults. *Cereb Cortex* 17: 1033–1046, 2007.

Verghese, J., Lipton, R.B., Katz, M.J., et al.: Leisure activities and the risk of dementia in the elderly. *New Engl J Med* 348: 2508–16, 2003.

Verhaeghen, P., Cerella, J., and Basak, C.: Aging, task complexity, and efficiency modes: The influence of working memory involvement on age differences in response times for verbal and visuospatial tasks. *Neuropsychol Dev Cogn B Aging Neuropsychol Cogn* 13(2): 254–280, 2006.

Wang, H.X., Karp, A., Winblad, B., and Fratiglioni, L.: Late-life engagement in social and leisure activities is associated with a decreased risk of dementia: A longitudinal study from the Kungsholmen project. *Am J Epidemiol* 155 (12): 1080–1087, 2002.

Wang, J.Y.J., Zhou, D.H.D., Li, J., et al.: Leisure activity and risk of cognitive impairment: the Chongqing aging study. *Neurology* 66: 911–913, 2006.

West, R.: In defense of the frontal lobe hypothesis of cognitive aging. *J Int Neuropsychol Soc* 6(6): 727–730, 2000.

West, R.: Visual distraction, working memory and aging. *Mem Cognit* 27 (6): 1064–72, 1999.

Weuve, J., Kang, J.H., Manson, J.E., et al.: Physical activity, including walking, and cognitive function in older women. *J Am Med Assoc* 292 (12): 1454–1461, 2004.

Wheeler, M.A., Stuss, D.T., and Tulving, E.: Toward a theory of episodic memory: The frontal lobes and autonoetic consciousness. *Psychol Bull* 121(3): 331–354, 1997.

White, K.K, and Abrams, L.: Does priming specific syllables during tip-of-the-tongue states facilitate word retrieval in older adults? *Psychol Aging* 17 (2): 226–235, 2002.

Wierenga, C.E., Benjamin, M., Gopinath, K., et al.: Age-related changes in word retrieval: Role of bilateral frontal and subcortical networks. *Neurobiol Aging* 29: 436–451, 2008.

Wilson, R.S., Hebert, L.E., Scherr, P.A., et al.: Educational attainment and cognitive decline in old age. *Neurology* 72: 460–465, 2009.

Wilson, R.S., Mendes de Leon, C.F., Barnes, L.L., et al.: Participation in cognitively stimulating activities and risk of incident Alzheimer disease. *J Am Med Assoc* 287 (6): 742–748, 2002.

Wright, R.M., Roumani, Y.F., Boudreau, R., et al.: Effect of central nervous system medication use on decline in cognition in community-dwelling older adults: Findings from the health, aging and body composition study. *J Am Geriatr Soc* 57: 243–250, 2009.

Yaffe, K., Barnes, D., Nevitt, M., et al.: A prospective study of physical activity and cognitive decline in elderly women: women who walk. *Arch Intern Med* 161(14): 1703–1708, 2001.

Yonelinas, A.P.: The nature of recollection and familiarity: a review of 30 years of research. *J Mem Lang* 46: 441–517, 2002.

Zamarian, L., Stadelmann, E., Nurk, H.-C., et al.: Effects of age and mild cognitive impairment on direct and indirect access to arithmetic knowledge. *Neuropsychologia* 45: 1511–1521, 2007.

Zarahn, E., Rakitin, B., Abela, D., et al.: Age-related changes in brain activation during a delayed item recognition task. *Neurobiol Aging*, 28(5): 784–798, 2007.

Zimprich, D. and Martin, M.: Can longitudinal changes in processing speed explain longitudinal age changes in fluid intelligence? *Psychol Aging* 17 (4): 690–695, 2002.

15 Mild Cognitive Impairment

Jennifer R. Molano and Ronald C. Petersen

Introduction

Mild cognitive impairment (MCI) is considered to be an intermediate state between normal cognition and dementia. MCI has become an important area of research over the past decade, due to its potential impact on public health. Alzheimer's disease (AD), the most common cause of dementia due to a neurodegenerative process, is predicted to affect at least 11 million people by 2050 if no therapeutic advances are made (Sloane 2002; Alzheimer's Association 2009). The economic burden of AD is substantial; longitudinal analyses have shown that the direct cost of caring for an AD patient can increase from $9,239 per patient during the early stages of the disease to $19,925 by fourth year after diagnosis (Zhu 2006).

In individuals over 65 years old without dementia, prevalence rates for MCI have ranged from 4–27% (Bennett 2002; Unverzagt 2001; Palmer 2002; Busse 2006; Plassman,2008; Manly 2008; Lopez 2003; Fischer 2007; Hanninen 2002; DiCarlo 2007; Ganguli 2004; Das 2007; Roberts 2008). Incidence rates for AD are approximately 1–2% per year in the general population; however, these figures are higher in MCI, with progression to dementia ranging from approximately 10–20% per year (Busse 2006; DiCarlo 2007; Das 2007; Fischer 2007; Tschanz 2006; Roberts 2008). As the general population is living longer, identifying early cognitive decline is essential. Early detection of cognitive impairment presumably can assist in developing treatments that may delay the onset, slow the progression, or reduce the severity of dementia.

Those with dementia have impairment in cognitive function and activities of daily living. On the other hand, those with MCI have (a.) a subject cognitive complaint, preferably corroborated by an informant, (b.) normal general cognitive function, (c.) cognitive impairment in one or more domains as identified on objective neuropsychological measurements, (d.) essentially normal activities of daily living, and (e.) are not demented (Petersen 2004). Though the original criteria for MCI were designed to characterize an early AD process and centered on memory impairment (Petersen 1999), the concept has evolved to incorporate other cognitive domains, such as attention-executive function, visuospatial skills, and language (Petersen 2004; Winbald 2004). With the incorporation of these domains, MCI now can be broadly classified into amnestic and non-amnestic subtypes. Amnestic MCI (aMCI) refers to cognitive impairment in which memory is affected; non-amnestic MCI (naMCI) refers to impairment in any of the other domains with preservation of memory.

Once the MCI subtype has been determined, it is equally important to consider the possible etiology of the cognitive impairment to finalize the diagnosis. Just as a vast number of causes may lead to dementia, these etiologies of MCI are also heterogeneous. The main goal for the clinician is to utilize the history, exam, and ancillary data in order to determine the most likely outcome in a patient diagnosed with MCI.

Clinical Presentation

The clinical presentation of a patient with MCI typically involves a cognitive complaint. Patients or family members commonly report difficulties with "short term memory" (by which most people mean recent memory), but detailed history-taking should also ask about symptoms in other cognitive domains. Motor, neuropsychiatric, autonomic, and sleep symptoms also may be present and should be elicited specifically during the initial evaluation.

Diagnosis: History, Exam, Imaging, Laboratory Tests, Exclusionary Conditions

Diagnostic Criteria

Figure 1 shows the MCI diagnostic algorithm (Petersen 2004). Three aspects of the criteria are important to appreciate. First, a cognitive concern should be made by a patient or an informant who knows the individual well and can indicate a change in performance (Daly 2000). The second criterion requires objective demonstration of cognitive impairment relative to age- and education-adjusted expectations (Ivnik 1992; Smith 1996), and finally, the individual should be maintaining essentially normal functional status. Determining whether a patient meets these criteria is based on the history, examination, and ancillary findings.

History

The clinical history is paramount in the diagnosis of MCI. While individuals are typically mildly affected and have insight to their deficits, obtaining a history from both the patient and an informant may provide further support that a cognitive *decline* exists (Daly 2000).

Questions about cognition should address all major domains, including memory, attention-executive functioning, visuospatial skills, and language. Common memory symptoms include frequent repetition or forgetfulness for recent events. Those with attention-executive functioning impairment may have problems in making decisions, planning activities, and multitasking. Visuospatial difficulties may be elicited by asking about a tendency to get lost while driving or an inability to track the lines on a page while reading. Word finding difficulty, paraphasias, and/or anomia may indicate language dysfunction.

The history-taking also should focus on functional status, including the ability to drive, manage finances, and maintain basic activities of daily living. Possible neuropsychiatric, motor, and sleep issues should be addressed, as the presence of these symptoms may suggest a possible etiology of an MCI subtype. Language difficulties, disinhibition, or socially inappropriate behavior, for example, may be seen in those with frontotemporal dementia. REM sleep behavior disorder, characterized

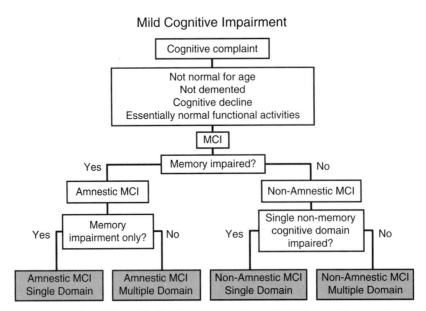

Figure 1 Algorithm for diagnosing and subtyping mild cognitive impairment. From (Petersen 2004). Reprinted by permission.

by a tendency to act out dreams, has been associated in MCI patients who develop dementia with Lewy bodies (DLB) (Molano 2009). A thorough past medical history always should be obtained, as cerebrovascular disease, seizures, head trauma, systemic cancer, or infections may be contributing to the cognitive impairment.

The time course of symptoms is also important. A gradual, insidious progression of symptoms may suggest a degenerative cause, while a more acute onset may indicate a vascular, inflammatory, or infectious etiology.

Examination

After a history has been obtained, a general neurological examination should be performed. While the examination may be normal, abnormalities could suggest a potential etiology for the cognitive deficits. Parkinsonism may be seen with DLB as well as other neurodegenerative disorders, motor neuron signs may be associated with FTD, and focal deficit consistent with a specific vascular distribution may suggest a vascular cause for the cognitive impairment.

In addition to a general neurological examination, a screening mental status examination, such as the Mini-Mental State Examination (MMSE), the Montreal Cognitive Assessment, (MoCA) or Kokmen Short Test of Mental Status (Folstein 1975; Nasreddine 2005; Kokmen 1991), should be administered. Severity of symptoms may be determined using assessments such as the Clinical Dementia Rating scale (CDR) (Morris 1993). A formal neuropsychological battery also can be performed and should include tests that sufficiently challenge a patient in each cognitive domain.

After adjusting for age and education, scores 1–2 standard deviations below the mean on formal neuropsychological testing typically indicate cognitive impairment (Ivnik 1992; Smith 1996). Learning and recall tasks may differentiate subjects with MCI from those experiencing normal aging. Figure 2 illustrates typical neuropsychological testing profiles of individuals with MCI, normal aging, and very mild clinically probable AD. On measures of general cognitive function such as the MMSE and full scale IQ, the individual with MCI performs similarly to a normal elderly subject, while memory function on delayed verbal recall (Logical Memory II) and non-verbal delayed recall (Visual Reproductions II) more closely resembles mild AD (Petersen 1999).

Though the screening mental status examination and neuropsychological battery may be useful, it is important to remember that these tests may not be sensitive to cognitive impairment. Individuals may score within the "normal" range, particularly those with high premorbid intellectual functioning. Despite normal scores, these patients may have MCI if the clinician determines that there has been a change from baseline functioning. In these circumstances, it is usually best to follow these patients clinically, with repeat evaluations at regular intervals.

Laboratory Tests

Medical laboratory tests used in the evaluation of dementia may identify medical issues that could affect cognitive function (Knopman 2001). Basic laboratory tests that look for reversible causes of cognitive impairment include a complete blood count, basic metabolic panel, thyroid function tests, vitamin B12 levels and folate levels. Neuroimaging with magnetic resonance imaging (MRI) or computerized tomography (CT) of the brain is also recommended to look for any structural abnormalities that may be contributing to symptoms.

Diagnosis

Following the algorithm of Figure 1, information from the history, screening mental status exam, neuropsychological testing and ancillary studies should be used to determine if cognitive function is normal or impaired. Functional status can be obtained from the individual, the informant, or both. If the patient has experienced cognitive decline but has maintained most daily activities, then that individual can be given an MCI diagnosis.

Once an individual has been diagnosed as having MCI, the clinician can determine the MCI subtype based on which cognitive domains are impaired. From this determination, the MCI subtype can be made. If memory impairment is present, then the individual has an aMCI subtype. If memory is preserved but evidence of decline is seen in other cognitive domains, then the subtype is naMCI.

After indicating the subtype as aMCI or naMCI, the next step is to determine if one or more cognitive domains are affected. If memory is the only domain affected then the subtype would be aMCI-single domain; if at least one other cognitive domain is also affected, then the subtype would be an aMCI-multiple domain. If the impairment was

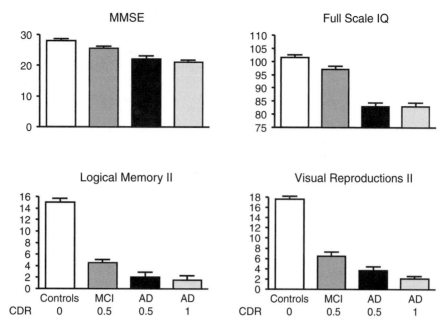

Figure 2 Cognitive profiles comparing individuals having mild cognitive impairment with performance of normal subjects and AD subjects. The Mini-Mental State Exam (MMSE) and Full Scale IQ represent measures of general intellectual function (top two panels). Measures of verbal memory function (Logical Memory II) and non-verbal memory function (Visual Reproductions II) are shown in the bottom two panels. From (Petersen et al., 1999). Reprinted by permission.

isolated to one of the non-memory domains, then the subtype would be naMCI-single domain; if two or more non-memory domains were affected, then the subtype would be naMCI-multiple domain as illustrated in the case below. Again, function must be essentially preserved to differentiate multiple-domain MCI from dementia.

Case #1

A 72-year-old right-handed man presents with a two-year history of progressive cognitive difficulties. His wife reports that he does not multitask and make decisions as well as he did during his years as a skilled engineer. He also takes longer to complete tasks and finds it challenging to fix items around the house. Otherwise, he maintains all activities of daily living independently and has been driving without any accidents or near-accidents. Both he and his wife reported no problems with his memory. On examination, he scores a 33/38 on the Kokmen Short Test of Mental Status. Though he lost two points on learning, two points on calculation, and one point on construction, he was able to state all four words on the delayed recall task. His general neurological examination was significant for mild bradyphrenia, bradykinesia, and hypomimia. He did not have any signs for motor neuron disease or corticospinal tract involvement. Formal neurological testing showed impairment in attention-executive functioning and visuospatial skills, with above average performance on measurements that tested the memory and language domains. Screening laboratory tests did not reveal a reversible cause for his cognitive difficulties. MRI brain also was unremarkable, without any evidence of cerebral or hippocampal atrophy. The patient was diagnosed with non-amnestic mild cognitive impairment-multiple domain, affecting the attention-executive functioning and visuospatial skills.

The goal of such subtyping in clinical practice is to accurately describe the individual's clinical syndrome and then to determine the possible etiology of the patient's symptoms. Using the history, examination, and ancillary data as illustrated in the following case example, the clinician can begin to deduce whether the cause of impairment is degenerative, vascular, psychiatric, or secondary to concomitant

medical disorders (Figure 3). Such deductions may assist in providing treatment options for each patient.

Case #2

A 70-year-old right-handed man presents with a two-year history of memory complaints. His wife mentions that he tends to misplace items, forget conversations, and repeat himself. He maintains all activities of daily living. Though he finishes tasks with accuracy, he takes a slightly longer time to finish activities such as balancing the checkbook. He does not have a history of depression. On the Kokmen Short Test of Mental Status, he scores a 34/38, losing all four points on recall. His general neurological examination is within normal limits, without any evidence of parkinsonism, motor neuron disease, or corticospinal tract signs. Formal neuropsychological testing shows impairment only in the memory domain, with difficulties on delayed verbal recall. Performance on tests of attention-executive functioning, visuospatial skills, and language is in the above-average range. Screening laboratory tests did not reveal a reversible cause for his cognitive difficulties. His MRI brain is significant for mild bilateral hippocampal atrophy. The patient was diagnosed with single-domain amnestic mild cognitive impairment. Since hippocampal atrophy on MRI is considered to be a potential biomarker for the conversion of MCI to Alzheimer's disease, the etiology for the patient's cognitive symptoms is most likely to be associated with Alzheimer's pathology.

Natural Progression of Disease and Outcomes

Since MCI is considered to be an intermediate state between normal aging and dementia, the etiologies for dementia theoretically could be applied to MCI as shown in Figure 3. While the construct in Figure 3 has yet to be validated, amnestic MCI due to a degenerative etiology is thought to progress most likely to AD—an assertion that has been endorsed in a practice parameter from the American Academy of Neurology (Petersen 2001).

While a diagnosis of MCI places an individual at higher risk for developing dementia, it does not indicate that the patient necessarily

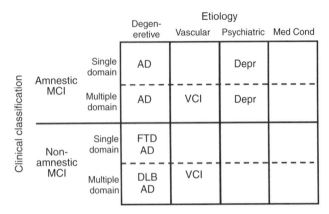

Figure 3 Predicted outcome of mild cognitive impairment subtypes according to presumed etiology. Adapted from (Petersen 2004). Reprinted by permission.

will progress to a dementia state. Though the majority of the MCI subjects in one large prospective trial progressed to AD at a rate of 7–10 % per year, a small percentage of these individuals improved to normal (Busse 2006). Others have been known to remain clinically stable for many years and may not develop dementia (Panza 2005). These potential outcomes should be discussed with patients and their families after a diagnosis of MCI has been made.

Identification of factors that predict progression to dementia is a major area of research interest, especially with AD. Several possible predictors have emerged, including features seen clinically, changes on structural and functional neuroimaging, and surrogate biomarkers in the CSF and plasma. Recent studies also have suggested that the use of combined biomarkers with neuroimaging may be useful in identifying MCI patients who are at risk for developing a neurodegenerative disorder such as AD (Petersen 2009; Jack 2009).

Predictors of Progression

Clinical Markers

The clinical severity of cognitive impairment and MCI subtype may be useful in predicting outcomes. Individuals with more severe memory impairment progress to AD more rapidly than those having less severe memory impairment (Dickerson 2007). In addition, those with an aMCI-multiple domain subtype have been found to have poorer overall survival than those with an aMCI-single domain subtype (Hunderfund 2006). These results suggest that the MCI subtype may predict the rate of progression to dementia, with individuals having the aMCI-multiple domain subtype progressing more rapidly than those having aMCI-single domain.

Structural and Functional Neuroimaging

MRI Volumetric Studies

In addition to clinical severity and MCI subtype, changes seen on structural and functional neuroimaging may assist in identifying those at risk for developing dementia. Cross-sectional volumetric MRI analyses have shown that differences in mesial temporal volume may distinguish between cognitively normal subjects from those with MCI (Ries 2008), and longitudinal studies have shown that hippocampal atrophy is an important predictor of progression from MCI to dementia and AD (Jack 1999) (Figure 4). A higher rate of hippocampal atrophy over a two-year period has been associated with older age, worse baseline cognitive performance, ApoE4 carrier status, and baseline hippocampal volumes (van de Pol 2007). Potential predictive utility also has been seen with whole brain, ventricular and entorhinal cortex volumes, subjective visual assessments of the hippocampal formation, as well as combined entorhinal and hippocampal measurements (Jack 2005; Devanand 2007; DeCarli 2007).

Functional Neuroimaging

Fluorodeoxyglucose positron emission tomography (FDG-PET) imaging studies have suggested that metabolic changes in the brain may precede structural changes in AD (Jagust 2009). FDG-PET changes that suggest evolving AD have been shown in cognitively normal subjects with a genetic predisposition to AD (Small 1995; Reiman 1996). Further, AD patterns of PET at the MCI stage may predict progression to AD (Anchisi 2005; Drzezga 2005). One more recent longitudinal study showed that hippocampal hypometabolism predicted cognitive decline prior to the onset of a clinical diagnosis of MCI or dementia (Mosconi 2008).

Newer imaging techniques using molecular imaging techniques also have been developed, targeting the proteins that have been implicated in AD pathology. Pittsburgh compound B (PiB), for example, is a tracer that binds to amyloid (Klunk 2004). Due to limited longitudinal studies, the clinical meaning of PiB retention has not been well-defined, as MCI subjects may have patterns similar to either normal or AD subjects (Wolk 2009). The technique also may not be specific to AD, as increased PiB retention has been reported in those with cerebral amyloid angiopathy (Johnson 2007; Lockhart 2007). More recent studies, however, have shown that combining PiB-PET with other methodologies such as MRI may provide complimentary information in distinguishing between cognitively normal subjects and those with MCI or AD (Jack et al. 2008).

FDDNP, a newer tracer that labels both amyloid and tau, theoretically indicates neuritic plaque and neurofibrillary tangle burden (Small 2006). As with PiB, future longitudinal studies on these ligand-bound agents more clearly will determine the utility of these techniques in predicting progression from MCI to AD (Ryu 2008).

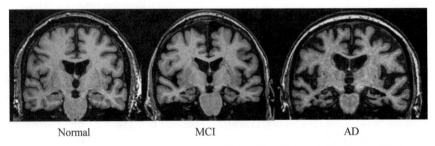

Normal   MCI   AD

Figure 4 Coronal MRI showing degrees of hippocampal atrophy in normal (left), MCI (middle), and AD (right) subjects. From (Petersen 2004). Reprinted by permission.

Surrogate Biomarkers

Plasma Biomarkers

Since abnormal protein processing of amyloid is thought to lead to the development of neuritic plaques, plasma Aβ levels may be potentially useful biomarkers for AD (van Oijen 2006; Graff-Radford 2007). Cognitively normal older adults with lower AB42/AB40 ratios were found to have a significantly greater risk of progressing to MCI or AD (Graff-Radford 2007). However, other studies have found that plasma AB levels are less effective predictors of progression to AD (Hansson 2008; Lopez 2008). Given these conflicting results, more research needs to be performed to determine the utility of plasma biomarkers in predicting disease progression. Current studies are investigating the biochemical analysis of plasma signaling proteins to identify those most at risk (Ray 2007).

CSF Biomarkers

In addition to the abnormal protein processing of amyloid, the pathophysiology of AD is also thought to be due to the abnormal protein processing of tau. As a result, CSF levels of amyloid βeta (Aβ), total tau (T-tau), and phosphorylated tau have been studied as potential biomarkers for AD (Borroni 2007). In those with AD, lower Aβ and higher tau measurements in the CSF may be seen (Shaw 2009), and CSF Aβ and tau measurements also may differentiate MCI subjects from those with normal cognition (Galasko 1997; Galasko 1998; Growdon 1999). Pathological studies of AD have shown a correlation between neocortical neurofibrillary pathology and tau phosphorylated at threonine 231 (p-tau$_{231}$), though this correlation may not be associated with tau phosphorylated at threonine 181 (p-tau$_{181}$) (Buerger 2006).

Longitudinal studies have also suggested that CSF levels may have predictive utility in the progression from MCI to AD (Sunderland 1999; Stefani 2006). Baseline CSF levels of tau phosphorylated at threonine 231 have been correlated with both cognitive decline and conversion from MCI to AD (Buerger 2002; Brys 2007), and CSF T-tau/ Aβ$_{42/40}$ and T-tau/ Aβ$_{42/40}$ ratios also have been studied as possible predictors (Brys 2007). Other studies have shown that progression from MCI to AD is more likely to be seen in those with lower AB42 and higher phosphorylated tau and/or T-tau levels in the CSF (Hansson 2006; Mattson 2009), and more recent research has shown that the CSF profile of AB1-42 and T-tau levels not only may be a biomarker signature for AD but also may identify conversion from MCI to AD (Shaw 2009). Amnestic MCI patients who have a CSF profile that is characteristic of AD also may progress to a dementia syndrome more rapidly (deLeon 2006).

CSF isoprostane has been studied as another potential marker, especially since oxidative stress has been thought to contribute to the pathogenesis of AD (deLeon 2007). The use of proteomics also may assist in determining a protein pattern in the CSF that might distinguish AD from control subjects (Finehout 2007).

Use of Combined Biomarkers

Though there has not been enough data to recommend one specific predictor in the progression from MCI to dementia, recent research has started to combine biomarkers to create a potential predictive profile for those who might develop AD (Borroni 2007; Visser 1999). One study demonstrated that combination of cognitive test performance, informant report of functional impairment, apoE genotyping, olfactory identification deficit, and MRI hippocampal and entorhinal volume may predict conversion from MCI to AD (Devanand 2007).

Researchers more recently have investigated the utility of combining biomarkers with neuroimaging techniques (Petersen 2009). Lower AB42 and higher phosphorylated tau CSF levels, for example, have been correlated with medial temporal lobe atrophy in those who progressed from MCI to AD (Herukka 2008). However, by the time that atrophy is seen on structural neuroimaging, the process of neurodegeneration is thought to already have occurred (Petersen 2009; Jack, 2009; Jack 2010). Since amyloid deposition may be the precipitating event in AD process and may occur many years prior to neurodegeneration and cognitive symptom onset (Petersen 2009; Jack 2009), neuroimaging techniques that bind to amyloid, such as Pib-PET, may complement the medial temporal atrophy seen on structural MRI in MCI patients (Jack 2009). The combination of neuroimaging with biomarkers such as CSF AB and tau levels may further increase the ability to identify MCI patients most at risk for developing AD (Petersen 2009). While such studies are promising, further longitudinal investigations will be necessary to determine a profile that most accurately will predict which MCI patients progress to AD or another type of dementia.

Pathophysiology

The clinical construct implies that an individual with MCI is at a higher risk of developing dementia. Figure 3 shows the number of possible outcomes for MCI and its various subtypes. In addition to AD patients, those with vascular disease, depression, and other neurodegenerative disorders such as frontotemporal dementia and dementia with Lewy bodies also may pass through an MCI state (Molano 2009). The outcomes for both amnestic and non-amnestic subtypes of MCI are still under investigation, but the neuropathological substrate particularly for aMCI continues to be a source of discussion.

Amnestic MCI is thought to be a risk factor for AD. Neuritic plaques and neurofibrillary tangles are the neuropathological hallmarks of AD, resulting from abnormal protein processing of amyloid and tau. Some investigators contend that aMCI individuals should be given a clinical diagnosis of early AD because they have the changes associated with its pathological diagnosis (Markesbery 2006; Morris 2001).

However, other studies have suggested that aMCI may not simply be a manifestation of early AD. An intermediate pathology between normal aging and early AD has been seen in those who died with the clinical classification of MCI (Bennett 2005; Petersen 2006). With some medial temporal neurofibrillary tangles but sparse diffuse neocortical plaques, these individuals have shown mostly low probability scores for meeting AD neuropathological criteria (Petersen 2006).

Heterogenous findings, such as combined neurodegenerative and vascular pathologies, also may contribute the clinical picture of MCI (Bennett 2005), and one study showed that approximately 20% of aMCI patients had pathological diagnoses other than AD on autopsy, including frontotemporal dementia, dementia with Lewy bodies, progressive supranuclear palsy and vascular dementia (Figure 5) (Jicha 2006). While the majority of aMCI subjects may evolve to AD, other potential etiologies therefore should be considered in the evaluation of these patients.

Other processes, such as cholinergic system dysfunction and oxidative stress, have been associated with AD (Bowen 1976; Davies 1976; Petersen 1977; Whitehouse 1981; Goodwin 1983; Gale 1996; La Rue 1997; Perrig 1997; Morris 1998). While both of these processes also may be involved with aMCI, more research needs to be performed in order to determine the pathophysiological factors that may lead to each MCI subtype.

Possible Genetic Contributions

Amnestic MCI due to a degenerative cause most likely has similar features to clinically probable AD, with risk factors such as age, hypertension,

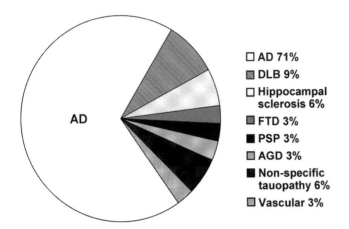

Figure 5 Neuropathological outcome of subjects with history of MCI. Adapted from (Jicha 2006). Reprinted by permission.

and diabetes (Reitz 2007; Luchsinger 2007; Kryscio 2006). Apolipoprotein E4 (ApoE4) carrier status is a recognized genetic risk factor for the development of AD (Corder 1993), but its value for detecting progression to cognitive impairment is less clear.

Some studies have suggested that ApoE4 carrier status may assist in predicting those more likely to convert from MCI to AD (Petersen 1995; Tierney 1996; Aggarwal 2005), and a synergistic effect with depression has been seen in cognitively normal individuals at risk for developing MCI. ApoE4 carrier status also may be associated both with hippocampal atrophy in MCI subjects and with higher rates of cognitive decline in cognitively normal adults (Jak 2007; Caselli 2007). However, others have shown that ApoE4 carrier status itself has not been shown to predict cognitive decline or conversion to AD (Devanand 2005), and its routine use is not recommended (Farrer 1997); the diagnosis of MCI is made clinically.

Treatment

Early detection of cognitive decline theoretically may lead to the implementation of therapies that slow the progression of impairment. However, there currently is no FDA-approved treatment intervention for MCI. Since the etiologies of MCI can be heterogeneous, medications targeting a neurodegenerative cause theoretically would be different than those targeting cognitive impairment due to vascular, psychiatric or other medical disorders. Clinical trials nevertheless have focused on the aMCI subtype, with the goal of slowing the progression to AD.

As summarized in Table 1, studies have targeted medications used in the symptomatic treatment of clinically probable AD. These medications have included three of the cholinesterase inhibitors—donepezil, galantamine, and rivastigmine (Petersen 2005; Winbald 2008; Feldman 2007). Additionally, vitamin E and rofecoxib have been studied (Petersen 2005; Thal 2005), as both oxidative damage and inflammation have been implicated in the pathophysiology of AD (Goodwin 1983; Gale 1996; La Rue 1997; Perrig 1997; Morris 1998). Unfortunately, none of the medications have shown a significant reduction in conversion rates of aMCI to AD, ranging from 6–17 % in the medication arms vs. 4–21% with placebo. However, one study did find that donepezil reduced the progression risk for 12 months in those with aMCI—an effect that persisted up to 24 months in apolipoprotein E4 carriers (Petersen 2005).

Despite the results of clinical trial data, these studies do support the construct that aMCI of a degenerative etiology is an intermediate state between normal cognition and AD. The overall progression rates for MCI in these studies ranged from 5% to 16%, which are higher than the incidence rate for AD in the general population (Petersen 1999, Petersen 2005). These rates suggest that patients who meet MCI criteria are at a higher risk of developing AD. Since not all of those with MCI develop AD pathology, more accurate identification of these subjects is essential. Incorporating potential predictive biomarkers in clinical trials may assist in testing compounds that target the underlying disease process of AD (Cummings 2007).

Rehabilitative/Psychological Aspects as Pertinent

Patients and families should be aware that those who have aMCI due to a degenerative cause may have a 10–15% chance of developing AD; however, it also should be noted that MCI is heterogeneous with a number of potential outcomes (Panza 2005). Although some patients may not develop dementia, the label of "mild cognitive impairment" nevertheless may lead to psychological consequences, such as a feeling of uncertainty or concerns of becoming burdensome to others (Joosten-Weyn Banningh 2008). Neuropsychiatric symptoms such as depression, anxiety, apathy and/or irritability also may be seen in those with MCI and may be associated with progression to AD (Lyketsos 2002; Hwang TJ 2004; Muangpaisan 2008; Rozzini 2008; Teng 2007; Apostolova 2008).

Encouraging patients and families to consider decisions about advance directives, future planning, and finances is essential, especially if the cognitive impairment is thought to be due to a degenerative cause. Though definitive data are limited, patients should be encouraged to follow a heart-healthy diet and to remain active physically, intellectually, and socially (Fratiglioni 2004; Rovio 2005). Participation in a

Table 1 MCI Clinical Trials

Sponsor	Compound	Number Enrolled	Duration (Years)	Primary Outcome	Progression Rate	Result	Reference
ADCS	Donepezil Vitamin E	769	3	AD	16%	Partially Positive	(Petersen et al. 2005)
Johnson and Johnson*	Galantamine	2048	2	CDR 1	5%	Negative	(Winblad et al. 2008)
Novartis	Rivastigmine	1018	4	AD	5%	Negative	(Feldman et al. 2007)
Merck	Rofecoxib	1457	3-4	AD	5%	Negative	(Thal et al. 2005)

* Two trials
CDR: clinical dementia rating scale

cognitive rehabilitation program also may be useful in MCI subjects, with improvements in activities of daily living, mood, and memory (Kurz 2008). While these modifications may improve their overall quality of life, there has not been enough research to support a decreased progression from aMCI to AD.

Future Directions

The MCI construct has become useful in the early detection of those at risk for developing dementia. Given the heterogeneity of the MCI subtypes and their potential etiologies, identifying these individuals with more accuracy is essential. One area of future research is in developing a predictive profile for these patients. With aMCI, for example, a combination of ApoE4 genotypes, CSF biomarkers, and neuroimaging findings on MRI, FDG-PET, and Pib-PET may identify those who are more likely to progress to AD, as opposed to some other pathology.

Longitudinal studies also need to be performed on the various MCI subtypes. While there has been a plethora of research on aMCI and its association with AD, there is a lack of information on the outcomes of naMCI; some research even has suggested that both aMCI and naMCI subtypes may progress to AD (Fischer 2007). Similar to AD, other neurodegenerative disorders such as dementia with Lewy bodies and frontotemporal dementia may pass through an MCI state, though this presumption has not yet been validated.

Finally, neuropsychological tests that are more sensitive in detecting cognitive impairment should be developed, as they may assist in identifying those with early MCI. In those with high intellectual premorbid functioning, scores on screening mental status examinations and formal neuropsychological batteries may be within normal limits. Nevertheless, these patients may still be diagnosed with MCI, especially if the clinician believes that there has been a decline from the individual's baseline cognition. More research is starting to be performed in this population of patients (O'Bryant 2008)

Being able to identify patients at risk for developing dementia is essential for clinical trials. Possible disease-modifying agents for AD currently are at various stages of investigation, including modulators of amyloid processing, active and passive immunization strategies, and monoclonal antibodies. More accurate identification of MCI individuals may structure enrollment procedures and endpoints in future studies (Cummings 2007) and hopefully will lead to better outcomes in subsequent treatment trials.

Summary

The MCI construct implies an intermediate state between normal cognition and dementia. Individuals with MCI have (a) a subjective cognitive complaint that is usually corroborated by an informant, (b) preserved general cognitive functioning, (c) impairment in one or more of the cognitive domains (memory, attention-executive function, visuospatial skills, and/or language), (d) essentially normal activities of daily living, and (e) are not demented. Once the diagnosis of MCI has been made, the specific subtype can be determined, with amnestic MCI referring to the presence of memory impairment and non-amnestic MCI referring to the presence of impairment in one or more of the other domains with relative preservation of memory.

MCI remains a clinical diagnosis, aided by a thorough history, neurological examination, screening mental status examination, and formal neuropsychological testing. Though an individual with high premorbid intellectual functioning may score within the normal range on bedside and formal testing, that patient may still be considered to have MCI based on the judgment of the clinician.

Since there is subjectivity in the clinical diagnosis, creating an operational definition for clinical trials has been a challenge. In addition, a number of etiologies can be associated with MCI, including degenerative and vascular processes, psychiatric causes, and comorbid medical conditions.

The most researched subtype has been aMCI. Thought to be a risk factor for AD, the aMCI subtype has been associated with increased rates of progression to AD compared to the general population. A great deal of research has been performed to determine factors that may predict this progression, with more recent studies combining data on clinical, genetic, neuroimaging, and surrogate biomarkers. While further studies clearly need to be performed in order to refine the MCI construct and its potential etiologies, the ultimate goal is to use this construct as a tool in developing treatments that will potentially prevent or delay the progression of dementia. If a profile of neuroimaging and surrogate biomarkers can be used in conjunction with an MCI diagnosis and if that profile accurately can indicate which patients with MCI are most at risk of progressing to AD, then perhaps there is the potential of moving the AD diagnosis to an earlier stage and subsequently treating these patients even before they develop dementia.

References

Aggarwal, N.T., Wilson, R.S., Beck, T.L., et al.: The apolipoprotein E epsilon4 allele and incident Alzheimer's disease in persons with mild cognitive impairment. *Neurocase* 11(1):3–7, 2005.

Alzheimer's Association. 2009 Alzheimer's disease facts and figures. *Alzheimer's and Dementia* 5(3)234–270, 2009.

Anchisi, D., Borroni, B., Franceschi, M., et al.: Heterogeneity of brain glucose metabolism in mild cognitive impairment and clinical progression to Alzheimer disease. *Arch Neurol* 62(11):1728–1733, 2005.

Apostolova, L.G. and Cummings, J.L.: Neuropsychiatric manifestations in mild cognitive impairment: A systematic review of the literature. *Dement Geriatr Cogn Disord* 25(2):115–26, 2008.

Bennett, D.A., Schneider, J.A., Bienias, J.L., et al.: Mild cognitive impairment is related to Alzheimer disease pathology and cerebral infarctions. *Neurology* 64(5):834–841, 2005.

Bennett, D.A., Wilson, R.S., Schneider, J.A., et al.: Natural history of mild cognitive impairment in older persons. *Neurology* 59(2):198–205, 2002.

Borroni B, Premi E, DiLuca M, and Padovani A.: Combined biomarkers for early Alzheimer disease diagnosis. *Current Medicinial Chemistry* 14(11):1171–1178, 2007.

Bowen, D.M., Smith, C.B., White, P., et al.: Neurotransmitter-related enzymes and indices of hypoxia in senile dementia and other abiotrophies. *Brain* 99(3):459–496, 1976.

Brys, M., Pirraglia, E., Rich, K., et al.: Prediction and longitudinal study of CSF biomarkers in mild cognitive impairment. *Neurobiol Aging* [epub ahead of print], 2007.

Buerger, K., Ewers, M., Pirttila, T., et al.: CSF phosphorylated tau protein correlates with neocortical neurofibrillary pathology in Alzheimer's disease. *Brain* 129(Pt 11):3035–3041, 2006.

Buerger, K., Teipel, S.J., Zinkowski, R., et al.: CSF tau protein phosphorylated at threonine 231 correlates with cognitive decline in MCI subjects. *Neurology* 59(4):627–629, 2002.

Busse, A., Hensel, A., Guhne, U., et al.: Mild cognitive impairment: long-term course of four clinical subtypes. *Neurology* 67(12):2176–2185, 2006.

Caselli, R.J., Reiman, E.M., Locke, D.E., et al.: Cognitive domain decline in healthy apolipoprotein E epsilon4 homozygotes before the diagnosis of mild cognitive impairment. *Arch Neurol* 64(9):1306–1311, 2007.

Corder, E.H., Saunders, A.M., Strittmatter, W.J., et al.: Gene dose of apolipoprotein E type 4 allele and the risk of Alzheimer's disease in late onset families. *Science* 261(5123):921–923, 1993.

Cummings, J.L., Doody, R. and Clark, C.: Disease-modifying therapies for Alzheimer disease: challenges to early intervention. *Neurology* 69(16):1622–1634, 2007.

Daly, E., Zaitchik, D., Copeland, M., et al. Predicting conversion to Alzheimer disease using standardized clinical information. *Arch Neurol* 57(5):675–680, 2000.

Das, S.K., Bose, P., Biswas, A., et al.: An epidemiologic study of mild cognitive impairment in Kolkata, India. *Neurology* 68(23):2019–2026, 2007.

Davies, P. and Maloney, A.J.: Selective loss of central cholinergic neurons in Alzheimer's disease. *Lancet* 2(8000):1403, 1976.

DeCarli, C., Frisoni, G.B., Clark, C. M., et al.: Qualitative estimates of medial temporal atrophy as a predictor of progression from mild cognitive impairment to dementia. *Arch Neurol* 64(1):108–115, 2007.

deLeon, M.J., Mosconi, L., Li, J., et al.: Longitudinal CSF isoprostanes and MRI atrophy in the progression to AD. *J Neurol* 254(12):1666–75, 2007.

deLeon, M.J., DeSanti S., Zinkowski, R., et al.: Longitudinal CSF and MRI biomarkers improve the diagnosis of mild cognitive impairment. *Neurobiology of Aging*, 27(3):384–401, 2006.

Devanand, D.P., Pelton, G.H., Zamora, D., et al.: Predictive utility of apolipoprotein E genotype for Alzheimer disease in outpatients with mild cognitive impairment. *Arch Neurol* 62(6):975–80, 2005.

Devanand, D.P., Pradhaban, G., Liu, X., et al.: Hippocampal and entorhinal atrophy in mild cognitive impairment: prediction of Alzheimer disease. *Neurology* 68(11):828–836, 2007.

DiCarlo, A., Lamassa, M., Baldereschi, M., et al.: CIND and MCI in the Italian elderly: frequency, vascular risk factors, progression to dementia. *Neurology* 68(22):1909–1916, 2007.

Dickerson, B.C., Sperling, R.A., Hyman, B.T., et al.: Clinical prediction of Alzheimer disease dementia across the spectrum of mild cognitive impairment. *Arch Gen Psychiatry* 64(12):1443–50, 2007.

Drzezga, A., Grimmer, T., Riemenschneider, M., et al.: Prediction of individual clinical outcome in MCI by means of genetic assessment and (18)F-FDG PET. *J Nucl Med* 46(10):1625–1632, 2005.

Farrer, L.A., Cupples, L.A., Haines, J.L., et al.: Effects of age, sex, and ethnicity on the association between apolipoprotein E genotype and Alzheimer disease. A meta-analysis. APOE and Alzheimer Disease Meta Analysis Consortium. *JAMA* 278(16):1349–1356, 1997.

Feldman, H.H., Ferris, S., Winblad, B., et al.: Effect of rivastigmine on delay to diagnosis of Alzheimer's disease from mild cognitive impairment: the InDDEx study. *Lancet Neurol* 6(6):501–512, 2007.

Finehout, E.J., Franck, Z., Choe, L.H., et al.: Cerebrospinal fluid proteomic biomarkers for Alzheimer's disease. *Ann Neurol* 61(2):120–9, 2007.

Fischer, P., Jungwirth, S., Zehetmayer, S., et al.: Conversion from subtypes of mild cognitive impairment to Alzheimer dementia. *Neurology* 68(4):288–291, 2007.

Folstein, M., Folstein, S. and McHugh, P.: "Mini-mental state". A practical method for grading the cognitive state of patients for the clinician. *J Psychiatr Res* 12:189–198, 1975.

Fratiglioni, L., Paillard-Borg, S. and Winblad, B.: An active and socially integrated lifestyle in late life might protect against dementia. *Lancet Neurol* 3(6):343–353, 2004.

Galasko, D., Chang, L., Motter, R., et al.: High cerebrospinal fluid tau and low amyloid beta42 levels in the clinical diagnosis of Alzheimer disease and relation to apolipoprotein E genotype. *Arch Neurol* 55(7):937–945, 1998.

Galasko, D., Clark, C., Chang, L., et al.: Assessment of CSF levels of tau protein in mildly demented patients with Alzheimer's disease. *Neurology* 48(3):632–635, 1997.

Gale, C.R., Martyn, C.N. and Cooper, C.: Cognitive impairment and mortality in a cohort of elderly people. *BMJ* 312(7031):608–611, 1996.

Ganguli, M., Dodge, H.H., Shen, C., et al.: Mild cognitive impairment, amnestic type: an epidemiologic study. *Neurology* 63:115–121, 2004.

Geda, Y.E., Knopman, D.S., Mrazek, D.A., et al.: Depression, apolipoprotein E genotype, and the incidence of mild cognitive impairment: a prospective cohort study. *Arch Neurol* 63(3):435–40, 2006.

Gold, M., Francke, S., Nye, J.S., et al.: Impact of APOE genotype on the efficacy of galantamine for the treatment of mild cognitive impairment. *Neurobiol Aging* 25(Sup 2):S521, 2004.

Goodwin, J.S., Goodwin, J.M. and Garry, P.J.: Association between nutritional status and cognitive functioning in a healthy elderly population. *JAMA* 249(21):2917–2921, 1983.

Graff-Radford, N.R., Crook, J.E., Lucas, J., et al.: Association of low plasma Abeta42/Abeta40 ratios with increased imminent risk for mild cognitive impairment and Alzheimer disease. *Arch Neurol* 64(3):354–362, 2007.

Growdon, J.H.: Biomarkers of Alzheimer disease. *Arch Neurol* 56(3):281–283, 1999.

Hanninen T., Hallikainen, M., Tuomainen, S., et al.: Prevalence of mild cognitive impairment: A population-based study in elderly subjects. *Acta Neurologica Scandinavica* 160:148–154, 2002.

Hansson, O., Zetterberg, H., Buchhave, P., et al.: Association between CSF biomarkers and incipient Alzheimer's disease in patients with mild cognitive impairment: a follow-up study. *Lancet Neurol* 5(3):228–234, 2006.

Hansson, O., Zetterberg, H., Vanmechelen, E., et al.: Evaluation of plasma Abeta(40) andAbeta(42) as predictors of conversion to Alzheimer's disease in patients with mild cognitive impairment. *Neurobiol Aging* Epub May 16, 2008.

Herukka, S.K., Pennanen, C., Soininen, H., et al.: CSF Abeta42, tau, and phosphorylated tau correlate with medial temporal lobe atrophy. *J Alzheimers Dis* 14(1): 51–57, 2008.

Hunderfund, A.L., Roberts, R.O., Slusser, T.C., et al.: Mortality in amnestic mild cognitive impairment: a prospective community study. *Neurology* 67(10):1764–1768, 2006.

Hwang, T.J., Masterman, D.L., Ortiz, F., et al.: Mild cognitive impairment is associated with characteristic neuropsychiatric symptoms. *Alzheimer Dis Assoc Disord* 18(1):17–21, 2004.

Ivnik, R.J., Malec, J.F., Smith, G.E., et al.: Mayo's Older Americans Normative Studies: WAIS-R, WMS-R and AVLT norms for ages 56 to 97. *Clin Neuropsychol* 6(Suppl):1104, 1992.

Jack, C.R., Knopman, D.S., Jagust, W.J., et al.: Hypothetical model of dynamic biomarkers of the Alzheimer's pathological cascade. *The Lancet Neurology* 9(1):119128, 2010.

Jack, C.R., Jr, Lowe, V.J., Senjem, M.L., et al.: 11C PiB and structural MRI provide complementary information in imaging of Alzheimer's disease and amnestic mild cognitive impairment. *Brain.* 131(Pt3):665–80, 2008.

Jack, C.R., Jr., Lowe, V.J., Weigand, S.D., et al.: Serial PIB and MRI in normal, mild cognitive impairment, and Alzheimer's disease: Implications for sequence of pathological events in Alzheimer's disease. *Brain* 132(Pt5):1355–1365, 2009.

Jack, C.R., Jr., Petersen, R.C., Xu, Y.C., et al.: Prediction of AD with MRI-based hippocampal volume in mild cognitive impairment. *Neurology* 52(7):1397–1403, 1999.

Jack, C.R., Jr., Shiung, M.M., Weigand, S.D., et al.: Brain atrophy rates predict subsequent clinical conversion in normal elderly and amnestic MCI. *Neurology* 65(8):1227–1231, 2005.

Jagust, W.J., Landau, S.M., Shaw, L.M., et al.: Relationships between biomarkers in aging and dementia. *Neurology* 73(15):1193–1199, 2009.

Jak, A.J., Houston, W.S., Nagel, B.J., et al.: Differential Cross-Sectional and Longitudinal Impact of APOE Genotype on Hippocampal Volumes in Nondemented Older Adults. *Dement Geriatr Cogn Disord* 23(6):282–289, 2007.

Jicha, G.A., Parisi, J.E., Dickson, D.W., et al.: Neuropathologic outcome of mild cognitive impairment following progression to clinical dementia. *Arch Neurol* 63(5):674–681, 2006.

Johnson, K.A., Gregas, M., Becker, J.A., et al.: Imaging of amyloid burden and distribution in cerebral amyloid angiopathy. *Ann Neurol* 62(3):229–234, 2007.

Joosten-Weyn Banningh L., Vernooij-Dassen, M., Rikkert, M.O., et al.: Mild cognitive impairment: Coping with an uncertain label. *Int J Geriatr Psychiatry* 23(2):148–54, 2008.

Klunk, W.E., Engler, H., Nordberg, A., et al.: Imaging brain amyloid in Alzheimer's disease with Pittsburgh Compound-B. *Ann Neurol* 55(3):306–319, 2004.

Knopman, D.S., DeKosky, S.T., Cummings, J.L., et al.: Practice parameter: diagnosis of dementia (an evidence-based review). Report of the Quality Standards Subcommittee of the American Academy of Neurology. *Neurology* 56(9):1143–53, 2001.

Kokmen, E., Smith, G.E., Petersen, R.C., et al.: The short test of mental status. Correlations with standardized psychometric testing. *Arch Neurol* 48(7):725–728, 1991.

Kryscio, R.J., Schmitt, F.A., Salazar, J.C., et al.: Risk factors for transitions from normal to mild cognitive impairment and dementia. *Neurology* 66(6):828–32, 2006.

Kurz, A., Pohl, C., Ramsenthaler, M., et al.: Cognitive rehabilitation in patients with mild cognitive impairment. *Int J Geriatr Psychiatry* Epub Jul 17, 2008.

La Rue, A., Koehler, K.M., Wayne, S.J., et al.: Nutritional status and cognitive functioning in a normally aging sample: A 6-y reassessment. *Am J Clin Nutr* 65(1):20–29, 1997.

Lockhart, A., Lamb, J.R., Osredkar, T., et al.: PIB is a non-specific imaging marker of amyloid-beta (Abeta) peptide-related cerebral amyloidosis. *Brain* 130(Pt 10):2607–2615, 2007.

Lopez, O.L., Jagust, W.J., DeKosky, S.T., et al.: Prevalence and classification of mild cognitive impairment in the Cardiovascular Health Study Cognition Study: part 1. *Arch Neurol* 60(10):1385–1389, 2003.

Lopez, O.L., Kuller, L.H., Mehta, P.D., et al.: Plasma amyloid levels and the risk of AD in normal subjects in the Cardiovascular Health Study. *Neurology* 70(19):1664–71, 2008.

Luchsinger, J.A., Reitz, C., Patel, B., et al.: Relation of diabetes to mild cognitive impairment. *Arch Neurol* 64(4):570–5, 2007.

Lyketsos, C.G., Lopez, O., Jones, B., et al.: Prevalence of neuropsychiatric symptoms in dementia and mild cognitive impairment: Results from the Cardiovascular Health Study. *JAMA* 288(12):1475–83, 2002.

Manly, J.J., Tang M.X., Schupf N., et al.: Frequency and course of mild cognitive impairment in a multiethnic community. *Ann Neurol* 63(4):494–506, 2008.

Markesbery, W.R., Schmitt, F.A., Kryscio, R.J., et al.: Neuropathologic substrate of mild cognitive impairment. *Arch Neurol* 63(1):38–46, 2006.

Mattsson, N., Zetterberg, H., Hansson, O., et al.: CSF biomarkers and incipient Alzheimer's disease in patients with mild cognitive impairment. *JAMA* 302(4):385–393, 2009.

Molano, J., Boeve, B., Ferman, T., et al.: Mild cognitive impairment associated with limbic and neocortical lewy body disease: A clinicopathological study. *Brain* advance online publication doi:10.1093/brain/awp280, 4 November 2009.

Morris, J.C.: The clinical dementia rating (CDR): Current version and scoring rules. *Neurology* 43:2412–2414, 1993.

Morris, J.C., Storandt, M., Miller, J.P., et al.: Mild cognitive impairment represents early-stage Alzheimer disease. *Arch Neurol* 58(3):397–405, 2001.

Morris, M.C., Beckett, L.A., Scherr, P.A., et al.: Vitamin E and vitamin C supplement use and risk of incident Alzheimer disease. *Alzheimer Dis Assoc Disord* 12(3):121–126, 1998.

Mosconi, L., De Santi, S., Li, J., et al.: Hippocampal hypometabolism predicts cognitive decline from normal aging. *Neurobiol Aging* 29(5):676–92, 2008.

Muangpaisan, W., Intalapaporn, S., and Assantachai, P.: Neuropsychiatric symptoms in the community-based patients with mild cognitive impairment and the influence of the demographic factors. *Int J Geriatr Psychiatry* 23(7):699–703, 2008.

Mueller, S.G., Weiner, M.W., Thal, L.J., et al.: The Alzheimer's disease neuroimaging initiative. *Neuroimaging Clin N Am* 15(4):869–877, xi–xii, 2005.

Nasreddine, Z.S., Phillips N.A., Bedirian, V., et al.: The Montreal Cognitive Assessment, MoCA: A brief screening tool for mild cognitive impairment. *J Am Geriatr Soc* 53(4):695–699, 2005.

O'Bryant S.E., Humphreys J.D., Smith G.E., et al.: Detecting dementia with the mini-mental state examination in highly educated individuals. *Arch Neurol* 65(7):963–967, 2008.

Palmer K., Wang H.X., Backman L., et al.: Differential evolution of cognitive impairment in nondemented older persons: Results from the Kungsholmen Project. *Am J Psychiatry*. 159:436–442, 2002.

Panza, F., D'Introno A., Colacicco, A.M., et al.: Current epidemiology of mild cognitive impairment and other predementia syndromes. *Am J Geriatr Psychiatry* 13(8):633–44, 2005.

Perrig, W.J., Perrig, P. and Stahelin, H.B.: The relation between antioxidants and memory performance in the old and very old. *J Am Geriatr Soc* 45(6):718–724, 1997.

Petersen, R.C., Aisen, P.S., Beckett, L.A., et al.: Alzheimer's Disease Neuroimaging Initiative: Clinical characterization. *Neurology* advance online publication doi:10.1212/WNL.0b013e3181cb3e25, 30 December 2009.

Petersen, R. and Jack, C. Imaging and biomarkers in early Alzheimer's disease and mild cognitive impairment. *Clinical Pharmacology and Therapeutics* advance online publication doi:10.1038/clpt.(2009).166, 26 August 2009.

Petersen, R.C.: Scopolamine induced learning failures in man. *Psychopharmacology (Berl)* 52(3):283–289, 1977.

Petersen, R.C.: Mild cognitive impairment as a diagnostic entity. *J Intern Med* 256(3):183–194, 2004.

Petersen, R.C.: Mild Cognitive Impairment. *Continuum: Lifelong Learning in Neurology* 10:9–28, 2004.

Petersen, R.C., Doody, R., Kurz, A., et al.: Current concepts in mild cognitive impairment. *Arch Neurol* 58(12):1985–1992, 2001.

Petersen, R.C., Parisi, J.E., Dickson, D.W., et al.: Neuropathologic features of amnestic mild cognitive impairment. *Arch Neurol* 63(5):665–672, 2006.

Petersen, R.C., Smith, G.E., Ivnik, R.J., et al.: Apolipoprotein E status as a predictor of the development of Alzheimer's disease in memory-impaired individuals. *JAMA* 273(16):1274–1278, 1995.

Petersen, R.C., Smith, G.E., Waring, S.C., et al.: Mild cognitive impairment: clinical characterization and outcome. *Arch Neurol* 56(3):303–308, 1999.

Petersen, R.C., Stevens, J.C., Ganguli, M., et al.: (2001). Practice parameter: early detection of dementia: Mild cognitive impairment (an evidence-based review). Report of the Quality Standards Subcommittee of the American Academy of Neurology. *Neurology* 56(9):1133–1142, 2001.

Petersen, R.C., Thomas, R.G., Grundman, M., et al.: Vitamin E and donepezil for the treatment of mild cognitive impairment. *N Engl J Med* 352(23):2379–2388, 2005.

Plassman B.L., Langa K.M., Fisher G.G., et al.: Prevalence of cognitive impairment without dementia in the United States. *Ann Intern Med*. 148(6):427–434, 2008.

Ray, S., Britschgi, M., Herbert, C., et al.: Classification and prediction of clinical Alzheimer's diagnosis based on plasma signaling proteins. *Nat Med* 13(11):1359–1362, 2007.

Reiman, E.M., Caselli, R.J., Yun, L.S., et al.: Preclinical evidence of Alzheimer's disease in persons homozygous for the epsilon 4 allele for apolipoprotein E. *N Engl J Med* 334(12):752–758, 1996.

Reitz. C., Tang, M.X., Manly, J., et al.: Hypertension and the risk of mild cognitive impairment. *Arch Neurol* 64(12):1734–40, 2007.

Ries, M.L., Carlsson, C.M., Rowley, H.A., et al.: Magnetic resonance imaging characterization of brain structure and function in mild cognitive impairment: a review. *J Am Geriatr Soc* 56(5):920–34, 2008.

Roberts, R.O., Geda, Y.E., Knopman, D., et al.: The Mayo Clinic Study of Aging: Design and sampling, participation, baseline measures and sample characteristics. *Neuroepidemiology* 30:58–69, 2008.

Rovio, S., Kareholt, I., Helkala, E.L., et al.: Leisure-time physical activity at midlife and the risk of dementia and Alzheimer's disease. *Lancet Neurol* 4(11):705–711, 2005.

Rozzini, L., Chilovi, B.V., Peli, M., et al.: Anxiety symptoms in mild cognitive impairment. *Int J Geriatr Psychiatry* Epub Sept 1, 2008.

Ryu, E.K. and Chen, X.: Development of Alzheimer's disease imaging agents for clinical studies. *Front Biosci* 13:777–789, 2008.

Shaw, L.M., Vanderstichele, H., Knappik-Czajka, M., et al.: Cerebrospinal fluid biomarker signature in Alzheimer's Disease Neuroimaging Initiative subjects. *Ann Neurol* 65:403–413, 2009.

Sloane, P.D., Zimmerman, S., Suchindran, C., et al.: The public health impact of Alzheimer's disease, 2000-2050: Potential implication of treatment advances. *Annu Rev Public Health* 23:213–231, 2002.

Small, G.W., Kepe, V., Ercoli, L.M., et al.: PET of brain amyloid and tau in mild cognitive impairment. *N Engl J Med* 355(25):2652–2663, 2006.

Small, G.W., Mazziotta, J.C., Collins, M.T., et al.: Apolipoprotein E type 4 allele and cerebral glucose metabolism in relatives at risk for familial Alzheimer disease. *JAMA* 273(12):942–947, 1995.

Smith, G.E., Petersen, R.C., Parisi, J.E., et al.: Definition, course, and outcome of mild cognitive impairment. *Aging Neuropsychology & Cognition* 3(2):141–147, 1996.

Teng, E., Lu, P.H., and Cummings, J.L.: Neuropsychiatric symptoms are associated withprogression from mild cognitive impairment to Alzheimer's disease. *Dement Geriatr Cogn Disord* 24(4):253–259, 2007.

Thal, L.J., Ferris, S.H., Kirby, L., et al.: A randomized, double-blind, study of rofecoxib in patients with mild cognitive impairment. *Neuropsychopharmacology* 30(6):1204–1215, 2005.

Tierney, M.C., Szalai, J.P., Snow, W.G., et al.: A prospective study of the clinical utility of ApoE genotype in the prediction of outcome in patients with memory impairment. *Neurology* 46(1):149–154, 1996.

Tschanz, J.T., Welsh-Bohmer, K.A., Lyketsos, C.G., et al.: Conversion to dementia from mild cognitive disorder: The Cache County Study. *Neurology* 67(2):229–234, 2006.

Unverzagt, F.W., Gao, S., Baiyewu, O., et al.: Prevalence of cognitive impairment: Data from the Indianapolis Study of Health and Aging. *Neurology* 57(9):1655–1662, 2001.

van de Pol, L.A., van der Flier, W.M., Korf, E.S., et al.: Baseline predictors of rates of hippocampal atrophy in mild cognitive impairment. *Neurology* 69(15):1491–1497, 2007.

van Oijen, M., Hofman, A., Soares, H.D., et al.: Plasma Abeta(1-40) and Abeta(1-42) and the risk of dementia: A prospective case-cohort study. *Lancet Neurol* 5(8):655–660, 2006.

Visser, P.J., Scheltens, P., Verhey, F.R., et al.: Medial temporal lobe atrophy and memory dysfuction as predictors for dementia in subjects with mild cognitive impairment. *J Neuro.* 246(6):477–485, 1999.

Whitehouse, P.J., Price, D.L., Clark, A.W., et al.: Alzheimer disease: Evidence for selective loss of cholinergic neurons in the nucleus basalis. *Ann Neurol* 10(2):122–126, 1981.

Winblad, B., Gauthier, S., Scinto, L., et al.: Safety and efficacy of galantamine in subjects with mild cognitive impairment. *Neurology* 70(22):2024–35, 2008.

Winblad, B., Palmer, K., Kivipelto, M., et al.: Mild cognitive impairment—beyond controversies, towards a consensus: Report of the International Working Group on Mild Cognitive Impairment. *J Intern Med* 256(3):240–246, 2004.

Wolk, D.A., Price, J.C., Saxton, J.A., et al.: Amyloid imaging in mild cognitive impairment subtypes. *Ann Neurol* 65(5):557–568, 2009.

Zhu C.W., Scarmeas N., Torgan R., et al.: Longitudinal study of effects of patient characteristics on direct costs in Alzheimer's disease. *Neurology* 67;998–1005, 2006.

16 Alzheimer's Disease

David A. Bennett

Introduction

As a result of declining fertility and increasing life expectancy, the 20th century witnessed a remarkable increase in the number and proportion of older persons. These demographic trends will continue well into this century. The aging of the population has wide ranging health-related consequences, as older persons are at risk for a number of chronic conditions that are relatively rare among younger persons. These conditions impair the ability of older persons to function optimally in the community, reduce wellbeing for both the individuals and their families, and are associated with significant health care costs that must be borne by individuals, their families, and society at large. Dementia, which refers to a significant loss of cognition relative to a previous level of performance, is among the most common and devastating conditions of old age. While loss of cognitive abilities in old age has been recognized since antiquity, the disease that bears his name was described by Dr. Alois Alzheimer barely 100 years ago.

In 1906, Dr. Alzheimer described the case of a 51-year-old woman, Auguste D. She died following a four year course of progressive dementia. He examined her brain and ascribed her dementia to the neuritic plaques and neurofibrillary tangles that now characterize the disease. Over the next several decades, Alzheimer's disease (AD) was thought to be a relatively rare progressive dementia of mid-life; a condition quite separate from the all too common senility of old age. However, a series of clinical-pathologic studies conducted in the 1960s and 1970s demonstrated that AD was also the most common cause of dementia in old age. It was soon recognized that a combination of the high prevalence of AD in old age coupled with the changing demographics would result in a major public health burden. These predictions, unfortunately, have come true, making AD the subject of intense clinical, scientific, public health, and public policy interest in the United States and other nations around the world.

Epidemiology

Epidemiology is the study of the distribution and causes of disease in human populations. It is often separated into descriptive epidemiology, which refers to studies that describe the distribution, correlates, and consequences of disease; observational analytic epidemiology, either case control or cohort studies, which refers to studies designed to identify putative causes of disease; and experimental analytic epidemiology, or clinical trials, which refer to cohort studies that randomize the exposure.

Descriptive Epidemiology

Descriptive epidemiology is important for determining the scope of a disease and is important for public health planning. There are a number of key indicators including incidence, mortality, prevalence, and economic impact which are used to establish the public health importance of a disease. Because many people with AD do not come to the attention of the health care system (as opposed to some other diseases such as glioblastoma), descriptive epidemiologic data is best obtained from population-based studies conducted in geographically defined communities.

Incidence

Incidence refers to the number of new cases of a condition that occur in a population over a given period of time. Because the number of new cases depends on the length of follow-up and follow-up time varies across studies and persons, incidence rates usually refer to the number of new cases per 1000 person-years. The incidence of AD has been examined in several populations around the world. In general, the results suggest that the incidence of disease increases markedly with age beginning in the seventh decade of life and continues to increase exponentially until at least the tenth decade of life (Tang et al. 2001). The incidence effectively doubles with every five additional years of age after age 65, such that about one person out of every hundred persons between the ages of 65 and 74 will get the disease each year, whereas about four out of every hundred persons between the ages of 75 and 84 will get the disease each year, and about nine out of every hundred persons over age 85 will get the disease each year. Given the increasing number of persons expected in the at-risk older age group, the incidence of AD is expected to increase correspondingly and more than double from 1995 to 2050.

Some data suggest that women may be at increased risk. However, the number of women that live to the age of highest risk far outnumber men such that it is difficult to make stable comparisons. There is also evidence that African Americans and Hispanics are at greater risk. However, making a diagnosis of AD in a similar fashion among whites and racial and ethnic minorities can be difficult due to pre-morbid differences on cognitive performance.

Mortality

Survival with AD depends on a variety of factors, especially age and sex. However, most data regarding survival with the disease comes from persons who come to the attention of the health care system who have the disease for some time. These persons tend to be younger, and thus tend to survive longer. Further, most data is from persons with prevalent disease. This tends to overestimate survival because persons with more rapidly progressive dementia are under-represented among prevalent cases (prevalence bias). Little data is available regarding survival from incident cases. Disease duration from diagnosis is more than 4 years for men and nearly 6 years for women (Larson et al. 2004). Disease duration is more than 8 years for persons diagnosed at age 65 but only about 3.5 years for persons diagnosed at age 90 (Brookmeyer et al. 2002). However, survival may be as short as 3.5 years among community dwelling elderly from the time of disease onset. Overall, persons with the disease are at greater risk of death after adjusting for age and sex. Among persons with AD, several factors have been consistently associated with risk of death including severity of cognitive impairment, parkinsonian signs, and more years of formal education.

Prevalence

Prevalence refers to the number of cases of a condition in a population at a particular time. Thus, it is essentially a combination of incidence plus disease duration. There have been a number of population-based prevalence studies, some of which have been used to estimate the prevalence of AD in the United States (Hebert et al. 2003). The numbers range from nearly 3 million to about 4.5 million persons with the disease at the turn of the last century. The reasons behind these discrepancies are not completely understood. However, a number of factors are known to alter prevalence estimates, especially the extent to which persons with mild disease are included, the use of laboratory tests, and the use of weights to estimate the prevalence from a sample of the population. The number of persons with dementia in the world has been estimated to be between 25–30 million persons (Ferri et al. 2005). While the numbers vary, in some cases widely, what is clear is the number is large and all estimates forecast a large increase in the number of cases, essentially doubling every several years such that the number of persons with AD worldwide will exceed 100 million by the middle of this century.

Economic Impact

The cost of care for persons with dementia due to AD and other conditions is borne by the individual, her family, and society as a whole. Some of the costs are direct health care expenditures such as health care professionals' fees, medications, and hospitalization, while others reflect costs of in-home and long-term care, and still others reflect indirect costs such as donation of care-giving time, lost wages to businesses, and reduced tax revenues to governments (Langa et al. 2001). Worldwide, costs for dementia in 2003 approached $250 billion annually. This is larger than the gross national product of more than 90% of the countries in the world. According to an estimate by the Lasker Foundation published in 2002, AD was the third most costly disease in the United States, with an estimated direct and indirect cost of about $100 billion annually.

Future Trends: There are now about 40 million persons over age 65 in the US. By 2030, more than 70 million persons, or about one in five Americans, will be over age 65. These demographic changes are expected to result in a marked increase in the absolute number and proportion of persons with AD. In the United States, the number of persons with AD is expected to double or triple by the middle of this century, depending on census projections, to an estimated 8.5–13 million persons (Hebert et al. 2003). Similar demographic changes are occurring across the globe. Worldwide, the population over the age of 65 was about 550 million in 2000; the number of older persons is expected to nearly double to about one billion by 2030. By mid century, more than 100 million persons worldwide will have AD (Brookmeyer et al. 2007). Given the large numbers and costs, the prevention of AD is among the must urgent major public health issues of this century.

Analytic Epidemiology

Analytic epidemiology is important for identifying factors associated with risk (increased or decreased) of disease. Risk factor data are generated from observational case-control or cohort studies. In general, the associations from such studies are correlational and do not imply causation. For example, while age is the most robust risk factor for AD, it is not clear that age causes disease. It is much more likely that age is a proxy for unknown factors related to age that cause disease. In some

cases, a combination of robust and consistent associations from observational studies, and ethical, financial or methodological concerns precluding clinical trials, can result in some associations being considered causal. For example, despite the absence of clinical trial data, the medical community and policy makers have come to accept the fact that smoking causes lung cancer. Finally, for diseases that develop slowly over years such as AD, early signs of disease will predict the development of disease and appear to be risk factors. For example, mild cognitive impairment and hippocampal volume are associated with risk of AD. However, they are really just early signs of the disease.

Risk Factors: Numerous factors have been associated with risk of AD. A partial list is provided in Table 1. Perhaps the most robust factor

Table 1 Factors Associated with Risk of Alzheimer's Disease

Author (year)	Demographic Factors
Evans et al. (1989)	Age
Tang et al. (1998)	African American
Tang et al. (1998)	Hispanic
Experiential Factors	
Stern et al. (1994)	Years of education
Wilson et al. (2007)	Early life cognitive activities
Stern et al. (1994)	Occupational status
Wilson et al. (2002)	Late-life cognitive activites
Podewils et al. (2005)	Physical activities
Scarmeas et al. (2007)	Leisure activities
Bennett et al. (2006)	Social networks
Vascular Factors	
Snowdon et al. (1997)	Cerebrovascular disease (cerebral infarction)
Newman et al. (2005)	Cardiovascular disease
Arvanitakis et al. (2004)	Diabetes
Kivipelto et al. (2001)	Hypertension
Merchant et al. (1999)	Smoking
Personality and Psychological Factors	
Wilson et al. (2003)	Distress proneness
Wilson et al. (2007)	Loneliness
Wilson et al. (2007)	Conscientiousness
Devanand et al. (1996)	Depressive symptoms
Other Factors	
Schofield et al. (1997)	Head trauma
Luchsinger et al. (2007)	Diet and nutrition
in t' Veld et al. (2001)	Anti-inflammatories
Early Non-cognitive Signs	
Wilson et al. (2003)	Parkinsonian signs
Buchman et al. (2005)	Loss of body mass index (weight loss)
Buchman et al. (2007)	Physical frailty
Wang et al. (2006)	Physical function
Devanand et al. (2000)	Olfactory identification

is age. While tertiary care medical centers often see patients in their fifth or sixth decade of life, in community populations AD is uncommon under the age of 65. By contrast, between a third and a half of persons over the age of 85 have the disease. While some data suggest that women and racial and ethnic minorities are at increased risk, this remains controversial.

A number of experiential factors have been related to risk of AD. Most studied is years of formal education, which is associated with a reduced risk of disease in many but not all studies. Factors related to education such as perceived occupational status are also associated with reduced risk. Cognitive, physical, and leisure activity, and social networks have all been associated with a reduced risk of AD.

Cerebrovascular disease and factors associated with risk of cerebrovascular disease have been related to risk of clinical AD. These include cardiovascular disease, diabetes, hypertension, and smoking. In some cases, the associations were strongest when the exposure was measured in mid-life rather than in the few years prior to disease onset.

Several psychological factors and personality traits have been related to risk of AD. Proneness to psychological distress (i.e., neuroticism) has been associated with increased risk. Perceived social isolation (i.e., loneliness) has also been associated with increased risk. By contrast, conscientiousness has been associated with reduced risk. Depressive symptoms have been associated with an increased risk in many but not all studies.

A number of other factors have been related to risk of AD. In particular, head trauma has been associated with AD risk. A number of dietary and nutritional factors such as vitamin E, folate, omega-3 fatty acids, and fish also have been related to risk of AD in some studies but not others. In addition, medications such as statins and anti-inflammatories have been associated with disease risk in some studies but not in clinical trials. Studies that examine these factors are prone to numerous biases making it difficult to draw delimitative conclusions in the absence of a clinical trial.

Early Non-cognitive Signs of Alzheimer's Disease

A number of factors related to the occurrence of clinical AD are probably early signs of disease rather than true risk factors. For example, parkinsonian (extra pyramidal) signs, loss of body mass index (weight loss), physical frailty, and physical function are common non-cognitive features of AD (see below). It is likely that these signs are developing in conjunction with cognitive decline and are detectable before some people meet the threshold for the diagnosis of dementia. In this way they can predict the clinical syndrome.

Pathophysiology

The pathologic hallmarks of AD are the accumulation of extracellular deposits of amyloid-β peptide and the intracellular accumulation of hyperphosphorylated tau proteins. Pathologically, these are visualized as neuritic and diffuse plaques and neurofibrillary tangles, most commonly using a silver stain such as modified Bielshowsky (Figure 1). Thioflavin S, which binds to beta pleated sheets and exhibits birefringence under polarized light, is also used to identify plaques.

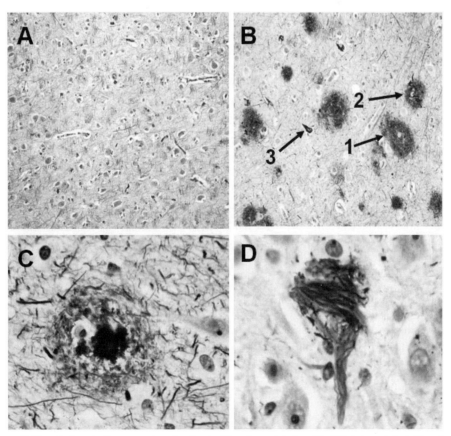

Figure 1 Alzheimer's disease (AD) pathology in the neocortex visualized with a silver stain (modified Bielschowsky). A. The absence of AD pathology. B. AD pathology illustrating (1) diffuse plaques, (2) neuritic plaques, and (3) neurofibrillary tangles. C. High power view of classic neuritic plaque. D. High power view of neurofibrillary tangle.

Currently, there are two sets of criteria in common use for the pathologic diagnosis of AD. One, developed by the Consortium to Establish a Registry for Alzheimer's Disease (CERAD), is based on the density of neocortical neuritic plaques (Mirra et al. 1991). These criteria are often used to confirm a diagnosis of AD since they require that dementia be present in order for the "clinical-pathologic" diagnosis of AD to be made. The second is based on both the density of neocortical neuritic plaques and the presence and distribution of neurofibrillary tangles (Consensus recommendations 1997). These criteria make probabilistic statements about the likelihood of dementia based on the distribution and severity of AD pathology. It should be noted that while nearly all persons who meet clinical criteria for AD also meet pathologic criteria (Bennett et al. 2006), many persons without dementia, including those with mild cognitive impairment (Bennett et al. 2005) and even those without cognitive impairment (Bennett et al. 2006), have sufficient pathology to meet current pathologic thresholds for the disease. This has led to the idea of neural or cognitive reserve whereby some persons have factors protecting them from expressing AD as cognitive impairment (Stern 2002). The identification of such factors has important implications for the prevention of clinical dementia. For example, several of the risk factors for AD listed in Table 1 do not appear to be directly related to the development of AD pathology (Bennett et al. 2006; Wilson et al. 2007; Wilson et al. 2007).

The pathology of AD is not uniformly distributed across the brain. Rather, there are certain brain regions that are selectively vulnerable to the accumulation of the pathology, including the hippocampus and entorhinal cortex, neocortical association areas, and the cholinergic basal forebrain. This observation has been used to develop staging schemes for neurofibrillary tangles which are based on the geographic distribution of the pathology and which correlate, to some extent, with the severity of cognitive impairment (Braak et al. 1991). This selective vulnerability, and the resultant pattern of brain atrophy, has also been used to identify structural neuroimaging indicators of the disease. Finally, it has been nearly three decades since deficits in the basal forebrain cholinergic system in AD led to the cholinergic hypothesis. Manipulation of the cholinergic system remains one of the few approved therapeutic strategies for the symptomatic treatment of AD.

Amyloid Metabolism: Much has been learned about amyloid metabolism over the past two decades which have had important implications for therapeutic strategies for the treatment and prevention of AD (Golde 2006). Brain amyloid deposits are composed of fibrillar aggregates of primarily 40 to 42 amino acid peptides called amyloid-β. Brain deposits of amyloid-β result from endoproteolysis of a large transmembrane protein called the amyloid precursor protein (APP). APP is cleaved by three enzymes known as α-, β-, and γ-secretase. The initial cleavage is β-secretase, which is β-site, APP-cleaving enzyme 1 (BACE1) (Cole and Vassar 2008). Following this cleavage, the resulting fragment is further cleaved by either α- or γ-secretase. γ-secretase, an enzyme complex that includes the protein presenilin, cleaves APP resulting in amyloid-β via the γ-secretase pathway (Selkoe and Wolfe 2007). The accumulation of amyloid begins with soluble monomers which then coalesce into oligomers, followed by insoluble fibrils, and ultimately amyloid plaques that can be visualized under a microscope. Deposited amyloid can now be visualized by positron emission tomography (PET). By contrast, α-secretase cleaves APP in the middle of the amyloid-β sequence, resulting in innocuous APP fragments via the α-secretase pathway.

While deposited amyloid plaques correlate, to some extent, with cognitive status (Bennett et al. 2004), it is not clear that these deposits are toxic. This is important because one strategy being advanced for the treatment of AD is administration of an active vaccine which would remove amyloid. Evidence from preclinical studies suggests that the soluble species may, in fact, represent the neurotoxic aspect of amyloid (Lesne et al. 2006). Either way, the primacy of altered amyloid metabolism in the sequence of events leading to dementia is called the amyloid hypothesis (Hardy and Selkoe 2002). Numerous therapeutic strategies have been developed and have been or are currently being tested to prevent the formation and accumulation of amyloid, and to enhance its degradation and clearance.

Tau Metabolism: Tau is a microtuble binding protein involved in the formation and stabilization of microtubules, a structural component of cells (Ballatore et al. 2007). Tau function is regulated by phosphorylation catalyzed by protein kinases. In the AD brain, tau is hyperphosphorylated, which via mechanisms as yet unknown, results in aggregation and the formation of filaments that can be visualized under a microscope. Recently, PET can also visualize these lesions. As tangles generally correspond much more closely than amyloid to dementia severity, considerable efforts are being expended, with limited success, to identify therapeutic strategies to alter tau metabolism.

Other: There are a number of other findings in the brains of persons with AD such as inflammation and oxidative stress. The extent to which these contribute to cognitive impairment is not well established. However, they represent other therapeutic targets that have been the subject of clinical trials.

Genetic Contributions

It has long been known that genetic factors play an important role in the development of AD (Table 2). Familial aggregation studies report that first degree relatives of probands with AD are more likely to have or develop AD compared to relatives of controls (Farrer et al. 1990). Twin studies report a higher concordance of AD among monozygotic compared to dizygotic twins, with heritability estimates between 60% and 80% (Gatz et al. 2006). Variants in four genes are now accepted as increasing the risk of or causing AD (Ertekin-Taner 2008).

Mutations: Mutations in three genes are known to cause early-onset AD. There are about 25 mutations in the amyloid precursor protein (APP) gene on chromosome 21. This is the APP that is the precursor to the deposited amyloid-β peptide. In addition, there are about 150 mutations in the presenilin 1 gene (*PSEN1*) on chromosome 14 and about 10 mutations in the presenilin 2 gene (*PSEN2*) on chromosome 1. Presenilin is part of the complex of proteins that comprise γ-secretase. Thus, all three mutations for early-onset AD are involved in the metabolism of amyloid, providing strong support for the amyloid hypothesis. While these mutations account for the majority of cases of autosomal dominant transmission of AD, autosomal dominant AD is a rare form of AD and they probably account for less than 1% of all cases of the disease.

Table 2 Genetic Factors Associated with Risk of Alzheimer's Disease

Author (year)	Genetic Mutations
Goate et al. (1991)	Amyloid precursor protein, chromosome 21
Sherrington et al. (1995)	Presenilin 1, chromosome 14
Levy-Lahad et al. (1995)	Presenilin 2, chromosome 1
Genetic Polymorphisms	
Corder et al. (1993)	Apolipoprotein E ε4 allele, chromosome 19
Corder et al. (1994)	Apolipoprotein E ε2 allele, chromosome 19

Genetic Polymorphisms: A polymorphism in the gene coding for apolipoprotein E (*APOE*) on chromosome 19 is associated with risk of late-onset AD (LOAD). With *APOE* 3/3 as the reference group, persons with one or two 4 alleles are at increased risk of AD and those with the 2 allele are at a reduced risk (Farrer et al. 1997). These associations have been confirmed in numerous studies of European ancestry, although results among racial and ethnic minorities have been conflicting. Like the mutations, considerable evidence implicates APOE in the metabolism of amyloid, but other mechanisms also appear important. The population attributable risk of AD due to these polymorphisms has been estimated to be about 10% to 15%, suggesting that many other genetic risk factors remain to be identified (Evans et al. 2003). Numerous other polymorphisms have been reported to be associated with risk of AD, but none of these have been consistently replicated (Bertram et al. 2007). This is partly due to the difficulty of identifying and confirming polymorphisms that likely have small effect sizes for complex diseases (Kennedy et al. 2003). It is also due, in part, to phenotypic heterogeneity such that the clinical AD phenotype is often the result of both AD pathology and other pathology (Bennett et al. in press; Schneider et al. 2009). A number of polymorphisms remain to be identified and gene discovery efforts are ongoing worldwide.

Clinical Characteristics

Clinically, AD is defined by progressive loss of memory and other cognitive abilities with impairment documented by neuropsychological performance tests (McKhann et al. 1984). However, the disease is frequently accompanied by changes in mood, behavior, and impaired motor function.

Cognitive Function

Memory is the recording, retention, and retrieval of information. It accounts for all knowledge gained through experience, including the memories of specific events, knowledge of facts, and the acquisition of skills. Memory is not a unitary process as diseases such as AD, or focal brain lesions such as stroke, can impair some forms of memory while leaving others relatively intact. Thus memory represents dissociable systems that mediate different types of mnemonic processing including episodic memory, semantic memory, working memory, perceptual speed, and implicit memory. All of these memory systems can be impaired from AD pathology (Schneider et al. 2007; Fleischman et al. 2005).

Episodic memory: Episodic memory refers to learning and retention of specific events, or episodes, embedded within the autobiographical, temporal context, of one's life. Progressive loss of episodic memory is the clinical hallmark of AD and may often be the sole deficit early in the disease process. This memory system requires an intact hippocampal formation, an area of the brain almost universally affected by AD pathology. Episodic memory is assessed by asking the patient to learn new information such as a brief story or list of unrelated words, and then testing retention after a short delay that includes a distraction (e.g., another cognitive test inserted between the learning phase and recall phase). In such a paradigm, one is testing learning and free recall. A recognition procedure is typically added to these tests.

Semantic memory: Semantic memory refers to previously acquired general knowledge such as facts and language abilities. In contrast to episodic memory, semantic memory is unconcerned with the context in which the facts were learned. Whereas the hippocampal formation is required for encoding new information, it is not required for information retrieval. Rather, general knowledge is thought to be stored in domain-specific neocortical association regions. When one of these regions is damaged, information stored in the area is lost and the patient is unable to acquire new knowledge of that type. As AD progresses, deficits in semantic memory occur that are thought to reflect the involvement of AD pathology in these regions. Semantic memory is assessed by asking the patient to name public figures, pictured objects (visual confrontation naming), or to define a list of words (vocabulary test).

Working memory: Working memory refers to the ability to hold and manipulate information in short-term, limited-capacity memory stores. This type of memory is similar to attention and is well known to decline with age separately from its decline in AD. Working memory is hypothesized to be mediated by a frontal-striatal dopaminergic system. Working memory is assessed by asking the patient to repeat a random series of numbers in reverse (digits backward) or in ascending order (digit ordering). Other experimental paradigms require simultaneous performance of two tasks.

Perceptual speed: Perceptual speed is also related to attention and is impaired early in AD. It refers to the speed with which simple perceptual comparisons can be made. Similar to working memory, perceptual speed also may be mediated by a frontal-striatal dopaminergic system and declines with age as well as AD. It also appears to be highly susceptible to damage from cerebrovascular disease. Perceptual speed can be assessed with symbol substitution tasks in which the patient is provided with a key consisting of a series of symbols with corresponding digits. The patient is subsequently given a list of symbols in random order and is asked to match each with the corresponding digit within a given time limit (symbol digit).

Implicit memory: Implicit memory refers to a change in task performance attributable to prior experience in the absence of explicit instructions to remember the experience. In contrast to the cognitive abilities outlined above, implicit memory is typically measured as the unconscious change in speed, accuracy, or response bias in the processing of study-phase stimuli. Implicit memory skills are thought to involve domain-specific regions. For example, AD pathology has been related to conceptual (i.e., meaning-based) cognitive processing but not perceptual (i.e., sensory-based) cognitive processing. Another example of implicit memory is skill learning (procedural or motor) which is thought to require the basal ganglia.

Affective Disturbances

Depressive symptoms are common in AD and typically precede the diagnosis. About a third of persons with AD have depression (Lyketsos et al. 2002). The diagnosis of major depression can be problematic, as vegetative signs such as poor appetite, early morning awakening, reduced energy level, inability to concentrate, restlessness and agitation, and disinterest may result from impaired cognition. However, dysphoria is also common and indicative of depression. The extent to which depressive symptoms are associated with risk of AD or represent an early sign of disease remains controversial (Steffans et al. 2006). The biology of depression in AD is also controversial as AD pathology has been related to depression in some studies (Rapp et al. 2006) but not others (Bennett et al. 2004).

Behavioral Disturbances

Most AD patients display one or more of a wide variety of behavioral disturbances (Lyketsos et al. 2002). Apathy, agitation, and aggression are the most common behavioral disturbances, each present in about a third of patients. Agitation and aggression are primarily motor overactivities and include fidgetiness and pacing, with or without physical aggression such as hitting, biting, and scratching, or verbally aggressive behavior such as threats or obscenities. Many AD patients pace, but this is only a concern if the patient wanders out of the immediate environment. Less common are psychotic symptoms including visual and auditory hallucinations, misperceptions, and delusions. These occur in about a quarter of patients and may be more common early in the disease. Common formed delusions include thinking that someone is stealing from them, that their caregiver will abandon them, or that their spouse is unfaithful. Visual hallucinations are more common than auditory ones and appear to be more common in advanced disease. Misperceptions include the inability to recognize oneself in the mirror, conversing with a person in a photograph or mirror, and thinking that people on television are real. Patients may also appear to have a fear of being alone. It is not unusual for patients to follow their caregivers from room to room, including into the bathroom, allowing them little privacy or rest. Little is known about the neurobiology of behavioral disturbances. AD pathology in the orbital frontal cortex and cingulate gyrus has been related to agitation (Tekin et al. 2001). The pathology of psychotic symptoms is less secure (Sweet et al. 2000). However, the association of psychotic symptoms with parkinsonian signs raises the possibility of involvement of the dopamine system.

Sleep Disturbance

Altered sleep behavior is a common problem in AD. Nocturnally disrupted sleep may manifest as nighttime agitation, early awakening, excessive daytime sleepiness, and disrupted chronology, altering sleep-wake cycles with patients sleeping much of the day. While sleep disturbances are more common in AD compared to persons without dementia, it should be noted that older patients with AD also experience other age-related sleep problems, including sleep-disordered breathing such as sleep apnea. Further, the cholinesterase inhibitors commonly used to treat cognition in AD are associated with insomnia and vivid dreams and represent an iatrogenic cause of sleep disturbance in AD. On polysomnography, AD patients show decreased rapid eye movement (REM) sleep which is related to the severity of cognitive impairment. Little is known about the neurobiology of sleep disturbance in AD. However, some observations suggest that it is related to synucleinopathies such as the association of REM sleep disturbance with Lewy body disease (Boeve et al. 2007) and the fact that sleep disturbance in AD is related to parkinsonian signs (Park et al. 2006).

Motoric Dysfunction

AD is accompanied by a wide range of changes in motor structure and function, especially Parkinsonian or extrapyramidal signs. These signs include bradykinesia, gait disturbance, rigidity, and tremor. They are not uncommon early in the disease and become more common as the severity of cognitive impairment increases. Pathology in the substantia nigra, especially neurofibrillary tangles (Schneider et al. 2006) and Lewy bodies (Burns et al. 2005) are related to parkinsonian signs. Weight loss and loss of body mass index is also common in AD and is also related to AD pathology (Buchman et al. 2006). Physical frailty, composed of grip strength, timed walk, body composition, and fatigue is also common and progressive in AD and is also related to AD pathology (Buchman et al. 2008). Myoclonus is another motor sign that becomes more common as the disease advances (Chen et al. 1991).

Disability and Driving

Disability refers to a physical or mental impairment that substantially limits life activity. Disability is among the most important public health consequences of cognitive decline due to AD and is considered a defining feature of dementia. For relatively young persons with AD, disability may be due to loss of occupational ability. This is especially true for persons with occupations that have high cognitive demands.

However, most people with AD are older persons who are not working and suffer from one to several co-morbidities. In these persons, AD will initially result in loss of higher order functional abilities such as driving. Eventually, AD will impair instrumental activities of daily living such as managing finances, shopping, preparing meals, taking medications, and using the phone. As the disease advances, basic activities of daily living including eating, dressing, bathing, and toileting, become problematic.

Diagnosis

Currently, the clinical diagnosis of AD requires the presence of a dementia syndrome. However, the dementia syndrome of AD develops over many months or even years and most if not all persons with AD pass through a phase when cognitive impairment is present but dementia is not. This phase is called mild cognitive impairment (Gauthier et al. 2006). Thus, as more is learned about the early stages of AD, as disease biomarkers become available, and as effective therapeutic strategies are developed, a diagnosis will be possible and prudent prior to the development of overt dementia (Dubois, et al. 2007). At this time, however, the clinical evaluation should focus first on determining the presence of dementia and subsequently on the presence of AD. It should be noted that for many years, AD was considered a "diagnosis of exclusion." In other words, following determination of dementia, causes of dementia were sought and if none could be found, a diagnosis of AD was made. This approach is no longer acceptable. Most importantly, the presence of AD does not prevent the occurrence of other common age-related problems and it turns out that the most common cause of AD in the elderly is AD pathology plus another condition, in particular cerebrovascular disease and Lewy body disease (Schneider et al. 2009). Thus, the clinical evaluation should focus on determining whether the history, clinical evaluation, and laboratory tests are consistent with AD.

Medical History

The medical history should be obtained from a knowledgeable informant when one is available. This could be a spouse, adult child, sibling or other relative, or a close friend. In some cases informants are not available, or they are available but not knowledgeable. Thus, a history also should be obtained from the patient. Self-report cognitive complaints from older persons should be taken seriously as they have been shown to be related to AD pathology (Barnes et al. 2006). The medical history should focus on documenting loss of memory and other cognitive abilities as the defining features of AD. However, it should also elicit evidence of changes in mood, behavior, sleep disturbance, and disturbances in motor function as these contribute to the patient's function and to caregiver distress.

Cognitive Decline: Prior to obtaining information about decline in cognitive abilities, it is important to establish the patient's pre-morbid level of functioning. Thus, the history should start by documenting years of education, occupation, and other pre-morbid activities and abilities. The history should focus on the nature, timing, and evolution of cognitive decline, with an emphasis on decline in episodic memory. Thus, after documenting the first problem noticed by the informant, the physician should inquire into other areas, such as whether the patient was repeating questions, had difficulty recollecting events, misplaced important items, and got lost, especially when out of town. The informant will sometimes recollect some event that triggered the cognitive problems. However, the clinician should take care to differentiate an abrupt recognition of the problem by the observer from an actual abrupt onset. Informants will also assign cognitive deficits to other medical problems. For example, you may be told: She repeats questions because she is hard of hearing; she no longer does the crossword puzzles because of her macular degeneration; she finds it hard to cook because of her arthritis. Evidence of impairment in other cognitive abilities such as language, executive function, calculations, and visuospatial ability should be sought. This includes asking about word finding difficulties, difficulty making detailed plans, balancing a checkbook, and impaired facial recognition. The clinical hallmark of AD is the insidious onset and progression of memory deficits followed by deficits in other cognitive abilities. The presence of slowly progressive and profound deficits in episodic memory is nearly always the beginning of AD. Unfortunately, because AD often coexists with other conditions, the episodic memory impairment may be less pronounced relative to other problems. Care should be taken to separate the onset and progression from other dementing illnesses which are discussed elsewhere in this volume.

There are few brief formal interviews designed and validated to identify mild dementia. One is the AD8 (Galvin et al. 2005). There are eight questions including changes in memory such as repeating stories, statements or questions, forgetting the month or year, forgetting appointments, and difficulty learning the use of new technology; impaired judgment and difficulty handling complicated financial matters; and loss of interest in hobbies and activities. While not necessarily specific for AD, it is heavily laden with episodic memory and is likely to identify early AD.

Changes in Mood, Behavior, and Sleep: The Neuropsychiatric Inventory (NPI) is among the most widely used informant-based instruments to assess a range of psychopathology in persons with AD (Cummings et al. 1994). It can be used to rapidly determine the presence of psychotic features including hallucinations and delusions, and it assesses dysphoria and euphoria, anxiety, agitation/aggression, disinhibition, irritability/lability, apathy, and aberrant motor activity. The informant should also be asked whether the patient seems sad, cries, or has voiced any passive or active suicidal ideation (Barak and Aizenberg 2002). Vegetative signs in the absence of dysphoria may be due to cognitive impairment in the absence of depression. However, as depression in AD is generally thought to be treatable, one should be vigilant. One clue to the possibility of depression in the absence of significant dysphoria is an apparent mismatch between the severity of cognitive deficits and the severity of functional impairment as depression is related to disability separate from cognition (Benoit et al. 2008). Informants should be asked if the patient is physically or verbally abusive. Has the patient ever hit or spit at the caregiver? They also should be asked if the patient wanders. Informants should be asked how the patient is sleeping. Does she sleep through the night? Is she sleepy during the day?

Changes in Motor Function: The informant should be asked if the patient has difficulty walking. In particular, is she slow, unsteady, and has she fallen? If the patient has changes in gait, the interview should focus on determining the timing and severity of the gait disturbance relative to the onset of cognitive decline. While parkinsonian signs often precede the development of AD, these signs tend to be relatively mild and slowly progressive (Wilson et al. 2003). By contrast, significant and more rapidly progressive parkinsonian signs prior to or concurrent with cognitive decline should raise the possibility of Lewy body disease. The history should also elicit evidence of unintended weight loss. A stroke can also contribute to impaired motor function and its presence should be considered a coexisting condition when it occurs in the context of a progressive and profound loss of episodic memory.

Functional Ability and Driving: A careful interview regarding the patient's functional abilities is essential to proper clinical management. This will need to be tailored to each patient's age, gender, living situation and available social support, and severity of cognitive impairment. For patients who are employed, a careful assessment of disability is essential to ensure that the patient receives the appropriate social care benefits, if appropriate, before she loses her job due to poor performance. For patients living alone, it is necessary to ensure that they are not a hazard to themselves or others. For example, is the patient leaving food in the oven or on a hot stove? If so, one might want to disconnect the gas or electricity and ensure that the facility has adequate fire alarms. Disability can be assessed with the Functional Activities Questionnaire (FAQ) (Pfeffer et al. 1982).

Driving is a higher level functional ability frequently affected by AD. While many patients with AD curtail their driving on their own or from pressure from family members (Foley et al. 2000), some patients with AD continue to drive. The extent to which these persons are at greater motor vehicle crash risk compared to other high risk groups (e.g., 16–24 year old males) remains controversial as the risk estimates differ markedly whether one considers absolute crash risk vs. crash risk per mile driven. However, many patients will continue to drive. Thus, it is important to know whether the patient is driving, and whether he is having accidents and represents a hazard to himself or others, as some patients with mild AD may in fact be able to operate a motor vehicle (Ott et al. 2008).

Neurologic Evaluation

The neurologic examination should focus on the assessment of cognition and look for evidence of stroke and parkinsonian signs, which may suggest diagnoses other than AD. Though, other conditions typically coexist with AD.

Bedside Cognitive Testing: A number of brief cognitive screening tools are available for the evaluation of persons with possible dementia (Table 3). None are specific for AD and all have significant limitations related to sensitivity and specificity. Nonetheless, they are an important adjunct to the medical history in order to document the presence of cognitive impairment.

The Mini-Mental Status Examination (MMSE) is perhaps the most widely used bedside mental status test. It takes 10–15 minutes to administer. There are a total of 30 points. Orientation to time and place is worth 10 points. There is an immediate and delayed recall of three words worth three points each. The distracter prior to administration of the delayed recall is a five point measure of attention which is typically spelling the word "WORLD" backwards or counting backwards by 7 from 100. Eight of the remaining nine points are language function and include naming, repetition, a three-step verbal command, reading, andwriting. Finally there is one point for copying a design (intersecting pentagons).

Table 3 Cognitive Screening Tests

Author (year)	Test
Folstein et al. (1975)	Mini-Mental Status Examination
Sunderland et al. (1989)	Clock Drawing Test
Borson et al. (2000)	Mini-Cog
Solomon et al. (1998)	7-Minute Screen
Nasreddine et al. (2005)	Montreal Cognitive Assessment

A screening cognitive test that takes less time than the MMSE is the Mini-Cog. The Mini-Cog combines a three word recall with the clock drawing test. The 7-minute screen is comprised of four tests, including a cued recall, category fluency, orientation, and the clock drawing test. All of these tests are somewhat insensitive to mild dementia. The Montreal Cognitive Assessment is a 10-minute screening test that is thought to be sensitive to very mild dementia. It includes short-term recall, the clock drawing test and figure copying, trails, verbal fluency, a verbal abstraction test, a serial subtraction task and digits forward and backward, naming and repetition, and orientation.

Assessment of Mood: The patient should be interviewed about dysphoria in addition to asking for an informant report. A number of instruments are available for the rapid assessment of depressive symptoms and clinical depression. A ten-item version of the Center for Epidemiologic Studies Depression Scale (CES-D) is a rapid tool to assess depressive symptoms (Kohout et al. 1993). The Geriatric Depression Scale (GDS) is a more comprehensive 15-item tool designed to determine the presence of major depression (Yesavage et al. 1982).

Neurologic Examination: There are no specific findings of AD on the neurologic examination. However, a number of motoric signs including parkinsonian signs of bradykinesia, gait disturbance, rigidity, and tremor are commonly found. These can be quantified with modifications of the Unified Parkinson's Disease Rating Scale (Bennett et al. 1997). Low body mass index and physical frailty are also found in persons with AD (Buchman et al. 2005; Buchman et al. 2007). Frontal release signs and myoclonus are found in late stage AD (Chen et al. 1992). Focal neurologic signs suggestive of stroke or brain tumor are unusual in AD, although AD is a common disease and may mimic other conditions such as cortico-basal degeneration with alien hand syndrome (Chand et al. 2006), and progressive aphasia (Mesulam et al. 2008).

Laboratory Testing

Cognitive Test Batteries: In many cases, the history of cognitive decline in conjunction with bedside mental status testing is sufficient to document dementia and make a diagnosis of AD with great confidence. However, in some cases, especially situations in which there is no or only a poor informant, the history is atypical, or there is only mild cognitive difficulties, formal neuropsychological testing is needed to document the type and severity of cognitive deficits. A number of batteries have been developed for use to document dementia. These include the Consortium to Establish a Registry for Alzheimer's Disease (Morris et al. 1989) and the Unified Data Set developed by the Clinical Task Force for the Alzheimer's Disease Centers funded by the National Institute on Aging (Morris et al. 2006).

Repeat cognitive testing also is essential to the conduct of clinical trials for AD. The most widely used measure for clinical trials is the Alzheimer's Disease Assessment Scale (ADAS-Cog) (Rosen et al. 1984). There are 11 tasks for a total of 70 points, including 35 points for learning and memory, 25 points for language, and 10 points for praxis. A higher score denotes worsening cognition. At the time when large scale AD clinical trials were first being launched, a consensus opinion was that a four point difference between the placebo and control group, a difference equivalent to about six months of change, was clinically significant.

The ADAS-Cog continues to be one of the primary outcome measures for clinical trials. However, other more comprehensive batteries have been developed and are currently in use as adjunct measures (Harrison et al. 2007; Randolph et al. 1998). Whether these newer and ostensibly more robust measures will supplant the ADAS-Cog in the near future is not clear.

Structural Neuroimaging: Structural neuroimaging is primarily used in the differential diagnosis of AD to find evidence of co-morbid conditions that present as memory loss and mimic AD or be present as a second complicating condition (Knopman et al. 2001). The routine evaluation of dementia, therefore, continues to employ magnetic resonance imaging (MRI) or non-contrast computed tomography (CT) when MRI is contraindicated or not available, to identify cerebral infractions, brain tumors, hydrocephalus, and other conditions that may present as dementia. A number of quantitative MRI parameters are being investigated for diagnostic use, such as the volume of the hippocampus or entorhinal cortex, in addition to other measurements (Small et al. 2008). Changes in MRI measures such as brain or hippocampal volume, or cerebrospinal fluid (CSF) volume, are now being investigated for use as surrogate outcome measures of clinical trials (Schott et al. 2005). They would be used in conjunction with cognitive endpoints to provide evidence of potential disease-modifying effects of pharmacotherapy.

MRI scans can also be used to obtain a variety of other measures which may eventually prove useful in the evaluation of persons with AD. These include functional MRI (fMRI), diffusion tensor imaging (DTI), and magnetic resonance spectroscopy (MRS) (Small et al. 2008). These are all experimental procedures at this time but some of them show great promise for eventual clinical utility.

Functional Neuroimaging: Functional imaging procedures have a limited role in the evaluation of dementia. Single photon emission computed tomography (SPECT) measures blood flow and is widely available at a relatively low cost. Although there are characteristic patterns of blood flow deficits in persons with AD, SPECT is used primarily to support the diagnosis of fronto-temporal dementia (FTD). Positron emission tomography (PET) measures glucose utilization with the 2-deoxy-2-2^{18}fluoro-D-glucose (FDG) tracer. It has much greater resolution than SPECT and is the preferred test when available. Although there are characteristic patterns of glucose utilization in persons with AD, PET is not approved for use to support a diagnosis of AD. Rather, PET is approved, with a number of restrictions, for the diagnosis of FTD.

Among the most exciting recent advances in functional imaging is the emergence of *in vivo* imaging of AD pathology. Pittsburgh Compound B (PIB) is the most extensively studied to date (Klunk et al. 2004). This agent is relatively specific for amyloid. Its use is limited by its relatively short half-life such that it can only be used at medical centers with a cyclotron on site. Newly developed fluorine-18 (F-18) PET ligands are now being evaluated and have the potential for clinical use due to their longer half-life (Rowe et al. 2008). Other PET ligands are under evaluation, including some that identify both plaques and tangles (Small et al. 2008).

Blood Testing: There are no routine blood tests that aid the diagnosis of AD. Routine blood tests are used as clinically indicated to identify co-morbid conditions that may be contributing to or mimicking AD (Knopman et al. 2001).

While controversial, there is considerable interest in quantifying amyloid in peripheral blood for use as diagnostic marker or a biomarker that tracks with disease (Ertekin-Taner, et al. 2008). Plasma amyloid has a complicated relationship with the presence of AD and severity of dementia precluding its clinical use at this time. As yet, there are no peripheral markers of tau proteins.

Cerebrospinal Fluid Testing: Both amyloid and different tau proteins can be quantified in CSF (Clark et al. 2003). These markers correlate with the presence of AD and the severity of cognitive impairment and show promise for use as both a diagnostic test and a biomarker to monitor progression of disease. However, they are not recommended in clinical settings at this time.

Prognosis and Natural History

The clinical hallmark of AD is progressive loss of cognitive abilities over time. On average, people with AD decline about three points per year on the MMSE (Wilson et al. 2000c). However, there is substantial between-person variability in the rate of decline. Some of the variability is due to the limited psychometric properties of the MMSE such that there is little change at the high and low end of the scales. However, even with the use of sophisticated composite measures of cognition, some persons experience little decline while others experience marked decline over three to five years of follow-up. A number of factors are related to rate of cognitive decline including parkinsonian signs, psychotic features, earlier age at onset, and higher educational attainment (Wilson et al. 2000a–d; Stern et al. 1999). Parkinsonian signs, psychotic features, and educational attainment are also related to nursing home placement, functional decline, and death (Stern et al. 1994; Stern et al. 1995; Bennett et al. 1998). Severity of cognitive impairment is also related to risk of hospitalization (Albert et al. 1999).

Approved Pharmacologic Treatment

There are now five medications approved by the United States Food and Drug Administration (US FDA) for the symptomatic treatment of AD (Table 4). Four of these medications are acetylcholinesterase inhibitors and one is an N-methyl-D-aspartate (NMDA) receptor antagonist.

Acetylcholinesterase Inhibitors: The basal forebrain, the major source of cholinergic innervation of the hippocampus and neocortex, is highly vulnerable to the pathology of AD, and its neurons atrophy and degenerate as part of the disease. Acetylcholinesterase is the enzyme that degrades acetylcholine at the synaptic junction. The therapeutic rationale for these agents is that inhibition of acetylcholinesterase would allow enhanced cholinergic transmission. All four agents result in modest improvement in cognitive function. However, response is variable and difficult to detect on a case by case basis as the studies were designed, in general, to identify the equivalent of six months of improvement over the course of a six month trial. Thus, stabilization of cognition is the typical observed clinical outcome over a six month period. However, there is a remarkable degree of heterogeneity of cognitive decline over this period making it difficult to ascribe the lack of change to a drug.

The first agent to be approved was tacrine (Davis et al. 1992). This agent is no longer in widespread use as a result of side effects including elevated liver enzymes and cholinergic symptoms including nausea, vomiting, and diarrhea. The second agent approved for the symptomatic treatment was donepezil. It was initially approved for mild to moderate AD but the labeling was later modified to include severe AD. The initial dose is 5 mg per day. It is usually increased to 10 mg per day after 4 weeks. The titration is intended to reduce cholinergic side effects. Donepezil is available as a tablet. The third agent was galantamine. It is now available as an extended release (ER). The initial dose is 8 mg daily. It is usually increased to 16 mg daily after 4 weeks. It can be increased by 8 mg increments every 4 weeks to a maximum of 24 mg daily. The most recent acetylcholinesterase inhibitor is rivastigmine. It is approved for mild to moderate AD and also for Parkinson's disease dementia. The initial dose is 1.5 mg twice daily and it can be increased by 1.5 mg twice daily every 4 weeks. The maximum dose is 6 mg twice a day. Rivastigmine is available as a capsule, oral solution, and a patch.

NMDA Receptor Antagonist: Memantine is an NMDA receptor antagonist. Stimulation of the NMDA receptor by the excitatory amino acid glutamate is thought to contribute to neurodegeneration through the prolonged influx of calcium ions. Blocking this pathway may be the mechanism through which memantine exerts its effects. Memantine is approved for the treatment of moderate to severe AD and is often used in conjunction with an acetylcholinesterase inhibitor. The initial dose is 5 mg daily and it may be increased by 5 mg every 1 to 4 weeks to a maximum of 10 mg twice daily. Memantine is available as a tablet and oral solution.

Other Agents: No other agents are approved by the US FDA for the treatment of cognitive or non-cognitive symptoms of AD. While a number of agents are used off label for the treatment of psychosis, agitation, sleep disturbance, and depression associated with AD, the reader is referred elsewhere for a discussion of these agents (Carson et al. 2006; Farlow et al. 2008; Schneider et al. 2006). While it is possible that off label use provides some benefit, there is good evidence that it is also associated with significant risks (Ballard et al. 2009). Thus, physicians should familiarize themselves with both the potential benefits and risks.

Experimental Pharmacotherapy

A variety of agents are under active investigation. Perhaps the most promising are agents that alter amyloid metabolism. The strategies range widely. One strategy involves altering the accumulation of amyloid by inhibition or modulation of β- or γ- secretase. A second strategy involves interfering with deposition. Finally, a third approach involves removing deposited amyloid by active or passive immunization against

Table 4 Pharmacotherapy for Alzheimer's Disease

Author (year)	Cholinesterase Inhibitors	Indication	Start Dose	Max Dose
Rogers et al. (1998)	Donepezil	Mild-Mod AD	5 mg q d	10 mg q d
Feldman et al. (2001)		Mod-Sev AD		
Raskind et al. (2000)	Galantamine	Mild-Mod AD	8 mg q d	24 mg q d
Rösler et al. (1999)	Rivastigmine	Mild-Mod AD	1.5 mg bid	6 mg bid
McKeith et al. (2000)		PD Dementia		
NMDA Anatagonist				
Reisberg et al. (2003)	Memantine	Mod-Sev AD	5 mg q d	10 mg bid

the deposited amyloid-β peptide. Other exciting approaches are agents targeting the kinases involved in tau phosphorylation. Finally, numerous other approaches are being investigated that do not directly involve amyloid or tau.

Caregiver Stress

Stress, anxiety, and depression commonly affect caregivers of persons with dementia (Schultz et al. 2004). It is beyond the scope of this review to discuss interventions directed at the caregiver. However, it is important to be aware that caregiver characteristics including age and perceived burden are associated with important patient outcomes, including nursing home placement (Yaffe et al. 2002).

Driving

States vary in terms of reporting dementia patients to the department of motor vehicles and the extent to which medical professionals are given immunity from civil liability. Thus, it is prudent for physicians to be aware of their own state laws (American Medical Association 2008). While a 2000 practice guideline from the American Academy of Neurology recommends that persons with AD refrain from driving, it is increasingly recognized that some persons with mild AD maintain driving competence (Bacon et al. 2007).

Advance Directives

Many patients with AD eventually become incompetent and are unable to make their own financial and health care decisions (Moye and Marson 2007). Thus, early in the disease patients should be encouraged to complete advance directives specifying the extent of heroic care that should be taken in the event they become incompetent. They should also sign a durable power of attorney for health care and financial decisions specifying an individual (proxy) that can make medical and financial decisions on the patient's behalf. These need not be the same individual. In the event the patient becomes incompetent and unable to sign such documents, the family may need to have the court appoint a legal guardian.

Summary and Future Directions

Much has been learned about AD over the past two decades. Because of the magnitude of the public health problem posed by the disease, prevention is the most urgent need. This will require a combination of observational and experimental cohort studies. Such studies are ongoing and have resulted in the identification of numerous environmental and genetic factors that are associated with disease risk. However, considerable efforts are currently being expended to identify additional factors associated with the occurrence of the disease. For example, like many common chronic diseases of aging, it is becoming increasingly clear that AD is a disease of a lifetime with early- and mid-life factors being associated with the development of disease decades later. In addition, there are now a number of ongoing initiatives to identify the remaining genetic variants associated with disease risk. Eventually, it will be important to identify the neurobiologic mechanisms underlying the association of risk factors with clinical disease, as such information is likely to be highly relevant to the rational development of strategies to delay disease onset. In the meantime, many people currently have the disease and many more will develop AD while prevention efforts are sought. Thus, better therapeutic strategies are needed to improve cognition and delay cognitive decline and other consequences of the disease. There is considerable excitement that the era of disease-modifying agents may be in the near future. However, the success of all of these efforts will depend on the cooperation of funding

Table 5 Physician, Patient, and Family Resources on the Web

Website	Information
http://www.clinicaltrials.gov/	Registry of federally and privately supported clinical trials
http://www.nia.nih.gov/Alzheimers/	Alzheiemr's Disease Education & Referral Center
http://www.alzforum.org/	Alzheimer Research Forum includes news; drugs in development; Alzgene (published AD candidate genes); Alzrisk (published AD epidemiologic database)
http://www.alz.org/istaart/	Alzheimer's Association International Society to Advance Alzheimer Research and Treatment (ISTAART) professional society
http://www.alz.org/	Alzheimer's Association
http://www.alzfdn.org/	Alzheimer's Foundation

agencies, academic and industry researchers, patients and their family members, and practicing physicians. A variety of online sources are available for physicians, patients, and their families to learn about AD, the latest treatment, research, and clinical trials (Table 5).

Acknowledgments

The author thanks the patients and staff of the Rush Alzheimer's Disease Center. This work was supported in part by National Institute on Aging grants P30AG10161 and R01AG17918.

References

Albert SM, Costa R, Merchant C, Small S, Jenders RA, and Stern Y. Hospitalization and Alzheimer's disease: Results from a community-based study. *J Gerontol A Biol Sci Med Sci.* 1999;54:M267–71.

American Medical Association. Physician's guide to assessing and counseling older drivers. http://www.ama-assn.org/ama/pub/category/10791.html

Arvanitakis Z, Bienias JL, Wilson RS, Evans DA, and Bennett DA. Diabetes and risk of Alzheimer's disease and decline in cognitive function. *Archives of Neurology.* 2004;61:661–666.

Bacon D, Fisher RS, Morris JC, Rizzo M, and Spanaki MV. American Academy of Neurology position statement on physician reporting of medical conditions that may affect driving competence. *Neurology.* 2007;68:1174–7.

Ballard C, Hanney ML, Theodoulou M, Douglas S, McShane R, Kossakowski K, et al; for the DART-AD investigators. The dementia antipsychotic withdrawal trial (DART-AD): Long-term follow-up of a randomised placebo-controlled trial. *Lancet Neurol.* 2009;8:151–157.

Ballatore C, Lee VM, and Trojanowski JQ. Tau-mediated neurodegeneration in Alzheimer's disease and related disorders. *Nat Rev Neurosci.* 2007;8:663–72.

Barak Y, Aizenberg D. Suicide amongst Alzheimer's disease patients: A 10-year survey. *Dement Geriatr Cogn Disord.* 2002;14:101–3.

Barnes LL, Schneider JA, Boyle PA, Bienias JL, and Bennett DA. Memory complaints are related to Alzheimer's disease pathology in older persons. *Neurology.* 2006;67:1581–1585.

Bennett DA, Shannon KM, Beckett LA, Goetz CG, and Wilson RS. Metric properties of nurses' ratings of parkinsonian signs with a modified

Unified Parkinson's Disease Rating Scale. *Neurology.* 1997;49:1580–1587.

Bennett DA, Beckett LA, Wilson RS, Murray AM, and Evans DA. Parkinsonian signs and mortality from Alzheimer's disease. *Lancet.* 1998;351:1631.

Bennett DA, Schneider JA, Wilson RS, Bienias JL, and Arnold SE. Neurofibrillary tangles mediate the association of amyloid load with clinical Alzheimer disease and level of cognitive function. *Arch Neurol.* 2004;61:378–384.

Bennett DA, Wilson RS, Schneider JA, Bienias JL, and Arnold SE. Cerebral infarctions and the relation of depressive symptoms to level of cognitive function in older persons. *American Journal of Geriatric Psychiatry.* 2004;12:211–219.

Bennett DA, Schneider JA, Bienias JL, Evans DA, and Wilson RS. Mild cognitive impairment is related to Alzheimer disease pathology and cerebral infarctions. *Neurology.* 2005;64:834–841.

Bennett DA, Schneider JA, Aggarwal NT, Arvanitakis Z, Shah R, Kelly JF, et al. Decision rules guiding the clinical diagnosis of Alzheimer's disease in two community-based cohort studies compared to standard practice in a clinic-based cohort study. *Neuroepidemiology.* 2006;27:169–176.

Bennett DA, Schneider JA, Arvanitakis Z, Kelly JF, Aggarwal NT, Shah R, and Wilson RS. Neuropathology of older persons without cognitive impairment from two community-based clinical-pathologic studies. *Neurology.* 2006;66:1837–1844.

Bennett DA, Schneider JA, Tang Y, Arnold SE, and Wilson RS. The effect of social networks on the relation between Alzheimer's disease pathology and level of cognitive function in old people: A longitudinal cohort study. *Lancet Neurol.* 2006;5:406–412.

Bennett DA, De Jager PL, Leurgans SE, and Schneider JA. Neuropathologic intermediate phenotypes enhance association to Alzheimer susceptibility alleles. *Neurology.* In press.

Benoit M, Andrieu S, Lechowski L, Gillette-Guyonnet S, Robert PH, and Vellas B; REAL-FR group. Apathy and depression in Alzheimer's disease are associated with functional deficit and psychotropic prescription. *Int J Geriatr Psychiatry.* 2008;23:409–14.

Bertram L, McQueen MB, Mullin K, Blacker D, and Tanzi RE. Systematic meta-analyses of Alzheimer disease genetic association studies: The AlzGene database. *Nat Genet.* 2007;39:17–23.

Borson S, Scanlan J, Brush M, Vitaliano P, and Dokmak A. The mini-cog: A cognitive 'vital signs' measure for dementia screening in multi-lingual elderly. *Int J Geriatr Psychiatry.* 2000;15:1021–7.

Boeve BF, Silber MH, Saper CB, Ferman TJ, Dickson DW, Parisi JE, et al. Pathophysiology of REM sleep behaviour disorder and relevance to neurodegenerative disease. *Brain.* 2007;130:2770–88.

Braak H and Braak E. Neuropathological staging of Alzheimer-related changes. *Acta Neuropathol (Berl).* 1991;82:239–259.

Brookmeyer R, Corrada MM, Curriero FC, and Kawas C. Survival following a diagnosis of Alzheimer disease. *Arch Neurol.* 2002; 59:1764–1767.

Brookmeyer R, Johnson E, Ziegler-Graham K, and Arrighi HM. Forecasting the global burden of Alzheimer's disease. *Alzheimer Dementia.* 2007; 3:186–191.

Buchman AS, Wilson RS, Bienias JL, Shah R, Evans DA, and Bennett DA. Change in body mass index (BMI) and risk of incident Alzheimer's disease (AD). *Neurology.* 2005;65:892–897.

Buchman AS, Boyle PA, Wilson RS, Tang Y, and Bennett DA. Frailty is associated with incident Alzheimer's disease and cognitive decline in the elderly. *Psychosomatic Medicine.* 2007;69:483–489.

Burns JM, Galvin JE, Roe CM, Morris JC, and McKeel DW. The pathology of the substantia nigra in Alzheimer disease with extrapyramidal signs. *Neurology.* 2005;64:1397–403.

Carson S, McDonagh MS, and Peterson K. A systematic review of the efficacy and safety of atypical antipsychotics in patients with psychological and behavioral symptoms of dementia. *J Am Geriatr Soc.* 2006;54:354–361.

Chand P, Grafman J, Dickson D, Ishizawa K, and Litvan I. Alzheimer's disease presenting as corticobasal syndrome. *Mov Disord.* 2006;21:2018–22.

Chen JY, Stern Y, Sano M, and Mayeux R. Cumulative risks of developing extrapyramidal signs, psychosis, or myoclonus in the course of Alzheimer's disease. *Arch Neurol.* 1991;48:1141–3.

Clark CM, Xie S, Chittams J, Ewbank D, Peskind E, Galasko D, et al. Cerebrospinal fluid tau and beta-amyloid: How well do these biomarkers reflect autopsy-confirmed dementia diagnoses? *Arch Neurol.* 2003;60:1696–702.

Cole SL and Vassar R. The role of amyloid precursor protein processing by BACE1, the beta-secretase, in Alzheimer disease pathophysiology. *J Biol Chem.* 2008;283:29621–5.

Consensus recommendations for the postmortem diagnosis of Alzheimer's disease. The National Institute on Aging and Reagan Institute Working Group on Diagnostic Criteria for the Neuropathological Assessment of Alzheimer's Disease. *Neurobiol Aging.* 1997;18(suppl 4):S1–S2.

Corder EH, Saunders AM, Strittmatter WJ, Schmechel DE, Gaskell PC, Small GW, et al. Gene dose of apolipoprotein E type 4 allele and the risk of Alzheimer's disease in late onset families. *Science.* 1993;261:921–3.

Corder EH, Saunders AM, Risch NJ, Strittmatter WJ, Schmechel DE, Gaskell PC Jr, et al. Protective effect of apolipoprotein E type 2 allele for late onset Alzheimer disease. *Nat Genet.* 1994;7:180–4.

Cummings JL, Mega M, Gray K, Rosenberg-Thompson S, Carusi DA, and Gornbein J. The Neuropsychiatric Inventory: Comprehensive assessment of psychopathology in dementia. *Neurology.* 1994;44:2308–14.

Davis KL, Thal LJ, Gamzu ER, Davis CS, Woolson RF, Gracon SI, et al. A double-blind, placebo-controlled multicenter study of tacrine for Alzheimer's disease. The Tacrine Collaborative Study Group. *N Engl J Med.* 1992;327:1253–9.

Devanand DP, Sano M, Tang MX, Taylor S, Gurland BJ, Wilder D, et al. Depressed mood and the incidence of Alzheimer's disease in the elderly living in the community. *Arch Gen Psychiatry.* 1996;53: 175–82.

Devanand DP, Michaels-Marston KS, Liu X, Pelton GH, Padilla M, Marder K, et al. Olfactory deficits in patients with mild cognitive impairment predict Alzheimer's disease at follow-up. *Am J Psychiatry.* 2000;157:1399–1405.

Dubois B, Feldman HH, Jacova C, Dekosky ST, Barberger-Gateau P, Cummings J, et al. Research criteria for the diagnosis of Alzheimer's disease: Revising the NINCDS-ADRDA criteria. *Lancet Neurol.* 2007;6:734–46.

Ertekin-Taner N. Genetics of Alzheimer's disease: A centennial review. *Neurol Clin.* 2007;25:611–67.

Ertekin-Taner N, Younkin LH, Yager DM, Parfitt F, Baker MC, Asthana S, et al. Plasma amyloid beta protein is elevated in late-onset Alzheimer disease families. *Neurology.* 2008;70:596–606.

Evans DA, Funkenstein HH, Albert MS, Scherr PA, Cook NR, Chown MJ, et al. Prevalence of Alzheimer's disease in a community population of older persons. Higher than previously reported. *JAMA.* 1989;262:2551–2556.

Evans DA, Bennett DA, Wilson RS, et al. Incidence of Alzheimer disease in a biracial urban community: Relation to apolipoprotein E allele status. *Arch Neurol.* 2003;60:185–9.

Farlow MR, Miller ML, and Pejovic V. Treatment options in Alzheimer's disease: Maximizing benefit, managing expectations. *Dement Geriatr Cogn Disord.* 2008;25:408–22.

Farrer LA, Myers RH, Cupples LA, St George-Hyslop PH, Bird TD, Rossor MN, et al. Transmission and age-at-onset patterns in familial

Alzheimer's disease: Evidence for heterogeneity. *Neurology*. 1990;40:395–403.

Farrer LA, Cupples LA, Haines JL, et al. Effects of age, sex, and ethnicity on the association between apolipoprotein E genotype and Alzheimer disease. A meta-analysis. APOE and Alzheimer Disease Meta Analysis Consortium. *JAMA*. 1997;278:1349–56.

Feldman H, Gauthier S, Hecker J, Vellas B, Subbiah P, Whalen E; Donepezil MSAD Study Investigators Group. A 24-week, randomized, double-blind study of donepezil in moderate to severe Alzheimer's disease. *Neurology*. 2001;57:613–20.

Ferri CP, Prince M, Brayne C, Brodaty H, Fratiglioni L, Ganguli M, et al.; Alzheimer's Disease International. Global prevalence of dementia: A Delphi consensus study. *Lancet*. 2005;366:2112–7.

Fleischman DA, Wilson RS, Gabrieli JDE, Schneider JA, Bienias JL, and Bennett DA. Implicit memory and Alzheimer's disease neuropathology. *Brain*. 2005;128:2006–2015.

Foley DJ, Masaki KH, Ross GW, and White LR. Driving cessation in older men with incident dementia. *J Am Geriatr Soc*. 2000;48:928–30.

Folstein MF, Folstein SE, and McHugh PR. Mini-mental state. A practical method for grading the cognitive state of patients for the clinician. *J Psychiatr Res*. 1975;12:189–98.

Galvin JE, Roe CM, Powlishta KK, Coats MA, Muich SJ, Grant E, et al. The AD8: A brief informant interview to detect dementia. *Neurology*. 2005;65:559–64.

Gatz M, Reynolds CA, Fratiglioni L, Johansson B, Mortimer JA, Berg S, et al. Role of genes and environments for explaining Alzheimer disease. *Arch Gen Psychiatry*. 2006;63:168–174.

Gauthier S, Reisberg B, Zaudig M, Petersen RC, Ritchie K, Broich K, et al.; International Psychogeriatric Association Expert Conference on mild cognitive impairment. Mild cognitive impairment. *Lancet*. 2006;367:1262–70.

Goate A, Chartier-Harlin MC, Mullan M, Brown J, Crawford F, Fidani L, et al. Segregation of a missense mutation in the amyloid precursor protein gene with familial Alzheimer's disease. *Nature*. 1991;349:704–6.

Golde TE. Disease modifying therapy for AD? *J Neurochem*. 2006;99:689–707.

Hardy J and Selkoe DJ. The amyloid hypothesis of Alzheimer's disease: Progress and problems on the road to therapeutics. *Science*. 2002;297:353–6.

Harrison J, Minassian SL, Jenkins L, Black RS, Koller M, and Grundman M. A neuropsychological test battery for use in Alzheimer disease clinical trials. *Arch Neurol*. 2007;64:1323–9.

Hebert LE, Scherr PA, Bienias JL, Bennett DA, and Evans DA. Alzheimer disease in the US population: Prevalence estimates using the 2000 census. *Arch Neurol*. 2003;60:1119–22.

Veld BA, Ruitenberg A, Hofman A, Launer LJ, van Duijn CM, Stijnen T, Breteler MM, Stricker BH. Nonsteroidal antiinflammatory drugs and the risk of Alzheimer's disease. *N Engl J Med*. 2001;345:1515–21.

Kennedy JL, Farrer LA, Andreasen NC, Mayeux R, and St George-Hyslop P. The genetics of adult-onset neuropsychiatric disease: Complexities and conundra? *Science*. 2003;302:822–826.

Kivipelto M, Helkala EL, Laakso MP, Hänninen T, Hallikainen M, Alhainen K, et al. Midlife vascular risk factors and Alzheimer's disease in later life: Longitudinal, population based study. *BMJ*. 2001;322:1447–51.

Klunk WE, Engler H, Nordberg A, et al. Imaging brain amyloid in Alzheimer's disease with Pittsburgh Compound-B. *Ann Neurol*. 2004; 55: 306–19.

Knopman DS, DeKosky ST, Cummings JL, Chui H, Corey-Bloom J, Relkin N, et al. Practice parameter: Diagnosis of dementia (an evidence-based review). Report of the Quality Standards Subcommittee of the American Academy of Neurology. *Neurology*. 2001;56:1143–53.

Kohout FJ, Berkman LF, Evans DA, and Cornoni-Huntley J. Two shorter forms of the CES-D (Center for Epidemiological Studies Depression) depression symptoms index. *J Aging Health*. 1993;5: 179–93.

Langa KM, Chernew ME, Kabeto MU, Herzog AR, Ofstedal MB, Willis RJ, et al. National estimates of the quantity and cost of informal caregiving for elderly with denetia. *J Gen Intern Med*. 2001; 16:770-778.

Larson EB, Shadlen MF, Wang L, McCormick WC, Bowen JD, Teri L, and Kukull WA. Survival after initial diagnosis of Alzheimer disease. *Ann Intern Med*. 2004; 140:501–509.

Lesné S, Koh MT, Kotilinek L, Kayed R, Glabe CG, Yang A, et al. A specific amyloid-beta protein assembly in the brain impairs memory. *Nature*. 2006;440:352–7.

Levy-Lahad E, Wasco W, Poorkaj P, Romano DM, Oshima J, Pettingell WH, et al. Candidate gene for the chromosome 1 familial Alzheimer's disease locus. *Science*. 1995;269:973–7.

Luchsinger JA, Noble JM, and Scarmeas N. Diet and Alzheimer's disease. *Curr Neurol Neurosci Rep*. 2007;7:366–72.

Lyketsos CG, Lopez O, Jones B, Fitzpatrick AL, Breitner J, and DeKosky S. Prevalence of neuropsychiatric symptoms in dementia and mild cognitive impairment: Results from the cardiovascular health study. *JAMA*. 2002;288:1475–83.

McKeith I, Del Ser T, Spano P, Emre M, Wesnes K, Anand R, et al. Efficacy of rivastigmine in dementia with Lewy bodies: A randomised, double-blind, placebo-controlled international study. *Lancet*. 2000;356:2031–6.

McKhann G, Drachman D, Folstein M, Katzman R, Price D, and Stadlan E. Clinical diagnosis of Alzheimer's disease: Report of the NINCDS-ADRDA Work Group under the auspices of Department of Health and Human Services Task Force on Alzheimer's Disease. *Neurology*. 1984;34:939–944.

Merchant C, Tang MX, Albert S, Manly J, Stern Y, and Mayeux R. The influence of smoking on the risk of Alzheimer's disease. *Neurology*. 1999;52:1408–12.

Mesulam M, Wicklund A, Johnson N, Rogalski E, Léger GC, Rademaker A, et al. Alzheimer and frontotemporal pathology in subsets of primary progressive aphasia. *Ann Neurol*. 2008;63:709–19.

Mirra SS, Heyman A, McKeel D, Sumi SM, Crain BJ, Brownlee LM, et al. The Consortium to Establish a Registry for Alzheimer's Disease (CERAD). Part II. Standardization of the neuropathologic assessment of Alzheimer's disease. *Neurology*. 1991;41:479–86.

Morris JC, Heyman A, Mohs RC, Hughes JP, van Belle G, Fillenbaum G, et al. The Consortium to Establish a Registry for Alzheimer's Disease (CERAD). Part I. Clinical and neuropsychological assessment of Alzheimer's disease. *Neurology*. 1989;39:1159–65.

Morris JC, Weintraub S, Chui HC, Cummings J, Decarli C, Ferris S, et al. The Uniform Data Set (UDS): Clinical and cognitive variables and descriptive data from Alzheimer Disease Centers. *Alzheimer Dis Assoc Disord*. 2006;20:210–6.

Moye J and Marson DC. Assessment of decision-making capacity in older adults: An emerging area of practice and research. *J Gerontol B Psychol Sci Soc Sci*. 2007;62:P3–P11.

Nasreddine ZS, Phillips NA, Bédirian V, Charbonneau S, Whitehead V, Collin I, et al. The Montreal Cognitive Assessment, MoCA: A brief screening tool for mild cognitive impairment. *J Am Geriatr Soc*. 2005;53:695–9.

Newman AB, Fitzpatrick AL, Lopez O, Jackson S, Lyketsos C, Jagust W, et al. Dementia and Alzheimer's disease incidence in relationship to cardiovascular disease in the Cardiovascular Health Study cohort. *J Am Geriatr Soc*. 2005;53:1101–1107.

Ott BR, Heindel WC, Papandonatos GD, Festa EK, Davis JD, Daiello LA, and Morris JC. A longitudinal study of drivers with Alzheimer disease. *Neurology*. 2008;70:1171–8.

Park M, Comella CL, Leurgans SE, Fan W, Wilson RS, and Bennett DA. Association of daytime napping and Parkinsonian signs in Alzheimer's disease. *Sleep Med.* 2006;7:614–8.

Pfeffer RI, Kurosaki TT, Harrah CH Jr, Chance JM, and Filos S. Measurement of functional activities in older adults in the community. *J Gerontol.* 1982;37:323–9.

Podewils LJ, Guallar E, Kuller LH, Fried LP, Lopez OL, Carlson M, and Lyketsos CG. Physical activity, APOE genotype, and dementia risk: Findings from the Cardiovascular Health Cognition Study. *Am J Epidemiol.* 2005;161:639–51.

Randolph C, Tierney MC, Mohr E, and Chase TN. The Repeatable Battery for the Assessment of Neuropsychological Status (RBANS): Preliminary clinical validity. *J Clin Exp Neuropsychol.* 1998;20:310–9.

Rapp MA, Schnaider-Beeri M, Grossman HT, Sano M, Perl DP, Purohit DP, et al. Increased hippocampal plaques and tangles in patients with Alzheimer disease with a lifetime history of major depression. *Arch Gen Psychiatry.* 2006;63:161–7.

Raskind MA, Peskind ER, Wessel T, and Yuan W. Galantamine in AD: A 6-month randomized, placebo-controlled trial with a 6-month extension. The Galantamine USA-1 Study Group. *Neurology.* 2000;54:2261–8.

Reisberg B, Doody R, Stöffler A, Schmitt F, Ferris S, Möbius HJ; Memantine Study Group. Memantine in moderate-to-severe Alzheimer's disease. *N Engl J Med.* 2003;348:1333–41.

Rogers SL, Farlow MR, Doody RS, Mohs R, and Friedhoff LT. A 24-week, double-blind, placebo-controlled trial of donepezil in patients with Alzheimer's disease. Donepezil Study Group. *Neurology.* 1998;50:136–45.

Rosen WG, Mohs RC, and Davis KL. A new rating scale for Alzheimer's disease. *Am J Psychiatry.* 1984;141:1356–64.

Rösler M, Anand R, Cicin-Sain A, Gauthier S, Agid Y, Dal-Bianco P, et al. Efficacy and safety of rivastigmine in patients with Alzheimer's disease: International randomised controlled trial. *BMJ.* 1999;318:633–8.

Rowe CC, Ackerman U, Browne W, Mulligan R, Pike KL, O'Keefe G, et al. Imaging of amyloid beta in Alzheimer's disease with 18F-BAY94-9172, a novel PET tracer: Proof of mechanism. *Lancet Neurol.* 2008;7:129–35.

Scarmeas N, Levy G, Tang MX, Manly J, and Stern Y. Influence of leisure activity on the incidence of Alzheimer's disease. *Neurology.* 2001;57:2236–42.

Schneider JA, Li JL, Li Y, Wilson RS, Kordower JH, and Bennett DA. Neurofibrillary tangles in the substantia nigra are related to gait impairment in older persons. *Annals of Neurology.* 2006;59:166–173.

Schneider JA, Boyle PA, Arvanitakis Z, Bienias JL, and Bennett DA. Subcortical cerebral infarcts, episodic memory, and AD pathology in older persons. *Annals of Neurology.* 2007;62:59–66.

Schneider JA, Arvanitakis Z, Leurgans SE, and Bennett DA. Neuropathology of probable AD and amnestic and non-amnestic MCI. *Annals of Neurology.* 2009;66:200–208.

Schneider LS, Dagerman K, and Insel PS. Efficacy and adverse effects of atypical antipsychotics for dementia: Meta-analysis of randomized, placebo-controlled trials. *Am J Geriatr Psychiatry.* 2006;14:191–210.

Schofield PW, Tang M, Marder K, Bell K, Dooneief G, Chun M, et al. Alzheimer's disease after remote head injury: An incidence study. *J Neurol Neurosurg Psychiatry.* 1997;62:119–24.

Schott JM, Price SL, Frost C, Whitwell JL, Rossor MN, et al. Fox NC. Measuring atrophy in Alzheimer disease: A serial MRI study over 6 and 12 months. *Neurology.* 2005; 65: 119–24.

Schulz R, Belle SH, Czaja SJ, McGinnis KA, Stevens A, and Zhang S. Long-term care placement of dementia patients and caregiver health and well-being. *JAMA.* 2004;292:961–7.

Selkoe DJ and Wolfe MS. Presenilin: Running with scissors in the membrane. *Cell.* 2007;131:215–21.

Sherrington R, Rogaev EI, Liang Y, Rogaeva EA, Levesque G, Ikeda M, et al. Cloning of a gene bearing missense mutations in early-onset familial Alzheimer's disease. *Nature.* 1995;375:754–60.

Small GW, Bookheimer SY, Thompson PM, Cole GM, Huang SC, Kepe V, and Barrio JR. Current and future uses of neuroimaging for cognitively impaired patients. *Lancet Neurol.* 2008;7:161–72.

Snowdon DA, Greiner LH, Mortimer JA, Riley KP, Greiner PA, and Markesbery WR. Brain infarction and the clinical expression of Alzheimer disease. The Nun Study. *JAMA.* 1997;277:813–817.

Solomon PR, Hirschoff A, Kelly B, Relin M, Brush M, DeVeaux RD, and Pendlebury WW. A 7 minute neurocognitive screening battery highly sensitive to Alzheimer's disease. *Arch Neurol.* 1998;55:349–55.

Steffens DC, Otey E, Alexopoulos GS, Butters MA, Cuthbert B, Ganguli M, et al. Perspectives on depression, mild cognitive impairment, and cognitive decline. *Arch Gen Psychiatry.* 2006;63:130–8.

Stern Y. What is cognitive reserve? Theory and research application of the reserve concept. *J Int Neuropsychol Soc.* 2002;8:448–60.

Stern Y, Albert M, Brandt J, Jacobs DM, Tang MX, Marder K, et al. Utility of extrapyramidal signs and psychosis as predictors of cognitive and functional decline, nursing home admission, and death in Alzheimer's disease: Prospective analyses from the Predictors Study. *Neurology.* 1994;44:2300–7.

Stern Y, Gurland B, Tatemichi TK, Tang MX, Wilder D, and Mayeux R. Influence of education and occupation on the incidence of Alzheimer's disease. *JAMA.* 1994;271:1004–1010.

Stern Y, Tang MX, Denaro J, and Mayeux R. Increased risk of mortality in Alzheimer's disease patients with more advanced educational and occupational attainment. *Ann Neurol.* 1995;37:590–5.

Stern Y, Albert S, Tang MX, and Tsai WY. Rate of memory decline in AD is related to education and occupation: Cognitive reserve? *Neurology.* 1999;53:1942–7.

Sunderland T, Hill JL, Mellow AM, Lawlor BA, Gundersheimer J, Newhouse PA, and Grafman JH. Clock drawing in Alzheimer's disease. A novel measure of dementia severity. *J Am Geriatr Soc.* 1989;37:725–9.

Sweet RA, Hamilton RL, Lopez OL, Klunk WE, Wisniewski SR, Kaufer DI, et al. Psychotic symptoms in Alzheimer's disease are not associated with more severe neuropathologic features. *Int Psychogeriatr.* 2000;12:547–58.

Tang MX, Stern Y, Marder K, et al. The APOE-epsilon4 allele and the risk of Alzheimer disease among African Americans, whites, and Hispanics. *JAMA.* 1998;279:751–5.

Tang MX, Cross P, Andrews H, Jacobs DM, Small S, Bell K, et al. Incidence of AD in African-Americans, Caribbean Hispanics, and Caucasians in northern Manhattan. *Neurology.* 2001;56:49–56.

Tekin S, Mega MS, Masterman DM, Chow T, Garakian J, Vinters HV, and Cummings JL. Orbitofrontal and anterior cingulate cortex neurofibrillary tangle burden is associated with agitation in Alzheimer disease. *Ann Neurol.* 2001;49:355–61.

Wang L, Larson EB, Bowen JD, and van Belle G. Performance-based physical function and future dementia in older people. *Arch Intern Med.* 2006;166:1115–20.

Wilson RS, Bennett DA, Gilley DW, Beckett LA, Barnes LL, and Evans DA. Premorbid reading activity and patterns of cognitive decline in Alzheimer's disease. *Arch Neurol.* 2000a;57:1718–23.

Wilson RS, Bennett DA, Gilley DW, Beckett LA, Schneider JA, and Evans DA. Progression of parkinsonism and loss of cognitive function in Alzheimer's disease. *Arch Neurol.* 2000b;57:855–60.

Wilson RS, Gilley DW, Bennett DA, Beckett LA, and Evans DA. Person-specific paths of cognitive decline in Alzheimer's disease and their relation to age. *Psychology & Aging.* 2000c;15:18–28.

Wilson RS, Gilley DW, Bennett DA, Beckett LA, and Evans DA. Hallucinations, delusions, and cognitive decline in Alzheimer's disease. *J Neurol Neurosurg Psychiatry.* 2000d;69:172–7.

Wilson RS, Mendes de Leon CF, Barnes LL, Schneider JA, Bienias JL, Evans DA, and Bennett DA. Participation in cognitively stimulating activities and risk of incident Alzheimer's disease. *JAMA*. 2002;287:742–748.

Wilson RS, Evans DA, Bienias JL, Mendes de Leon CF, Schneider JA, and Bennett DA. Proneness to psychological distress and risk of Alzheimer's disease. *Neurology*. 2003;61:1579–1585.

Wilson RS, Schneider JA, Bienias JL, Evans DA, and Bennett DA. Parkinsonian-like signs and risk of incident Alzheimer's disease in older persons. *Archives of Neurology*. 2003;60:539–544.

Wilson RS, Krueger KR, Arnold SE, Schneider JA, Kelly JF, Barnes LL, et al. Loneliness and risk of Alzheimer's disease. *Archives of General Psychiatry*. 2007;64:234–40.

Wilson RS, Scherr PA, Schneider JA, Tang Y, and Bennett DA. The relation of cognitive activity to risk of developing Alzheimer's disease. *Neurology*. 2007;69:1911–20.

Wilson RS, Schneider JA, Arnold SE, Bienias JL, and Bennett DA. Conscientiousness and the incidence of Alzheimer's disease and mild cognitive impairment. *Archives of General Psychiatry*. 2007;64: 1204–12.

Yaffe K, Fox P, Newcomer R, Sands L, Lindquist K, Dane K, and Covinsky KE. Patient and caregiver characteristics and nursing home placement in patients with dementia. *JAMA*. 2002;287:2090–7.

Yesavage JA, Brink TL, Rose TL, Lum O, Huang V, Adey M, and Leirer VO. Development and validation of a geriatric depression screening scale: A preliminary report. *J Psychiatr Res*. 1982-1983;17:37–49.

17 Frontotemporal Dementia and Related Syndromes

Mario F. Mendez, Harry V. Vinters, and Jeffrey L. Cummings

Introduction

Frontotemporal dementia (FTD) syndromes comprise a group of related disorders with degeneration of the frontal lobes, anterior temporal lobes, or both. Arnold Pick originally described a patient with left anterior temporal degeneration in 1892 and published a series of three patients with left anterior temporal atrophy in 1904 (Baldwin et al. 1993; Pick 1892). Seven years later, Alois Alzheimer described the neuropathology of what came to be known as "Pick's disease." Little subsequent research occurred in FTD syndromes until the late 1980s when investigators in Lund, Sweden reported on a large autopsy series of patients with dementia (Brun and Passant 1996; Gustafson 1993). They found 20 (13%) patients with frontal lobe degeneration among a total of 158 patients. From then on, developments began to accelerate quickly with several clinicopathological studies of FTD (Knopman et al. 1990; Mendez et al. 1993) and the eventual demonstration of a linkage of some cases to the tau gene region on chromosome 17 (Wilhelmsen et al. 1994). More recently, in 2006, researchers discovered an association of FTD with mutations in the progranulin gene (PGRN) and identified one of the major ubiquitinated proteins in FTD as the TAR DNA-binding protein 43 (TDP-43) (Arai et al. 2006; Baker et al. 2006; Cruts et al. 2006; Neumann et al. 2006).

The three main FTD syndromes are the behavioral variant (bvFTD), which comprises over half of these patients, and the language-predominant syndromes of progressive non-fluent aphasia (PNFA) and semantic dementia (SD). Although often underdiagnosed (Kertesz and Munoz 2002; Mendez et al. 2002, 2007), bvFTD is the third most common neurodegenerative dementia after Alzheimer's disease (AD) and dementia with Lewy bodies (DLB). In the largest clinic-based series, there were 74 (5%) patients diagnosed with FTD syndromes among 1517 consecutive outpatients attending a memory disorders program (Pasquier et al. 1999). Other reports, particularly from Japan, describe frequencies of FTD of 7–13% among dementia outpatients (Ikeda et al. 2004; Imamura et al. 1999). In possibly the best population-based series, there was a calculated annual (1990–1994) incidence of FTD in Rochester, MN, of 2.2 per 100,000 in the age group 40–49 years, 3.3 for 50–59, and 8.9 for 60–69 (Knopman et al. 2004).

The FTD syndromes usually have a presenile onset, occur about equally among men and women, and have no proven ethnic predisposition. The age of onset of bvFTD averages around 57 years with a usual range of 51 to 63 years, but patients have presented as early as the 20s and as late as the 80s (Coleman et al. 2002; Johnson et al. 2005; Pasquier and Delacourte 1998). The age of onset of SD is similar to that of bvFTD, but PNFA patients are often slightly older (Johnson et al. 2005). FTD syndromes are common among dementia patients with an age of onset of less than 65 years, accounting for 20% or more of neurodegenerative dementias (The Lund and Manchester Groups 1994; Pasquier and Delacourte 1998; Ratnavalli et al. 2002; Robert et al. 1999) with prevalences in the 45–64 year age group of 15 per 100,000 in the U.K. and 6.7 per 100,000 in the Netherlands (Harvey et al. 2003; Ratnavalli et al. 2002; Rosso et al. 2003).

Pathology and Pathophysiology

On gross pathology, "frontotemporal lobar degeneration" primarily characterizes the brains of patients with FTD syndromes. The ventromedial frontal region and the anterior temporal areas show the most severe atrophic changes. The cortical degeneration is usually initially asymmetric and involves mainly the gray matter, including the insula and the anterior cingulate gyrus (Gustafson et al. 1992; Hooten and Lyketsos 1996). There is neuronal and synaptic loss and astrogliosis with spongiosis (minute cavities or microvacuolation) of the outer, supragranular (II–III) layers of the frontotemporal cortex, with variable involvement of subcortical and limbic structures (Hooten and Lyketsos 1996; Schmitt et al. 1995). Neurochemical investigations reveal that serotonergic and dopaminergic systems are decreased with relative sparing of cholinergic systems (Rinne et al. 2002; Sparks et al. 1994).

The FTD syndromes include pathological variants that are either due primarily to the neuronal accumulation of TAR DNA-binding protein-43 (TDP-43) protein, with tau-negative, ubiquitin-positive inclusions, or of tau protein, with tau-positive inclusions (See Figure 1). Among 74 bvFTD patients from North America, 55% were associated with a TDP-43 proteinopathy (Josephs et al. 2006d; Kertesz et al. 2005), and among 26 bvFTD patients from the U.K. and Australia there were equal numbers with tau-positive and tau-negative pathology (Hodges et al. 2004). TDP-43 is a nuclear protein that functions in the regulation of transcription and mRNA splicing (Buratti and Baralle 2008). TDP-43 is a normal nuclear protein when ubiquinated but it is abnormal when phosphorylated (Buratti and Baralle 2008). Tau is a microtubule-associated protein that functions to stabilize microtubules and promote microtubule assembly by binding to tubulin (Hirokawa et al 1994). If tau is hyperphosphorylated, microtubules break down and there is impairment of axonal transport.

The majority of FTD patients have tau-negative, ubiquitin-positive inclusions which contain TDP-43 (Freeman et al. 2008; Lipton et al. 2004; Mackenzie et al. 2007). In neuronal injury, there is an increased expression of TDP-43, which undergoes caspase dependent cleavage and then forms insoluble neuronal inclusions. Investigators have categorized these ubiquitin-positive inclusions into different ubiquitin subtypes (U1-U5) depending on the distribution of ubiquitin positivity (See Table 1) (Cairns et al. 2007; Grossman et al. 2007; Mackenzie et al. 2006; Snowden et al. 2007). About one-half are U2, a quarter U1, and another quarter U3. Many FTD cases formerly described as "dementia lacking distinctive histology" have now been shown to have ubiquinated inclusions and evidence of neuronal loss with or without hippocampal sclerosis (Josephs et al. 2004a,b; Lipton et al. 2004;

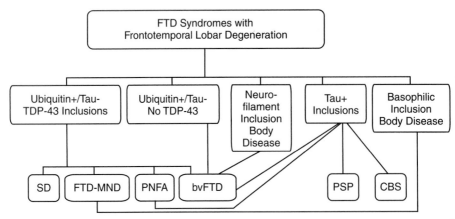

Figure 1 FTD syndromes with frontotemporal lobar degeneration. This figure demonstrates the relationships among the different pathologic and clinical variants.

Mackenzie et al. 2007). In addition to over half of the bvFTD patients, a ubiquitin positive, TDP-43 proteinopathy underlies the SD variant and FTD patients who develop associated motor neuron disease (MND) (Hodges et al. 2004; Josephs et al. 2006d; Kertesz et al. 2005; Knibb et al. 2006). Finally, abnormal TDP-43 immunoreactivity may occur in AD and other neurodegenerative disorders (Amador-Ortiz et al. 2007; Josephs et al. 2008b).

At least a third of patients with FTD syndromes have the accumulation of another abnormal protein, the microtubule-associated protein tau (MAPT) (Adamec et al. 2001; Neary et al. 2000; Poorkaj et al. 2001). Tau has six different isoforms generated by alternative splicing, particularly of exon 10, which affects the number of carboxyl-terminal repeats (Andreadis et al. 1992; Goedert et al. 1989). "Tauopathy" results from tau-positive inclusions from filaments formation due to either an imbalance in the ratio of tau isoforms with three or four microtubular binding repeats or to the abnormal hyperphosphorylation of tau. In addition to a portion of the bvFTD patients, tauopathy underlies most of those with the PNFA variant and those who develop parkinsonism, including the related disorders of progressive supranuclear palsy (PSP)

and corticobasal degeneration (CBD) (Boeve et al. 2003; Josephs et al. 2006a,d; Kertesz et al. 2005; Hodges et al. 2004).

Although more than 90% of FTD syndromes are either a TDP-43 proteinopathy or a tauopathy, a small proportion of FTD cases are associated with other pathologies. One such pathology is neurofilament inclusion body disease (Cairns et al. 2004a,b; Josephs et al. 2003), which is due to the accumulation of intraneuronal inclusions that are immunoreactive to neurofilament and α-internexin. Another rare pathology is basophilic inclusion disease which results in the identification of basophilic round neuronal inclusions that show variable immunoreactivity to ubiquitin but are unreactive to other stains (Aizawa et al. 2000). Basophilic inclusion body disease tends to be associated with bvFTD with MND (Matsumoto et al. 1992; Munoz-Garcia and Ludwin. 1984).

Genetic Contribution

A positive family history of a similar dementia in a first-degree relative is present in 38–50% of patients with an FTD syndrome (Stevens et al.

Table 1 Ubiquitin-Positive Inclusions

Type	TDP-43 Histopathology	Clinical Syndromes	Genetic Association
U1	Yes	Dystrophic neurites (elongated, long), Semantic Dementia	None known
		Neuronal cytoplasmic inclusions (few)	
U2	Yes	Dystrophic neurites (few, short), FTD-MND, MND	Intraflagellar
U3	Yes	Neuronal cytoplasmic inclusions	transport 74
		Dystrophic neurites (short), bvFTD, PNFA PRGN	transport 74
		Neuronal cytoplasmic inclusions,	
		Neuronal intranuclear inclusions	
U4	Yes	Dystrophic neurites, bvFTD	VCP
		Neuronal cytoplasmic inclusions (very few),	
		Neuronal intranuclear inclusions	
U5	No	None	bvFTD CHMP2B

Reference: Cairns et al. 2007

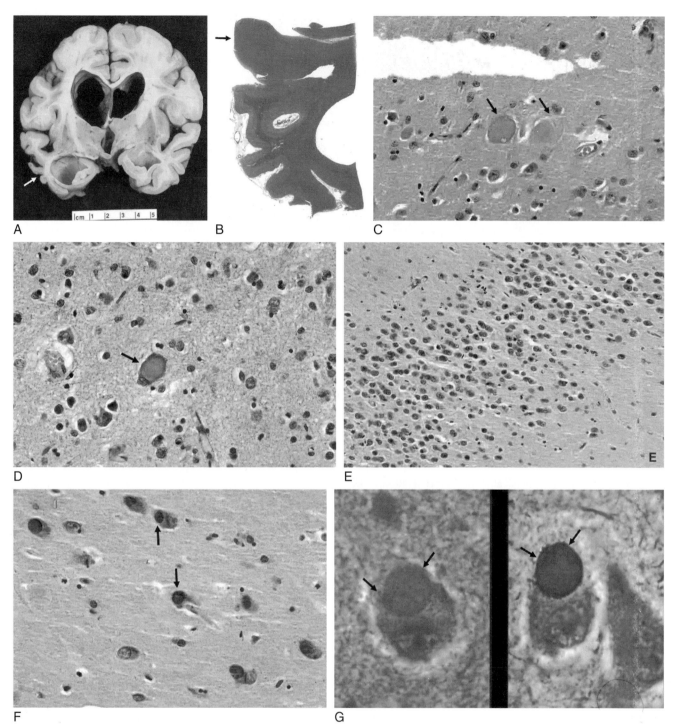

Figure 2 FTLD Neuropathology with Pick Bodies. Panel A shows representative coronal section of a fixed brain with asymmetrical cerebral cortical atrophy, affecting left cerebral hemisphere more prominently than right, and compensatory enlargement of the lateral ventricles (left greater than right). The arrow indicates marked atrophy of the left middle and inferior temporal gyri. In contrast, the entire right temporal lobe appears relatively intact. (Note that, in this and other images of fixed brain, left side of brain is "on the left," and right is "on the right," i.e. the reverse of how neuroradiographic images are usually presented). Panel B shows whole mount from a similar case to that illustrated in panel A. Arrow indicates preserved superior temporal gyrus, but atrophic middle and inferior temporal gyri. Panel C. Balloon-like neurons (arrows) in the cerebral cortex (Hematoxylin & Eosin or H&E stain). Neuron at left shows granulovacuolar-like change. Panel D. A cortical balloon cell (arrow) immunostained with primary antibody to tau. Panels E, F. Hippocampal granule cell layer neurons (E) and pyramidal neurons (F) immunostained with primary antibody to tau. Note prominent Pick bodies in most neurons (highlighted by arrows in panel F). Panel G. Pick bodies-H&E (left) and silver stain (right). Magnified view of Pick bodies, photographed from and H&E-stained section (at left) and a silver (Bodian) stained section (at right). Pick bodies are indicated by arrows in both panels.

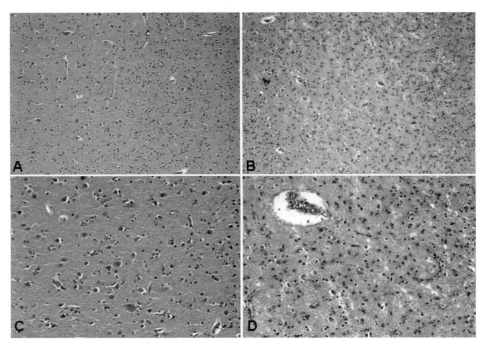

Figure 3 Some cases of FTLD show relatively non-specific histopathology, manifest as subtle neuron loss, astrocytic gliosis and slight spongy change, the latter much more subtle than in cases of spongiform encephalopathy (CJD). All micrographs are from H&E-stained sections; panels A, C are from 'control' cortex photographed at low and high magnification; panels B, D are from cortex of a patient with FTLD photographed a comparable magnification to images at left. See Figure 17.3 on the color insert.

1998; Chow et al. 1999), and direct autosomal dominant inheritance may be present in about 15% (Josephs 2008). Among familial cases, 5–26% are PGRN mutations and 7–21% are MAPT mutations, both linked to chromosome 17 (Cruts et al. 2006; Gass et al. 2006; LeBer et al. 2007; Pickering-Brown et al. 2008).

In 2006, two groups of researchers reported the identification of mutations in the progranulin (PGRN) gene that were associated with FTD and ubiquitin-positive (U3) inclusions (Cruts et al. 2006; Baker et al. 2006; Josephs et al. JNEN07; Mackenzie et al. Br07). Since then, investigators have described from 40 to 50 different PGRN mutations that led to degradation of mutant RNA (Baker et al, 2006; Gass et al, 2006; Rademakers and Hutton, 2007). Progranulin is a 593 amino acid, secreted glycosolated protein that is a growth factor, plays a role in brain development, has anti-inflammatory properties, and functions in wound healing. Its relationship to TDP-43 is, as yet, not definitely established.

MAPT mutations may result in neurodegeneration from hyperphosphorylation of tau and tau aggregation in neurons and glia resulting in interference with axonal transport (Foster et al. 1997; Hutton et al. 1998). One common mechanism leading to this abnormal tau function and aggregation is missplicing of exon 10 and the surrounding intronic "stem-loop." Investigators have reported over 40 different potential pathogenic MAPT mutations including 27 missense mutations, 4 silent mutations, 2 in-frame single codon deletions, and 8 intronic mutations (Rademakers and Hutton 2007).

In addition to PGRN and MAPT, there are a few rare genetic mutations associated with FTD syndromes. Mutations in the charged multi-vesicular body protein 2B (CHMP2B) linked to chromosome 3 results in early onset bvFTD with severe cognitive deficits (Skibinski et al. 2005). CHMP2B plays a role in efficient autophagy. Neuropathologically, there are ubiquitinated inclusions that were not immunoreactive to TDP-43 (U5) (Holm et al. 2007). Mutations in the valosin-containing protein (VCP) linked to chromosome 9 results in bvFTD with

inclusion body myopathy or Paget's disease (Watts et al. 2004). VCP is an ATPase associated with multiple cellular activity. At autopsy, there are widespread ubiquitin- and TDP-43-positive intranuclear inclusions (U4) (Cairns et al. 2007; Neumann et al. 2007). Interestingly, investigators have identified mutations in the gene encoding for TDP-43 in familial amyotrophic lateral sclerosis, but not in FTD-MND families (Gitcho et al. 2008; Sreedharan et al. 2008). Finally, the clinical bvFTD phenotype can result from an alternative transcription of the presenilin 1 mutation associated with familial AD (Mendez et al. 2006).

Clinical Presentations

Behavioral Variant FTD

The main clinical syndrome of FTD usually presents with several specific personality and behavioral changes in mid-life (See Table 2) (Bathgate et al. 2001; Bozeat et al. 2000; Mendez et al. 2008). Most commonly, there is apathy or abulia with decreased spontaneity and interest. Second, there is disinhibition and impulsivity. Third, patients lose insight into these personality and behavioral changes and lack self-referential behaviors such as embarrassability or shame. Fourth, they manifest "emotional blunting" with a loss of empathy and awareness of the needs of others. Basic emotional appreciation is diminished as well with decreased perception of facial or vocal emotions (Keane et al. 2002; Lavenu et al. 1999; Lough et al. 2006). Fifth, bvFTD patients violate social and moral norms or conventions. They may readily touch others or violate their personal space, talk to children that they don't know, make sexual comments, forego tact or table manners, and even manifest sociopathic behavior. Sixth, they may have changes in dietary or eating behavior, most commonly a carbohydrate craving. Finally, bvFTD patients have a range of repetitive behaviors from simple motor stereotypies to more complex compulsive-like acts. A further supportive criterion is neglect or loss of interest in personal hygiene with failure to wash, bathe, groom, or

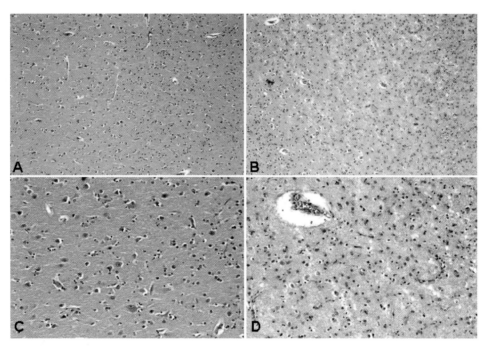

Figure 17.3 Some cases of FTLD show relatively non-specific histopathology, manifest as subtle neuron loss, astrocytic gliosis and slight spongy change, the latter much more subtle than in cases of spongiform encephalopathy (CJD). All micrographs are from H&E-stained sections; panels A, C are from 'control' cortex photographed at low and high magnification; panels B, D are from cortex of a patient with FTLD photographed a comparable magnification to images at left.

dress appropriately. In comparison, psychotic symptoms such as delusions and hallucinations are uncommon in FTD.

Cognitive Functions

Patients with bvFTD develop a frontal "dysexecutive" syndrome. Abnormal executive behavior is reflected in their lack of insight and loss of awareness or distress at their disability or the consequences of their behavior. Judgment is abnormal, and bvFTD patients are often concrete on idiom and proverb interpretation. Some patients have stimulus-bound behavior such as echolalia and utilization behavior (grasping and repeatedly using objects that they see or tending to read aloud anything they see). On language assessment, bvFTD patients tend towards progressively decreased verbal output, reiterative speech or verbal stereotypies, and progression to complete mutism. In contrast,

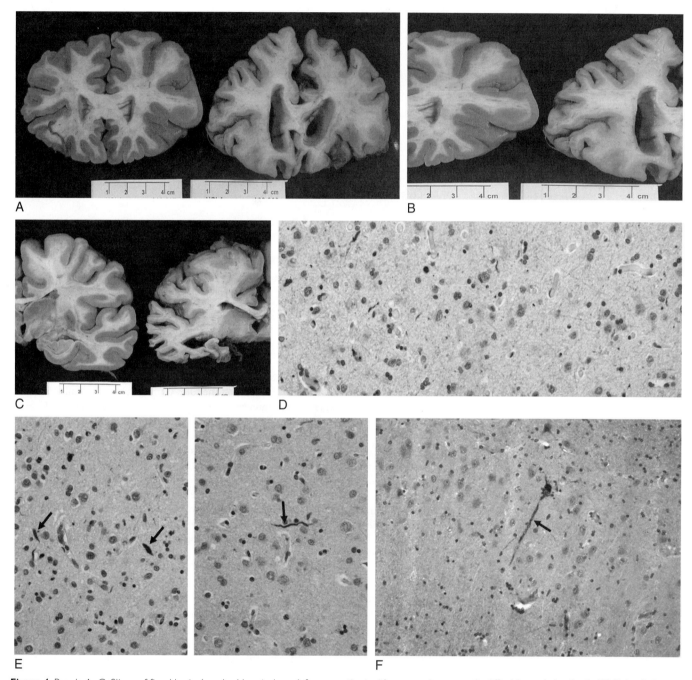

Figure 4 Panels A–C. Slices of fixed brain (cerebral hemispheres) from a patient with progressive semantic difficulties, culminating in FTLD. In all three panels, a control specimen is at left of the image, the patient's brain is at right. In all regions, note diffuse frontotemporal atrophy of a severe degree, with compensatory enlargement of the lateral ventricles (hydrocephalus *ex vacuo*). Especially prominent enlargement of the left temporal horn is noted in panel C. Cortical ribbon in the affected gyri is thinned, though underlying subcortical white matter is relatively preserved. Panels D & E show anti-ubiquitin immunostained sections from this patient's cortex, with rod-like ubiquitin immunoreactivity scattered throughout cortex in multiple regions (patient was thought to have "FTLD-U"). Ubiquitin positive "neurites" are highlighted by arrows in panel E. Panel F shows a rare tau-immunoreactive neurofibrillary tangle in pyramidal cell layer of the hippocampus.

Table 2 Behavioral Variant Frontotemporal Dementia: Consensus Criteria

I. Core diagnostic features (all must be present)

    A. Insidious onset and gradual progression

    B. Early decline in social interpersonal conduct

    C. Early impairment in regulation of personal conduct

    D. Early emotional blunting

    E. Early loss of insight

II. Supportive diagnostic features

    A. Behavioral disorder

        1. Decline in personal hygiene and grooming

        2. Mental rigidity and inflexibility

        3. Distractibility and impersistence

        4. Hyperorality and dietary changes

        5. Perseverative and stereotyped behavior

        6. Utilization behavior

    B. Speech and language: Altered speech output (aspontaneity and economy of speech, press of speech), stereotypy of speech, echolalia, perseveration, mutism

    C. Physical signs: Primitive reflexes, incontinence, akinesia, rigidity, tremor, low and labile blood pressure

    D. Investigations

        1. Neuropsychology: impaired frontal lobe tests; no amnesia or perceptual deficit

        2. EEG: normal on conventional EEG despite clinically evident dementia

        3. Brain imaging: predominant frontal and/or anterior temporal abnormality

(Reprinted from Neary et al. 1998.)

Table 3 Progressive Nonfluent Aphasia: Consensus Criteria

I. Core diagnostic features

    A. Insidious onset and gradual progression

    B. Nonfluent spontaneous speech with at least one of the following: agrammatism, phonemic paraphasias, anomia

II. Supportive diagnostic features

    A. Speech and language

        1. Stuttering or oral apraxia

        2. Impaired repetition

        3. Alexia, agraphia

        4. Early preservation of word meaning

        5. Late mutism

    B. Behavior

        1. Early preservation of social skills

        2. Late behavioral changes similar to FTD

    C. Physical signs: late contralateral primitive reflexes, akinesia, rigidity, and tremor

    D. Investigations

        1. Neuropsychology: nonfluent aphasia without amnesia or pereeptual disorder

        2. EEG: normal or minor asymmetric slowing

        3. Brain imaging (structural and/or functional): asymmetric abnormality predominantly affecting dominant (usually left) hemisphere

(Reprinted from Neary et al. 1998.)

bvFTD patients are not classically amnesic and have better free recall, cued recall, and recognition than do Alzheimer's disease patients (Glosser et al. 2002; Nestor et al. 2002; Pasquier et al. 2001). Furthermore, they have relatively preserved visuospatial abilities such as spatial localization and orientation in familiar surroundings (Hodges and Gurd. 1994; Neary. 1995). Some bvFTD patients may even have a facilitation of artistic and musical ability (Miller et al. 2000).

On neurological examination, most bvFTD patients are normal early in their course but can develop primitive reflexes and motor changes as the disease progresses. Some develop parkinsonism, dystonia and ideomotor apraxia, or fasciculations and muscle wasting. Many of those who develop parkinsonism eventually meet criteria for the related syndromes of PSP and CBD (Boeve et al. 2002; Jendroska et al. 1995; Kertesz et al. 1994, 2000; Henderson et al. 2001; Mathuranath et al. 2000; Miyamoto et al. 2001). Finally, 10–15% of bvFTD patients develop MND, primarily with bulbar and proximal upper extremity impairment (Caselli et al. 1993; Ferrer et al. 1991; Neary et al. 1990; Sam et al. 1991). Conversely, up to 10% of patient with MND might show features of dementia or aphasia (Murphy et al. 2007).

On neuropsychological testing, bvFTD patients perform particularly poorly on tests of executive functions (Hodges 2001; Hodges and Miller 2001). They are often impaired on Trailmaking Test B, verbal fluency, and the Wisconsin Card Sort Test (fewer categories, greater perseverations). They are poor on the Iowa Gambling Test and fail to improve when offered monetary rewards (Graham 2005; Torralva et al. 2007). Patients with the bvFTD syndrome cannot do tasks of abstraction and have poor verb comprehension relative to nouns (Cappa et al. 1998; Rhee et al. 2001; Snowden et al. 2003). Patients may be impaired on paradigms where they must infer other people's mental states, thoughts, and feelings, referred to as "theory of mind" (Gregory et al. 2002), and the ability to process social rule violations is impaired along with their sense of "personal' morality (Lough et al. 2006; Mendez et al. 2005). In comparison, there is an absence of severe amnesia or visuospatial impairments on neuropsychological measures.

Progressive Nonfluent Aphasia

PNFA is characterized by an initial two or more year period of relatively isolated difficulty in verbal expression with anomia, shortened phrase length, and agrammatism in the presence of relatively preserved comprehension (See Table 3) (Gorno-Tempini et al. 2004; Kertesz et al. 2005; Neary et al. 1998). Patients have particular difficulty with verbs and with sentence processing (Grossman 2002). Motor speech is also disturbed. The patients have apraxia of speech with hesitant, broken, and effortful output and phonologic (phonemic paraphasic) errors, particularly in repetition of polysyllabic words. Additional speech changes include progressive dysarthria with stuttering and oral apraxia (Santens et al. 1999). Reading and writing is correspondingly impaired. Patients with PNFA are aware of their language and speech deficits.

Table 4 Semantic Dementia: Consensus Criteria

I. Core diagnostic features

 A. Insidious onset and gradual progression

 B. Language disorder characterized by

  1. Progressive, fluent, empty spontaneous speech

  2. Loss of word meaning, manifest by impaired naming and comprehension

  3. Semantic paraphasias *and/or*

 C. Perceptual disorder characterized by

  1. Prosopagnosia: impaired recognition of identity of familiar faces *and/or*

  2. Object agnosia: impaired recognition of object identity

 D. Preserved perceptual matching and drawing reproduction

 E. Preserved single-word repetition

 F. Preserved ability to read aloud and write to dictation orthographically regular words

II. Supportive diagnostic features

 A. Speech and language: Press of speech, idiosyncratic word usage, absence of phonemic paraphasias, surface dyslexia and dysgraphia, preserved calculation

 B. Behavior: Loss of sympathy and empathy, narrowed preoccupations, parsimony

 C. Physical signs: Absent or late primitive reflexes, akinesia, rigidity, and tremor

 D. Investigations: Neuropsychology: Profound semantic loss, manifest in failure of word comprehension and naming and/or face and object recognition; preserved phonology, syntax, perceptual/spatial skills, memorizing. EEG: normal; Brain imaging: predominant anterior temporal abnormality-symmetric or asymmetric

(Reprinted from Neary et al. 1998.)

In PNFA, atrophy is asymmetric, involving chiefly the left frontotemporal lobes (Neary et al. 1998). Magnetic resonance imaging (MRI) with voxel-based morphometry (VBM) and functional imaging reveal marked atrophic changes or hypometabolism and decreased blood flow localized to the left perisylvian, inferior frontal, and anterior insular regions (Gorno-Tempini et al. 2004; Rosen et al. 2002; San Pedro et al. 2000). PNFA tends to progress anteriorly and is usually associated with FTD pathology, but some patients have had a focal form of AD at postmortem (Green et al. 1990).

Semantic Dementia

This FTD variant results in multimodal loss of conceptual knowledge, particularly in word comprehension and in facial recognition (See Table 4). In contrast to PNFA patients, those with SD are fluent and have normal grammatical speech output but cannot understand words (Adlam et al. 2006). Their speech output becomes empty as they progressively lose substantive words and their meanings from their vocabulary. Testing involves evaluating single word comprehension with pointing commands, asking for word definitions, and having them match objects or pictures with words. There is relative preservation of repetition, phonology, syntax, the ability to read aloud, and the ability to write orthographically regular words. On reading, there is "surface dyslexia" with inability to read irregularly spelled words but preserved ability to sound them out from their spelling (Noble et al. 2000). The rest of the cognitive profile in SD reflects semantic loss in other domains. In particular, there may be an impairment in the recognition of familiar faces (prosopagnosia) and impairment of object meaning or identity (object agnosia) that cannot be attributed to naming difficulties. Despite these deficits, SD patients can learn (episodic or autobiographical memory) and have intact visuospatial skills (Galton et al. 2001; Nestor et al. 2006).

SD is associated with circumscribed atrophy of the anterior inferior temporal gyri bilaterally (Mummery et al. 2000). From a neuropsychological perspective, the function of this region is to bind information together. Most SD patients have asymmetric involvement with greater atrophy in the left anterior temporal region compared to the right. Cortical atrophy involves the left inferolateral temporal lobe and fusiform gyrus, right temporal pole, bilateral ventromedial frontal cortex, and the amygdaloid complex with sparing of the hippocampus, entorhinal, or caudal perirhinal cortex (Mummery et al. 2000). The asymmetric involvement of the left and right temporal lobes is often evident on MRI imaging and correlates with relative impairments for word meaning versus prosopagnosia or object recognition, respectively (Hodges et al. 1999; Rosen et al. 2002).

Diagnosis

The FTD syndromes are clinical diagnoses. There are as yet no definitive laboratory tests for these disorders (except for those with identifiable mutations). In bvFTD, behavioral changes usually precede or overshadow their cognitive disabilities (Mendez et al. 1993; Miller et al. 1991; Pasquier and Delacourte 1998; The Lund and Manchester Groups 1994), and suspicion of bvFTD arises when there is a gradual personality change usually in mid-life (Knopman et al. 1989; Neary et al. 1993, 1998; The Lund and Manchester Groups 1994). In contrast, suspicion of the PNFA or SD variants of FTD arises when there is new speech or word-finding difficulty in mid-life. Clinical criteria for diagnosing the three main FTD syndromes are the FTD Consensus Criteria (See Tables 2–4) (Galante et al. 1999; Neary et al. 1998). Despite selected reports of high sensitivities and specificities for these criteria (Lopez et al. 1999), clinicians frequently misdiagnose or fail to recognize the FTD syndromes (Halliday et al. 2002; Litvan et al. 1997; McKhann et al. 2001; Mendez et al. 1993).

Structural neuroimaging, particularly MRI, can help confirm the presence of an FTD syndrome (See Figure 5) (Knopman et al. 1998). Although not sensitive to early clinical changes (Kirshner 1999; Rossor 1999), most FTD patients eventually show frontal and anterior temporal atrophy, enlargement of the Sylvian fissures, and anterior callosal atrophy (Duara et al. 1999; Friedland et al. 1993; Frisoni et al. 1999; Kaufer et al. 1997; Kitagaki et al. 1998; Rosen et al. 2002; Yamauchi et al. 2000). Hippocampal atrophy is less severe than for AD, and there is more temporal polar, amygdalar, and lateral temporal and fusiform gyral involvement (Frisoni et al. 1999; Galton et al. 2001a,b; Jack et al. 2002; Laakso et al. 2000). Some FTD patients may have additional MRI evidence of bilateral caudate atrophy, and others have changes in the substantia nigra and putamen or high signal changes in white matter (Varma et al. 2002). VBM studies in autopsy-confirmed cohorts have confirmed the mesial frontal, anterior insular, and anterior temporal regional atrophy (Josephs et al. 2006a, 2008a,b; Whitwell et al. 2005, 2007d). Among patients with the related syndromes of PSP and CBD, there is posterior frontal and parietal lobe involvement (Josephs et al. 2008a). Finally, both the TDP-43 proteinopathies and the tauopathies appear to have frontal atrophy, but there may be more anterior

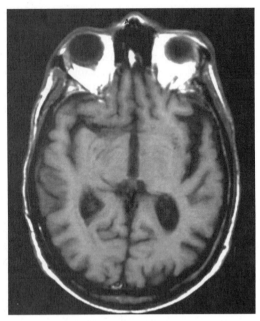

Figure 5 MRI (T2-weighted) image of progressive nonfluent aphasia (PNFA). Asymmetric atrophy of the left Sylvian fissure with reciprocal enlargement of the left frontal horn.

temporal involvement among the TDP-43 proteinopathies (except in the presence of MND) (Whitwell et al. 2005; 2007).

Functional imaging is more sensitive than structural imaging for the diagnosis of FTD. Single-photon emission tomography and positron emission tomography (PET) scans show decreased regional cerebral blood flow and hypometabolism in the frontal cortex and anterior temporal lobes, respectively (see Figure 6) (Alexander et al. 1995; Charpentier et al. 2000; Friedland et al. 1993; Miller et al. 1991). Using fluorodeoxyglucose (FDG)-PET, Jeong et al. (2005a) demonstrated significant frontal and anterior temporal hypometabolism in 29 bvFTD cases. Glucose uptake is reduced primarily in dorsolateral and ventrolateral prefrontal cortices and in frontopolar and anterior cingulate regions (Garraux et al. 1999). Although the lack of specificity limits the contribution of functional imaging for diagnosis (Pasquier et al. 1997), worsening of cerebral blood flow or of hypometabolism over time favors the diagnosis of a neurodegenerative dementia such as FTD (Golan et al. 1996; Sjogren et al. 2000). Furthermore, 90% of cases had significant discordance between left and right hemispheric involvement emphasizing that asymmetry, in particular, may help discriminate FTD from other degenerative disorders. Finally, the use of new functional imaging technologies, such as Pittsburgh Compound B (PIB), holds great promise for distinguishing FTD syndromes from AD and other neurodegenerative disorders with amyloid-related pathology (Cummings 2008).

There are compelling relationships between symptoms and regions of involvement in FTD. Cases with right greater than left-sided atrophy have a higher prevalence of bvFTD (Rosen et al. 2005; Williams et al. 2005). The initial locus of pathology in bvFTD typically involves the ventromedial frontal cortices (Broe et al. 2003; Ibach et al. 2004; Kril and Halliday 2004), and functional imaging particularly implicates this region when there are significant abnormalities in social conduct (Hornak et al. 2003). Apathy correlates with the degree of mesial frontal atrophy near the frontal pole on both MRI VBM and on FDG-PET, whereas disinhibition correlates with atrophy of the subcallosal part of the mesial frontal lobe (Franceschi et al. 2005; Rosen et al.

2005). Left peri-Sylvian and anterior insular involvement correlates with PNFA and apraxia of speech (Josephs et al. 2006), and anterior temporal atrophy correlates with SD and the loss of the ability to form semantic associates (Galton et al. 2001; Snowden et al. 2004). In SD, worse atrophy in the left anterior temporal atrophy corresponds to impaired word comprehension and worse right temporal atrophy corresponds to impaired recognition of faces (see Figure 7).

Biomarker studies, such as plasma TDP-43 or tau levels, have not yet proven to be clinically useful, but plasma levels of the progranulin protein are decreased in FTD patients with PRGN mutations (Coppola et al. 2008; Ghidoni et al. 2008). Cerebrospinal fluid (CSF) biomarkers may help distinguish FTD from AD (Ingelson et al. 1999). Among patients with bvFTD, one study found a significant decrease of CSF tau (Roks et al. 1999), others found normal or increased CSF total tau and phospho-tau levels, but lower than that for AD (Fabre et al. 2001; Green et al. 1999; Riemenschneider et al. 2002; Rosengren et al. 1999; Sjogren et al. 2000a,b; Sjogren and Wallin. 2001). In the only autopsy-verified study to date, low CSF total tau occurred among 52% of FTD patients compared to 24% of AD, along with a lower tau/Aβ42 amyloid ratio with 1.9 cut-off (Hu et al. 2008). Although requiring further study, it appears that there are significantly lower total tau and tau/Aβ42 amyloid ratios in FTD compared to AD. Finally, an increase in CSF neurofilament protein occurs early in FTD and late in AD (Sjogren et al. 2000a,b). Differences between tauopathies and other forms of FTD are to be anticipated.

Treatment

The management of bvFTD, a disorder characterized by varied behavioral symptoms, involves primarily the use of psychoactive medications. Although there are no approved treatments for the disorder, selective serotonin-receptor inhibitors, such as sertraline, paroxetine, or fluoxetine, can decrease disinhibition-impulsivity, repetitive behaviors, and eating disorders in bvFTD (Swartz et al. 1997). Low doses of trazodone or an atypical antipsychotic such as aripriprazole can also help manage significantly disturbed or agitated behavior, disinhibition, or verbal outbursts. Antipsychotics, however, carry some risk in dementia and in bvFTD. Occasionally, similar to patients with dementia with Lewy bodies, patients with bvFTD may manifest unusual neuroleptic hypersensitivity (Janssen et al. 2002; Mendez and Lipton 2001), and the US Food and Drug Administration has required warning labels on antipsychotic medications that they may increase mortality in elderly patients. The acetylcholinesterase inhibitors used for patients with AD have not had significant efficacy for patients with bvFTD and may worsen disinhibition or compulsions (Mendez et al. 2006. One major study of the acetylcholinesterase inhibitor galantamine found no improvement except in progressive aphasia subgroups on language scores (Kertesz et al. 2007). Memantine, another dementia medication, is under investigation for the treatment of this disorder (Diehl-Schmidt et al. 2008). Most recently, investigators have initiated steps toward rational drug therapy with the development of outcome measures for clinical drug trials in FTD and the characterization of treatment targets such the TDP-43 or tau protein (Knopman et al. 2008). This approach holds great promise for an eventual treatment for this devastating early-onset dementia.

In addition to drug therapy, the non-pharmacological management of patients with FTD syndromes focuses on behavioral interventions and care of the caregivers. Some behavioral disturbances such as social misconduct and stereotypy may respond to retraining or to rehabilitation techniques (Ikeda et al. 1995; Robinson. 2001). Speech therapy may benefit PNFA and SD patients; physical and occupational therapy may benefit those with motor difficulties. Special attention is needed

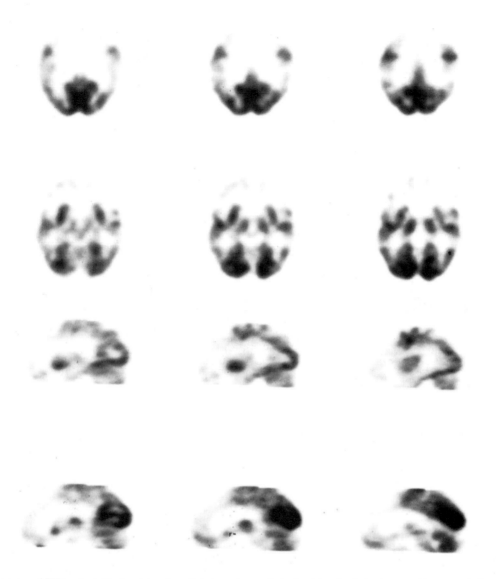

Figure 6 FDG-PET imaging of FTD patient. Horizontal and saggital views demonstrate frontal and anterior temporal hypometabolism.

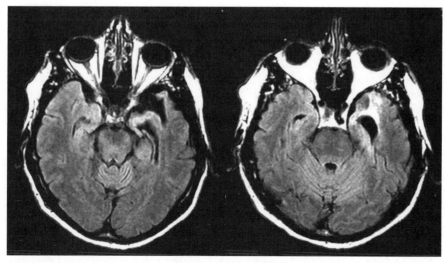

Figure 7 MRI (T2-weighted) images from patient with semantic dementia (SD). There is bilateral anterior temporal atrophy disproportionately affecting the left temporal lobe and associated with impaired word comprehension.

SECTION 3 COGNITIVE DISORDERS IN AGING

for safety issues among behaviorally-disturbed FTD patients (Talerico and Evans 2001). When hyperorality is present, restrictions may be necessary to prevent excessive weight gain or lethal ingestion behaviors (Mendez and Foti 1997). As immobility occurs, FTD patients become susceptible to pulmonary emboli, aspiration pneumonia, urinary tract infections, and decubitus ulcers. Finally, FTD is very stressful to families, and caregiver and family support and education is critical, including the availability of psychosocial support and community resources.

Natural Progression of Disease

The usual duration of FTD is 8 to 11 years (Mendez et al. 1993; Snowden et al. 2003), although variants such as those with MND have a shorter, more malignant course (Pasquier and Delacourte 1998). There is no apparent relationship between impairment level and illness duration, indicating considerable individual variation in the clinical course of FTD (Elfgren et al. 1993). As the disease progresses from its initial syndrome, there is an accumulation of cognitive deficits and an evolution towards mutism. Syndromes may transform from one phenotype to another. For example, patients may begin with language syndromes and evolve to PSP-like disorders. Impairment of all spheres of cognition becomes apparent, and the patients become profoundly demented. Death usually results from a terminal pulmonary, urinary tract, or decubitus ulcer infection. Some studies report a decreased survival if there is tau pathology (Xie et al. 2008). Finally, a small enigmatic group of patients fulfilling criteria for bvFTD show little progression in their symptoms over time (Josephs et al. 2006; Davies et al. 2006).

Future Directions and Summary

FTD syndromes are fascinating brain-behavior disorders that are just beginning to be understood. They are heterogeneous in clinical, pathological, and genetic relationships. The main clinical syndromes are bvFTD, with apathy, disinhibition, and other changes in behavior and personality; and PNFA and SD, with prominent language or word comprehension difficulty. These FTD syndromes can be associated or evolve into related neurodegenerative disorders, including PSP, CBD, and MND. In recent years, there has been an explosion of basic scientific discoveries, including the characterization of the underlying neuropathology as predominately TDP-43 or tau proteinopathies and the discovery of mutations of the PRGN, MAPT, and other genes. The current rapid pace of discovery suggests that disease-modifying therapies may be developed targeting FTD syndromes.

References

Adamec, E., Chang, H.T., Stopa, E.G., et al.: Tau protein expression in frontotemporal dementias. Neurosci Lett 315:21–24, 2001.

Adlam, A.L., Patterson, K., Rogers, T.T., et al.: Semantic dementia and fluent primary progressive aphasia: Two sides of the same coin? Brain 129:3066–3080, 2006.

Aizawa, H., Kimura, T., Hashimoto, K., et al.: Basophilic cytoplasmic inclusions in a case of sporadic juvenile amyotrophic lateral sclerosis. J Neurol Sci 176:109–113, 2000.

Alexander, G.E., Prohovnik, I., Sackeim, H.A., et al.: Cortical perfusion and gray matter weight in frontal lobe dementia. J Neuropsychiatry Clin Neurosci 7:188–196, 1995.

Amador-Ortiz, C., Lin, W.L., Ahmed, Z., et al.: TDP-43 immunoreactivity in hippocampal sclerosis and Alzheimer's disease. Ann Neurol 61:435–445, 2007.

Andreadis, A., Brown, W.M., Kosik, K.S.: Structure and novel exons of the human tau gene. Biochemistry 31:10626–10633, 1992.

Arai, T., Hasegawa, M., Akiyama, H., et al.: TDP-43 is a component of ubiquitin-positive tau-negative inclusions in frontotemporal lobar degeneration and amyotrophic lateral sclerosis. Biochem Biophys Res Commun 351:602–611, 2006.

Baker, M., Mackenzie, I.R., Pickering-Brown, S.M., et al.: Mutations in progranulin cause tau-negative frontotemporal dementia linked to chromosome 17. Nature 442:916–919, 2006.

Baldwin, B. and Forstl, H.: 'Pick's disease'—101 years on still there, but in need of reform. Br J Psychiatry 163:100–104, 1993.

Bancher, C., Lassmann, H., Budka, H., et al.: Neurofibrillary tangles in Alzheimer's disease and progressive supranuclear palsy: antigenic similarities and differences. Microtubule-associated protein tau antigenicity is prominent in all types of tangles. Acta Neuropathol 74:39–46, 1987.

Bathgate, D., Snowden, J.S., Varma, A., et al.: Behaviour in frontotemporal dementia, Alzheimer's disease and vascular dementia. Acta Neurol Scand 103:367–378, 2001.

Boeve, B.F., Lang, A.E., Litvan, I.: Corticobasal degeneration and its relationship to progressive supranuclear palsy and frontotemporal dementia. Ann Neurol 54(suppl 5):S15–S19, 2003.

Boeve, B.F., Maraganore, D.M., Parisi, J.E., et al.: Corticobasal degeneration and frontotemporal dementia presentations in a kindred with nonspecific histopathology. Dement Geriatr Cogn Disord 13:80–90, 2002.

Bozeat, S., Gregory, C.A., Ralph, M.A., Hodges, J.R.: Which neuropsychiatric and behavioural features distinguish frontal and temporal variants of frontotemporal dementia from Alzheimer's disease? J Neurol Neurosurg Psychiatry 69:178–186. 2000.

Broe, M., Hodges, J.R., Schofield, E., et al.: Staging disease severity in pathologically confirmed cases of frontotemporal dementia. Neurology 25;60:1005–1011, 2003.

Brun, A., Passant, U.: Frontal lobe degeneration of non-Alzheimer type. Structural characteristics, diagnostic criteria and relation to other frontotemporal dementias. Acta Neurol Scand Suppl 168:28–30, 1996.

Buratti, E. and Baralle, F.E.: Multiple roles of TDP-43 in gene expression, splicing regulation, and human disease. Front Biosci 13:867–878. 2008.

Cairns, N.J., Bigio, E.H., Mackenzie, I.R., et al.: Neuropathologic diagnostic and nosologic criteria for frontotemporal lobar degeneration: consensus of the Consortium for Frontotemporal Lobar Degeneration. Acta Neuropathol 114:5–22. 2007.

Cairns, N.J., Grossman, M., Arnold, S.E., et al.: Clinical and neuropathologic variation in neuronal intermediate filament inclusion disease. Neurology 63:1376–1384, 2004a.

Cairns, N.J., Zhukareva, V., Uryu, K., et al.: alpha-Internexin is present in the pathological inclusions of neuronal intermediate filament inclusion disease. Am J Pathol 164:2153–2161, 2004b.

Cappa, S.F., Binetti, G., Pezzini, A., Padovani, A., Rozzini, L., and Trabucchi, M.: Object and action naming in Alzheimer's disease and frontotemporal dementia. Neurology 50:351–355, 1998.

Caselli, R.J., Windebank, A.J., Petersen, R.C., et al.: Rapidly progressive aphasic dementia and motor neuron disease. Ann Neurol 1993;33:200–207, 1993.

Charpentier, P., Lavenu, I., Defebvre, L., et al.: Alzheimer's disease and frontotemporal dementia are differentiated by discriminant analysis applied to (99m)Tc HmPAO SPECT data. J Neurol Neurosurg Psychiatry 69:661–663, 2000.

Chow, T.W., Miller, B.L., Hayashi, V.N., and Geschwind, D.H.: Inheritance of frontotemporal dementia. Arch Neurol 56:817–822, 1999.

Coleman, L.W., Digre, K.B., Stephenson, G.M., and Townsend, J.J.: Autopsy-proven, sporadic pick disease with onset at age 25 years. Arch Neurol 59:856–859, 2002.

Cummings, J.L.: Progrtessive aphasia and the growing role of biomarkers in neurologic diagnosis. *Ann Neurol*, 2008 (in press).

Cruts, M., Gijselinck, I., van der Zee, J., et al.: Null mutations in progranulin cause ubiquitin-positive frontotemporal dementia linked to chromosome 17q21. *Nature* 442:920–924, 2006.

Davies, R.R., Kipps, C.M., Mitchell, J., et al.: Progression in frontotemporal dementia: Identifying a benign behavioral variant by magnetic resonance imaging. *Arch Neurol* 63:1627–1631, 2006.

Diehl-Schmid, J., Förstl H., Perneczky R., et al.: A 6-month, open-label study of memantine in patients with frontotemporal dementia. *Int J of Geriatric Psychiatry* 23:754–759, 2008.

Duara, R., Barker, W., and Luis, C.A.: Frontotemporal dementia and Alzheimer's disease: Differential diagnosis. *Dement Geriatr Cogn Disord* 1 10 Suppl 1:37–42, 1999.

Elfgren, C., Passant, U., and Risberg, J.: Neuropsychological findings in frontal lobe dementia. *Dementia* 4:214–219, 1993.

Fabre, S.F., Forsell, C., Viitanen, M., et al.: Clinic-based cases with frontotemporal dementia show increased cerebrospinal fluid tau and high apolipoprotein E epsilon4 frequency, but no tau gene mutations. *Exp Neurol* 168:413–418, 2001.

Ferrer, I., Roig, C., Espino, A., et al.: Dementia of frontal lobe type and motor neuron disease. A Golgi study of the frontal cortex. *J Neurol Neurosurg Psychiatry* 54:932–934, 1991.

Forman, M.S., Farmer, J., Johnson, J.K., et al.: Frontotemporal dementia: Clinicopathological correlations. *Ann Neurol* 59:952–962, 2006.

Foster, N.L., Wilhelmsen, K., Sima, A.A., et al.: Frontotemporal dementia and parkinsonism linked to chromosome 17: A consensus conference. Conference participants. *Ann Neurol* 41:706–715, 1997.

Freeman, S.H., Spires-Jones, T., Hyman, B.T., et al.: TAR-DNA binding protein 43 in Pick disease. *J Neuropathol Exp Neurol* 67:62–67, 2008.

Friedland, R.P., Koss, E., Lerner, A., et al.: Functional imaging, the frontal lobes, and dementia. *Dementia* 4:192–203, 1993.

Frisoni, G.B., Laakso, M.P., Beltramello, A., et al.: Hippocampal and entorhinal cortex atrophy in frontotemporal dementia and Alzheimer's disease. *Neurology* 52:91–100, 1999.

Galante, E., Muggia, S., Spinnler, H., and Zuffi, M.: Degenerative dementia of the frontal type. Clinical evidence from 9 cases. *Dement Geriatr Cogn Disord* 10:28–39, 1999.

Galton, C.J., Gomez-Anson, B., Antoun, N., et al.: Temporal lobe rating scale: application to Alzheimer's disease and frontotemporal dementia. *J Neurol Neurosurg Psychiatry* 70:165–173, 2001a.

Galton, C.J., Patterson, K., Graham, K., et al.: Differing patterns of temporal atrophy in Alzheimer's disease and semantic dementia. *Neurology* 57:216–225, 2001b.

Garraux, G., Salmon, E., Degueldre, C., et al.: Comparison of impaired subcortico-frontal metabolic networks in normal aging, subcortico-frontal dementia, and cortical frontal dementia. *Neuroimage* 10:149–162, 1999.

Gass, J., Cannon, A., Mackenzie, I.R., et al.: Mutations in progranulin are a major cause of ubiquitin-positive frontotemporal lobar degeneration. *Hum Mol Genet* 15:2988–3001, 2006.

Gitcho, M.A., Baloh, R.H., Chakraverty, S., et al.: TDP-43 A315T mutation in familial motor neuron disease. *Ann Neurol* 63:535–538, 2008.

Glosser, G., Gallo, J.L., Clark, C.M., and Grossman, M.: Memory encoding and retrieval in frontotemporal dementia and Alzheimer's disease. *Neuropsychology* 16:190–196, 2002.

Goedert, M., Spillantini, M.G., Potier, M.C., et al.: Cloning and sequencing of the cDNA encoding an isoform of microtubule-associated protein tau containing four tandem repeats: differential expression of tau protein mRNAs in human brain. *Embo J* 8:393–399, 1989.

Golan, H., Kremer, J., Freedman, M., Ichise, M.: Usefulness of follow-up regional cerebral blood flow measurements by single-photon emission computed tomography in the differential diagnosis of dementia. *J Neuroimaging* 6:23–28, 1996.

Gorno-Tempini, M.L., Dronkers, N.F., Rankin, K.P., et al.: Cognition and anatomy in three variants of primary progressive aphasia. *Ann Neurol* 55:335–346, 2004.

Graham, K.S., Patterson, K., and Hodges, J.R.: Episodic memory: New insights from the study of semantic dementia. *Curr Opin Neurobiol* 9:245–250, 1999.

Green, A.J., Harvey, R.J., Thompson, E.J., and Rossor, M.N.: Increased tau in the cerebrospinal fluid of patients with frontotemporal dementia and Alzheimer's disease. *Neurosci Lett* 259:133–135, 1999.

Green, J., Morris, J.C., Sandson, J., et al.: Progressive aphasia: A precursor of global dementia? *Neurology* 40:423–429, 1990.

Gregory, C., Lough, S., Stone, V., et al.: Theory of mind in patients with frontal variant frontotemporal dementia and Alzheimer's disease: Theoretical and practical implications. *Brain* 125:752–764, 2002.

Grossman, M., Wood, E.M., Moore, P., et al.: TDP-43 pathologic lesions and clinical phenotype in frontotemporal lobar degeneration with ubiquitin-positive inclusions. *Arch Neurol* 64:1449–1454, 2007.

Grossman, M.: Progressive aphasic syndromes: Clinical and theoretical advances. *Curr Opin Neurol* 15:409–413, 2002.

Gustafson, L., Brun, A., and Passant, U.: Frontal lobe degeneration of non-Alzheimer type. *Baillieres Clin Neurol* 1:559–582, 1992.

Gustafson, L.: Clinical picture of frontal lobe degeneration of non-Alzheimer type. *Dementia* 4:143–148. 1993.

Halliday, G., Ng, T., Rodriguez, M. et al.: Consensus neuropathological diagnosis of common dementia syndromes: Testing and standardising the use of multiple diagnostic criteria. *Acta Neuropathol (Berl)* 104:72–78, 2002.

Harvey, R.J., Skelton-Robinson, M., and Rossor, M.N.: The prevalence and causes of dementia in people under the age of 65 years. *J Neurol Neurosurg Psychiatry* 74:1206–1209, 2003.

Henderson, J.M., Gai, W.P., Hely, M.A., et al.: Parkinson's disease with late Pick's dementia. *Mov Disord* 16:311–319, 2001.

Hirokawa, N.: Microtubule organization and dynamics dependent on microtubule-associated proteins. *Curr Opin Cell Biol* 6:74–81, 1994.

Hodges, J.R., Davies, R.R., Xuereb, J.H., et al.: Clinicopathological correlates in frontotemporal dementia. *Ann Neurol* 56:399–406, 2004.

Hodges, J.R. and Gurd, J.M.: Remote memory and lexical retrieval in a case of frontal Pick's disease. *Arch Neurol* 51:821–827, 1994.

Hodges, J.R. and Miller, B.: The classification, genetics and neuropathology of frontotemporal dementia. Introduction to the special topic papers: Part I. *Neurocase* 7:31–35. 2001.

Hodges, J.R. and Miller, B.: The neuropsychology of frontal variant frontotemporal dementia and semantic dementia. Introduction to the special topic papers: Part II. *Neurocase* 7:113–121, 2001.

Hodges, J.R., Patterson, K., Ward, R., et al.: The differentiation of semantic dementia and frontal lobe dementia (temporal and frontal variants of frontotemporal dementia) from early Alzheimer's disease: A comparative neuropsychological study. *Neuropsychology* 13:31–40, 1999.

Hodges, J.R.: Frontotemporal dementia (Pick's disease): Clinical features and assessment. *Neurology* 2001;56:S6–10.

Holm, I.E., Englund, E., Mackenzie, I.R., et al.: A reassessment of the neuropathology of frontotemporal dementia linked to chromosome 3. *J Neuropathol Exp Neurol* 66:884–891, 2007.

Hooten, W.M. and Lyketsos, C.G.: Frontotemporal dementia: A clinicopathological review of four postmortem studies. *J Neuropsychiatry Clin Neurosci* 8:10–19, 1996.

Hutton, M., Lendon, C.L., Rizzu, P., et al.: Association of missense and 5'-splice-site mutations in tau with the inherited dementia FTDP-17. *Nature* 393:702–705, 1998.

Ikeda, M., Ishikawa, T., and Tanabe, H.: Epidemiology of frontotemporal lobar degeneration. *Dement Geriatr Cogn Disord* 17:265–268, 2004.

Ikeda, M., Tanabe, H., Horino, T., et al.: [Care for patients with Pick's disease—by using their preserved procedural memory]. *Seishin Shinkeigaku Zasshi* 97:179–192, 1995.

Ingelson, M., Blomberg, M., Benedikz, E., et al.: Tau immunoreactivity detected in human plasma, but no obvious increase in dementia. *Dement Geriatr Cogn Disord* 10:442–445, 1999.

Jack, C.R., Jr., Dickson, D.W., Parisi, J.E., et al.: Antemortem MRI findings correlate with hippocampal neuropathology in typical aging and dementia. *Neurology* 58:750–757, 2002.

Janssen, J.C., Warrington, E.K., Morris, H.R., et al.: Clinical features of frontotemporal dementia due to the intronic tau 10(+16) mutation. *Neurology* 58:1161–1168, 2002.

Jendroska, K., Rossor, M.N., Mathias, C.J., and Daniel, S.E.: Morphological overlap between corticobasal degeneration and Pick's disease: A clinicopathological report. Mov Disord 10:111–114, 1995.

Johnson, J.K., Diehl, J., Mendez, M.F., et al.: Frontotemporal lobar dementia: Demographic characteristics of 353 patients. *Arch Neurol* 62:925–930, 2005.

Josephs, K.A. Frontotemporal dementia and related disorders: Deciphering the enigma. *Ann Neurol* 64:4–14, 2008.

Josephs, K.A., Ahmed, Z., Katsuse, O., et al.: Neuropathologic features of frontotemporal lobar degeneration with ubiquitin-positive inclusions with progranulin gene (PGRN) mutations. *J Neuropathol Exp Neurol* 66:142–151, 2007.

Josephs, K.A., Duffy, J.R., Strand, E.A., et al.: Clinicopathological and imaging correlates of progressive aphasia and apraxia of speech. *Brain* 129:1385–1398, 2006a.

Josephs KA, Holton JL, Rossor MN, et al.: Frontotemporal lobar degeneration and ubiquitin immunohistochemistry. *Neuropathol Appl Neurobiol* 30: 369–373, 2004a.

Josephs, K.A., Holton, J.L., Rossor, M.N., et al.: Neurofilament inclusion body disease: A new proteinopathy? *Brain* 126:2291–2303, 2003.

Josephs, K.A., Jones, A.G., and Dickson, D.W.: Hippocampal sclerosis and ubiquitin-positive inclusions in dementia lacking distinctive histopathology. *Dement Geriatr Cogn Disord* 17:342–345, 2004b.

Josephs, K.A., Katsuse, O., Beccano-Kelly, D.A., et al.: Atypical progressive supranuclear palsy with corticospinal tract degeneration. *J Neuropathol Exp Neurol* 65:396–405, 2006b.

Josephs, K.A., Parisi, J.E., Knopman, D.S., et al.: Clinically undetected motor neuron disease in pathologically proven frontotemporal lobar degeneration with motor neuron disease. *Arch Neurol* 63:506–512, 2006c.

Josephs, K.A., Petersen, R.C., Knopman, D.S., et al.: Clinicopathologic analysis of frontotemporal and corticobasal degenerations and PSP. *Neurology* 66:41–48, 2006d.

Josephs, K.A., Whitwell, J.L., Dickson, D.W., et al.: Voxel-based morphometry in autopsy proven PSP and CBD. *Neurobiol Aging* 29:280–289, 2008a.

Josephs KA, Whitwell JL, Duffy JR, et al.: Progressive aphasia secondary to Alzheimer disease vs. FTLD pathology. *Neurology* 70:25–34, 2008b.

Josephs, K.A., Whitwell, J.L., Jack, C.R., et al.: Frontotemporal lobar degeneration without lobar atrophy. *Arch Neurol* 63:1632–1638, 2006e.

Kaufer, D.I., Miller, B.L., Itti, L., et al.: Midline cerebral morphometry distinguishes frontotemporal dementia and Alzheimer's disease. *Neurology* 48:978–985, 1997.

Keane, J., Calder, A.J., Hodges, J.R., and Young, A.W.: Face and emotion processing in frontal variant frontotemporal dementia. *Neuropsychologia* 40:655–665, 2002.

Kertesz, A., Hudson, L., Mackenzie, I.R., and Munoz, D.G.: The pathology and nosology of primary progressive aphasia. *Neurology* 44:2065–2072, 1994.

Kertesz, A., Kawarai, T., Rogaeva, E. et al.: Familial frontotemporal dementia with ubiquitin-positive, tau-negative inclusions. *Neurology* 54:818–827, 2000.

Kertesz, A., Martinez-Lage, P., Davidson, W., and Munoz, D.G.: The corticobasal degeneration syndrome overlaps progressive aphasia and frontotemporal dementia. *Neurology* 55:1368–1375, 2000.

Kertesz, A., McMonagle, P., Blair, M., et al.: The evolution and pathology of frontotemporal dementia. *Brain* 128:1996–2005, 2005.

Kertesz, A. and Munoz, D.G.: Frontotemporal dementia. *Med Clin North Am* 86:501–518, 2002.

Kertesz, A. and Munoz, D.G.: Primary progressive aphasia: a review of the neurobiology of a common presentation of Pick complex. *Am J Alzheimers Dis Other Demen* 17:30–36, 2002.

Kertesz, A., Nadkarni, N., Davidson, W., and Thomas, A.W.: The Frontal Behavioral Inventory in the differential diagnosis of frontotemporal dementia. *J Int Neuropsychol Soc* 6:460–468, 2000.

Kirshner, H.S.: Frontotemporal dementia. *Neurology* 52:1516, 1999.

Kitagaki, H., Mori, E., Yamaji, S., et al.: Frontotemporal dementia and Alzheimer disease: Evaluation of cortical atrophy with automated hemispheric surface display generated with MR images. *Radiology* 208:431–439, 1998.

Knibb, J.A., Xuereb, J.H., Patterson, K., Hodges, J.R.: Clinical and pathological characterization of progressive aphasia. *Ann Neurol* 59:156–165, 2006.

Knopman, D.S., Christensen, K.J., Schut, L.J., et al.: The spectrum of imaging and neuropsychological findings in Pick's disease. *Neurology* 39:362–368, 1989.

Knopman, D.S., Kramer, J.H., Boeve, B.S., et al. Development of methodology for conducting clinical trials in frontotemporal lobar degeneration. *Brain* 131:2957-2968, 2008. .

Knopman, D.S., Mastri, A.R., Frey, W.H. 2nd, et al.: Dementia lacking distinctive histologic features: A common non-Alzheimer degenerative dementia. *Neurology* 40:251–256, 1990.

Knopman D.S.: The initial recognition and diagnosis of dementia. *Am J Med* 1998;104:2S–12S; discussion 39S-42S.

Knopman, D.S., Petersen, R.C., Edland, S.D., et al.: The incidence of frontotemporal lobar degeneration in Rochester, Minnesota, 1990 through 1994. *Neurology* 10;62:506–588, 2004.

Kril, J.J. and Halliday, G.M.: Clinicopathological staging of frontotemporal dementia severity: correlation with regional atrophy. *Dement Geriatr Cogn Disord* 17:311–315, 2004.

Laakso, M.P., Frisoni, G.B., Kononen, M., et al.: Hippocampus and entorhinal cortex in frontotemporal dementia and Alzheimer's disease: A morphometric MRI study. *Biol Psychiatry* 47:1056–1063, 2000.

Lavenu, I., Pasquier, F., Lebert, F., et al.: Perception of emotion in frontotemporal dementia and Alzheimer disease. *Alzheimer Dis Assoc Disord* 13:96–101, 1999.

Le Ber, I., van der Zee, J., Hannequin, D., et al.: Progranulin null mutations in both sporadic and familial frontotemporal dementia. *Hum Mutat* 28:846–855, 2007.

Lipton, A.M., White, C.L. 3rd, and Bigio, E. H.: Frontotemporal lobar degeneration with motor neuron disease-type inclusions predominates in 76 cases of frontotemporal degeneration. *Acta Neuropathol* 108:379–385, 2004

Litvan, I., Agid, Y., Sastry, N., et al.: What are the obstacles for an accurate clinical diagnosis of Pick's disease? A clinicopathologic study. *Neurology* 49:62–69, 1997.

Lopez, O.L., Litvan, I., Catt, K.E., et al.: Accuracy of four clinical diagnostic criteria for the diagnosis of neurodegenerative dementias. *Neurology* 53:1292–1299, 1999.

Lough, S., Kipps, C.M., Treise, C., et al.: Social reasoning, emotion and empathy in frontotempora dementia. *Neuropsychologia* 44:980–988, 2006.

Lough, S., Gregory, C., and Hodges, J.R.: Dissociation of social cognition and executive function in frontal variant frontotemporal dementia. *Neurocase* 7:123–130, 2001.

Mackenzie, I.R., Baborie, A., Pickering-Brown, S., et al.: Heterogeneity of ubiquitin pathology in frontotemporal lobar degeneration: Classification and relation to clinical phenotype. *Acta Neuropathol* 112:539–549, 2006a.

Mackenzie, I.R., Baker, M., Pickering-Brown, S., et al.: The neuropathology of frontotemporal lobar degeneration caused by mutations in the progranulin gene. *Brain* 2006; 129:3081–3090, 2006b.

Mackenzie IR, Baker M, Pickering-Brown S et al.: The neuropathology of frontotemporal lobar degeneration caused by mutations in the progranulin gene. *Brain* 129(Pt11):3081–90, 2006c.

Mackenzie I.R., Bigio E.H., Ince P.G., et al.: Pathological TDP-43 distinguishes sporadic amyotrophic lateral sclerosis from amyotrophic lateral sclerosis with SOD1 mutations. *Ann Neurol* 61(5):427–34, 2007.

Mackenzie, I.R., Foti, D., Woulfe, J., et al.: Atypical frontotemporal lobar degeneration with ubiquitin-positive, TDP-43 negative neuronal inclusions. *Brain* 131:1282–1293, 2008.

Mackenzie, I.R., Shi, J., Shaw, C.L., et al.: Dementia lacking distinctive histology (DLDH) revisited. *Acta Neuropathol* 112:551–559, 2006d.

Mathuranath, P.S., Nestor, P.J., Berrios, G.E., et al.: A brief cognitive test battery to differentiate Alzheimer's disease and frontotemporal dementia. *Neurology* 55:1613–1620, 2000.

Mathuranath, P.S., Xuereb, J.H., Bak, T., Hodges, J.R.: Corticobasal ganglionic degeneration and/or frontotemporal dementia? A report of two overlap cases and review of literature. *J Neurol Neurosurg Psychiatry* 68:304–312, 2000.

Matsumoto S, Kusaka H, Murakami N, et al.: Basophilic inclusions in sporadic juvenile amyotrophic lateral sclerosis: An immunocytochemical and ultrastructural study. *Acta Neuropathol* 83:579–583, 1992.

McKhann, G.M., Albert, M.S., Grossman, M., et al.: Clinical and pathological diagnosis of frontotemporal dementia: Report of the Work Group on Frontotemporal Dementia and Pick's Disease. *Arch Neurol* 58:1803–1809, 2001.

Mendez, M.F.and Foti, D.J.: Lethal hyperoral behaviour from the Kluver-Bucy syndrome. *J Neurol Neurosurg Psychiatry* 62:293–294, 1997.

Mendez, M.F., Lauterbach, E.C., Sampson, S.M., et al.: An evidence-based review of the psychopathology of frontotemporal dementia: A Report of the ANPA Committee on Research. *J Neuropsychiatry Clin Neurosci* 20:130–149, 2008.

Mendez, M.F. and Lipton, A.: Emergent neuroleptic hypersensitivity as a herald of presenile dementia. *J Neuropsychiatry Clin Neurosci* 13:347–356, 2001.

Mendez, M.F., Selwood, A., Mastri, A.R., and Frey, W.H., 2nd.: Pick's disease versus Alzheimer's disease: A comparison of clinical characteristics. *Neurology* 43:289–292, 1993.

Mendez, M.F. and Perryman, K.M.: Neuropsychiatric features of frontotemporal dementia: evaluation of consensus criteria and review. *J Neuropsychiatry Clin Neurosci* 14:424–429, 2002.

Mendez, M.F., Shapira, J.S., McMurtray, A., et al.: Accuracy of the clinical evaluation for frontotemporal dementia. *Arch Neurol* 64:830–835, 2007.

Mendez, M.F., Anderson, E., and Shapira, J.S.: An investigation of moral judgment in frontotemporal dementia. *Cogn Behav Neurol* 18:193–197, 2005.

Mendez, M.F., McMurtray, A.: Frontotemporal dementia-like phenotypes associated with presenilin-1 mutations. *Am J Alzheimers Dis Other Demen* 21:281–286, 2006.

Mendez, M.F., Shapira, J.S., McMurtray, A., and Licht, E: Preliminary report: Behavioral worsening on donepezil in patients with frontotemporal dementia. *Am J Geriatr Psychiatry* 15:84–87, 2007.

Miller, B.L., Boone, K., Cummings, J.L., et al.: Functional correlates of musical and visual ability in frontotemporal dementia. *Br J Psychiatry* 176:458–463, 2000.

Miller, B.L., Cummings, J.L., Villanueva-Meyer, J., et al.: Frontal lobe degeneration: Clinical, neuropsychological, and SPECT characteristics. *Neurology* 41:1374–1382, 1991.

Miyamoto, K., Ikemoto A, Akiguchi, I., et al.: A case of frontotemporal dementia and parkinsonism of early onset with progressive supranuclear palsy-like features. *Clin Neuropathol* 20:8–12, 2001.

Miyamoto, K., Kowalska, A., Hasegawa, M., et al.: Familial frontotemporal dementia and parkinsonism with a novel mutation at an intron 10+11-splice site in the tau gene. *Ann Neurol* 50:117–120, 2001.

Mori, H., Nishimura, M., Namba, Y., Oda, M.: Corticobasal degeneration: A disease with widespread appearance of abnormal tau and neurofibrillary tangles, and its relation to progressive supranuclear palsy. *Acta Neuropathol* 88:113–121, 1994.

Mummery, C.J., Patterson, K., Price, C.J., et al.: A voxel-based morphometry study of semantic dementia: Relationship between temporal lobe atrophy and semantic memory. *Ann Neurol* 47:36–45, 2000.

Munoz-Garcia, D., Ludwin, S.K.: Classic and generalized variants of Pick's disease: A clinicopathological, ultrastructural, and immunocytochemical comparative study. *Ann Neurol* 16:467–480, 1984.

Murphy, J.M., Henry, R.G., Langmore, S., et al.: Continuum of frontal lobe impairment in amyotrophic lateral sclerosis. *Arch Neurol* 64:530–534, 2007.

Neary, D., Snowden, J.S., Gustafson, L., et al.: Frontotemporal lobar degeneration: A consensus on clinical diagnostic criteria. *Neurology* 51:1546–1554, 1998.

Neary, D., Snowden, J.S., Mann, D.M., et al.: Frontal lobe dementia and motor neuron disease. *J Neurol Neurosurg Psychiatry* 53:23–32, 1990.

Neary, D., Snowden, J.S., and Mann, D.M.: Classification and description of frontotemporal dementias. *Ann N Y Acad Sci* 920:46–51, 2000.

Neary, D., Snowden, J.S., and Mann, D.M.: Familial progressive aphasia: Its relationship to other forms of lobar atrophy. *J Neurol Neurosurg Psychiatry* 56:1122–1125, 1993.

Neary, D.: Neuropsychological aspects of frontotemporal degeneration. *Ann N Y Acad Sci* 769:15–22, 1995.

Nestor, P.J., Graham, K.S., Bozeat, S., et al.: Memory consolidation and the hippocampus: Further evidence from studies of autobiographical memory in semantic dementia and frontal variant frontotemporal dementia. *Neuropsychologia* 40:633–654, 2002.

Nestor P.J., Fryer T.D., and Hodges J.R.: Declarative memory impairments in Alzheimer's disease and semantic dementia. *Neuroimage* 30:1010–1020, 2006.

Neumann, M., Mackenzie, I.R., Cairns, N.J., et al.: TDP-43 in the ubiquitin pathology of frontotemporal dementia with VCP gene mutations. *J Neuropathol Exp Neurol* 66:152–157, 2007.

Neumann, M., Sampathu, D.M., Kwong, L.K., et al.: Ubiquitinated TDP-43 in frontotemporal lobar degeneration and amyotrophic lateral sclerosis. *Science* 314:130–133, 2006.

Noble, K., Glosser, G., and Grossman, M.: Oral reading in dementia. *Brain Lang* 74:48–69, 2000.

Pasquier, F. and Delacourte, A.: Non-Alzheimer degenerative dementias. *Curr Opin Neurol* 11:417-427, 1998.

Pasquier F, Grymonprez, L., Lebert, F., and Van der Linden, M.: Memory impairment differs in frontotemporal dementia and Alzheimer's disease. *Neurocase* 7:161–171, 2001.

Pasquier, F., Lavenu, I., Lebert, F., et al.: The use of SPECT in a multidisciplinary memory clinic. *Dement Geriatr Cogn Disord* 8:85–91, 1997.

Pasquier, F. and Petit, H.: Frontotemporal dementia: Its rediscovery. *Eur Neurol* 38:1–6, 1997.

Pick, A.: Über die Beziehungen der senilen Hirnatrophie zur Aphasie. *Prag Med Wochenschr* 17:165–167, 1892.

Pickering-Brown, S.M., Rollinson, S., Plessis, D.D., et al.: Frequency and clinical characteristics of progranulin mutation carriers in the Manchester frontotemporal lobar degeneration cohort: Comparison with patients with MAPT and no known mutations. *Brain* 131:721–731, 2008.

Poorkaj P., Grossman M., Steinbart E., et al.: Frequency of tau gene mutations in familial and sporadic cases of non-Alzheimer dementia. *Arch Neurol* 2001;58:383–387, 2001.

Rademakers, R. and Hutton, M.: The genetics of frontotemporal lobar degeneration. *Curr Neurol Neurosci Rep* 7:434–442, 2007.

Ratnavalli, E., Brayne, C., Dawson, K., and Hodges, J.R.: The prevalence of frontotemporal dementia. *Neurology* 58:1615–1621, 2002.

Rhee, J., Antiquena, P., and Grossman, M.: Verb comprehension in frontotemporal degeneration: The role of grammatical, semantic and executive components. *Neurocase* 7:173–184, 2001.

Riemenschneider, M., Diehl, J., Muller, U., et al.: Apolipoprotein E polymorphism in German patients with frontotemporal degeneration. *J Neurol Neurosurg Psychiatry* 72:639–641. 2002.

Riemenschneider, M., Wagenpfeil, S., Diehl, J., et al.: Tau and Abeta42 protein in CSF of patients with frontotemporal degeneration. *Neurology* 58:1622–1628, 2002.

Rinne, J.O., Laine, M., Kaasinen, V., et al.: Striatal dopamine transporter and extrapyramidal symptoms in frontotemporal dementia. *Neurology* 58:1489–1493, 2002.

Robert, P.H., Lafont, V., Snowden, J.S., and Lebert, F.: Criteres diagnostiques des degenerescences lobaires fronto-temporales. *Encephale* 25:612–621, 1999.

Robinson, K.M.: Rehabilitation applications in caring for patients with Pick's disease and frontotemporal dementias. *Neurology* 56:S56–58, 2001.

Roks, G., Dermaut, B., Heutink, P., et al.: Mutation screening of the tau gene in patients with early-onset Alzheimer's disease. *Neurosci Lett* 277:137–139, 1999.

Rosen, H.J., Gorno-Tempini, M.L., Goldman, W.P., et al.: Patterns of brain atrophy in frontotemporal dementia and semantic dementia. *Neurology* 58:198–208, 2002.

Rosen, H.J., Hartikainen, K.M., Jagust, W., et al.: Utility of clinical criteria in differentiating frontotemporal lobar degeneration (FTLD) from AD. *Neurology* 58:1608–1615, 2002.

Rosen, H.J., Kramer, J.H., Gorno-Tempini, M.L., et al.: Patterns of cerebral atrophy in primary progressive aphasia. *Am J Geriatr Psychiatry* 10:89–97, 2002.

Rosen H.J., Allison S.C., Schauer G.F., et al.: Neuroanatomical correlates of behavioural disorders in dementia. *Brain* 128:2612–2625, 2005.

Rosengren, L.E., Karlsson, J.E., Sjogren, M., et al.: Neurofilament protein levels in CSF are increased in dementia. *Neurology* 52:1090–1093, 1999.

Rosso, S.M., Landweer, E.J., Houterman, M., et al.: Medical and environmental risk factors for sporadic frontotemporal dementia: a retrospective case-control study. *J Neurol Neurosurg Psychiatry* 74:1574–1576, 2003.

Rossor, M.N.: Differential diagnosis of frontotemporal dementia: Pick's disease. *Dement Geriatr Cogn Disord* 10 Suppl 1:43–45, 1999.

Sam, M., Gutmann, L., Schochet, S.S., Jr., and Doshi, H.: Pick's disease: A case clinically resembling amyotrophic lateral sclerosis. *Neurology* 41:1831–1833, 1991.

San Pedro, E.C., Deutsch, G., Liu, H.G., and Mountz, J.M.: Frontotemporal decreases in rCBF correlate with degree of dysnomia in primary progressive aphasia. *J Nucl Med* 41:228–233, 2000.

Santens, P., Van Borsel, J., Foncke, E. et al.: Progressive dysarthria. Case reports and a review of the literature. *Dement Geriatr Cogn Disord* 10:231–236, 1999.

Schmitt, H.P., Yang, Y., and Forstl, H.: Frontal lobe degeneration of non-Alzheimer type and Pick's atrophy: Lumping or splitting? *Eur Arch Psychiatry Clin Neurosci* 245:299–305, 1995.

Sjogren, M., Gustafson, L., Wikkelso, C., and Wallin, A.: Frontotemporal dementia can be distinguished from Alzheimer's disease and subcortical white matter dementia by an anterior-to-posterior rCBF-SPET ratio. *Dement Geriatr Cogn Disord* 11:275–285, 2000.

Sjogren, M., Minthon, L., Davidsson, P., et al.: CSF levels of tau, beta-amyloid(1-42) and GAP-43 in frontotemporal dementia, other types of dementia and normal aging. *J Neural Transm* 107:563–579, 2000a.

Sjogren, M., Rosengren, L., Minthon, L., et al.: Cytoskeleton proteins in CSF distinguish frontotemporal dementia from AD. *Neurology* 54:1960–1964, 2000b.

Sjogren, M. and Wallin, A.: Pathophysiological aspects of frontotemporal dementia—emphasis on cytoskeleton proteins and autoimmunity. *Mech Ageing Dev* 122:1923–1935, 2001.

Skibinski, G., Parkinson, N.J., Brown, J.M., et al.: Mutations in the endosomal ESCRTIII-complex subunit CHMP2B in frontotemporal dementia. *Nat Genet* 37:806–808, 2005.

Snowden, J., Neary, D., and Mann, D.: Frontotemporal lobar degeneration: Clinical and pathological relationships. *Acta Neuropathol* 114:31–38, 2007.

Snowden J.S., Gibbons Z.C., Blackshaw A., et al.: Social cognition in frontotemporal dementia in Huntington's disease. *Neuropsychologia* 41:688–701, 2003.

Snowden J.S., Thompson J.C., and Neary D.: Knowledge of famous faces and names in semantic dementia. *Brain* 127: 860–872, 2004.

Sparks, D.L., Danner, F.W., Davis, D.G., et al.: Neurochemical and histopathologic alterations characteristic of Pick's disease in a non-demented individual. *J Neuropathol Exp Neurol* 53:37–42, 1994.

Sreedharan, J., Blair, I.P., Tripathi, V.B., et al.: TDP-43 mutations in familial and sporadic amyotrophic lateral sclerosis. *Science* 319:1668–1672, 2008.

Stevens, M., van Duijn, C.M., Kamphorst,W. et al.: Familial aggregation in frontotemporal dementia. *Neurology* 50:1541–1545, 1998.

Swartz, J.R., Miller, B.L., Lesser, I.M., and Darby, A.L.: Frontotemporal dementia: Treatment response to serotonin selective reuptake inhibitors. *J Clin Psychiatry* 58:212–216, 1997.

Talerico, K.A. and Evans, L.K.: Responding to safety issues in frontotemporal dementias. *Neurology* 56:S52–55, 2001.

Tanemura, K., Akagi, T., Murayama, M., et al.: Formation of filamentous tau aggregations in transgenic mice expressing V337M human tau. *Neurobiol Dis* 8:1036–1045, 2001.

The Lund and Manchester Groups. Clinical and neuropathological criteria for frontotemporal dementia. *J Neurol Neurosurg Psychiatry* 57:416–418, 1994.

Torralva T., Kipps C.M., Hodges J.R., et al.: The relationship between affective decision-making and theory of mind in the frontal variant of fronto-temporal dementia. *Neuropsychologia* 45:342–349, 2007.

Varma, A.R., Laitt, R., Lloyd, J.J., et al.: Diagnostic value of high signal abnormalities on T2 weighted MRI in the differentiation of Alzheimer's, frontotemporal and vascular dementias. *Acta Neurol Scand* 105:355–364, 2002.

Watts, G.D., Wymer, J., Kovach, M.J., et al.: Inclusion body myopathy associated with Paget disease of bone and frontotemporal dementia is caused by mutant valosin-containing protein. *Nat Genet* 36:377–381, 2004.

Williams, G.B., Nestor, P.J., and Hodges, J.R.: Neural correlates of semantic and behavioural deficits in frontotemporal dementia. *Neuroimage* 24:1041–1051, 2005.

Whitwell J.L., Petersen R.C., Negash S., et al.: Patterns of atrophy among specific subtypes of mild cognitive impairment. *Arch Neurol* 64:1130–1138, 2007a.

Whitwell J.L., Przybelski S.A., Weigand S.D., et al.: 3D maps from multiple MRI illustrate changing atrophy patterns as subject progress from mild cognitive impairment to Alzheimer's disease. *Brain* 130:1777–1786, 2007b.

Whitwell J.L., Jack C.R. Jr, Parisi J.E., et al.: Rates of cerebral atrophy differ in different degenerative pathologies. *Brain* 130:1148–1158, 2007c.

Whitwell J.L., Josephs K.A., Rossor M.N., et al.: Magnetic resonance imaging signatures of tissue pathology in frontotemporal dementia. *Arch Neurol* 62:1402–1408, 2005.

Whitwell, J.L., Jack, C.R. Jr., Baker, M., et al.: Voxel-based morphometry in frontotemporal lobar degeneration with ubiquitin-positive inclusions with and without progranulin mutations. *Arch Neurol* 64:371–376, 2007d.

Wilhelmsen, K.C., Lynch, T., Pavlou, E., et al.: Localization of disinhibition-dementia-parkinsonism-amyotrophy complex to 17q21–22. *Am J Hum Genet* 55:1159–1165, 1994.

Williams G.B., Nestor P.J., and Hodges J.R.: Neural correlates of semantic and behavioural deficits in frontotemporal dementia. *Neuroimage* 24:1042–1051, 2005.

Xie S.X., Forman M.S., Farmer J., et al.: Factors associated with survival probability in autopsy-proven frontotemporal lobar degeneration. *J Neurol Neurosurg Psychiatry* 79:126–129, 2008.

Yamauchi, H., Fukuyama, H., Nagahama, Y. et al.: Comparison of the pattern of atrophy of the corpus callosum in frontotemporal dementia, progressive supranuclear palsy, and Alzheimer's disease. *J Neurol Neurosurg Psychiatry* 69:623–629, 2000.

18 Vascular Cognitive Impairment

John C. Adair, Branko Huisa-Garate, and Gary A. Rosenberg

Introduction

Vascular disease was considered the major cause of dementia prior to recognizing the importance of Alzheimer's disease (AD) in the 1970s. As the population ages and the incidence of age-related cerebrovascular disease increases, resurgent interest in vascular cognitive impairment (VCI) has yielded several important insights. First, clinical paradigms appropriate for AD prove less useful for VCI because amnesia, a major and early symptom of AD, is often less conspicuous in VCI. Other neuropsychological findings, transparent to familiar cognitive screening tasks, may be more salient. Second, patients' sensorimotor deficits may dominate their clinical presentation and intellectual problems may be overlooked (Knopman 2006). Patients with VCI may thus be underrepresented in dementia or memory disorders clinics. Third, neuroimaging developments have greatly advanced VCI evaluation. Because of growing interest, a recent consensus conference was convened to propose a framework for using multimodal methods to diagnose and classify VCI (Hachinski et al. 2006).

Cognitive dysfunction that develops in the setting of signs and symptoms of cerebrovascular disease suggests VCI, a diagnosis that comprises several subtypes. Vascular dementia (VaD) refers to stroke patients who develop subsequent cognitive impairments that cause impaired self-care ability. The category VCI-no dementia (VCI-ND) includes patients with cerebrovascular injury whose cognitive dysfunction is not severe enough to qualify for dementia. The VCI concept also includes the particularly challenging but not infrequent patients in whom stroke coexists with other causes of dementia (Bowler 2007). Like other age-related cognitive disorders, VCI is common and costly to patients, their caregivers, and society. In contrast, VCI may represent the most readily preventable or modifiable cause of cognitive decline in the elderly (Moorehouse and Rockwood 2008).

Because of VCI's heterogeneous nature, many investigators have focused on cases associated with small vessel injury, referred to as subcortical ischemic vascular dementia (SIVD) or Binswanger's disease. Compared with other types of VCI, SIVD may be more consistent in terms of clinical manifestations and natural history and, thus, be more suitable for clinical trials (Erkinjuntti et al. 2000). For maximal effectiveness, however, interventions will likely need to start in early stages of disease. Therefore, as with other dementias, the development of biomarkers to confirm diagnosis and monitor course will be critical for identifying patients early in the disease course. The following review discusses VCI with an emphasis on SIVD. Several excellent reviews have also appeared recently on this topic (Bowler 2007; Chui 2007; Gorelick and Bowler 2008).

Epidemiology

Most authorities consider VCI the second most common type of dementia in the elderly. Prevalence estimates for VCI vary widely, however, reflecting the sample from which investigators recruit subjects and differences in case definitions. Population-based samples usually yield prevalence figures exceeding those from memory disorder clinics (Knopman 2007). The Framingham Study, for example, found that dementia frequency doubled (to 19.3%) up to 10 years following stroke (Ivan et al. 2004). In turn, hospital-based series tend to report higher prevalence rates than population-based studies, particularly when evaluating cognition early in the course of recovery (Desmond et al. 2000). Combining VCI-ND patients with VaD further escalates prevalence. In the Sydney Stroke Study, 60% of patients evaluated 3–6 months after stroke were diagnosed as either VaD or VCI-ND (Sachdev et al. 2006). Autopsy series typically show even higher VCI frequency. Although population prevalence data remain inexact, recent estimates suggest that about 5% of individuals older than 65 have VCI in some form (Rockwood et al. 2000).

Advanced age is the most significant risk factor for dementia due to either degenerative or vascular conditions (Bowler et al. 2007). Treatable disorders that increase risk of systemic atherosclerosis, such as diabetes and hypertension, also raise cerebrovascular risk. Numerous investigations thus identify the same conditions as independent contributors to VCI risk (Curb et al. 1999; Desmond et al. 2000; Posner et al. 2002). Other modifiable predisposing factors include smoking and dyslipidemia (Suryadevara et al. 2003; Chui 2007). Some research indicates that the number of concurrent systemic disorders might be a more important determinant of cognitive decline than any individual factor (Sachdev et al 2006). Data also suggests that vascular risk profiles may vary between different types of VCI. For example, Khan and associates (2008) recently reported that hypertension was more commonly associated with small vessel ischemia while smoking and dyslipidemia were more strongly linked to VCI due to large vessel stroke.

A patient's ethnic origin may also influence VCI risk. Several, but not all, studies document an increased VCI prevalence among Asians, African Americans, and Hispanics (Desmond et al. 2000; Kuller et al. 2005; Hou et al. 2006). In Asian countries, VCI may actually surpass AD as the most common cause of dementia. Population-based imaging studies also identify a greater burden of abnormal white matter and subclinical cerebral infarcts in non-demented African Americans and Hispanics (Brickman et al. 2008; Prabhakaran et al. 2008). Whether biological or socioeconomic determinants, or both, mediate the relationship between ethnicity and vascular disease remains an important area of ongoing investigation.

Pathology and Pathophysiology
Pathological Studies

A number of postmortem studies in VCI patients have been published (Esiri et al. 1997; Fernando et al. 2006; Jagust et al. 2008; Jellinger 2005). Pathological findings range from large vessel strokes in major vascular territories to subtle ischemic changes affecting subcortical white matter. A recent report on the prevalence of different VCI pathologies showed that most lesions were due to small vessel ischemia (Andin et al. 2005). Even among patients with territorial infarcts, a significant proportion also exhibited small vessel injury. Small vessel disease primarily affects the subcortical nuclei and hemispheric white matter and is thought to result from less severe ischemia, referred to as "hypoxic-hypoperfusion," over protracted periods (Andin et al. 2006). In these regions, the white matter demonstrates extensive astrogliosis and demyelination without frank infarction (Esiri et al. 1997).

Patients with VCI due to large vessel injury show ischemic encephalomalacia, often involving several vascular territories. Other brains may reveal a single infarct in cortical or subcortical sites (e.g., paramedian thalamus) that strategically impact multiple cognitive processes. A number of autopsy studies also identify microscopic cortical infarcts invisible on gross inspection (Vinters et al. 2000). Referred to as "cortical granular atrophy," the clinical relevance of these small defects is disputed. Some authorities assert that cortical micro-infarcts have "little or no clinical relevance" (Andin et al. 2005). Conversely, recent studies claim that such lesions were significant independent predictors of cognitive decline and dementia (Kovari et al. 2004; Kovari et al. 2007; Troncoso et al. 2008). Segmental hippocampal gliosis with neuronal loss (i.e., sclerosis) may be present, though the etiologic role of vascular disease to hippocampal sclerosis remains controversial (Jagust et al. 2008). Lastly, dilated perivascular spaces represent another commonly observed abnormality. Dilated perivascular spaces share predisposing factors with lacunar infarcts and show similar associations with cognitive decline and late-onset depression (Patankar et al. 2005).

Typical small artery (100–400 μm) and arteriolar pathology consists of replacement of normal structures with material that thickens the wall and narrows the lumen. Hyalinosis refers to accumulation of homogenous eosinophilic substance in the tunica media, often including fibrillar connective tissue, while lipohyalinosis describes the presence of lipid-laden macrophages within hyalinized segments (Zhang et al. 1994). Cerebral vessels undergo similar alterations with normal senescence (Farkas et al. 2006). Age-associated microvascular changes include basal lamina thickening with accumulation of adventitial collagen and degeneration of myocytes in the media. Advanced age also increases the extent of amyloid deposition in leptomeningeal and penetrating vessels (Greenberg and Vonsattel 1997).

Brains of SIVD patients reveal other pathologies. Inflammatory cells surround blood vessels in tissue without completed infarction, suggesting an ongoing reaction to vascular stress (Rosenberg et al. 2001). White matter pallor, indicating myelin loss and oligodendrocyte injury, can be observed in tissue adjacent to inflammatory cells (Simpson et al. 2007). Demyelination is often, but not universally, found in proximity to hyalinized vessels. In SIVD with white matter involvement, ischemic white matter shows extensive gliosis with demyelination and inflammation (Figure 1). Reactive astrocytes replace damaged oligodendrocytes. In addition to myelin disruption, some white matter lesions also show microscopic axonal loss (O'Sullivan 2008).

The presence of serum-derived proteins in SIVD brains suggests that blood-brain-barrier (BBB) disruption is associated with microvascular disease (Tomimoto et al. 1996). Further evidence of BBB dysfunction comes from an autopsy series that found serum components (e.g., IgG, C3d, Clq, fibrinogen) deposited in periventricular and subcortical white matter in 42% of cases (Tomimoto et al. 2000). Another recent study identified potential histopathological correlates of defective BBB function (Young et al. 2008). Evaluating abnormal white matter identified on post-mortem magnetic resonance imaging (MRI), demyelination was most strongly associated with reduced reactivity to CD31 and P-gp, endothelial proteins important for BBB integrity.

Medullary End-arteries and Subcortical Hypoperfusion

The subcortical blood supply comes from medullary vessels, small arteries and arterioles arising from larger pial surface vessels (De Reuck et al. 1980). Medullary vessels traverse subcortical U fibers in the direction of the ventricles. These end-arteries lack anastomoses and create a subcortical "watershed" that renders deep structures vulnerable to hypoxic/ischemic injury. Medullary arterioles in subcortical white matter show more fibrinoid degeneration with stenosis than vessels of similar caliber in the basal ganglia. Arteriolar narrowing is also more pronounced in SIVD than in AD or normal aging (Tomimoto et al. 1999).

A number of mechanisms probably contribute to chronic "subthreshold" ischemia in SIVD. Cerebral microvessels are active metabolically. Fibrosis may thus impede nutrient transport into the brain and removal of metabolic products out of the brain, the process Binswanger originally proposed to explain white matter lesions. Besides flow limitation due to stenosis or occlusion, recent research also provides evidence that altered endothelial function may exacerbate hypoperfusion. Markers of endothelial activation have been identified in postmortem tissue and detected in peripheral blood of patients with SIVD (Hassan et al. 2003; Fernando et al. 2006). Endothelial activation promotes leukocyte adhesion and produces a prothrombotic state. Endothelial dysfunction may also compromise circulation hemodynamically. A number of studies demonstrate impaired cerebrovascular autoregulatory capacity in elderly subjects with abnormal white matter on MRI (Marstrand et al. 2002; Mandell et al. 2008) and patients with lacunar infarcts (Pretnar-Oblak et al. 2006). Such mechanisms may account for white matter lesions without spatially concordant vascular stenosis. Venous changes, including venule collagenization, are observed histologically in abnormal white matter and could further affect circulation (Moody et al. 1995). Beyond effects on outflow resistance, less distensible venules fail to accommodate transmitted arterial pulsations, secondarily raising inflow impedance (Mills et al. 2007).

Disorders that expose the nervous system to protracted, low-level hypoperfusion or hypoxia also injure subcortical myelin. For example, MRI scans from patients with compromised cerebral blood flow due to reduced cardiac output or severe carotid stenosis show abnormal white matter signal (Pico et al. 2002; Vogels et al. 2007). Chronic, recurrent hypoxia may also be responsible for the occurrence of white matter lesions in patients with obstructive sleep apnea.

Mechanisms of Myelin Injury

The way chronic hypoperfusion damages myelin without infarction remains uncertain. However, perivascular inflammatory cells may signify a reparative reaction. Extracellular matrix-degrading proteases (matrix metalloproteinases, MMPs) and free radicals continuously remodel the microvasculature and contribute to adaptive responses to many classes of brain injury (Liu and Rosenberg 2005). Evidence suggests that reduced tissue oxygen tension impels an injury response in SIVD. A recent autopsy series found elevated immunostaining for hypoxia-inducible factor-1α (HIF-1α) in abnormal white matter (Fernando et al. 2006). HIF-1α turns on genes involved in injury as well as repair. The disrupted BBB may result from activation of a gelatinase, matrix metalloproteinase-2 (MMP-2), by membrane type metalloproteinase (MT-MMP). Another gelatinase, MMP-9, may also be induced and activated by stromelysin-1 (MMP-3). On the other hand, HIF-1α initiates angiogenesis and neurogenesis, promoting repair.

Blood vessels damaged by hypertension, diabetes, amyloid, and genetic factors undergo remodeling. When vascular remodeling is associated with microglial activation and macrophage infiltration, an

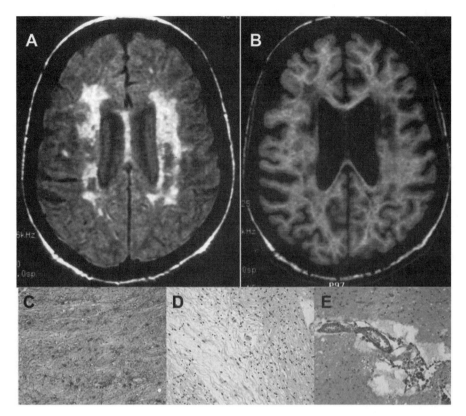

Figure 1 MRI and histology from autopsy tissue in 54 year-old patient with SIVD. A) FLAIR image showing the extensive damage to the periventricular white matter. B) T1-weighted image showing "black holes" consistent with tissue loss. C) Glial fibrillary acidic protein (GFAP)-stained tissue from white matter showing extensive gliosis. D) Myelin stain demonstrating myelin loss. E) Inflammatory cells around a damaged blood vessel in the deep white matter. Image compiled from Rosenberg (2009) and from Dr. Ross Reichert, Neuropathology, UNM. See Figure 18.1 on the color insert.

inflammatory process occurs with release of cytokines, proteases and free radicals. Macrophages secrete MMPs into the extracellular space; this induction can be amplified *in vivo* by high glucose and low oxygen concentrations (Death et al. 2003). Deposition of amyloid in the blood vessels activates astrocytes, which produce MMPs. *In vitro* cultured astrocytes exposed to amyloid-β (1-40), the predominant peptide in amyloid angiopathy, secrete MMP-9 (Deb and Gottschall 1996). Exposure of myelin to MMPs and plasmin *in vitro* results in the breakdown of myelin. This *in vitro* evidence of myelin damage suggests that a similar mechanism may occur *in vivo* when proteases released in proximity to myelinated fibers result in a non-immunological attack termed "by-stander" demyelination (Cammer et al. 1978).

Adaptive remodeling due to chronic hypoperfusion may further exacerbate perivascular white matter injury via BBB dysfunction. Active MMPs degrade tight junction proteins (occludin, claudin-5) important for BBB integrity (Yang et al. 2007). Leakage of serum-derived proteins (e.g., fibrin) incites a microglial response with cyclooxygenase-2 production and free radical generation. Interstitial plasmin within vascular walls or brain parenchyma also activates MT-MMP, an enzyme that determines the balance between collagenase activation and inhibition. In the absence of MT-MMP, a tissue inhibitor checks MMP-2 activity; when present, MT-MMP forms a trimolecular complex with the tissue inhibitor to activate latent MMP-2. Active MMP-2 may in turn promote a deleterious positive feedback cycle through activating endothelin-1, a potent vasoconstrictor that would further compromise subcortical perfusion. Autopsy studies that document increased endothelin-1 in VCI white matter support this potential cause of white matter injury (Zhang et al. 1994).

Genetic Contributions

Common causes of atherosclerosis, responsible for most VCI cases, represent polygenic disorders. However, less frequent monogenic conditions can be considered in the differential diagnosis.

Cerebral autosomal dominant arteriopathy with subcortical infarcts and leukoencephalopathy (CADASIL) presents a fairly consistent clinical profile. The disorder strikes young and middle-aged adults with few or no cerebrovascular risk factors and follows an autosomal dominant inheritance pattern. Patients most commonly present with recurrent strokes or transient ischemic attacks; other phenotypic features include migraine-like headache, seizure, and sensorineural hearing loss (Dichgans et al. 1998). Intellectual capacity declines later and primarily relates to executive dysfunction and reduced processing speed (Peters et al. 2005a; Charlton et al. 2006).

Brain MRI in CADASIL reveals multiple small regions or confluent zones of abnormal subcortical white matter. Abnormal signal in anterior temporal and external capsule white matter may be relatively characteristic (O'Sullivan et al. 2001). Lacunar infarcts and punctate hemosiderin deposits, consistent with remote hemorrhage, can also be detected. Other routine diagnostic tests, including cerebral angiogram, fail to clarify the diagnosis. Commercially available genetic tests to detect NOTCH3 gene mutations can confirm the disease's identity (Peters et al. 2005b).

The neuropathology of CADASIL resembles more common causes of SIVD. Vascular damage predominantly involves medullary arteries, causing small infarcts in the periventricular and deep subcortical white matter, basal ganglia, and thalamus (Miao et al. 2004). White matter shows diffuse demyelination with relative axonal preservation. Other features are relatively characteristic of CADASIL. Arterioles show degeneration of medial smooth muscle with deposition of granular eosinophilic and osmiophilic material in the basal lamina (Glusker et al. 1998). The extracellular domain of the NOTCH3 receptor accumulates at the cytoplasmic membrane of vascular smooth muscle cells.

Less frequent hereditable causes of VCI occur in association with autosomal dominant cerebral amyloid angiopathy (CAA). One clinical variant presents in the fifth or sixth decade of life with progressive dementia, ataxia, and spastic quadriparesis. Referred to by country of origin, familial British dementia and familial Danish dementia result from mutations in the ABri gene on chromosome 13 (Revesz et al. 2003). Another family of disorders, known as hereditary cerebral hemorrhage with amyloidosis, is associated with mutation of genes encoding amyloid precursor protein (Dutch and Iowa types) or cystain C (Icelandic type).

Brain MRI features of hereditary CAA consist of multiple regions of abnormal white-matter signal and lacunar infarctions (Mead et al. 2000). Besides severe subcortical myelin pallor, post-mortem examination shows other similarities to more common forms of SIVD and CADASIL. All three disorders disrupt medial smooth muscle and increase arteriolar wall diameter. Meningeal arteries and intracerebral arterioles exhibit marked expression of fibrillar collagen type III and basement membrane component collagen type IV (Spzak et al. 2007). In contrast to arteriosclerotic luminal obstruction, microvessels frequently remain patent in both CAA and CADASIL, suggesting that the hereditary angiopathies exact their circulatory toll through altering vasoreactivity and impairing autoregulation (Stopa et al. 2008).

Clinical Presentations

The nomenclature to describe vascular disease associated with loss of intellect has evolved over the past 10 years. In VCI due to multiple large vessel strokes, previously referred to as multi-infarct dementia (MID), or a single strategic stroke, the cause of cognitive decline is clinically evident. Until relatively recently, MID was considered the predominant form of VCI. Early concepts of VCI thus described a course clearly distinguishable from degenerative dementia, with cognitive change developing abruptly, often but not always associated with other cerebrovascular symptoms (Knopman 2006). Intellectual decline that starts within a short time after clinical stroke unequivocally links the two events, a feature used as a primary criterion in proposed diagnostic schemes (Chui et al. 1992; Roman et al. 1993). The subsequent course of multiple-infarct or single strategic infarct forms of VCI is erratic and less predictable. Symptoms might improve or stabilize over time. Alternatively, recurrent vascular injury may cause further discrete episodes of decline, resulting in "step-wise" progression.

Early VCI criteria relied on historical and physical features to determine the likelihood of a vascular etiology for cognitive decline. For years, tools like the Hachinski Ischemic Scale or the Diagnostic and Statistical Manual served as standards for both clinical and research purposes (Moroney et al. 1997). The subsequent introduction of computerized tomographic (CT) scans and MRI revealed many people with vascular disease thought previously to have degenerative dementia. More recently published consensus criteria retain many elements of earlier approaches and incorporate brain imaging to supplement clinical examination for detecting vascular lesions (Roman et al. 1993; Chui et al. 1992). Available criteria differ regarding the definition of dementia, the temporal relationship between clinical stroke and cognitive decline, which physical exam findings support the diagnosis, and whether neuroimaging is required to substantiate clinical impressions. Data suggest that, compared to earlier standards, recently proposed

criteria possess somewhat higher specificity but lower sensitivity and poor inter-rater reliability (Gold et al. 1997; Chui et al. 2000). Furthermore, none of the criteria clearly specify the basis for SIVD diagnosis.

Diagnostic confusion relates to protean clinical symptoms at the onset of SIVD, which may mimic other neurological conditions. Because small vessel ischemia involves the basal ganglia and subcortical white matter, gait and balance problems often appear earliest. In one study, gait dysfunction in the setting of mild dementia was diagnostic of non-AD disorders, including VaD, with 78% sensitivity and 100% specificity (Allan et al. 2005). Other data from a recent multi-center clinical trial revealed that 97% of VCI patients showed at least one of the sixteen graded exam findings. The most frequently observed sign was reflex asymmetry (49%), presumably related to disruption of subcortical pyramidal pathways. Patients with SIVD frequently exhibited few focal signs, however, demonstrating dysarthria, hypokinesia, rigidity, and parkinsonian gait (Staekenborg et al. 2008).

Diagnosis

No single diagnostic test can substantiate a clinical impression of VCI. The lack of confirmatory studies necessitates judgments based on a "preponderance of evidence" from several sources, including cognitive measures and biomarkers such as brain imaging. Although no test in isolation is diagnostic, improved certainty may result from different modalities considered together.

Cognitive and Behavioral Features

Compared to AD, cognitive disorders attributed to VCI vary across an immense spectrum. Vascular injury may occur anywhere in the central nervous system. Hence, VCI may present with virtually any cognitive impairment, either alone or in combination (Looi and Sachdev 1999; Knopman 2006). Early concepts attributing dementia to multiple territorial infarcts (i.e., MID) largely disregarded cases that resulted from single strokes in strategic locations. As summarized in Table 1, however, such "strategic infarct" syndromes may be the most readily identified variety of VCI, causing relatively distinctive cognitive deficits by virtue of the function and connectivity of involved structures.

The variable distribution of vascular lesions makes a reliable description of "typical" neurobehavioral features of VCI unrealistic (McPherson and Cummings 1996). When VCI results from small vessel injury, however, findings may be relatively more consistent (Erkinjuntti et al. 2000). Because SIVD does not specifically involve medial temporal regions, patients may exhibit relatively minimal episodic memory disturbance. When present, memory deficits result from ineffective retrieval, leading to impaired free recall with relative sparing of recognition or cued-recall (Tierney et al. 2001). Ischemic lesions in SIVD predominate in regions that link prefrontal areas to subcortical nuclei in parallel circuits critical for regulation of other cognitive processes, collectively termed "executive function" (Cummings 1993; Chui 2007). Accordingly, many authorities consider disproportionate executive function impairment as the most salient cognitive distinction between SIVD and AD (Tierney et al 2001; Graham et al 2004).

Empiric evidence that a dysexecutive syndrome supports VCI diagnosis remains relatively modest, however. One study compared clinically diagnosed AD and VCI patients on a comprehensive neuropsychological battery (Graham et al. 2004). From nine executive function measures, VCI patients' performance was worse than AD on only four and did not differ on the remainder. A number of other investigators report either no or minimal discrepancy between executive and memory performance in clinically diagnosed VCI (Paul et al.

Table 1 Strategic Single Infarcts Causing Multiple Cognitive Deficits

Vascular Territory	Cognitive Features
Left PCA	Verbal memory deficit, alexia without agraphia, dysnomia, achromatopsia
Right PCA	Nonverbal memory deficit, hemispatial neglect, prosopagnosia, visual hallucination
Left ACA	Transcortical aphasia, memory deficit, bilateral ideomotor apraxia, alien hand
Right ACA	Abulia, hemispatial neglect, contralateral ideomotor apraxia, alien hand
Left MCA (posterior)	Fluent aphasia, auditory agnosia or pure word deafness, alexia with agraphia, Gerstmann's syndrome, ideomotor apraxia, contralateral tactile agnosia/anomia
Right MCA (posterior)	Hemispatial neglect, constructional disorders, psychosis, contralateral tactile agnosia
Tuberothalamic	Memory deficit, aphasia, hemispatial neglect, ideomotor apraxia
Paramedian thalamic	Abulia, executive dysfunction, memory deficit, aphasia, hemispatial neglect

MCA: middle cerebral artery; PCA:posterior cerebral artery; ACA:anterior cerebral artery

2001; Schmidtke and Hull 2002). Recent longitudinal observations indicate that cognitive testing may afford discriminative value only before dementia is established. In the Canadian Study of Health and Aging, cognitively normal older subjects with incident VCI performed worse at baseline on a test of abstract reasoning compared to incident AD. Conversely, the incident AD group performed significantly worse on baseline memory tasks (Ingles et al., 2007).

Given advanced subject age, however, contrasts between clinically diagnosed groups likely misclassified patients with degenerative dementia as VCI and vice versa. Hence, one recent study contrasted cognitive function of patients separated based on brain imaging features rather than clinical diagnosis (Libon et al. 2008). Across groups, patients with minimal subcortical white matter abnormality obtained lower scores on episodic memory tests while the group with severe scan abnormalities performed worst on mental control tests. Similarly, Carey and associates (2008) examined a large group of normal older subjects for imaging correlates of executive function and episodic memory. Results demonstrated that the number of clinically silent lacunar infarcts, present in 33% of their subjects, was the only significant predictor of poorer executive function.

Misclassification error can, of course, also be minimized through analyzing cognitive profiles in diagnostic groups based on autopsy. Reed and colleagues (2007) recently examined whether composite cognitive domain scores could distinguish between groups separated by burden of vascular injury versus AD pathology. Consistent with previous research based on clinical diagnosis, the AD patient groups exhibited disproportionately poor memory. Executive function deficit with memory sparing was found in less than half (45%) of patients in the vascular group, however. Accordingly, some authorities express skepticism that cognitive profiles help substantiate whether cerebrovascular disease contributes to diagnosis (Knopman 2006).

Psychiatric symptoms also frequently complicate VCI. An extensive literature links subcortical white matter hyperintensity (WMH) with late-life affective disorders (Kales et al. 2005; Hoptman et al. 2006).

A number of studies report that depression occurs more commonly in VaD than AD (Ballard et al. 2000). However, like overlap in cognitive profiles, the frequent occurrence of affective disorders, as well as anxiety and psychosis, in both VCI and AD negates their value as reliable diagnostic clues.

Neuroimaging

Advances in neuroimaging raised awareness of the contribution of vascular injury to late-life cognitive disorders. Despite extensive research, however, standardized and validated radiographic criteria for VCI diagnosis are not available. Recent VCI criteria describe the distribution and extent of injury compatible with diagnosis. For example, NINDS-AIREN criteria consider MRI consistent with VaD if more than 25% of total white matter shows abnormal signal (Roman et al. 2003). Unfortunately, subsequent studies found poor reliability for the proposed standards (van Straaten et al. 2003). In addition, autopsy series show that extensive cerebrovascular disease is frequently not accompanied by significant cognitive impairment (Bennett et al. 2006; Reed et al. 2008). The clinical challenge is thus determining which, if any, radiographic findings account for cognitive decline in the individual patient.

Brain MRI identifies WMH on T2-weighted and FLAIR sequences more sensitively than CT. Some AD patients show similar MRI findings, making distinction from SIVD challenging (Figure 2). Large cohort studies suggest that WMH, also termed leukoaraiosis, is associated with lacunar strokes and dementia (Vermeer et al. 2003). White matter abnormalities on MRI have thus been proposed as a reliable marker for VCI (Schmidt et al. 2004). However, depending upon the study population being investigated and the screening methods, approximately 30% of normal individuals over 65 years of age have moderate WMH, limiting the usefulness of routine MRI sequences for diagnosis (Hunt et al. 1989).

Other factors make the relationship between lacunar infarcts or WMH and their cognitive consequences extremely complex. Subcortical nucleus or tract injury can disrupt function in anatomically remote sites, possibly through diaschisis (Reed et al. 2004). Hence, the clinical correlates of MRI findings may be transparent without further assessment of brain metabolism or activity. Furthermore, not all WMH results from ischemic injury (O'Sullivan 2008). Standard imaging sequences can not determine the extent to which tissue in WMH functions improperly due to myelin or axonal damage. Despite the foregoing caveats, most authorities believe that some clinically relevant information may be gleaned from measuring WMH severity.

Quantitative WMH measures, favored by researchers, entail time- and resource-intensive image processing. Clinicians, on the other hand, can most readily apply one of several available visual scales to grade WMH severity. The Fazekas scale, for example, codes lesions from 0 (no abnormality) to 3 (marked abnormality) and divides findings into periventricular and subcortical locations (Fazekas et al. 1987). Anatomic precision varies from instruments that simply make separate ratings for anterior versus posterior regions (van Swieten et al. 1990) to those summing scores in lobar, infratentorial, and basal ganglia sites (Junque et al. 1990; Scheltens et al. 1992; Wahlund et al. 2001). Although conclusions vary, studies provide evidence that visual rating scales demonstrate good inter-rater reliability and correlate well with quantitative measures (Kapeller et al. 2003; Prins et al. 2004).

Extensive research supports several general principles to judge the clinical relevance of MRI findings. First, WMHs increase with age and some degree can be found in more than 90% of the elderly (de Groot et al. 2001). The same extent of WMH is thus less clinically significant in the ninth decade of life than the sixth. One series showed that 7% of carefully selected normal subjects over 65 years of age had extensive

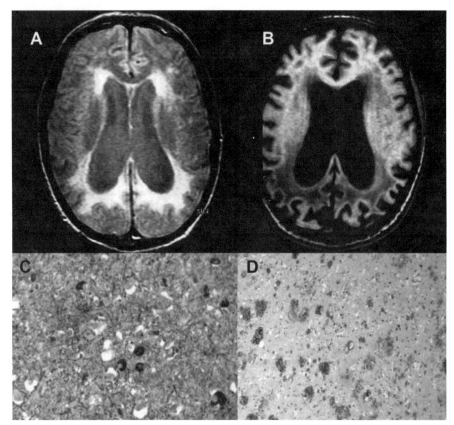

Figure 2 Patient with Alzheimer's disease and extensive white matter hyperintensities demonstrates the overlap between MRI findings in VCI and AD. A) FLAIR image showing the white matter hyperintensities involving the entire white matter. B) T1-weighted image showing loss of tissue around the ventricles. C) Tau immunostaining in the cortex. D) amyloid-β immunostaining in the cortex. Courtesy of Dr. Ross Reichart, Neuropathology, UNM. See Figure 18.2 on the color insert.

WMH and, in this population, there was no relationship between cognitive test scores and the extent of white matter abnormality (Hunt et al. 1989). Second, large confluent WMHs more likely reflect injured white matter compared to smaller, punctate lesions (Fazekas et al. 1993). Whether this generality applies equivalently to normal elderly versus clinic-based samples is unclear; at least one post-mortem study documented ischemic changes in small WMHs from patients but not control subjects (Thomas et al. 2002). Third, substantial WMH burden predicts future progression regarding both worsening scan appearance and cognitive function (Smith et al. 2008). Fourth, advanced cortical and medial temporal atrophy, considered "phenotypic" for AD, do not contradict a VCI diagnosis. Numerous investigations link VCI to global cortical volume loss as well as reduced hippocampal volume (Fein et al. 2000; Du et al. 2002; Bastos-Leite et al. 2007). Lastly, conventional imaging sequences may be useful in separating different types of VCI (Figure 3), but fail to detect the entire spectrum of small vessel injury (Schmidt et al. 2007). Cortical microinfarcts, for example, thus far escape detection with any available imaging modality.

Several more contemporary imaging modalities may clarify the functional impact of white matter abnormality. One approach uses proton magnetic resonance spectroscopy (^{1}H-MRS) to identify WMHs that are ischemic in origin (Brooks et al. 1997; Sappey Marinier et al. 1992). In areas of neuronal or axonal loss, ^{1}H-MRS shows reduced levels of n-acetylaspartate (NAA), a neuronal marker; increased myoinositol (MI) is considered to reflect gliosis (Figure 4). Schuff and associates (2003) examined patients with cognitive impairment or dementia, many of whom had lacunar infarcts on MRI. In patients with lacunes and cognitive impairment, frontal cortex NAA correlated inversely with WMH volume, linking subcortical fiber tract injury to neurochemical abnormality. Several investigations have contrasted ^{1}H-MRS characteristics between clinically diagnosed VCI and AD groups. Both patient groups show lower NAA and higher MI measures compared to normal elderly controls; the topographic distribution of ^{1}H-MRS findings may help distinguish VCI from AD. Specifically, AD patients exhibit abnormal NAA and MI in mesial temporal and parieto-occipital cortex, particularly in posterior cingulate, while similar changes predominantly occur in subcortical structures in VCI (Jones and Waldman 2004).

Other novel MRI applications may improve the future diagnostic value of neuroimaging. For example, diffusion tensor imaging (DTI) quantifies axonal integrity through measuring anisotropy of water diffusion. Studies document reduced fractional anisotropy (FA) and increased mean diffusivity (MD) in patients with WMH that extends into regions with normal radiographic appearance (O'Sullivan et al. 2001). A recent investigation that combined ^{1}H-MRS with DTI showed that voxels with damaged axons on DTI exhibit an ischemic spectroscopic pattern (Nitkunan et al. 2006). Importantly, DTI measures demonstrate much stronger correlations with cognitive function than morphological and ^{1}H-MRS parameters. Furthermore, changes in FA and MD more sensitively follow clinical decline than other morphological indicators (e.g., WMH volume) and thus may serve as a surrogate endpoint for clinical trials (Nitkunan et al. 2008). To this point, however, little data exist to contrast DTI characteristics between VCI and AD. While these and other MRI methods are still in the experimental phase, many show great promise for extending the value of MRI findings.

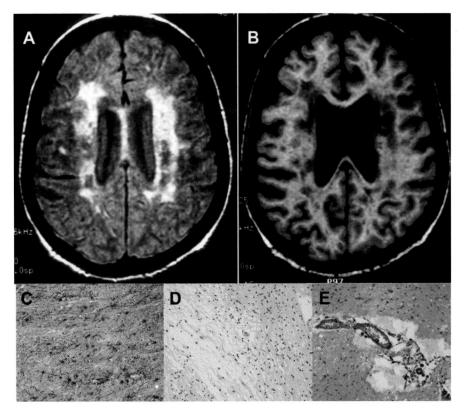

Figure 18.1 MRI and histology from autopsy tissue in 54 year-old patient with SIVD. A) FLAIR image showing the extensive damage to the periventricular white matter. B) T1-weighted image showing "black holes" consistent with tissue loss. C) Glial fibrillary acidic protein (GFAP)-stained tissue from white matter showing extensive gliosis. D) Myelin stain demonstrating myelin loss. E) Inflammatory cells around a damaged blood vessel in the deep white matter. Image compiled from Rosenberg (2009), and from Dr. Ross Reichert, Neuropathology, UNM.

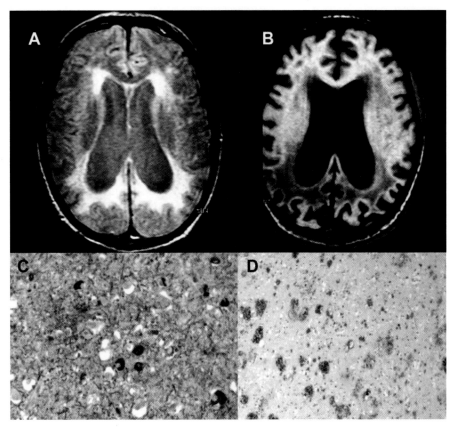

Figure 18.2 Patient with Alzheimer's disease and extensive white matter hyperintensities demonstrates the overlap between MRI findings in VCI and AD. A) FLAIR image showing the white matter hyperintensities involving the entire white matter. B) T1-weighted image showing loss of tissue around the ventricles. C) Tau immunostaining in the cortex. D) amyloid-β immunostaining in the cortex. Courtesy of Dr. Ross Reichart, Neuropathology, UNM.

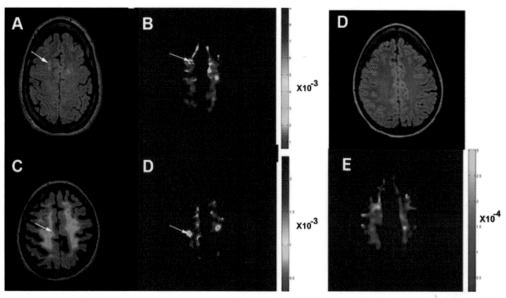

Figure 18.5 Multiple time graphical plots (Patlak plots) of BBB permeability with Gd-DTPA in two VCI patients. A) FLAIR image from one patient with early changes in the white matter. B) White matter permeability maps with gray matter removed. The red regions represent increased BBB permeability in a region of white matter hyperintensity on the MRI (arrows). C) FLAIR image from patient with advanced Binswanger disease and extensive changes in the white matter with relative sparing of the gray matter. D) Corresponding permeability map showing several smaller regions of increased permeability within the extensive white matter changes (arrows). D) FLAIR image from normal elderly control without white matter hyperintensities. E) Permeability map showing absence of increased permeability. Note that the color coding is not comparable in the patients and controls since the permeability scale is $\times 10^{-3}$ (mmol/kgmin) in the patients and $\times 10^{-4}$ (mmol/kg-min) in controls, indicating the lack of enhancement in the controls.
(From Rosenberg, *Stroke* in press; used with permission from Wolters Kluwer Health.)

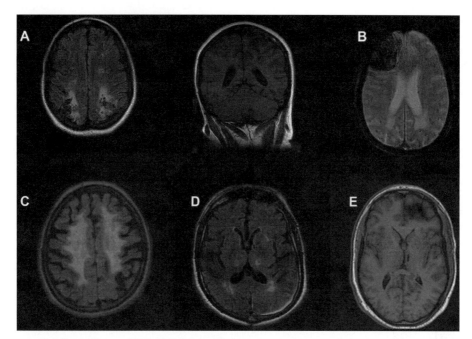

Figure 3 MRIs from patients with different forms of VCI. A) FLAIR and T1 MRI in patient with large vessel disease with bilateral parietal strokes. B) T2 MRI of amyloid angiopathy associated white matter disease (SIVD). C) FLAIR MRI of patient with extensive SIVD or Binswanger's disease. D) FLAIR MRI showing SIVD with multiple lacunar. E) T1 MRI showing a single strategic thalamic stroke next to the third ventricle.

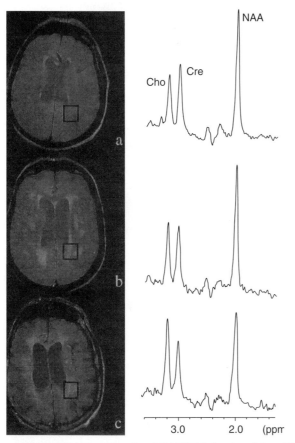

Figure 4 FLAIR MRI (right column) and 1H-MRS (left column) from VCI patients. A) FLAIR shows minimal white matter involvement and ^{1}H-MRS is normal. B) Moderate white matter hyperintensities with slight reduction in NAA. C) Severe white matter hyperintensities with greater reduction in NAA indicating ischemic injury. (From Brooks et al. Stroke 1997, permission pending.)

Imaging BBB Permeability

As mentioned above, autopsy studies indicate abnormal BBB associated with VCI. Novel MRI methods can assess BBB integrity *in vivo*, though data regarding human diseases remains preliminary. One study in patients with various age-related cognitive disorders failed to find contrast leak consistent with BBB dysfunction (Wahlund and Bronge 2000). Using more sensitive techniques, however, increased BBB permeability was demonstrated in older diabetic patients without dementia (Starr et al. 2003). Greater WMH also correlated with contrast leak in both diabetic and control subjects. Small vessel cerebral ischemia may be particularly associated with BBB disruption. Compared to cortical stroke, patients with lacunar infarcts showed more ventricular and white matter post-contrast enhancement, consistent with greater BBB permeability (Wardlaw et al. 2008). Recently, we have developed a more quantitative method to measure BBB integrity (Figure 5). Preliminary data from VCI patients demonstrate that values vary considerably within radiographically indistinguishable areas of WMH, but patients with SIVD exhibit the highest permeability values (Rosenberg 2009).

Cerebrospinal Fluid (CSF) Analysis

A number of investigators have found higher CSF/serum albumin ratios in individuals with WMH compared to controls, consistent with BBB damage identified in postmortem and radiographic studies. However, elevated CSF/serum albumin values are not specific and thus fail to differentiate VCI from AD or from non-demented elderly with MRI abnormalities (Blennow 2004).

Measures of tau and amyloid-β in CSF, proposed to distinguish AD from other age-related dementias, have been evaluated in clinically diagnosed VCI. While the majority of published research usually incorporates VCI into larger "neurological control" groups for comparison to AD, some preliminary data directly contrasts AD and VCI. Two studies found that phosphorylated tau was significantly lower and amyloid-β significantly higher in VCI patients (Jia et al. 2005; Stefani et al. 2005). Another recent investigation also reported that median levels of total and phosphorylated tau were significantly lower in VCI than AD (Boban et al. 2008).

Other CSF biomarkers with potential relevance to VCI pathophysiology may contribute to diagnosis. For example, the light neurofilament subunit is mainly localized to large myelinated axons and increased CSF concentrations correlate with WMH. However, studies to date have revealed elevated CSF light neurofilament in several types of age-related dementia without clear discriminating value (Hu et al. 2002). Other research has examined CSF levels of inflammatory markers. Some, but not all, studies demonstrate higher CSF interleukin-6 in VCI compared to AD and other neurological conditions (Wada-Isoe et al. 2004). Another investigation detected higher CSF TNF-α concentrations from VCI patients than AD and age-matched controls (Jia et al. 2005). Higher levels of MMP-9, but not MMP-2, were also found in VCI compared to AD and control subjects in one study (Adair et al. 2004). Within the VCI group, individuals with SIVD more frequently exhibited higher values of both MMPs. The diagnostic value of these novel CSF assays is unproven, though some investigators assert that normal CSF tau/amyloid measures might be successfully combined with more pathology-specific indicators to support VCI diagnosis.

Therapeutic Strategies

No treatment specifically targeted to VCI presently exists. Reasonable measures include treatments to reduce risk of future stroke. Other interventions aim to improve or maintain function. The most relevant trials treated established VCI patients and assessed clinical outcome measures. However, pertinent data also come from at-risk populations that assessed treatment effects on both clinical and imaging endpoints.

Several longitudinal studies provide evidence that risk factor modification reduces radiographic indicators of white matter damage. In the Rotterdam Scan Study, patients with successfully controlled hypertension showed reduced relative risk of WMH (de Leeuw et al. 2002). The Epidemiology of Vascular Ageing study also found that risk for severe WMH was significantly reduced in normotensive subjects, including treated hypertensive patients, compared to those with high blood pressure despite treatment (Dufouil et al. 2001). In the PROGRESS trial, patients randomized to perindopril with or without indapamide showed a significant reduction in emergent WMH number and volume compared to placebo (Dufouil et al. 2005).

Several prospective antihypertensive trials analyzed the impact of treatment on cognitive decline, though conclusions remain discrepant. The Study on Cognition and Prognosis in the Elderly trial assessed the effect of an angiotensin receptor blocker on cognitive outcomes in older hypertensive patients (Lithell et al. 2003). Results showed no difference between treatment groups with regard to incidence of cognitive decline or dementia. In contrast, the Systolic Hypertension in Europe trial found that diuretic or calcium channel blocker therapy reduced the incidence of dementia by 50%, but did not modify lesser degrees of cognitive decline (Forette et al. 1998). Similarly, hypertensive therapy in the Honolulu Asia Aging Study modestly reduced the risk of incident dementia (Peila et al. 2006). Most recently, preliminary observations from the Observational Study on Cognitive function and systolic blood pressure reduction reported cognitive benefits after only six months of treatment (Shlyakhto 2007).

Substantial uncertainties about blood pressure management in VCI await further investigation, however. Low diastolic blood pressure actually increases risk of dementia as well as WMH (Qiu et al. 2003; de Leeuw et al. 1999). Because lower blood pressure may compromise

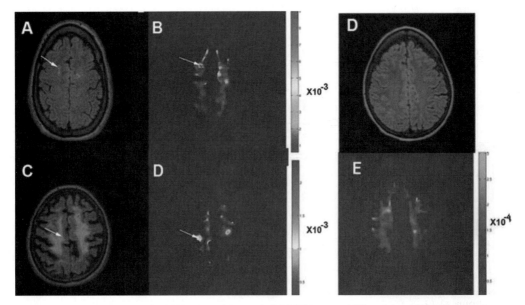

Figure 5 Multiple time graphical plots (Patlak plots) of BBB permeability with Gd-DTPA in two VCI patients. A) FLAIR image from one patient with early changes in the white matter. B) White matter permeability maps with gray matter removed. The red regions represent increased BBB permeability in a region of white matter hyperintensity on the MRI (arrows). C) FLAIR image from patient with advanced Binswanger disease and extensive changes in the white matter with relative sparing of the gray matter. D) Corresponding permeability map showing several smaller regions of increased permeability within the extensive white matter changes (arrows). D) FLAIR image from normal elderly control without white matter hyperintensities. E) Permeability map showing absence of increased permeability. Note that the color coding is not comparable in the patients and controls since the permeability scale is $\times 10^{-3}$ (mmol/kgmin) in the patients and $\times 10^{-4}$ (mmol/kg-min) in controls, indicating the lack of enhancement in the controls. (From Rosenberg, Stroke in press; used with permission from Wolters Kluwer Health.) See Figure 18.5 on the color insert.

cerebral perfusion in the setting of established cerebrovascular disease, some investigators raise concerns about the timing and intensiveness of blood pressure control in preventing or treating VCI (Birns et al. 2005).

Less data exist regarding lipid-lowering therapies. The Cardiovascular Health Study found that statin use, in patients for whom lipid-reduction was indicated, was associated with smaller decline in cognitive test scores compared to other cohort members (Bernick et al. 2005). Conversely, the PROSPER trial failed to demonstrate reduced risk of WMH or cognitive and functional decline in elderly at-risk subjects treated with pravastatin (Bowler 2007). Similar to lipid-lowering agents, the role of antiplatelet drugs, clearly accepted for secondary prevention of ischemic stroke, remains essentially unestablished for preventing VCI progression. The utility of treatments approved for AD in patients with VCI remains unclear.

Cholinergic deficits have been demonstrated *ex vivo* in VCI (Tomimoto et al. 2005; Keverne 2007). Several large clinical trials have thus examined the effect of cholinesterase inhibitors. Patients with VCI who received galantamine showed improved cognitive performance compared to placebo, though functional measures were unchanged (Erkinjuntti et al. 2002). In another double-blind, placebo-controlled trial of donepezil for VaD, statistically significant gains occurred for cognitive outcomes, dementia severity and global clinician-based improvement ratings (Wilkinson et al. 2003). However, favorable effects on functional status were again not obtained. In fact, only one study to date has reported benefit for activities of daily living (Black et al. 2003). A recent placebo-controlled study compared donepezil to placebo in patients with CADASIL (Dichgans et al. 2008). No significant effect was found on the primary outcome measure, though treatment improved some secondary endpoints. The lack of benefit for functional outcomes or dementia severity again indicated uncertain clinical efficacy, a conclusion reinforced in a recent meta-analysis (Kavirajan and Schneider 2007).

Relatively less is published about treatment of VCI patients with memantine, an N-methyl-D-aspartate antagonist approved for moderate-to-severe AD. Two large, placebo-controlled studies found statistically significant drug-placebo differences on cognitive outcome measures (Orgogozo et al. 2002; Wilcock et al. 2002). No effect on global or functional outcomes was demonstrated, however, undermining their clinical significance in a manner similar to cholinesterase inhibitors.

Future Directions

Research in VCI remains hampered by the lack of an acceptable definition of the illness. A growing consensus exists that SIVD, the progressive form of VCI, presents the most tractable opportunity for further investigation. A major obstacle remains the poor specificity of standard MRI sequences. While large cohort studies demonstrate that "silent strokes" in the basal ganglia and white matter correlate with a variety of cognitive disorders, a substantial number of older people exhibit similar findings without clinical manifestations.

The key to unraveling this complex problem requires improved detection and classification in early stages when a particular etiology may predominate. Diagnosing VCI will likely require a staged, multimodal approach. When clinical and cognitive observations suggest cerebrovascular injury, routine clinical MRI provides a rough marker of vascular disease burden and excludes other diagnostic considerations (e.g., hydrocephalus). For patients with imaging consistent with VCI, supplemental MRI modalities (e.g., ^{1}H-MRS and DTI) may eventually afford a more precise determination of whether, or plausibly which, abnormalities are ischemic in nature. The utility of CSF for

evaluating age-related cognitive disorders may become more widely adopted and, if confirmed in additional studies, may further substantiate the value of novel biomarkers. While concentrations of CSF tau and amyloid-β consistent with AD do not exclude a role for vascular injury, normal levels might point toward VCI. Adjunctive analysis of CSF cytokine and protease levels may further raise diagnostic specificity by distinguishing VCI from other conditions with normal tau and amyloid-β.

Research implicates hypoxic hypoperfusion of the medullary end-artery circulation as a major source of white matter injury. Acute ischemia associated with small vessel occlusion leads to acute elevation of MMP-9, while long-term astrogliosis, associated with protracted hypoxia, results in chronic increases of MMP-2. We thus propose that normal vascular repair responses, involving phagocytosis and digestion of damaged proteins by proteases, leads to myelin damage near small arteries. In addition, blood vessels exposed to chronic stress (e.g., hypertension, diabetes) remodel their walls, beginning with the extracellular matrix and resulting in "extravascular coagulation." Ongoing investigations that correlate MRI-based measures of BBB disruption with protease activity and ^{1}H-MRS indicators of tissue integrity may provide important insight into the temporal evolution of small vessel injury in VCI.

Improved understanding of the pathophysiology of subcortical damage in VCI will facilitate parallel prevention and treatment studies. Research aimed at unraveling the impact of hypoxia on white matter astrocytes and microvascular repair mechanisms that secondarily damage myelin could lead to novel treatments. For example, modulation of the inflammatory response may be beneficial. Clearer knowledge of VCI pathogenesis will also permit stratification of patients into etiologically valid subgroups, a strategy that will greatly reduce the numbers of subjects needed for an adequately powered clinical trial.

References

Adair JC, Charlie J, Dencoff J, et al. Measurement of gelatinase B (MMP-9) in the cerebrospinal fluid of patients with vascular dementia and Alzheimer's disease. *Stroke* 2004;35: 159–162.

Allan LM, Ballard CG, Burn DJ, and Kenny RA. Prevalence and severity of gait disorders in Alzheimer's and non-Alzheimer's dementias. *J Am Geriatr Soc* 2005;53:1681–1687.

Andin U, Gustafson L, Passant U, and Brun A. A clinico-pathological study of heart and brain lesions in vascular dementia. *Dement Geriatr Cogn Disord* 2005;19:222–228.

Andin U, Gustafson L, Brun A, and Passant U. Clinical manifestations in neuropathologically defined subgroups of vascular dementia. *Int J Geriatr Psychiatry* 2006;21:688–697.

Ballard C, Neill D, O'Brien J, et al. Anxiety, depression and psychosis in vascular dementia: Prevalence and associations. *J Affect Disord* 2000;59:97–106.

Bastos-Leite AJ, van der Flier WM, van Straaten EC, et al. The contribution of medial temporal lobe atrophy and vascular pathology to cognitive impairment in vascular dementia. *Stroke* 2007;38: 3182–3185.

Bennett DA, Schneider JA, Arvanitakis Z, et al. Neuropathology of older persons without cognitive impairment from two community-based studies. *Neurology* 2006;66:1837–1844.

Bernick C, Katz R, Smith NL, et al. Statins and cognitive function in the elderly. The Cardiovascular Health Study. *Neurology* 2005:65: 1388–1394.

Birns J, Markus H, and Kalra L. Blood pressure reduction for vascular risk: Is there a price to be paid? *Stroke* 2005;36: 1308–1313.

Black S, Román GC, Geldmacher DS, et al; Donepezil 307 Vascular Dementia Study Group. Efficacy and tolerability of donepezil in vascular dementia. Positive results of a 24-week, multicenter, international, randomized, placebo-controlled clinical trial. *Stroke* 2003;34:2323–2330.

Blennow K. Cerebrospinal fluid protein biomarkers for Alzheimer's disease. *Neuro Rx* 2004;1:213–225.

Boban M, Grbic K, Mladinov M, et al. Cerebrospinal fluid markers in differential diagnosis of Alzheimer's disease and vascular dementia. *Coll Antropol* 2008;32:31–36.

Bowler JV. Modern concept of vascular cognitive impairment. *Br Med Bull* 2007;83:291–305.

Brickman AM, Schupf N, Manly JJ, et al. Brain morphology in African Americans, Caribbean Hispanics and whites from northern Manhattan. *Arch Neurol* 2008;65:1053–1061.

Brooks WM, Wesley MH, Kodituwakku PW, et al. 1H-MRS differentiates white matter hyperintensities in subcortical arteriosclerotic encephalopathy from those in normal elderly. *Stroke* 1997;28:1940–1943.

Cammer W, Bloom BR, Norton WT, and Gordon S. Degradation of basic protein in myelin by neutral proteases secreted by stimulated macrophages: A possible mechanism of inflammatory demyelination. *Proc Natl Acad Sci USA* 1978; 75:1554–1558.

Carey CL, Kramer JH, Josephson SA, et al. Subcortical lacunes are associated with executive dysfunction in cognitively normal elderly. *Stroke* 2008;39:397–402.

Charlton RA, Morris RG, Nitkunan A, and Markus HS. The cognitive profiles of CADASIL and sporadic small vessel disease. *Neurology* 2006;66:1523–1526.

Chui HC, Victoroff JI, Margolin D, et al. Criteria for the diagnosis of ischemic vascular dementia proposed by the State of California Alzheimer's Disease Diagnostic and Treatment Centers. *Neurology* 1992;42:473–480.

Chui HC, Mack W, Jackson JE, et al. Clinical criteria for the diagnosis of vascular dementia: A multicenter study of comparability and inter-rater reliability. *Arch Neurol* 2000;57:191–196.

Chui HC. Subcortical ischemic vascular dementia. *Neurol Clin* 2007;25:717–740.

Cummings JL. Frontal-subcortical circuits and human behavior. *Archives of Neurology* 1993;50:873–880.

Curb JD, Rodriguez BL, Abbott RD, et al. Longitudinal association of vascular and Alzheimer's dementia, diabetes, and glucose tolerance. *Neurology* 1999;52:971–975.

Death AK, Fisher EJ, McGrath KC, and Yue DK. High glucose alters matrix metalloproteinase expression in two key vascular cells: Potential impact on atherosclerosis in diabetes. *Atherosclerosis* 2003;168:263–269.

Deb S and Gottschall PE. Increased production of matrix metalloproteinases in enriched astrocyte and mixed hippocampal cultures treated with beta-amyloid peptides. *J Neurochem* 1996;66:1641–1647.

de Groot JC, de Leeuw FE, Oudkerk M, et al. Cerebral white matter lesions and subjective cognitive dysfunction: The Rotterdam Scan Study. *Neurology* 2001;56:1539–1545.

de Leeuw FE, de Groot JC, Oudkerk M, et al. A follow-up study of blood pressure and cerebral white matter lesions. *Ann Neurol* 1999;46:827–833.

de Leeuw FE, de Groot JC, Oudkerk M, et al. Hypertension and cerebral white matter lesions in a prospective cohort study. *Brain* 2002;125:765–772.

de Reuck J, Crevits L, De Coster W, et al. Pathogenesis of Binswanger chronic progressive subcortical encephalopathy. *Neurology* 1980;30:920–928.

Desmond DW, Moroney JT, Paik MC, et al. Frequency and determinants of dementia after ischemic stroke. *Neurology* 2000;54:1124–1131.

Dichgans M, Mayer M, Uttner I, et al. The phenotypic spectrum of CADASIL: Clinical findings in 102 cases. *Ann Neurol* 1998;44:731–739.

Dichgans M, Markus HS, Salloway S, et al. Donepezil in patients with subcortical vascular cognitive impairment: A randomized double-blind trial in CADASIL. *Lancet Neurol* 2008;7:310–318.

Du AT, Schuff N, Laakso MP, et al. Effects of subcortical ischemic vascular dementia and AD on entorhinal cortex and hippocampus. *Neurology* 2002;58:1635–1641.

Dufouil C, de Kersaint-Gilly A, Besancon V, et al. Longitudinal study of blood pressure and white matter hyperintensities. The EVA MRI cohort. *Neurology* 2001;56:921–926.

Dufouil C, Chalmers J, Coskun O, et al; PROGRESS MRI Substudy Investigators. Effects of blood pressure lowering on cerebral white matter hyperintensities in patients with stroke: The PROGRESS magnetic resonance imaging substudy. *Circulation* 2005;112:1644–1650.

Erkinjuntti T, Inzitari D, Pantoni L, et al. Research criteria for subcortical vascular dementia in clinical trials. *J Neural Transm* 2000 Suppl;59:23–30.

Erkinjuntti T, Kurz A, Gauthier S, et al. Efficacy of galantamine in probable vascular dementia and Alzheimer's disease combined with cerebrovascular disease: A randomized trial. Lancet 2002;359:1283–1290.

Esiri MM, Wilcock GK, and Morris JH. Neuropathological assessment of the lesions of significance in vascular dementia. *J Neurol Neurosurg Psychiatry* 1997;63:749–753

Farkas E, de Vos RAI, Donka G, et al. Age-related microvascular degeneration in the human cerebral periventricular white matter. *Acta Neuropathol* 2006;111:150–157.

Fazekas F, Chawluk JB, Alavi A, et al. MR signal abnormalities at 1.5 T in Alzheimer's dementia and normal aging. *Am J Roentgenol* 1987;149:351–356.

Fazekas F, Kleinert R, Offenbacher H, et al. Pathologic correlates of incidental MRI white matter signal hyperintensities. *Neurology* 1993;43:1683–1689.

Fein G, Di Sclafani V, Tanabe J, et al. Hippocampal and cortical atrophy predict dementia in subcortical ischemic vascular disease. *Neurology* 2000;55;1626–1635.

Fernando MS, Simpson JE, Matthews F, et al. White matter lesions in an unselected cohort of the elderly: Molecular pathology suggests origin from chronic hypoperfusion injury. *Stroke* 2006;37:1391–1398.

Forette F, Seux ML, Staessen JA, et al. Prevention of dementia in randomised double-blind placebo-controlled Systolic Hypertension in Europe (Syst-Eur) trial. *Lancet* 1998;352:1347–1351.

Glusker P, Horoupian DS, and Lane B. Familial arteriopathic leukoencephalopathy: imaging and neuropathologic findings. *Am J Neuroradiol* 1998;19:469–475.

Gold G, Giannakopoulous P, Montes-Paixao C, et al. Sensitivity and specificity of newly proposed clinical criteria for possible vascular dementia. *Neurology* 1997;49:690–694.

Gorelick PB and Bowler JV. Advances in vascular cognitive impairment 2007. *Stroke* 2008;39:279–282.

Graham NL, Emery T, and Hodges JR. Distinctive cognitive profiles in Alzheimer's disease and subcortical vascular dementia. *J Neurol Neurosurg Psychiatry* 2004;75:61–71.

Greenberg SM and Vonsattel JP. Diagnosis of cerebral amyloid angiopathy. Sensitivity and specificity of cortical biopsy. *Stroke* 1997;28:1418–1422.

Hachinski V, Iadecola C, Petersen RC, et al. National Institute of Neurological Disorders and Stroke-Canadian Stroke Network vascular cognitive impairment harmonization standards. *Stroke* 2006;37:2220–2241.

Hassan A, Hunt BJ, O'Sullivan M, et al. Markers of endothelial dysfunction in lacunar infarction and ischaemic leukoaraiosis. *Brain* 2003;126:424–432.

Hoptman MJ, Gunning-Dixon FM, Murphy CF, Lim KO, and Alexopoulos GS. Structural neuroimaging research methods in geriatric depression. *Am J Geriatr Psychiatry* 2006;14:812–822.

Hou CE, Yaffe K, Pérez-Stable EJ, and Miller BL. Frequency of dementia etiologies in four ethnic groups. *Dement Geriatr Cogn Disord* 2006;22:42–47.

Hu YY, He SS, Wang XC, et al. Elevated levels of phosphorylated neurofilament proteins in cerebrospinal fluid of Alzheimer disease patients. *Neurosci Lett* 2002;320:156–160.

Hunt AL, Orrison WW, Yeo RA, et al. Clinical significance of MRI white matter lesions in the elderly. *Neurology* 1989;39:1470–1474.

Ingles JL, Boulton DC, Fisk JD, and Rockwood K. Preclinical vascular cognitive impairment and Alzheimer disease: Neuropsychological test performance 5 years before diagnosis. *Stroke* 2007;38:1148–1153.

Ivan CS, Seshadri S, Beiser A, et al. Dementia after stroke: The Framingham Study. *Stroke* 2004;35:1264–1268.

Jagust WJ, Zheng L, Harvey DJ, et al. Neuropathological basis of magnetic resonance images in aging and dementia. *Ann Neurol* 2008;63:72–80.

Jellinger KA. Understanding the pathology of vascular cognitive impairment. *J Neurol Sci* 2005;229-230:57–63.

Jia JP, Meng R, Sun YX, et al. Cerebrospinal fluid tau, Abeta1-42 and inflammatory cytokines in patients with Alzheimer's disease and vascular dementia. *Neurosci Lett* 2005;383:12–16.

Jones RS and Waldman AS. 1H-MRS evaluation of metabolism in Alzheimer's disease and vascular dementia. *Neurol Res* 2004;26:488–495.

Junque C, Pujol J, Vendrell P, et al. Leuko-araiosis on magnetic resonance imaging and speed of mental processing. *Arch Neurol* 1990;47:151–156.

Kales HC, Maixner DF, and Mellow AM. Cerebrovascular disease and late-life depression. *Am J Geriatr Psychiatry* 2005;13:88–98.

Kapeller P, Barber R, Vermeulen RJ, et al. White matter changes. Visual rating of age-related white matter changes on magnetic resonance imaging: Scale comparison, interrater agreement, and correlations with quantitative measurements. *Stroke* 2003;34:441–445.

Kavirajan A and Schneider LS. Efficacy and adverse effects of cholinesterase inhibitors and memantine in vascular dementia: A meta-analysis of randomized controlled trials. *Lancet Neurol* 2007;6:782–792.

Keverne JS, Low WCR, Ziabreva I, et al. Cholinergic neuronal deficits in CADASIL. *Stroke* 2007;38:188–191.

Khan U, Porteous L, Hassan A, and Markus HS. Risk factor profile of cerebral small vessel disease and its subtypes. *J Neurol Neurosurg Psychiatry* 2007;78:702–706.

Knopman DS. Dementia and cerebrovascular disease. *Mayo Clin Proc* 2006;81:223–230.

Knopman DS. Cerebrovascular disease and dementia. *Br J Radiol* 2007;80:S121–S127.

Kovari E, Gold G, Herrman FR, et al. Cortical microinfarcts and demyelination affect cognition in cases at high risk for dementia. *Neurology* 2007;68:927–931.

Kovari E, Gold G, and Herrman FR. Cortical microinfarcts and demyelination significantly affect cognition in brain aging. *Stroke* 2004;35:410–414.

Kuller LH, Lopez OL, Jagust WJ, et al. Determinants of vascular dementia in the Cardiovascular Health Cognition Study. *Neurology* 2005;64:1548–1552.

Libon DJ, Price CC, Giovannetti T, et al. Linking MRI hyperintensities with patterns of neuropsychological impairment. Evidence for a threshold effect. *Stroke* 2008;39:806–813.

Lithell H, Hansson L, Skoog I, et al. The Study on Cognition and Prognosis in the Elderly (SCOPE): Principal results of a randomized double-blind intervention trial. *J Hypertens* 2003;21:873–886.

Liu KJ and Rosenberg GA. Matrix metalloproteinases and free radicals in cerebral ischemia. *Free Radic Biol Med* 2005;39:71–80.

Looi JC and Sachdev PS. Differentiation of vascular dementia from AD on neuropsychological tests. *Neurology* 1999;53:670–678.

Mandell DM, Han JS, Poublanc J, et al. Selective reduction of blood flow to white matter during hypercapnia corresponds with leukoaraiosis. *Stroke* 2008;39:1993–1998.

Marstrand JR, Garde E, Rostrup E, et al. Cerebral perfusion and cerebrovascular reactivity are reduced in white matter hyperintensities. *Stroke* 2002;33:972–976.

McPherson SE and Cummings JL. Neuropsychological aspects of vascular dementia. *Brain Cogn* 1996;3:269–282.

Mead S, James-Galton M, Revesz T, et al. Familial British dementia with amyloid angiopathy. Early clinical, neuropsychological and imaging findings. *Brain* 2000;123:975–991.

Miao Q, Paloneva T, Tuominen S, et al. Fibrosis and stenosis of the long penetrating cerebral arteries: The cause of the white matter pathology in cerebral autosomal dominant arteriopathy with subcortical infarcts and leukoencephalopathy. *Brain Pathol* 2004;14:358–364.

Mills S, Cain J, Purandare N, and Jackson A. Biomarkers of cerebrovascular disease in dementia. *Br J Radiol* 2007;80:S128–S145.

Moody DM, Brown WR, Challa VR, and Anderson RL. Periventricular venous collagenosis: Association with leukoaraiosis. *Radiology* 1995;194:469–476.

Moorehouse P and Rockwood K. Vascular cognitive impairment: Current concepts and clinical developments. *Lancet Neurology* 2008;7:246–255.

Moroney JT, Bagiella E, Desmond DW, et al. Meta-analysis of the Hachinski Ischemic Score in pathologically verified dementias. *Neurology* 1997;49:1096–1105.

Nitkunan A, McIntyre DJ, Barrick TR, et al. Correlations between MRS and DTI in cerebral small vessel disease. *NMR Biomed* 2006;19:610–616.

Nitkunen A, Barrick TR, Charlton RA, et al. Multimodal MRI in cerebral small vessel disease: Its relationship with cognition and sensitivity to change over time. *NMR Stroke* 2008;39:1999–2005.

Orgogozo JM, Rigaud AS, Stöffler A, et al. Efficacy and safety of memantine in patients with mild to moderate vascular dementia: A randomized, placebo-controlled trial (MMM 300). *Stroke* 2002;33:1834–1839.

O'Sullivan M, Jarosz JM, Martin RJ, et al. MRI hyperintensities of the temporal lobe and external capsule in patients with CADASIL. *Neurology* 2001;56:628–634.

O'Sullivan M. Leukoariosis. *Pract Neurol* 2008;8:26–38.

Patankar TF, Mitra D, Varma A, et al. Dilatation of the Virchow-Robin space is a sensitive indicator of cerebral microvascular disease: Study in elderly patients with dementia. *Am J Neuroradiol* 2005;26:1512–1520.

Paul R, Moser D, Cohen R, et al. Dementia severity and pattern of cognitive performance in vascular dementia. *Appl Neuropsychol* 2001;8:211–217.

Peila R, White LR, Masaki K, et al. Reducing the risk of dementia. Efficacy of long-term treatment of hypertension. *Stroke* 2006;37:1165–1170.

Peters N, Opherk C, Bergmann T, et al. Spectrum of mutations in biopsy-proven CADASIL: Implications for diagnostic strategies. *Arch Neurol* 2005;62:1091–1094.

Peters N, Opherk C, Danek A, et al. The pattern of cognitive performance in CADASIL: A monogenic condition leading to subcortical ischemic vascular dementia. *Am J Psychiatry* 2005;162:2078–2085.

Pico F, Dufouil C, Lévy C, et al. Longitudinal study of carotid atherosclerosis and white matter hyperintensities: The EVA-MRI cohort. *Cerebrovasc Dis* 2002;14:109–115.

Posner HB, Tan MX, Luchsinger J, et al. The relationship of hypertension in the elderly to AD, vascular dementia and cognitive function. *Neurology* 2002;58:1175–1181.

Prabhakaran S, Wright CB, Yoshita M, et al. Prevalence and determinants of subclinical brain infarction: The Northern Manhattan Study. *Neurology* 2008;70:425–430.

Pretnar-Oblak J, Sabovic M, Sebestjen M, et al. Influence of atorvastatin treatment on L-arginine cerebrovascular reactivity and flow-mediated dilatation in patients with lacunar infarctions. *Stroke* 2006;37: 2540–2545.

Prins ND, van Straaten EC, van Dijk EJ, et al. Measuring progression of cerebral white matter lesions on MRI: Visual rating and volumetrics. *Neurology* 2004;62:1533–1539.

Qiu C, von Straus E, Fastbom J, et al. Low blood pressure and risk of dementia in the Kungsholmen project. A 6-year follow-up study. *Arch Neurol* 2003;60:223–229.

Reed BR, Eberling JL, Mungas D, et al. Effects of white matter lesions and lacunes on cortical function. *Arch Neurol* 2004;61:1545–1550.

Reed BR, Mungas DM, Kramer JH, et al. Profiles of neuropsychological impairment in autopsy-defined Alzheimer's disease and cerebrovascular disease. *Brain* 2007;130:731–739.

Revesz T, Ghiso J, Lashley T, et al. Cerebral amyloid angiopathies: A pathologic, biochemical, and genetic view. *J Neuropathol Exp Neurol* 2003;62:885–898.

Rockwood K, Wentzel C, Hachinski V, et al. Prevalence and outcomes of vascular cognitive impairment. Vascular cognitive impairment investigators of the Canadian Study of Health and Aging. *Neurology* 2000; 54:447–451.

Roman GC, Tatemichi TK, Erkinjuntti T, et al. Vascular dementia: Diagnostic criteria for research studies. Report of the NINDS-AIREN International Workshop. *Neurology* 1993;43:250–260.

Rosenberg GA, Sullivan N, Esiri MM. White matter damage is associated with matrix metalloproteinases in vascular dementia. *Stroke* 2001;32:1162–1168.

Rosenberg, GA. Inflammation and white matter damage in vascular cognitive impairment. *Stroke* 2009;40:S20–23.

Rosenberg, GA. Matrix metalloproteinases and their multiple roles in neurodegenerative diseases. *Lancet Neurology* 2009;8:205–216.

Sachdev PS, Brodaty H, Valenzuela MJ, et al. Clinical determinants of mild cognitive impairment and dementia following ischemic stroke: The Sydney Stroke Study. *Dement Geriatr Cogn Disord* 2006;21: 275–283.

Sappey Marinier D, Calabrese G, Hetherington HP, et al. Proton magnetic resonance spectroscopy of human brain: Applications to normal white matter, chronic infarction, and MRI white matter signal hyperintensities. *Magn Reson Med* 1992;26:313–327.

Scheltens PH, Barkhof F, Valk J, et al. White matter lesions on magnetic resonance imaging in clinically diagnosed Alzheimer's disease. *Brain* 1992;115:735–748.

Schmidt R, Scheltens P, Erkinjuntti T, et al. White matter lesion progression: A surrogate endpoint for trials in cerebral small-vessel disease. *Neurology* 2004;63:139–144.

Schmidt R, Petrovic K, Ropele S, et al. Progression of leukoaraiosis and cognition. *Stroke* 2007;38:2619–2625.

Schmidtke K, Hull M. Neuropsychological differentiation of small vessel disease, Alzheimer's disease and mixed dementia. *J Neurol Sci* 2002;203-204;17–22.

Schuff N, Capizzano AA, Du AT, et al. Different patterns of N-acetylaspartate loss in subcortical ischemic vascular dementia and AD. *Neurology* 2003;61:358–364.

Shlyakhto E. Observational study on cognitive function and systolic blood pressure reduction. *Current Medical Research & Opinion* 2007;23:S13–S18.

Simpson JE, Ince PG, Higham CE, et al.; MRC Cognitive Function and Ageing Neuropathology Study Group. Microglial activation in white matter lesions and nonlesional white matter of ageing brains. *Neuropathol Appl Neurobiol* 2007;33:670–683.

Smith EE, Egorova S, Blacker D, et al. Magnetic resonance imaging white matter hyperintensities and brain volume in the prediction of mild cognitive impairment and dementia. *Arch Neurol* 2008;65:94–100.

Spzak GM, Lewandowska E, Wierzba-Bobrowicz T, and Bertrand E. Small cerebral vessel disease in familial amyloid and non-amyloid angiopathies: FAD-PS-1 (P117L) mutation and CADASIL. Immunohistochemical and ultrastructural studies. *Folia Neuropathol* 2007;45:192–204.

Staekenborg SS, va der Flier WM, van Straaten EC, et al. Neurologic signs in relation to type of cerebrovascular disease in vascular dementia. *Stroke* 2008;39:317–322.

Starr JM, Wardlaw J, Ferguson K, et al. Increased blood-brain barrier permeability in type II diabetes demonstrated by gadolinium magnetic resonance imaging. *J Neurol Neurosurg Psychiatry* 2003;74:70–76.

Stefani A, Bernardini S, Panella M, et al. AD with subcortical white matter lesions and vascular dementia: CSF markers for differential diagnosis. *J Neurol Sci* 2005;237:83–88.

Stopa EG, Butala P, Salloway S, et al. Cerebral cortical arteriolar angiopathy, vascular beta-amyloid, smooth muscle actin, Braak stage, and APOE genotype. *Stroke* 2008;39:814–21.

Suryadevara V, Storey SG, Aronow WS, Ahn C. Association of abnormal serum lipids in elderly persons with atherosclerotic vascular disease and dementia, atherosclerotic vascular disease without dementia, dementia without atherosclerotic vascular disease, and no dementia or atherosclerotic vascular disease. *J Gerontol A Biol Sci Med Sci* 2003;58:M859–861.

Thomas AJ, O'Brien JT, Davis S, et al. Ischemic basis for deep white matter hyperintensities in major depression. A neuropathologic study. *Arch Gen Psychiatry* 2002;59:785–792.

Tierney MC, Black SE, Szalai JP, et al. Recognition memory and verbal fluency differentiate probable Alzheimer disease from subcortical ischemic vascular dementia. *Arch Neurol* 2001;58:1654–1659.

Tomimoto H, Akiguchi I, Suenaga T, et al. Alterations of the blood-brain barrier and glial cells in white-matter lesions in cerebrovascular and Alzheimer's disease patients. *Stroke* 1996;27:2069–2074.

Tomimoto H, Akiguchi I, Akiyama H, et al. Vascular changes in white matter lesions of Alzheimer's disease. *Acta Neuropathol* 1999;97:629–634.

Tomimoto H, Akiguchi I, Wakita H, et al. Cyclooxygenase-2 is induced in microglia during chronic cerebral ischemia in humans. *Acta Neuropathol* 2000;99:26–30.

Tomimoto H, Ohtani R, Shibata M, et al. Loss of cholinergic pathways in vascular dementia of the Binswanger type. *Dement Geriatr Cogn Disord* 2005;19:282–288.

Troncoso JC, Zonderman AB, Resnick SM, et al. Effects of infarcts on dementia in the Baltimore longitudinal study of aging. *Ann Neurol* 2008;64:168–176.

van Straaten EC, Scheltens P, Knol DL, et al. Operational definitions for the NINDS-AIREN criteria for vascular dementia. An interobserver study. *Stroke* 2003;34:1907–1912.

van Swieten JC, van den Hout JH, van Ketel BA, et al. Periventricular lesions in the white matter on magnetic resonance imaging in the elderly. A morphometric correlation with arteriolosclerosis. *Brain* 1991; 114:761–774.

Vermeer SE, Hollander M, van Dijk EJ, et al. Silent brain infarcts and white matter lesions increase stroke risk in the general population: The Rotterdam Scan Study. Stroke 2003;34:1126–1129.

Vinters HV, Ellis WG, Zarow C, et al. Neuropathologic substrates of ischemic vascular dementia. *J Neuropathol Exp Neurol* 2000;59:931–945.

Vogels RL, van der Flier WM, van Harten B, et al. Brain magnetic resonance imaging abnormalities in patients with heart failure. *Eur J Heart Fail* 2007;9:1003–1009.

Wada-Isoe K, Wakutani Y, Urakami K, and Nakashima K. Elevated interleukin-6 levels in cerebrospinal fluid of vascular dementia patients. *Acta Neurol Scand* 2004;110:124–127.

Wahlund LO and Bronge L. Contrast-enhanced MRI of white matter lesions in patients with blood-brain barrier dysfunction. *Ann NY Acad Sci* 2000;903:477–481.

Wahlund LO, Bakhof F, Fazekas F, et al. A new rating scale for age-related white matter changes applicable to MRI and CT. *Stroke* 2001;32:1318–1322.

Wardlaw JM, Farrall A, Armitage PA, et al. Changes in background blood-brain barrier integrity between lacunar and cortical ischemic stroke subtypes. *Stroke* 2008;39:1327–1332.

Wilcock G, Möbius HJ, Stöffler A; MMM 500 group. A double-blind, placebo-controlled multicentre study of memantine in mild to moderate vascular dementia (MMM500). *Int Clin Psychopharmacol* 2002;17:297–305.

Wilkinson D, Doody R, Helme R, et al. Donepezil in vascular dementia: A randomized, placebo-controlled study. *Neurology* 2003;61: 479–486.

Yang Y, Estrada EY, Thompson JF, et al. Matrix metalloproteinase-mediated disruption of tight junction proteins in cerebral vessels is reversed by synthetic matrix metalloproteinase inhibitor in focal ischemia in rat. *J Cereb Blood Flow Metab* 2007;27:697–709.

Young V, Halliday GM, and Kril JJ. Neuropathologic correlates of white matter hyperintensities. *Neurology* 2008;71:804–811.

Zhang WW, Badonic T, Hoog A, et al. Structural and vasoactive factors influencing intracerebral arterioles in cases of vascular dementia and other cerebrovascular disease: A review. *Dementia* 1994;5: 153–192.

19 Synucleinopathies

Michael S. Rafii and Jody Corey-Bloom

The synucleinopathies are a group of neurodegenerative disorders that share a pathological lesion composed of fibrillary aggregates of insoluble α-synuclein (AS) protein in selective populations of neurons and glia. These disorders include Parkinson's disease (PD) and dementia with Lewy bodies (DLB), where α-synuclein accumulates as Lewy bodies (LBs) and dystrophic neurite (Lewy neuritis), in addition to multiple system atrophy (MSA), where abnormal α-synuclein is a major component of the glial cytoplasmic inclusions found in oligodendrocytes (Baba et al. 1998).

The AS protein family consists of three members: α-, β-, and γ-synuclein. The AS gene is located on chromosome 4, whereas the β- and γ-synuclein genes are found on chromosomes 5 and 10, respectively. AS is a natively unfolded protein that becomes structured upon binding in lipid membranes, and the unfolded form is degraded by the proteosome in a Ubiquitin-independent manner (Tofaris et al. 2001). In diseases where it accumulates, the so-called synucleinopathies, AS changes conformation and aggregates with fibrils of β-sheet structure similar to other amyloid proteins. These are called Lewy bodies (LBs). The three main synucleinopathies (DLB, PD, MSA)—will be discussed in this chapter.

Dementia with Lewy Bodies

DLB was first described as a clinical entity in 1984 by Kosaka and colleagues (Kosaka et al. 1984). These authors reported finding LBs throughout the cortices of some patients with dementia, rather than the neuritic plaques and neurofibrillary tangles characteristic of Alzheimer's disease (AD). Subsequently, DLB has come to be recognized as the second most common cause of dementia in the elderly.

The relationship between DLB, PD, and AD is an area of considerable controversy, particularly because dementia occurs frequently in PD. Additionally, there are patients with dementia who, at autopsy, demonstrate pathological hallmarks consistent with both DLB and AD. Many investigators therefore believe that a spectrum of LB disorders exists. Although our understanding of DLB is still evolving, it appears that the clinical course, treatment, and prognosis differ considerably from those of AD, PD with dementia, and the vascular dementias. The clinical criteria for DLB were originally proposed in 1996 (McKeith et al. 1996) and modified in subsequent DLB Consortium reports. Several clinicopathological studies have assessed the sensitivity and specificity of these clinical criteria; the most recent criteria are detailed in Table 1.

Epidemiology

DLB is the second most common cause of dementia in the elderly, exceeded only by AD (McKeith et al. 2004). At least 5% of non-institutionalized adults 85 years and older are believed to have DLB, and the disease represents approximately 22% of all patients with dementia.

Table 1 Consensus Criteria for DLB, Modified after McKeith et al. (2005)

1. *Central Feature* (essential for a diagnosis of possible or probable DLB)

Dementia defined as progressive cognitive decline of sufficient magnitude to interfere with normal social or occupational function. Prominent or persistent memory impairment may not necessarily occur in the early stages but is usually evident with progression. Deficits on tests of attention, executive Function, and visuospatial ability may be especially prominent.

2. *Core Features* (two core features are sufficient for a diagnosis of probable DLB, one for possible DLB)

Fluctuating cognition with pronounced variations in attention and alertness

Recurrent visual hallucinations that are typically well formed and detailed

Spontaneous features of parkinsonism

3. *Suggestive Features* (one or more of these in the presence of one or more core features is sufficient for a diagnosis of probable DLB. In the absence of any core features, one or more suggestive features is sufficient for a diagnosis of possible DLB. Probable DLB should not be diagnosed on the basis of suggestive features alone)

REM sleep behavior disorder

Severe neuroleptic sensitivity

Low dopamine transporter uptake in basal ganglia demonstrated by SPECT or PET imaging

4. *Supportive Features* (commonly present but proven to have diagnostic specificity)

Repeated falls and syncope

Transient, unexplained loss of consciousness

Severe autonomic dysfunction

Hallucinations in other modalities

Systematized delusions

Depression

Relative preservation of MTL structures on CT/MRI

Reduced occipital activity on SPECT/PET

Low uptake MIBG myocardial scintigraphy

Prominent slow wave activity on EEG with temporal lobe transient sharp waves

DLB = dementia with Lewy bodies; REM = rapid eye movement; SPECT = single positron emission computed tomography; PET = positron emission tomography; MTL=medial temporal lobe; CT = computed tomography; MRI = magnetic resonance imaging; MIBG = iodine-131-meta-iodobenzylguanidine; EEG = electroencephalogram

The number of cases is expected to increase as the population ages and as DLB is increasingly recognized in the differential diagnosis of dementia. To date, no specific risk factors for DLB have been identified. Age of onset is typically between 60 to 90 years and it is slightly more common among men.

Pathology

The relationships among DLB, AD, and PD with dementia are difficult to define because the current evidence supports different points of view. Some experts believe that DLB is related to AD or PD with dementia, but the emerging consensus is that DLB is a distinct pathologic entity somewhere between the two.

Pathologically, classical AD is associated with amyloid plaques and neurofibrillary tangles distributed in the frontal, parietal, and temporal cortices, whereas PD is associated with LBs primarily in the subcortical regions of the brain, and in the substantia nigra and locus ceruleus. In contrast, the central histopathologic features of DLB include LBs and Lewy neurites (LNs) in the subcortical and cortical (frontotemporal) regions of the brain, neuronal loss in brainstem nuclei, and spongiform change in the transentorhinal cortex. There may or may not be associated AD pathology. Compared to classical brainstem LBs, the cortical LBs of DLB are smaller, lack a halo, and may be difficult to see with routine staining. LBs and LNs are eosinophilic cytoplasmic inclusions that contain deposits of the alpha-synuclein protein (Galvin et al. 2001).

Biochemically, DLB is associated with deficits in both acetylcholine and dopamine, which are the primary neurotransmitter deficits in AD and PD, respectively (Leverenz et al. 2001). Thus, clinically, pathologically, and biochemically, DLB appears to fall somewhere in the middle of a disease spectrum ranging from AD to PD (Table 2). LBs are, in fact, found pathologically in numerous neurodegenerative diseases, but their role in pathophysiology remains unclear (Table 3).

Clinical Features and Diagnosis

The most widely accepted clinical criteria for DLB are found in the consensus guidelines from the recent international consortium on

Table 2 Comparison of Clinical Symptoms, Pathological Features, and Biochemical Features in AD, DLB, and PD

	AD	DLB	PD
Clinical Symptoms			
Delirium	Occasional	Frequent	Rare
Visual hallucinations	Occasional	Frequent	Occasional
Delusions	Frequent	Frequent	Occasional
Parkinsonism	Rare	Frequent	Frequent
Autonomic dysfunction	Rare	Occasional	Frequent
Bradykinesia	Rare	Frequent	Frequent
Tremor	Rare	Occasional	Frequent
Pathologic Features			
Neuritic plaques	Frequent	Frequent	Rare
Neurofibrillary tangles	Frequent	Occasional	Rare
Subcortical Lewy bodies	Rare	Frequent	Occasional
Cortical Lewy bodies	Rare	Frequent	Frequent
Biochemical Features			
Cholinergic Deficit	Frequent	Frequent	Occasional
Dopaminergic Deficit	Rare	Frequent	Frequent

Table 3 Synucleinopathies

Parkinson's disease

Dementia with Lewy bodies (DLB)

Lewy body variant of Alzheimer's disease (LBV-AD)

Sporadic AD

Familial Alzheimer's disease (AD)

Down's syndrome

Neuroaxonal dystrophies

Hallervorden-Spatz disease

Amyotrophic lateral sclerosis

   Sporadic

   Familial

ALS-dementia complex of Guam

Tauopathies

   Frontotemporal degeneration/dementia

   Pick's disease

   Progressive supranuclear palsy

   Corticobasal degeneration

Multiple system atrophy (MSA)

Shy-Drager syndrome

Striatonigral degeneration (MSA-P)

Olivopontocerebellar atrophy (MSA-C)

DLB (Table 1). The clinical symptoms of DLB can be similar to those of AD, making the differentiation difficult. However, according to consortium criteria, there are certain 'Central Features' essential for a clinical diagnosis of DLB. First, there must be a dementia with progressive cognitive decline of sufficient magnitude to interfere with social or occupational function or both. Memory impairment may not necessarily occur early but usually develops with progression. Patients with DLB tend to have more problems with attention, executive functioning (e.g., planning, prioritizing, sequencing) and visuospatial ability, but do better with verbal memory than patients with AD. Thus, memory changes on the Mini-Mental State Examination may be more prominent with AD, whereas difficulties in clock drawing or figure copying may be more indicative of DLB.

The "Core Features" (two or more of which would be indicative of "probable" DLB) include fluctuating cognition, which is a pronounced variation in attention and alertness, reminiscent of delirium; recurrent visual hallucinations, typically well formed and detailed; and spontaneous parkinsonism. Fluctuating cognition occurs in 50 to 75% of patients with DLB. These fluctuations may occur over minutes, hours, or days, and their presence may be particularly helpful in differentiating DLB from AD. The fluctuating cognitive state closely mimics delirium. The features of such fluctuations include daytime drowsiness and lethargy, daytime sleep of two or more hours, staring into space for long periods, and episodes of disorganized thought and speech. Input about the patient's cognitive state should be sought from family members and caregivers. Physicians should not rely on clinical impressions at a single visit, because the patient's cognitive function may range from near normal to severe confusion on different days.

The visual hallucinations of DLB are recurrent, complex, and occur early in the course of the disease. They are often vivid and colorful, involving humans or animals (Mosimann et al. 2003). Although these hallucinations may upset family and caretakers, they often are not particularly distressing to the patient. Nevertheless, because patients who have DLB can experience severe reactions to antipsychotic medications, it is important to recognize these hallucinations as part of the disease process and not as evidence of a superimposed psychotic illness.

Extrapyramidal signs (EPS), including bradykinesia, facial masking, and rigidity, are the most frequent signs of parkinsonism in DLB patients. Resting tremor is distinctly uncommon. Parkinsonism is usually bilateral and occurs with the onset of dementia, although the onset and the severity of the parkinsonism are highly variable. There is often more axial rigidity and facial masking in DLB than in idiopathic PD. Although conventional teaching suggests that DLB may be poorly responsive to levodopa, small trials have shown that DLB patients tolerate this medication and, in some cases, show a beneficial response.

In addition to these core items, the recent DLB consortium identified additional "Suggestive Features" that, in combination with core features, could point to a diagnosis of DLB (one core symptom and one suggestive feature would indicate probable DLB; one or more suggestive symptoms alone would indicate possible DLB). These suggestive features include rapid-eye-movement (REM) sleep disorder, severe neuroleptic sensitivity, and low dopamine transporter uptake in basal ganglia demonstrated by SPECT or PET imaging. REM sleep behavior disorder (RBD) consists of particularly vivid (and sometimes violent) dreams during REM sleep, without the normal muscle atonia that prevents movements (other than eye movements) during dreams. Patients literally act out their dreams, manifested by talking and moving, sometimes with goal-oriented violence (Boeve et al. 2004). Interestingly, the sleep disorder may be present many years before the onset of dementia (Britton et al. 2009). Neuroleptic sensitivity to D2 receptor blockers is a feature of about half of DLB patients and, when present, is considered suggestive of DLB. Functional imaging of the dopamine transporter (DAT) defines the integrity of the nigrostriatal dopaminergic system and, using specific ligands (e.g., beta-CIT, FP-CIT), provides a marker for presynaptic neuronal degeneration. Low striatal DAT activity occurs in DLB but not in AD and, thus, may be helpful in distinguishing between the two disorders.

Commonly present but not specific ("supportive") features of DLB include repeated falls and syncope, transient, unexplained loss of consciousness, severe autonomic dysfunction, hallucinations in other modalities, systematized delusions, depression, relative preservation of medial temporal lobe structures on structural neuroimaging, reduced occipital activity on functional neuroimaging, prominent slow wave activity on EEG, and low uptake iodine-123 metaiodobenzylguanidine (MIBG) myocardial scintigraphy. Scintigraphy with [I-123] MIBG, which enables quantification of post-ganglionic sympathetic cardiac innervation, is reduced in DLB and may have high sensitivity and specificity in differentiating it from AD.

Unfortunately, DLB has no characteristic laboratory findings that distinguish it from other forms of dementia. Diagnosis primarily relies on the history and exam to meet the criteria outlined above. History obtained from a caretaker is essential as those with early dementia often have little insight or memory for the symptoms of their disease. Appropriate laboratory investigations are identical to those for other forms of dementia and should include routine screening for depression, vitamin B_{12} deficiency, and hypothyroidism. Magnetic resonance imaging in DLB shows relative preservation of hippocampal and medial temporal lobe volumes compared with AD. Single photon emission CT (SPECT) may reveal occipital hypoperfusion and positron emission tomography (PET) may show occipital hypometabolism. MIBG imaging of the heart, as mentioned above, has demonstrated decreased sympathetic innervation in subjects with DLB, but is not yet widely used for this clinical purpose.

Treatment

Developing a problem list of cognitive, psychiatric, and motor disabilities may be helpful in managing patients with DLB. Working with the patient and family, the physician can help prioritize target symptoms such as cognitive impairment; neuropsychiatric features (e.g., hallucinations, depression, sleep disorder, associated behavioral disturbances); extrapyramidal motor features; or autonomic dysfunction. Identifying the most disabling and distressing symptoms is especially helpful because successful treatment in one area may come at the expense of losses in another (McKeith et al. 1999). For example, use of cholinesterase inhibitors for dementia may exacerbate parkinsonian features such as drooling and postural instability.

Pharmacologic management of DLB can be challenging (Table 4). In patients with acute psychotic symptoms, other causes of psychosis such as pain, intercurrent infection, subdural hematoma, or adverse drug reaction must be excluded. Differentiating pseudo-delirium caused by DLB from a superimposed delirium can be difficult, and a diagnostic medical evaluation is still necessary for any abrupt increase in confusion. Patients with significant visual hallucinations are reported to have better response to cholinesterase inhibitor therapy than other patients with dementia (Doody et al. 2001); these medications improve fluctuating cognition, hallucinations, apathy, anxiety, and sleep disturbances.

Table 4 Pharmacologic Management of Symptoms of Dementia with Lewy Bodies

Symptom	Preferred Medication	Medications to Avoid	Goal of Therapy	Possible Adverse Effects
Delirium	Cholinesterase inhibitors	Antipsychotics (especially neuroleptics with high D2 affinity, such as haloperidol	Decrease fluctuations in cognition	GI symptoms, rare worsening of EPS
Dementia	As above	As above	Improve cognition	As above
Parkinson's disease symptoms	Levodopa with carbidopa	Anticholinergics, antimuscarinics	Improve mobility	Visual hallucinations, delusions, orthostatic hypotension, GI upset
REM sleep behavior disorder	Clonazepam	None	Improve sleep	Ataxia, morning sedation
Visual hallucinations	Cholinesterase inhibitors	Antipsychotics (especially neuroleptics with high D2 affinity, such as haloperidol)	Reduce number of hallucinations	GI symptoms, rare worsening of EPS

GI = gastrointestinal; EPS = extrapyramidal symptoms; REM = rapid eye movement.

The results of a trial of rivastigmine (Exelon) compared with placebo in 120 DLB patients reported statistically and clinically significant behavioral effects at 20 weeks (McKeith et al. 2000).

Patients with DLB should not be given the older, typical D2-antagonist antipsychotic agents such as haloperidol, fluphenazine, and chlorpromazine since up to half of DLB patients who receive neuroleptic medications experience life-threatening adverse effects (including sedation, rigidity, postural instability, falls, increased confusion, and neuroleptic malignant syndrome), and there is an associated two- to threefold increase in mortality (McKeith et al. 1992). Atypical antipsychotics may be tried in low doses, but these can cause similar adverse effects and increase the risk of stroke (Sink et al. 2005).

If antiparkinsonian drugs are prescribed, the lowest possible dose of levodopa with carbidopa should be used, and monotherapy is preferred. The effect on parkinsonian symptoms is probably less than in classic Parkinson's disease, and potential side effects include visual hallucinations, delusions, orthostatic hypotension, and GI upset. The goal of antiparkinsonian medication is to improve mobility without inducing or exacerbating psychotic symptoms or confusion.

Information is not yet available about the use of cholinesterase inhibitors in combination with antiparkinsonian or atypical antipsychotic medications in DLB, although this is a common clinical situation. Anticholinergic agents should be strictly avoided. Orthostatic hypotension can be treated with vigorous hydration, ample dietary sodium, avoidance of prolonged bed rest, efforts to stand up slowly, and avoidance of medications that contribute to orthostasis. Constipation can be treated with exercise, increased dietary fiber, and hydration.

Parkinson's Disease

Although the motor syndrome of PD is extensively reviewed elsewhere in this book, we will briefly describe some of the salient features of this synucleinopathy with special attention to its cognitive and nonmotor symptoms.

Epidemiology

PD is the most frequent neurodegenerative movement disorder, with a prevalence of 1 to 3% in people older than 55 years of age, and a slight male preponderance. The majority of cases of PD are sporadic, but more than 10% of cases are familial. The familial cases may show autosomal dominant inheritance, as in the rare cases with α-synuclein mutations, or autosomal recessive inheritance, as in cases with the Parkin gene or the DJ-1 gene mutations of juvenile parkinsonism (Gasser 2007).

Pathology

The main pathologic feature of PD is deposition of LBs in the substantia nigra. Frederick Lewy first described LBs in cells of the substantia nigra in patients with idiopathic PD in 1914, but it was not until the mid 1980s that sensitive immunocytochemical methods to identify LBs were developed.

Clinical Features and Diagnosis

Motor Syndrome

The cardinal clinical features of PD include bradykinesia, rigidity, rest tremor, and gait and postural reflex abnormalities. Based on clinicopathological studies, diagnosis of PD is highly probable in a patient presenting with slowing of movements (bradykinesia) with either the classic pill-rolling tremor or rigidity and an excellent and sustained levodopa response. Asymmetric parkinsonism at onset and absence of atypical features improve the accuracy of the diagnosis. The course of the disease can be influenced by the clinical presentation and the age at onset of the disease. At least two different types of PD have been proposed: one characterized by postural instability and gait disorder (PIGD) and another where tremor is dominant. The tremor subtype is associated with preserved mental status, earlier age at onset, and a slower progression compared with the PIGD subtype. Patients with young-onset progress at a slower rate than those with late-onset but develop levodopa-induced dyskinesias earlier in the course of treatment (Post et al. 2008). Clinical features supporting the diagnosis of PD include absence of atypical features for PD (e.g., early marked autonomic disturbance, early severe dementia, corticospinal tract dysfunction, supranuclear gaze palsy); absence of possible causes for secondary parkinsonism (such as use of neuroleptic drugs, history of cerebrovascular events or encephalitis); asymmetric onset; and tremor-dominant pattern.

Cognitive and Non-motor Syndrome

In addition to the characteristic motor syndrome, PD patients demonstrate various non-motor manifestations, including neuropsychiatric disturbances, autonomic dysfunction, abnormalities in olfactory perception, sensory symptoms, and sleep disorders.

Disturbances of cognition and emotion are common in PD (Simuni et al. 2008). The most frequent neuropsychiatric symptom is depression, followed by visual hallucinations and anxiety. In general, depression is mild or moderate but can present as a chronic major depression or fluctuating dysthymia. It often begins several years before the motor symptoms. The lack of association between depression and disease stage suggests that mood changes in PD are not due to motor disability but rather reflect a primary neurobiological dysfunction.

Specific cognitive domains, such as visuospatial and executive function, are frequently affected in PD; language is usually spared. The prevalence of frank dementia has been estimated at 25 to 30% and it appears more often in patients in whom postural instability and gait disturbances are prominent (Goetz et al. 2008). The dementia of PD has been characterized as "ubcortical" in type, but in some patients, the features can be difficult to distinguish from Alzheimer's disease (Merims et al. 2008). As one of the classic subcortical dementias, Parkinson's dementia is characterized by cognitive slowing, depression and absence of aphasia, as well as by difficulties in working memory and problem-solving due to disruption of frontal-subcortical circuits (Zgaljardic et al. 2003).

Cognitive fluctuations seem to be less frequent than in DLB, but prevalence of visual hallucinations is similar in both DLB and PD with dementia. Although the neuropathological basis of dementia in PD is heterogeneous, recent reports suggest that diffuse cortical Lewy bodies may be an important pathological substrate in the majority.

Apathy is present in approximately 30% of patients with Parkinson disease (Kirsch-Darrow et al. 2006). Apathy can be very difficult to differentiate from depression, as the two disorders can occur together. Apathy can also be present without signs or symptoms of depressed mood. Apathy is commonly conceptualized as involving three domains: cognitive (lack of interest), behavioral (lack of initiation and drive), and affective (lack of emotion).

Anxiety disorders commonly accompany depression in Parkinson disease, but they can also occur independently. They most often present in the setting of wearing-off or on-off fluctuations associated with medication status. Anxiety disorders in patients with Parkinson disease include generalized anxiety and panic attacks. Classic obsessive-compulsive disorder is less common, but obsessive behaviors and impulse control difficulties can occur in up to 7% of patients with

Parkinson disease and presumably reflect dopamine dysregulation, most often associated with dopamine agonists. Impulsive behavior can include gambling, hypersexuality, and bingeing. One form of obsessive-compulsive disorder is punding, a behavior characterized by intense fascination with repetitive handling and examining of objects, most often mechanical objects. Behaviors can include assembling and disassembling, collecting, or sorting of objects.

Many patients with Parkinson disease have visual hallucinations as a side effect of dopaminergic drugs. At first, the patient realizes that they are hallucinations, but this insight may be lost as the disease progresses. The clinician should also consider other potential causes such as dementia, systemic illness, or psychosocial stress.

Nearly all PD patients experience some degree of autonomic disturbances during the course of their illness. By far the most frequent complaints are urinary and intestinal symptoms. Constipation is a common problem that can become quite serious in PD, occasionally leading to intestinal pseudo-obstruction and toxic megacolon. The basis of the constipation has been attributed to reduced colonic mobility secondary to PD, because Lewy bodies have been observed within the myenteric plexuses of the gastrointestinal tract (Kupsky et al. 1987). In fact, Lewy bodies are most frequent in the plexus of the lower esophagus, which may explain the frequent swallowing difficulties that some PD patients experience. Sexual dysfunction, due to both loss of libido and impotence, in addition to urinary symptoms, such as urgency, frequency, and incontinence, are also common complaints.

Treatment

PD is not considered to be a fatal disease by itself, but it is clearly a progressive one. The average life expectancy of a PD patient is generally lower than for people who do not have the disease. In the late stages, PD may cause complications such as choking, pneumonia, and falls that can lead to death. The progression of symptoms in PD may take 20 years or more. In some people, however, the disease progresses more quickly. There is no way to predict what course the disease will take for an individual person. With appropriate treatment, most people with PD can live productive lives for many years after diagnosis.

The most widely used treatments for the motor symptoms of PD include levodopa (L-dopa) in various forms, including the combination preparation of carbidopa/levodopa, controlled release versions of carbidopa/levodopa, COMT (catechol-O-methyltransferase) inhibitors such as entacapone, the combination of entacapone/carbidopa/levodopa, monoamine oxidase–B (MAO-B) inhibitors such as selegiline and rasagiline, and dopamine agonists, including bromocriptine, pramipexole, ropinirole, cabergoline, and apomorphine.

For the apathy of PD, bupropion and methylphenidate can be tried for their activating or stimulant properties although efficacy data are limited. Depression, generalized anxiety, and panic attacks are usually responsive to SSRIs and benzodiazepines. Because of its long half-life, some clinicians prefer clonazepam (Klonopin®) for the anxiety associated with wearing off or unpredictable off periods. Conversely, a long half-life and depressive effects may limit its usefulness in advanced age. Cholinesterase inhibitors appear to moderately improve cognition and, to a lesser extent, activities of daily living in patients with PD dementia. A randomized, double-blind, placebo-controlled study (Emre et al. 2004) involving 541 patients with PD dementia found statistically significant improvements in the primary cognitive measure, the ADAS-Cog, and a functional measure, the ADCS-ADL Scale, in rivastigmine-treated subjects compared to placebo.

Multiple System Atrophy

Multiple system atrophy (MSA) is a progressive sporadic neurodegenerative disorder, characterized clinically by parkinsonism, autonomic failure, and cerebellar and pyramidal dysfunction, in any combination. The historical terms striatonigral degeneration (SND), olivopontocerebellar atrophy (OPCA), and Shy-Drager syndrome (SDS) refer to neuropathological descriptions of patients with a combination of symptoms with predominant parkinsonism (SND), cerebellar dysfunction (OPCA), or autonomic failure (SDS), which have been embraced under the term MSA (Graham and Oppenheimer 1969). As practically all patients with MSA have some degree of autonomic dysfunction, the terms MSA-P and MSA-C are currently used to refer to the parkinsonism-predominant or cerebellar-predominant subtypes, respectively (Table 5).

Epidemiology

The prevalence of MSA is estimated to be between 2.3 and 310 per 100,000 in different studies. Annual incidence was 3 per 100,000 people over the age of 50 in a single study in Olmsted County (Minnesota). It is slightly more common in men (ratio 1.3:1). In a review of 203 autopsy-confirmed cases (Bower et al. 2002), the mean age at onset was 54.3 years (range, 33–78 years) and the mean disease duration was 6.1 years (range, 0.3–24 years) from the onset of symptoms.

Pathology

The pathologic hallmark of MSA is the presence of alpha-synuclein-rich cytoplasmic inclusions in glial cells of the basal ganglia, motor cortex, reticular formation, and pontocerebellar system. In MSA-P, neurodegeneration is most prominent in the striatonigral system; in MSA-C, neurodegeneration is most prominent in the olivopontocerebellar system.

Clinical Features and Diagnosis

The clinical presentation of MSA is variable (Gilman et al. 2008). Parkinsonism is the predominant symptom in more than 80% of cases

Table 5 Consensus Criteria for MSA, Modified after Gilman et al. 2008

Possible MSA-P or MSA-C

—Babinski sign with hyperreflexia

—Stridor

Possible MSA-P

—Rapidly progressive parkinsonism

—Poor response to levodopa

—Postural instability within 3 years of motor onset

—Gait ataxia with cerebellar dysarthria, limb ataxia, or cerebellar oculomotor dysfunction

—Dysphagia within 5 years of motor onset

—Atrophy on MRI of putamen, middle cerebellar peduncle, pons, or cerebellum

—Hypometabolism on FDG-PET in putamen, brainstem, or cerebellum

Possible MSA-C

—Parkinsonism

—Atrophy on MRI of putamen, middle cerebellar peduncle, pons, or cerebellum

MSA = multiple system atrophy

(MSA-P). A cerebellar syndrome predominates in less than 20% (MSA-C), but cerebellar features ultimately develop in approximately half of patients. Autonomic dysfunction is present in almost every patient to a certain extent. In addition to these key features, a variety of accompanying symptoms may also develop, including cognitive impairment (Kawai et al. 2008).

Parkinsonism

As mentioned, parkinsonism is the predominant symptom in more than 80% of MSA patients and also the initial feature in approximately half of cases. It is usually asymmetric, and akinesia and rigidity are the most common features. Tremor is present in two-thirds of patients, and manifests as rest tremor in one-third, sometimes of pill-rolling type. Other parkinsonian signs are postural instability and hypokinetic speech. Dyskinesias develop in half of the treated patients and are less common and severe than in Parkinson's disease (PD). In contrast to PD, they are characterized by a predominant involvement of face, jaw, and neck muscles and are usually dystonic.

Cerebellar Signs

Cerebellar dysfunction develops in approximately half of the MSA patients but is predominant (MSA-C) in less than 20% of cases in Western populations. In the Japanese population, prevalence of MSA-C type has been reported as high as 67% (Watanabe et al. 2002). It manifests mainly with ataxia of gait, instability, and falls but also with ataxia of limbs and speech, intention tremor, and disorders of extraocular movements such as square wave jerks, saccadic pursuit, nystagmus, overshoot or undershoot dysmetria, or slow pursuit. It is frequently difficult to recognize cerebellar involvement in patients with MSA-P who have marked akinesia and rigidity, when limb dysmetria or intention tremor is not present.

Autonomic Dysfunction

The most common manifestations of autonomic failure are impotence, affecting the majority of male patients, and urinary incontinence. These signs may begin 5 to 10 years before the onset of other symptoms and may be considered by the patient to be a consequence of normal aging. Urinary incontinence and frequency are due to multiple factors: involuntary detrusor contraction, loss of ability to initiate the micturition reflex, and urethral sphincter dysfunction (Papatsoris et al. 2008).

Orthostatic hypotension is found in more than half of the patients and is usually mild and asymptomatic. It is defined as a reduction of systolic blood pressure of at least 20 mmHg, or diastolic blood pressure of at least 10 mmHg, within 3 minutes of standing from recumbent position, although decreases of 30 and 15 mmHg, respectively, were used for the definition of MSA criteria. In some cases, it can be severe and manifest as recurrent syncopes. Other signs of autonomic failure, such as severe constipation, fecal incontinence, decreased sweating, or iris atrophy, are also found (Mathias et al. 2006).

Cognitive Impairment

A recent study of 35 patients confirmed earlier reports of cognitive difficulties in MSA and found that patients with MSA-P showed more severe impairment compared to patients with MSA-C (Kawai et al. 2008). Although patients with MSA-C showed visuospatial and constructional difficulties, patients with MSA-P showed more wide-ranging cognitive difficulties such as visuospatial and constructional dysfunction, impairment of verbal fluency, dysexecutive syndrome, and depression, likely reflective of prefrontal involvement.

Diagnostic Criteria

The criteria for diagnosis of MSA were recently updated following a second consensus conference (Gilman et al. 2008). According to the criteria, a diagnosis of definite MSA requires neuropathologic confirmation. A diagnosis of probable MSA requires progressive adult-onset disease, autonomic failure, poorly levodopa-responsive parkinsonism, and a cerebellar syndrome. A diagnosis of possible MSA requires parkinsonism OR a cerebellar syndrome, at least one feature suggestive of autonomic dysfunction, and at least one additional supportive feature.

Treatment

There is currently no specific therapy for MSA, although patients may experience benefit from symptomatic treatment of their parkinsonism with levodopa and their orthostatic hypotension with a high salt diet or with agents such as fludrocortisone and midodrine.

Future Directions

Undoubtedly, the development of transgenic animal models that recapitulate the key pathologic aspects of human synucleinopathies will help answer questions regarding the fundamental mechanisms leading to this group of neurodegenerative diseases. Further studies will be necessary to determine how alpha-synuclein aggregates into Lewy bodies and leads to the demise of neurons. In addition, advanced neuroimaging tools are needed for more accurate diagnosis of synucleinopathies. In particular, ligands, much the same as Pittsburgh-compound B has been for amyloid imaging in Alzheimer's disease, will likely be needed to visualize the buildup of the misfolded protein as the disease progresses. Finally, biomarkers, whether blood or CSF-based, will be of great utility in managing patients and evaluating potential therapies that target the underlying pathology.

References

Baba M, Nakajo S, Tu PH, Tomita T, Nakaya K, Lee VM, et al. Aggregation of alpha-synuclein in Lewy bodies of sporadic Parkinson's disease and dementia with Lewy bodies. *Am J Pathol* 152:879–84, 1998.

Boeve BF, Silber MH, and Ferman TJ. REM sleep behavior disorder in Parkinson's disease and dementia with Lewy bodies. *J Geriatr Psychiatry Neurol* 17:146–57, 2004.

Bower JH, Maraganore DM, McDonnell SK, et al. Incidence of progressive supranuclear palsy and multiple system atrophy in Olmsted County, Minnesota, 1976 to 1990. *Neurology* 49:1284–8, 1997.

Britton TC and Chaudhuri KR. REM-sleep behavior disorder and the risk of developing Parkinson disease or dementia. *Neurology* (15):1294–5, 2009.

Doody RS, Stevens JC, Beck C, et al. Practice parameter: Management of dementia (an evidence-based review). Report of Quality Standards Subcommittee of the American Academy of Neurology. *Neurology* 56:1154–66, 2001.

Driver-Dunckley E, Samanta J, and Stacy M. Pathological gambling associated with dopamine agonist therapy in Parkinson's disease. *Neurology* 61:422–3, 2003.

Emre M, Aarsland D, Albanese A, Byrne EJ, Deuschl G, De Deyn PP, et al. Rivastigmine for Dementia Associated with Parkinson's Disease. *NEJM* 351:2509–2518, 2004.

Galvin JE, Lee VM, and Trojanowski JQ. Synucleinopathies: Clinical and pathological implications. *Arch Neurol* 58:186–90, 2001.

Gasser T. Update on the genetics of Parkinson's disease. *Mov Disord* 17:S343–50, 2007.

Gilman S, Wenning GK, Low PA, et al. Second consensus statement on the diagnosis of multiple system atrophy. *Neurology* 71:670–6, 2008.

Goetz CG, Emre M, and Dubois B. Parkinson's disease dementia: Definitions, guidelines, and research perspectives in diagnosis. *Ann Neurol* 2:S81–92, 2008.

Goetz CG, et al.; Movement Disorder Society UPDRS Revision Task Force. Movement Disorder Society-sponsored revision of the Unified Parkinson's Disease Rating Scale (MDS-UPDRS): Scale presentation and clinimetric testing results. *Mov Disord* 23:2129–70, 2008.

Graham JG and Oppenheimer DR. Orthostatic hypotension and nicotine sensitivity in a case of multiple system atrophy. *J Neurol Neurosurg Psychiatry*. 32:28–34, 1969.

Hoehn MM and Yahr MD. Parkinsonism: Onset, progression and mortality. *Neurology*. 17:427-42, 1967.

Kawai Y, Suenaga M, Takeda A, Ito M, Watanabe H, Tanaka F, et al. Cognitive impairments in multiple system atrophy, MSA-C vs. MSA-P. *Neurology* 70:1390–1396, 2008.

Kirsch-Darrow L, Fernandez HH, Marsiske M, et al. Dissociating apathy and depression in Parkinson disease. *Neurology* 67:33–38, 2006.

Kosaka K, Yoshimura M, Ikeda K, and Budka H. Diffuse type of Lewy body disease: Progressive dementia with abundant cortical Lewy bodies and senile changes of varying degree-a new disease? *Clin Neuropathol* 3:185–92, 1984.

Kupsky WJ, Grimes MM, Sweeting J, et al. Parkinson's disease and megacolon: Concentric hyaline inclusions (Lewy bodies) in enteric ganglion cells. *Neurology* 37:1253–5,1987.

Leverenz JB and McKeith IG. Dementia with Lewy bodies. *Med Clin North Amer* 86:519–35, 2002.

Lozano AM and Snyder BJ. Deep brain stimulation for parkinsonian gait disorders. *J Neurol* 4:30–1, 2008.

Mathias CJ. Multiple system atrophy and autonomic failure. *J Neural Transm* 70:343–7, 2006.

McKeith I, Del Ser T, Spano P, et al. Efficacy of rivastigmine in dementia with Lewy bodies: A randomised, double-blind, placebo-controlled international study. *Lancet* 356:2031–6, 2000.

McKeith I, Fairbairn A, Perry R, et al . Neuroleptic sensitivity in patients with senile dementia of Lewy body type. *BMJ* 305:673–8, 1992.

McKeith I, Mintzer J, Aarsland D, Burn D, Chiu H, Cohen-Mansfield J, et al. Dementia with Lewy bodies. *Lancet Neurol* 3:19–28, 2004.

McKeith IG, Ballard CG, Perry RH, et al. Prospective validation of consensus criteria for the diagnosis of dementia with Lewy bodies. *Neurology* 54:1050–1058, 2000.

McKeith IG, Dickson DW, Lowe J, et al. Diagnosis and management of dementia with Lewy bodies: Third report of the DLB Consortium. *Neurology* 65:1863–72, 2005.

McKeith IG, Galasko D, Kosaka K, Perry EK, Dickson DW, Hansen LA, et al. Consensus guidelines for the clinical and pathologic diagnosis of dementia with Lewy bodies (DLB): Report of the consortium on DLB international workshop. *Neurology* 47:1113–24, 1996.

McKeith IG, Perry EK, and Perry RH. Report of the second dementia with Lewy body international workshop: Diagnosis and treatment. *Neurology* 53:902–5, 1999.

Merims D and Freedman M. Cognitive and behavioural impairment in Parkinson's disease. *Int Rev Psychiatry* 20:364–73, 2008.

Mosimann UP and McKeith IG. Dementia with Lewy bodies diagnosis and treatment. *Swiss Med Wkly* 133:131–42, 2003.

Okun MS and Vitek JL. Lesion therapy for Parkinson's disease and other movement disorders: Update and controversies. *Mov Disord* 19:375–89, 2004.

Papatsoris AG, Papapetropoulos S, Singer C, and Deliveliotis C. Urinary and erectile dysfunction in multiple system atrophy (MSA). *Neurourol Urodyn* 27:22–7, 2008.

Simuni T and Sethi K. Nonmotor manifestations of Parkinson's disease. *Ann Neurol* Suppl 2:S65–80, 2008.

Sink KM, Holden KF, and Yaffe K. Pharmacological treatment of neuropsychiatric symptoms of dementia: A review of the evidence. *JAMA* 293:596–608, 2005.

Song YJ, Lundvig DM, Huang Y, et al. p25 alpha relocalizes in oligodendroglia from myelin to cytoplasmic inclusions in multiple system atrophy. *Am J Pathol* 171:1291–303, 2007.

Tofaris GK, Layfield R, and Spillantini MG. Synuclein metabolism and aggregation is linked to ubiquitin-independent degradation by the proteasome. *FEBS Lett* 509: 22–26, 2001.

Watanabe H, Saito Y, Terao S, et al. Progression and prognosis in multiple system atrophy: An analysis of 230 Japanese patients. *Brain* 125:1070–83, 2002.

Zgaljardic DJ, Borod JC, Foldi NS, et al. A review of the cognitive and behavioral sequelae of Parkinson's disease: Relationship to frontostriatal circuitry. *Cogn Behav Neurol* 16:193–210, 2003.

20 Alcohol and Toxin-related Dementias

Sachio Matsushita and Masaru Mimura

Introduction

The relationship between alcohol abuse and dementia is complex. Although some authors insist that alcohol has direct neurotoxic effects leading to the characteristic dementia syndrome of alcohol related dementia (ARD) as a neuropathologic entity, other authors claim that a large proportion of ARD individuals are probably unrecognized cases of Wernicke-Korsakoff syndrome (WKS). Additionally, some individual cases of dementia in the setting of alcohol use may possibly be attributed to other conditions, including chronic hepatocerebral degeneration, communicating hydrocephalus, Alzheimer's disease (AD), ischemic infarction, and vascular dementia (VaD) (Torvik et al. 1982; Victor 1993; Victor and Adams 1985; Lishman 1990).

Concerning other substances of abuse, the association between chronic use of benzodiazepines and cognitive impairment is inconclusive. The Kungsholmen study examined the association between long-term use of benzodiazepines and cognitive impairment in a prospective manner and found no significant relationship between benzodiazepine use and dementia (Fastbom 1998). However, a recent nested case-control study demonstrated increased risk of dementia in older persons who ever used benzodiazepine (Lagnaoui 2002). The chronic use of cannabis may impair intellectual abilities but data on this topic remain sparse and difficult to interpret (Hulse 2005).

Another neuropathology entity related to toxin exposure is toxic leukoencephalopathy, which is a structural alteration of cerebral white matter wherein the myelin sheath suffers the most severe damage. Toxic leukoencephalopathy may be caused by exposure to a wide variety of agents, drugs of abuse, and environmental toxins (Table1). Toxic leukoencephalopathy particularly involves white-matter tracts devoted to higher cerebral function, causing clinical features that range from inattention, forgetfulness, and changes in personality to dementia, coma, and death (Filley and Kleinschmidt-DeMasters 2009).

In this chapter, we will discuss mainly the alcohol and toxin-related dementias.

Table 1 Toxins that Cause Leukoencephalopathy

1) Antineoplastic agents (cranial irradiation, methotrexate, carmustine, cisplatin, cytarabine, fluorouracil, levamisole, fludarabine, thiotepa, interleukin-2, interferon alpha)
2) Immunosuppressive drugs (cyclosporine, tacrolimus)
3) Antimicrobial agents (amphotericin B, hexachlorophene)
4) Drugs of abuse (toluene, ethanol cocaine, 3,4-methylenedioxymethamphetamine, intravenous heroin, inhaled "heroin" pyrolysate, psilocybin)
5) Environmental toxins (carbon monoxide, arsenic, carbon tetrachloride)

Modified from the article by Filley 2001.

Epidemiology

Most studies focus on the prevalence of the comorbidity between alcohol use or abuse and dementia or cognitive impairment. Among community dwelling adults over 55 years old assessed in the Epidemiologic Catchment Area Study, the prevalence of a lifetime history of alcohol abuse or dependence was 1.5 times greater among persons with mild to severe cognitive impairment than those with no cognitive impairment (George 1991). Furthermore, the Liverpool Longitudinal Study of mental health in community dwelling elderly, found that dementia was 4.6 times more likely to occur in men aged 65 and older who had a lifetime history of heavy drinking (Saunders 1991). Thomas and Rockwood (2001) reported the results of a cross-sectional analysis of the Canadian Study of Health and Aging that included 2873 older adults. Subjects with questionable or definite alcohol abuse were more likely to have cognitive impairment or dementia than older adults with no such history (OR = 1.5, 95% CI = 1.2-2.0).

There are several studies examining the prevalence of alcohol use problems in patients with dementia. Rains and Ditzler studied 383 men and women with dementia, 9% of whom had a history of heavy alcohol use (Rains 1993). The study by King reported the prevalence of heavy alcohol use to be 21% in patients presenting to a dementia clinic (King 1986). In one of the few studies of alcohol use among demented long-term care residents, Carlen and colleagues determined that 29% of 130 residents with dementia met criteria for ARD (Carlen 1994).

Studies have also suggested high prevalence rates of dementia among patients with alcohol use disorders seeking for treatment. Finlayson and colleagues (1988) found 49 of 216 (23%) elderly alcoholics presenting for addiction treatment to have a comorbid dementia. Similarly, in a study of older alcoholic veterans presenting for mental health treatment, Blow and colleagues (1992) found 9% of the 60 to 69 year old age group (n = 3986) and 18.4% of those over 70 (n = 543) to have a comorbid dementia.

In contrast to the higher rates of heavy alcohol use associated with dementia, the prevalence of WKS has been estimated to occur in only 0.4% to 2.8% of autopsies regardless of the clinical history (Harper 1995). Although community-based prevalence rates of WKS are difficult to ascertain, the comparison of prevalence between dementia in subjects with alcohol abuse and WKS suggests an association between alcohol use, especially heavy use or alcohol dependence, and the development of dementia regardless of WKS.

On the other hand, the prevalence of toxic leukoencephalopathy is unknown.

Pathophysiology

Even after excluding specific alcohol-related disorders, such as WKS, hepatic encephalopathy, and pellagra, there is still a group of heavy alcohol consumers exhibiting cognitive impairment (Harper and

Corbett 1997). A direct toxic effect of ethanol on the brain has been suggested as the primary cause of ARD (Sun and Sun 2001). There are several studies reporting neuropathological findings in brains of alcoholic patients without neurological complications such as WKS. For example, reduction of volume/weight ratios of white matter and of archicortex (Badsberg Jensen 1993), selective loss of neurons from the superior frontal association cortex (Kril 1997), and an association between atrophy of cerebellum and alcoholism (Torvik 1982) are reported.

Moreover, results of neuroimaging studies indicate that people with alcohol-related disorders have thinner gyri and wider sulci, as well as loss of gray and white matter (Ding et al. 2004). Reduction in brain volume is unlikely to be the result of simple dehydration, but rather due to alcohol-induced reduction of the dentritic arbor, a precursor of cellular death, which is possibly reversible in the early stages of alcohol neurotoxicity (Harper and Corbett 1990). Recent MRI study using diffusion tensor imaging found disruption of the microstructure of white matter in patients with alcoholism (Pfefferbaum 2000) that might indicate the leukotoxicity of ethanol (Filley 2009).

However, the lack of consistent neuropathologic findings associated with alcohol use has led many researchers to cast doubt on the clinical relevance of any direct neurotoxic effects of alcohol use. This line of argument is that alcohol per se is unlikely to be the causal agent of dementia, but is instead a probable contributing factor that can only cause or result in dementia when acting with other agents (i.e., thiamine insufficiency, chronic hepatocerebral degeneration, communicating hydrocephalus, AD, ischemic infarction). For example, people who drink excessively may develop nutritional deficiencies such as folate and vitamin B_{12} deficiency (Laufer et al. 2004), which in turn may increase the risk of cognitive impairment and dementia. Moreover, excessive alcohol consumption (more than 60g of ethanol per day) has been shown to double the risk of strokes [relative risk (RR) = 1.69, 95% CI = 1.34–2.15 for ischemic stroke and RR = 2.18, 95% CI = 1.48–3.20 for hemorrhagic stroke] (Reynolds 2003), which substantially increases the risk of cognitive impairment and dementia (Ivan et al. 2004). Other common factors associated with alcoholism, such as smoking, increase the risk of cognitive impairment and dementia (Almeida et al. 2002).

Finally, the relationship between WKS and cognitive decline is well established. Wernicke's encephalopathy represents the abrupt clinical manifestation of severe thiamine deficiency and is characterized by nystagmus, ophthalmoplegia (conjugated gaze palsies), gait ataxia and confusion. Although Wernicke's encephalopathy is most commonly seen in malnourished persons with alcoholism, it is not caused by alcohol per se. Wernicke's encephalopathy is caused by a thiamine diphosphate deficiency, which is a biologically active form of thiamine (vitamin B_1), a cofactor in several enzyme reactions involved in the biosynthesis of cell constituents, neurotransmitters, production of antioxidants, catabolism of carbohydrates and synthesis of nucleic acid precursors (Singleton 2001). Approximately 80% to 90% of alcoholics with Wernicke's encephalopathy develop Korsakoff's syndrome (Victor 1989), which is characterized by marked memory impairment, in particular a striking loss of episodic memory with relative preservation of other cognitive functions. Typically, patients are unable to learn new information, and may also have some difficulty recalling past events. Severe thiamine deficiency, and the consequent WKS, is associated with lesions to the mamillary bodies, thalamus, hypothalamus, brainstem, and cerebellum (particularly the vermis) (Harper 1998).

Cranial irradiation and anticancer chemotherapy are well-established causes of toxic leukoencephalopathy. Radiation produces three stages of leukoencephalopathy: an acute reaction involving patchy, reversible edema of the white matter, a more sustained delayed reaction involving wide-spread edema and demyelination, and a severe delayed reaction involving the loss of myelin and axons as a result of vascular necrosis and thrombosis (Sheline 1980). Methotrexate and carmustine are the most commonly implicated anticancer drugs. Leukoencephalopathy may occur in less than 10 percent of those who are treated intravenously with methotrexate (Mahoney 1998), but in up to 40 percent of those who are treated by the intrathecal route (Asato 1992). Therefore, the incidence of neurotoxicity is suggested to depend on the route of delivery, the dose, and the drug used (Filley 2009).

Prolonged inhalation of toluene, which is a highly lipophilic white-matter toxin, results in dementia, ataxia, brain-stem dysfunction, and corticospinal deficits (Hormes 1986). Findings at autopsy include diffuse pallor of the cerebral and cerebellar white matter, with clusters of trilaminar inclusions within the cytoplasm of mononuclear cells and increased numbers of very-long-chain fatty acids, as are found in patients with adrenoleukodystrophy (Rosenberg 1988; Kornfeld 1994). These findings suggest that myelin is the target of toluene.

Genetic Contributions

As far as the authors know, there are no studies examining genetic risk factors of ARD. However, recent epidemiologic studies examining the genetic and environmental risk factors of dementia are reporting the effect of apolipoprotein E (APOE) ε4 allele on the relationship between alcohol and dementia. Mukamal et al. (2003) reported that protective action of moderate alcohol use against dementia may be more pronounced among persons without an APOE ε4 allele, as subjects with an APOE ε4 allele were found to be prone to the deleterious effects of high alcohol intake. In the same way, Dufoil et al. (2000) reported APOE ε4 carriers who consumed five or more glasses of alcohol per day were at increased risk of cognitive deterioration over a follow-up period of four years compared to nondrinkers who were noncarriers (RR=8.3, 95% CI = 1.0–66.0). Moreover, another study reported that risk of dementia increased with increasing alcohol consumption only in those individuals carrying the APOE ε4 allele (Anttila 2004) and a recent cohort study also reported the alcohol drinking increased the risk of AD among the subjects with APOE ε4 allele [odds ratio (OR) = 7.42, 95% CI = 1.51–36.38 in APOE ε4 allele carrier, OR = 0.62, 95% CI = 0.17–2.33, in APOE ε4 allele non-carrier] (Kivipelto 2008).

On the other hand, in WKS, biochemical study showed that transketolase extracted from WKS patients' fibroblast had decreased affinity for thiamine pyrophosphate (Blass 1977). However, because no specific genetic variations which cause amino acid substitution are found (McCool 1993), other mechanisms such as post-translational modifications or aberrant assembly of proteins have been postulated to explain the difference in biochemical activity of transketolase in WKS. Furthermore, although genetic variations coding for the high-affinity thiamine transporter protein SLC19A2 has been implicated in the pathophysiology of WKS (Guerrini 2005), other studies are needed to draw firm conclusions.

Several genetic variations in alcohol metabolizing enzyme might be a risk factor for WKS. There is a study reporting an association between alcohol dehydrogenase-2 (ADH2) gene polymorphism and WKS (Matsushita 2000), showing the slow metabolizing type of ADH2 allele (ADH2*2) predominant in alcoholic WKS patients compared with alcoholics without WKS and non-alcoholic controls. Another study reported that alcoholic WKS patients with global intellectual deficits had higher APOE 4 allele frequency compared with WKS patients without global intellectual deficits, suggesting the involvement of APOE ε4 allele in the intellectual decline of WKS (Muramatsu 1997).

Clinical Presentations

Clinical presentation of ARD is heterogeneous and includes mild cognitive impairment, amnesia, and dementia.

The onset of ARD is usually gradual while WKS presents with acute onset with nystagmus, ataxia, and disturbance in consciousness (Cutting 1978). However, neuropathological study found that WKS may occur with gradual onset, without the apparent acute clinical signs of Wernicke encephalopathy (Harper 1983).

Patients with ARD are impaired in memory tests, and have difficulty with tasks requiring speed or frontal lobe function (Tarter 1973). The deficits typically reported include difficulty with complex reasoning, planning, abstract reasoning, judgment, attention, and memory (Fein et al. 1990). This pattern of deficits, in comparison with other dementing disorders, such as Alzheimer's disease and vascular dementia, suggests an association between ARD with both cortical and subcortical neuropathology (Schmidt 2005). On the other hand, areas that are spared include language and verbal skills.

There is ample evidence of recovery of some deficits in some patients, usually in a few weeks to months after cessation of drinking. However, for some patients the deficits persist or only slowly improve after years of sobriety; but, at the very least, these deficits usually show an arrest of progression with prolonged abstinence (Smith 1995). Such reversibility of dementia is used as supportive evidence for the presence of ARD, as opposed to Alzheimer's disease or vascular dementia.

Neurological examination reveals that patients with ARD often show evidence of ataxia or peripheral sensory neuropathy (Smith 1995). However, Victor reported more than 80% of patients with WKS also showed some impairment of stance and gait, and polyneuropathy as well as nystagmus was quite common (Victor 1989). These neurological symptoms might suggest an association of ARD with WKS.

The clinical spectrum of toxic leukoencephalopathy generally parallels the severity of white-matter damage as well as its distribution, which is usually diffuse. In contrast to disorders of cortical gray matter such as Alzheimer's disease, toxic leukoencephalopathy does not primarily affect language, praxis, or perception. Neurologic signs such as hemiparesis, sensory deficits, and visual loss are less prominent than changes in mental status unless focal necrosis of white matter also occurs.

Diagnosis

Although alcohol-induced persisting dementia is included in the Diagnostic and Statistical Manual of Mental Disorders, 4th edition (DSM-IV) (Table 2), studies examining validity or reliability of this criterion have not been published. The criteria are controversial in the following points: Terms describing abnormal alcohol use such as 'heavy alcohol use' or 'problem alcohol use' are ambiguous; duration of abstinence may also be uncertain; and the qualitative differences between alcohol-induced persisting dementia and Alzheimer's disease or vascular dementia are unclear (Moriyama 2006).

Based on these critical problems and in an effort to reduce subjective bias, Oslin (1998) proposed diagnostic criteria of the diagnosis of ARD (Table 3). The proposed criteria were modeled after those of the National Institute of Neurologic and Communicative Disorders and Stroke/Alzheimer's Disease and Related Disorders Association (NINCDS/ADRDA) (McKhann 1984) for Alzheimer's disease, proving the categories 'definite,' 'probable,' and 'possible.' The criteria exclude dementia secondary to focal vascular lesions and head trauma, cases with multiple risk factors and multiple brain infarctions, and those that occur after more than ten years of abstinence from alcohol use. These include WKS, Marchiafava-Bignami disease, pellagrous encephalopathy, acquired hepatocerebral degeneration, and primary alcoholic dementia.

The diagnosis of toxic leukoencephalopathy requires that there be documented exposure to a toxin and the presence of neurobehavioral deficits, and neuroradiologic abnormalities in the patient. The clinician must have a high index of suspicion for a diagnosis of toxic leukoencephalopathy in this setting. Physical examination typically reveals neurologic findings referable to the cerebrum, although cerebellar, peripheral-nerve, hepatic, cardiac, or hematologic injury may also be present. Documentation of changes in mental status is essential for the diagnosis of toxic leukoencephalopathy. Useful tests include the digit span and serial sevens tests to detect inattention, the three-word delayed recall test to identify deficits of recent memory, clock drawing to assess visuospatial dysfunction, and alternating motor sequences to assess executive function (Filley 2009). Toxic leukoencephalopathy should not be diagnosed in the absence of corroborating neuroradiologic evidence. T2-weighted MRI is the procedure of choice because of its superior ability to display white matter (Council on Scientific Affairs 1988). There is a broad differential diagnosis of genetic, demyelinating, infectious, metabolic, vascular, traumatic, and hydrocephalic disorders.

Table 2 Criteria for Alcohol-induced Persisting Dementia in the *Diagnostic and Statistical Manual of Mental Disorders (DSM-IV)*, 4th edition

---

A. The development of multiple cognitive deficits manifested by both:

   (1) Memory impairment (impaired ability to learn new information or to recall previously learned information)

   (2) One (or more) of the following cognitive disturbances:

      a. Aphasia (language disturbance)

      b. Apraxia (impaired ability to carry out motor activities despite intact motor function)

      c. Agnosia (failure to recognize or identify objects despite intact sensory function)

      d. Disturbance in executive functioning (i.e., planning, organizing, sequencing, abstracting)

B. The cognitive deficits in Criteria A1 and A2 each cause significant impairment in social or occupational functioning and represent a significant decline from a previous level of functioning.

C. The deficits do not occur exclusively during the course of a delirium and persist beyond the usual duration of substance intoxication or withdrawal.

D. There is evidence from the history, physical examination, or laboratory findings that the deficits are etiologically related to the persisting effects of substance use (e.g., a drug of abuse, a medication).

Modified from the American Psychiatric Association 1994.

Table 3 Proposed Clinical Criteria of Alcohol-related Dementia

Definite Alcohol-related Dementia

At the current time there are no acceptable criteria to definitively define alcohol-related dementia.

Probable Alcohol-related Dementia

A. The criteria for the clinical diagnosis of probable alcohol-related dementia include the following.

1. A clinical diagnosis of dementia at least 60 days after the last exposure to alcohol.
2. Significant alcohol use as defined by a minimum average of 35 standard drinks per week for men (28 for women) for greater than a period of 5 years. The period of significant alcohol use must occur within 3 years of the initial onset of dementia.

B. The diagnosis of alcohol-related dementia is supported by the presence of any of the following:

1. Alcohol-related hepatic, pancreatic, gastrointestinal, or renal disease, i.e., other end-organ damage.
2. Ataxia or peripheral sensory polyneuropathy (not attributable to other specific causes).
3. Beyond 60 days of abstinence, the cognitive impairment stabilizes or improves.
4. After 60 days of abstinence, any neuroimaging evidence of ventricular or sulcal dilatation improves.
5. Neuroimaging evidence of cerebellar atrophy, especially of the vermis.

C. The following clinical features cast doubt on the diagnosis of alcohol-related dementia.

1. The presence of language impairment, especially dysnomia or anomia.
2. The presence of focal neurologic signs or symptoms (except ataxia or peripheral sensory polyneuropathy).
3. Neuroimaging evidence for cortical or subcortical infarction, subdural hematoma, or other focal brain pathology.
4. Elevated Hachinski Ischemia Scale score.

D. Clinical features that are neither supportive nor cast doubt on the diagnosis of alcohol-related dementia.

1. Neuroimaging evidence of cortical atrophy.
2. The presence of periventricular or deep white matter lesions on neuroimaging in the absence of focal infarct(s).
3. The presence of the apolipoprotein ε4 allele.

Possible Alcohol-related Dementia

1. A clinical diagnosis of dementia at least 60 days after the last exposure to alcohol.
2. Either: Significant alcohol use as defined by a minimum average of 35 standard drinks per week for men (28 for women) for 5 or more years. However, the period of significant alcohol use occurred more than 3 years but less than 10 years prior to the initial onset of cognitive deficits. Or Possibly significant alcohol use as defined by a minimum average of 21 standard drinks per week for men (14 for women) but no more than 34 drinks per week for men (27 for women) for 5 years. The period of significant alcohol use must have occurred within 3 years of the onset of cognitive deficits.

Modified from the article by Oslin 1998.

Clinical features (e.g., the patient's age, the presence or absence of a family history, and systematic disease manifestations) and MRI findings (e.g., the distribution of the lesions and the appearance of the ventricles) most often suggest the correct diagnosis.

In summary, the relationship between alcohol/toxin abuse and dementia is complex but diagnosable, given adequate clinical history, clinical suspicion, neurological and cognitive examinations, and findings in the supporting laboratory tests and neuroimaging.

References

Almeida, O.P., Hulse, G., Lawrence, D., et al: Smoking as a risk factor for Alzheimer's disease: Contrasting evidence from a systematic review of case-control and cohort studies. *Addiction* 97: 15–28, 2002.

American Psychiatric Association: *Diagnostic criteria from DSM-IV.* Washington, D.C.: American Psychiatric Association, 1994.

Anttila, T., Helkala, E-L., Viitanen, M., et al.: Alcohol drinking in middle age and subsequent risk of mild cognitive impairment and dementia in old age: A prospective population based study. *BMJ* 329: 539–542, 2004.

Asato, R., Akiyama, Y., Ito, M., et al.: Nuclear magnetic resonance abnormalities of the cerebral white matter in children with acute lymphoblastic leukemia and malignant lymphoma during and after central nervous system prophylactic treatment with intrathecal methotrexate. *Cancer* 70: 1997–2004, 1992.

Badsberg Jensen, G., Pakkenberg, B.: Do alcoholics drink their neurons away? *Lancet* 342: 1201–1204, 1993.

Blass, J.P., Gibson, G.E.: Abnormality of a thiamine requiring enzyme in patients with Wernicke-Korsakoff syndrome. *N Engl J Med* 297: 1367–1370, 1977.

Blow, F., Cook, C.L., Booth, B., et al.: Age-related psychiatric comorbidities and level of functioning in alcoholic veterans seeking outpatient treatment. *Hosp Commun Psychiatr* 43: 990–995, 1992.

Brandt, J., Butters, N., Ryan, C., et al.: Cognitive loss and recovery in long-term alcohol abusers. *Arch Gen Psychiatry* 40: 435–442, 1983.

Buffett-Jerrott, S.E. and Stewart, S.H.: Cognitive and sedative effects of benzodiazepine use. *Curr Pharm Des* 8: 45–58: 2002.

Carlen, P.L., McAndrews, M.P., Weiss, R.T., et al.: Alcohol-related dementia in the institutionalized elderly. *Alcohol Clin Exp Res* 18: 1330–1334, 1994.

Council on Scientific Affairs: Magnetic resonance imaging of the central nervous system: Report of the Panel on Magnetic Resonance Imaging. *JAMA* 259: 1211–1222, 1988.

Cutting, J.: The relationship between Korsakov's syndrome and 'alcoholic dementia'. *Br J Psychiat* 132: 240–251, 1978.

Ding, J., et al.: Alcohol intake and cerebral abnormalities on magnetic resonance imaging in a community-based population of middle-aged adults: The Atherosclerosis Risk in Communities (ARIC) study. *Stroke* 35: 16–21, 2004.

Dufoil, C., Tzourio, C., Brayne, C., et al.: Influence of apolipoprotein E genotype on the risk of cognitive deterioration in moderate drinkers and smokers. *Epidemiology* 11: 280–284, 2000.

Fastbom, J., Forsell, Y., Winblad, B.: Benzodiazepines may have protective effects against Alzheimer disease. *Alzheimer Dis Assoc Disord* 12: 14–17, 1998.

Fein, G., Bachman, L., Fisher, S., et al.: Cognitive impairment in abstinent alcoholics. *West J Med* 152: 531–537, 1990.

Filley, C.M. and Kleinschmidt-DeMasters, B.K.: Toxic leukoencephalopathy. *N Engl J Med* 345: 425–432, 2001.

Finlayson, R., Hurt, R., Davis, L., et al.: Alcoholism in elderly persons: A study of the psychiatric and psychosocial features of 216 inpatients. *Mayo Clinics Proc* 63: 761–768, 1988.

George, L.K., Landerman, R., Blazer, D.G., and Anthony, J.C.: Cognitive impairment. In L.N. Robins & D.A. Regier (Eds), Psychiatric disorders in America: The Epidemiologic Catchment Area Study. The Free Press, New York, 1991, pp.291–327.

Guerrini, I., Thomson, A.D., Cook, C. C., et al.: Direct genomic PCR sequencing of the high affinity thiamine transporter (SLC19A2) gene identifies three genetic variants in Wernicke-Korsakoff syndrome (WKS). *Am J Med Genet B Neuropsychiatr Genet* 137: 17–19, 2005.

Harper, C.: The incidence of Wernicke's encephalopathy in Australia – a neuropathological study of 131 cases. *J Neurol Neurosurg Psychiatry* 46: 593–598, 1983.

Harper, C. and Corbett, D.: Changes in the basal dendrites of cortical pyramidal cells from alcoholic patients—a quantitative Golgi study. *J Neurol Neurosurg Psychiatry* 53: 856–861, 1990.

Harper, C., Fornes, P., Duyckaerts, C., et al.: An international perspective on the prevalence of the Wernicke-Korsakoff syndrome. *Metabol Brain Dis* 10: 17–24, 1995.

Harper, C.: The neuropathology of alcohol-specific brain damage, or does alcohol damage the brain? *J Neuropathol Exp Neurol* 57: 101–110, 1998.

Hormes, J.T., Filley, C.M., and Rosenberg, N.L.: Neurologic sequelae of chronic solvent vapor abuse. *Neurology* 36: 698–702, 1986.

Hulse, G.K., Lautenschlager, N.T., Tait, R. J., et al.: Dementia associated with alcohol and other drug use. *International Psychogeriatrics* 17: Suppl., S109–127, 2005.

Ivan, C.S., Seshadri, S., Beiser, A., et al: Dementia after stroke: the Framingham study. *Stroke* 35: 1264–1269, 2004.

King, M.B.: Alcohol abuse and dementia. *Int J Geriatr Psychiatry* 1: 31–36, 1986.

Kivipelto, M., Rovio, S., Ngandu, T., et al.: Apolipoprotein E 4 magnifies lifestyle risks for dementia: a population-based study. *J Cell Mol Med* 12: 2762–2771, 2008.

Kornfeld, M., Moser, A.B., Moser H.W., et al.: Solvent vapor abuse leukoencephalopathy: Comparison to adrenoleukodystrophy. *J Neuropathol Exp Neurol* 53: 389–398, 1994.

Kril, J.J., Halliday, G.M., Svoboda, M.D., et al: The cerebral cortex is damaged in chronic alcoholics. *Neuroscience* 79: 983–998, 1997.

Launer, L.J., Andersen, K., Dewey, M.E., et al: Rates and risk factors for dementia and Alzheimer's disease: Results from EURODEM pooled analyses. *Neurology* 52: 78–84, 1999.

Lagnaoui, R., Bégaud, B., Moore, N., et al.: Benzodiazepine use and risk of dementia: A nested case–control study. *J Clin Epidemiol* 55: 314–318, 2002.

Lishman, W.A.: Alcohol and the brain. *Br J Psychiatry* 156: 635–644, 1990.

Mahoney, D.H., Shuster, J.J., Nitschke, R., et al.: Acute neurotoxicity in children with B-precursor acute lymphoid leukemia: An association with intermediate-dose intravenous methotrexate and intrathecal triple therapy- a Pediatric Oncology Group Study. *J Clin Oncol* 16: 1712–1722, 1998.

Matsushita, S., Kato, M., Muramatsu, T., et al.: Alcohol and aldehyde dehydrogenase genotypes in Korsakoff syndrome. *Alcohol Clin Exp Res* 24: 337–340, 2000.

McCool, B.A., Plonk, S.G., Martin, P.R., et al.: Cloning of human transketolase cDNAs and comparison of the nucleotide sequence of the coding region in Wernicke-Korsakoff and non-Wernicke-Korsakoff individuals. *J Biol Chem* 268: 1397–1404, 1993.

McKhann, G., Drachman, D., Folstein, M., et al.: Clinical diagnosis of Alzheimer's disease: Report of the NINCDS-ADRDA Work Group under the auspices of Department of Health and Human Service Task Force on Alzheimer's Disease. *Neurology* 34: 939–944, 1984.

Moriyama, Y., Mimura, M., Kato, M., et al.: Primary alcoholic dementia and alcohol-related dementia. *Psychogeriatrics* 6: 114–118, 2006.

Mukamal, K.J., Kuller, L.H., Fitzpatrick, A.L., et al.: Prospective study of alcohol consumption and risk of dementia in older adults. *Journal of the American Medical Association* 289: 1405–1413, 2003.

Muramatsu, T., Kato, M., Matsui, T., et al.: Apolipoprotein E 4 allele distribution in Wernicke-Korsakoff syndrome with or without global intellectual deficits. *J Neural Transm* 104: 913–920, 1997.

Oslin, D., Atkinson, R.M., Smith, D.M., et al.: Alcohol related dementia: Proposed clinical criteria. *International Journal of Geriatric Psychiatry* 13:203–212, 1998.

Ott, A., Slooter, A.J., Hofman, A. et al.: Smoking and risk of dementia and Alzheimer's disease in a population-based cohort study: The Rotterdam Study. *Lancet* 351: 1840–1843, 1998.

Pfefferbaum, A., Sullivan, E.V., Hedehus, M., et al.: In vivo detection and functional correlation of white matter microstructure disruption in chronic alcoholism. *Alcohol Clin Exp Res* 24: 1214–1221, 2000.

Rains, V. and Ditzler, T.: Alcohol use disorders in cognitively impaired patients referred for geriatric assessment. *J Addictive Dis* 12: 55–64, 1993.

Reynolds, K., Lewis, B.L., Nolen J.D.L., et al.: Alcohol consumption and risk of stroke: A meta-analysis. *JAMA* 289: 579–588, 2003.

Rosenberg, N.L., Kleinschmidt-DeMasters, B.K., Davis, K.A., et al.: Toluene abuse causes diffuse central nervous system white matter changes. *Ann Neurol* 23: 611–614, 1988.

Saunders, P.A., Copeland, J.R., Dewey, M.E., et al.: Heavy drinking as a risk factor for depression and dementia in elderly men. *Br J Psychiatry* 159: 213–216, 1991.

Saxton, J., Munro, C.A., Butters, M.A., et al.: Alcohol, dementia, and Alzheimer's disease: Comparison of neuropsychological profiles. *J Geriatr Psychiatry Neurol* 13: 141–149, 2000.

Schmidt, K.S., Gallo, J.L., Ferri, C., et al.: The neuropsychological profile of alcohol-related dementia suggests cortical and subcortical pathology. *Dement Geriatr Cogn Disord* 20: 286–291, 2005.

Sheline, G.E., Wara, W.M., Smith, V.: Therapeutic irradiation and brain injury. *Int J Radiat Oncol Biol Phys* 6: 1215–1228, 1980.

Singleton, C.K. and Martin, P.R.: Molecular mechanisms of thiamine utilization. *Curr Mol Med* 1: 197–207, 2001.

Smith, D.M. and Atkinson, R.M.: Alcoholism and dementia. *Int J Addict* 30: 1843–1869, 1995.

Tarter, R.E.: An analysis of cognitive deficits in alcoholics. *J Nerv Ment Dis* 157: 138–147, 1973.

Thomas, V.S., Rockwood, K.J.: Alcohol abuse, cognitive impairment, and mortality among older people. *J Am Geriatr Society* 49: 415–420, 2001.

Torvik, A., Lindboe, C.F., and Rogde, S.: Brain lesions in alcoholics. A neuropathological study with clinical correlations. *J Neurol Sci* 56: 233–248, 1982.

Victor, M.: Persistent altered mentation due to ethanol. *Neurologic Clinics* 11:639–661, 1993.

Victor, M., Adams, R.D.: The alcoholic dementias. In P.J. Vinken, G.W. Bruyn and H.L. Klawans (Eds.) Handbook of clinical neurology (Vol. 2). Elsevier Science, Amsterdam, 1985, pp. 335–352.

Victor, M., Adams, R.C., and Collins, G.H.: *The Wernicke-Korsakoff syndrome and related neurological disorders due to alcoholism and malnutrition*, 2nd ed. Philadelphia: F.A. Davis, 1989.

21 Delirium in the Elderly

Teneille E. Gofton and G. Bryan Young

Case Vignette

A 75-year-old widow with low-output cardiac failure due to ischemic heart disease lived at home with her mentally challenged son. She was on long-term therapy with warfarin for atrial fibrillation, furosemide, and digoxin. She managed reasonably independently and was of normal mental status until the evening of presentation when she became agitated and confused, wandering about the apartment calling for her deceased husband. Her son summoned an ambulance, which took her to a community general hospital in a small city. She continued to be agitated, so physical restraints were applied. She was noted to be febrile and a urine culture revealed an infection with *E. coliform*. After antibiotic therapy for one day she returned to her normal, sedate mental status and was discharged home a few days later.

About a year later an acute confusional state recurred, similar to the first and again apparently due to a urinary tract infection. She escaped her physical restraints one night, fell over the side of the bed and suffered a scalp laceration. After it was sutured she was returned to bed and was given 4 mg of lorazepam orally. She remained quiet through the rest of the night, but was found comatose in the morning with a dilated, fixed left pupil. A CT scan of the head revealed a large, acute left subdural hematoma with midline shift of 12 mm. While being transported to a tertiary care hospital, the other pupil became unreactive. It was felt that no treatment would improve the patient's condition and life support measures were discontinued.

Introduction

Delirium in the elderly is a common problem, whether patients present in a community setting, in hospital for medical illness or surgical intervention, or in the intensive care unit (ICU) (Engel and Romano 2004). The condition is referred to by multiple terms and definitions including cerebral insufficiency, acute confusional state, and encephalopathy among others. Throughout this chapter, the term delirium will be used. The gold standard, four-part definition for delirium is outlined within the Diagnostic and Statistical Manual of Mental Disorders, version IV-text revision (Association 2000): a disturbance of consciousness (attention and awareness), a change in cognition and perception not due to a preexisting dementia, a short course with characteristic fluctuation under circumstances in which the change is due to a general medical condition, substance intoxication, substance withdrawal or is multifactorial (see Table 1 for full diagnostic criteria). Three important elements of cognition are impacted in delirium: perception, mental data processing, and memory (Guidotti et al. 2006).

Delirium is frequently encountered in elderly patients, especially in an acute setting (10–60% of older adults) (Lindesay et al. 2002). In elderly patients from either the community and or the hospital, delirium impacts morbidity and mortality and has been associated with increased

rates of cognitive impairment. Delirium in the elderly is associated with longer hospitalization and increased nursing home admissions (Inouye et al. 1998; McCusker et al. 2001; Samuels and Evers 2002). Furthermore, elderly patients who develop delirium have been shown to be at increased risk for developing dementia over the 2 years subsequent to hospital discharge (Girard chapter). In elderly patients with dementia, as many as 13% have delirium superimposed on dementia (Fick et al. 2005). Delirium in this population is associated with increased six month mortality following hospital discharge (Adamis et al. 2007). For all of these reasons, delirium is an important consideration in the elderly populations and effective identification and management of delirium in the elderly has the potential to impact patient outcomes in a positive manner.

Clinically, elderly patients with delirium can present in many ways. Most commonly, patients may be classified as manifesting a hyperactive, hypoactive, or mixed delirium, which will be discussed further in the clinical features section. In the first episode in the above case vignette, a 75-year-old woman develops an acute delirium secondary to infection. The case highlights several features of delirium that are important to consider clinically. This patient has an acute mental status change and agitation (hyperactive delirium) associated with a systemic infection, which presents in an atypical manner, likely due to the patient's age and comorbidities. Effective management of the underlying etiology resulted in clearing of the mental status. With a second episode of hyperactive delirium, further issues such as the judicious use of psychoactive medications, physical restraints, monitoring (e.g., neuro-checks), and supervision became important. Delirious patients require close supervision to detect and manage complications.

Clinical Presentation of Delirium

Delirium presents a challenge in clinical practice, as multitude etiologies produce delirium as a final common pathway. A high index of suspicion as well as a broad approach to the elderly patient with delirium is essential. In general, elderly patients with delirium present in one of three ways: hyperactive delirium, hypoactive delirium, or mixed delirium (Bourgeois and Seritan 2006).

Hyperactive delirium is the most easily recognized of the three presentations. Patients with hyperactive delirium are frequently agitated, angry, or euphoric. They rapidly come to the attention of health care workers due to their disruptive, incongruous, and agitated or anxious behavior (Bourgeois and Seritan 2006). Patients with hyperactive delirium often require supervision and pharmacological or physical restraints in order to ensure their safety. Fluctuating, increased motor activity and agitation are the hallmarks of hyperactive delirium.

A hypoactive delirium is much more difficult to diagnose. Patients may appear depressed or unmotivated. Key features that differentiate hypoactive delirium from depression are the cognitive and attentional

Table 1 Diagnostic Criteria for Delirium. DSM-IV TR

Diagnostic Criteria

A. Disturbance of consciousness (i.e., reduced clarity of awareness of the environment) with reduced ability to focus, sustain, or shift attention

B. A change in cognition (such as memory deficit, disorientation, language disturbance) or the development of a perceptual disturbance that is not better accounted for by a preexisting, established, or evolving dementia

C. The disturbance develops over a short period of time (usually hours to days) and tends to fluctuate during the course of the day

For delirium due to a general medical condition:

D. There is evidence from the history, physical examination, or laboratory findings that the disturbance is caused by the direct physiological consequences of a general medical condition

For substance intoxication delirium:

D. There is evidence from the history, physical examination, or laboratory findings of either (1) the symptoms in Criteria A and B developed during substance intoxication, or (2) medication use is etiologically related to the disturbance

For substance withdrawal delirium:

D. There is evidence from the history, physical examination, or laboratory findings that the symptoms in Criteria A and B developed during, or shortly after, a withdrawal syndrome

For delirium due to multiple etiologies:

D. There is evidence from the history, physical examination, or laboratory findings that the delirium has more than one etiology (e.g., more than one etiological general medical condition, a general medical condition plus substance intoxication or medication side effect).

*From the DSM-IV-TR (American Psychiatric Association 2000).

All four criteria (A-D) are required to diagnose delirium.
(Table 1 from Girard chapter)

disturbances accompanying the former (Bourgeois and Seritan 2006). It is important to identify such patients, as hypoactive delirium is associated with worse outcomes (Samuels and Evers 2002). Patients with a mixed delirium present with fluctuating features typical of both hyperactive and hypoactive delirium.

The elderly may present with delirium in many different settings, e.g., the community, palliative care wards, surgical or medical units, or the ICU. In cognitively intact, community-dwelling elderly, delirium is rare, presenting less than 0.5% of the time (Andrew et al. 2006). It is much more common in elderly patients with known dementia (13%) (Fick et al. 2005). In hospitalized elderly, delirium is most often seen in the more frail patients. It develops due to an altered environment, concomitant acute medical or surgical illnesses, fear and anxiety, sleep deprivation, and a sense of lack of freedom (Guidotti et al. 2006). Delirium is very common in ICUs (in over 80% of our ICU patients!) and occurs primarily due to frequent use of psychoactive and sedative medications and toxic or metabolic insults to the brain (Khan and Harrison 2008). Risk factors for the development of delirium include preexisting neurological disease, acute or subacute central nervous system lesions, advancing age, male gender, preexisting comorbidities, medications, dehydration, use of restraints, dysregulation of sleep, preexisting cognitive impairment, visual or hearing impairment, history of heavy substance use or abuse, fever, hypothermia, and social isolation (Bourgeois and Seritan 2006; Inouye and Charpentier 1996).

Diagnosis of Delirium

The differential diagnosis for delirium is broad (Table 2). It is important to rule out other conditions with similar clinical presentations such as depression, psychosis, mania, dementia, aphasia, or anxiety (Bourgeois and Seritan 2006; Guidotti et al. 2006).

The most effective approach to the management of elderly patients with delirium is to identify and treat the underlying cause of delirium promptly and effectively. However, as discussed throughout this chapter, each case is different and the possible causes of delirium in any one patient seem innumerable. Thus, a systematic approach is important (Figure 1). A recent review by Guidotti et al. presents a comprehensive approach to the patient with delirium (Guidotti et al. 2006). Because delirium manifests itself as a cognitive and behavioral disturbance, a complete history of the onset and course of delirium should be obtained. Reliable collateral history from a family member or friend can be very helpful since they are best acquainted with the patient's usual behavior. In the absence of such history, or if the delirium develops in hospital, collateral history from allied health workers and the physician andclose observation of the patient on the ward should be obtained. A comprehensive review of the medications administered prior to the onset of delirium must be done, especially those that were recently introduced, discontinued, or altered. Many classes of drugs can impact cerebral function (Table 3). Assessment of the patient's

Table 2 Differential Diagnosis of Delirium

Drugs	Hyperglycemia and hypoglycemia
Prescribed drugs See Table 3.	Electrolyte disturbance (elevated or depressed): sodium, calcium, magnesium, phosphate
Drugs of abuse, e.g., alcohol intoxication or withdrawal, narcotics, cocaine, LSD, phencyclidine	Endocrine disturbance (depressed or increased): thyroid, parathyroid, pancreas, pituitary, adrenal
Poisons: ethylene glycol, methanol, insecticides, carbon monoxide, etc.	Infection: sepsis, CNS infections
Inborn errors of metabolism: porphyria, Wilson's disease, etc.	Trauma: with systemic inflammatory response syndrome, *head injury, fat embolism,
Hypoxemia	*Epileptic seizures, especially nonconvuslive status epilepticus
Hypercarbia	*Psychiatric disorders:
Cardiac failure	Nutritional: Wernicke's encephalopathy, vitamin B12 deficiency, possibly folate and niacin deficiencies
Liver failure: acute, chronic	Hypertensive encephalopathy
Renal failure: acute, chronic	Physical disorders: hyperthermia, hypothermia, electrocution, burns
Hematological: thrombocytosis, hypereosinophilia, blast cell crisis in leukemias, polychythemia	Hyperosmolar and hypo-osmolar states

*Indicates those disorders that, while not truly systemic or "medical," may produce the clinical picture of delirium in all other aspects.
(table from Uptodate)

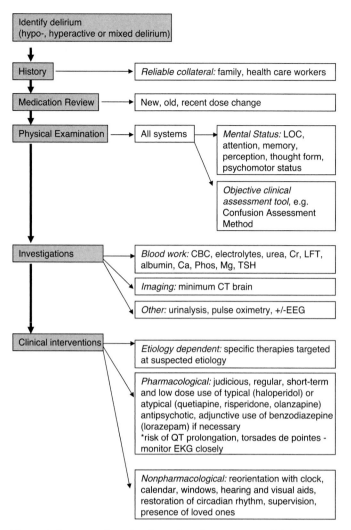

Figure 1 An approach to the diagnosis and management of delirium.

level of attention and perception of the environment will help to determine the type of delirium (Table 4). A complete neurological exam including careful testing of attention (serial 7's, spelling 'world' backwards, 'A' random letter test [selectively striking out or noting the letter 'A'], etc.) and language will help to identify other conditions that may present in a similar manner, such as a dominant cerebral hemisphere stroke presenting with Wernicke's aphasia (Guidotti et al. 2006).

Clinical assessment tools are useful in the setting of delirium. A complete review of the numerous existing assessment tools is beyond the scope of this chapter. However, the frequently encountered tools include the Confusion Assessment Method (CAM), the Memorial Delirium Assessment Scale, the Delirium Rating Scale, the Confusional State Evaluation, the Delirium Symptom Interview, the Cognitive Test for Delirium, the Intensive Care Delirium Screening Test, the NEECHAM Confusion Scale and the Delirium Inventory. The CAM is widely used and has a version, the I-CAM, for use in the ICU (Ely et al. 2001; Inouye et al. 1990). The CAM is a two-part assessment tool designed to screen for cognitive impairment and features that differentiate delirium from other forms of cognitive impairment. It requires approximately five minutes to administer and has a sensitivity of 94% for delirium (Inouye et al. 1990). Whichever method for assessment of delirium is chosen, patients require frequent reassessment to monitor the progress of the delirium.

Investigations should be tailored to the findings on history and physical examination, keeping in mind that elderly patients, especially those with dementia, may not manifest as robust clinical symptoms and signs as younger patients. At a minimum, blood work including complete blood count, electrolytes, urea, creatinine, liver function tests, calcium, albumin, magnesium, phosphate, and thyroid stimulating hormone levels should be checked. Urinalysis and pulse oximetry may be of assistance (Bourgeois and Seritan 2006; Guidotti et al. 2006). Most patients will require intracranial imaging, such as computed tomography, in order to rule out an intracranial cause. Inclusion of electroencephalogram in the initial work up may or may not be helpful or feasible, especially in the agitated patient. Most often the EEG will show nonspecific changes, either a low voltage fast pattern or nonspecific slowing. Triphasic waves are suggestive of a metabolic or septic encephalopathy. The mixture of beta (>13 Hz waves) and theta (>4 but < 8Hz) or delta (4 Hz or less) is suggestive of intoxication with benzodiazepines or barbiturates. Nonconvulsive seizures are a rare cause of delirium, but usually require an EEG for their detection or confirmation.

Table 3 Medications Reported to Cause Delirium

Medications and Medication Classes Commonly Implicated in Delirium

Benzodiazepines (e.g., lorazepam)	H1 blockers (e.g., diphenhydramine)
Narcotics (e.g., morphine)	Antiparkonisonian agents (e.g., levodopa)
Antipsychotics (e.g., haloperidol)	Tricyclic antidepressants (e.g., amitripyline)
H2 blockers (e.g., ranitidine)	Warfarin
NSAIDS (e.g., ibuprofen)	Digoxin
Promethazine	Theophyline
Antibiotics (e.g., ceftriaxone)	Nifedipine
Phenytoin	Oxybutynin
Corticosteroids (e.g., methylprednisolone)	Isosorbide dinitrate
Furosemide	Captopril

Modified from Girard chapter.

Table 4 Neuropsychological Signs in Delirium

Disturbed Function	Resulting Problems
Disturbance of consciousness	—Quantitatively: diminished arousal, somnolence, stupor, coma —Qualitatively: awareness
Orientation	time, place, situation, self
Alertness and memory	Short and long-term memory
Thought (form and content)	Perseveration, incoherence, concept formation, problem solving
Perception	Illusions, hallucinations
Drive and affect	Mood, emotion, anxiety
Psychomotor activity	—Increased or decreased motoric activity, restlessness, apathy

Modified from Kunze 2002.

The fluctuating nature of delirium means that a single isolated assessment will be inadequate to detect delirium and to follow its course. If the delirium is not resolving, as would be expected based on clinical interventions, then reassessment of the patient, reanalysis of the laboratory investigations and reconsideration of the cause of delirium are important. The varied causes and clinical presentations of delirium in elderly patients make delirium a challenge to diagnose and manage.

Pathophysiology of Delirium

The exact pathophysiology of delirium remains to be established. Since the recognition of delirium as an important clinical phenomenon, however, multiple pathophysiological theories have surfaced. Also, delirium is known to occur as a manifestation of a number of clinical conditions, such as infection and hepatic impairment among others (Table 2). Many factors predispose to developing delirium, all of which involve disruptions in the normal homeostasis of the central nervous system. As discussed previously, preexisting acute or chronic neurological disease, medications that alter CNS function, and systemic metabolic disturbances that alter the chemical milieu of the CNS are among the most important predisposing factors for the development of delirium (Bourgeois and Seritan 2006).

Currently, the most popular pathophysiological model for delirium is that of a disturbance in neurotransmitter balance (Bourgeois and Seritan 2006; Gaudreau and Gagnon 2005; Samuels and Evers 2002). It is proposed that imbalances between cholinergic and dopaminergic neurotransmission, namely a cholinergic deficit and a dopaminergic excess, leads to more global neurotransmitter imbalances and delirium (Samuels and Evers 2002). Building on this theory, Gaudreau et al. suggest a model of thalamic gating to explain delirium. They propose that in addition to the cholinergic and dopaminergic imbalance, altered gluatamatergic and GABAergic signaling lead to altered thalamic function and decreased cerebral oxidative metabolism (Gaudreau and Gagnon 2005). While this theory for the genesis of delirium suggests a mechanism for global cerebral dysfunction, it does not explain delirium in the context of specific systemic illness such as sepsis, or cardiovascular or hepatic dysfunction.

Cardiac Delirium

In the case of cardiac encephalopathy, it has been proposed that cardiac failure leads to increased systemic venous pressures, which are in turn transmitted to the cerebral venous system (Caplan 2006). Increased pressure within the intracranial venous system may decrease cerebrospinal fluid (CSF) absorption and cause elevations in CSF pressures. However, we have observed patients with thrombosis of the superior vena cava who are not confused. It seems more likely that cardiac failure may lead to reduced oxygen availability to the brain via hypoperfusion or hypo-oxygenation of the blood. Decreased cerebral perfusion pressures and poor gas exchange in the pulmonary vasculature secondary to pulmonary edema will both reduce oxygen availability to the brain (Francis Tang and Sonnenblick 2004; Victor and Ropper 2001). This may explain reductions in cognitive function, alertness, and level of consciousness seen in delirium accompanying cardiac disease.

Interestingly, patients with cardiac failure may also develop a clinical syndrome similar to hydrocephalus (Caplan 2006). It is thought that fluid shifts secondary to cardiac failure may result in increased intracranial pressures leading to apathy and abulia, resembling a hypoactive delirium. Removal of excess CSF via lumbar puncture can result in clinical improvement. In addition, low ejection fractions and cardiac surgery have been associated with cognitive deficits (Lee and Wijdicks 2008; Zuccala et al. 1997).

In addition to delirium secondary to heart failure, patients having undergone cardiopulmonary bypass procedures or open-heart surgery (the average age in our unit is 75 years) are at risk of developing a post-pump delirium. It has been hypothesized that this is due to a lack of pulsatile blood flow and to periods of hypoxia (Lee and Wijdicks 2008). Furthermore, cardiac bypass has an inherent risk of embolic phenomena, both gaseous and particulate. Studies demonstrate that aortic cannulation, cross-clamping, and the release of side clamp are most associated with microemboli. Pugsley et al. have shown that post-cardiopulmonary bypass neurologic outcome is associated with the quantity of cerebral micro-emboli during bypass (Pugsley et al. 1994). "Off pump" techniques for cardiac surgery are now being used and reduce the number of intraoperative microemboli. However, studies have not yet proven there to be a difference in neurological outcomes.

Seizures affect about 0.3% of adult post-cardiac surgery patients (Kuroda et al. 1993). Focal seizures correlate with areas of embolic cerebral infarction in such patients, while primary generalized seizures are associated with negative MRI scans and a benign course (Young et al. in press.)

Hepatic Delirium

Delirium associated with hepatic insufficiency occurs frequently. The main pathophysiological cause of hepatic encephalopathy is thought to be an overload of ammonia from the gastrointestinal tract (Khan and Harrison 2008). Normally, ammonia absorbed from the gastrointestinal tract is metabolized by the liver. However, in the case of hepatic insufficiency, liver metabolism of ammonia is impaired and the brain is exposed to out-of-the-ordinary levels of ammonia. The brain is unable to metabolize the ammonia due to a lack of the urea synthesis pathway. Instead, astrocytes utilize the ammonia in a glutamine synthesis pathway, which leads to accumulation of glutamine in astrocytes and to altered neuronal function (Khan and Harrison 2008). Excess cerebral ammonia is also thought to increase the availability of reactive oxygen species, which result in mitochondrial dysfunction. Typically, the basal ganglia and cerebellum are very sensitive to hepatic insufficiency. This is likely due to a rich blood supply to these areas and therefore relatively more exposure to excess ammonia.

Renal Delirium

With acute or chronic renal insufficiency, the accumulation of toxic substances leads to cerebral dysfunction and delirium. The specific pathophysiological mechanisms for renal delirium have not been identified. However, there is some evidence in animal models that, in addition to uremia, increased levels of parathyroid hormone lead to increased circulating calcium and accumulation of calcium within the cortex (Kunze 2002).

Septic Delirium

In the setting of sepsis, delirium is known to influence mortality. Sprung et al. demonstrated that delirium secondary to sepsis is associated with higher mortality (49%) when compared to septic patients without delirium (26%) (Sprung et al. 1991). Research has shown that altered cerebral amino acid concentrations paired with compromised blood brain barrier function all contribute to the development of sepsis-associated delirium (Jeppsson et al. 1981; Mizock et al. 1990). Furthermore, there is a glutamate excess in patients with sepsis and delirium (Wilson and Young 2003), which contributes to altered cerebral function. More recent data also suggests that oxidative stress and neuronal cytoskeletal changes contribute to cerebral dysfunction and delirium (Voigt et al. 2001). Delirium can present as the first clinical sign of sepsis and early recognition is important.

ICU Delirium

Although delirium is very common in the ICU, there has been little research specific to the pathophysiology of ICU delirium. Similar mechanisms to those invoked above are discussed in the literature. Patients in the ICU frequently have multiple predisposing factors for delirium as well as multi-organ dysfunction, all of which contribute to the genesis of delirium. Thus, the pathophysiology of ICU delirium is often multifactorial.

Delirium at the End of Life

There is little data available specific to the presentation, management, or pathophysiology of delirium in terminal cancer and other terminal diseases. This is an important subtype of patients to consider because end-of-life delirium can be distressing to patients, families, and caregivers alike and comprises an under-recognized aspect of palliative care. End-of-life delirium is of increasing interest to the research community and it is likely that emerging research will enhance the current state of knowledge in this area, thereby improving patient care.

Delirium in the Elderly

In the elderly, it is important to contrast delirium presenting in a cognitively normal person versus delirium presenting in the setting of a preexisting dementia. While there is data to suggest that delirium alone in patients with or without dementia does not influence 6-month mortality in medical patients (Adamis et al. 2007), more recent data suggests that delirium superimposed on dementia increases mortality (Bellelli et al. 2008). Bellelli et al. hypothesize that the adverse metabolic changes leading to delirium in previously demented patients sets up a self-sustaining chain of not yet identified pathophysiological events leading to increased mortality (Bellelli et al. 2008).

While delirium in the elderly shares many characteristics with delirium in other populations of patients, it is also has unique features. There are important considerations in elderly patients with delirium including the variety of predisposing factors, the presence of multiple risk factors, and the possibility of previously impaired cognition or nervous system disease. Taken together, all aspects of the elderly patient's prior medical history and present clinical condition must be considered.

Management of Delirium

As the cause of delirium is being identified and therapies are being targeted to the underlying cause, other interventions should be ongoing. General management approaches applicable to most elderly patients with delirium include avoiding the use of psychoactive medications (antipsychotics, benzodiazepines, anticholinergics, dopaminergics, opioids, etc.) and restoring a more normal physical environment. Patients may be fearful and anxious due to new surroundings or due to restraints that may be required. Attempts should be made to reorient patients frequently, using clocks, calendars, windows, hearing and visual aids, as well as the presence of loved ones to help. Restoration of the sleep-wake cycle is also challenging, but helpful. Dimming lights at the appropriate hours and maintaining a quiet environment at night are important (Bourgeois and Seritan 2006; Inouye et al. 1999).

Despite the above strategies, pharmacological intervention is often required to stabilize and to maintain the safety of elderly patients with delirium. It is known that chronic use of antipsychotics may be detrimental in elderly patients with dementia as per the 2005 FDA Public Health Advisory (Administration 2005); there is little data behind the use of antipsychotic medications in an acute delirium in the elderly with or without preexisting dementia. The regular use of low dose

haloperidol throughout the period of acute delirium may be necessary (note the risk of QT prolongation and *torsades de pointes*). Recommended starting doses are as low as 0.5–1.0 mg q12h with dose escalation only if required (Bourgeois and Seritan 2006). Olanzapine, risperidone, and quetiapine have a growing literature supporting use in acute delirium in the elderly. These should also be administered at regular intervals at comparably low doses and escalated only as required (Bourgeois and Seritan 2006). In most types of delirium, benzodiazepines should be avoided because they may take longer for elderly patients to metabolize and they often have metabolically active metabolites that remain in circulation for extended periods of time. Other medications with recent supportive data include cholinergic medications, propofol, valproic acid, and serotonin blockers (Bourgeois and Seritan 2006).

Close monitoring of the clinical course of delirium is essential. In elderly patients, delirium may herald a change in clinical status, such as sepsis, that alters patient outcome if not detected and treated early. Also, a delirium not resolving as expected should alert clinicians to further evaluate the patient for other contributing factors. The ongoing assessment of patients with delirium allows physicians and health care workers to assess the efficacy of the clinical approach and to determine if further interventions are necessary (Sleiman et al. 2008).

Hepatic Delirium

The targeted therapy of hepatic delirium, specifically, is to reduce the amount of circulating ammonia. The most commonly used compounds used with this aim are the nonabsorbable disaccharides such as lactulose. These compounds reduce the gastrointestinal absorption of proteins and bacterial production of ammonia because of their cathartic effects, their action to acidify the gastrointestinal contents, and to interfere with the uptake of glutamine. The therapeutic target when using disaccharides is two to three soft bowel movements per day (Weissenborn 2008). Other agents used to reduce plasma ammonia levels include L-ornithine-L-aspartate and zinc administration.

ICU Delirium

The management of elderly patients with delirium in the ICU is similar to the management of other causes of delirium. The underlying cause must be identified and corrected. Reinforcement of circadian rhythms and early mobilization may also be helpful (Khan and Harrison 2008).

Overall, the management goals for elderly patients with delirium are to identify the precipitating cause and to address all contributing modifiable factors. The emergence of delirium in a previously cognitively well patient should alert health care workers to the decline of the patient and the need to determine the cause of the decline.

Prognosis Following Delirium

As discussed earlier, delirium in the elderly has negative prognostic implications. Delirium has several possible outcomes outlined by Lipowski et al.: full recovery, progression to stupor and coma, transitional cognitive affective or mixed abnormality with gradual full recovery, progression to an irreversible mental syndrome and a posttraumatic stress syndrome (Lipowski 1990). In the elderly, delirium is associated with poor functional recovery following hip fracture (Marcantonio et al. 2000), contributes to poor in-hospital outcomes (McCusker et al. 2001), and may be associated with subsequent cognitive decline (Inouye et al. 1998).

While not specific to elderly patients, research demonstrates that in the ICU, delirium is associated with prolonged ICU and hospital length of stay, increased risk of death over the 2-year period following hospital discharge and increased costs (Girard chapter). Furthermore, data suggest that in-hospital delirium is an independent risk factor for the development of long-term cognitive impairment (Jackson et al. 2004). Patients with delirium in the ICU not only self-extubate more often, but also fail planned extubation attempts more frequently (Dubois et al. 2001).

Andrew et al. provide further supportive evidence for the deleterious effects of delirium in the elderly in a study of community-dwelling patients presenting with delirium (Andrew et al. 2006). Although their analysis is on a small number of patients, Andrew et al. demonstrate that the development of delirium in community-dwelling older patients resulted in lower five year survival than those without delirium (18% versus 70%). These elderly patients also presented with higher rates of incontinence and at a younger age than those without delirium or those with dementia. Andrew et al. concluded that the impact of delirium on survival in elderly patients is equivalent to that of severe dementia. Fortunately, delirium is uncommon in the community-dwelling elderly population (<0.5%).

Taken together, the effects of delirium on an elderly population are significant and therefore must be taken very seriously.

Future Directions in Delirium

Because delirium occurs secondary to metabolic or physical disturbances, the mainstay in the management of delirium will likely remain management of the triggering condition. However, emerging research assessing cerebral neurotransmitter imbalances in the setting of delirium will lead to further, more targeted, interventions to reduce the severity and duration of delirium. Furthermore, new developments in clinical medicine for managing the various triggers for delirium will likely also serve to reduce the impact of delirium in the elderly. Medications with shorter half-lives and fewer pharmacologically active metabolites would be ideal for use in elderly patients with delirium with a variety of comorbidities. Further development of guidelines applicable to elderly patients with delirium would be beneficial. Guidelines are helpful to ensure that a broad differential is considered, to limit the use of detrimental medications such as sedatives and other medications with cognitive side effects and to remind the clinician to apply multiple approaches to patient management (pharmacological, nonpharmacological, and social).

Summary of Key Points in Delirium

- Delirium is an acute confusional state in which there are disturbances in cognition (attention and memory) and perceptions (hallucinations and illusions) of the environment.

- Delirium is caused by medical illness and its course is fluctuating in nature.

- Delirium in the elderly is common.

- An acute onset of delirium in the elderly should prompt clinical assessment and investigations aimed at determining the cause and subsequent management.

- Elderly patients may present with different types of delirium: hypoactive delirium, hyperactive delirium, or mixed delirium.

- The clinical management of delirium consists of modifying existing risk factors, treating the underlying cause, reorienting the patient (clocks, calendars, sleep, loved ones), and restoring a reassuring and nonthreatening environment.

- The main pathophysiological theory of delirium involves neurotransmitter imbalances, most importantly the cholinergic and dopaminergic systems. GABAergic and serotonergic system are also likely to play a role.

References

Adamis, D., Treloar, A., Darwiche F.Z., et al.: Associations of delirium with in-hospital and in 6-months mortality in elderly medical inpatients. *Age Ageing* 36: 644–649, 2007.

Administration, UFaD. FDA Public Health Advisory: Deaths with antipsychotics in elderly patients with behavioural disturbances. 2005: Available from: http://www.fda.gov/cder/drug/advisory/antipsychotics.htm, cited August 10, 2008.

Andrew M.K., Freter, S.H. and Rockwood, K.: Prevalence and outcomes of delirium in community and non-acute care settings in people without dementia: A report from the Canadian Study of Health and Aging. *BMC Med* 4: 15, 2006.

American Psychiatric Association: *Diagnostic and statistical manual of mental disorders DSM-IV-TR (Text Revision)*. American Psychiatric Association Press. Washington, DC, USA. 2000: 943.

Bellelli, G., Morghen, S., Turco, R. and Trabucchi, M.: Delirium in older people: An epiphenomenon of incipient death or a separate biological process? *Age Ageing* 37: 353–354, 2008.

Bourgeois J.A. and Seritan, A.: Diagnosis and management of delirium. *Continuum* 12: 18, 2006.

Caplan L.R.: Cardiac encephalopathy and congestive heart failure: A hypothesis about the relationship. *Neurology* 66: 99–101, 2006.

Dubois, M.J., Bergeron, N., Dumont, M., Dial, S. et al.: Delirium in an intensive care unit: A study of risk factors. *Intensive Care Med* 27: 1297–304, 2001.

Ely, E.W., Margolin, R., Francis, J., May, L. et al.: Evaluation of delirium in critically ill patients: Validation of the Confusion Assessment Method for the Intensive Care Unit (CAM-ICU). *Crit Care Med* 29: 1370–1379, 2001.

Engel, G.L. and Romano, J.: Delirium, a syndrome of cerebral insufficiency. *J Neuropsychiatry Clin Neurosci* 16: 526–538, 2004.

Fick, D.M., Kolanowski, A.M., Waller, J.L. and Inouye, S.K.: Delirium superimposed on dementia in a community-dwelling managed care population: A 3-year retrospective study of occurrence, costs, and utilization. *J Gerontol A Biol Sci Med Sci* 60: 748–753, 2005.

Francis Tang, W.H.M. and Sonnenblick, E.H.: *Pathophysiology of heart failure. Hurst's the heart*, 11th ed. McGraw Hill 39, 2004.

Gaudreau, J.D. and Gagnon, P.: Psychotogenic drugs and delirium pathogenesis: The central role of the thalamus. *Med Hypotheses* 64: 471–475, 2005.

Guidotti, M., Chiveri, L. and Mauri, M.: Acute encephalopathies. *Neurol Sci* 27 Suppl 1: S55–S56, 2006.

Inouye, S.K., Bogardus, S.T., Jr., Charpentier, P.A., Leo-Summers, L., et al.: A multicomponent intervention to prevent delirium in hospitalized older patients. *N Engl J Med* 340: 669–676, 1999.

Inouye, S.K. and Charpentier, P.A.: Precipitating factors for delirium in hospitalized elderly persons. Predictive model and interrelationship with baseline vulnerability. *JAMA* 275: 852–857, 1996.

Inouye, S.K., Rushing, J.T., Foreman, M.D., Palmer, R. M., et al.: Does delirium contribute to poor hospital outcomes? A three-site epidemiologic study. *J Gen Intern Med* 13: 234–342, 1998.

Inouye, S.K., van Dyck, C.H., Alessi, C.A., Balkin, S. et al.: Clarifying confusion: The confusion assessment method. A new method for detection of delirium. *Ann Intern Med* 113: 941–948, 1990.

Jackson, J.C., Gordon, S.M., Hart, R.P., Hopkins, R. O., et al.: The association between delirium and cognitive decline: A review of the empirical literature. *Neuropsychol Rev* 14: 87–98, 2004.

Jeppsson, B., Freund, H.R., Gimmon, Z., James, J. H., et al.: Blood-brain barrier derangement in sepsis: Cause of septic encephalopathy? *Am J Surg* 141: 136–142, 1981.

Khan, J. and Harrison, T.: Central and peripheral neurologic manifestations of critical medical illness. *Continuum* 14: 19, 2008.

Kuroda, Y., Urchimoto R., Kaieda, R., Shinohara, K. et al.: Central nervous system complications after cardiac surgery: A comparison between coronary artery bypass grafting and valve surgery. *Anesthe Analg* 76:222–227, 1993.

Kunze, K.: Metabolic encephalopathies. *J Neurol* 249: 1150–1159, 2002.

Lee, V.H. and Wijdicks, E.F.: Neurologic complications of cardiac surgery. *Continuum* 14: 19, 2008.

Lindesay, J., Rockwood, K. and Rolfson, D.: *The epidemiology of delirium. Delirium in old age.* New York: Oxford University Press. 13, 2002.

Lipowski, Z.J.L. *Delirium: Acute confusional states.* Rev Ed. Oxford University Press, New York 1990.

Marcantonio, E.R.– Flacker, J.M., Michaels, M. and Resnick, N.M.: Delirium is independently associated with poor functional recovery after hip fracture. *J Am Geriatr Soc* 48: 618–624, 2000.

McCusker, J., Cole, M., Dendukuri, N. and Belzile, E.: Delirium in older medical inpatients and subsequent cognitive and functional status: A prospective study. *CMAJ* 165: 575–583, 2001.

Mizock, B.A., Sabelli, H.C., Dubin, A. and Javaid JI et al.: Septic encephalopathy. Evidence for altered phenylalanine metabolism and comparison with hepatic encephalopathy. *Arch Intern Med* 150: 443–449, 1990.

Pugsley, W., Klinger, L., Paschalis, C. and Treasure, T. et al.: The impact of microemboli during cardiopulmonary bypass on neuropsychological functioning. *Stroke* 25: 1393–1399, 1994.

Samuels, S.C. and Evers, M.M.: Delirium. Pragmatic guidance for managing a common, confounding, and sometimes lethal condition. *Geriatrics* 57: 33–38, 2002.

Sleiman, I., Rozzini, R. and Trabucchi, M.: Delirium in older patients in intensive care units. *Arch Intern Med* 168: 1229, 2008.

Sprung, C.L., Cerra, F.B., Freund, H.R. and Schein, R.M.: Amino acid alterations and encephalopathy in the sepsis syndrome. *Crit Care Med* 19: 753–757, 1991.

Victor, M., Ropper, A.H.: *Adam's and Victor's principles of neurology,* 7th ed. McGraw-Hill.: 21, 2001.

Voigt, K., Schweizer, M., Sturenburg, H. and Hansen, H.: Damage to the neuronal cytoskeleton in septic encephalopathy. *ANIM* 43, 2001.

Weissenborn, K.: Neurologic manifestations of liver disease. *Continuum* 14: 15, 2008.

Wilson, J.X. and Young, G.B.: Progress in clinical neurosciences. Sepsis-associated encephalopathy: Evolving concepts. *Can J Neurol Sci* 30: 98–105, 2003.

Zuccala, G., Cattel, C., Manes-Gravina, E. and Di Niro, M.G., et al.: Left ventricular dysfunction: A clue to cognitive impairment in older patients with heart failure. *J Neurol Neurosurg Psychiatry* 63: 509–512, 1997.

4

Motor Disorders in Aging

22 Parkinson's Disease

Stanley Fahn

Introduction

Parkinson's disease (PD) was first described by James Parkinson in 1817; it took over 100 years before the substantia nigra was recognized as the major site of neuronal loss and another 50 years for the discovery of the marked reduction of the neurotransmitter, dopamine, in the basal ganglia (Fahn and Jankovic 2007). In less than another ten years, effective therapy with levodopa, the precursor of dopamine, was developed (Cotzias et al. 1969). Since then, levodopa has remained the most effective treatment for the motor symptoms of PD. Levodopa is most effective in the early stages of the illness, but PD is a progressively worsening neurodegenerative disease, and new motor symptoms develop that do not respond to levodopa. These later-appearing features impact posture, balance, and gait, resulting in falls. Making matters worse, levodopa, even when it is still beneficial, commonly causes complications that can be very troublesome to patients; these are dyskinesias (abnormal involuntary movements) and motor fluctuations (wearing-off of levodopa's benefit in less than four hours). Fortunately, other medications and surgical approaches have been introduced that can mitigate some of these motor complications from levodopa.

Nonmotor features are also seen in patients with PD. These consist of behavioral changes, cognitive impairment, autonomic dysfunction, sleep disturbances, sensory complaints and fatigue. Each of the nonmotor symptoms needs it own specific treatments to improve quality of life for both the patient and the care-provider, who has the burden in the advanced stages of PD. The fact that both the motor and nonmotor features of PD can be treated to some extent makes it important for clinicians to recognize the disorder and apply therapeutic strategies to keep the patient independent as long as possible. Efforts to find means to slow the rate of worsening of PD have led to some success in clinical trials, and the clinician should weigh how effective these results are and if they should play a role in therapy.

Parkinson's disease is primarily a disease of aging, although young onset cases are seen. The lifetime risk is about 2%. The mean age at onset is 55 years, and the prevalence and incidence rates climb with increasing age. The prevalence of PD in the general population is approximately 160 per 100,000, and the incidence is about 20 per 100,000/year. At age 70, the prevalence is approximately 550 per 100,000, and the incidence is 120 per 100,000/year. The male-to-female ratio is 3:2. Prior to the levodopa era, mortality from PD was about 3-fold greater than an age-matched control population. The mortality rate was cut in half after the introduction of levodopa, but as dopa-unresponsive symptoms accumulate with advanced disease, the mortality rate in this advanced-stage group has risen back to 3-fold greater than normal (Hely et al. 2008). PD is the second most common neurodegenerative disease after Alzheimer's disease.

Pathophysiology

Pathology

The characteristic pathologic feature of PD is the loss of dopamine-containing neurons in the substantia nigra and norepinephrine-containing neurons in the locus ceruleus. The resulting effect is a reduction of these neurotransmitters in the target areas for these neurons, particularly dopamine in the striatum. There is a correlation of severity of clinical signs with the reduction of dopamine concentration. Moreover, there is a clinical benefit by restoring dopamine by treatment with levodopa. In addition to neuronal loss, there is the presence of cytoplasmic inclusions, known as Lewy bodies, in surviving neurons, and an accompanying gliosis.

Etiology

The causes of PD are largely unknown with the exception of specific gene mutations, discussed later. Twin studies indicate that PD with an onset under the age of 50 years is more likely to have a genetic relationship than for patients with an older age at onset (Tanner et al. 1999). Thus, the more typical older-onset patients are suspected of more likely having PD due to unknown environmental factors. No specific environmental toxicant has been identified, although exposure to pesticides appears to increase the risk of developing PD (Tanner et al. 2009). A few factors have been associated with a reduced risk for PD. Multiple studies have consistently shown that cigarette smoking reduces the risk of developing PD (Hernan et al. 2002). The lower risk correlates with a) more years smoked, b) smoking more cigarettes per day, c) older age at quitting smoking, and 4) fewer years since quitting smoking (Thacker et al. 2007). Coffee consumption has also been found to be associated with a lower risk of developing PD, as has a higher serum urate level.

Pathogenesis

Factors implicated in leading to the death of the susceptible neurons in the substantia nigra are the presence of toxic proteins, oxidative stress, mitochondrial dysfunction, and inflammation. Each of these factors cross-interact with the others to add to the pathogenesis of cell death. Toxic proteins accumulate because of insufficient degradation or an excess synthesis of protein not sufficiently handled by the normal mechanisms of protein degradation by the proteasome and lysosome. One protein, in particular, appears to play a prominent role. Alpha–synuclein is present in Lewy bodies and also accumulates in other neurons, beginning in the lower brainstem and progresses in a caudal-to-rostral direction, starting in the medulla, then pons, midbrain, thalamus and eventually cerebral cortex (Braak et al. 2006).

Endogenous factors within catecholamine neurons can render these cells particularly susceptible. These neurons fire autonomously at a rate of 2 Hz, utilizing calcium rather than sodium as the entering ions to trigger neuronal firing (Surmeier 2007). Increased intracellular calcium can impair mitochondrial function. In the nigral neurons, dopamine interacts with alpha–synuclein to block protein degradation in the lysosome (Martinez-Vicente et al. 2008) and also increases cytosolic dopamine to increase oxidative stress (Mosharov et al. 2009).

Genetic Contributions

A major advance in improving our understanding of the etiology and pathogenesis of PD in the past decade has been the discovery of a number of gene mutations that can cause this disease (Table 1) (Klein and Schlossmacher 2007). These have been given the PARK label, beginning with PARK1 and numbered successively in chronologic order of their discovery. Shortly after PARK1 was found to be a mutation in the gene for alpha-synuclein, insoluble aggregates of this protein were discovered to be present in Lewy bodies. PARK4 is not a mutation, but triplications and duplications of the gene for alpha-synuclein, leading to an excess formation of normal (wild-type) alpha-synuclein. This emphasizes that too much of this protein can cause PD. Three autosomal recessive mutations (PARK2, PARK6, and PARK7) for the proteins of parkin, PINK1 and DJ-1 cause a younger onset, even juvenile onset, form of PD, with a slower rate of worsening, compared to typical older-onset PD. The most common mutation causing PD is PARK8, in which certain ethnic groups (North African Arabs, Ashkenazi Jews, and inhabitants of the Iberian Peninsula) are particularly prone to carry the G2019S mutation. The mutations in the beta-glucocerebrosidase gene causing autosomal recessive Gaucher's disease have been found to be a world-wide risk in all ethnic groups for developing PD, with just a single (autosomal dominant) mutation (Sidransky et al. 2009). Despite the large number of genes whose mutations are able to cause PD, only about 10% of patients with PD are considered to have a genetic etiology.

Table 1 Gene Alterations Causing Parkinsonism

Gene	Locus	Protein	Mode of Inheritance	Mean Age at Onset	Progression; Clinical Features	Protein Function
SCNA (PARK1)	4q21.3	α-synuclein; A53T, A30P, and E46K mutations	AD	45 (20–85)	Rapid; dementia, hypoventilation, myoclonus, abnl EOM, incontinence	Possibly synaptic vesicle trafficking; elevated in bird song learning
PRKN (PARK2)	6q25.2–q27	Parkin	AR in juvenile onset; AD in older onset	Young (3–64); usually below 20	Very slow; dystonia at onset; sleep benefit; no Lewy bodies	Ubiquitin E3 ligase, attaches short ubiquitin peptide chains to proteins for degradation
PARK3	2p13	Unknown	AD	59 (37–89)	Slow; indistinguishable from idiopathic PD	——
SCNA (formerly PARK4)	4q21 region duplication & triplication	Excess wild-type α-synuclein	AD	33	Rapid; wide range of symptoms from idiopathic PD to dementia with Lewy bodies	Same as PARK1
UCH–L1 (PARK5)	4p14	Ubiquitin-C-terminal hydrolase L1	AD	~50	Indistinguishable from idiopathic PD	Removes polyubiquitin in ubiquitin-proteasomal cycle
PINK1 (PARK6)	1p35–p36	PTEN-induced putative kinase 1	AR	40 (30–68)	Slow	Mitochondrial serine-threonine kinase; modulates mitochondrial dynamics
DJ-1 (PARK7)	1p36	DJ-1	AR	33 (27–40)	Slow; as in parkin, but with behavioral problems and focal dystonia	Possible atypical peroxiredoxin; protects against oxidative stress
LRRK2 (PARK8)	12p11.2–q13.1	Leucine rich repeat kinase 2 (dardarin)	AD	~60	Indistinguishable from idiopathic PD; ↓ penetrance	Probably a cytoplasmic kinase
ATP13A2 (PARK9)	1p36	Lysosomal ATPase	AR	12–16	Kufor-Rakeb syndrome, similar to PD and to pallidopyramidal syndrome (PARK15)	Maintain acid pH in lysosome
PARK10	1p32	Unknown	AR	Typical late onset	Standard PD; Families in Iceland	——

Table 1 Continued

Gene	Locus	Protein	Mode of Inheritance	Mean Age at Onset	Progression; Clinical Features	Protein Function
PARK11	2q21.2	unknown	AD	Typical late onset	Indistinguishable from idiopathic PD	——
PARK12	Xq21–q25	unknown	X-linked recessive	Typical late onset	Indistinguishable from idiopathic PD	——
HTRA2 (PARK13)	2p12	High temperature requirement protein A2 (HTRA2)	AD	Typical late onset	Indistinguishable from idiopathic PD	Serine protease primarily localized in the endoplamic reticulum and mitochondria
PLA2G6 (PARK14)	22q13.1	Phospholipase A2	AR	Infants, children, and adults	1) Infantile neuroaxonal dystrophy with spasticity, ataxia and iron accumulation (NBIA2); 2) dystonia-parkinsonism in adults without iron	Phospholipase A2, releases fatty acids from phospholipids
FBXO7 (PARK15)	22q12–q13	F-box only protein 7	AR	Childhood onset	Pallidopyramidal disease; parkinsonian-pyramidal syndrome	Component of modular E3 ubiquitin protein ligases; functions in phosphorylation-dependent ubiquitination
GBA	1q21	β-glucocerebro-sidase	AD	Slightly younger than average	Indistinguishable from idiopathic PD; all ethnic groups; most common in Ashkenazi Jews; homozygotes → Gaucher disease	Lysosomal enzyme; Metabolizes membrane lipid glucosylceramide to ceramide and glucose

Table adapted and expanded from Fahn and Jankovic (2007).

Clinical Presentation

Parkinsonism is a clinical syndrome defined by its motor phenomenology of any combination of six distinct and independent motor features: tremor-at-rest, rigidity, bradykinesia, flexed posture, loss of postural reflexes, and the freezing phenomenon (in which the feet are transiently "stuck" to the ground) (Table 2). A number of diseases can present as parkinsonism (Table 3), and PD (primary parkinsonism) is the one most commonly encountered by the general clinician and is the one discussed in this chapter. Of the six cardinal motor symptoms of parkinsonism, tremor, bradykinesia, and rigidity occur early, and the other three appear late, usually not before three years after onset. PD can be familial (as described in the genetics section) but is usually sporadic.

The symptoms of PD begin insidiously and worsen gradually over time. They typically begin on one side of the body, rather than bilaterally and symmetrically, and eventually spread to involve both sides of the body. The most common initial symptom recognized by the patient is tremor of a hand or foot when that limb is at rest, called tremor-at-rest or resting tremor, with a frequency of about 4 Hz. The tremor can be intermittent at the beginning, being present only in stressful situations. Later, tremor tends to be more constant. The tremor involving the fingers in the hand has been called a "pill-rolling" tremor. Tremor is not present in everyone with PD. When tremor is absent, the initial symptom is usually a reduced arm swing or a decreased stride length and speed when walking. In some patients, a sensory complaint of aching in the shoulder of the soon-to-be-affected side can precede the motor features of tremor and bradykinesia.

Bradykinesia is slowness and reduced amplitude of movement. In the cranial area, there is decreased frequency in blinking with a staring expression (facial hypomimia), and soft voice with loss of prosody. Features of limb bradykinesia are a smaller and slower handwriting (micrographia), and difficulty cutting food and putting on make-up. Walking becomes slow, with a shortened stride length and decreased

Table 2 Cardinal Motor Features of Parkinsonism

Tremor-at-rest

Bradykinesia/hypomimia/akinesia

Rigidity

Flexed posture of neck, trunk & limbs

Loss of postural reflexes

Freezing of gait

These motor features are independent clinical phenomena that comprise the syndrome of parkinsonism. In primary parkinsonism (Parkinson's disease) the first three on this list appear early in the illness, and the last three appear late. If any of these last three features appear in the first three years, some other parkinsonian state, rather than PD, is more likely.

Table 3 Classification of the Parkinsonian States

I. Primary parkinsonism (Parkinson disease)

   Sporadic

   Known genetic etiology

II. Secondary parkinsonism (environmental etiology)

   A. Drugs

      1. Dopamine receptor blockers (most commonly antipsychotic medications)

      2. Dopamine storage depletors (reserpine)

   B. Postencephalitic

   C. Toxins—Mn, CO, MPTP, cyanide

   D. Vascular

   E. Brain tumors

   F. Head trauma

   G. Normal pressure hydrocephalus

III. Parkinsonism—plus syndromes

   A. Progressive supranuclear palsy (PSP)

   B. Multiple system atrophy (MSA)

   C. Cortical-basal ganglionic degeneration (CBGD)

   D. Diffuse Lewy body disease (DLBD)

   E. Parkinson-dementia-ALS complex of Guam

   F. Progressive pallidal atrophy

IV. Heredodegenerative disorders

   A. Alzheimer disease

   B. Wilson disease

   C. Huntington disease

   D. Frontotemporal dementia on chromosome 17

   E. X-linked dystonia-parkinsonism (in Filipino men; known as lubag)

arm swing. Difficulty arising from a deep chair, getting out of automobiles, and turning in bed are symptoms of truncal bradykinesia. Rigidity of muscles is detected by the examiner when he/she moves the patient's limbs, neck, or shoulders and experiences increased resistance. There is often a ratchet-like feel to the muscles, so-called cogwheel rigidity.

These early features of PD, especially bradykinesia and rigidity, usually respond to levodopa and appear to be manifestations of striatal dopamine deficiency. However, the three later motor symptoms of flexed posture, loss of postural reflexes, and freezing of gait do not respond well to levodopa, suggesting that they are the result of non-dopaminergic defects. As PD worsens over time, bradykinesia becomes less responsive to levodopa. When the motor symptoms fail to adequately respond to levodopa, disability ensues. Walking and balance are impaired, resulting in falls, and the patient may need to use a walker or a wheelchair.

Most patients with PD have nonmotor features in addition to their motor problems (Chaudhuri et al. 2006). Their personality slowly becomes more passive and dependent; decisions are difficult to make, and there is a loss of motivation. Mental function becomes slow (bradyphrenia), and eventually dementia usually develops as the patient ages (Buter et al. 2008). Depression and anxiety are often present, often preceding the onset of motor symptoms. Fragmented sleep is common. REM sleep behavior disorder is characterized by a lack of atonia when dreaming; thus, the patient acts out his dreams. The patient is unaware of this problem, but the bed partner is affected by the patient's thrashing about. Autonomic disturbances are many (constipation, urinary urgency and incontinence, impaired sexual function, and sometimes orthostatic hypotension). There are also sensory complaints, including pain, numbness, tingling and burning in the affected limbs. One of the fairly common sensory problems is restless legs syndrome with its accompanying periodic leg movements in sleep that can cause sleep disturbance. The nonmotor features can be more disabling than the motor ones, particularly if the latter still respond to levodopa. The nonmotor aspects can largely be treated. Table 4 lists some of the medications for mitigating these problems. Some nonmotor features in PD are due to the medications used to treat the motor problems. These will be dealt with during the discussion of those treatments.

Diagnosis

The diagnosis of PD depends on the clinical examination and not on laboratory tests, for the most part. Required is the presence of at least two of the three early motor features (tremor, bradykinesia, and rigidity) that signify parkinsonism, along with the absence of features that would implicate some other form of parkinsonism (Table 3) instead of PD. These other features are loss of postural reflexes or freezing of gait within three years of onset of symptoms, the presence of ataxia, and spasticity or supranuclear gaze palsy. Dementia at the onset would

Table 4 Treatment Approaches to the Non-motor Symptoms in Parkinson's Disease

Condition	Treatment
Insomnia	Bedtime hypnotic
REM sleep behavior disorder	Clonazepam h.s
Fragmented sleep	Short-acting hypnotic such as zolpidem if unable to fall back asleep
Excessive daytime sleepiness	Modafinil
Restless legs syndrome	Dopaminergic; if already on a dopaminergic, add an opioid in the evening
Dementia	Cholinesterase inhibitors, such as rivastigmine or donepezil
Depression	Selective serotonin reuptake inhibitors or tricyclics
Anxiety	Benzodiazepines
Orthostatic hypotension	Midodrine; fludrocortisone
Sialorrhea	Propantheline; atropine oral drops; scopolamine transdermal patch; botulinum toxin injections into the salivary glands
Constipation	High fiber diet; polyethylene glycol; pyridostigmine

indicate a disorder such as Alzheimer's, dementia with Lewy bodies, or frontotemporal dementia. Also, there should be absence of a history that suggests secondary parkinsonism, such as severe head trauma, encephalitis, or recent exposure to antipsychotic medication that blocks dopamine receptors. Supportive features for a diagnosis of PD are asymmetry of motor signs and a very good response to levodopa therapy. The Parkinson-plus syndromes (except for cortical basal degeneration) typically show symmetric signs; they also typically do not respond to levodopa.

Occasionally, severe essential tremor (ET) (which typically presents with postural and action tremor instead of resting tremor) can cause confusion because some patients with PD have had a prior development of ET, and some ET patients can have resting tremor if the tremor is severe, and some patients with PD can have postural and action tremors in addition to or instead of resting tremor. When the diagnosis is confusing, functional neuroimaging studies such as fluor-odopa positron emission tomography (FDOPA PET) and dopamine transporter single photon emission tomography (SPECT scans) that can detect reduced striatal dopamine might help. In PD, there is a reduction in striatal binding that can be detected with these scans, and this scan would be normal in ET. However, such scans would not distinguish between PD and Parkinson-plus syndromes. The clinical features that suggest an atypical parkinsonian syndrome rather than PD are presented in Table 5.

Table 5 Features Favoring Another Cause of Parkinsonism, Rather than Parkinson's Disease

	Likely Diagnosis
1. History of:	
encephalitis	Postencephalitic
exposure to carbon monoxide, manganese, or other toxins	Toxin-induced
recent exposure to neuroleptic medication	Drug-induced
2. Onset of parkinsonian symptoms following:	
head trauma	Posttraumatic
stroke	Vascular
3. Presence on examination of:	
cerebellar ataxia	OPCA, MSA
loss of downward ocular movements	PSP
pronounced postural hypotension not due to concurrent medication	MSA
pronounced unilateral rigidity	CBD
unilateral dystonia, apraxia, cortical sensory loss, alien limb	CBD
myoclonus	CBD, MSA
falling or freezing of gait early in the course of the disease	PSP
autonomic dysfunction not due to medications	MSA
excessive drooling of saliva	MSA
early dementia or hallucinations	DLB
dystonia induced with low dose levodopa	MSA
4. Neuroimaging (MRI or CT scan) revealing	
lacunar infarcts	Vascular
capacious cerebral ventricles	NPH
cerebellar atrophy	OPCA, MSA
atrophy of the midbrain or other parts of the brainstem	PSP, MSA
5. Effect of medication:	
poor response to levodopa	PSP, MSA, CBD, Vascular, NPH
no dyskinesias despite high dosage levodopa	same as above

Abbreviations used: CBD, cortical-basal degeneration; DLB, dementia with Lewy bodies; MSA, multiple system atrophy; NPH, normal pressure hydrocephalus; OPCA, olivo-ponto-cerebellar atrophy, which can be one form of MSA.

Treatment

The various treatments of the nonmotor problems in PD are listed in Table 4. This section discusses the approach to treat the motor problems. Keeping the patient physically active is important in all stages of the illness. This includes an exercise program to stretch the muscles and joints; balance and gait training with a physiotherapist or trainer may be required as the disease worsens. The mainstay of treatment is the use of medications. Brain surgery known as deep brain stimulation (DBS) can be appropriate for selected patients with advanced disease who respond to levodopa but have disabling motor complications from medications, such as dyskinesias and motor fluctuations (wearing-off phenomenon).

Medical Therapy

The treatment of PD should be tailored for each individual, taking into account the specific symptoms affecting the patient and their severity. The age of the patient is important. Younger patients are more likely to develop motor fluctuations and dyskinesias from levodopa; older patients are more likely to develop confusion, excessive daytime sleepiness, and psychosis from dopamine agonists. The clinician needs to weigh the potential benefit and the possible adverse effects.

Neuroprotective Therapy

There have been clinical trials testing agents for their potential to slow the progression of the disease. So far no drug or surgical approach has unequivocally been shown to be neuroprotective. Two drugs that have suggested evidence in slowing the rate of clinical worsening are selegiline (Shoulson et al. 2002; Palhagen et al. 2006) and rasagiline (Olanow et al. 2009). Both drugs are irreversible MAO-B inhibitors, and are approved to treat the symptoms of PD. When used at the recommended dose, they do not cause the "cheese effect" from tyramine-rich foods. They can be used at the time the diagnosis of PD is made in the hope they will slow clinical worsening somewhat. Selegiline has been shown to delay the onset of freezing of gait, in the presence or absence of levodopa therapy. Coenzyme Q10 is currently being tested in a controlled clinical trial to determine if it has neuroprotective effects.

Symptomatic Therapy

With the discovery of striatal dopamine deficiency to correlate with severity of bradykinesia, the major medical approach to treating PD has been dopamine replacement therapy. Several dopaminergic agents are available (Table 6). The most powerful symptomatic drug is levodopa, the immediate precursor of dopamine. Levodopa is an amino acid and can enter the brain, whereas dopamine cannot. Levodopa is usually administered combined with a peripheral decarboxylase inhibitor (carbidopa or benserazide) to prevent formation of dopamine in the peripheral tissues, thereby increasing levodopa's bioavailability and also markedly reducing gastrointestinal side effects. Carbidopa/levodopa and benserazide/levodopa are available in standard (i.e., immediate-release) and extended–release formulations. The former allows a more rapid and predictable "on," and the latter allows for a slightly longer plasma half–life, but with a slower and less predictable "on." The combination of the two release formulations can be administered in an attempt to smooth out and extend plasma levels of levodopa. There is a formulation of carbidopa/levodopa that dissolves in the patient's mouth and enters the stomach with swallowed saliva. Its usefulness is for patients who have swallowing difficulties or who need to take a dose of carbidopa/levodopa quickly, without delay by a search for liquid to swallow with a tablet.

Unfortunately, the majority of patients develop troublesome complications of disabling response fluctuations ("wearing-off" effect) and dyskinesias after five years of levodopa therapy. Duration of treatment,

Table 6 Drugs Used to Treat Motor Features of Parkinson's Disease

Dopaminergic Agents	Non-Dopaminergic Agents
Dopamine precursor: levodopa	Antimuscarinics: trihexyphenidyl, benztropine
Peripheral decarboxylase inhibitors: carbidopa, benserazide	Antihistaminics: diphenhydramine, orphenadrine
Dopamine agonists: pramipexole, ropinirole, rotigotine, apomorphine	Antiglutamatergics (to reduce dyskinesia): amantadine
Catechol-O-methyltransferase inhibitors: tolcapone, entacapone	Muscle relaxants: cyclobenzaprine, diazepam, baclofen
Dopamine releaser: amantadine	Mitochondrial enhancer: coenzyme Q10
Peripheral dopamine receptor blocker: domperidone	Benzodiazepines to reduce stress-activated tremor
MAO type B inhibitor: selegiline, Zydis selegiline, rasagiline	Antipsychotics: clozapine and quetiapine to treat psychosis without worsening parkinsonism

severity of PD, dosage of levodopa, and age of the patient are important risk factors. Younger patients (less than 60 years of age) are particularly prone to develop these problems. Thus, younger patients are often started with a dopamine agonist rather than levodopa. Older patients over age 70, who are less likely to develop motor complications from levodopa and more likely to develop confusion and hallucinations from dopamine agonists, are often started with levodopa. Discontinuing levodopa suddenly can induce the neuroleptic malignant syndrome of fever, sweating, rigidity, and mental confusion and obtundation. Therefore it is safer to reduce the dose over a 3-day period if the drug needs to be discontinued.

Because starting levodopa "starts the clock" for developing motor complications, many clinicians delay the onset of therapy until the symptoms are sufficient to warrant treatment. A dopa-sparing strategy can be employed, namely utilizing other agents prior to levodopa. This strategy would employ dopamine agonists, antimuscarinic agents, amantadine, and MAO-B inhibitors prior to introducing levodopa to those with high risk for developing motor complications. When levodopa is introduced, build the dose up slowly, avoiding gastrointestinal adverse effects. Start with carbidopa/levodopa one-half of a 25/100 mg tablet once a day. Add another dose weekly until a dose of 25/100 mg tid is reached. If necessary, the dose can be increased again as needed to control symptoms.

Levodopa is metabolized by aromatic amino acid decarboxylase (commonly known as dopa decarboxylase) to form dopamine. Inhibiting this enzyme peripherally avoids gastrointestinal adverse effects from peripheral dopamine, and also allows more of the administered levodopa to enter the brain. Levodopa is also metabolized by catechol–O–methyltransferase (COMT) to form 3-O-methyldopa. COMT inhibitors (entacapone and tolcapone) extend the plasma half–life of levodopa and slightly increase its peak plasma concentration. Although useful to reduce the amount of wearing-off, they can induce dyskinesias and worsen the dyskinesias in those patients who already have them. The dosage of levodopa may need to be lowered to avoid this problem.

Entacapone is very short-acting, and each 200 mg tablet is taken simultaneously with levodopa; entacapone has been combined with carbidopa/levodopa into a single tablet, known as Stalevo. Tolcapone (100 and 200 mg tablets) is more potent and has a longer duration of action; it is taken three times daily, but it is encumbered with a greater likelihood to cause diarrhea and hepatic toxicity. Liver function must be monitored and the drug stopped if abnormal liver chemistries are seen. Tolcapone is therefore given only if entacapone has been found to be ineffective in controlling motor fluctuations.

The second most powerful drugs in treating PD symptoms are the dopamine agonists. The ergot compounds of pergolide, bromocriptine, and cabergoline have the potential to induce fibrosis (cardiac valvulopathy and retroperitoneal, pleuropulmonary, and pericardial fibrosis), so these agents are not recommended, and indeed pergolide has been withdrawn from the U.S. market. Pramipexole and ropinirole appear to be equally effective at therapeutic levels. As mentioned above, dopamine agonists are more likely than levodopa to cause hallucinations, confusion, and psychosis, especially in the elderly,. Thus, it is safer to utilize levodopa in patients over the age of 70 years. On the other hand, many clinical trials have shown dopamine agonists to be less likely to produce dyskinesias than levodopa. But those trials also showed that levodopa provided greater symptomatic benefit than the agonists. Other problems more likely to occur with dopamine agonists than levodopa are sudden sleep attacks, including falling asleep at the wheel, daytime drowsiness, ankle edema, and impulse control problems such as hypersexuality, pathologic gambling, compulsive shopping, and binge eating.

Pramipexole is available only in an immediate-release formulation, while ropinirole is available in both immediate-release and extend-release formulations. The latter may be useful in treating nocturnal akinesia and possibly motor fluctuations. Rotigotine dermal patch is a weak dopamine agonist that is applied to the upper torso or arms. Rotigotine penetrates the epidermis and dermis and enters the subcutaneous fat where it slowly enters the blood stream. The skin patch is applied once daily, usually after the morning shower, and is removed the next day before the shower; a new patch is applied to a different surface of the skin to reduce the chance of a rash, a not uncommon adverse effect. Absorption is steady over 24 hours, and three dose strengths (four in Europe) are available: 2, 4 and 6 mg/day (plus 8 mg/day in Europe). It is useful for those with swallowing difficulties, and may help smooth out motor fluctuations and nocturnal akinesia. The rotigotine leaked out of the patch to form crystals, so it has been withdrawn temporarily until the manufacturer has solved the problem.

Apomorphine is the most powerful dopamine agonist, but it needs to be injected subcutaneously. It is used to provide faster relief to overcome a deep "off" state, a so-called rescue effect. In Europe, subcutaneous infusion of apomorphine is being applied to patients with motor fluctuations.

Amantadine has several actions; its ability to enhance the release of dopamine from nerve terminals, block dopamine reuptake into the nerve terminals, and its antimuscarinic effects give amantadine an antiparkinsonian effect. It is more commonly used to reduce levodopa-induced dyskinesias by blocking glutamate NMDA receptors. It is the only known effective antidyskinetic agent. The dose of amantadine for its anti-PD effect is usually 100 mg twice daily, but its antidyskinetic effect requires higher dosages, usually 300 to 400 mg/day. Unfortunately, the antidyskinetic effect tends to lessen over time. Its adverse effect profile includes the induction of livedo reticularis (reddish mottling of the skin around the knees), ankle edema, visual hallucinations, and confusion. The elderly do not tolerate amantadine well because of mental adverse effects of confusion and hallucinations.

Domperidone is a peripherally–active dopamine receptor blocker and is useful in preventing gastrointestinal upset from levodopa and the dopamine agonists. It is not available in the U.S., but is available in other countries. Monoamine oxidase type B (MAO-B) inhibitors (selegiline, rasagiline, and Zydis selegiline) have been mentioned above as possible modest neuroprotective agents. They also have mild symptomatic benefit and enhance the potency of levodopa. Selegiline, but not rasagiline, is metabolized to L-amphetamine and methamphetamine. Zydis selegiline is a formulation of selegiline that dissolves under the tongue and is absorbed via the oral mucosa directly into the blood stream, thereby by-passing the gut and liver and not generating the amphetamines. All these drugs can reduce the severity of motor fluctuations with levodopa. They are more likely, however, to increase dyskinesias.

Non-dopaminergic agents are useful to treat both motor (Table 6) and nonmotor (Table 4) symptoms in PD. Antimuscarinic drugs have been used widely for over a half century, but are less effective than the dopaminergic agents, including amantadine. They can induce adverse effects of forgetfulness, dry mouth, dilated pupils with blurred vision, and urinary hesitancy and inability to void. They can be helpful in reducing the severity of tremor when other medications have failed to do so. Because of sensitivity to memory impairment and hallucinations in the elderly population, antimuscarinics should be avoided in patients over the age of 70 years. Antihistaminics have mild anticholinergic properties and can serve as alternatives to antimuscarinic drugs in the elderly population. Another alternative agent is the tricyclic amitriptyline because it also has anticholinergic properties. Muscle relaxants can sometimes reduce muscle tightness and cramping, and might help overcome "off" dystonia and peak–dose dystonia that patients sometimes develop on levodopa therapy. Coenzyme Q10 is undergoing a controlled clinical trial to determine if it has a disease-modifying effect. Because excitement and stress activate tremor, in situations where stress is predicted, taking a short-acting benzodiazepine, such as alprazolam, can often be helpful. Most antipsychotics block D2 dopamine receptors and worsen the symptoms of PD. But the two atypical antipsychotics, clozapine and quetiapine, can be used in patients with PD without worsening the parkinsonism while ameliorating drug-induced psychosis. Other antipsychotic agents are more likely to worsen the parkinsonism and should be avoided.

Treatment of Motor Complications from Levodopa Therapy

Motor complications from levodopa are common. They fall into two categories: abnormal involuntary movements (dyskinesias) and motor fluctuations (most commonly, wearing-off) (Table 7). As mentioned above, young patients almost always develop these problems; not all older patients do, and if they do, it takes longer before these complications appear. Levodopa-induced dyskinesias are most commonly choreic (brief, irregular, non-rhythmic movements), but can also be dystonic (sustained, twisting contractions). Combinations of chorea and dystonia are common.

Peak-dose dyskinesias are present when plasma and brain levels of levodopa are high. Reducing the individual dosage can resolve this problem, but the patient may need to take more frequent doses at this lower amount because reducing the amount of an individual dose also reduces the duration of benefit. More frequent dosings of levodopa tends to lead to delayed "ons" and dose failures eventually. A simple approach is to add amantadine, which suppresses the severity of dyskinesias, possibly because of its antiglutamatergic action. Start with a dose of 100 mg b.i.d. and increase up to 200 mg b.i.d. if necessary. Another approach is to add or substitute higher doses of a dopamine agonist while lowering the dose of carbidopa/levodopa. But adding the

Table 7 Common Complications of Levodopa Therapy

Motor Complications	Non-motor Complications
DYSKINESIAS (chorea and dystonia)	**LOSS OF ALERTNESS**
Peak-dose dyskinesias	Drowsy from a dose of levodopa
Diphasic dyskinesias (beginning and end-of-dose dyskinesias)	Excessive daytime sleepiness
End-of-day dyskinesias	Reversal of sleep-wake cycle
FLUCTUATIONS	**BEHAVIORAL AND COGNITIVE**
Wearing-off	Vivid dreams
Delayed "ons"	Hallucinations
Dose failures	Delusions
Sudden, unpredictable "offs" (on-offs)	Paranoia
Early morning "off" dystonia	Confusion
"Off" dystonia during day	Dementia
Behavioral-sensory-autonomic "offs"	

agonist while maintaining the levodopa dosage will usually result in an increase of dyskinesias. If lowering the dose of levodopa results in more severe "off" states, then the agonists become more important.

Diphasic dyskinesias are dyskinesias that occur at the beginning and end of a dose, not during the time of peak plasma and brain levels of levodopa. They tend to affect particularly the legs with a mixture of chorea and dystonia. Because the mechanism is unclear, treatment of diphasic dyskinesias is difficult. In this situation, one should use a dopamine agonist as the major pharmacologic agent with supplementary levodopa. End-of-the-day dyskinesias are end-of-dose dyskinesias. There is some dose that is the last dose of the day, and after that dose, severe dyskinesias can appear. Treatment has not been satisfactory, and many patients just "ride out" these dyskinesias for a couple of hours. When they resolve, the patient is comfortable again.

When levodopa is initiated and an effective dose is reached, the benefit lasts a few days; this is called the long-duration response. Eventually, the long-duration response becomes lost, and only a short-duration response occurs; patients then develop the wearing-off phenomenon. This can be defined as when an adequate dosage of levodopa does not last at least four hours. The "offs" tend to be mild at first, but over time become deeper with more severe parkinsonism; simultaneously, the duration of the "on" response becomes shorter. Some patients develop random, sudden "offs" in which the deep state of parkinsonism develops over minutes rather than tens of minutes, and they are less predictable in terms of timing with the doses of levodopa. Many patients who develop response fluctuations also develop peak-dose dyskinesias.

When mild, the wearing-off phenomenon may be ameliorated by moving the doses of levodopa closer together. Alternatively, one can 1) add an MAO-B inhibitor, which potentiates the action of levodopa, 2) add entacapone with each dose of levodopa to extend the plasma half-life, or 3) switch immediate-release carbidopa/levodopa to the extended-release formulation. If a patient is underdosed, one can add extended-release carbidopa/levodopa along with the standard immediate-release carbidopa/levodopa. Multiple doses of levodopa per day, with short intervals between doses, make it more likely that

some doses may fail to turn the patient "on;" these are called dose failures and are due to poor gastric emptying. Levodopa is absorbed only in the proximal small intestine. If a patient has dose failures or a delayed time in turning "on" after a dose, the patient can grind the tablet of carbidopa/levodopa in his or her teeth before swallowing it with lots of water. Getting the medication dissolved will aid it being passed into the small intestine.

An alternative to adding more levodopa or regulating its method of administration is to add a long-acting dopamine agonist, such as ropinirole XL or rotigotine dermal patch. The addition of this type of dopamine agonist tends to make the "off" state less severe when used in combination with carbidopa/levodopa. The addition of the dopamine agonist, however, will likely increase dyskinesias; in this situation the dosage of levodopa would need to be reduced. One must also be careful of the adverse side effects of the dopamine agonists, such as hallucinations in the elderly and excessive daytime sleepiness and the rarer sudden onset of sleep without warning (sleep attacks) in young and old. About 20% of users of dopamine agonists may develop an impulse control problem, discussed later.

Instead of a return of parkinsonism whenever the patient is "off," some patients will have dystonic "offs," which are painful muscle cramps. The most common form of these "off" dystonias are in the early morning as the patient wakes up and as the last pre-bedtime dose of levodopa has worn off. Early-morning dystonia manifests as painful foot and toe cramps, which are relieved when the next dose of levodopa begins to take effect. Dystonic "offs" can occur at other times of the day, as well. Some peak-dose dystonias can be identical in appearance, and it is not always easy to distinguish these from "off" dystonia. Preventing "offs" is the best way to control these painful dystonias. An effective treatment is to use a dopamine agonist as the major pharmacologic agent with supplementary levodopa. Here is where ropinirole XL or the rotigotine dermal patch can be particularly useful, by keeping a steady pharmacokinetic level of active drug throughout the day and night. Baclofen has also been reported to symptomatically benefit some patients. An alternative is to set the alarm early to take a dose of standard carbidopa/levodopa in the middle of the night and then fall back to sleep and awaken at the usual time.

Largely unrecognized by clinicians are behavioral-sensory-autonomic "offs" if they occur in the absence of a motor "off." Behavioral-sensory-autonomic "offs" can consist of pain, akathisia, depression, anxiety, dysphoria, panic, drenching sweats, abdominal bloating, dyspnea, and urinary urgency. Usually there is a mixture of more than one of these clinical features. Like dystonic "offs," behavioral-sensory-autonomic "offs" are extremely poorly tolerated. It is often the presence of one of these sensory and behavioral phenomena—more so than motoric parkinsonian or dystonic "offs"—that drives the patient to take more and more levodopa, turning the patient into a "levodopa addict." Treatment depends on utilizing ropinirole XL or rotigotine dermal patch to keep the dopamine receptors activated.

Treatment of Non-motor Complications from Levodopa Therapy

Mental changes of psychosis, confusion, agitation, hallucinations, paranoid delusions, and excessive sleeping are probably related to activation of dopamine receptors in non-striatal regions, particularly the cortical and limbic structures. Elderly patients and patients with concomitant dementia are extremely sensitive to small doses of levodopa, and even more so to dopamine agonists. Regardless of age, all patients with PD can develop psychosis if they take excess amounts of levodopa as a means to overcome "off" periods, such as the behavioral-sensory-autonomic "offs" described above.

If hallucinations are mild and not frightening, treatment can begin with the addition of quetiapine, starting with 25 mg at bedtime. The dose should be increased steadily until the hallucinations are brought under control. If quetiapine is ineffective or if the hallucinations are frightening, clozapine needs to be initiated instead because it is much more effective than quetiapine. Clozapine is not the first drug of choice in dopaminergic-induced hallucinations because clozapine causes agranulocytosis in approximately 1–2% of patients. Patients must have their blood counts monitored weekly for this potential complication, and then discontinue the drug if leukopenia develops. Both quetiapine and clozapine often cause drowsiness, so bedtime dosing is recommended. Quetiapine can cause falling, and clozapine, seizures with high doses. The dosing regimen for clozapine is similar to that for quetiapine. Quetiapine and clozapine are labeled as "atypical antipsychotics" because they usually do not induce or worsen parkinsonism, and therefore can be used in patients with PD.

If the psychosis is severe or if the patient is in an acute delirious state, hospitalization is necessary, with immediate initiation of high dosages of clozapine, and some reduction in anti-PD medication. These medications could even be withdrawn temporarily to overcome the psychosis, but this should be done stepwise over a 3-day period to avoid the neuroleptic-malignant-like syndrome that could occur with sudden withdrawal of levodopa.

Regardless of the severity of the hallucinations, if the patient does not respond well or is unable to tolerate quetiapine and clozapine, then the physician needs to reduce one or more anti-PD medication. All antiparkinson drugs have the potential to induce psychosis, so the less efficacious drugs should be withdrawn first. Accordingly, COMT inhibitors, MAO-B inhibitors, amantadine, anticholinergics, and dopamine agonists should be withdrawn in that order, reserving levodopa as the most effective agent.

Levodopa can induce irresistible drowsiness after a dose, particularly in patients who have cognitive impairment. Excessive daytime sleepiness can lead to being awake at night. This altered sleep–wake cycle is fairly common in the elderly. If a patient becomes drowsy after each dose of levodopa, reducing the individual dose may correct this problem. Once an altered sleep–wake cycle has developed, the care provider often needs to remain awake at night, making it extremely difficult for her or him. It is important to get the patient onto a sleep–wake schedule that fits with the rest of the household. Efforts must be made to stimulate the patient physically and mentally during the daytime and force him or her to remain awake. It may be necessary to use stimulants in the morning and sedatives at night in order to reverse the altered state back towards normal. Modafinil can sometimes be helpful to overcome daytime drowsiness, and one or two doses in the morning and early afternoon can be employed. Drugs such as methylphenidate and amphetamine are usually also well tolerated by patients with PD, and can be considered if modafinil fails. A 10 mg dose of either of these two drugs, repeated once if necessary, may be helpful. To encourage sleep at night, a hypnotic may be necessary in addition to using daytime stimulants. It should be noted that strong sedatives, such as barbiturates, are poorly tolerated by patients with PD. Milder hypnotics, such as benzodiazepines and zolpidem, are usually taken without difficulty. Taking advantage of the soporific effects of quetiapine, clozapine, mirtazapine, and amitriptyline is a good strategy if a patient can also benefit from the other actions of these antipsychotics and antidepressants.

Orthostatic hypotension can be caused by levodopa, dopamine agonists, and other drugs taken by the patient, such as tricyclic antidepressants. These other drugs should be discontinued. If orthostatic hypotension remains, it can sometimes be managed by using support stockings, NaCl, midodrine (ProAmatine), and fludrocortisone (Florinef).

Impulse control problems have been recognized as a complication of dopamine agonists. These consist of behavioral changes such as pathologic gambling, compulsive shopping, binge eating with weight gain, and unpleasant hypersexual drive. These can be serious problems for the patient and family. So far, the only remedy has been to reduce the dose of the dopamine agonists or stop them altogether.

Surgical Therapy

Stereotaxic deep brain stimulation (DBS) has replaced the older technique of producing a lesion in the brain because the latter is more risky for inducing permanent neurological deficits. With DBS, the parameters of stimulation, such as voltage and frequency, can be adjusted, and the electrodes could be removed if required. However, DBS is more costly, and frequent adjustments of the stimulators are usually needed. The location of the stereotaxic target is a major factor that needs to be individualized for each patient. The subthalamic nucleus (STN) is the favored target because this location reduces bradykinesia and tremor, allowing for a reduction of levodopa dosage, thus reducing the severity of dyskinesias as well. The internal segment of the globus pallidus (GPi) is a more satisfactory target for controlling choreic and dystonic dyskinesias, which in turn would allow a higher dose of levodopa to be used to control the major symptoms of PD. Also, for those patients who already have behavioral-sensory-autonomic "offs," a reduction of levodopa with STN stimulation may not be tolerated, and the GPi may be a better target. The thalamus, particularly the ventral intermediate nucleus, is the target most successful for controlling tremor, but this target does not eliminate bradykinesia as well as the STN does, so the thalamus is not a preferred choice today.

Surgical procedures for patients with PD are best performed at specialty centers with an experienced team of a neurosurgeon, neurophysiologist to monitor the target during the operative procedure, and a neurologist to program the stimulators. The patient needs close follow-up to adjust the stimulator settings to their optimum. Patients with cognitive decline should not have DBS because cognition can be further impaired. Also, intractable symptoms of freezing of gait, loss of postural reflexes, and falling are not benefited. The major benefits of STN stimulation are those symptoms that respond to levodopa. Adverse effects include surgical complications, mechanical problems with the stimulator and leads to the electrodes, infections attacking any of the inserted hardware, and neurologic and behavioral changes. The latter include troubles with speech, dystonic postures, depression, suicide attempts, and cognitive decline. The best candidates are younger patients who can tolerate the penetration of the brain and who have uncontrollable motor fluctuations and dyskinesias.

Summary

Parkinson's disease (PD) is the second most common neurodegenerative disorder. The early symptoms primarily due to a loss of dopaminergic neurons can be largely ameliorated by medications that restore dopamine or act on dopamine receptors. Besides the typical motor manifestations of tremor, rigidity, and bradykinesia, most patients also have accompanying nonmotor symptoms, involving cognitive, sensory, autonomic, and emotional problems. These need to be treated as well. Treatment is often accompanied by adverse effects, and these can be the most important problem. New surgical techniques can often benefit the motor complications induced by levodopa therapy. The pathology, genetics, clinical features, diagnosis, and treatment of PD are reviewed in this chapter.

References

Braak, H., Bohl, J.R., Muller, C.M., et al.: Stanley Fahn Lecture 2005: The staging procedure for the inclusion body pathology associated with sporadic Parkinson's disease reconsidered. *Mov Disord* 21:2042–2051, 2006.

Buter, T.C., van den Hout, A., Matthews, F.E., et al.: Dementia and survival in Parkinson disease: A 12-year population study. *Neurology* 70(13):1017–1022, 2008.

Chaudhuri, K.R., Healy, D.G., and Schapira, A.H.: Non-motor symptoms of Parkinson's disease: diagnosis and management. *Lancet Neurol* 5:235–245, 2006.

Cotzias, G.C., Papavasiliou, P.S., and Gellene, R.: Modification of parkinsonism—chronic treatment with L–dopa. *N Engl J Med* 280:337–345, 1969.

Fahn, S.: The history of dopamine and levodopa in the treatment of Parkinson's disease. *Mov Disord* 23 Suppl 3:S497–508, 2008.

Fahn, S. and Jankovic, J. *Principles and practice of movement disorders.* Churchill Livingstone Elsevier, Philadelphia, 2007, p. 107.

Hely, M.A., Reid, W.G., Adena, M.A., et al.: The Sydney multicenter study of Parkinson's disease: The inevitability of dementia at 20 years. *Mov Disord* 23(6):837–844, 2008.

Hernan, M.A., Takkouche, B., Caamano-Isorna, F., and Gestal-Otero, J.J.: A meta-analysis of coffee drinking, cigarette smoking, and the risk of Parkinson's disease. *Ann Neurol* 52(3):276–284, 2002.

Klein, C. and Schlossmacher, M.G.: Parkinson disease, 10 years after its genetic revolution: Multiple clues to a complex disorder. *Neurology* 69(22):2093–104, 2007.

Martinez-Vicente, M. and Cuervo, A.M.: Autophagy and neurodegeneration: When the cleaning crew goes on strike. *Lancet Neurol* 6(4):352–361, 2007.

Mosharov, E.V., Larsen, K.E., Kanter, E., et al.: Interplay between cytosolic dopamine, calcium, and alpha-synuclein causes selective death of substantia nigra neurons. *Neuron* 62(2):218–229, 2009.

Olanow, C.W., Rascol, O., Hauser, R., et al.: A double-blind, delayed-start trial of rasagiline in Parkinson's disease. *N Engl J Med* 361(13):1268–1278, 2009.

Palhagen, S., Heinonen, E., Hagglund, J., et al.: Selegiline slows the progression of the symptoms of Parkinson disease. *Neurology* 66(8):1200–1206, 2006.

Shoulson, I., Oakes, D., Fahn, S., et al. Impact of sustained deprenyl (selegiline) in levodopa-treated Parkinson's disease: A randomized placebo-controlled extension of the deprenyl and tocopherol antioxidative therapy of parkinsonism trial. *Ann Neurol* 51(5):604–612, 2002.

Sidransky, E., Nalls, M.A., Aasly, J.O., et al.: Multicenter analysis of glucocerebrosidase mutations in Parkinson's disease. *N Engl J Med* 361(17):1651–1661, 2009.

Surmeier, D.J.: Calcium, ageing, and neuronal vulnerability in Parkinson's disease. *Lancet Neurol* 6(10):933–938, 2007.

Tanner, C.M., Ross, G.W., Jewell, S.A., et al.: Occupation and risk of parkinsonism: A multicenter case-control study. *Arch Neurol* 66:1106–1113, 2009.

Tanner, C.M., Ottman, R., Goldman, S.M., et al.: Parkinson disease in twins. An etiologic study. *JAMA* 281(4):341–346, 1999.

Thacker, E.L., O'Reilly, E.J., Weisskopf, M.G., et al.: Temporal relationship between cigarette smoking and risk of Parkinson disease. *Neurology* 68(10):764–768, 2007.

23 Other Parkinsonian Disorders

Nabila Dahodwala, Amy Colcher, and Matthew B. Stern

Introduction

Parkinsonian disorders are characterized by a combination of at least two of the following cardinal signs: bradykinesia, rigidity, tremor, and gait or balance problems. Among community-dwelling older adults, these signs are highly prevalent and lead to increased morbidity and mortality. One study found that over 14% of adults between the ages of 65 and 74, 29% of adults between the ages of 75 and 84, and 50% of adults over the age of 85 had evidence of parkinsonism on examination (Bennett et al. 1996). However, while parkinsonian signs are common among older adults, only a small fraction of these individuals are diagnosed and treated in clinical centers for known causes. The etiologies for parkinsonian signs can vary from neurodegenerative diseases, neurovascular disease, medication side-effects, and structural brain lesions (see Table 1).

In the following section, we will discuss the principal primary and secondary causes of parkinsonian disorders. Primary causes of parkinsonian disorders include neurodegenerative disorders in older adults. The most common syndrome, Parkinson's disease (see Chapter 22) is followed by Lewy body dementia (see Chapter 19) in prevalence. Other less common neurodegenerative diseases associated with parkinsonism or atypical parkinsonian disorders are progressive supranuclear palsy (PSP), multiple system atrophy (MSA), and corticobasal degeneration (CBD).

There are also numerous secondary causes of parkinsonism, but the most common include drug-induced and vascular parkinsonism. There has also been a growing recognition that normal pressure hydrocephalus (NPH) can present with parkinsonian signs. Other, infrequent causes of secondary parkinsonism can occur after exposure to certain toxins, for example, manganese, carbon monoxide, and 1-methyl-4-phenyl-1,2,3,6-tetrahydropyridine (MPTP), a synthetic opioid (Bove et al. 2005). From 1915–1930 post-encephalitic cases of parkinsonism occurred in epidemic proportions, but are now rarely reported (Rail, Scholtz, and Swash 1981). Structural lesions to the basal ganglia due to trauma and hydrocephalus, and metabolic disturbances such as hypoparathyroid or pseudohypoparathyroid which lead to basal ganglia calcifications, all can result in a secondary parkinsonian syndrome (Stern and Koller 1993). Lastly, in rare instances, parkinsonism may be psychogenic in nature.

Pathophysiology

Any structural or metabolic derangement of the nigro-striatal/dopaminergic system can lead to parkinsonism. In the cases of PSP, MSA, and CBD, the accumulation of abnormal protein aggregates within the basal ganglia are thought to play some role in the development of these neurodegenerative diseases either through direct neuro-toxicity or as a secondary marker. MSA is characterized by the abnormal aggregation of the alpha synuclein protein. For a definite diagnosis of MSA, neuropathologic findings of widespread and abundant central nervous system glial cytoplasmic inclusions that are positive for alpha synuclein in association with neurodegeneration in striatonigral or olivopontocerebellar structures is required (Trojanowski and Revesz 2007).

PSP and CBD, on the other hand, have abnormal tau protein pathology. There is neuronal loss, gliosis, and accumulation of tau protein in the cerebral areas affected by the disease process. The tau protein builds up in the cells and is apparent as neurofibrillary tangles. The paraprotein in PSP is highly phosphorylated (Albers et al. 2000). The dopaminergic, GABA-ergic, cholinergic, and neuroadrenergic pathways are also affected and this leads to the typical symptoms of PSP (Rajput and Rajput 2001). In CBD, tau-immunoreactive lesions are seen in neurons, glia, and cell processes within the cortex and striatum, which leads to neuronal loss in focal cortical regions and the substantia nigra in addition to astrocytic plaques (Dickson et al. 2002).

Vascular parkinsonism has evidence of white matter ischemic damage in conjunction with ischemic infarcts within the striatum in the absence of other pathology (Zijlmans, Daniel et al. 2004). Typical neurovascular risk factors, especially hypertension, appear to contribute to the development of vascular parkinsonism.

Idiopathic NPH is suspected to represent a unique reversible form of neuronal injury that is poorly understood (Gallia, Rigamonti, and

Table 1 Causes of Parkinsonism in Older Adults

Primary parkinsonism	Secondary Parkinsonism
◆ Parkinson's disease	◆ Medications
◆ Lewy body dementia	◆ Structural lesion of basal ganglia
◆ Progressive supranuclear palsy (PSP)	◆ tumor
◆ Multiple system atrophy (MSA)	◆ vascular malformation
◆ Corticobasal degeneration (CBD)	◆ stroke
◆ Other neurodegenerative diseases	◆ hydrocephalus
◆ Alzheimer's disease	◆ trauma
◆ Frontotemporal dementia	◆ Toxins
◆ Neurodegeneration with brain iron accumulation	◆ MPTP
	◆ manganese
	◆ carbon monoxide
	◆ Infectious
	◆ post-encephalitis
	◆ Metabolic
	◆ hypoparathyroid
	◆ pseudohypoparathyroid
	◆ Psychogenic

MPTP = 1-methyl-4-phenyl-1,2,3,6-tetrahydropyridine

Williams 2006). However, NPH may occur also secondarily to other disease processes such as subarachnoid hemorrhage, traumatic brain injury, stroke, and meningitis.

Genetics

Most of the primary parkinsonian disorders are sporadic in nature. In a subset of individuals with PSP and CBD, though, there is growing evidence of the association of mutations in the tau gene, *Microtubule associated protein tau (MAPt)*, and increased risk of developing either disease (Pittman, Fung, and de Silva 2006). Additionally, mutations in the *progranulin* gene, a multifunctional growth factor believed to promote neuronal survival, have been found in familial cases of corticobasal degeneration (Masellis et al. 2006). Testing for these genetic mutations is performed in research settings only as we learn more about their clinical significance.

Clinical Presentation

In addition to the cardinal features of parkinsonism: tremor, rigidity, bradykinesia, and gait or postural instability, other clinical features are present in parkinsonian disorders which will help distinguish one cause of parkinsonism from another (see Table 2).

Progressive Supranuclear Palsy (PSP)

PSP is a rapidly progressive disorder combining early gait and eye movement abnormalities in patients with bradykinesia and rigidity. PSP typically begins in patients in their 60s. Of the atypical parkinsonian syndromes, it has the highest prevalence, which is estimated to be 6–6.4 per 100,000 persons (Schrag, Ben-Shlomo, and Quinn 1999).

Most patients' early symptoms include problems with balance, frequent falling, dysarthria, and bradykinesia (Litvan and Hutton 1998). The clinical hallmark of progressive supranuclear palsy is the supranuclear gaze palsy where initially vertical eye movements and later horizontal eye movements are impaired. Cognitive difficulties occur later in the course of the disease. There is proximal axial muscle rigidity which leads patients with PSP to stand erect and when they lose their balance they fall with no postural reflexes to correct themselves. There is much more axial rigidity than limb rigidity in this disease, which helps to differentiate it from idiopathic Parkinson's disease.

Other associated features include a pseudobulbar affect with dysarthria, dysphagia, and emotional incontinence (Gomez-Haro et al. 1999). The supranuclear gaze palsy usually appears within three to four years of diagnosis but can take as many as six years for the complete syndrome to be clinically evident. Initially there is slowing of vertical saccades followed by difficulty with downgaze and a complete palsy of vertical gaze. Pursuit movements can be preserved at the beginning of the disease but eventually disappear entirely. Horizontal saccadic intrusion or square wave jerks occur when patients are staring at an object in primary gaze. Oculovestibular reflexes are preserved in these patients.

Behavioral and emotional disorders such as depression, dementia, and frontal release signs as well as sleep disturbance may coexist with the movement disorder. The dementia that can be seen in PSP patients is of the subcortical type with slowness of information processing and difficulty planning tasks.

Multiple System Atrophy (MSA)

Multiple system atrophy (MSA) is a neurodegenerative disease involving, as its name implies, multiple systems in the brain. It is characterized by parkinsonism, cerebellar ataxia, autonomic failure, and corticospinal dysfunction. The symptoms may overlap, but, in general, patients present with both autonomic dysfunction and either cerebellar dysfunction or parkinsonism. Typically, patients present with this disorder in the sixth decade of life. The prevalence has been reported to be 4.4 per 100,000 cases (Schrag, Ben-Shlomo, and Quinn 1999). However, many patients are undiagnosed during their lifetime, so the prevalence may actually be higher.

The autonomic dysfunction is usually the earliest clinical symptom of this disorder. Typical autonomic symptoms are orthostatic hypotension; erectile dysfunction in males; urinary dysfunction including urgency, frequency, and incomplete bladder emptying; constipation; fecal incontinence; and anhidrosis. Orthostatic hypotension is defined as a drop of at least 30 mmHg systolic or 15 mmHg diastolic when standing.

There are two motor subsets of MSA—MSA-P (parkinsonism) and MSA-C (cerebellar) (Wenning et al. 2003). In almost 80% of cases parkinsonism is the predominant feature (MSA-P). The parkinsonism in MSA can be atypical. The tremor is less often a classic rest tremor, but more often irregular and observed with posture. Furthermore, postural instability occurs earlier than in idiopathic Parkinson's disease. In the other 20% of cases, ataxia or cerebellar dysfunction predominates (MSA-C). The hallmarks of the cerebellar dysfunction present in MSA consist of gait and limb ataxia, scanning dysarthria, and oculomotor disorders.

Other features that are seen in MSA include oral facial dystonia, dysphagia, dysphonia, contractures or dystonic posturing of the hands or feet, camptocormia, inspiratory sighing, snoring, REM sleep behavior disorder, cold hands and feet, myoclonus, hyperreflexia, and pseudobulbar affect (i.e. pathologic laughter or crying). Over time, patients with MSA develop severe dysphagia and immobility which leads to increased risk of aspiration and falls.

Corticobasal Degeneration (CBD)

CBD is a highly asymmetric parkinsonism that is associated early on with cognitive impairment and certain, subtle characteristic signs. This disorder also typically presents in the sixth decade of life. Its incidence and prevalence are unknown; however, estimates based on the prevalence of associated parkinsonian disorders conclude that the prevalence of CBD would be 4.9–7.3 per 100,000 (Togaski and Tanner 2000).

An early and common sign of CBD is a clumsy or "useless arm" due to rigidity, dystonia, akinesia, or motor apraxia in some combination. Other early features include gait impairment, if onset is in the leg, due to lateralized stiffness or apraxia (Mahapatra et al. 2004). In addition to dementia, other higher cortical signs are ideational apraxia, aphasia, cortical sensory abnormalities (e.g. loss of spatial orientation), and

Table 2 Distinguishing Clinical Features among the Primary Parkinsonian Disorders

Clinical Feature	MSA	CBD	PSP
Vertical gaze palsy	Absent	Absent	Present
Early falls	Absent	Absent	Present
Autonomic dysfunction	Early onset and severe	Absent	Absent
Cerebellar signs	Present	Absent	Absent
Limb apraxia or dystonia	Absent	Present	Absent
Gait	Shuffling, ataxic	Shuffling, apraxic	Unsteady, ataxic

alien-limb phenomenon. Additional hyperkinetic movements include coarse action tremor and myoclonus (Kompoliti et al. 1998). Rest tremor is less likely to be present in CBD than in idiopathic Parkinson's disease, but when it does manifest it can be differentiated from parkinson tremor because it occurs mainly with action, is coarser and higher in frequency, and is associated with marked rigidity of the affected limb or limbs. Neuropsychiatric features of depression, anxiety, apathy, and irritability frequently co-exist.

As CBD progresses, dysphagia can develop, which increases the risk of aspiration and pneumonia. Worsening dementia and increased fall risk ultimately contribute to the high morbidity and mortality of the disease.

Vascular Parkinsonism

Parkinsonism can occur rarely after a single stroke in the basal ganglia or brainstem, or as the cumulative result of several strokes. Patients with vascular parkinsonism usually have a long history of hypertension and may present with a step-wise progression of symptoms. Evidence for stroke may be noted on examination; for example, hemiparesis, hemisensory loss, aphasia, ataxia, or hyperreflexia. Gait may be shuffling or magnetic, a term used to describe the phenomenon of difficulty lifting feet from the floor and may include transient freezing. Patients should have evidence of extensive subcortical cerebrovascular disease on computed tomography (CT) scan or magnetic resonance imaging (MRI), although asymptomatic ischemic changes are common in older patients and do not independently make the diagnosis of vascular parkinsonism (Hurtig 1993). Unfortunately, there are no specific diagnostic criteria for this entity, but additional features may support the diagnosis.

Other supporting features of a neurovascular etiology of a parkinsonian disorder include pseudobulbar affect, pyramidal or cerebellar signs, and dementia. Some clues that may help differentiate vascular parkinsonism from idiopathic Parkinson's disease include lack of resting tremor, symmetric onset, and minimal response to levodopa.

Normal Pressure Hydrocephalus (NPH)

Hydrocephalus can cause parkinsonian signs and symptoms. Normal pressure hydrocephalus (NPH) is a syndrome characterized by the triad of gait instability, urinary incontinence, and cognitive dysfunction (Krauss et al. 1997; Shannon 1993). Symptoms generally develop slowly between the sixth and eight decades of life. As with vascular parkinsonism, gait in NPH is classically magnetic, but many gait disturbances, especially "gait ignition failure" and "frontal gait" (Nutt 2001), have been described in NPH; the gait disturbance often leads to falls. The clinical presentation, however, can vary in severity and progression, and all three symptoms of gait, cognitive, and urinary dysfunction are not required. Brain imaging (CT or MRI) shows communicating hydrocephalus with ventricles enlarged out of proportion to atrophy of the cerebral cortical sulci. This is an important disorder to consider in any patient with a parkinsonian gait, cognitive impairment, and urinary frequency or incontinence because ventriculo-peritoneal shunting may lead to marked improvement in symptoms.

Drug-induced Parkinsonism

Drug-induced parkinsonism (Table 3) is a critically important disorder to recognize because it is one of the few reversible causes of parkinsonism. It also the most prevalent form of secondary parkinsonism. In one community, 9% of all cases of parkinsonism identified were due to medications (Morgante et al. 1996). The most common culpable medications that lead to parkinsonism are the antipsychotics, or neuroleptics, which disrupt the nigro-striatal pathway because of their

Table 3 Medications that Can Cause Secondary Parkinsonism

Neuroleptics	Antiemetics	Other
◆ Phenothiazines	◆ Metoclopramide	◆ Reserpine
◆ Butrophenones	◆ Prochlorperazine	◆ Verapamil
◆ Thioxanthenes		◆ Valproic Acid

dopamine receptor blocking properties. These include the typical neuroleptics: phenothiazines, butyrophenones, and thioxanthenes and several atypical neuroleptics, including olanzapine, risperidone, ziprasidone, and aripiprazole, although these may have lower affinity for the dopamine receptor than the typical neuroleptics (Jankovic 1995). The antiemetic prochlorperazine; gastrointestinal promotility agent metoclopramide; the antihypertensives methyldopa, verapamil, and reserpine; and the antiepileptic valproic acid, can all affect the dopamine system and have the potential to induce parkinsonism (Indo and Ando 1982; Hubble 1993).

Clozapine, an atypical neuroleptic, mediates its anti-psychotic effects via non-dopaminergic neural circuits. Therefore it relieves symptoms of psychosis without a resulting side-effect of causing parkinsonism. Quetiapine is one of the more recently developed atypical neuroleptics with an extrapyramidal side effect profile similar to clozapine, and thus less likely to cause a drug-induced parkinsonism.

Diagnosis

The diagnosis of specific parkinsonian disorders early in their course can be difficult due to the overlap of symptoms and lack of clinically available definitive diagnostic tests. However, the accuracy of clinical diagnoses has improved over time. The positive predictive value for a parkinsonian disorder diagnosis among movement disorder specialists range from 33.3 to 98.6 (Hughes et al. 2002).

Distinguishing features based on history, exam, neuroimaging, and ancillary tests can aid in the diagnostic certainty. All patients should undergo a complete history with thorough past medical history, medication history (past and current) and exposure history, general examination, and neurological examination. Special focus should be placed on cognitive testing, cranial nerve testing, especially eye movements, motor speed and tone, tremor evaluation, coordination, reflexes, and gait. Subsequent select neuroimaging and ancillary testing can aid in the diagnosis.

History/Physical. Several components of the patient's history and physical can give clues to the type of parkinsonian disorder present and subsequent treatment options.

1. *Clinical course.* The clinical course will be chronic and progressive in primary neurodegenerative diseases and more likely to be subacute to acute in drug-induced parkinsonism, vascular parkinsonism, and NPH.

2. *Symmetry of onset.* CBD tends to present asymmetrically, while PSP, MSA, and most forms of secondary parkinsonism will present with bilateral symptoms.

3. *Associated symptoms.* Key distinguishing associated symptoms include: early falls (PSP, NPH), early dementia (PSP, CBD), any autonomic or cerebellar symptoms (MSA), early urinary incontinence (NPH, MSA), limb apraxia or alien limb (CBD), and vascular risk factors or prior stroke (vascular parkinsonism).

4. *Medication history.* Treatment with a dopamine antagonist (see Table 3) up to 6 months prior to presentation can cause drug-induced parkinsonism.

5. *Exposure history.* A history of exposure to certain toxins such as manganese or carbon monoxide suggests a secondary toxin-related parkinsonism.

6. *Gait evaluation.* Certain characteristic gaits can be observed in parkinsonian disorders. In NPH, while the gait will be slow and shuffling like other parkinsonian disorders, step height may be smaller and arm swing relatively normal with normal posture. An apraxic gait also seen in NPH, in addition to CBD, will have short shuffling steps with start hesitation and frequent freezing in the absence of motor or sensory impairment (Rinne et al. 1994). The ataxic gait of MSA-C will be wide-based and unsteady.

7. *Lower body parkinsonism.* In cases of vascular parkinsonism and NPH, the legs are often affected with more severe rigidity and bradykinesia than the arms, leading to gait impairment as a primary complaint.

Neuroimaging. Imaging of the brain with either CT or MRI scan can provide supportive evidence in the diagnosis of some parkinsonian disorders. In cases of suspected CBD, an MRI scan may show asymmetric shrinkage of one half of the parietofrontal cortex. MRI scans of patients with PSP demonstrate atrophy of the tegmentum and tectum with dilation of the aqueduct at the level of the midbrain. In MSA, MRI findings can include putaminal atrophy, a hyperintense putaminal rim and a cruciform hyperintensity in the pons (Savoiardo 2003). To make the diagnosis of NPH, neuroimaging showing ventriculomegaly out of proportion to sulcal enlargement is needed (Figure 1). Unfortunately, ventriculomegaly is a common, non-specific finding on CT scans of the head in older adults.

Neuroimaging may also reveal evidence of prior ischemic changes, specifically in the basal ganglia, which would support a diagnosis of vascular parkinsonism. However, this is another common, non-specific finding on head CT scans of older adults.

Ancillary tests. Laboratory tests may be appropriate in certain settings such as history of toxic exposures (e.g. manganese, carboxyhemoglobin), tremor (e.g. thyroid stimulating hormone), cerebellar ataxia (e.g. genetic screening for inherited cerebellar degeneration), or dementia (e.g. vitamin B12, thyroid stimulating hormone). It is important in these cases to rule out other reversible causes of the patient's symptoms.

Temporary relief of symptoms after cerebrospinal fluid drainage may be a more specific indicator of the presence of NPH; however, diagnostic criteria remain controversial. Cerebrospinal fluid drainage can be achieved through either a large-volume lumbar puncture, that is, withdrawal of 40–50 ml of cerebrospinal fluid, or prolonged cerebrospinal fluid drainage via a spinal catheter. These supplemental tests increase the predictive accuracy of the NPH diagnosis (Marmarou et al. 2005).

Researchers are investigating serum and cerebrospinal fluid biomarkers and advanced neuroimaging techniques to help better diagnose causes of primary parkinsonism. Measurement of CSF tau forms may prove to be a reliable biomarker for PSP in the future (Borroni et al. 2008).

Treatment

PSP, MSA, and CBD usually respond poorly to the typical Parkinson's disease treatment of dopamine replacement with levodopa. In fact, levodopa can worsen orthostatic hypotension, particularly in MSA, and can worsen cognitive function or cause hallucinations. However, a trial of levodopa of as much as 1000 mg per day may be needed to exclude Parkinson's disease with a high response threshold. Failure to respond is strong evidence that an atypical parkinsonian disorder is the probable diagnosis.

If patients have no response to levodopa, there is no reason to try other dopaminergic agents, since they have less therapeutic potency and usually cause more side effects than levodopa. However, other treatments can provide symptomatic relief (Table 4). Botulinum toxin (BTX) injections may treat focal dystonias, such as eyelid opening apraxia, and spasticity or sialorrhea. Orthostatic hypotension can be treated non-pharmacologically with salt tablets, increased fluid intake, sleeping with the head of the bed elevated at 30 degrees, compression stockings, and abdominal binders. Specific drugs such as midodrine or fludrocortisone can also increase blood pressure when standing. It is important to note that supine hypertension can be a complication of therapy for orthostatic hypertension. Urinary incontinence can be managed with anticholinergic medications and constipation with a combination of high fiber diet, laxatives and stool softeners. The pseudobulbar aspects of parkinsonian disorders such as PSP can be effectively treated with tricyclic antidepressants, selective serotonin reuptake inhibitors, and guanfacine. Common sleep disorders like REM behavior disorder are effectively treated with low-dose clonazepam and sleep apnea with continuous positive airway pressure.

Nonpharmacologic therapies should be included in the management of patients with parkinsonian disorders. These include speech therapy for dysarthria or hypophonia, swallowing therapy and diet modification for dysphagia, and physical therapy for gait and mobility.

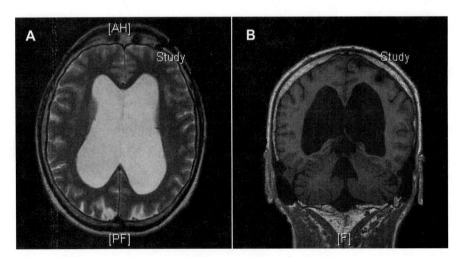

Figure 1 A) Axial T2-weighted brain MRI demonstrating enlarged ventricles out of proportion to sulcal loss as seen in idiopathic normal pressure hydrocephalus. B) Corresponding coronal T1-weighted brain MRI demonstrating same. Images courtesy of Dr. Roy H. Hamilton.

Table 4 Symptomatic Therapy for Primary Parkinsonian Disorders

Symptom	Treatment Options	Side Effects
Focal dystonias	Botulinum toxin injections	Excess weakness
Orthostatic hypotension	Salt tablets, increased fluid intake, sleeping with head of bed at 30 degrees, compression stockings, abdominal binders Midodrine, fludrocortisone	Supine hypertension
Urinary incontinence	Anticholinergic medications	Dry mouth, blurry vision, constipation, confusion
Constipation	High fiber diet Stool softeners Laxatives	Diarrhea, electrolyte disturbances
Pseudobulbar affect	Tricyclic antidepressants Selective serotonin reuptake inhibitors Guanfacine	Cardiac arrhythmia Serotonin syndrome Dizziness, fatigue
Sleep disorders ◆ Sleep apnea ◆ REM behavior disorder	Continuous positive airway pressure Clonazepam	Excess sedation
Depression	Tricyclic antidepressants Selective serotonin reuptake inhibitors	Cardiac arrhythmia Serotonin syndrome
Psychosis	Quetiapine Clozapine	Metabolic syndrome Agranulocytosis
Dementia	Memantine Cholinesterase inhibitors	Stevens-Johnson syndrome Worsening parkinsonism

Comorbid psychiatric conditions including depression and psychosis are frequently seen with the neurodegenerative disorders that cause parkinsonism: PSP, MSA, and CBD. It is important to treat depression with an antidepressant. Both tricyclic antidepressants and selective serotonin reuptake inhibitors are common first-line agents. If behavioral modification is insufficient, anti-psychotics may be needed for disorientation, hallucinations, or agitation. Atypical antipsychotics with the least extrapyramidal side effects such as quetiapine or clozapine are the best options, although clozapine will require frequent blood count monitoring given the increased risk of agranulocytosis with its use. Lastly, memantine or cholinesterase inhibitors are frequently used in the treatment of co-existing dementia. However, there have been no placebo-controlled trials of their efficacy in atypical parkinsonian disorders.

Treatment is also available for parkinsonism that is secondary to vascular disease. There is evidence that this form of parkinsonism may have some response to levodopa therapy (Zijlmans, Katzenschlager et al. 2004) or cerebrospinal fluid drainage (Ondo, Chan, and Levy 2002); however, rehabilitation is the most effective treatment (Guerini et al. 2004). The most important intervention is the initiation of secondary stroke prevention to prevent further brain injury (Sacco et al. 2006).

In cases of NPH, treatment with cerebrospinal drainage through a ventriculo-peritonial shunt is most effective if initiated early to prevent irreversible injury to the brain.

Treatment of parkinsonism in the setting of medication side effect includes the careful withdrawal of the offending drug or, if this is not possible, addition of an anti-cholinergic such as trihexyphenidyl.

Prognosis

PSP, CBD, and MSA are all chronic, progressive diseases that lead to increased morbidity due to dementia, falls, aspiration and immobility, and high mortality. Survival from time of diagnosis to death is less than nine years in MSA (Ben-Shlomo et al. 1997), five to ten years in PSP (Nath et al. 2003) and an average of seven years in CBD (Litvan, Grimes, and Lang 2000). Symptoms are relentlessly progressive and most patients become wheelchair bound, dysarthric, and dysphagic over a period of years. They lose their ability to communicate and lose their ability to swallow safely without aspiration. The discussion of potential feeding tube placement with the patient and the family is worthwhile before a feeding tube becomes necessary. End-of-life planning is essential.

On the other hand, drug-induced parkinsonism is generally reversible within 6–12 months, shunt placement for NPH has variable effectiveness, and secondary stroke prevention in the case of vascular parkinsonism can help prevent progression. Furthermore, intensive physical therapy can help improve walking and prevent falls.

Rehabilitation/Psychological Aspects

In all cases of parkinsonism, therapy should be considered. Physical therapy can help with gait, transfers, posture, balance, reaching and grasping, and overall mobility (Keus et al. 2009). In conjunction with physical therapy, occupational therapy may provide additional benefits. Specifically, weighted utensils or wrist weights may dampen tremor; many other assistive devices are available for home care.

Depression is a frequent co-morbidity in older adults with multiple medical conditions, especially parkinsonian disorders. In addition to the psychiatric treatment discussed above, supportive psychotherapy may be indicated. Changes in behavior, executive dysfunction, and memory loss may respond to cognitive/behavioral therapy.

Lastly, local patient support groups and national disease-specific organizations can provide additional resources and education for both the patient and family members. Counseling services are a useful, but oftentimes difficult to find, resource for patients and families dealing with a new diagnosis and potentially poor prognosis.

Future Directions

While parkinsonian signs in older adults are very common and lead to increased disability and mortality, we still do not understand who is at risk for developing subsequent parkinsonian disorders. We need better diagnostic tools to understand the mechanisms underlying the pathogenesis of parkinsonism which can, in turn, lead to the development of targeted treatment. Researchers are investigating the genetic and causal pathways, identifying potential cerebrospinal biomarkers, and using advanced neuroimaging to help in the timely and appropriate identification of primary parkinsonian disorders. Furthermore, potential curative, neuroprotective, or disease-modifying therapies to treat these primary neurodegenerative disorders are needed, and once established, will need to be initiated at the earliest stages for maximum benefit. Currently, clinical trials directed at the treatment of symptoms of parkinsonian disorders are in progress.

Summary

Parkinsonian disorders comprise a heterogeneous group of disorders which have a common presentation of bradykinesia, rigidity, tremor, and/or postural instability. A thorough history, examination and diagnostic work-up can help differentiate the cause and determine the best treatment and accurate prognosis.

References

Albers, D.S., S.J. Augood, L.C. Park, S.E. Browne, D.M. Martin, J. Adamson, et al. 2000. Frontal lobe dysfunction in progressive supranuclear palsy: Evidence for oxidative stress and mitochondrial impairment. *J Neurochem* 74:871–881.

Ben-Shlomo, Y., G. Wenning, F. Tison, N.P. Quinn. 1997. Survival of patients with pathologically proven multiple systems atrophy: A meta-analysis. *Neurology* 48:384–393.

Bennett, D. A., L. A. Beckett, A. M. Murray, K. M. Shannon, C. G. Goetz, D. M. Pilgrim, D. A. Evans. 1996. Prevalence of Parkinsonian signs and associated mortality in a community population of older people. *New England Journal of Medicine* 334 (2):71–76.

Borroni, B., M. Malinverno, F. Gardoni, A. Alberici, L. Parnetti, E. Premi, et al. 2008. Tau forms in CSF as a reliable biomarker for progressive supranuclear pasly. *Neurology* 71:1796–1903.

Bove, J., D. Prou, C. Perier, and S. Przedborski. 2005. Toxin-induced models of Parkinson's disease. *NeuroRx* 2 (3):484–494.

Dickson, D. W., C. Bergeron, S. S. Chin, C. Duyckaerts, D. Horoupian, K. Ikeda, K. et al. 2002. Office of Rare Diseases neuropathologic criteria for corticobasal degeneration. *J Neuropathol Exp Neurol* 61 (11):935–46.

Gallia, G.L., D. Rigamonti, and M.A. Williams. 2006. The diagnosis and treatment of idiopathic normal pressure hydrocephalus. *Nat Clin Prac Neurol* 2 (7):375–381.

Gomez-Haro, C., R. Espert-Tortajada, M. Gadea-Domenech, and J.F. Navarro-Humanes. 1999. Progressive Supranuclear Palsy: Neurological, neuropathological and neuropsychological aspects. *Rev Neurol* 29:936–956.

Guerini, F., G. B. Frisoni, C. Bellwald, R. Rossi, G. Bellelli, and M. Trabucchi. 2004. Subcortical vascular lesions predict functional recovery after rehabilitation in patients with L-dopa refractory parkinsonism. *J Am Geriatr Soc* 52 (2):252–6.

Hubble, J. 1993. Drug-induced parkinsonism. In *Parkinsonian syndromes*, edited by M. B. Stern, W. C. Koeller. New York: Marcel Dekker.

Hughes, A.J., S.E. Daniel, Y. Ben-Shlomo, and A.J. Lees. 2002. The accuracy of diagnosis of parkinsonian syndromes in a specialist movement disorder service. *Brain* 125:861–870.

Hurtig, H.I. 1993. Vascular parkinsonism. In *Parkinsonian syndromes*, edited by M. B. Stern, W. C. Koeller. New York: Marcel Dekker.

Indo, T., and K. Ando. 1982. Metoclopramide-induced Parkinsonism. Clinical characteristics of ten cases. *Arch Neurol* 39 (8):494–6.

Jankovic, J. 1995. Tardive syndromes and other drug-induced movement disorders. *Clin Neuropharmacol* 18 (3):197–214.

Keus, S.H.J., M. Munneke, M.J. Nijkrake, G. Kwakkel, and B.R. Bloem. 2009. Physical therapy in Parkinson's disease: Evolution and future challenges. *Mov Disord* 24 (1):1–14.

Kompoliti, K., C. G. Goetz, B. F. Boeve, D. M. Maraganore, J. E. Ahlskog, C. D. Marsden, K. P. et al. 1998. Clinical presentation and pharmacological therapy in corticobasal degeneration. *Archives of Neurology* 35:957–961.

Krauss, J. K., J. P. Regel, D. W. Droste, M. Orszagh, J. J. Borremans, and W. Vach. 1997. Movement disorders in adult hydrocephalus. *Mov Disord* 12 (1):53–60.

Litvan, I., D. Grimes, and A.E. Lang. 2000. Phenotypes and prognosis: clinicopathologic studies of corticobasal degeneration. *Adv Neurol* 82:183–196.

Litvan, I. and M. Hutton. 1998. Clinical and genetic aspects of progressive supranuclear palsy. *J Geriatr Psychiatry Neurol* 11:107–114.

Mahapatra, R. K., M. J. Edwards, J. M. Schott, and K. P. Bhatia. 2004. Corticobasal degeneration. *Lancet Neurol* 3 (12):736–43.

Marmarou, A., M. Bergsneider, P. Klinge, N. Relkin, and P.M. Black. 2005. The value of supplemental prognostic tests for the perioperative assessment of idiopathic normal-pressure hydrocephalus. *Neurosurgery* 57:S17–S28.

Masellis, M., P. Momeni, W. Meschino, R Jr. Heffner, J. Elder, C. Sato, et al. 2006. Novel splicing mutation in the progranulin gene causing familial corticobasal syndrome. *Brain* 129:3115–3123.

Morgante, L., A.E. Di Rossi, G. Savettieri, A. Reggio, F. Patti, G. Salemi, et al. 1996. Drug-induced parkinsonism: Prevalence, clinical features and follow-up in three Sicilian communities. *J. Neurol* 243:293–301.

Nath, U., Y. Ben-Shlomo, R.G. Thompson, A. J. Lees, and D. J. Burn. 2003. Clinical features and natural history of progressive supranuclear palsy: A clinical cohort study. *Neurology* 60:910–916.

Nutt, J. G. 2001. Classification of gait and balance disorders. *Adv Neurol* 87:135–141.

Ondo, W. G., L. L. Chan, and J. K. Levy. 2002. Vascular parkinsonism: Clinical correlates predicting motor improvement after lumbar puncture. *Mov Disord* 17 (1):91–7.

Pittman, A. M., H. C. Fung, and R. de Silva. 2006. Untangling the tau gene associations with neurodegenerative disorders. *Human Molecular Genetics* 15 (2):188–195.

Rail, D., C. Scholtz, and M. Swash. 1981. Post-encephalitic parkinsonism: Current experiences. *J Neurol Neurosurg Psychiatry* 44:670–676.

Rajput, A., and A. H. Rajput. 2001. Progressive supranuclear palsy: Clinical features, pathophysiology and management. *Drugs Aging* 18:913–925.

Rinne, J. O., M. S. Lee, P. D. Thompson, and C. D. Marsden. 1994. Corticobasal degeneration: A clinical study of 36 cases. *Brain* 117:1183–1196.

Sacco, R. L., R. Adams, G. Albers, M. J. Alberts, O. Benavente, K. Furie, et al. 2006. Guidelines for prevention of stroke in patients with ischemic stroke or transient ischemic attack: A statement for healthcare professionals from the American Heart Association/ American Stroke Association Council on Stroke: co-sponsored by the Council on Cardiovascular Radiology and Intervention: The American Academy of Neurology affirms the value of this guideline. *Stroke* 37 (2):577–617.

Savoiardo, M. 2003. Differential diagnosis of Parkinson's disease and atypical parkinsonian disorders by magnetic resonance imaging. *Neurol Sci* 24(suppl 1):S35–S37.

Schrag, A., Y. Ben-Shlomo, and N. Quinn. 1999. Prevalence of PSP and MSA: A cross-sectional study. *Lancet* 354:1771–1772.

Shannon, K. M. 1993. Hydrocephalus and parkinsonism. In *Parkinsonian Syndromes*, edited by M. B. Stern and W. C. Koeller. New York: Marcel Dekker.

Stern, M. B., and W. C. Koller, eds. 1993. *Parkinsonian Syndromes*. New York: Marcel Dekker.

Togaski, D. M., and C. M. Tanner. 2000. Epidemiologic aspects. *Adv Neurol* 82:53–59.

Trojanowski, J. Q., and T. Revesz. 2007. Proposed neuropathological criteria for the post mortem diagnosis of multiple system atrophy. *Neuropathol Appl Neurobiol* 33:615–620.

Wenning, G. K., F. Geser, M. Stampfer-Kountchev, and F. Tison. 2003. Multiple system atrophy: An update. *Mov Disord* 18: S34–S42.

Zijlmans, J. C., S. E. Daniel, A. J. Hughes, T. Revesz, and A. J. Lees. 2004. Clinicopathologic investigation of vascular parkinsonism, including clinical criteria for diagnosis. *Mov Disord* 19 (6): 630–640.

Zijlmans, J. C., R. Katzenschlager, S. E. Daniel, and A. J. Lees. 2004. The L-dopa response in vascular parkinsonism. *J Neurol Neurosurg Psychiatry* 75 (4):545–7.

24 Essential Tremor

Elizabeth Haberfeld and Elan D. Louis

Introduction

Essential tremor (ET) is one of the most common neurological disorders seen by general practitioners, geriatricians, and neurologists. The traditional view has been that ET is a relatively benign, monosymptomatic condition of little consequence. This view, however, has undergone revision in recent years. The emerging view is that ET is a progressive and often disabling neurological disorder characterized by a number of motor and non-motor features that accompany the readily recognizable action tremor.

Tremor in Human History: From Past to Present

Descriptions of human tremor phenomena, as well as evidence of their geographic ubiquity, are present in writings as old as those of ancient India (5000–3000 BC), Egypt (700 BC), Greece (~400 BC), and Israel (200 BC) (Louis 2000). These early records evidenced an awareness of tremor and the connection between heightened emotional states and emergence or worsening of tremors. The important distinction between kinetic tremor (occurring during visually-guided voluntary movements) and rest tremor (occurring when a limb is fully relaxed) (Table 1) was first noted by Galen of Pergamon (130–200 AD), and later by Sylvius de la Boe (1680), Van Swieten (1745), and Sauvages (1768) (Louis 2000). Among the most complete early accounts of ET was that of the New York neurologist Charles Dana (Dana 1887), who in the late nineteenth century described a pervasive action tremor in several large New York families. The term "essential" entered the lexicon in that era and gained greater usage during in the mid-twentieth century (Louis 2000; Louis et al 2008).

Epidemiology and Genetics

More than twenty studies have attempted to estimate the number of ET cases in populations around the world (Louis et al. 1998), but

Table 1 Glossary of Common Tremor Terms

Action tremor: tremor that occurs during voluntary contraction of skeletal muscle. Action tremor is sub-divided into kinetic tremor and postural tremor.

Kinetic tremor: tremor occurring during visually-guided voluntary movements like writing or touching finger to nose.

Postural tremor: tremor occurring in a body part that is maintained against gravity (e.g., arm tremor during sustained arm extension).

Rest tremor: tremor occurring when a limb is fully relaxed.

Intentional tremor: tremor that is present with visually-guided movement and increases in amplitude with approach to the target.

methodology has been inconsistent, and estimates have varied as a consequence. According to a recent population-based study that used improved methods (i.e., direct examination of all participants rather than use of a screening questionnaire), the prevalence of ET was 4.0% among individuals age > 40 years (Dogu et al. 2003b) making ET the most common tremor disorder. In this and other studies (Louis et al. 1998; Dogu et al. 2003b) prevalence increased with advancing age; ET was highly prevalent in the sixth through eighth decades of life, with prevalence estimates in the range of 6%–9% (Dogu et al. 2003b). The rate at which new ET cases arise (incidence) has been estimated in a population-based study in Spain: the adjusted incidence was 619 cases per 100,000 person-years (Benito-Leon et al. 2005a).

Although it is often stated that there is no increased risk of mortality in ET cases compared to similarly-aged controls, only a single retrospective cohort study supported that view (Rajput et al. 1984). Indeed, a recent three-year prospective, population-based study of the mortality risk in ET patients vs. controls found that the risk of mortality was increased by 45% (Louis et al. 2007e). The cause of this possible increased risk of mortality is unclear, but there is an association between ET and both prevalent and incident dementia (see below), suggesting at least one possible mechanism (Benito-Leon et al. 2006c; Bermejo-Pareja et al. 2007b).

Several risk factors for ET have been identified. First and most salient is age. Multiple epidemiological studies have shown an age-associated rise in incidence and prevalence of ET (Rajput et al. 1984; Louis et al. 1998; Dogu et al. 2003b; Mancini et al. 2007). Second, ethnicity may be a risk factor for ET, with a higher prevalence in whites than in African-Americans in some studies (Haerer et al. 1992; Louis et al. 1995). Third, a family history of ET is a risk factor for ET, as the disease is often familial (Tanner et al. 2001; Louis 2001b). Finally, although ET is predominantly seen in adults, it can begin in childhood, and is more common in boys than girls in that age group (Louis et al. 2005h). In adults, however, the prevalence is the same in both sexes (Louis et al. 1998).

Genetic factors have long been considered important in the etiology of ET because the disease can aggregate in families, many of which show an autosomal dominant pattern of inheritance (Gulcher et al. 1997; Higgins et al. 1998; Tanner et al. 2001; Louis 2001b; Louis et al. 2001k). Specific genes for ET have not yet been identified although linkage has been reported on three different chromosomes: 3q13 (ETM1), 2p22-p25 (ETM2), and 6p (Gulcher et al. 1997; Higgins et al. 1998; Shatunov et al. 2006). Other investigators have demonstrated the absence of linkage in ET families to any of these loci, indicating that there is further genetic heterogeneity (Kovach et al. 2001).

Twin studies have shown pairwise concordance ranging between 60% and 63% among monozygotic twins in two studies (Tanner et al. 2001; Lorenz et al. 2004), suggesting that environmental factors are important as well (Louis 2001b). Recent epidemiological studies have implicated several specific environmental factors (toxicants), namely β-carboline alkaloids (e.g., harmine and harmane, a group of highly tremorogenic dietary chemicals; Louis et al. 2002s; Louis et al. 2007n) and lead (Louis et al. 2003q; Dogu et al. 2007a) in ET. Further studies of putative environmental toxins are needed. Interestingly, one environmental factor, the Mediterranean diet, has been associated with lowered odds of ET (Scarmeas and Louis 2007); this is consistent with the lower prevalence of ET that some investigators have reported in Mediterranean countries (Mancini et al. 2007).

Clinical Presentation

The following diagnostic criteria for ET were proposed in the Consensus Statement of the Movement Disorder Society: (i) bilateral action tremor of the arm for five or more years (ii) either head tremor or action tremor of at least one arm that is moderate or severe (i.e., arm tremor resulting in difficulty with two or more activities of daily living or requiring medication), and (iii) action tremor is not the result of other movement disorders, medical conditions, or medications (Deuschl et al. 1998a).

As the criteria indicate, the hallmark feature of ET is an action tremor (Table 1) of the arms. It typically appears when the patient is performing activities of daily living such as writing, eating, or pouring (Figure 1). This tremor often has an intentional component as well (Table 1), meaning that it increases as the patient's limb approaches a target, as during the finger-nose finger test. Patients with more severe ET may also have a postural tremor (Table 1) (Brennan et al. 2002). A subset of patients with ET develop tremor at rest (Koller and Rubino 1985c; Rajput et al. 1993). The prevalence of rest tremor has been documented to be as high as 18.8% at one tertiary care center (Cohen et al. 2003). In that study, patients with longer disease duration and greater tremor severity were more likely to manifest rest tremor. The kinetic tremor of ET has a 4–12Hz frequency. The frequency tends to slow with advancing age (Brennan et al. 2002). It is usually seen in the arms, but the head and/or voice are frequently involved. Head tremor occurs

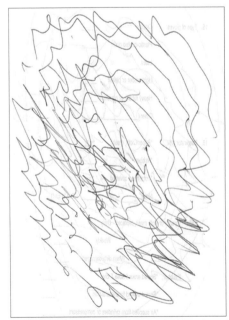

Figure 1 An ET patient's attempt to draw an Archimedes spiral. Regular oscillations are apparent.

in 30% to 50% of patients, with greater prevalence in women (Louis et al. 2000i; Louis et al. 2003j). Occasionally, the chin, tongue and legs are affected (Critchley 1949). Interestingly, a characteristic somatotopic spread over time occurs in ET. Head tremor typically evolves several years after the onset of arm tremor and the converse (spread of tremor from the head to the arms) is distinctly unusual (Critchley 1949; Larsson and Sjogren1960; Louis et al. 2003j; Rajput et al. 2004).

In general, the tremor in ET is gradually progressive (Critchley 1949; Rautakorpi 1978; Bain 1994; Louis et al. 2003o); however, longitudinal data are few. In one study (Elble 2000), patients were followed prospectively for a four-year period and there was a 7% increase in tremor amplitude each year, confirming the clinical anecdotal sense that the kinetic tremor in ET worsens gradually over time.

Indeed, despite the often held view of ET as a benign entity, more than 90% of patients who come to medical attention report disability (Louis et al. 2001c) and severely-affected end-stage patients are physically unable to feed or dress themselves (Louis et al. 2001c). Between 15% and 25% of clinic patients are forced to retire prematurely, and 60% choose not to apply for a job or promotion because of uncontrollable shaking (Rautakorpi 1978; Bain 1994). Most patients with this disorder must make adjustments in the way they perform their daily activities.

There is mounting evidence that the clinical features of this disease are not limited to the kinetic tremor alone, and that additional clinical features, both motor and non-motor, exist in patients with ET. Motor features beyond tremor can include cerebellar signs. Several studies (Singer et al. 1994; Stolze et al. 2000; Deuschl et al. 2000b) have observed postural instability and ataxic gait in patients with ET. Another observed subtle eye movement abnormalities in these patients (Helmchen et al. 2003). Non-motor features are predominantly cognitive and psychiatric. Multiple studies have described mild cognitive difficulties with deficits in verbal fluency, recent memory, and mental set-shifting, suggesting involvement of the frontal cortical or frontal cortical-cerebellar pathways (Gasparini et al. 2001; Lombardi et al. 2001; Vermilion et al. 2001; Lacritz et al. 2002; Duane and Vermilion 2002; Benito-Leon et al. 2006b). Beyond this, several recent studies have reported increased odds or risk of dementia in patients with ET compared to controls (Benito-Leon et al. 2006c; Bermejo-Pareja et al. 2007b). In one study of personality, patients with ET scored higher on measures of harm-avoidance (Chatterjee et al. 2004), suggesting that the non-motor features could involve the domain of personality. In another study (Louis et al. 2007d), depressive symptoms were more common in ET cases than controls, and these symptoms seemed to precede the onset of the motor manifestations, suggesting that they could be a primary manifestation of the disease. Finally, as in Parkinson's disease, an olfactory deficit has been reported in some studies of ET patients, although it is milder in ET than in PD (Louis and Jurewicz 2002m; Louis et al. 2003f; Applegate and Louis 2005).

Pathophysiology

For most of its history, ET was thought to be a disease lacking specific brain pathology. Until 2007, there were only 25 published postmortem studies of ET brains. Many were published 50–100 years ago, most did not use rigorous methodologies, and none used age-matched control brains (Frankl-Hochwart 1903; Bergamasco 1907; Hassler 1939; Mylle and Van Bogaert 1940; Mylle and Van Bogaert 1948; Herskovitz and Blackwood 1969; Lapresle et al. 1974; Boockvar et al. 2000; Rajput et al. 2004). No consistent pathological abnormality had been identified. The Essential Tremor Centralized Brain Repository was established in 2003 at Columbia University to collect postmortem tissue from ET patients, enabling researchers to assemble the largest-ever

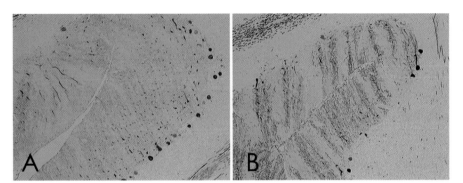

Figure 24.2 Degenerative changes in patients with cerebellar ET include a significant reduction in Purkinje cell number.

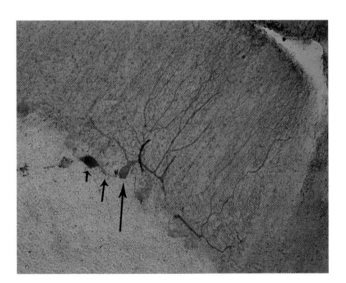

Figure 24.3 Purkinje cell torpedoes (swellings of the proximal portion of the Purkinje cell axon) occur in abundance in patients with cerebellar ET.

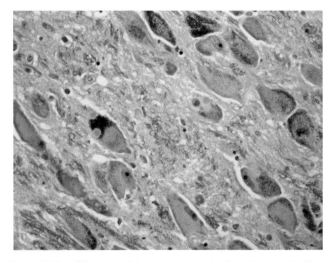

Figure 24.4 In ET cases with brain stem Lewy bodies, the Lewy bodies are distributed primarily in the locus ceruleus (in the pons).

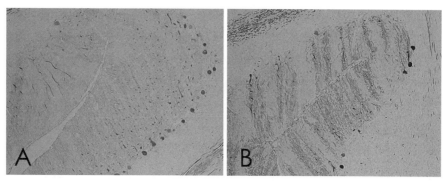

Figure 2 Degenerative changes in patients with cerebellar ET include a significant reduction in Purkinje cell number. See Figure 24.2 on the color insert.

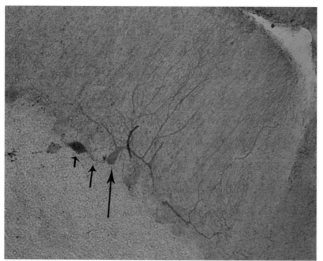

Figure 3 Purkinje cell torpedoes (swellings of the proximal portion of the Purkinje cell axon) occur in abundance in patients with cerebellar ET. See Figure 24.3 on the color insert.

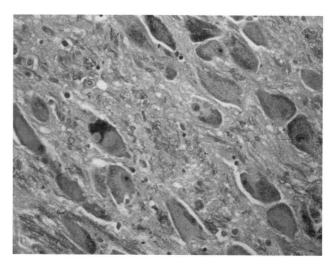

Figure 4 In ET cases with brain stem Lewy bodies, the Lewy bodies are distributed primarily in the locus ceruleus (in the pons). See Figure 24.4 on the color insert.

series of ET brains for study. A 2007 study (Louis et al. 2007g) of 33 ET brains and 21 controls demonstrated that ET brains are divisible into two groups, namely, a majority (75.8%) with cerebellar degenerative changes ("ET with cerebellar pathology") and no Lewy bodies, and a minority (24.2%) with brain stem Lewy bodies ("Lewy body variant of ET") and relatively normal cerebellae (Louis et al. 2005l; Louis et al. 2006p; Louis et al. 2007g; Louis 2007q; Axelrad et al. 2008).

In those with cerebellar pathology, degenerative changes include a significant loss of Purkinje cells (Figure 2) and an increase in Purkinje cell torpedoes (swellings of the proximal portion of the Purkinje cell axon, presumably in response to injury) (Figure 3), with Purkinje cell heterotopia and dendrite swellings (Louis and Vonsattel 2007q; Axelrad et al. 2008). In the cases showing brain stem Lewy bodies (Figure 4), the Lewy bodies are distributed primarily in the locus ceruleus (in the pons). This differs from Parkinson's disease, in which Lewy bodies form in the substantia nigra pars compacta (in the midbrain) as well as other structures. This restricted Lewy body deposition pattern is unlike that seen in normal aging or incidental Lewy body disease (Louis et al. 2005l; Louis and Vonsattel 2007q).

The 2007 series helped localize the possible source of the ET tremor to alterations in the cerebellum and its connecting pathways. The primary cerebellar pathology is most direct, but the Lewy body variant is also a logical pathological pattern to produce the ET tremor, given the connections involved. The neurons of the locus ceruleus are the major source of norepinephrine in the brain; they also synapse with cerebellar Purkinje cells. Impaired activity in the locus ceruleus could result in a diminution of stimulatory output from that locus to the Purkinje cells. The cerebellar Purkinje cells are inhibitory output neurons. Thus, the net result would be reduction in the normal inhibitory output from the cerebellum (Louis and Vonsattel 2007w). Whether through primary cerebellar degeneration, or secondary effects on cerebellar outflow as a result of locus ceruleus involvement, the consequence is de-regulation (through decreased cerebellar inhibitory output) of the neuronal pathway that involves the cerebellum, thalamus, and motor cortex (i.e., the cerebellar-thalamic-cortical pathway).

Clinical Investigations and Differential Diagnosis

The diagnosis of ET is largely clinical and based on the history and physical examination; laboratory tests are indicated in select instances. Important questions to ask in the history are those regarding location of the tremor, age of onset, and progression over time. Amelioration of the tremor with ethanol is a particularly useful diagnostic clue. The clinician should inquire about a family history of shaking, the patient's current use of caffeine, cigarettes, and ethanol, and should elicit a thorough medication history. Numerous medications (e.g., valproate, lithium, prednisone, tacrolimus, asthma inhalers) can exacerbate enhanced physiologic tremor, which resembles the early stages of ET. Because hyperthyroidism can also cause kinetic tremor, one should inquire about its symptoms (diarrhea, weight loss, and heat intolerance).

Physical examination of the patient with tremor comprises an assessment of tone (by passively moving the patient's wrist and elbow while the arm is relaxed), bradykinesia (by having the patient perform rapid finger taps, repeated grip movements, or rapid alternating movements, with each hand individually), followed by evaluation of the tremor. A tremor is by definition oscillatory, alternating around a central plane; and rhythmic, meaning regularly recurring. It is important to focus on the features of the tremor, which the following physical maneuvers facilitate: (1) postural tremor: the patient should hold the arms extended palms-down in front of the body for ten seconds (2) kinetic tremor: finger-nose-finger maneuver, or ask the patient to pour water between two cups (3) rest tremor: examine the arms while they are resting in the patient's lap or while he or she is walking or lying down. An assessment of balance and gait is necessary.

By using the maneuvers outlined above, ET usually can be distinguished from several other diseases that also involve tremor. Primary among these is Parkinson's disease. Mild to moderate postural or kinetic tremor may be present in both ET and PD (Koller et al. 1989e; Jankovic et al. 1999). However, rest tremor is present in approximately 85% of patients with autopsy-proved Parkinson's disease (Louis et al. 1997). Rest tremor can accompany ET, but usually only in the setting of longstanding kinetic tremor. The postural tremor of ET also tends to involve wrist flexion and extension whereas in Parkinson's disease, wrist rotation often occurs. Further, unlike ET patients, Parkinson's disease patients exhibit other signs of Parkinsonism, including rigidity and bradykinesia.

It is generally true that the kinetic tremor in ET has a higher amplitude and lower frequency than that of enhanced physiological tremor, although this is not always the case. Hence, distinguishing mild ET from pronounced enhanced physiologic tremor may be difficult. Head tremor, when present, is a sign of ET and is not a feature of enhanced physiological tremor. If needed, some tertiary centers offer quantitative computerized tremor analysis, with accelerometers attached to the arms: inertial loading of the limbs during tremor analysis leads to a reduction in tremor frequency in ET tremor but not in enhanced physiological tremor.

ET patients may have gait ataxia and an intentional component to their tremor, as do patients with spinocerebellar ataxia. However, the two groups can be distinguished by other features. ET patients seldom exhibit nystagmus or scanning or dysarthric speech.

Finally, laboratory tests are sometimes indicated. Thyroid function tests are appropriate for patients with symptoms or signs of hyperthyroidism. Patients under 40 with kinetic tremor should have a serum ceruloplasmin to check for possible Wilson's disease. In truly ambiguous cases, striatal dopamine transporter imaging can help distinguish patients with ET (generally similar to those of controls) from those with Parkinson's disease (generally reduced values) (Benamer 2000; Antonini 2001). Such testing is seldom necessary however, after a thorough clinical assessment by an experienced clinician.

Treatment

The treatment of ET involves pharmacotherapy (Table 2) and surgery. Medications are appropriate if there is functional disability or embarrassment (Louis 2005; Zesiewicz et al. 2005). Surgery has a role in severe, disabling cases that are refractory to medications.

Current data suggest that two neurochemical systems may play a role in the pathophysiology and modulation of ET: the gamma amino-butyric acid (GABA)-ergic system in the central nervous system (CNS) and the adrenergic system (beta-2 muscular adrenoreceptors) on the muscle spindles (Rincon and Louis 2005). Cerebellar Purkinje

Table 2 Oral Medications Used in the Treatment of ET

Medication	Usual Starting Dose	Therapeutic Doses	Side Effects
Propranolol	10 mg per day	10 to 320 mg per day	Fatigue, bradycardia, hypotension, depression, exercise intolerance
Primidone	50 mg per day	50 to 1,000 mg per day	Sedation, nausea, vomiting, unsteadiness
Gabapentin	300 mg per day	300 to 3,600 mg per day	Drowsiness, nausea, dizziness, unsteadiness
Topiramate	25 mg per day	25–400 mg per day	Paresthesias, weight loss, taste perversion, fatigue, nausea, somnolence
Alprazolam	0.25 mg per day	0.25 to 2.75 mg per day	Sedation, fatigue

cells are densely GABA-ergic, and GABA is the major inhibitory neurotransmitter in the CNS. Thus, it is plausible that a disturbance of the GABA system underlies the tremor of ET, and as plausible that GABA-enhancing medications would ameliorate it. Primidone, benzodiazepines, and barbiturates (all GABA-ergic) have therapeutic value in patients with ET. Notably, so does ethanol, which binds to the GABA-$_A$ receptor, facilitating GABA-ergic neurotransmission (Rincon and Louis 2005). Adrenoreceptors are located deep in the striated muscle outside of the nervous system; they probably play a role in the peripheral modulation of ET. Propranolol and other beta-adrenergic receptor blocking medications for ET appear to work through this mechanism.

Several treatment issues require special emphasis. First, a large proportion of patients do not benefit from any medication; factors that predict this lack of response have not been identified. Second, patients who respond to medications are often only partial responders, and tremor is rarely reduced to asymptomatic levels. The discussion that follows is largely limited to medications that have undergone scrutiny in double-blind trials. Propranolol and primidone are the two front line agents (Table 2).

Peripheral beta-adrenergic receptors (Jefferson et al. 1979) most probably mediate the effects of beta-adrenergic blocking agents like propranolol. Propranolol, given in doses of 120 mg/day or more, significantly reduces tremor severity (Tolosa and Loewenson 1975). In the elderly these doses may be difficult to achieve because of dose-dependent bradycardia. In addition, the following relative contraindications (Packer et al. 1999) do not preclude the use of propranolol, but make its use more difficult: asthma, congestive heart failure, diabetes mellitus, and atrioventricular block. Several beta-1 selective beta-blockers, including sotalol and atenolol, appear to be effective in the management of ET but propranolol, a non-selective antagonist, has been the most consistently studied and is more effective than relatively selective beta-1 antagonists (Jefferson et al. 1979). One crossover study found arotinolol to be as effective as propranolol (Lee et al. 2003). One study demonstrated that sustained-release propranolol is as effective as conventional propranolol (Cleeves and Findley 1988).

Primidone is an anti-convulsant medication that is partially metabolized to phenylethylmalonamide and phenobarbital. Both the barbiturate metabolite and the parent compound are thought to mediate most of the therapeutic effect (Findley et al. 1985; Sasso et al. 1990; Gorman et al. 1986), and primidone is superior to phenobarbital alone in reducing tremor (Sasso et al. 1988). In doses of up to 750 mg/day, primidone significantly reduces tremor compared with placebo (Findley et al. 1985; Gorman et al. 1986; Sasso et al. 1988; Sasso et al. 1990). However, tolerability is a common problem. Even at a low starting dose (62.5 mg/day), an acute toxic reaction, consisting of nausea, vomiting, or ataxia has been reported in 22.7% (Findley et al. 1985) to 72.7% (Sasso et al. 1990) of patients. One study found that the use of a very low initial dose (2.5 mg in suspension) and a graduated titration schedule did not appear to improve primidone tolerability (O'Suilleabhain and Dewey 2002). However, pre-medicating patients with phenobarbital (30 mg bid for three days) may improve tolerability by activating the liver's P450 system. Sedation is another side effect that often limits the attainable dose in the elderly.

The two front-line agents, propranolol and primidone, have been compared to one another in several studies (Gorman et al. 1986; Koller and Royse 1986b), but neither has been conclusively shown to be superior to the other. While initial tolerability is a sizeable problem with primidone, one study provides tentative evidence that long-term tolerability of primidone is superior to that of propranolol. In a study of 25 ET patients, acute adverse reactions occurred in 8% with propranolol and 32% with primidone; however, "significant" side effects after one year occurred in 0% with primidone compared with 17% taking propranolol (Koller et al. 1989e).

Several additional agents have been used with variable efficacy in the treatment of patients with ET. Gabapentin is an anticonvulsant medication that is structurally similar to the inhibitory neurotransmitter GABA. In two of three clinical trials, gabapentin (1,200 to 3,600 mg/day) resulted in a significant reduction in tremor compared with placebo, and in one of the two its effect was similar to that of propranolol (Gironell et al. 1999; Pahwa et al. 1998; Ondo et al. 2000). Gabapentin is generally well-tolerated. Pregabalin, a GABA isomer, was tested in a pilot randomized placebo-controlled trial that demonstrated its efficacy at reducing tremor as measured by accelerometry (mean dose, 287 +/− 100 mg/day) (Zesiewicz et al. 2007). Topiramate, an anticonvulsant agent with mixed effects (including effects of GABA-$_A$ receptors) was administered to 24 patients at a single center and that study demonstrated a significant anti-tremor effect (Connor 2000). A multi-center double-blind trial in which 208 patients were randomized found that topiramate (mean maintenance dose = 292 mg/day) was more effective than placebo in treating ET, although side effects (paresthesia, fatigue, somnolence) were very common (Ondo et al. 2006). Benzodiazepines potentiate the effect of GABA by binding to the GABA-$_A$ receptor. In one trial (Huber and Paulson 1988), alprazolam (dose ranging from 0.75 to 2.75 mg/day) resulted in significant reduction in tremor compared with placebo, and 75% of patients demonstrated at least some improvement. However, another agent, clonazepam, has shown variable efficacy in clinical trials (Thompson et al. 1984; Biary and Koller 1987b), with one of these trials demonstrating no improvement compared with placebo (Thompson et al. 1984). One problem with the benzodiazepines is that their anti-tremor effect often comes at a dose that is associated with sedation and/or cognitive slowing. Sodium oxybate (Frucht et al. 2005) has demonstrated some efficacy in open-label studies of ET. Its mechanism of action may involve the GABA system, as its precursor is GABA.

A number of other agents have also been used on an empirical basis. Calcium channel blockers have had variable success in treating ET. In one trial, flunarizine resulted in a significant reduction in tremor compared with placebo; 13 of 15 patients improved; however, none of the patients improved in a second trial (Curran and Lang 1993). In one trial (Biary et al. 1995a), nimodipine (30 mg/day) resulted in a significant reduction in tremor compared with placebo; 8 of 15 patients improved, however there are no further data regarding its efficacy. Clozapine, an atypical neuroleptic agent, effectively reduced tremor in one clinical trial (Ceravolo et al. 1999), although there are no further data and the possibility of agranulocytosis has limited the use of this agent. More recently, zonisamide, an anticonvulsant with multiple mechanisms of action, was used in a cross-over trial (zonisamide or arotinolol). Zonisamide resulted in significant tremor reduction (Mortia et al. 2005). It was also effective at controlling tremor in a small, uncontrolled sample of patients with features of both ET and PD (Bermejo 2007a). Levetiracetam is another anticonvulsant whose exact mechanism of action is unknown. In a recent double-blind, placebo-controlled trial, a single 1,000 mg dose of levetiracetam produced a significant reduction of hand tremor for at least two hours (Bushara et al. 2005b).

In summary, propranolol and primidone remain the two front-line agents in the treatment of ET. Several other agents have shown promise and further studies are needed to examine their efficacies and compare them with the two front line agents.

Intramuscular botulinum toxin injections have the potential to reduce arm tremor by producing weakness. Patients with ET received 50–100 U per arm in trials (Jankovic et al. 1996). These studies have shown a significant reduction in tremor amplitude but have not always demonstrated a significant improvement in function; in addition, moderate hand and finger weakness is a common side effect. Intramuscular botulinum toxin injections may play more of a role in the treatment of head tremor, particularly because oral medications tend to be less effective in treating the head than the arm tremor of ET.

For advanced, disabling and medication-refractory cases, surgery with deep brain stimulation may be the best option. Because ET appears to be mediated by neuronal loops that pass from the cerebellum to the cortex by way of the ventral intermediate nucleus of the thalamus, the main surgical approach that is currently used is continuous deep-brain stimulation through an electrode implanted in the ventral intermediate nucleus of the thalamus. The procedure is effective in reducing tremor. Patients with moderate to severe tremor at baseline demonstrate marked improvement of tremor after treatment (Schuurman et al. 2000). The clinician has the ability to adjust the stimulator settings during follow-up care (Hariz et al. 2002). Several studies also have evaluated the use of gamma knife thalamotomy, reporting favorable results (Niranjan et al. 2000; Young et al. 2000), particularly in reducing action tremor and ameliorating handwriting. It may be useful for patients unable to undergo open surgery (Kondziolka et al 2008). However, deep-brain stimulation remains the surgical treatment of choice.

Non-prescription agents such as ethanol also traditionally have played a role in the treatment of ET. The effect of ethanol on tremor has been demonstrated in several studies (Growden et al. 1975; Koller and Biary 1984a). However, several factors limit its use. Older patients take medications with which the concurrent use of ethanol is often contraindicated; many have concerns about dependence as well as the social stigma of ethanol use. 1-octanol is an alcohol that is currently used as a food-flavoring agent. In a recent randomized, placebo-controlled trial of 12 ET patients, a single 1mg/kg oral dose of 1-octanol significantly decreased tremor amplitude for up to 90 minutes and no significant side effects or signs of intoxication were observed (Bushara et al. 2004a). Further studies are warranted.

Conclusion

ET is one of the most commonly-encountered neurological diseases among the elderly. The traditional view of ET as a trivial mono-symptomatic condition of little consequence is being replaced with a more scientific and comprehensive account of the entire disease process, its physiology, pathology, clinical features, and treatment.

Increasingly, it appears that ET shares features with other recognized neurodegenerative diseases. As our understanding of neurodegenerative disease changes, conditions once thought to be monolithic are now conceptualized as varying pathologies sharing overlapping clinical features. Our understanding of ET is evolving in this direction. The emerging pathological evidence, as well as observed clinical, genetic, and pharmacological heterogeneity, suggests that this entity may be a composite of several disease processes: a family of diseases unified by the presence of kinetic tremor. Ultimately, ET might represent a complex of diseases rather than a single disease entity. These may eventually be more appropriately classified as "the essential tremors."

References

Antonini A, Moresco RM, Gobbo C, et al. The status of dopamine nerve terminals in Parkinson's disease and essential tremor: A PET study with the tracer [11-C]FE-CIT. *Neurol Sci* 2001;22:47–48.

Applegate LM and Louis ED. Essential tremor: Mild olfactory dysfunction in a cerebellar disorder. *Parkinsonism Related Disord* 2005;11:399–402.

Ashenhurst EM. The nature of essential tremor. *CMAJ* 1973;109:876–878.

Axelrad JE, Louis ED, Honig LS, et al. Reduced Purkinje cell number in essential tremor: A postmortem study. *Arch Neurol* 2008;65:101–107.

Bain PG, Findley LJ, Thompson PD, et al. A study of heredity of essential tremor. *Brain* 1994;117:805–824.

Benamer TS, Patterson J, Grosset DG, et al. Accurate differentiation of parkinsonism and essential tremor using visual assessment of [123I]-FP-CIT SPECT imaging: The [123I]-FP-CIT study group. *Mov Disord* 2000;15:503–510.

Benito-Leon J, Bermejo-Pareja F, and Louis ED. Incidence of essential tremor in three elderly populations of central Spain. *Neurology* 2005;64:1721–1725.

Benito-Leon J, Louis ED, and Bermejo-Pareja F. Population-based case-control study of cognitive function in essential tremor. *Neurology* 2006;66:69–74.

Benito-Leon J, Louis ED, and Bermejo-Pareja F. Elderly onset essential tremor is associated with dementia. The NEDICES study. *Neurology* 2006;66:1500–1505.

Bergamasco I. Intorno ad un caso di tremore essenziale simulant in parte il quadro della sclerosi multipla. *Riv Pat Nerv Ment* 1907;115:80–90.

Bermejo PE. Zonisamide in patients with essential tremor and Parkinson's disease. Mov Disord. 2007 Oct 31;22(14):2137–8.

Bermejo-Pareja F, Louis ED, and Benito-Leon J. Risk of incident dementia in essential tremor: A population-based study. *Mov Disord* 2007;22:1573–1580.

Biary N, Bahou Y, Sofi MA, Thomas W, and Al Deeb SM. The effect of nimodipine on essential tremor. *Neurology* 1995;45:1523–1525.

Biary N and Koller W. Kinetic predominant essential tremor: Successful treatment with clonazepam. *Neurology* 1987;37:471–474.

Boockvar J, Telfeian A, and Baltuch GH. Long-term deep brain stimulation in a patient with essential tremor: Clinical response and postmortem correlation with stimulator termination sites in ventral thalamus. *J Neurosurg* 2000;93:140–144.

Brennan KC, Jurewicz E, Ford B, Pullman SL, and Louis ED. Is essential tremor predominantly a kinetic or a postural tremor? A clinical and electrophysiological study. *Mov Disord* 2002;17:313–316.

Bushara KO, Goldstein SR, Grimes GJ, JR., Burstein AH, and Hallett M: Pilot trial of 1-octanol in essential tremor. *Neurology* 2004;62:122–124.

Bushara KO, Malik T, and Exconde RE. The effect of levetiracetam on essential tremor. *Neurology* 2005;64:1078–1080.

Ceravolo R, Salvetti S, Piccini P, et al. Acute and chronic effects of clozapine in essential tremor. *Mov Disord* 1999;14:468–472.

Chatterjee A, Jurewicz EC, Applegate LM, and Louis ED. Personality in essential tremor. *J Neurology Neurosurg Psychiatry* 2004;75:958–961.

Cleeves L and Findley LJ. Propranolol and propranolol-LA in essential tremor: A double blind comparative study. *J Neurology Neurosurg Psychiatry* 1988;51:379–384.

Cohen O, Pullman S, Jurewicz E, Watner D, and Louis ED. Rest tremor in essential tremor patients: Prevalence, clinical correlates, and electrophysiological characteristics. *Arch Neurol* 2003;60:405–410.

Connor GS. Efficacy of topiramate in treatment of essential tremor: A randomized, double-blind, placebo-controlled, cross-over study. *Ann Neurol* 2000;48:486.

Constantino AEA and Louis ED. Unilateral disappearance of essential tremor after cerebral hemispheric infarct. *J Neurol* 2003;250:354–355.

Critchley M. Observations on essential tremor (heredofamilial tremor). *Brain* 1949;72:113–139.

Curran T and Lang AE. Flunarizine in essential tremor. *Clin Neuropharm* 1993;16: 460–463.

Dana CL. Hereditary tremor, a hitherto undescribed form of motor neurosis. *Amer J Med Sci* 1887;94:386–389.

Deuschl G, Bain P, Brin M. Consensus statement of the movement disorder society on tremor. Ad Hoc scientific committee. *Mov Disord* 1998;13 Suppl 3:2–23.

Deuschl G, Wenzelburger R, Loffler K, Raethjen J, Stolze H. Essential tremor and cerebellar dysfunction. Clinical and kinematic analysis of intention tremor. *Brain* 2000;123:1568–1580.

Dogu O, Louis ED, Tamer L, Unal O, Yilmaz A, Kaleagasi H. Elevated blood lead concentrations in essential tremor: A case-control study in Mersin, Turkey. *Environ Health Perspect* 2007 Nov; 115(11):1564–8.

Dogu O, Sevim S, Camdeviren H, et al. Prevalence of essential tremor: Door-to-door neurological exams in Mersin Province, Turkey. *Neurology* 2003;61:1804–1807.

Duane DD and Vermilion KJ. Cognitive deficits in patients with essential tremor. *Neurology* 2002;58:1706.

Elble RJ. Essential tremor frequency decreases with time. *Neurology* 2000;55:1547–1551.

Findley LH, Cleeves L, and Calzetti S. Primidone in essential tremor of the hands and head: A double blind controlled clinical study. *J Neurology Neurosurg Psychiatry* 1985;48:911–915.

Frankl-Hochwart. *La degenerescence hepato-lenticulaire (maladie de Wilson, pseudo-sclerose)*. Masson et Cie, Paris 1903.

Frucht SJ, Houghton WC, Bordelon Y, Louis ED, and Greene PE. Sodium oxybate (Xyrem®) for myoclonus and essential tremor: Tolerability and efficacy. *Mov Disord* 2005;20:1240.

Gasparini M, Bonifati V, Fabrizio E, et al. Frontal lobe dysfunction in essential tremor. A preliminary study. *J Neurol* 2001;248:399–402.

Gironell A, Kulisevsky J, Barbanoj M, Lopez-Villegas D, Hernandez G, Pascual-Sedano B. A randomized placebo-controlled comparative trial of gabapentin and propranolol in essential tremor. *Arch Neurol* 1999;56:475–480.

Gorman WP, Cooper R, Pocock P, and Campbell MJ. A comparison of primidone, propranolol, and placebo in essential tremor, using quantitative analysis. *J Neurology Neurosurg Psychiatry* 1986;49:64–68.

Growden JH, Shahani BT, and Young RR. The effect of alcohol on essential tremor. *Neurology* 1975;25:259–262.

Gulcher JR, Jonsson P, Kong A, et al. Mapping of a familial essential tremor gene, FET1, to chromosome 3q13. *Nature Genetics* 1997;17:84–87.

Haerer AF, Anderson DW, and Schoenberg BS. Prevalence of essential tremor. Results from the Copiah county study. *Arch Neurol* 1992;39:750–751.

Hariz GM, Lindberg M, and Bergenheim AT. Impact of thalamic deep brain stimulation on disability and health-related quality of life in patients with essential tremor. *J Neurol Neurosurg Psychiatry* 2002;72:47–52.

Hassler R. Zur pathologischen anatomie des senilen und des parkinsonistischen tremor. *J Psychol Neurol* 1939;49:193–230.

Helmchen C, Hagenow A, Miesner J, et al. Eye movement abnormalities in essential tremor may indicate cerebellar dysfunction. *Brain* 2003;126:1319–1332.

Herskovitz E and Blackwood W. Essential (familial, hereditary) tremor: A case report. *J Neurology Neurosurg Psychiatry* 1969;32:509–511.

Higgins JJ, Loveless JM, Jankovic J, and Patel PI. Evidence that a gene for essential tremor maps to chromosome 2p in four families. *Mov Disord* 1998;13:972–977.

Higgins JJ, Pho LT, and Nee LE. A gene (ETM) for essential tremor maps to chromosome 2p22-p25. *Mov Disord* 1997;12:859–864.

Hubble J P, Busenbark KL, Pahwa R, Lyons K, and Koller WC. Clinical expression of essential tremor: Effects of gender and age. *Mov Disord* 1997;12:969–972.

Huber SJ and Paulson GW. Efficacy of alprazolam for essential tremor. *Neurology* 1988;38:241–243.

Jankovic J, Schwartz K, Clemence W, Aswad A, and Mordunt J. A randomized, double-blind, placebo-controlled study to evaluate botulinum toxin type A in essential hand tremor. *Mov Disord* 1996;11:250–256.

Jankovic J, Schwartz KS, and Ondo W. Re-emergent tremor of Parkinson's disease. *J Neurol Neurosurg Psychiatry* 1999;67:646–650.

Jefferson D, Jenner P, and Marsden CD. B-Adrenoreceptor antagonists in essential tremor. *J Neurology Neurosurg Psychiatry* 1979;42:904–909.

Koller WC and Biary N. Effect of alcohol on tremors: Comparison with propranolol. *Neurology* 1984;34:221–222.

Koller WC and Royse VL. Efficacy of primidone in essential tremor. *Neurology* 1986;36:121–124.

Koller WC and Rubino FA. Combined resting postural tremors. *Arch Neurol* 1985;42:683–684.

Koller WC, and Vetere-Overfield B. Acute and chronic effects of propranolol and primidone in essential tremor. *Neurology* 1989;39:1587–1588.

Koller WC, Vetere-Overfield B, and Barter R. Tremors in early Parkinson disease. *Clin Neuropharmacol* 1989;12:293–297.

Kondziolka D, Ong JG, Lee JY, et al. Gamma knife thalamotomy for essential tremor. *J Neurosurg* 2008 Jan; 255(1): 103–11.

Kovach MJ, Ruiz J, and Kimonis K. Genetic heterogeneity in autosomal dominant essential tremor. *Genet Med* 2001;3:197–199.

Lacritz LH, Dewey R Jr., Giller C, and Cullum CM. Cognitive functioning in individuals with "benign" essential tremor. *J Int Neuropsychol Soc* 2002;8:125–9.

Lapresle J, Rondot P, and Said G. Tremblement idopathique de repos, d'attitude et d'action. Etude anatomo-clinique d'une observation. *Rev Neurol* 1974;130:343–348.

Larsson T and Sjogren T: Essential tremor: A clinical and genetic population study. *Acta Psychiatrica Et Neurologica Scandinavica* 1960:36 (S 144);1–176.

Lee KS, Kim JS, et al. A multicenter randomized crossover multiple-dose comparison study of arotinolol and propranolol in essential tremor. *Parkinsonism Relat Disord* 2003; 9:341–347.

Lombardi WJ, Woolston DJ, Roberts WJ, and Gross RE. Cognitive deficits in patients with essential tremor. *Neurology* 2001;57:785–790.

Lorenz D, Frederiksen H, Moises H, Kopper F, Deuschl G, and Christensen K. High concordance for essential tremor in monozygotic twins of old age. *Neurology* 2004;62:208–211.

Lou JS and Jankovic J. Essential tremor: Clinical correlates in 350 patients. *Neurology* 1991;41:234–238.

Louis ED. Essential tremor (Seminal Citations Section). *Arch Neurol* 2000;57:1522–1524.

Louis ED. Essential tremor. *N Engl J Med* 2001a;345:887–891.

Louis ED. Etiology of essential tremor: Should we be searching for environmental causes? *Mov Disord* 2001b;16:822–829.

Louis ED. Essential tremor. *Lancet Neurology* 2005;4:100–110.

Louis ED, Barnes LF, Albert SM, et al. Correlates of functional disability in essential tremor. *Mov Disord* 2001c;16:914–920.

Louis ED, Benito-Leon J, Bermejo-Pareja F. Self-reported depression and anti-depressant medication use in essential tremor: Cross-sectional and prospective analyses in a population-based study. *Eur J Neurol* 2007d;14:1138–1146.

Louis ED, Benito-Leon J, Ottman R, and Bermejo-Pareja F. A population-based study of mortality in essential tremor. *Neurology* 2007e;69:1982–1989.

Louis ED, Bromley SM, Jurewicz EC, Watner D. Olfactory dysfunction in essential tremor: A deficit unrelated to disease duration or severity. *Neurology* 2002f;59:1631–1633.

Louis ED, Broussolle E, Goetz CG, Krack P, Kaufmann P, Mazzoni P. Historical underpinnings of the term "essential tremor" in the late nineteenth century. *Neurology* 2008;71:856–859.

Louis ED, Faust PL, Vonsattel JPG, Honig LS, Rajput A, Robinson CA, et al. Neuropathological changes in essential tremor: 33 cases compared with 21 controls. *Brain* 2007g;130:3297–3307.

Louis ED, Fernandez-Alvarez E, Dure LS 4th, Frucht S, Ford B. Association between male gender and pediatric essential tremor. *Mov Disord* 2005h Jul;20(7):904–6.

Louis ED, Ford B, and Barnes LF. Clinical subtypes of essential tremor. *Arch Neurol* 2000i;57:1194–1198.

Louis ED, Ford B, and Frucht S. Factors associated with increased risk of head tremor in essential tremor: A community-based study in northern Manhattan. *Mov Disord* 2003j;18:432–436.

Louis ED, Ford B, Frucht S, Barnes LF, Tang M-X, and Ottman R. Risk of tremor and impairment from tremor in relatives of patients with essential tremor: A community-based family study. *Ann Neurol* 2001k;49: (6):761–9.

Louis ED, Honig LS, Vonsattel JPG, Maraganore DM, Borden S, and Moskowitz CB. Essential tremor associated with focal non-nigral Lewy bodies: A clinical-pathological study. *Arch Neurol* 2005l;62:1004–1007.

Louis ED, and Jurewicz EC. Olfaction in essential tremor patients with and without isolated rest tremor. *Mov Disord* 2003m;18: 1387–1389.

Louis ED, Jurewicz EC, Applegate L, et al. Association between essential tremor and blood lead concentration. *Environ Health Perspect* 2003n;111:1707–1711.

Louis ED, Jurewicz EC, and Watner D. Community-based data on associations of disease duration and age with severity of essential tremor: Implications for disease pathophysiology. *Mov Disord* 2003o;18:90–93.

Louis ED, Klatka LA, Lui Y, and Fahn S. Comparison of extrapyramidal features in 31 pathologically confirmed cases of diffuse Lewy body disease and 34 pathologically confirmed cases of Parkinson disease. *Neurology* 1997;48:376–380.

Louis ED, Marder K, Cote L, et al. Differences in the prevalence of essential tremor among elderly African-Americans, whites and Hispanics in Northern Manhattan, NY. *Arch Neurol* 1995;52:1201–1205.

Louis ED, Ottman R, and Hauser WA. How common is the most common adult movement disorder?: Estimates of the prevalence of essential tremor throughout the world. *Mov Disord* 1998;13:5–10.

Louis ED, Vonsattel JPG, Honig LS, Ross GW, Lyons KE, and Pahwa R. Neuropathological findings in essential tremor. Neurology 2006p;66:1756–1759.

Louis ED, and Vonsattel JP. The emerging neuropathology of essential tremor. *Mov Disord* 2007q;23:174–182.

Louis ED, Zheng W, Jurewicz EC, et al. Elevation of blood β-carboline alkaloids in essential tremor. *Neurology* 2002r;59:1940–1944.

Louis ED, Zheng W, Mao X, and Shungu DC. Blood harmane is correlated with cerebellar metabolism in essential tremor: a pilot study. *Neurology* 2007s Aug 7;69(6):515–20.

Mancini ML, Stracci F, Tambasco N, et al. Prevalence of essential tremor in the territory of Lake Trasimeno, Italy: Results of a population-based study. *Mov Disord* 2007 Mar 15;22(4):540–5.

Mortia S, Miwa H, and Kondo T. Effect of zonisamide on essential tremor: A pilot crossover study in comparison with arotinolol. *Parkinsonism Relat Disord* 2005;11:101–103.

Mylle G and Van Bogaert L. Etudes anatomo-cliniques de syndromes hypercinetiques complexes. I. Sur le tremblement familial. *Mschr Psychiatr Neurol* 1940;103:28–43.

Mylle G andVan Bogaert L. Du tremblement essentiel non familial. *Monatsschr Psychiatr Neurol* 1948;115:80–90.

Niranjan A, Kondziolka D, Baser S, Heyman R, and Lunsford LD. Functional outcomes after gamma knife thalamotomy for essential tremor and MS-related tremor. *Neurology* 2000 55:443–446.

Ondo W, Hunter C, Dat Vuong K, Schwartz K, and Jankovic J. Gabapentin for essential tremor: A multiple-dose, double-blind, placebo-controlled trial. *Mov Disord* 2000;15:678–682.

Ondo WG, Jankovic J, Connor GS, et al. Topiramate in essential tremor. A double-blind, placebo-controlled trial. *Neurology* 2006 Mar 14;66(5):672.

O'Suilleabhain P and Dewey RB Jr. Randomized trial comparing primidone initiation schedules for treating essential tremor. *Mov Disord* 2002;17:382–386.

Packer M, Cohn JN, Abraham WT, et al. Consensus recommendations for the management of chronic heart failure. *Am J Cardiology* 1999;83:1A–38A.

Pahwa R, Lyons K, Hubble JP, et al. Double-blind controlled trial of gabapentin in essential tremor. *Mov Disord* 1998;13:465–467.

Rajput AH, Offord KP, Beard CM, and Kurkland LT. Essential tremor in Rochester, Minnesota: A 45-year study. *J Neurol Neurosurg Psychiatry* 1984;466–470.

Rajput A, Robinson C, and Rajput AH. Essential tremor course and disability: A clinicopathologic study of 20 cases. *Neurology* 2004;62:932–936.

Rajput AH, Rozdilsky B, Ang L, and Rajput A. Significance of Parkinsonian manifestations in essential tremor. *Can J Neurol Sci* 1993;20:114–117.

Rautakorpi I. *Essential Tremor. An epidemiological, clinical and genetic study.* Research Reports from the Department of Neurology, University of Turku, Finland 1978;12

Rincon F, and Louis ED. Benefits and risks of pharmacological and surgical treatments for essential tremor: Disease mechanisms and current management. *Expert Opin Drug Saf* 2005;4:899–913.

Rocca WA, Bower JH, Ahlskog JE, et al. Increased risk of essential tremor in first-degree relatives of patients with Parkinson's disease. *Mov Disord* 2007 Aug 15;22(11):1607–14.

Sasso E, Perucca E, and Calzetti S. Double-blind comparison of primidone and phenobarbitol in essential tremor. *Neurology* 1988;38:808–810.

Sasso E, Perucca E, Fava R, Calzetti S. Primidone in the long-term treatment of essential tremor: A prospective study with computerized quantitative analysis. *Clin Neuropharm* 1990;13:67–76.

Scarmeas N and Louis ED. Mediterranean diet and essential tremor: A case-control study. *Neuroepidemiology* 2007;29(3-4):170–7.

Schuurman PR, Bosch DA, Bossuyt PMM, et al. A comparison of continuous thalamic stimulation and thalamotomy for suppression of severe tremor. *N Engl J Med* 2000;432:461–468.

Shahed J and Jankovic J. Exploring the relationship between essential tremor and Parkinson's disease. *Parkinsonism Realt Disord* 2007 Mar;13(2)67–76.

Shatunov A, Sambuughin N, Jankovic J, et al. Genomewide scans in North American families reveal genetic linkage of essential tremor to a region on chromosome 6p23. *Brain* 2006;129:2318–2331.

Singer C, Sanchez-Ramos J, and Weiner WJ. Gait abnormality in essential tremor. *Mov Dis* 1994;9:193–196.

Stolze H, Petersen G, Raethjen J, Wenzelburger R, and Deuschl G. Gait analysis in essential tremor- further evidence for a cerebellar dysfunction. *Mov Disord* 2000;15 (Suppl 3):87.

Tan EK, Lee SS, Fook-Chong S, and Lum SY. Evidence of increased odds of essential tremor in Parkinson's disease. *Mov Disord* 2008 May 15;23(7):993–7.

Tanner CM, Goldman SM, Lyons KE, et al. Essential tremor in twins: An assessment of genetic vs. environmental determinants of etiology. *Neurology* 2001;57:1389–1391.

Thompson C, Lang A, Parkes JD, and Marsden CD. A double-blind trial of clonazepam in benign essential tremor. *Clin Neuroparm* 1984;7:83–88.

Tolosa ES and Loewenson RB. Essential tremor: Treatment with propranolol. *Neurology* 1975;25:1041–1044.

Vermilion K, Stone A, and Duane D. Cognition and affect in idiopathic essential tremor. *Mov Disord* 2001;16:S30.

Young RF, Jacques K, Mark R, et al. Gamma knife thalamotomy for treatment of tremor: Long-term results. *J Neursurg* 2000;93: 128–135.

Zesiewicz TA, Elble R, Louis ED, et al. Practice parameter: Therapies for essential tremor. Report of the Quality Standards Subcommittee of the American Academy of Neurology. *Neurology* 2005;64:2008–2020.

Zesiewicz TA, Ward CL, Hauser RA, et al. A pilot, double-blind, placebo-controlled trial of pregabalin (Lyrica) in the treatment of essential tremor. *Mov Disord* 2007 Aug 15;22(11):1660–3.

25   Gait Disturbances in Aging

Ron Ben-Itzhak, Talia Herman,
Nir Giladi, and Jeffrey M. Hausdorff

Background and Epidemiology

Mobility limitations and gait disturbances often have devastating consequences, especially among older adults. These limitations involve a complex interaction of multiple systems that often reflect the integrated effects of aging on health and function. Gait problems associated with aging may lead to injury, disability, loss of independence, and institutionalization. Falls are one of the most serious complications of gait disturbances (Figure 1). According to figures released in 2006 by the United States Centers for Disease Control and Prevention (CDC), about 5.8 million (15.9%) persons aged 65 years and older reported falling at least once during just a three month period, and 1.8 million (31.3%) of those who fell sustained an injury that resulted in a doctor's visit or restricted activity for at least one day (Stevens et al. 2006).

Gait disturbances are also a bio-marker for the future development of cardiovascular disease and dementia (Verghese et al. 2002; Bloem et al. 2000) (Figure 2), possibly reflecting an early, pre-clinical underlying cerebrovascular and/or neurodegenerative disease. Gait disorders among the elderly are associated with reduced survival, reduced cardiovascular fitness, and death from underlying disease

(Wilson et al. 2002). Although there is no clear standard for "normal" gait in older adults, abnormal gait patterns can often be easily identified, even by an untrained observer (Alexander 1996). Given the predictive nature of gait alterations, some have suggested that observational analysis of gait may be viewed as a gross, general marker of neuromuscular function, analogous to a "mini" neurological assessment.

Regardless of the underlying mechanisms, gait disorders are common in elderly populations and their prevalence increases with age. At the age of 60 years, about 85% of the population have a normal gait, but at the age of 85 years or older, some estimate that less than 20% have a normal gait (Sudarsky 2001; Sudarsky 1990). In a sample of non-institutionalized older adults aged 85 years or more, the incidence of limitation in walking was over 54% (Ostchega et al. 2000). Similarly, Bloem et al. (1992) evaluated 142 elderly subjects over 88 years of age; 61% claimed distinct diseases as a cause of gait impairment, while only 18% of all responders had a completely normal gait. In addition, they stated that many elderly have a gait disturbance of variable clinical nature and unclear pathologic basis, which may represent the so called "idiopathic senile gait." In the Einstein Aging Study of 488

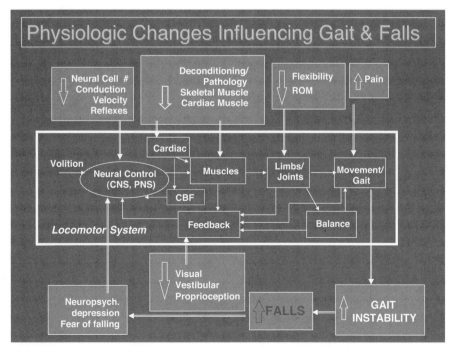

Figure 1 Simplified block diagram of the locomotor system and some of changes that occur with aging and disease that affect gait instability and fall risk. Modified from Hausdorff et al. 2001.

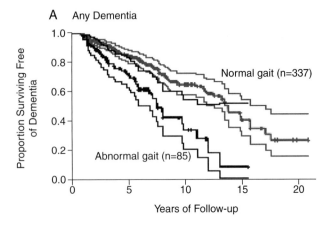

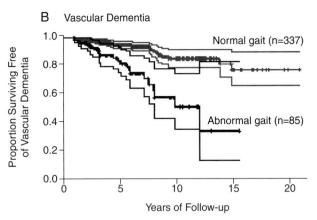

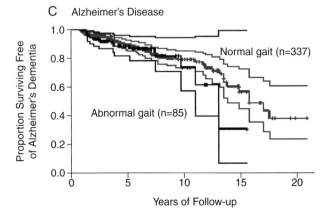

Figure 2 Kaplan-Meier curves for the cumulative risk of any dementia (Panel A), vascular dementia (Panel B), and Alzheimer's disease (Panel C) according to baseline gait status. Dotted lines represent 95 percent confidence intervals. Adapted from Verghese et al. 2002.

community-residing older adults, the prevalence of abnormal gait was 35% and the incidence of abnormal gait was 168.6 per 1,000 person-years and increased with age (Verghese et al. 2006). These abnormal gait patterns were associated with greater risk of institutionalization and death (Verghese et al. 2006).

A growing body of evidence suggests that gait disorders are not an inevitable consequence of aging but rather they reflect the increased prevalence of age-associated diseases (Bloem et al. 1992) (Figure 3).

Indeed, many gait disorders among the elderly appear in connection with underlying diseases (e.g., stroke, hip fracture, Parkinson's disease), particularly as disease severity increases (Tables 1 and 2). Similar gait abnormalities are common to many diseases. It is, therefore, often difficult to attribute the gait disorder in older adults to one disease etiology (Alexander 1996) rather than underlying neurological and non-neurological diseases.

The highest incidence of falls in older persons occurs *while walking*, although falls in older individuals can also result from sudden loss of postural stability (e.g., falling from a ladder, postural hypotension) (Lipsitz et al. 1991). This is especially true in more demanding or less familiar environments, such as settings with many distractions, environmental hazards, or obstacles (Hill et al. 1999; Sehested and Severinnielsen 1977; Tinetti et al. 1986; Nyberg and Gustafson 1995; Blake et al. 1988; Connell and Wolf 1997). Gait changes and falls in the elderly have been associated with a range of biomechanical, vestibular/sensory, and disease-related mechanisms that accompany aging, including progressive degeneration of sensory systems and diminished sensory input from the lower extremities (Calne 1980). These changes, however, are often not sufficient to explain the age-associated increase in poor balance and fall risk (Alexander 1994), implicating the role of additional factors. For example, as detailed further below, cognitive deficits also likely independently contribute to this process (Buchner and Larson 1987; Yogev-Seligmann, Hausdorff and Giladi, 2008).

To summarize, gait disorders are common in older adults and are predictors of several factors critical to health-related quality of life, including, for example, mobility, cognitive decline, morbidity and mortality. The etiology of these disorders in the elderly is usually multi-factorial, thus requiring a comprehensive assessment of different sensorimotor levels including medical, functional, and cognitive performance, and as needed, laboratory and imaging assessments.

Effects of Normal Aging on Gait

Normal gait requires constant balancing of interacting motor, sensory, and neuronal systems and consists of three primary domains: locomotion, equilibrium, and interrelations with the environment (Nutt and Marsden 1993). Before any motor response is determined, including execution of gait, there are three basic components or dimensions that provide input into the system. These components reflect physiological, cognitive, and affective processes.

Physiological Dimension

This component refers to the range of basic motor/skeletal/sensory processes that are involved in movement. These include (but are not limited to) factors such as biomechanical processes (e.g., muscle strength, range of motion, nerve conduction velocity), sensory processes (e.g., vision and proprioception), and vestibular functioning.

Cognitive Dimension

This component encompasses fundamental cognitive processes, including basic attention skills such as alertness and arousal, language, episodic and semantic memory, visual spatial skills and related navigation ability, and information processing speed. The degree to which any one of these domains is involved in a response is determined by the task itself, though attention has been shown to be involved in even the most basic postural stability tasks (Teasdale et al. 1993; Teasdale, Stelmach, and Breunig 1991). Working memory abilities may be important in the recall of motor schemas and retention of task instructions, as well as recalling directions and routes while walking. Visual spatial skills and navigation are involved in maneuvering successfully

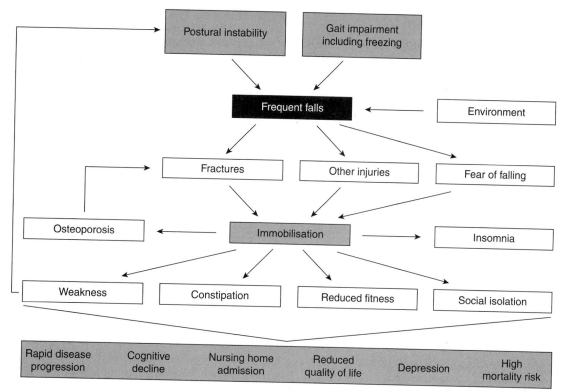

Figure 3 Clinical impact of instability and falls. Note the vicious cycle that arises as a result of gait instability and impairment. Adapted from Bloem, Hausdorff et al. 2004.

Table 1 Classification of Gait Syndromes

Peripheral Origin

- Musculo-skeletal disturbances
- Joint, bones, or neuromuscular
- Sensory disturbances: position, vestibular, or visual

Central, System Predominant

- Pyramidal—Plegic/paretic
- Cerebellar—Ataxic
- Extrapyramidal—Parkinsonian, dyskinetic
- Frontal
  - Disequilibrium
  - "Apractic"
  - Anxious, fear of falling
- **Unclassified**

Adapted from Giladi et al., 2007

Table 2 Temporal Characteristics of Gait Disturbances

Continuous	Episodic
• Hemiparetic gait	• Freezing of gait
• Antalgic gait	• Start/turning hesitation
• Spastic gait	• Tight quarters hesitation
• Bradykinetic gait	• Hesitation while reaching destination
• Hypotonic gait	• Hesitation during mental over-load or stressful situations
• Ataxic gait	
• Shuffling gait	
• Disequilibrium gait	• Festinating gait
• Fear of falling gait	• Paroxysmal disequilibrium—vestibular
• Disrhythmic gait	• Psychogenic gait
• Dyskinetic gait	• Light headed, pre-fainting, sudden weakness episodes
• Stiffed gait	
• Hypokinetic gait with/without increased cadence	

Adapted from Giladi et al., 2007.

in space, while language skills may be important to understand the thread of concurrent conversations while walking or verbal directions.

Behavioral/Affective Dimension

This component emphasizes the importance of studying the impact of both cognitive and emotional factors on gait and motor performance, especially in older individuals (Tinetti, Speechley, and Ginter 1988). Affective states at the time of completing tasks, as well as perceptions of task demands and inherent risks, can be very essential in understanding variability found across studies attempting to identify significant predictors of fall risk. Moreover, self-perception of motor abilities

can have a direct influence on outcomes (Alexander et al. 2000; Cress et al. 1995).

One area that has been studied in some detail is the role of anxiety on balance impairment leading to falls (Yardley and Redfern 2001; Balaban and Thayer 2001). Even in healthy, young adults, links between anxiety experienced in the laboratory setting, and balance and postural sway have been found (Wada, Sunaga, and Nagai 2001; Bolmont et al. 2002). Cautiousness or hesitation in a response, often attributed to behavioral change with aging (Woollacott and Shumway-Cook 2002), may also affect motor outcomes. For example, among older individuals, there is a strong link between fear of falling (see further below) and both mobility performance in the laboratory and fall risk in the community (Hill et al. 1999; Tinetti, Richman, and Powell 1990; Tinetti et al. 1994). In a study of older adults living in the community, scores on the Falls Efficacy Scale (FES), as well as self-ratings for anxiousness, depressed mood, and general willingness to take risks, were significantly related to both self-report and performance-based measures of functional status (Alexander et al. 2000; Giordani et al. 1995; Giordani et al. 1995). In addition, more global mood disturbances such as clinical depression have been shown to impact mobility-related factors, including gait speed, in older individuals (Cress et al. 1995).

It is well documented that aging has detrimental effects on many aspects of these three basic dimensions. As sensory and other physiological systems decline with age, individuals demonstrate increased reliance on already limited sensory systems, such as vision. For example, older persons require longer periods of direct visual information (look down more often) when walking over simple or more complex walkways (Anderson 1993; Patla and Vickers 1997). As a result of this increased reliance on already taxed sensory systems, the cognitive control demands for completing even relatively simple tasks increase with age due to the need to compensate for these age-associated changes. Increased attention is necessary in order to "heighten" the signal coming from peripheral sensory systems, and executive control processes are required to effectively interpret and combine the sensory information that is available to integrate the necessary information for proper motor planning to maintain postural control (Shumway-Cook et al. 1997).

Concomitant with physical and sensory changes with aging, mechanisms related to cognitive control and supervision also decrease in efficiency, and some are disproportionately compromised by older age (Albert and Moss 1984). The decline in executive function in older adults often includes changes in inhibitory control, mental flexibility, problem solving skills, divided attention, and working memory. These represent skills that the executive control dimension relies upon to integrate information and compensate for age-related changes to other physical systems. Essentially, with advancing age, cognitive control mechanisms are more and more called for but less and less able to counteract wide-ranging adverse consequences of sensory, motor, basic cognitive and affective changes (Welford 1958). This can lead to inefficient interpretation and integration of already compromised incoming information and result in an impaired ability to efficiently allocate these resources, resulting in inappropriate motor programs that potentially exacerbate fall risk.

Affective changes also occur with age, including a tendency to approach tasks in a more cautious way that often results in an altered response (Li, Meyer, and Thornby 2001). Only minimal research has been directed to describe the different approaches that younger and older persons take when facing complex mobility tasks. Aging does appear to affect the selection of different responses in successfully adjusting to competing cognitive and motor demands while walking (Kemper, Herman, and Lian 2003). Older persons' adjustments, however, although initially appearing to be more cautious, could actually lead to increased risk of tripping or falls (e.g., early step initiation to clear obstacles may increase the risk of later foot contact with an obstacle during final foot placement) (Chen et al. 1996; Schrodt et al. 2004).

Age-associated physiological changes (specifically in gait characteristics) generally appear between the 6th to 7th decade of life (Whittle 1996) (Table 3). These changes may include: prolongation of gait cycle time, thus increasing stride time, reduced gait speed by 10–20%, reduced cadence (number steps per minute) and shorter step length. In addition, prolonged double limb support time was found as well as slight widening of the base of support (Whittle 1996; Elble 1997; Jancovic, Nutt, and Sudarsky 2001; Watelain 2000). With aging, there is a reduced range of motion especially in the lower extremities, flatter

Table 3 Gait Changes that are Common with Aging

Although slight changes occur in "successful," healthy aging, the healthy gait pattern is largely intact

Decrease	Increase
Gait speed	Double limb support
Stride length	Hip strategy for balance control
Cadence	Widening of the base of support
Flexibility and range of motion	Stride-to-stride variability
	Reaction time
Muscle strength	

foot meets the ground, reduced range of plantar flexion, reduced push power developing while pushing off and general weakness within total body muscles, mostly the foot extensors muscles (Whittle 1996; Elble 1997; Jancovic, Nutt, and Sudarsky 2001; Watelain 2000). These changes may enable better adaptation of the older adult with respect to a safer and more stable gait, controlling more efficiently the equilibrium during walking. One of the implicit motivations for this adaptation is to reduce the time of the single leg support (which is very challenging to equilibrium), and reduce gait speed in order to better interact with environmental hazards and external factors (Jancovic, Nutt, and Sudarsky 2001). The stride dynamics (i.e., stride-to-stride variability) are also affected by subtle age-associated changes in physiology in older adults (Yogev-Seligman et al. 2008; Hausdorff et al. 1997) and may serve as a marker for instability and reduced automaticity, thus explaining the association with increasing fall risk (Hausdorff, Edelberg et al. 1997; Hausdorff, Rios, Edelberg 2001).

To summarize, gait changes associated with age are sometimes difficult to differentiate from disease-related gait disturbances because many functions that are utilized during normal walking inevitably deteriorate over the years as part of the aging process. Aging-associated gait disturbances can be affected by deterioration of vision, proprioception, or vestibular function and may reflect weakening of skeletal muscles, as well as degenerative joint changes in the limbs or in the spinal column. In addition to alterations in the motor system, cognitive changes with disturbances in executive functions, attention, visuospatial orientation, and reaction time all can lead to changes in locomotion. Awareness of deterioration in the quality of responses is a common cause for insecurity, which is a characteristic of nonspecific gait disturbances in the elderly (e.g., cautious gait). Overall, it is good practice to look for a specific cause for any gait disturbance, even in an elderly person, and not to relate it to normal aging.

Balance and Equilibrium in the Elderly

Traditionally, postural control was considered an automatic process, though recent studies have shown that such basic neuropsychological or cognitive processes as attention are necessary for balance maintenance (Macpherson et al. 1989; McIlroy and Maki 1993; Nashner and Woollacott 1979). Across the age range, increasing motor demand (e.g., rising from sitting to standing, transfers) has been shown to require increased attentional control (Woollacott and Shumway-Cook 2002). Walking is even a more complex process than standing itself, with different postural and balance requirements (Lajoie et al. 1996). Specifically, walking has been described as essentially a series of episodes of loss of balance and recovery (during the different phases of the gait cycle) in a continually changing environment (Downtown and Andrews 1990). Whereas aspects of attentional control may be critical for posture and balance, walking involves a range of cognitive systems for response selection, monitoring, and adjustment to environmental, as well as physical and other age-related changes.

It is widely recognized that older people with balance disorders typically suffer from multiple impairments, such as multi-sensory loss, weakness, orthopedic constraints and cognitive impairments. Postural control is no longer considered one system or a set of righting and equilibrium reflexes. Rather, postural control is considered a complex motor skill derived from the interaction of multiple sensorimotor processes (Horak, Shupert, and Mirka 1989). The two main functional goals of postural control are postural orientation and postural equilibrium. Postural orientation involves the active control of the body alignment and tone with respect to gravity, support surface, visual environment, and internal references. Spatial orientation in postural control is based on the interpretation of convergent sensory information from somatosensory, vestibular, and visual systems. Postural equilibrium involves the coordination of sensorimotor strategies to stabilize the body's center of mass (CoM) during both self-initiated and externally triggered disturbances in postural stability. There are several important resources required for postural stability and orientation:

Biomechanical Constraints

These are: degrees of freedom, strength, and limits of stability. The most important biomechanical constraint on balance is the size and quality of the base of support: the feet. Any limitations in size, strength, range, pain, or control of the feet will affect balance. Control of the body (CoM) with respect to its base of support is the most important biomechanical constraint on balance control. In stance, the limits of stability is the area within which the individual can move his body (CoM) and maintain equilibrium without changing the base of support. It is a cone-shaped space. Equilibrium is not a particular position but a space determined by the size of the support base (feet in stance) and the limitations on joint range, muscle strength, and sensory information available to detect the limits. The CNS has an internal representation of this cone space of stability that it uses to determine how to move to maintain equilibrium. In many elderly people with balance disorders, this cone of stability is often very small or their central neural representations of this cone of stability are distorted, both of which affect their selection of movement strategies to maintain equilibrium. Subjects prone to falls tend to have small limits of stability. It is important for the CNS to have an accurate central representation of the stability limits of the body. Basal ganglia disorders, such as Parkinson's disease, may result in abnormal representation of limits of stability, leading to postural instability.

Cognitive Processing

Many cognitive resources are required in postural control. Standing quietly requires cognitive processing as can be seen by increased reaction times in persons standing, compared to persons sitting with support. The more difficult the postural task, the more cognitive processing is generally required. Reaction times and performance in a cognitive task decline as the difficulty of the postural task increases (Teasdale and Simoneau 2001; Teasdale et al. 1993). Much of the cognitive processing is executive function (EF), in particular attention and concentration. Control of posture as well as cognitive processing share cognitive resources; performance of postural tasks is also impaired by a secondary cognitive task (dual task). Individuals who have limited cognitive processing due to neurological deficits may use more of their available processing capabilities to control posture. Falls can result from insufficient cognitive processing to control posture while occupied with a secondary cognitive task (Melzer, Benjuya, and Kaplanski 2001).

Control of Dynamics

Three main types of movement strategies can be used to return the body to equilibrium in a stance position: Two strategies keep the feet in place and the other strategy changes the base of support through stepping or reaching. The ankle strategy, in which the body moves at the ankle as a flexible inverted pendulum, is appropriate to maintain balance for small amounts of sway when standing on a firm surface. The hip strategy, in which the body exerts torque at the hips to quickly move the body CoM, is used when the individual stands on a narrow or compliant surface that does not allow adequate ankle torque or when the CoM must be moved quickly. Taking a step to recover equilibrium is common, especially during gait and when keeping the feet in place is not important. However, even when individuals step in response to an external perturbation, they first attempt to return the CoM to the initial position by exerting angle toque. An elderly individual at risk of falling tends to use the stepping, reaching, and hip strategies more than an individual with a low risk of falling who uses the ankle strategy to maintain postural stability. Anticipatory postural adjustments, prior to voluntary movement, also help to maintain stability by compensating for anticipated destabilization associated with moving a limb. Subjects with poorly coordinated automatic postural reflexes show postural instability in response to external perturbations whereas subjects with poorly coordinated anticipatory postural adjustments show postural instability during self-initiated movements (Horak, Shupert, and Mirka 1989).

Orientation in Space

These are: perception, gravity, surfaces vision, and verticality. The ability to orient the body parts with respect to gravity, the support surface, visual surround, and internal references is a critical component of postural control. Healthy individuals can identify gravitational vertical in the dark to within 0.5 degrees. Studies have shown that perception of verticality, or upright, may have multiple neural representations (Karnath, Ferber, and Dichgans 2000). The perception of visual verticality, the ability to align a line to gravitational vertical in the dark, is independent of the perception of postural (or proprioceptive) verticality. The internal representation of visual but not postural, verticality is tilted in persons with unilateral vestibular loss, whereas the internal representation of postural, but not visual, verticality is tilted in persons with hemi-neglect due to stroke. A tilted or inaccurate internal representation of verticality will result in automatic postural alignment that is not aligned with gravity and, therefore, renders a person unstable.

Sensory Strategies

Sensory integration and sensory reweighing are the main sensory strategies. Sensory information from somatosensory, visual, and vestibular systems must be integrated to interpret complex sensory environments. In a well-lit environment with a firm base of support, healthy persons rely on somatosensory (70%), vision (10%), and vestibular (20%) information (Horak, 2006). However, when they stand on an unstable surface, they increase sensory weighting to vestibular and visual information as they decrease their dependence on surface somatosensory inputs for postural orientation. The ability to re-weight sensory information depending on the sensory context is important for maintaining stability when an individual moves from one sensory context to another, such as from a well-lit sidewalk to a dimly lit garden. Individuals with peripheral vestibular loss or somatosensory loss from neuropathy are limited in their ability to re-weight postural sensory dependence and, thus, are at risk of falling in particular sensory contexts. Some CNS disorders, such as

Alzheimer's disease, may impair the ability of the CNS to quickly re-weight sensory dependence, even when the peripheral sensory system is intact.

Age-associated Changes in Cognitive Function: Effects on Gait

It is well established that healthy older adults generally undergo age-related decline in cognition (Robbins et al. 1998). The *Diagnostic and Statistical Manual of Mental Disorders (DSM)-IV* defines age-related cognitive decline as an objectively identified decline in cognitive functioning consequent to the aging process that is within normal limits given the person's age. Individuals with this condition may report problems remembering names or appointments or may experience difficulties in solving complex problems.

One of the keys to age-associated change in cognitive function that impact on gait is executive function (EF). EF refers to a variety of higher cognitive processes that utilize and modify information from posterior cortical sensory systems to modulate and produce behavior. These integrative functions include both cognitive and behavioral components that are necessary for effective, goal-directed actions and for the control of attentional resources which are at the basis of the ability to manage independent activities of daily living (Yogev-Seligmann, Hausdorff, and Giladi 2008). Lezak (1995) divided executive function into several major components: volition, planning, self-awareness, response inhibition, purposive action, and effective performance (action monitoring). Impairment of one or more of these components of EF may impact one's ability to walk efficiently and

safely. For example, one aspect of volition, impaired self-awareness of limitations, might be a critical risk factor for falling. Impaired planning skills could result in getting lost or choices that produce inefficient pathways or unnecessary effort to arrive at the destination (Table 4).

EF and Aging Process

The frontal lobes are apparently highly susceptible to age-associated changes (Craik and Grady 2002; Lorenz-Reuter 2000; Dorfman 1998). There is, however, a great variability of these frontal brain changes among aging individuals in terms of the magnitude, time of performance, and the influence of education and lifestyle (Buckner 2004; Kramer 2003). Although it is generally agreed that there is an overall cognitive slowing with aging, and that there is a decline in some aspects of EF, such as mental flexibility, abstract thinking, and attention, this does not necessarily reach the level of "dysfunction" and there is no consensus regarding the precise pattern of altered executive function that results from age-associated changes (Lezak 1995). Therefore, in a clinical setting, the determination of EF impairment should be carried out with caution, since decline in some EF domains should not lead to sweeping generalizations.

Attention may be viewed as a sub-type of EF. It includes a number of different processes that are related aspects of how the organism becomes receptive to stimuli. Attention may be further classified into separate functions: focused or selective, sustained, divided, and alternating, although these distinctions are somewhat artificial. Selective attention, which enables filtering of stimulus information and suppression of distractors, is commonly referred to as "concentration." Sustained attention refers to the ability to maintain attention to a task

Table 4 Executive Function (EF) Components and their Possible Effects on Gait Disorders: A Theoretical View

EF Component	Description of Component	Effect on Gait (when this component is impaired)
Volition	The capacity for intentional behavior, for formulation of a goal or intention, and for initiation of activity[1]	Loss of mobility due to reduced motivation. Decreased inner drive to move. May be mistaken for bradykinesia.
Self-awareness	The ability to place oneself (psychologically and physically) in the physical environment and the on-going situation[1]	Careless walking: Poor or inaccurate estimation of one's physical limitations may lead to inappropriate evaluation of environmental hazards and increase the risk of falling.
Planning	"The identification and organization of the steps and elements needed to carry out an intention"[1]. This may rely on other cognitive skills such as the ability to conceptualize changes from present circumstances, conceiving alternatives, weighing and making choices, controlling impulses and using memory.[1,2]	Deficits in decision-making abilities while walking in a complex environment. Inefficient, faulty or even risky choices. Losing the way or wasting time or effort to arrive at the desired destination.
Response inhibition	Allows one to ignore irrelevant sensory inputs, overcome primary reflexes, and filter out distractions in order to solve problems and respond discriminatively to important features in the environment[2,3]. This ability is closely related to selective attention.	When walking in complex, everyday environments, response inhibition allows one to focus on gait and give it the appropriate attention and priority, despite numerous distractions.
Response monitoring	Enables one to compare ongoing actions with an internal plan and to detect errors[3,4]. This skill facilitates decision making and the flexible adjustment of behavior.[3]	This EF component may also be important for walking in complex environments. Demented patients may walk too fast, increasing their risk of falls, because of reduced inhibition[5]. Performance on classical tests of response inhibition and response monitoring, the Stroop and the Go No-Go tests, have been associated with gait variability[6,7].
Attention/dual tasking	The ability to appropriately allocate attention among tasks that are performed simultaneously.	

Adapted from Yogev-Seligmann et al; 2008
[1] Lezak 1995; [2] Craik and Grady 2002; [3] Ridderinkhof et al. 2004; [4] Menon et al. 2001; [5] van Iersel et al. 2006; [6] Springer et al. 2006; [7] Yogev et al. 2005.

over a period of time. Divided attention refers to the ability to carry out more than one task simultaneously. This specific type of attention plays an important role during walking in multi-tasking and changing situations, serves as a common tool for testing the attentional demands of various tasks, and has clinical implications for fall risk (Lezak 1995; Lezak 1983; Giladi et al. 2007).

Gait and Cognitive Function

Walking safely and efficiently requires more than flexible joints and strong muscles; cognitive and mental resources are also needed for achieving the objectives of the action in a safe and timely manner and with no risk of falls. The relationship between higher level cognitive function and gait disturbances has received much attention during the last decade. Gait is no longer considered as merely an automated motor activity that utilizes minimal higher-level cognitive input, rather than actions involving estimation of the destination, control of limb movements, and navigation in an obstacle-environment. The executive control dimensions include decision making, visuo-spatial perception, and attention combined with mental function: mood, cautiousness, and risk-taking behavior. These cognitive aspects of motor behavior involved in walking and their importance have been recently recognized (Yogev-Seligmann, Hausdorff, and Giladi 2008). This role of cognition may become even more apparent during different daily living activities, when individuals need to selectively attend to foot placement (e.g., stepping on an icy sidewalk, stepping up onto a curb), when performing actions simultaneously or quickly shifting attention and control from one task to another (e.g., walking while talking, walking across a busy road while watching for oncoming traffic). Central to such actions are the abilities to effectively monitor the environment, choose flexible response patterns to balance threats that may appear, and make appropriate motor responses in order to complete goals at hand (O'Shea, Morris, and Iansek 2002).

Several investigations have attempted to directly study the relationships between cognitive function, mainly EF, and gait abilities. In the InCHIANTI study, over 900 non-demented older adults walked at a self-selected and fast speed over an obstacle course. Based on their performance on the Trail Making Test (TMT), a classic test of EF, subjects were stratified into three groups. Poor and intermediate performance on the TMT was associated with decreased gait speed on the obstacle course. The authors concluded that EF is critical in complex gait situations. A follow-up study in this cohort also found associations between the effects of other dual tasks on walking performance and TMT scores (Ble et al. 2005; Coppin et al. 2006).

Dual Tasking and Gait

Does gait require attention? The ability to maintain normal walking while performing a secondary task (dual task paradigm) has become the classic way to assess the interaction between cognition and gait. The dual task paradigm involves challenging attentional capacities, specifically the ability to divide attention. These effects of dual tasking on gait have been studied in various populations, including healthy young and older adults, as well as in patients suffering from neurological disease (e.g., Parkinson's disease, Alzheimer's disease, post stroke).

The term "dual task" refers to two tasks performed simultaneously (e.g., cognitive task with motor task, or two motor or two cognitive tasks in parallel). In a healthy subject, one task may be performed automatically (unconsciously), requiring minimal attention reservoirs, while the person is attentive to the second task (Bond and Morris 2000). With aging or disease, however, performance may deteriorate, leading to the "dual-task decrement" (Figure 4). Although dual tasking has now been studied for several decades, it is important

to note that the understanding of the neurophysiology of dual tasking is still evolving and there are many questions about how it is controlled (Herath et al. 2001). The mechanisms responsible for the "dual-task" decrement (or interference) are not always clear. In fact, Herath et al. (2001) go so far as to state that the "neurophysiological basis of dual task interference is unknown." One hypothesis explaining this decrement is the cortical field hypothesis (CFH). According to this hypothesis, if two different brain tasks make use of the same cortical fields, the tasks cannot be performed simultaneously. A population of neurons or pathways may be locked to one task for a certain time, during which time these pathways are unavailable to other tasks. According to the CFH theory, a serious problem will occur if gait relies upon executive function and if divided attention relies upon executive function.

Lundin-Olsson and colleagues (Lundin-Olsson, Nyberg, and Gustafson 1997) were the first to note that failure to maintain a conversation while walking is a marker for future falls ("stops walking while talking"). Older adults who could not "walk and talk" subsequently fell, while those subjects who could walk and talk were much less prone to future falls. Holtzer et al. (2006) demonstrated associations between performance on cognitive test battery and gait speed. The cognitive battery assessed speed of processing, attention, memory, language and EF. Both EF and memory were correlated with gait speed under dual task conditions, while verbal IQ was not. Those authors suggested that gait in the elderly is a complex task requiring higher control of executive processing and memory. Springer et al. (Springer et al. 2006) reported weak associations between EF and gait variability under usual walking conditions that became stronger under dual tasks conditions among non-demented elderly fallers while such associations were not observed in healthy young adults (see Figure 5). Similarly, Hausdorff et al. (2005) showed that better gait performance (e.g. higher gait speed, lower stride time variability) was associated with better scores on a "catch game," a complex motor task, but this association did not exist for finger tapping, a relatively simple motor task. Lindenberger et al. (2000) demonstrated that the dual task costs increased with aging, especially when walking through a complex course, i.e., reduction in gait speed, increased number of missteps when walking over a narrow route, as well as reduction in performance of the cognitive task. Thus, most studies in healthy older adults observe some "normal" strategies in response to dual tasking (e.g., reducing gait speed or decreasing the reaction time of the secondary cognitive task) without widespread changes to the gait pattern. Idiopathic fallers as well as patients with Alzheimer's disease decrease their gait speed, demonstrate shorter strides, increase double support times, and increase stride-to-stride variability. Herman et al. (2010) showed that even among healthy older adults who reported no falls in the past, the decrease in the ability of dual tasking in walking predicted future falls. Interestingly, the dual tasking not only affects the gait pattern, but performance on the secondary, cognitive task is also reduced during dual tasking, an effect that is exacerbated with aging (Figure 6) (Srygley et al. 2009).

To summarize, in older adults, dual task abilities deteriorate in part because central resources decline, secondary to sub-clinical disease processes or medication. This deterioration may lead to a mismatch between the limited processing resources and the complexity of the demand. Dual task walking abilities, therefore, may be an especially sensitive predictor of fall risk capable of identifying deficits not seen during single task walking. Dual tasking also apparently increases the risk of falling among the frail older adults or those elderly who suffer from recurrent falls without any known organic reason, i.e., "idiopathic fallers" (see also Table 5).

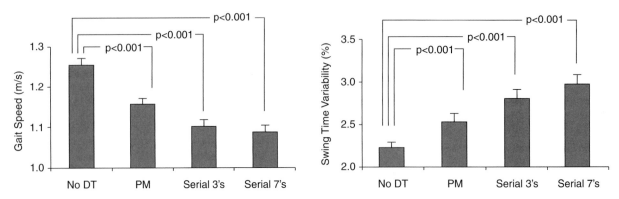

Figure 4 Gait speed and swing time variability during usual-walking (without any dual task, DT) and during three different dual tasks. Percentages shown in the columns are the % of subjects who showed a decrease in gait speed or an increase in swing time variability. For each dual task and each gait parameter, differences to the usual walking condition were highly significant (p<0.0001). PM: phoneme-monitoring. Adapted from Hausdorff et al. 2008.

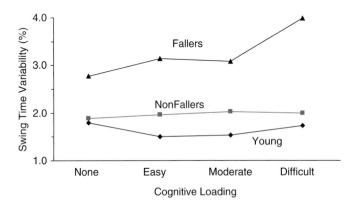

Figure 5 In fallers, but not in non-fallers or young adults, variability increased with the level of difficulty of the dual task, widening the gap between fallers and non-fallers. In contrast, gait speed (not shown) responded similarly in all three groups. Adapted from Springer et al. 2006.

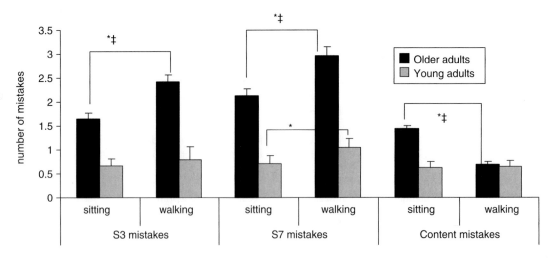

Figure 6 In older adults, walking apparently alters cognitive functioning, even during a relatively simple task such as listening to a story and recalling its content. In young adults, this effect is seen only during the more difficult serial 7 subtraction task. The number of mistakes performed on the three cognitive tests is shown during sitting and walking. Within group differences, i.e., sitting vs. walking, are indicated by *. Across group differences, which were present for all tasks, are indicated by ‡. The older adults made more subtraction mistakes during walking, for both serial 3's and serial 7's, while only serial 7 mistakes increased in the young adults. Content recall was similar in sitting and walking for the young adults, while it improved in the older adults during walking. Bars reflect the standard errors. Adapted from Srygley et al. 2008.

Table 5 Brief Summary of Disparate Effects of Dual Tasking on (average) Gait Speed and Gait Variability

Subjects	Average Gait Speed	Stride Time Variability	Swing Time Variability
Healthy young adults	↓	NS	NS
Elderly non-fallers	↓	NS	NS
Elderly Idiopathic Fallers	↓	↑	↑
Patients with Parkinson's disease	↓	↑	↑
Patients with Alzheimer's disease	↓	↑	↑

In the healthy young and elderly non-fallers, the relationship between dual tasking difficulty and the variability of stride and swing time was essentially flat (i.e., NS). For subjects with PD and fallers, the decline in gait speed with dual tasking difficulty paralleled that observed in the healthy subject groups.

High Level Gait Disorders (HLGD)

About 10–20% of older adults walk without any significant mobility impairment (Bloem et al. 2009; Bootsma-van der Weil et al. 2002; Sudarsky 2001). Among those older adults who do have a gait disturbance, the cause is often easily identifiable and attributable to underlying chronic disease (e.g., Parkinson's disease, stroke) (Sudarsky 2001; Bloem et al. 1992; Bootsma-van der Wiel et al. 2002; Jankovic, Nutt, and Sudarsky 2001; Nutt 2001). There are, however, many older adults who have an impaired gait that does not appear to be the result of any identifiable cause (Whitman et al. 1999). Various terms have been used to describe the changes in gait, common in older adults, that appear to be a result of "aging," including idiopathic senile gait and cautious gait of the elderly (Koller, Glatt, and Fox 1985). Using nomenclature based on the hierarchy of the nervous system organization to describe a clinical spectrum of gait disturbances in the elderly, Nutt et al. coined the termed "higher-level" gait disorders (HLGD) to refer to balance or walking difficulties that could not be fully explained by musculoskeletal, spastic, cerebellar, or extrapyramidal syndromes and could not be attributed to a well-defined chronic disease or any lesion in the brain (Koller, Glatt, and Fox 1985; Nutt, Marsden, and Thompson 1993).

The "cautious gait" type is one of the most common types of the HLGD spectrum, where patients look like they are very insecure and afraid of falling. These individuals walk slowly with small steps and a wider base of support (Nutt 2001; Bloem et al. 2000). Although this phenomena is fairly common and its association with reduced quality of life and future morbidity and mortality has been reported (Sudarsky 2001; Bloem et al. 2000; Suzuki et al. 2002; Verghese et al. 2002; Whitman et al. 2001), the pathophysiology of this subtype is poorly understood and the clinical characteristics of these patients are largely unknown. Subtle white matter changes and frontal atrophy of unknown origin have been reported in older adults with idiopathic disequilibrium and poor mobility (Baloh et al. 1995; Benson et al. 2002; Guttmann et al. 2000; Whitman et al. 1999; Whitman et al. 2001). Some have suggested that HLGD is related to premotor, motor, and supplementary motor cortex and neurological networks with subcortical areas such as the brain stem, basal ganglia, and cerebellum. These areas and the limbic systems may play an important role, to different degrees, in what can be viewed as a multi-system neurodegenerative syndrome clearly different from normal "aging" (Giladi et al. 2005; Huber-Machlin et al. 2010).

Bloem et al. suggested that sub-clinical, perhaps cerebrovascular, disease is the underlying cause (Bloem et al. 2000) and Fife et al. proposed that vestibular dysfunction may be involved (Fife and Baloh 1993). It has not been determined yet if this "primary central gait disorder" of the elderly is a result of a normal psychological and motor response to an objective functional deterioration, or a neurological syndrome with specific clinical, radiological, and possibly pathological features. It is unclear if the changes in gait are the product of a primary neuronal degeneration or if they are secondary to vascular changes. Others have suggested that HLGD may be caused mainly by vascular changes at the sub-cortical frontal lobe (Baloh et al. 1995; Benson et al. 2002; Guttmann et al. 2000; Nutt, Marsden, and Thompson 1993; Whitman et al. 2001). Based on the characterization of patients with HLGD, there might be another possibility that in a sub-group of those patients, primary neurodegeneration is an alternative pathophysiology.

Several clinical features were recently reported among those older adults with cautious gait of unknown origin (Giladi et al. 2005). In addition, freezing of gait is frequently observed in those HLGD patients especially with disease progression. Furthermore, it was suggested that freezing of gait is associated with significant functional disability and a specific frontal cognitive disturbance of initiation (Giladi et al. 2007). In addition, objective and susceptible measures demonstrate that gait variability is markedly increased among older adults with an HLGD and compared to control subjects of similar age (Herman et al. 2005).

Regarding HLGD, two parkinsonian syndromes should be considered in the differential diagnosis: progressive supranuclear palsy (PSP) and normal pressure hydrocephalus (NPH) (Zeilinger and Meier 1998). The early appearance of postural instability is a common feature of PSP, as is the involvement of the frontal lobe and the lack of response to levodopa (Rajput and Rajput 2001). However, in HLGD, normal eye movements and the lack of axial rigidity do not support the diagnosis of PSP. Nevertheless, only post-mortem pathological examination of the brain of such patients will be able to clearly exclude the diagnosis of PSP, or vascular PSP, considering that PSP is a heterogeneous syndrome (Factor et al. 2002). For the diagnosis of NPH, subjects must meet the clinical and radiological criteria for NPH. However, there is a possibility that in the future some of the patients with HLGD will develop dementia and will meet those criteria.

Cautious and Careless Gait

Typically, older adults with a cautious gait pattern move slowly, with a wide base and short strides, with little movement of the trunk, while the knees and elbows are bent. Cautious gait is common in elderly people and originates in part from fear of falling, which may sometimes be present even up to the degree of panic. There are two main subgroups. In one, fear of falling is the main manifestation; it is excessive and is relative to the degree of the actual instability (Giladi et al. 2005). Provision of external support or reassurance can substantially improve the gait pattern. In fact, balance abilities may be quite normal, as in people with pathological fear of falling (fall phobia) caused by a single random fall. In those individuals, the remaining neurological examination may be completely normal. In the second subgroup, fear of falling is justified by a recent history of recurrent falls or by a self-perceived instability due to overt or sometimes otherwise sub-clinical underlying disease. These individuals might show mild freezing of gait, occurring mainly with gait initiation (start hesitation) and while turning. Neurological examination may reveal mild extra-pyramidal signs, disturbed postural responses and frontal release signs. With time, these individuals may develop other sub-cortical or frontal disturbances or progress to a more severe gait impairment.

Careless gait is the counterpart of the cautious gait. Some individuals seem to be over confident and walk inappropriately fast, perhaps because of lack of insight or frontal lobe disinhibition. They seem to move abruptly, despite a severe balance deficit, are unable to properly judge the risk of their actions, and move recklessly. This kind of mobility correlates with high incidence of fall-related injuries. Confusion and delirium also can also contribute to a careless gait. van Iersel and colleagues (2006) showed that gait velocity should be judged in the context of the individual's physical capabilities. Although frail elderly individuals with dementia walked slowly, they still walked relatively too fast and put themselves at risk of falling, given their overall degree of physical impairment, which should have warranted an even slower gait.

Fear of Falling (FOF) and its Impact on Gait

The psychological consequences of falls in old age can be severe. Thus, it is important to assess whether a patient has fear of falling (FOF) and whether this fear is reasonable (in persons with extremely poor balance) or if it is inappropriate (a pathological fear induced by a single but otherwise innocent fall). "Self-confidence" (confidence in *not* falling) should also be evaluated as this provides valuable complementary information about the impact of falls on activities of daily living and independence. Note that some patients feel overly confident despite marked balance deficits, and they have a high risk of falling (Giladi, Bloem, and Hausdorff 2007).

Many older persons experience psychological difficulties following an innocent fall. These individuals can develop a "post fall syndrome," first described in 1982 in the classic essay by Murphy and Isaacs (Murphy and Isaacs 1982), who noticed that after a fall ambulatory patients developed an exaggerated fear and severe walking difficulties. This syndrome is a combination of anxiety, loss of self efficacy, pain, and immobility as a consequence, impinging severely on quality of life. Self-efficacy, first introduced in 1978 by Bandura, refers to "an individual's perception of capabilities within a particular domain of activities." For a long time, FOF was merely believed to be a result of psychological trauma of a fall (Legters 2002). Since that time, FOF has been recognized as a specific health problem among older adults.

Falls and fear of falling are associated with each other; however, development of FOF is not exclusive to the population of elderly people who experienced a fall. There is a population of elderly people who are fearful of falling even when they have not actually experienced a fall (Maki 1997). One study reported that over 50% of older adults who had not yet experienced a fall reported FOF (Suzuki et al. 2002). Prevalence of FOF seems to increase with age and to be higher in women. Dizziness and depression could also be an etiology to develop FOF. Consequences of FOF may lead to functional, psychological, and social changes in older adults, including avoidance of activities, social isolation, loss of functional independence, and falling (Cumming et al. 2000). The factors contributing to FOF in older adults are numerous, although the exact causes remain unclear. Poorer health status and functional decline, restriction of activity, decreased quality of life, and psychological factors, specifically depression and anxiety, are closely related to FOF (Legters 2002).

Reelick et al. (2009) examined the association between FOF and gait and balance in older people during walking with and without dual-tasking. Their findings show that FOF was significantly associated with gait velocity when walking at the two walking conditions. Stride-time variability and stride-length variability were also associated with FOF. Similarly, stride-to-stride variability was associated with the level of FOF in older adults with a "cautious" gait who walk fearfully (Herman et al. 2005). One could argue that fear of falling leads to instability and increased gait variability. Although this possibility cannot be completely ruled out, Maki's results suggest that fear of falling may be found without gait unsteadiness and gait unsteadiness may be found without fear of falling, at least in certain populations (Herman et al. 2005; Maki 1997).

Multiple interventions have been suggested for coping with FOF, including education and discussion of risk-taking behaviors, environmental safety considerations to reduce fall risk, assertiveness training, and maintaining or improving the physical fitness levels. These interventions have been recommended, with the optimal effect being a cognitive behavioral change in the older adult that results in bolstered self-confidence to perform daily activities (Legters 2002).

Comprehensive Assessment of Gait

Because multiple age-associated changes typically contribute to gait disorders in the elderly, a full comprehensive geriatric assessment should be made to evaluate gait and mobility. The anamnesis should include a history of medical, behavioral, and social status. Generally, history taking by interviewing the subject about the problems with gait or balance can be very challenging. When asking about gait problems, one has to estimate the amount of walking a person does in daily life. In addition, the nature of questions themselves should try to help the patient describe his difficulties in terms of walking speed, amount of effort required, confidence, or degree of fear from falling, and if any assistance or walking aids are used. The simple, short question, "have you fallen?" can be very informative. For patients presenting with gait disorders, it is important to try and distinguish between consistently present walking difficulties versus an episodic gait disorder, such as freezing of gait, festination, or sensory ataxia in the dark.

In addition, it is important to monitor medications and to perform a full physical examination including blood pressure in the supine as well as in the standing position and a brief neurological examination. The motor part (part III) of the Unified Parkinson's Disease Rating Scale (UPDRS) can be used to quantify extra-pyramidal signs, sometimes seen in older adults. Lower scores reflect fewer symptoms (Fahn S, Elton R, and Members of the UPDRS Development Committee 1987). Gait and posture should be assessed systematically as part of the routine clinical examination, along with static and dynamic balance in several positions, gradually increasing the difficulty (e.g., see Figure 7). Several aspects of gait should be checked:

- Assessment of the patient's ability to rise from a chair with his/her arms crossed, which enables testing of the strength of the hip and knee extensor muscles, as well as general postural control.

- Assessment of standing capacity, looking at the base of support, the ability to stand with the feet together, in a tandem stand (up to 30 seconds), on one leg (up to 5 seconds), and standing with both feet together and eyes closed (Romberg test). These tests provide valuable information about postural control, balance, vestibular function, and proprioception.

- Pulling backward (pull test) or pushing forward to probe the reactive and defensive balance reactions in order to score the severity of postural instability. This challenge test allows a more fine assessment of postural control/responses.

- Assessment of normal walking in an open space is informative with regard to locomotion, equilibrium, gross motor function, and interaction with the environment.

- Assessment of turning in place is informative in terms of general coordination, equilibrium, and gross motor function. Turning to both sides and sudden changes in direction, for example, are helpful for provoking "freezing" (turning hesitation).

◆ Assessment of the ability to perform another cognitive or motor task while walking (dual tasking) poses a challenge to the subject and can provide important information on fall risk during daily activities.

◆ If fear of falling and insecurity are suspected as contributing factors to the clinical syndrome, the effect of support by the examiner's hand, a walker, or a cane should be evaluated.

◆ When evaluating gait, other components of motor function should be assessed: muscle strength, tone, coordination, and range of motion. For testing cognition and affect, it is important to assess specifically attention, working memory, cognitive slowing, reaction time, executive functions, and visuospatial orientation because of their importance to the performance of daily walking (Giladi et al. 2007).

It is suggested to add several performance-based measures of balance and mobility. It is highly recommended to use the Timed Up and Go test (TUG) (Podsiadlo and Richardson 1991), a simple reliable measure of functional performance that captures transfers, walking, and turning components, and has been strongly associated with fall risk in the general elderly population. Recently, TUG performance has also been related to cognitive abilities (Herman et al. 2010). Subjects who perform the TUG test in more than 13.5 seconds are believed to have an increased risk of falls (Shumway-Cook, Brauer, and Woollacott 2000; AGS Guidelines 2001). The Berg Balance Test (BBT) can also be used to evaluate mobility and balance (Berg, Wood-Dauphinee, and Williams 1992). Performance is rated on 14 different tasks, e.g., tandem standing, single leg stand, reaching, 360°. The highest possible score is 56, while scores lower than 45 have been associated with a high risk of falls. The Tinetti Balance and Mobility scale (also known as the Performance Oriented Mobility Assessment—POMA) can be used to screen for balance and mobility skills in the aged population and to determine the risk for falls (Tinetti et al. 1994). It consists of two parts for evaluating balance (16 points) and gait (12 points). In addition, The Dynamic Gait Index (DGI), a more challenging but simple test, can be used to assess a subject's ability to modify gait in response to changing task demands (Shumway-Cook and Woollacott 1995).

Quantitative Assessment of Gait

Gait mats embedded with sensors provide a popular method for quantifying gait. Subjects walk across an instrumented carpet or walkway (e.g., GaitRite, Clifton, NJ) that is sensitive to the pressure changes caused by walking. The instrumented walkway quantifies stride length, stride width, stride time, and the timing of the gait cycle. A number of studies have demonstrated the validity, reliability, and clinical utility of these types of systems in various clinical populations.

Ambulatory monitoring systems enable the quantitative measurement of the timing of gait. The subject might be equipped with accelerometers and gyroscopes, footswitches, or other wearable sensors. A key advantage of such systems is the measurement of multiple strides, in almost any environment, thus enabling the evaluation of gait rhythmicity and the stride-to-stride fluctuations of gait timing. Several studies have shown that such measures of gait variability or dynamics are sensitive to subtle changes that occur with aging and neurodegenerative diseases, such as Parkinson's disease, Huntington's disease and Alzheimer's disease (Herman et al. 2005; Hausdorff, Ladin, and Wei 1995; Hausdorff et al. 1998; Hausdorff et al. 2003; Hausdorff 2004). Stride-to-stride fluctuations reflect the consistency or steadiness of gait and the ability of the locomotor system to regulate gait from one stride to the next. Such measures also have clinical efficacy in the identification and prospective prediction of elderly fallers (Hausdorff, Rios, and Edelberg 2001; Herman et al. 2010) (see, for example, Figure 8).

Gait laboratories offer the most comprehensive means of quantifying the walking pattern. Typically, a modern gait laboratory will include an array of 3-dimensional cameras or a marker-based system to measure the movement of various body segments (termed "kinematics"), force-platforms to measure the ground reaction forces, i.e., the forces exerted by the foot on the ground (termed "kinetics"), and electromyographic (EMG) equipment to measure muscle activity. Such systems provide a highly detailed assessment of walking, including the position, velocity, and acceleration of different joint segments and angles, muscle forces, and muscle timing. This combination can provide insightful information into changes in gait mechanics. Studies of children with cerebral palsy, especially when they are candidates for surgery, probably represent the most popular applications of a

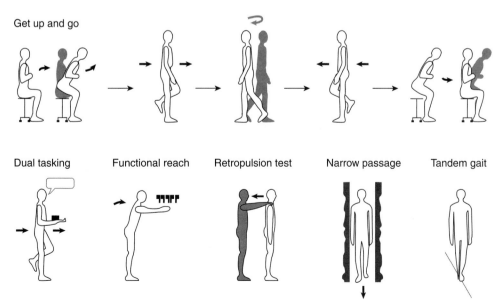

Figure 7 Examples of several performance-based tests of gait. Adapted from Voermans et al. 2007.

full-scale gait laboratory. For many clinical purposes, however, some of the simpler approaches described above may be sufficient (Giladi, Bloem, and Hausdorff 2007).

While gait assessment should focus on mobility and motor control, evaluation of gait should also include tests of cognitive function, mental well-being, and affect, factors that can contribute to or exacerbate gait disturbances in the elderly population. Tests that are commonly used include the Mini-Mental State Exam (MMSE) (Folstein, Folstein, and McHugh 1975) and the Montreal Cognitive Assessment (MoCA) (Nasreddine et al. 2005). Fear of falling can be measured using the Activities-specific Balance Confidence scale (ABC) (Powell and Myers 1995). In this questionnaire, the subject is given 16 activities and is asked to rate his/her confidence level when performing each activity, on a scale ranging from 0% to100%. The highest score (100%) represents full confidence, i.e., no FOF. ABC scores under 50% indicate a very low level of balance confidence; scores between 50%–80% indicate moderate confidence, and scores higher than 80% reflect high confidence and are typical for physically active older adults (Legters et al. 2005). The Geriatric Depression Scale (GDS) (Yesavage et al. 1982) may be used to assess emotional well-being. It includes 30 yes/no questions. A score of 0–10 is considered normal, while 21 and above suggests more severe depression. The State-Trait Anxiety Inventory (STAI) may be used to quantify the level of general and specific anxiety (Spielberger et al. 1983).

Therapeutic Interventions

The most commonly accepted approach to treatment of gait disorders in the elderly is based on a multi-factorial intervention that includes muscle strengthening, balance training, and gait training, among other things. Here we briefly describe several approaches that can be used individually or in combination, depending on the specifics of the impairment.

Pharmacological

A growing number of studies suggest that pharmacologic interventions may also help to improve gait among older adults. While large, randomized controlled trials are lacking, this possibility is supported by several reports. For example, a number of investigations have indicated that methylphenidate (MPH) (e.g., Ritalin®) apparently augments attention and that this carries over to gait and mobility in older adults (Ben-Itzhak et al. 2008; Ben-Itzhak et al. 2006; Auriel, Hausdorff,

and Giladi, 2009; Devos et al. 2007; Nutt, Carter, and Carlson 2007). To some degree, these studies may be viewed as parallel to the idea that intensive cognitive exercise may used as a way for improving dual task performance (Yogev-Seligmann, Hausdorff, and Giladi 2008). Amelioration of depressive symptoms via anti-depressive drugs also apparently improves gait in community-living depressed patients (Paleacu et al. 2007). Pilot studies also suggest that other drugs that are commonly used to treat dementia and improve cognitive function augment gait and mobility and reduce the risk of falls in the elderly and patients with neurodegenerative disease (Assal et al. 2008; Chung et al. 2010; Montero-Odasso et al. 2009; Montero-Odasso, Wells, and Borrie 2009). While these effects could be achieved via several different mechanistic pathways (e.g., enhanced attention may improve gait or they might more directly affect motor control), the results stand in contrast to the older notion that drugs, in general, typically increase the risk of falls in the elderly. Appropriate use of certain pharmacologic agents may actually enhance gait and reduce fall risk. Further work is needed, but the extant literature offers hope that pharmacologic therapies may soon become an accepted form of clinical care of certain types of gait disorders in the elderly.

Physical Therapy

Interventions designed to improve gait should take into account the objective of getting the individual back on his/her feet and walking again. Often, the ultimate goal is to give the subject appropriate tools to mobilize him/herself independently, but in a safe manner. By training and promoting regular exercise, physical therapy can lead to improvement of general fitness and reduce cardiovascular co-morbidity and mortality (Hakim et al. 1998).

Interventions for treating gait disturbances and preventing falls are designed to decrease intrinsic or extrinsic risk factors. Physical therapy may be helpful in dealing with several symptoms, such as muscle weakness, reduced range of motion, gait instability, and balance problems (Morris et al. 2006; Morris 2000; Pahor et al. 2006). Exercise has many proven benefits and appears to help reduce fall risk; however, the optimal type, duration, and intensity of exercise that is best to prevent falls remains uncertain (Carter, Kannus, and Khan 2001; Hausdorff et al. 2001; Gardner, Robertson, and Campbell 2000; Province et al. 2005; Robertson et al. 2001; American Geriatrics Society et al. 2001). Interventions that deal with extrinsic factors focus primarily on decreasing environmental demand and hazards. Examples include improving lighting, adding grab bars, raising the toilet seat, and finding

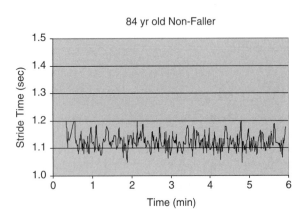
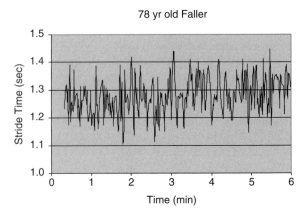

Figure 8 Quantification of step to step changes in gait rhythmicity. Stride-to-stride fluctuations in a non-faller older adult are much larger than those seen in an age-matched non-faller.

an appropriate bed height. Although commonly attempted, it is not clear how effective these environmental interventions are in ultimately reducing falls, perhaps due to the difficulty in ensuring patient compliance to these interventions and the complexity of fall causation (Sattin et al. 1998; Stevens et al. 2001).

Dance Therapy

Dancing is a mode of physical activity that may allow older adults to improve their physical function, health, and general well-being. Verghese (2006) studied the cognitive and mobility profiles of elderly social dancers compared with non-dancers. There were no differences in the frequency of participation in leisure activities, chronic illnesses, muscle strength, falls, or cognitive test performance between the two groups. However, the elderly social dancers had better balance than the non-dancers. On quantitative gait assessment, they showed a more stable pattern during walking, with reduced stance time, longer swing time, and shorter double support time. These results suggest that long-term social dancing may be associated with better balance and gait in older adults.

Recently, a review was published about the physical benefits of dancing for healthy older adults (Keogh et al. 2009). Moderate level of evidence indicated that older adults can significantly improve their aerobic power, lower body muscle endurance, strength and flexibility, balance, agility, and gait through dancing. It has been also suggested that dancing might improve older adults' lower body bone-mineral content and muscle power, as well as reduce the prevalence of falls and cardiovascular health risks. Dancing appears to be appropriate and effective also for other populations including patients with neurodegenerative diseases. For example, patients with Parkinson's disease may benefit from intensive tango or other dance lessons, thus improving several aspects of gait balance (Earhart 2009; Hackney and Earhart 2009).

Cueing

The use of external cueing is one of the most powerful modes of intervention to improve gait initiation and walking, at least in the presence of specifics types of gait disorders. Despite even severe locomotion disturbances, patients (classically those with Parkinson's disease, PD) can walk almost normally by adopting special behavioral techniques, by being exposed to special sensory stimulations or by using learned cognitive tricks (Rubenstein, Giladi, and Hausdorff 2002). Cueing training may be a useful therapeutic adjunct to the overall management of gait disturbance. The effect of rhythmic auditory stimulation (RAS) combined with gait training was studied in several population including patients following stroke, and patients with PD (Hausdorff et al. 2007; Hayden et al. 2009; Lim et al. 2005; McIntosh et al. 1994; Nieuwboer et al. 2007). There is strong evidence for improving walking speed with the help of auditory cues (Lim et al. 2005). Normal stride length can be elicited in Parkinson's disease using visual cues. Visual cues can improve stride length using gait training combined with attentional strategies with either visual floor markers or a mental picture of the appropriate stride size. The ability to generate a normal stepping pattern is not lost in Parkinson's disease and external auditory cues may be useful in reducing interference and maintaining gait performance even during more complicated functional activities. Clinical symptoms, such as depression and fatigue, often seen in PD, could influence the ability to focus attention and may increase gait interference during the performance of complex tasks, with subsequent implications for functional walking and safety (Morris et al. 1996; Rochester et al. 2005). Some investigators report that cueing is also efficacious in non-PD patients; the utility in the general elderly population remains to be seen.

Treadmill Training

Bodyweight-supported treadmill training (BWSTT) is often used to promote gait training in patients with spinal cord injuries and post-stroke (Hesse et al. 1995; Laufer et al. 2001; Behrman and Harkema 2000; Dietz, Colombo, and Jensen 1994; Dobkin et al. 2007; Dobkin 2005; van Hedel, Waldvogel, and Dietz 2006), allowing early intervention that enables patients who have difficulties standing to begin gait training. Recent studies have demonstrated the feasibility and safety, as well as the efficacy, of treadmill training and its potential therapeutic use for Parkinson's disease gait rehabilitation (Bello, Sanchez, and Fernandez-del-Olmo 2008; Frenkel-Toledo et al. 2005; Herman et al. 2002; Herman, Giladi, and Hausdorff 2009; Miyai et al. 2002). Following training, several aspects of gait improved, including over-ground walking speed, stride length, and gait variability, combined with improvements in other domains such as measures of disease severity (e.g., Unified Parkinson's Disease Rating Scale), reduced fall risk, and improved health-related quality of life. Long-term carryover effects were also found, raising the possibility that this training may be more than simply symptom relief, but elicit positive neural plastic changes (Fisher et al. 2008). While questions remain about its effect on non-aerobic gait deficits, it appears that this mode of training may enhance treatment option for older adults (Liston et al. 2000; Shimada et al. 2004) and for several patient populations.

Motor/Mental Imagery

Motor imagery is the mental representation of movement without any actual body movement. Evidence on the positive effects of motor imagery practice on motor performance and learning in athletes, people who are healthy, and people with neurological conditions (e.g., stroke, spinal cord injury) has been published (Sacco et al. 2006; Dunsky et al. 2008; Tamir, Dickstein, and Huberman 2007; Dickstein and Deutsch 2007). A positron emission tomography (PET) study was used to study the involvement of supraspinal structures in human locomotion. The findings suggest that higher brain centers become progressively engaged when demands of locomotor tasks require increasing cognitive and sensory information processing (Malouin et al. 2003).

The application of motor imagery practice in the treatment of Parkinson's disease (PD) is a relatively novel treatment approach for improving motor function. In a recent study by Tamir et al. (2007), following the intervention, the combined treatment group (regular physical therapy with motor imagery) exhibited significantly faster performance of movement sequences than the control group. In addition, the experimental subjects demonstrated higher gains in the mental and motor subsets of the UPDRS and in several cognitive tests. The combination of motor imagery and real practice may be effective in the treatment of PD, especially for reducing bradykinesia. The implementation of this treatment regimen allows for the extension of practice time with negligible risk and low cost. Additional work is needed to more fully evaluate the effects of motor imagery practice in community-living older adults with gait disorders.

Tai Chi

Mind-over-body training, such as in Tai Chi, appears to be a promising option for older adults (Li, Hong, and Chan 2001; Wolf et al. 1997; Wolf et al. 2001; Wu et al. 2007). Tai Chi-based interventions can impact favorably on defined biomedical and psychosocial indices of frailty, enhance balance and balance confidence, and have favorable effects upon the occurrence of falls. Tai Chi can prevent a decline in functional balance and gait among older people and improve the ability to tolerate unsteadiness. In addition, improvements in chair-rise and cardiovascular performance were found (Gatts and Woollacott 2007; Hackney and Earhart 2008; Hass et al. 2004; Lin et al. 2006; Wolf et al. 2007). Still, there are conflicting reports about the efficacy of Tai Chi in the literature, perhaps because not all patient groups or elderly have the same underlying balance and gait disorders.

Virtual Reality

Virtual reality (VR) is a relatively recently developed tool that can be used to treat gait disorders. VR is a simulation of a real world environment that is generated through computer software and is experienced by the user through a human-machine interface (Holden 2005). A wide variety of devices can be utilized to create VR simulations with a variety of equipment and display devices. The idea is to recreate a believable artificial environment that stimulates physical responses similar to those in real environments (Holden 2005). VR rehabilitation applications use visual, auditory, and haptic input, which allows the user to receive multi-sensory feedback. This feedback is a crucial aspect in motor learning and skill acquisition. Visual and haptic information are apparently an effective addition to increasing motor performance of challenging tasks while training with robotic–VR technologies (Jack et al. 2001).

VR can be used as an enhancement to conventional therapy for patients with conditions ranging from musculoskeletal problems (Girone et al. 2000), balance and gait disorders (Keshner and Weiss 2007; Mirelman, Bonato, and Deutsch 2009), stroke-induced paralysis (Deutsch and Merians 2004; Fung et al. 2006; Holden 2005; Jaffe et al. 2004; Mirelman, Bonato, Deutsch, in press; You et al. 2005), and cognitive deficits (Buckwalter and Rizzo 1997; Rizzo and Buckwalter 1997; Rizzo and Buckwalter 1997) and is often referred to as "VR-augmented rehabilitation" (Burdea et al. 2003). The use of this technology enables the creation of interventions in which the duration, intensity, and feedback given can be systematically manipulated and enhanced to create the most appropriate individualized exercise paradigm. With the use of virtual reality, the participant not only is given the opportunity to achieve multiple repetitions, but the repeated practice is linked to a task or a goal, which creates a motivating, engaging experience that is ideal for motor learning (Bisson et al. 2007; Bryanton et al. 2006). For example, in a study on obstacle negotiation while ambulating, 20 individuals post stroke were trained three times a week for two weeks using VR system. The subjects were randomized to either the VR group or the real world obstacle training group. Both groups demonstrated improvements; however, the VR group improved more on the percent of the gait speed increase and step length when tested at faster walking speeds as well as on obstacle navigation (Jaffe et al. 2004).

Research and Future Directions

Studies on gait disturbances in the elderly include many areas of research, ranging from physiology and biomechanics to brain physics and neuropsychology. Over the past several decades, we have learned many things about gait changes with aging. For example, refinements of the distinction between healthy aging and disease have been improved and the relationship between gait and cognitive function has increasingly been recognized. However, there are still many open questions. The optimal intervention programs to treat gait disorders and reduce falls risk have yet to be identified and large-scale RCT trials are lacking to provide high quality evidence for many of the proposed therapeutic options. It seems likely that genetics predispose to certain gait disorders, but only a few studies have begun to address this issue. Even norms and cut-offs to robustly distinguish frailty from normal

aging and from disease remain to be more fully established. While the understanding of age-associated changes in gait has improved dramatically over the past decades, additional work is needed to more fully understand these changes, to optimize diagnostic and tools, and to reduce the burden of gait disorders among the elderly.

References

AGS Guidelines. Guideline for the prevention of falls in older persons. American Geriatrics Society, British Geriatrics Society, and American Academy of Orthopaedic Surgeons Panel on Falls Prevention. *J Am Geriatr Soc.* 2001;49:664–672.

Albert M and Moss M. The assessment of memory disorders in patients with Alzheimer's disease. In: Squire LR and Butters N, eds. *Neduropsychology of memory.* New York: Guilford; 1984.

American Geriatrics Society, British Geriatrics Society, and American Academy of Orthopaedic Surgeons Panel on Falls Prevention. Guideline for the prevention of falls in older persons. *J Am Geriatr Soc.* 2001;49:664–672.

Alexander NB. Gait disorders in older adults. *J Am Geriatr Soc.* 1996;44:434–451.

Alexander NB. Postural control in older adults. *Journal of the American Geriatric Society.* 1994;42:93–108.

Alexander NB, Guire KE, Thelen DG, et al. Self-reported walking ability predicts functional mobility performance in frail older adults. *Journal of the American Geriatrics Society.* 2000;48:1408–1413.

Anderson PG, Nienhuis B, Mulder T, and Hulstijn W. Are older adults more dependent on visual information in regulating self-motion than younger adults? *Journal of Motor Behavior.* 1998;30:104–113.

Assal F, Allali G, Kressig RW, Herrmann FR, and Beauchet O. Galantamine improves gait performance in patients with Alzheimer's disease. *J Am Geriatr Soc.* 2008;56:946–947.

Auriel E, Hausdorf JM, and Giladi N. Methylphenidate for the treatment of Parkinson's disease and other neurological disorders. *Clinical Neuropharmacology.* 2009;32:75-81.

Auriel E, Hausdorff JM, Herman T, Simon ES, and Giladi N. Effects of methylphenidate on cognitive function and gait in patients with Parkinson's disease: A pilot study. *Clin Neuropharmacol.* 2006;29:15–17.

Balaban CD and Thayer JF. Neurological bases for balance-anxiety links. *Anxiety Disorders.* 2001;53–79.

Baloh RW, Yue Q, Socotch TM, and Jacobson KM. White matter lesions and disequilibrium in older people. I. Case-control comparison. *Arch Neurol.* 1995;52:970–974.

Behrman AL and Harkema SJ. Locomotor training after human spinal cord injury: A series of case studies. *Phys Ther.* 2000;80:688–700.

Bello O, Sanchez JA, and Fernandez-del-Olmo M. Treadmill walking in Parkinson's disease patients: Adaptation and generalization effect. *Mov Disord.* 2008;23:1243–1249.

Ben-Itzhak R, Giladi N, Gruendlinger L, and Hausdorff JM. Can methylphenidate reduce fall risk in community-living older adults? A double-blind, single-dose cross-over study. *J Am Geriatr Soc.* 2008;56:695–700.

Benson RR, Guttmann CR, Wei X, et al. Older people with impaired mobility have specific loci of periventricular abnormality on MRI. *Neurology.* 2002;58:48–55.

Berg KO, Wood-Dauphinee SL, Williams JI, and Maki B. Measuring balance in the elderly: Validation of an instrument. *Can J Public Health.* 1992;83 Suppl 2:S7–11.

Bisson E, Contant B, Sveistrup H, and Lajoie Y. Functional balance and dual-task reaction times in older adults are improved by virtual reality and biofeedback training. *Cyberpsychol Behav.* 2007;10:16–23.

Blake AJ, Morgan K, Bendall MJ, et al. Falls by elderly people at home: Prevalence and associated factors. *Age and Ageing.* 1988;17:365–372.

Ble A, Volpato S, Zuliani G, et al. Executive function correlates with walking speed in older persons: The InCHIANTI study. *J Am Geriatr Soc.* 2005;53:410–415.

Bloem BR, Gussekloo J, Lagaay AM, Remarque EJ, Haan J, and Westendorp RG. Idiopathic senile gait disorders are signs of subclinical disease. *J Am Geriatr Soc.* 2000;48:1098–1101.

Bloem BR, Haan J, Lagaay AM, van BW, Wintzen AR, and Roos RA. Investigation of gait in elderly subjects over 88 years of age. *J Geriatr Psychiatry Neurol.* 1992;5:78–84.

Bloem BR, Hausdorff JM, Visser JE, and Giladi N. Falls and freezing of gait in Parkinson's disease: A review of two interconnected, episodic phenomena. *Mov Disord.* 2004;19:871–884.

Bolmont B, Gangloff P, Vouriot A, and Perrin PP. Mood states and anxiety influence abilities to maintain balance control in healthy human subjects. *Neuroscience Letters.* 2002;329:96–100.

Bond JM and Morris M. Goal-directed secondary motor tasks: Their effects on gait in subjects with Parkinson disease. *Arch Phys Med Rehabil.* 2000;81:110–116.

Bootsma-van der Wiel A, Gussekloo J, De Craen AJ, Van Exel E, Bloem BR, and Westendorp RG. Common chronic diseases and general impairments as determinants of walking disability in the oldest-old population. *J Am Geriatr Soc.* 2002;50:1405–1410.

Bryanton C, Bosse J, Brien M, McLean J, McCormick A, and Sveistrup H. Feasibility, motivation, and selective motor control: Virtual reality compared to conventional home exercise in children with cerebral palsy. *Cyberpsychol Behav.* 2006;9:123–128.

Buchner DM and Larson EB. Falls and fractures in patients with Alzheimer-type dementia. *Journal of the American Medical Association.* 1987;257:1492–1495.

Buckner RL. Memory and executive function in aging and AD: Multiple factors that cause decline and reserve factors that compensate. *Neuron.* 2004;44:195–208.

Buckwalter JG and Rizzo AA. Virtual reality and the neuropsychological assessment of persons with neurologically based cognitive impairments. *Stud Health Technol Inform.* 1997;39:17–21.

Burdea GC. Virtual rehabilitation—benefits and challenges. *Methods Inf Med.* 2003;42:519–523.

Calne DB. Age and complexity hypothesis. In: Poon L, ed. *Aging in the 1980s.* Washington, D.C.: American Psychological Association; 1980:332–339.

Carter ND, Kannus P, and Khan KM. Exercise in the prevention of falls in older people: A systematic literature review examining the rationale and the evidence. *Sports Med.* 2001;31:427–438.

Chen HC, Schultz AB, AshtonMiller JA, Giordani B, Alexander NB, and Guire KE. Stepping over obstacles: Dividing attention impairs performance of old more than young adults. *Journals of Gerontology Series A-Biological Sciences and Medical Sciences.* 1996;51:M116–M122.

Chung KA, Lobb BM, Nutt JG, and Horak FB. Effects of a central cholinesterase inhibitor on reducing falls in Parkinson disease. *Neurology.* 2010 (epub ahead of print).

Connell BR and Wolf SL. Environmental and behavioral circumstances associated with falls at home among healthy elderly individuals. *Archives of Physical Medicine and Rehabilitation.* 1997;78: 179–186.

Coppin AK, Shumway-Cook A, Saczynski JS, et al. Association of executive function and performance of dual-task physical tests among older adults: Analyses from the InChianti study. *Age Ageing.* 2006;35:619–624.

Craik FIM and Grady CL. Aging, memory, and frontal lobe functioning. In: Stuss DT and Knight RT, eds. *Principles of frontal lobe function.* New York: Oxford University Press, Inc.; 2002.

Cress ME, Schectman KB, Mulrow CD, Fiatarone MA, Gerety MB, and Buchner DM. Relationship between physical performance and self-perceived physical function. *Journal of the American Geriatrics Society.* 1995;93–101.

Cumming RG, Salkeld G, Thomas M, and Szonyi G. Prospective study of the impact of fear of falling on activities of daily living, SF-36 scores, and nursing home admission. *J Gerontol A Biol Sci Med Sci.* 2000;55:M299–M305.

Deutsch JE, Merians AS, Adamovich S, Poizner H, and Burdea GC. Development and application of virtual reality technology to improve hand use and gait of individuals post-stroke. *Restor Neurol Neurosci.* 2004;22:371–386.

Devos D, Krystkowiak P, Clement F, et al. Improvement of gait by chronic, high doses of methylphenidate in patients with advanced Parkinson's disease. *J Neurol Neurosurg Psychiatry.* 2007;78:470–475.

Dickstein R and Deutsch JE. Motor imagery in physical therapist practice. *Phys Ther.* 2007;87:942–953.

Dietz V, Colombo G, and Jensen L. Locomotor activity in spinal man. *Lancet.* 1994;344:1260–1263.

Dobkin BH. Clinical practice. Rehabilitation after stroke. *N Engl J Med.* 2005;352:1677–1684.

Dobkin B, Barbeau H, Deforge D, et al. The evolution of walking-related outcomes over the first 12 weeks of rehabilitation for incomplete traumatic spinal cord injury: The multicenter randomized Spinal Cord Injury Locomotor Trial. *Neurorehabil Neural Repair.* 2007; 21:25–35.

Dorfman J. Problem solving, inhibition and frontal lobe function. In: Raz N, ed. *The other side of the error term: Aging and development as model systems in cognitive neuroscience.* Amsterdam, The Netherlands: Elsevier Science; 1998.

Downtown JH and Andrews K. Postural disturbance and psychological symptoms amongst elderly people living at home. *International Journal of Geriatric Psychiatry.* 1990;5:93–98.

Dunsky A, Dickstein R, Marcovitz E, Levy S, and Deutsch JE. Home-based motor imagery training for gait rehabilitation of people with chronic poststroke hemiparesis. *Arch Phys Med Rehabil.* 2008;89:1580–1588.

Earhart GM. Dance as therapy for individuals with Parkinson disease. *Eur J Phys Rehabil Med.* 2009;45:231–238.

Elble RJ. Changes in gait with normal aging. In: Masdeu JC SLWL, ed. *Gait disorders of aging. Falls and therapeutic strategies.* New York: Lippincott-Raven, 1997:93–105.

Factor SA, Jennings DL, Molho ES, and Marek KL. The natural history of the syndrome of primary progressive freezing gait. *Arch Neurol.* 2002;59:1778–1783.

Fahn S, Elton R, and Members of the UPDRS development committee. Unified Parkinson's disease rating scale. In: Fahn S, Marsden CD, Calne D, and Goldstein M, eds. *Recent developments in Parkinson's disease.* Florham Park, NJ: Macmillan Health Care Information; 1987:153–63.

Fife TD and Baloh RW. Disequilibrium of unknown cause in older people. *Ann Neurol.* 1993;34:694–702.

Fisher BE, Wu AD, Salem GJ, et al. The effect of exercise training in improving motor performance and corticomotor excitability in people with early Parkinson's disease. *Arch Phys Med Rehabil.* 2008;89:1221–1229.

Folstein MF, Folstein SE, and McHugh PR. "Mini-mental state." A practical method for grading the cognitive state of patients for the clinician. *J Psychiatr Res.* 1975;12:189–198.

Frenkel-Toledo S, Giladi N, Peretz C, Herman T, Gruendlinger L, and Hausdorff JM. Treadmill walking as an external pacemaker to improve gait rhythm and stability in Parkinson's disease. *Mov Disord.* 2005;20:1109–1114.

Fung J, Richards CL, Malouin F, McFadyen BJ, and Lamontagne A. A treadmill and motion coupled virtual reality system for gait training post-stroke. *Cyberpsychol Behav.* 2006;9:157–162.

Gardner MM, Robertson MC, and Campbell AJ. Exercise in preventing falls and fall related injuries in older people: A review of randomised controlled trials. *Br J Sports Med.* 2000;34:7–17.

Gatts SK and Woollacott MH. How Tai Chi improves balance: Biomechanics of recovery to a walking slip in impaired seniors. *Gait Posture.* 2007;25:205–214.

Giladi N., Bloem BR, and Hausdorff JM. Gait disturbances and falls. In: Schapira A, ed. *Neurology and clinical neurosceince*. Philadelphia: MOSBY; 2007:455–70.

Giladi N, Balash Y, Ruzicka E, and Jankovic J. Disorders of gait. In: J.Jankovic and E Tolosa, eds. *Parkinson's disease & movement disorders*. 5th ed. Philadelphia: Lippincott Williams & Wilkins; 2007:436–58.

Giladi N, Herman T, Reider-Groswasser II, Gurevich T, and Hausdorff JM. Clinical characteristics of elderly patients with a cautious gait of unknown origin. *J Neurol*. 2005;252:300–306.

Giladi N, Huber-Mahlin V, Herman T, and Hausdorff JM. Freezing of gait in older adults with high level gait disorders: Association with impaired executive function. *J Neural Transm*. 2007;114:1349–1353.

Giordani B, Miller AC, Alexander NB, Guire KE, Ashton-Miller JA, Berent S, et al. Neuropsychological factors relate to self-report and performance-based measures of functional mobility. Annual meeting of the Gerontological Society of America. Los Angeles, CA. 1995. Ref Type: Abstract

Giordani B, Persad CC, Miller AC, Alexander NB, Ashton-Miller JA, Guire KE, et al. Cognitive and personality measures as predictors of successful mobility performance. Annual Meeting of the American Psychological Association. Toronto, Ontario, Canada. 1996.

Girone M, Burdea G, Bouzit M, Popescu V, and Deutsch JE. Orthopedic rehabilitation using the "Rutgers ankle" interface. *Stud Health Technol Inform*. 2000;70:89–95.

Guttmann CR, Benson R, Warfield SK, et al. White matter abnormalities in mobility-impaired older persons. *Neurology*. 2000;54:1277–1283.

Hackney ME and Earhart GM. Tai Chi improves balance and mobility in people with Parkinson disease. *Gait Posture*. 2008;28:456–460.

Hackney ME and Earhart GM. Effects of dance on movement control in Parkinson's disease: A comparison of Argentine tango and American ballroom. *J Rehabil Med*. 2009;41:475–481.

Hakim AA, Petrovitch H, Burchfiel CM, et al. Effects of walking on mortality among nonsmoking retired men. *N Engl J Med*. 1998;338:94–99.

Hass CJ, Gregor RJ, Waddell DE, et al. The influence of Tai Chi training on the center of pressure trajectory during gait initiation in older adults. *Arch Phys Med Rehabil*. 2004;85:1593–1598.

Hausdorff JM. Stride variability: Beyond length and frequency. *Gait Posture*. 2004;20:304.

Hausdorff JM, Cudkowicz ME, Firtion R, Wei JY, and Goldberger AL. Gait variability and basal ganglia disorders: Stride-to-stride variations of gait cycle timing in Parkinson's disease and Huntington's disease. *Mov Disord*. 1998;13:428–437.

Hausdorff JM, Edelberg HK, Mitchell SL, Goldberger AL, and Wei JY. Increased gait unsteadiness in community-dwelling elderly fallers. *Arch Phys Med Rehabil*. 1997;78:278–283.

Hausdorff JM, Ladin Z, and Wei JY. Footswitch system for measurement of the temporal parameters of gait. *J Biomech*. 1995;28:347–351.

Hausdorff JM, Lowenthal J, Herman T, Gruendlinger L, Peretz C, and Giladi N. Rhythmic auditory stimulation modulates gait variability in Parkinson's disease. *Eur J Neurosci*. 2007;26:2369–2375.

Hausdorff JM, Mitchell SL, Firtion R, et al. Altered fractal dynamics of gait: Reduced stride-interval correlations with aging and Huntington's disease. *J Appl Physiol*. 1997;82:262–269.

Hausdorff JM, Nelson ME, Kaliton D, et al. Etiology and modification of gait instability in older adults: A randomized controlled trial of exercise. *J Appl Physiol*. 2001;90:2117–2129.

Hausdorff JM, Rios D, and Edelberg HK. Gait variability and fall risk in community-living older adults: A 1-year prospective study. *Arch Phys Med Rehabil*. 2001;82:1050–1056.

Hausdorff JM, Schaafsma JD, Balash Y, Bartels AL, Gurevich T, and Giladi N. Impaired regulation of stride variability in Parkinson's disease subjects with freezing of gait. *Exp Brain Res*. 2003;149:187–194.

Hausdorff JM, Schweiger A, Herman T, Yogev-Seligmann G, and Giladi N. Dual-task decrements in gait: Contributing factors among healthy older adults. *J Gerontol A Biol Sci Med Sci*. 2008;63: 1335–1343.

Hausdorff JM, Yogev G, Springer S, Simon ES, and Giladi N. Walking is more like catching than tapping: Gait in the elderly as a complex cognitive task. *Exp Brain Res*. 2005;164:541–548.

Hayden R, Clair AA, Johnson G, and Otto D. The effect of rhythmic auditory stimulation (RAS) on physical therapy outcomes for patients in gait training following stroke: A feasibility study. *Int J Neurosci*. 2009;119:2183–2195.

Herath P, Klingberg T, Young J, Amunts K, and Roland P. Neural correlates of dual task interference can be dissociated from those of divided attention: An fMRI study. *Cereb Cortex*. 2001;11:796–805.

Herman T, Mirelman A, Giladi N, Schweiger S, Hausdorff JM. Executive control deficits as a prodrome to falls in healthy older adults. A prospective study linking thinking, walking, and falling. Journal of Gerontology: Medical Sciences 2010 (ePub ahead of print).

Herman T, Giladi N, and Hausdorff JM. Properties of the 'Timed Up and Go' Test: More than Meets the Eye. *Gerontology*. 2010 (epub ahead of print).

Herman T, Giladi N, and Hausdorff JM. Treadmill training for the treatment of gait disturbances in people with Parkinson's disease: A mini-review. *J Neural Transm*. 2009;116:307–318.

Herman T, Giladi N, Gruendlinger L, and Hausdorff JM. Six weeks of intensive treadmill training improves gait and quality of life in patients with Parkinson's disease: A pilot study. *Arch Phys Med Rehabil*. 2007;88:1154–1158.

Herman T, Giladi N, Gurevich T, and Hausdorff JM. Gait instability and fractal dynamics of older adults with a "cautious" gait: Why do certain older adults walk fearfully? *Gait Posture*. 2005;21:178–185.

Hesse S, Bertelt C, Jahnke MT, et al. Treadmill training with partial body weight support compared with physiotherapy in nonambulatory hemiparetic patients. *Stroke*. 1995;26:976–981.

Hill K, Schwarz J, Flicker L, and Carroll S. Falls among healthy, community-dwelling, older women: A prospective study of frequency, circumstances, consequences and prediction accuracy. *Australian and New Zealand Journal of Public Health*. 1999;23: 41–48.

Holden MK. Virtual environments for motor rehabilitation: Review. *Cyberpsychol Behav*. 2005;8:187–211.

Holtzer R, Verghese J, Xue X, and Lipton RB. Cognitive processes related to gait velocity: Results from the Einstein Aging Study. *Neuropsychology*. 2006;20:215–223.

Horak FB. Postural orientation and equilibrium: what do we need to know about neural control of balance to prevent falls? *Age and Ageing*. 2006;35:ii7–ii11.

Horak FB, Shupert CL, and Mirka A. Components of postural dyscontrol in the elderly: A review. *Neurobiol Aging*. 1989;10:727–738.

Huber-Mahlin V, Giladi N, Herman T, Perez C, Gurevich T, Hausdorff JM. Progressive Nature of a Higher Level Gait Disorder: A 3 Year Prospective Study. *J Neurology* 2010 (ePub ahead of print).

Jack D, Boian R, Merians AS, et al. Virtual reality-enhanced stroke rehabilitation. *IEEE Trans Neural Syst Rehabil Eng*. 2001;9:308–318.

Jaffe DL, Brown DA, Pierson-Carey CD, Buckley EL, and Lew HL. Stepping over obstacles to improve walking in individuals with poststroke hemiplegia. *J Rehabil Res Dev*. 2004;41:283–292.

Jankovic J, Nutt JG, and Sudarsky L. Classification, diagnosis, and etiology of gait disorders. *Adv Neurol*. 2001;87:119–133.

Jancovic J, Nutt JG, and Sudarsky L. Classification, diagnosis, and etiology of gait disorders. In: Ruzicka E, ed. *Gait disorders*. Philadelphia: Lippincott Williams & Wilkins; 2001:119–133.

Karnath HO, Ferber S, and Dichgans J. The neural representation of postural control in humans. *Proc Natl Acad Sci U S A*. 2000;97:13931–13936.

Kemper S, Herman RE, and Lian CHT. The costs of doing two things at once for young and older adults: Talking while walking, finger tapping, and ignoring speech or noise. *Psychology and Aging.* 2003;18:181–192.

Keogh JW, Kilding A, Pidgeon P, Ashley L, and Gillis D. Physical benefits of dancing for healthy older adults: A review. *J Aging Phys Act.* 2009;17:479–500.

Keshner EA and Weiss PT. Introduction to the special issue from the proceedings of the 2006 International Workshop on Virtual Reality in Rehabilitation. *J Neuroeng Rehabil.* 2007;4:18.

Koller WC, Glatt SL, and Fox JH. Senile gait. A distinct neurologic entity. *Clin Geriatr Med.* 1985;1:661–669.

Kramer AF. Cognitive plasticity and aging. In: Ross BH, ed. *The psychology of learning and motivation.* 43 ed. NY: Academic Press.; 2003:267–302.

Lajoie Y, Teasdale N, Bard C, and Fleury M. Upright standing and gait: Are there changes in attentional requirements related to normal aging? *Experimental Aging Research.* 1996;22:185–198.

Laufer Y, Dickstein R, Chefez Y, and Marcovitz E. The effect of treadmill training on the ambulation of stroke survivors in the early stages of rehabilitation: A randomized study. *J Rehabil Res Dev.* 2001;38:69–78.

Legters K. Fear of falling. *Phys Ther.* 2002;82:264–272.

Legters K, Whitney SL, Porter R, and Buczek F. The relationship between the Activities-specific Balance Confidence Scale and the Dynamic Gait Index in peripheral vestibular dysfunction. *Physiother Res Int.* 2005;10:10–22.

Lezak MD. *Executive function.* New York: Oxford University Press; 1983.

Lezak MD. *Neuropsychological assessment.* New York: Oxford University Press, Inc.; 1995.

Li JX, Hong Y, and Chan KM. Tai Chi: Physiological characteristics and beneficial effects on health. *Br J Sports Med.* 2001;35:148–156.

Li YS, Meyer JS, and Thornby J. Longitudinal follow-up of depressive symptoms among normal versus cognitively impaired elderly. *International Journal of Geriatric Psychiatry.* 2001;16:718–727.

Lim I, Van Wegen E, de Goede C, et al. Effects of external rhythmical cueing on gait in patients with Parkinson's disease: A systematic review. *Clin Rehabil.* 2005;19:695–713.

Lin MR, Hwang HF, Wang YW, Chang SH, and Wolf SL. Community-based Tai Chi and its effect on injurious falls, balance, gait, and fear of falling in older people. *Phys Ther.* 2006;86:1189–1201.

Lindenberger U, Marsiske M, and Baltes PB. Memorizing while walking: Increase in dual-task costs from young adulthood to old age. *Psychol Aging.* 2000;15:417–436.

Lipsitz LA, Jonsson PV, Kelley MM, and Koestner JS. Causes and correlats of recurrent falls in ambulatory frail elderly. *Journals of Gerontology.* 1991;46:114–122.

Liston R, Mickelborough J, Harris B, Hann AW, and Tallis RC. Conventional physiotherapy and treadmill re-training for higher-level gait disorders in cerebrovascular disease. *Age Ageing.* 2000;29:311–318.

Lorenz-Reuter PA. Cognitive neuropsychology of the aging brain. In: Park DC and Schawartz N, eds. *Cognitive aging: A primer.* Philadelphia PA: Psychology Press, Taylor and Francis; 2000:93–114.

Lundin-Olsson L, Nyberg L, and Gustafson Y. "Stops walking when talking" as a predictor of falls in elderly people. *Lancet.* 1997;349:617.

Macpherson JM, Horak FB, Dunbar DC, and Dow RS. Stance dependence of automatic postural adjustments in humans. *Experimental Brain Research.* 1989;78:557–566.

Maki BE. Gait changes in older adults: Predictors of falls or indicators of fear. *J Am Geriatr Soc.* 1997;45:313–320.

Malouin F, Richards CL, Jackson PL, Dumas F, and Doyon J. Brain activations during motor imagery of locomotor-related tasks: A PET study. *Hum Brain Mapp.* 2003;19:47–62.

McIlroy WE and Maki BE. Changes in early automatic postural responses associated with the prior-planning and execution of a compensatory step. *Brain Research.* 1993;203–211.

McIntosh G, Thaut M, Rice R, and Miller R. Stride frequency modulation in Parkinsonian gait using rhythmic auditory stimulation. *Ann Neurol.* 1994;36(2):316.

Melzer I, Benjuya N, and Kaplanski J. Age-related changes of postural control: Effect of cognitive tasks. *Gerontology.* 2001;47:189–194.

Menon V, Adleman NE, White CD, Glover GH, and Reiss AL. Error-related brain activation during a Go/NoGo response inhibition task. *Hum Brain Mapp.* 2001;12:131–143.

Mirelman A, Bonato P, and Deutsch JE. Effects of training with a robot-virtual reality system compared with a robot alone on the gait of individuals after stroke. *Stroke.* 2009;40:169–174.

Miyai I, Fujimoto Y, Yamamoto H, et al. Long-term effect of body weight-supported treadmill training in Parkinson's disease: A randomized controlled trial. *Arch Phys Med Rehabil.* 2002;83:1370–1373.

Montero-Odasso M, Wells J, and Borrie M. Can cognitive enhancers reduce the risk of falls in people with dementia? An open-label study with controls. *J Am Geriatr Soc.* 2009;57:359–360.

Montero-Odasso M, Wells JL, Borrie MJ, and Speechley M. Can cognitive enhancers reduce the risk of falls in older people with mild cognitive impairment? A protocol for a randomised controlled double blind trial. *BMC Neurol.* 2009;9:42.

Morris ME. Movement disorders in people with Parkinson disease: A model for physical therapy. *Phys Ther.* 2000;80:578–597.

Morris ME, Iansek R, Matyas TA, and Summers JJ. Stride length regulation in Parkinson's disease. Normalization strategies and underlying mechanisms. *Brain.* 1996;119 (Pt 2):551–568.

Morris ME, Perry A, Bilney B, et al. Outcomes of physical therapy, speech pathology, and occupational therapy for people with motor neuron disease: A systematic review. *Neurorehabil Neural Repair.* 2006;20:424–434.

Murphy J and Isaacs B. The post-fall syndrome. A study of 36 elderly patients. *Gerontology.* 1982;28:265–270.

Nashner LM and Woollacott MH. The organization of rapid postural adjustments of standing humans: An experimental conceptual model. *Posture Movement.* 1979;243–257.

Nasreddine ZS, Phillips NA, Bedirian V, et al. The Montreal Cognitive Assessment, MoCA: A brief screening tool for mild cognitive impairment. *J Am Geriatr Soc.* 2005;53:695–699.

Nieuwboer A, Kwakkel G, Rochester L, et al. Cueing training in the home improves gait-related mobility in Parkinson's disease: The RESCUE trial. *J Neurol Neurosurg Psychiatry.* 2007;78:134–140.

Nutt JG. Classification of gait and balance disorders. *Adv Neurol.* 2001;87:135–141.

Nutt JG, Carter JH, and Carlson NE. Effects of methylphenidate on response to oral levodopa: A double-blind clinical trial. *Arch Neurol.* 2007;64:319–323.

Nutt JG, Marsden CD, and Thompson PD. Human walking and higher-level gait disorders, particularly in the elderly. *Neurology.* 1993;43:268–279.

Nyberg L and Gustafson Y. Patient falls in stroke rehabilitation - a challenge to rehabilitation strategies. *Stroke.* 1995;26:838–842.

O'Shea S, Morris ME, and Iansek R. Dual task interference during gait in people with Parkinson disease: Effects of motor versus cognitive secondary tasks. *Physical Therapy.* 2002;82:888–897.

Ostchega Y, Harris TB, Hirsch R, Parsons VL, and Kington R. The prevalence of functional limitations and disability in older persons in the US: Data from the National Health and Nutrition Examination Survey III. *J Am Geriatr Soc.* 2000;48:1132–1135.

Pahor M, Blair SN, Espeland M, et al. Effects of a physical activity intervention on measures of physical performance: Results of the lifestyle interventions and independence for Elders Pilot (LIFE-P) Study. *J Gerontol A Biol Sci Med Sci.* 2006;61:1157–1165.

Paleacu D, Shutzman A, Giladi N, Herman T, Simon ES, and Hausdorff JM. Effects of pharmacological therapy on gait and cognitive function in depressed patients. *Clin Neuropharmacol.* 2007;30:63–71.

Patla AE and Vickers JN. Where and when do we look as we approach and step over an obstacle in the travel path? *NeuroReport.* 1997;8:3661–665.

Podsiadlo D and Richardson S. The timed "Up & Go": A test of basic functional mobility for frail elderly persons. *J Am Geriatr Soc.* 1991;39:142–148.

Powell LE and Myers AM. The Activities-specific Balance Confidence (ABC) Scale. *J Gerontol A Biol Sci Med Sci.* 1995;50A:M28–M34.

Province MA, Hadley EC, Hornbrook MC, et al. The effects of exercise on falls in elderly patients. A preplanned meta-analysis of the FICSIT Trials. Frailty and Injuries: Cooperative Studies of Intervention Techniques. *JAMA.* 1995;273:1341–1347.

Rajput A and Rajput AH. Progressive supranuclear palsy: Clinical features, pathophysiology and management. *Drugs Aging.* 2001;18:913–925.

Reelick MF, van Iersel MB, Kessels RP, and Rikkert MG. The influence of fear of falling on gait and balance in older people. *Age Ageing.* 2009;38:435–440.

Ridderinkhof KR, van den Wildenberg WP, Segalowitz SJ, and Carter CS. Neurocognitive mechanisms of cognitive control: The role of prefrontal cortex in action selection, response inhibition, performance monitoring, and reward-based learning. *Brain Cogn.* 2004;56:129–140.

Rizzo AA and Buckwalter JG. The status of virtual reality for the cognitive rehabilitation of persons with neurological disorders and acquired brain injury. *Stud Health Technol Inform.* 1997;39:22–33.

Rizzo AA and Buckwalter JG. Virtual reality and cognitive assessment and rehabilitation: The state of the art. *Stud Health Technol Inform.* 1997;44:123–145.

Robbins TW, James M, Owen AM, et al. A study of performance on tests from the CANTAB battery sensitive to frontal lobe dysfunction in a large sample of normal volunteers: Implications for theories of executive functioning and cognitive aging. Cambridge Neuropsychological Test Automated Battery. *J Int Neuropsychol Soc.* 1998;4:474–490.

Robertson MC, Gardner MM, Devlin N, McGee R, and Campbell AJ. Effectiveness and economic evaluation of a nurse delivered home exercise programme to prevent falls. 2: Controlled trial in multiple centres. *BMJ.* 2001;322:701–704.

Rochester L, Hetherington V, Jones D, et al. The effect of external rhythmic cues (auditory and visual) on walking during a functional task in homes of people with Parkinson's disease. *Arch Phys Med Rehabil.* 2005;86:999–1006.

Rubenstein TC, Giladi N, and Hausdorff JM. The power of cueing to circumvent dopamine deficits: A review of physical therapy treatment of gait disturbances in Parkinson's disease. *Mov Disord.* 2002;17:1148–1160.

Sacco K, Cauda F, Cerliani L, Mate D, Duca S, and Geminiani GC. Motor imagery of walking following training in locomotor attention. The effect of "the tango lesson". *Neuroimage.* 2006;32:1441–1449.

Sattin RW, Rodriguez JG, DeVito CA, and Wingo PA. Home environmental hazards and the risk of fall injury events among community-dwelling older persons. Study to Assess Falls Among the Elderly (SAFE) Group. *J Am Geriatr Soc.* 1998;46:669–676.

Schrodt LA, Mercer VS, Giuliani CA, and Hartman M. Characteristics of stepping over an obstacle in community dwelling older adults under dual-task conditions. *Gait & Posture.* 2004;19:279–287.

Sehested P and Severinnielsen T. Falls by hospitalized elderly patients - causes, prevention. *Geriatrics.* 1977;32:101–108.

Shimada H, Obuchi S, Furuna T, and Suzuki T. New intervention program for preventing falls among frail elderly people: The effects of perturbed walking exercise using a bilateral separated treadmill. *Am J Phys Med Rehabil.* 2004;83:493–499.

Shumway-Cook A and Woollacott M. *Motor control: Theory and applications.* Baltimore, MD: Wilkins & Wilkins; 1995.

Shumway-Cook A, Brauer S, and Woollacott M. Predicting the probability for falls in community-dwelling older adults using the Timed Up & Go Test. *Phys Ther.* 2000;80:896–903.

Shumway-Cook A, Woollacott M, Kerns KA, and Baldwin M. The Effects of two types of cognitive tasks on postural stability in older adults with and without a history of falls. *Journal of Gerontology.* 1997;52A:M232–M240.

Spielberger, CD, et al. State-Trait Anxiety Inventory. Self-evaluation questionnaire (form Y). In: *Manual for the state-trait anxiety Inventory.* 1983. Palo Alto, CA.

Springer S, Giladi N, Peretz C, Yogev G, Simon ES, and Hausdorff JM. Dual-tasking effects on gait variability: The role of aging, falls, and executive function. *Mov Disord.* 2006;21:950–957.

Srygley JM, Mirelman A, Herman T, Giladi N, and Hausdorff JM. When does walking alter thinking? Age and task associated findings. *Brain Res.* 2009;1253:92–99.

Stevens M, Holman CDJ, and Bennett N. Preventing falls in older people: Impact outcome evaluation of a randomized controlled trial. *J Am Geriatr Soc.* 2001;49:1448–1455.

Stevens JA, Mack KA, Paulozzi LJ, and Ballesteros MF. Self-reported falls and fall-related injuries among persons aged>or=65 years–United States, 2006. *J Safety Res.* 2008;39:345–349.

Sudarsky L. Geriatrics: Gait disorders in the elderly. *N Engl J Med.* 1990;322:1441–1446.

Sudarsky L. Gait disorders: Prevalence, morbidity, and etiology. *Adv Neurol.* 2001;87:111–117.

Suzuki M, Ohyama N, Yamada K, and Kanamori M. The relationship between fear of falling, activities of daily living and quality of life among elderly individuals. *Nurs Health Sci.* 2002;4:155–161.

Tamir R, Dickstein R, and Huberman M. Integration of motor imagery and physical practice in group treatment applied to subjects with Parkinson's disease. *Neurorehabil Neural Repair.* 2007;21:68–75.

Teasdale N and Simoneau M. Attentional demands for postural control: The effects of aging and sensory reintegration. *Gait Posture.* 2001;14:203–210.

Teasdale N, Bard C, LaRue J, and Fleury M. On the cognitive penetrability of posture control. *Experimental Aging Research.* 1993;19:1–13.

Teasdale N, Stelmach GE, and Breunig A. Postural sway characteristics of the elderly under normal and altered visual and support surface conditions. *J Gerontol.* 1991;46:B238–B244.

Tinetti ME, Baker DI, McAvay G, et al. A multifactorial intervention to reduce the risk of falling among elderly people living in the community. *N Engl J Med.* 1994;331:821–827.

Tinetti ME, Richman D, and Powell L. Falls efficacy as a measure of fear of falling. *Journal of Gerontology: Psychological Sciences.* 1990;45:P239–P243.

Tinetti ME, Speechley M, and Ginter SF. Risk factors for falls among elderly persons living in the community. *The New England Journal of Medicine.* 1988;319:1701–1707.

Tinetti ME, Williams TF, and Mayewski R. Fall risk index for elderly patients based on number of chronic disabilities. *The American Journal of Medicine.* 1986;80:429–434.

Tinetti ME, Mendes de Leon CF, Doucette JT, and Baker DI. Fear of falling and fall-related efficacy in relationship to functioning among community-living elders. *Journal of Gerontology: Medical Sciences.* 1994;49:140–147.

van Hedel HJ, Waldvogel D, and Dietz V. Learning a high-precision locomotor task in patients with Parkinson's disease. *Mov Disord.* 2006;21:406–411.

van Iersel MB, Verbeek AL, Bloem BR, Munneke M, Esselink RA, and Rikkert MG. Frail elderly patients with dementia go too fast. *J Neurol Neurosurg Psychiatry.* 2006;77:874–876.

Verghese J. Cognitive and mobility profile of older social dancers. *J Am Geriatr Soc.* 2006;54:1241–1244.

Verghese J, Levalley A, Hall CB, Katz MJ, Ambrose AF, and Lipton RB. Epidemiology of gait disorders in community-residing older adults. *J Am Geriatr Soc.* 2006;54:255–261.

Verghese J, Lipton RB, Hall CB, Kuslansky G, Katz MJ, and Buschke H. Abnormality of gait as a predictor of non-Alzheimer's dementia. *N Engl J Med.* 2002;347:1761–1768.

Voermans NC, Snijders AH, Schoon Y, and Bloem BR. Why old people fall (and how to stop them). *Pract Neurol.* 2007;7:158–71.

Wada M, Sunaga N, and Nagai M. Anxiety affects the postural sway of the antero-posterior axis in college students. *Neuroscience Letters.* 2001;302:157–159.

Watelain E, Barbier F, Allard P, Thevenon A, and Angue JC. Gait pattern classification of healthy elderly men based on biomechanical data. *Arch Phys Med Rehabil.* 2000;81:579–586.

Welford AT. *Ageing and human skill.* London: Oxford University Press; 1958.

Whitman GT, DiPatre PL, Lopez IA, et al. Neuropathology in older people with disequilibrium of unknown cause. *Neurology.* 1999;53:375–382.

Whitman GT, Tang Y, Lin A, Baloh RW, and Tang T. A prospective study of cerebral white matter abnormalities in older people with gait dysfunction. *Neurology.* 2001;57:990–994.

Whittle MW. *Gait analysis: An introduction.* Second ed. ed. Oxford: Butterworth-Heinemann; 1996.

Wilson RS, Schneider JA, Beckett LA, Evans DA, and Bennett DA. Progression of gait disorder and rigidity and risk of death in older persons. *Neurology.* 2002;58:1815–1819.

Wolf SL, Barnhart HX, Ellison GL, and Coogler CE. The effect of Tai Chi Quan and computerized balance training on postural stability in older subjects. Atlanta FICSIT Group. Frailty and Injuries: Cooperative Studies on Intervention Techniques. *Phys Ther.* 1997;77: 371–381.

Wolf SL, Barnhart HX, Kutner NG, McNeely E, Coogler C, and Xu T. Reducing frailty and falls in older persons: An investigation of Tai Chi and computerized balance training. Atlanta FICSIT Group. Frailty and Injuries: Cooperative Studies of Intervention Techniques. *J Am Geriatr Soc.* 1996;44:489–497.

Wolf SL, Sattin RW, O'Grady M, et al. A study design to investigate the effect of intense Tai Chi in reducing falls among older adults transitioning to frailty. *Control Clin Trials.* 2001;22:689–704.

Woollacott M and Shumway-Cook A. Attention and the control of posture and gait: A review of an emerging area of research. *Gait & Posture.* 2002;16:1–14.

Wu G. Evaluation of the effectiveness of tai chi for improving balance and preventing falls in the older population-a review. *J Am Geriatr Soc.* 2002;50:746–754.

Yardley L and Redfern MS. Psychological factors influencing recovery from balance disorders. *Anxiety Disorders.* 2001;107–119.

Yesavage JA, Brink TL, Rose TL, et al. Development and validation of a geriatric depression screening scale: A preliminary report. *J Psychiatr Res.* 1982;17:37–49.

Yogev G, Giladi N, Peretz C, Springer S, Simon ES, and Hausdorff JM. Dual tasking, gait rhythmicity, and Parkinson's disease: Which aspects of gait are attention demanding? *Eur J Neurosci.* 2005;22:1248–1256.

Yogev-Seligmann G, Hausdorff JM, and Giladi N. The role of executive function and attention in gait. *Mov Disord.* 2008;23:329–342.

You SH, Jang SH, Kim YH, et al. Virtual reality-induced cortical reorganization and associated locomotor recovery in chronic stroke: An experimenter-blind randomized study. *Stroke.* 2005;36:1166–1171.

Zeilinger FS and Meier U. [Clinically suspected normal-pressure hydrocephalus diagnosis–current status of diagnosis and therapy]. *Z Arztl Fortbild Qualitatssich.* 1998;92:495–501.

26 Falls in Aging and Neurological Disease

Richard Camicioli

Introduction

Falls have been defined as unintentionally coming to the ground or some lower level other than as a consequence of sustaining a violent blow, loss of consciousness, sudden onset of paralysis as in stroke, or an epileptic seizure (Kellogg International Work Group 1987). Falls are a major public health problem. They occur in over 30% of older people with 10% of falls resulting in a serious injury. Falls can reliably be classified as intrinsic, due to factors directly related to the patient, or extrinsic, due to external environmental factors (Lach et al. 1991). While important consequences of falls include direct injury (including head and spinal cord injury and fractures) and death, falls can lead to restriction of activity and increased care needs, independent of injury. Fear of falling, beyond simple restriction due to pain or other factors, is another characteristic that can develop after a fall and inhibit normal activities (Zijlstra, van Haastregt, van Eijk et al. 2007).

Recognized risk factors for falls in older people include arthritis, depression, orthostatic blood pressure drop, cognitive impairment, visual impairment, balance impairment, gait disorder, weakness, and use of multiple medications (Ganz, Bao, Shekelle, and Rubenstein 2007). Age is one of the most important risk factor for falls and among older people neurological disorders compound this risk. A history of previous falls is an important factor that can readily be identified. Importantly, interventions can reduce the risk of falls, though the nature of interventions applied and their applicability to specific individuals with specific neurological requires consideration (Tinetti 2003). Quantitative screening assessments (i.e., timed balance or gait measures) may offer advantages over clinical assessments of risk factors in predicting falls risk, though approaches validated in the general population might not apply in specific neurological groups (Lamb, McCabe, Becker, Fried, and Guralnik 2008).

Falls in general, and injurious falls in particular, are accidents whose incidence increases in vulnerable individuals who place themselves in risky situations within an environment. Systems approaches, which have been applied to accidents such as airline crashes, may provide a more comprehensive view of falls, but are investigational (Zecevic, Salmoni, Lewko, and Vandervoort 2007). Even people with no intrinsic risk factors can fall if placed in risky situations. Specific neurological conditions, such as stroke, dementia, and Parkinson's disease, among others, lead to cognitive and physical impairment, which increase an individual's risk of falls when carrying out routine activities. Conditions such as osteoporosis can make it more likely that a fall might lead to a serious outcome such as a fracture. Complete elimination of extrinsic risk is impossible, though programs focusing on risk factor modification can be helpful. Just as the clinical features in an older person may be important in identifying at-risk individuals and tailoring treatment, the environment in which the person lives may also affect the approach to intervention. For example, people living at home may need different interventions compared to those living in institutional settings or acutely ill patients in a hospital.

Practice parameters for the assessment and treatment of falls in older people in general have been produced by the American Geriatrics Society (AGS) (American Geriatrics Society, British Geriatrics Society, and American Academy of Orthopaedic Surgeons 2001) (and the National Institute for Clinical Excellence (NICE) in the U.K. (www.nice.org.uk). The Cochrane collaborative has also published a systematic review of exercise in preventing falls (Gillespie et al. 2009). Recently, guidelines have been developed for application to neurological disorders (Thurman, Stevens, Rao, and Quality Standards Subcommittee of the American Academy of Neurology 2008).

The neurology guidelines systematically reviewed the literature with regards to non-syncopal falls in the setting of neurological disorders. Increased falls risk was clearly associated with dementia, stroke, and patients with gait and balance impairment, including the use of assistive devices (Level A). An increased risk of falls was also shown among patients with Parkinson's disease, peripheral neuropathy, sensory loss (including visual loss), and weakness (Level B). The utility of specific screening tests for refining falls risk, beyond the traditional neurological examination, required further evaluation. Thus, this chapter, while highlighting areas for future research, collated strong evidence for the importance of considering patients with neurological disease at high risk for falls. Among risk factors, a history of prior falls was strongly associated with subsequent falls. Thus the practice parameter suggested asking all patients with the neurological disorders associated with increased falls risk about prior falls. Semi-quantitative measurements such as assessing Timed Up and Go (Podsiadlo and Richardson 1989) or Tinetti's performance-based assessment of gait and balance (Tinetti 1986) may be considered, but their utility beyond standardized assessment requires further evaluation.

In a study that examined falls both with and without loss of consciousness in a neurological inpatient setting, one-third of patients with neurological disorders had fallen in the previous year, with a significant minority (22%) falling due to a disturbance of level of consciousness (including seizures and syncope) (Stolze et al. 2004). Diagnoses associated with falls were Parkinson's disease, syncope, polyneuropathy, epilepsy, motor neuron disease, multiple sclerosis, psychogenic disorders, stroke, and pain. Gait and posture disturbance was correlated with falls, with many falls associated with tripping over objects. Syncopal falls should be considered in the differential diagnosis of all neurological patients who have fallen, and appropriately investigated and treated.

Pathophysiology

A discussion of the pathophysiology of falls can be divided into consideration of intrinsic and extrinsic risk factors. As aging is a major risk factor, some investigators have examined age-related physiological changes associated with increased falls risk. Physiological changes associated with falls that have been examined include changes in vision, proprioception, strength, balance, and reaction time (Lord, Sherrington, Menz, and Close 2007). Gait impairment is also associated with increased falls risk (Verghese, Holtzer, Lipton, and Wang 2009). Decline in many of these intrinsic physiological factors are amplified as a consequence of neurological disorders.

The mechanism of falls may differ among neurological disorders. For instance, patients with dementia might exert poor judgment, placing themselves at risk for falls. Disorders associated with both physical and cognitive dysfunction, such as stroke, Parkinson's disease, Huntington disease, progressive supranuclear palsy, and corticobasal ganglionic degeneration may afford particular challenges. Patients with parkinsonian disorders (which include Parkinson's disease, progressive supranuclear palsy, and multiple system atrophy among others) are particularly prone to falls and fractures due to impaired protective responses (Williams, Watt, and Lees 2006).

Falls occur when the individual can't maintain upright posture against gravity, whatever the basis for the loss of ability to stand. Although by some definitions falls are not associated with loss of consciousness, practically speaking the first step in evaluation requires determination of whether consciousness was lost or not. Some older people, especially those with cognitive dysfunction, might not be able to reliably know if they lost consciousness or not. Therefore, falls associated with subject-centered risk can be divided into events associated with loss of consciousness and those not associated with loss of consciousness. Falls associated with loss of consciousness include events such as syncope, cardiac arrhythmias, or other factors that lead to impaired cardiopulmonary function and seizures and other disorders of consciousness (Thijs, Bloem, and van Dijk 2009). These mechanisms can interact as illustrated by the potential of seizures to lead to syncope (ictal syncope) (Schuele et al. 2007). Head injury can lead to amnesia for an event, even though the initial fall might not have been associated with initial loss of consciousness.

Drop attacks are a distinct type of fall associated with sudden loss of postural tone without loss of consciousness, often associated with diagnosable causes such as carotid sinus hypersensitivity and other cardiac and neurological causes (Parry and Kenny 2005). Thus, some causes of syncopal falls (such as cardiac arrhythmias or orthostatic hypotension) can lead to loss of postural tone without clear impairment of consciousness. Drop attacks can also be associated with otologic causes without clear vertigo (Ishiyama, Ishiyama, Jacobson, and Baloh 2001).

Maintenance of upright posture requires appropriate response to visual, proprioceptive, and vestibular sensory input, components of which can be assessed physiologically in the clinical (Matsumura and Ambrose 2006) and laboratory setting (Visser, Carpenter, van der Kooij, and Bloem 2008a). The ability to respond properly to such signals depends on an intact central nervous system for integration and processing, ultimately leading to an appropriate motor response. The musculoskeletal system is the final common pathway generating forces that counteract gravity in the situation of an extrinsic perturbation. Overlapping systems are involved in mobility.

Falls tend to occur while walking. Gait requires the same systems involved in balance. In addition, bipedal gait requires initiation, stepping, and adaptation to changing circumstances (Snijders, van de Warrenburg, Giladi, and Bloem 2007). Walking taxes balance, and hence places individuals at great risk for falls. In addition, walking requires that the cardio-respiratory system is functioning adequately. Abnormalities of balance and gait commonly occur in aging and particularly in the setting of neurological disease and disorders of the musculoskeletal system.

Extrinsic precipitants that are severe enough can overwhelm even optimally functioning individuals. However, factors such as dim lighting, obstacles, slippery or moving surfaces, and the need for rapid movement can synergize in increasing an individual's risk for falls.

Genetic Contribution

While falls in older people are often associated with conditions associated with aging, a family history of sudden death (suggesting cardiac arrhythmia or seizures) should be sought. Narcolepsy is associated with falls and genetic predisposition (Longstreth, Koepsell, Ton, Hendrickson, and van Belle 2007). Some degenerative neurological conditions can be associated with a family history (such as various dementias, including Alzheimer disease, Huntington disease, and frontotemporal dementias). Genetically mediated disorders such as myopathies, myotonic dystrophy, and some neuropathies are associated with weakness or sensory changes that predispose to falls. Apolipoprotein E4, which is associated with Alzheimer's disease, has been associated with fracture risk (Cauley et al. 1999; Johnston, Cauley, and Ganguli 1999). Genetic factors associated with pharmacokinetic or pharmacodynamic diversity (Salmen et al. 2002) or bone mineral density (Kannus, Palvanen, Kaprio, Parkkari, and Koskenvuo 1999) could be hypothesized as influencing falls and fracture risk, but are less thoroughly investigated.

Clinical Presentation and Approach

Patients may report falls to the clinician spontaneously, may acknowledge it when asked or can be identified as a consequence of injury. Whenever a fall has occurred it is important to obtain a detailed history from the patient, preferably corroborated by a witness. Specific issues include the patient's primary neurological diagnosis, co-morbid conditions, and medications. A general examination is important to rule out postural hypotension and systemic disease. The degree of neurological impairment from the patient's disease is important to document. Additionally, regardless of disease status, it is important to identify risk factors for falls, including altered mental status, sensory changes (visual, vestibular, peripheral sensory), and diminished strength, balance, or mobility. Assessment of specific neurological dysfunction and fall risk can follow the same approach utilized to classify gait impairment (Thompson and Nutt 2007), based on levels of the nervous system involved.

Lower Level Disorders

Disorders that affect primary sensory modalities such as vision (Coleman et al. 2007) and vestibular function (Jacobson, McCaslin, Grantham, and Piker 2008; Agrawal, Carey, Della Santina, Schubert, and Minor 2009) can increase falls risk. Evidence for these should be sought by history and screened for on examination. Lower level impairment would be expected to be associated with trips and slips. Patients with peripheral sensory impairment often complain of difficulty walking with diminished sensory input, such as walking in the dark; patients with weakness have difficulty rising from chairs or climbing stairs. Orthopedic problems should be kept in mind by neurologists assessing older people suspected of having lower level gait problems (Lim, Huang, Wu, Girardi, and Cammisa 2007). One study found that patients with lumbar radiculopathy were at risk for falls (Syrjala, Luukinen, Pyhtinen, and Tolonen 2003).

Neuromuscular Disorders

Disorders of peripheral nerves can affect balance both by impairment of afferent sensory input, but also through weakness. Such disorders are common in older people and associated with falls (DeMott,

Richardson, Thies, and Ashton-Miller 2007). Some disorders associated with neuropathy, such as diabetes (Patel et al. 2008), can also affect the brain and lead to falls by affecting both central and peripheral function. Another example of a cause of falls with both central and peripheral influences is alcohol use, which, along with medications, should be considered as contributing to falls.

Disorders of the neuromuscular junction and muscle can lead to weakness, which makes it difficult to rise from a chair, climb stairs, or reach for items. Impaired strength can reduce the individual's ability to respond if off-balance and decreases gait speed and floor clearance, all of which can increase falls risk. While specific disorders of muscle, such as acquired myopathy, or the neuromuscular junction, such as myasthenia gravis, cause weakness, quantitative strength testing shows that weakness also occurs in older people, without a clear cause, and is correlated with impaired gait and falls (Lloyd et al. 2009). Reasons for the loss of strength and muscle mass that occur in aging are not entirely clear, but at the extreme, the term sarcopenia is applied to the loss of muscle mass and subsequent weakness.

Myotonic dystrophy is a disease of muscle associated with falls (Wiles et al. 2006), which illustrates the difficulty with simply considering central versus peripheral aspects of neuromuscular diseases. Thought a muscle disorder, myotonic dystrophy is associated with visual and cognitive change, and cardiac abnormalities as well as sleep abnormalities, all of which might increase risk for falling.

Middle Level

Middle level pathologies lead to combined motor and sensory deficits, as well as impaired sensory integration and response to perturbation. These non-cortical central nervous system changes are often associated with more complex changes in motor abilities than simple peripheral or lower level changes placing people at especially high risk for falls.

Myelopathy

Myelopathy is associated with balance and gait impairment and weakness, which can lead to falls (Brotherton, Krause, and Nietert 2007). Given multiple potential causes, interventions need to be individualized. Recognition of falls risk is important to keep in mind, however. Spinal cord injury can be a consequence of falls and should be ruled out in the emergent assessment of falls.

Cerebellar Disorders

Cerebellar dysfunction can be seen in the setting of mass lesions, demyelinating disorders, degenerative disorders, and stroke. Hereditary and degenerative spinocerebellar disorders are also associated with falls (van de Warrenburg, Steijns, Munneke, Kremer, and Bloem 2005). Progressive disorders require ongoing adaptations by patients in attempting to continue to prevent falls.

Extrapyramidal System

Dysfunction of the extrapyramidal system can lead to hypo or hyperkinetic movements, exemplified by Parkinson's disease and Huntington disease, respectively, which we will discuss next. Dystonias and paroxysmal dyskinesias can also be associated with falls, but have not been as studied.

Parkinsonism and Parkinson's Disease

Falls and fracture risk are common in patients with Parkinson's disease and are even more common in people with parkinsonism from disorders other than idiopathic Parkinson's disease. In Parkinson's disease about a third to two-thirds experience a fall within a year of follow up

and 90% have a fall at some point during their life with the disease (Pickering et al. 2007). Clinical features associated with falling in patients with PD include previous falls, cognitive impairment, freezing of gait, and axial posture impairment; physiological measures such as imbalance and leg weakness may refine falls predictions (Latt, Lord, Morris, and Fung 2009). Other features seen in PD, such as postural hypotension, might also be predicted to be associated with falls, and while a recent study did not support this speculation, prospective study is indicated (Matinolli, Korpelainen, Korpelainen, Sotaniemi, and Myllyla 2009). The presence of early falls in a patient with parkinsonism raises the concern of an alternate diagnosis including dementia with Lewy bodies, progressive supranuclear palsy, multiple system atrophy, vascular parkinsonism, or normal pressure hydrocephalus (Wenning et al. 1999). Up to 90% of people with PSP will fall within a year of symptom onset. Since patients with parkinsonism don't have appropriate protective responses and refelxes, they are at particular risk of injury from their falls (Grimbergen, Munneke, and Bloem 2004).

Huntington Disease

Falls are common in patients with Huntington disease, where they are associated with impaired balance (using the Berg Balance Scale) and mobility (using the Timed Up and Go test) (Busse, Wiles, and Rosser 2009). Falls are a particular concern in older patients in whom age-related changes in balance and mobility and coexistent medical conditions may contribute to increasing falls risk (Lipe and Bird 2009). In addition, chorea may add to falls risk (Grimbergen et al. 2008). As in disorders associated with parkinsonism, the possible contribution of cognitive impairment to falls risk should be considered in patients with Huntington disease.

Higher Level Disorders
Mild Cognitive Impairment and Dementia

Dementia is clearly associated with an increased falls incidence. In a recent prospective study of various dementia subtypes, a diagnosis of a Lewy body dementia and prior falls were particular risk factors (Allan, Ballard, Rowan, and Kenny 2009). Multivariate predictors in this study were autonomic features, orthostatic hypotension, and depressive symptoms, while physical activity was protective. Features associated with dementia such as poor judgment, medications (which represents a modifiable risk factor), visuospatial impairment on a cognitive basis, and delirium can readily be envisaged as increasing falls risk.

While mild cognitive impairment (MCI) has not been studied in as much detail as dementia, there appears to be an association between subtypes of MCI and gait impairment (Verghese et al. 2008). Other studies have looked at the cognitive profile of people with falls and impairments of attention, and executive function seems to be particularly associated with falls risk (Holtzer et al. 2007). Given the high risk of dementia in people with MCI and related syndromes (cognitive impairment, not dementia; questionable dementia), identification of these subjects might provide a window of opportunity for falls prevention (Liu-Ambrose, Ashe, Graf, Beattie, and Khan 2008). This is particularly important given the lack of success of falls prevention interventions in people with established dementia (Shaw 2007a).

Based on the speculation that falls occur while conducting activities, investigators have examined the ability of dual task performance in predicting falls risk. While it is clear that performing a cognitive task and a motor task at the same time affects balance and walking, not all studies have shown and enhance ability to predict falls accurately (Zijlstra, Ufkes, Skelton, Lundin-Olsson, and Zijlstra 2008). In part, this might be due to study design, the specific subject groups examined, the nature of the dual tasks involved, and the parameters examined. For example, effects on gait variability may be particularly relevant in falls prediction (Kressig, Herrmann, Grandjean, Michel, and Beauchet 2008).

Multiple Level Disorders

Many neurological diseases can influence neurological dysfunction at multiple levels. As noted, some neuromuscular disorders, such as mytotonic dystrophy, can affect lower and higher levels. Multiple sclerosis and stroke typically affect higher and middle level systems. It should be noted that disorders affecting the basal ganglia, such as Parkinson's disease and Huntington disease, considered middle level disorders, have high-level effects on cognitive function that can contribute to increasing falls risk.

Stroke

A fall can be a consequence of an incident stroke, with one recent study showing that falls occurred in over one-third of patents in the six months following a stroke (Kerse et al. 2008). The mechanisms by which stroke increases falls risk is multi-factorial since stroke can reduce both cognitive function and mobility, which increase falls risk. White matter disease, in particular, is also associated with an increased risk of falls (Srikanth et al. 2009), possibly through cognitive and motor deficits combining to increase risk. Patients with white matter disease also often have depressive symptoms, which has also been associated with increased risk of falls. Patients with cerebrovascular disease are often on multiple medications that can further contribute to the risk of falling.

Demyelinating Disease

Multiple sclerosis commonly affects multiple levels of the nervous system, including the cortex, spinal cord, cerebellum and subcortical areas, hence it isn't surprising that this diagnosis is associated with increased falls risk (Finlayson, Peterson, and Cho 2006). In a retrospective study, Finlayson et al. have identified risk factors including male gender, fear of falling, variable or deteriorating MS status in the past year, never or occasional use of a wheelchair, problems with balance or mobility, poor concentration or forgetfulness, and incontinence of bladder. Some of these are amenable to specific interventions. Fear of falling may be present in MS patients and potentially is remediable (Peterson, Cho, and Finlayson 2007).

Diagnosis: History, Exam, Imaging, Laboratory Tests, Exclusionary Conditions

History

Obtaining an accurate history is the first and critical step in assessing falls. Regarding the fall itself, it is important to discern if there was loss of consciousness, though people who lose consciousness do not necessarily remember if they do. A reliable witness is critical to assist in clarifying the nature and circumstances of the fall. The history can identify precedent events, as well as the appearance of the faller after the falls. A history of a fall occurring after suddenly standing or postprandially, for example, might suggest syncope. A fall occurring after chest pain might raise concern of a pulmonary embolism, aortic dissection, or a myocardial infarction. A prolonged, post-event altered level of consciousness can be a consequence of a head injury or seizure, for instance. Incontinence and sustained or asymmetrical jerking movements suggest a seizure. New onset urgency or incontinence may suggest a urinary tract infection. An acute change in cognitive function might indicate a delirium and a search for an underlying cause such as a systemic infection should be considered in people who have fallen.

Environmental hazards can be identified by history, but inspection of the environment where the fall occurred will help target interventions. A fall can be the first manifestation of a neurological disorder, such as dementia with Lewy bodies, hence any history of progressive impairment is important to identify.

Visual impairment, hearing impairment, vestibular dysfunction or symptoms suggestive of a neuropathy can sometimes be elicited by history. Similarly a fall occurring in the setting of progressive functional impairment or declining mobility might raise the concern of a covert neurological condition.

Co-morbid conditions are important to identify. History of a neurological disorder, such as Parkinson's disease, helps focus the clinician on optimizing management. The presence of known dementia, while a risk factor for falls, also raises concern regarding the patient's ability to accurately render a history and participate actively in rehabilitation. Cardiovascular risk factors raise the probability of a vascular event as a direct cause or a contributing factor. A past medical history of a head injury or prior spell suggestive of a seizure makes another seizure more likely.

Since medications are a critical risk factor for falls, these should be reviewed in detail and part of any intervention will be focused on minimizing the use of unnecessary medications. In particular, antidepressants, sedative-hypnotics, and antipsychotic medication have been associated with falls.

Examination

Physical examination should include assessment of vision, hearing, and vital signs. Proper assessment of postural blood pressure changes is critical. A cardio-respiratory examination is important. Abdominal examination focuses on evidence for organomegaly and the presence of an abdominal aneurysm, the latter reflecting the presence of atherosclerosis. Musculoskeletal assessment is indicated.

Mental status is critical to assess. In addition to being a risk factor for falls, cognitive impairment requires special consideration in terms of planning intervention. Identification of patients with mild cognitive impairment may be relevant, even though not as clearly established a risk factor as dementia. To that end, more sensitive instruments such as the Montreal Cognitive Assessment (MOCA) may be useful (www.mocatest.org), but needs to be validated in the setting of falls prediction.

A psychiatric history to identify psychosis and depression is important. Behavioral difficulties such as impaired judgment can contribute to falls risk, while depression is a risk factor for falls.

The neurological examination is directed to the identification of focal neurological signs as well as determining the presence of parkinsonism. Clinical features arguing against a diagnosis of idiopathic Parkinson's disease are specifically sought. Such features include supranuclear gaze palsy suggesting progressive supranuclear palsy or cerebellar signs suggestive of multiple system atrophy. Pyramidal signs can also be seen in the latter disorder, or might suggest the presence of cerebrovascular disease or spinal cord dysfunction. Evidence for the presence of a neuropathy is important.

Balance and gait should be assessed. Both qualitative and quantitative features should be assessed (see chapters on balance and gait).

Special Investigations

Clinical assessment remains the cornerstone in the evaluation of falls; however, special studies can be useful in individual patients. Since some disorders associated with falls are associated with brain imaging changes, CT or MRI of the brain is often indicated. Normal pressure hydrocephalus and subdural hematomas are diagnosed by imaging in the appropriate setting. Given that silent cerebral infarctions are even more common than symptomatic events, patients with falls are good candidates for imaging (Tanne and Levine 2009). If there is a concern that the falls were associated with loss of consciousness, appropriate investigators for causes of loss of consciousness should be undertaken. These might include holter monitoring, electroencephalography, or even autonomic testing, including provocative testing such as tilt table assessment.

Vestibular complaints may be illuminated by vestibular testing. Quantitative balance assessment, or posturography, is widely available and complements the clinical assessment (Visser, Carpenter, van der Kooij, and Bloem 2008b). Many tools for posturography don't assess lateral stability, which may be an important predictor of falls (Hilliard et al. 2008). Similarly, quantitative gait assessment may be useful in measuring spatiotemporal gait characteristics, and though not often used in the clinical setting, can be used to quantify variability and asymmetry of gait, which may be more useful predictors of falls than simple spatiotemporal characteristics (Hausdorff 2007). More sophisticated gait laboratories are generally used only in the research setting.

Treatments Available, Recommended Prioritization of Treatments

Generic falls preventions strategies that have been successfully applied to older people at risk for falls may be applicable to patients with neurological disease. In the setting of neurological disorders, optimization of therapy targeted to the disease is obviously indicated. In addition, however, falls prevention strategies should be considered. As in older people, falls intervention can be single faceted (such as strength or gait training) or can be multifaceted. The latter approach makes sense in the setting of frail older people who don't have a single impairment, but also makes sense in most neurological disorders where multiple medications, cognitive impairment, physical impairment, and mood disturbance coexist in the context of an older individual. In addition, multifaceted approaches aim to alter the environment of the individual at risk. Assessment of the home environment by professionals, such as occupational therapists, may enhance its safety.

Natural Progression of Disease, Optimal Treatment Outcomes

The neurologist is ideally suited to understand the natural history of falls in patients with neurological disease. In addition to diagnosis, treatment, and establishment of prognosis (albeit imperfectly), neurological training allows assessment and understanding of the various levels of impairment that translate into functional limitations for patients. Interventions aimed at optimizing functional impairment will often translate into reducing falls risk. Attention to falls as a specific outcome to be avoided and monitored is also important.

In addition to proper disease management, management of specific co-morbid conditions, such as osteoporosis is critical. Bone mineral density is reduced in a number of neurological conditions, because of both restricted mobility and confinement, and increases the risk for fractures as a consequence of falls. Some recent studies found that treatment of osteoporosis in Parkinson's disease (Sato, Honda, and Iwamoto 2007), stroke (Sato, Iwamoto, Kanoko, and Satoh 2005d), and dementia (Sato, Kanoko, Satoh, and Iwamoto 2005a) prevented hip fractures. A study showed that vitamin D supplementation in stroke patients prevented both falls and injuries in a Japanese population (Sato, Iwamoto, Kanoko, and Satoh 2005c). While promising, these studies may not apply widely given selection biases. Pending disease-specific guidelines, current recommendations for assessment and prevention of osteoporosis should be applied to patients with neurological disorders (Marsden et al. 2008). It should be kept in mind that programs that increase mobility may also have a beneficial impact on bone mineral density and possibly fractures that can occur as a consequence of falls. Conversely, increased mobility can sometimes increase falls risk, hence measures designed to minimize the consequences of falls are important.

Drugs used in treating neurological disorders, notably antiepileptic agents (Sheth, Binkley, and Hermann 2008; Ensrud et al. 2008) and corticosteroids (Muley, Kelkar, and Parry 2008), are associated with osteoporosis and increased fracture risk. Levodopa increases homocysteine which was associated with an increased fracture rate in Japanese women with Parkinson's disease (Sato, Iwamoto, Kanoko, and Satoh 2005b).

Rehabilitative/Psychological Aspects

As noted, multifaceted interventions have been studied in the elderly, but their application to specific neurological disorders is not clear. Studies of community-dwelling elderly support exercise interventions (Gillespie, Robertson et al. 2009). In dementia, one well designed intervention study was negative (Shaw et al. 2003), consistent with the literature (Shaw 2007b). Stroke rehabilitation is well established in the setting of acute stroke, but patients with stroke remain at risk for falls. Therefore, it is important to identify high risk patients and implement measures to minimize risk and consequences of falls (Ashburn, Hyndman, Pickering, Yardley, and Harris 2008). Interventions to reduce falls in patients with Parkinson's disease are encouraging (Ashburn et al. 2007) but the role of specific interventions, such as exercise, requires further study. While the role of rehabilitation or multifaceted interventions is less well studied, it remains reasonable to consider measures to reduce risk of falls and fractures.

Few randomized studies exist in other neurological disorders. Novel interventions might be applicable to specific populations. For example, balancing-enhancing insoles might make sense in populations with diminished proprioceptive input such as those with neuropathy (Perry, Radtke, McIlroy, Fernie, and Maki 2008).

Fear of falling is a particular concern as it amplifies functional limitation beyond restriction based on physical impairment. Measures to reduce fear have falling have been successful in people without neurological disorders but need to be examined in many neurological diseases (Brouwer, Walker, Rydahl, and Culham, 2003; Zijlstra, van Haastregt, van Rossum et al. 2007).

Injury Prevention

While prevention of future falls is clearly important prevention of injuries in patients who fall is equally important. A study of patients with Alzheimer disease showed that risedronate, ergocalciferol and calcium prevented fractures, but not falls (Sato, Kanoko, Satoh, and Iwamoto 2005b). The same research group also showed that sunlight exposure with calcium supplementation could be effective in hospitalized patients with Alzheimer's disease (Sato, Iwamoto, Kanoko, and Satoh 2005a). While measures such as hip protectors have been examined preventing injuries, evidence for efficacy and compliance issues are a concern and few studies have examined well-defined populations with neurological disorders (Parker, Gillespie, and Gillespie 2006).

Future Directions

While a key to future studies is to identify at-risk individuals, this is unlikely to be completely successful. Nevertheless, targeting of interventions will be necessary to make them cost effective. The validation of specific interventions in selected patient populations is another area of future study. The evolution of technologies for home monitoring and perhaps to even treat patients at home is another trend that should have applications to falls preventions.

Summary

In summary, falls are important public health problems in generally and in patients with neurological disorders in particular. Neurologists, geriatricians and other clinicians who care for older people and people with these disorders should assess patients for falls risk and institute preventive measures.

References

Agrawal, Y., Carey, J. P., Della Santina, C. C., Schubert, M. C., and Minor, L. B. (2009). Disorders of balance and vestibular function in US adults: Data from the national health and nutrition examination survey, 2001–2004. *Archives of Internal Medicine, 169*(10), 938–944.

Allan, L. M., Ballard, C. G., Rowan, E. N., and Kenny, R. A. (2009). Incidence and prediction of falls in dementia: A prospective study in older people. *PloS One, 4*(5), e5521.

Ashburn, A., Fazakarley, L., Ballinger, C., Pickering, R., McLellan, L. D., and Fitton, C. (2007). A randomised controlled trial of a home based exercise programme to reduce the risk of falling among people with Parkinson's disease. *Journal of Neurology, Neurosurgery, and Psychiatry, 78*(7), 678–684.

Ashburn, A., Hyndman, D., Pickering, R., Yardley, L., and Harris, S. (2008). Predicting people with stroke at risk of falls. *Age and Ageing, 37*(3), 270–276.

Brotherton, S. S., Krause, J. S., and Nietert, P. J. (2007). Falls in individuals with incomplete spinal cord injury. *Spinal Cord, 45*(1), 37–40.

Brouwer, B. J., Walker, C., Rydahl, S. J., and Culham, E. G. (2003). Reducing fear of falling in seniors through education and activity programs: A randomized trial. *Journal of the American Geriatrics Society, 51*(6), 829–834.

Busse, M. E., Wiles, C. M., and Rosser, A. E. (2009). Mobility and falls in people with Huntington's disease. *Journal of Neurology, Neurosurgery, and Psychiatry, 80*(1), 88–90.

Cauley, J. A., Zmuda, J. M., Yaffe, K., Kuller, L. H., Ferrell, R. E., Wisniewski, S. R., et al. (1999). Apolipoprotein E polymorphism: A new genetic marker of hip fracture risk–the study of osteoporotic fractures. *Journal of Bone and Mineral Research, 14*(7), 1175–1181.

Coleman, A. L., Cummings, S. R., Yu, F., Kodjebacheva, G., Ensrud, K. E., Gutierrez, P., et al. (2007). Binocular visual-field loss increases the risk of future falls in older white women. *Journal of the American Geriatrics Society, 55*(3), 357–364.

DeMott, T. K., Richardson, J. K., Thies, S. B., and Ashton-Miller, J. A. (2007). Falls and gait characteristics among older persons with peripheral neuropathy. *American Journal of Physical Medicine & Rehabilitation / Association of Academic Physiatrists, 86*(2), 125–132.

Ensrud, K. E., Walczak, T. S., Blackwell, T. L., Ensrud, E. R., Barrett-Connor, E., Orwoll, E. S., et al. (2008). Antiepileptic drug use and rates of hip bone loss in older men: A prospective study. *Neurology, 71*(10), 723–730.

Finlayson, M. L., Peterson, E. W., and Cho, C. C. (2006). Risk factors for falling among people aged 45 to 90 years with multiple sclerosis. *Archives of Physical Medicine and Rehabilitation, 87*(9), 1274–9.

Ganz, D. A., Bao, Y., Shekelle, P. G., and Rubenstein, L. Z. (2007). Will my patient fall? *Journal of the American Medical Association, 297*(1), 77–86.

Gillespie, L. D., Robertson, M. C., Gillespie, W. J., Lamb, S. E., Gates, S., Cumming, R. G., et al. (2009). Interventions for preventing falls in older people living in the community. *Cochrane Database of Systematic Reviews (Online), (2)*(2), CD007146.

Grimbergen, Y. A., Knol, M. J., Bloem, B. R., Kremer, B. P., Roos, R. A., and Munneke, M. (2008). Falls and gait disturbances in Huntington's disease. *Movement Disorders, 23*(7), 970–976.

Grimbergen, Y. A., Munneke, M., and Bloem, B. R. (2004). Falls in Parkinson's disease. *Current Opinion in Neurology, 17*(4), 405–415.

Guideline for the prevention of falls in older persons. American Geriatrics Society, British Geriatrics Society, and American Academy of Orthopaedic Surgeons panel on falls prevention. (2001). *Journal of the American Geriatrics Society, 49*(5), 664–672.

Hausdorff, J. M. (2007). Gait dynamics, fractals and falls: Finding meaning in the stride-to-stride fluctuations of human walking. *Human Movement Science, 26*(4), 555–589.

Hilliard, M. J., Martinez, K. M., Janssen, I., Edwards, B., Mille, M. L., Zhang, Y., et al. (2008). Lateral balance factors predict future falls in community-living older adults. *Archives of Physical Medicine and Rehabilitation, 89*(9), 1708–1713.

Holtzer, R., Friedman, R., Lipton, R. B., Katz, M., Xue, X., and Verghese, J. (2007). The relationship between specific cognitive functions and falls in aging. *Neuropsychology, 21*(5), 540–548.

Ishiyama, G., Ishiyama, A., Jacobson, K., and Baloh, R. W. (2001). Drop attacks in older patients secondary to an otologic cause. *Neurology, 57*(6), 1103–1106.

Jacobson, G. P., McCaslin, D. L., Grantham, S. L., and Piker, E. G. (2008). Significant vestibular system impairment is common in a cohort of elderly patients referred for assessment of falls risk. *Journal of the American Academy of Audiology, 19*(10), 799–807.

Johnston, J. M., Cauley, J. A., and Ganguli, M. (1999). APOE 4 and hip fracture risk in a community-based study of older adults. *Journal of the American Geriatrics Society, 47*(11), 1342–1345.

Kannus, P., Palvanen, M., Kaprio, J., Parkkari, J., and Koskenvuo, M. (1999). Genetic factors and osteoporotic fractures in elderly people: Prospective 25-year follow-up of a nationwide cohort of elderly Finnish twins. *BMJ (Clinical Research Ed.), 319*(7221), 1334–1337.

Kerse, N., Parag, V., Feigin, V. L., McNaughton, H., Hackett, M. L., Bennett, D. A., et al. (2008). Falls after stroke: Results from the Auckland regional community stroke (ARCOS) study, 2002 to 2003. *Stroke, 39*(6), 1890–1893.

Kressig, R. W., Herrmann, F. R., Grandjean, R., Michel, J. P., and Beauchet, O. (2008). Gait variability while dual-tasking: Fall predictor in older inpatients? *Aging Clinical and Experimental Research, 20*(2), 123–130.

Lach, H. W., Reed, A. T., Arfken, C. L., Miller, J. P., Paige, G. D., Birge, S. J., et al. (1991). Falls in the elderly: Reliability of a classification system. *Journal of the American Geriatrics Society, 39*(2), 197–202.

Lamb, S. E., McCabe, C., Becker, C., Fried, L. P., and Guralnik, J. M. (2008). The optimal sequence and selection of screening test items to predict fall risk in older disabled women: The women's health and aging study. *The Journals of Gerontology. Series A, Biological Sciences and Medical Sciences, 63*(10), 1082–1088.

Latt, M. D., Lord, S. R., Morris, J. G., and Fung, V. S. (2009). Clinical and physiological assessments for elucidating falls risk in Parkinson's disease. *Movement Disorders, 24*(9), 1280–1289.

Lim, M. R., Huang, R. C., Wu, A., Girardi, F. P., and Cammisa, F. P.,Jr. (2007). Evaluation of the elderly patient with an abnormal gait. *The Journal of the American Academy of Orthopaedic Surgeons, 15*(2), 107–117.

Lipe, H., and Bird, T. (2009). Late-onset Huntington disease: Clinical and genetic characteristics of 34 cases. *Journal of the Neurological Sciences, 276*(1–2), 159–162.

Liu-Ambrose, T. Y., Ashe, M. C., Graf, P., Beattie, B. L., and Khan, K. M. (2008). Increased risk of falling in older community-dwelling women with mild cognitive impairment. *Physical Therapy, 88*(12), 1482–1491.

Lloyd, B. D., Williamson, D. A., Singh, N. A., Hansen, R. D., Diamond, T. H., Finnegan, T. P., et al. (2009). Recurrent and injurious falls in the year following hip fracture: A prospective study of incidence and risk factors from the sarcopenia and hip fracture study. *The Journals of Gerontology. Series A, Biological Sciences and Medical Sciences, 64*(5), 599–609.

Longstreth, W. T.,Jr, Koepsell, T. D., Ton, T. G., Hendrickson, A. F., and van Belle, G. (2007). The epidemiology of narcolepsy. *Sleep, 30*(1), 13–26.

Lord, S. R., Sherrington, C., Menz, H., and Close, J. (2007). *Falls in older people: Risk factors and strategies for prevention.* Cambridge University Press, New York.

Marsden, J., Gibson, L. M., Lightbody, C. E., Sharma, A. K., Siddiqi, M., and Watkins, C. (2008). Can early onset bone loss be effectively managed in post-stroke patients? an integrative review of the evidence. *Age and Ageing, 37*(2), 142–150.

Matinolli, M., Korpelainen, J. T., Korpelainen, R., Sotaniemi, K. A., and Myllyla, V. V. (2009). Orthostatic hypotension, balance and falls in Parkinson's disease. *Movement Disorders, 24*(5), 745–751.

Matsumura, B. A. and Ambrose, A. F. (2006). Balance in the elderly. *Clinics in Geriatric Medicine, 22*(2), 395–412.

Muley, S. A., Kelkar, P., and Parry, G. J. (2008). Treatment of chronic inflammatory demyelinating polyneuropathy with pulsed oral steroids. *Archives of Neurology, 65*(11), 1460–1464.

Parker, M. J., Gillespie, W. J., and Gillespie, L. D. (2006). Effectiveness of hip protectors for preventing hip fractures in elderly people: Systematic review. *BMJ (Clinical Research Ed.), 332*(7541), 571–574.

Parry, S. W., and Kenny, R. A. (2005). Drop attacks in older adults: Systematic assessment has a high diagnostic yield. *Journal of the American Geriatrics Society, 53*(1), 74–78.

Patel, S., Hyer, S., Tweed, K., Kerry, S., Allan, K., Rodin, A., et al. (2008). Risk factors for fractures and falls in older women with type 2 diabetes mellitus. *Calcified Tissue International, 82*(2), 87–91.

Perry, S. D., Radtke, A., McIlroy, W. E., Fernie, G. R., and Maki, B. E. (2008). Efficacy and effectiveness of a balance-enhancing insole. *The Journals of Gerontology. Series A, Biological Sciences and Medical Sciences, 63*(6), 595–602.

Peterson, E. W., Cho, C. C., and Finlayson, M. L. (2007). Fear of falling and associated activity curtailment among middle aged and older adults with multiple sclerosis. *Multiple Sclerosis (Houndmills, Basingstoke, England), 13*(9), 1168–1175.

Pickering, R. M., Grimbergen, Y. A., Rigney, U., Ashburn, A., Mazibrada, G., Wood, B., et al. (2007). A meta-analysis of six prospective studies of falling in Parkinson's disease. *Movement Disorders, 22*(13), 1892–1900.

Podsiadlo, D. and Richardson, S. (1989). The time "up and go" test. *Arch Phys Med Rehabil, (67),* 387–389.

The prevention of falls in later life. A report of the Kellogg international work group on the prevention of falls by the elderly. (1987). *Danish Medical Bulletin, 34 Suppl 4,* 1–24.

Salmen, T., Heikkinen, A. M., Mahonen, A., Kroger, H., Komulainen, M., Saarikoski, S., et al. (2002). Relation of estrogen receptor-alpha gene polymorphism and hormone replacement therapy to fall risk and muscle strength in early postmenopausal women. *Annals of Medicine, 34*(1), 64–72.

Sato, Y., Honda, Y., and Iwamoto, J. (2007). Risedronate and ergocalciferol prevent hip fracture in elderly men with Parkinson disease. *Neurology, 68*(12), 911–915.

Sato, Y., Iwamoto, J., Kanoko, T., and Satoh, K. (2005a). Amelioration of osteoporosis and hypovitaminosis D by sunlight exposure in hospitalized, elderly women with Alzheimer's disease: A randomized controlled trial. *Journal of Bone and Mineral Research, 20*(8), 1327–1333.

Sato, Y., Iwamoto, J., Kanoko, T., and Satoh, K. (2005b). Homocysteine as a predictive factor for hip fracture in elderly women with Parkinson's disease. *The American Journal of Medicine, 118*(11), 1250–1255.

Sato, Y., Iwamoto, J., Kanoko, T., and Satoh, K. (2005c). Low-dose vitamin D prevents muscular atrophy and reduces falls and hip fractures in women after stroke: A randomized controlled trial. *Cerebrovascular Diseases (Basel, Switzerland), 20*(3), 187–192.

Sato, Y., Iwamoto, J., Kanoko, T., and Satoh, K. (2005d). Risedronate therapy for prevention of hip fracture after stroke in elderly women. *Neurology, 64*(5), 811–816.

Sato, Y., Kanoko, T., Satoh, K., and Iwamoto, J. (2005a). The prevention of hip fracture with risedronate and ergocalciferol plus calcium supplementation in elderly women with Alzheimer disease: A randomized controlled trial. *Archives of Internal Medicine, 165*(15), 1737–1742.

Sato, Y., Kanoko, T., Satoh, K., and Iwamoto, J. (2005b). The prevention of hip fracture with risedronate and ergocalciferol plus calcium supplementation in elderly women with Alzheimer disease: A randomized controlled trial. *Archives of Internal Medicine, 165*(15), 1737–1742.

Schuele, S. U., Bermeo, A. C., Alexopoulos, A. V., Locatelli, E. R., Burgess, R. C., Dinner, D. S., et al. (2007). Video-electrographic and clinical features in patients with ictal asystole. *Neurology, 69*(5), 434–441.

Shaw, F. E. (2007). Prevention of falls in older people with dementia. *Journal of Neural Transmission (Vienna, Austria: 1996), 114*(10), 1259–1264.

Shaw, F. E., Bond, J., Richardson, D. A., Dawson, P., Steen, I. N., McKeith, I. G., et al. (2003). Multifactorial intervention after a fall in older people with cognitive impairment and dementia presenting to the accident and emergency department: Randomised controlled trial. *BMJ (Clinical Research Ed.), 326*(7380), 73.

Sheth, R. D., Binkley, N., and Hermann, B. P. (2008). Progressive bone deficit in epilepsy. *Neurology, 70*(3), 170–176.

Snijders, A. H., van de Warrenburg, B. P., Giladi, N., and Bloem, B. R. (2007). Neurological gait disorders in elderly people: Clinical approach and classification. *Lancet Neurology, 6*(1), 63–74.

Srikanth, V., Beare, R., Blizzard, L., Phan, T., Stapleton, J., Chen, J., et al. (2009). Cerebral white matter lesions, gait, and the risk of incident falls: A prospective population-based study. *Stroke, 40*(1), 175–180.

Stolze, H., Klebe, S., Zechlin, C., Baecker, C., Friege, L., and Deuschl, G. (2004). Falls in frequent neurological diseases–prevalence, risk factors and aetiology. *Journal of Neurology, 251*(1), 79–84.

Syrjala, P., Luukinen, H., Pyhtinen, J., and Tolonen, U. (2003). Neurological diseases and accidental falls of the aged. *Journal of Neurology, 250*(9), 1063–1069.

Tanne, D., and Levine, S. R. (2009). Capturing the scope of stroke: Silent, whispering, and overt. *Archives of Neurology, 66*(7), 819–820.

Thijs, R. D., Bloem, B. R., and van Dijk, J. G. (2009). Falls, faints, fits and funny turns. *Journal of Neurology, 256*(2), 155–167.

Thompson, P. D., and Nutt, J. G. (2007). Higher level gait disorders. *Journal of Neural Transmission (Vienna, Austria: 1996), 114*(10), 1305–1307.

Thurman, D. J., Stevens, J. A., Rao, J. K., and Quality Standards Subcommittee of the American Academy of Neurology. (2008). Practice parameter: Assessing patients in a neurology practice for risk of falls (an evidence-based review): Report of the quality standards subcommittee of the American Academy of Neurology. *Neurology, 70*(6), 473–479.

Tinetti, M. E. (1986). Performance-oriented assessment of mobility problems in elderly patients. *Journal of the American Geriatrics Society, 34*(2), 119–126.

Tinetti, M. E. (2003). Clinical practice: Preventing falls in elderly persons. *New England Journal of Medicine. 348*(1):42–49.

van de Warrenburg, B. P., Steijns, J. A., Munneke, M., Kremer, B. P., and Bloem, B. R. (2005). Falls in degenerative cerebellar ataxias. *Movement Disorders: Official Journal of the Movement Disorder Society, 20*(4), 497–500.

Verghese, J., Holtzer, R., Lipton, R. B., and Wang, C. (2009). Quantitative gait markers and incident fall risk in older adults. *The Journals of Gerontology. Series A, Biological Sciences and Medical Sciences, 64*(8), 896–901.

Verghese, J., Robbins, M., Holtzer, R., Zimmerman, M., Wang, C., Xue, X., et al. (2008). Gait dysfunction in mild cognitive impairment syndromes. *Journal of the American Geriatrics Society, 56*(7), 1244–1251.

Visser, J. E., Carpenter, M. G., van der Kooij, H., and Bloem, B. R. (2008a). The clinical utility of posturography. *Clinical Neurophysiology: Official Journal of the International Federation of Clinical Neurophysiology, 119*(11), 2424–2436.

Wenning, G. K., Ebersbach, G., Verny, M., Chaudhuri, K. R., Jellinger, K., McKee, A., et al. (1999). Progression of falls in postmortem-confirmed parkinsonian disorders. *Movement Disorders: Official Journal of the Movement Disorder Society, 14*(6), 947–950.

Wiles, C. M., Busse, M. E., Sampson, C. M., Rogers, M. T., Fenton-May, J., and van Deursen, R. (2006). Falls and stumbles in myotonic dystrophy. *Journal of Neurology, Neurosurgery, and Psychiatry, 77*(3), 393–396.

Williams, D. R., Watt, H. C., and Lees, A. J. (2006). Predictors of falls and fractures in bradykinetic rigid syndromes: A retrospective study. *Journal of Neurology, Neurosurgery, and Psychiatry, 77*(4), 468–473.

Zecevic, A. A., Salmoni, A. W., Lewko, J. H., and Vandervoort, A. A. (2007). Seniors falls investigative methodology (SFIM): A systems approach to the study of falls in seniors. *Canadian Journal on Aging = La Revue Canadienne Du Vieillissement, 26*(3), 281–290.

Zijlstra, A., Ufkes, T., Skelton, D. A., Lundin-Olsson, L., and Zijlstra, W. (2008). Do dual tasks have an added value over single tasks for balance assessment in fall prevention programs? A mini-review. *Gerontology, 54*(1), 40–49.

Zijlstra, G. A., van Haastregt, J. C., van Eijk, J. T., van Rossum, E., Stalenhoef, P. A., and Kempen, G. I. (2007). Prevalence and correlates of fear of falling, and associated avoidance of activity in the general population of community-living older people. *Age and Ageing, 36*(3), 304–309.

Zijlstra, G. A., van Haastregt, J. C., van Rossum, E., van Eijk, J. T., Yardley, L., and Kempen, G. I. (2007). Interventions to reduce fear of falling in community-living older people: A systematic review. *Journal of the American Geriatrics Society, 55*(4), 603–615.

27 The Ataxias

Katrina Gwinn

Introduction

The term *ataxia* refers to a relatively heterogeneous and large group of hereditary, acquired, or apparently idiopathic disorders which have in common jerky and uncoordinated movements and speech. Hence, ataxia is a symptom/sign, rather than a specific diagnosis per se. Many forms of ataxia are hereditary and due to single gene disorders. Many others are secondary to other central nervous system (CNS) conditions including alcohol abuse, stroke, tumor, and multiple sclerosis, or may be the result of paraneoplastic syndromes or vitamin deficiency. Apparent sporadic (idiopathic) ataxias can also occur. Ataxia may affect any part of the body (particularly gait, eye movements, and speech) and some types are associated with additional CNS, peripheral nervous system (PNS), or systemic findings. Most disorders that result in ataxia cause cells in the cerebellum to degenerate or atrophy. The age of onset of the resulting ataxia varies depending on the underlying cause of the degeneration; the scope of this chapter will remain focused on those disorders that affect adults. There is no interventional treatment currently available. Adaptive devices (such as walkers) are often utilized in combination with physical, occupational, and speech therapy. Treatment for most ataxia remains severely limited and translational research efforts are therefore of great importance.

Current epidemiologic studies of the inherited ataxias are limited by complex and confusing systems of nomenclature and by the lack of minimal diagnostic criteria. Despite the difficulties of comparing one study to another, most descriptive investigations provide a prevalence estimate of less than 6 cases/100,000. In isolated, inbred populations, a prevalence as high as 23 cases/100,000 has been reported for some forms of ataxia.

While informative epidemiological studies are sparse, the types of ataxia, depending on how they are grouped, are extensive. Traditionally, ataxia has been grouped by neuropathological criteria: spinocerebellar degeneration, cerebellar cortex degeneration, and olivopontocerebellar atrophy (Holmes classification). A subsequent classification by Harding groups the adult onset ataxias based on the clinical features. Autosomal dominant cerebellar ataxias (ADCAs) are a heterogeneous group of disorders that were classified clinically by Harding (1983). Progressive cerebellar ataxia is the primary feature. Currently, the Harding classification continues to be referenced, but as our molecular understanding of ataxias increases, it is increasingly apparent that there is a great deal of overlap across a given set of genetic disorders and they are not easily defined by their clinical features. Furthermore, it has been shown that in some instances (such as SCA2 and SCA3), the same genetic mechanism that leads to ataxia in one population may lead to another diagnosis, such as Parkinson's disease in a different population (in this example, ethnic Chinese and African origin people for SCA2 and SCA3 respectively). As laboratory-based discovery is translated into therapeutics, mechanistic categorization of ataxias is likely to become increasingly important.

Pathophysiology

A variety of insults to the cerebellum, both inherited and acquired, can result in ataxia. The cerebellum is the recognized location of gross or molecular lesions leading to ataxia; these processes can lead to isolated ataxia or ataxia combined with other symptoms and signs. The pathophysiology of ataxia depends on the underlying cause, and the causes are protean. In many patients, progressive ataxia results from environmental insults, other primary neurological disorders, and systemic disorders (Table 1). Many others are hereditary (see Table 2). Many patients are termed "sporadic" simply meaning the cause has not been identified.

Environmental insults which can lead to ataxia are numerous. The most common cause of both acute and chronic cerebellar dysfunction is ethyl alcohol (ethanol). When used acutely, alcohol can cause ataxic gait, speech, and eye movement abnormalities. Chronic abuse can also lead to a progressive ataxic gait disturbance speech and eye movement abnormalities, and rarely, upper extremity dysfunction. Upon imaging, chronic alcohol abuse can demonstrate isolated vermian atrophy, or generalized cerebellar atrophy, and also can cause atrophy of the olivary nucleus. Chemotherapeutic agents also can cause cerebellar toxicity with resultant ataxia, especially 5-fluorouracil (5-FU) and cytosine arabinioside. Heavy metal toxicity can lead to ataxia, especially mercury, manganese, and bismuth (the latter of which has been described following excessive intake of Pepto-Bismol®). Organic solvent-containing products such as paint thinner (especially those that contain toluene) are also possible causes of acute or chronic ataxia. Some anticonvulsants, especially phenytoin, cause cerebellar atrophy but may or may not cause clinical ataxia. In the supratherapeutic range, phenytoin and some other anticonvulsants can cause reversible cerebellar dysfunction. Interestingly, prior to laboratory-based testing of phenytoin levels, the presence of nystagmus was used as a clinical sign of compliance.

Infectious illnesses which can cause ataxia include HIV, Creutzfeldt Jakob disease (CJD), and encephalomyelitis sequelae. In addition to CJD, other prion diseases can cause ataxia including Gerstmann-Sträussler-Scheinker syndrome and variant CJD (including bovine spongiform encephalopathy, BSE). Systemic illnesses associated with ataxia include cancer, endocrine disorders, and vitamin deficiencies. Paraneoplastic antibodies can cause a pan-cerebellar syndrome usually within a few months of onset. Thyroid disease and vitamin E deficiency are reversible causes of ataxia which should not be overlooked in any evaluation of a patient with ataxia.

The autosomal dominant cerebellar degenerative disorders are generally referred to as 'spinocerebellar ataxias' (SCAs). The term 'spinocerebellar' refers to the fact that clinically there are often additional clinical features, including pyramidal, and that pathologically thinning of the upper spinal cord may be seen on gross examination. Neuropathologists have defined SCAs as cerebellar ataxias with

Table 1 Secondary or Acquired Causes of Ataxia in Adults

Disorder	Particular Features	Laboratory and Diagnostic Features
Cerebrovascular disease	Acute onset, risk factors for stroke, history of strokes or cardiac disease.	Typically localized lesion(s) seen on imaging.
Multiple sclerosis	History of prior motor or sensory waxing and waning symptoms.	Typically diagnosed clinically and supported with imaging, other diagnostic testing.
Hypoxic encephalopathy sequelae	History of hypoxic episode.	Evidence may be apparent on imaging.
Space-occupying lesion	Sub-acute or chronic onset of symptoms.	May have diagnosis of cancer if metastatic. Typically seen on imaging.
Medications leading to cerebellar toxicity	Aminoglycoside antibiotics, phenytoin and other anti-convulsants, lithium, chemotherapeutic agents.	Known by history.
Alcoholism	Concomitant features of alcohol abuse (liver disease, spider angiomas, esophageal varices)	Known by history.
Other Environmental exposures	Exposure to heavy metal (lead), organic solvents (toluene).	Known by history; heavy metal testing.
Post-infectious encephalomyelitis	Likely to be associated with a diffuse cerebral problem as well. More likely in children than adults.	CSF elevation in protein, mononuclear pleocytosis. MRI may reveal changes in cerebellum.
Prion disease (CJD, GSS, BSE)	Likely to have a rapidly progressive dementing illness. Myoclonus may be seen.	CSF serology.
Paraneoplastic syndromes	May have known history of cancer; however, this may be the presenting symptom of an occult malignancy. May be associated with sensory neuropathy (anti-Hu), opsoclonsus (anti-Ri).	Anti-Hu (SCC), anti-Yo (ovarian), anti-Ri (breast) antibodies, others
Hypothyroidism	Other features of hypothyroidism.	TFTs.
Vitamin E deficiency	Cystic fibrosis, cholestatic liver disease, or other malabsorption syndrome.	Known by history. Can also be inherited (childhood onset), genetic testing available.

GSS = Gerstmann-Sträussler-Scheinker syndrome; BSE = bovine spongiform encephalopathy; SCC = small cell lung cancer; TFTs = thyroid function tests.

variable involvement of the brainstem and spinal cord, and the clinical features of the disorders are caused by degeneration of the cerebellum and its afferent and efferent connections, which involve the brainstem and spinal cord.

Traditionally, three broadly defined mutational mechanisms are generally relevant to the pathophysiology of the hereditary adult onset ataxias.

The first mechanism is a trinucleotide expansion. The first to be described is a CAG repeat expansion resulting in expanded poly-glutamine tracts (the mechanism of SCA1, SCA2, SCA3, and SCA7, Tables 2, 3). In addition to ataxia, CAG repeat expansions have been associated with Huntington disease (HD; Online Mendelian Inheritance in Man, OMIM number 143100) and X-linked spinobulbar muscular atrophy (Kennedy disease, OMIM 313200). The CAG repeat arrays in these diseases are located in the coding region of the involved gene and are translated into polyglutamine tracts in the protein product. It is postulated that an expansion of the polyglutamine tract produces a gain of function in the protein product in each disease, accounting for the dominant inheritance. Microscopically, these disorders are characterized by neuronal intranuclear inclusions of unknown function. These inclusions include not only the polyglutamine expansion but also a number of other proteins. Expansion of repeat sequences involving the trinucleotides CAG, CTG, CGG, or GAA is the primary cause of several other inherited ataxias as well (Table 2).

The second mechanism implicated in the adult onset hereditary ataxias is that of mutations in genes coding ion channels (channelopathies) (including EA-1/SCA6, EA-2, Table 2, 3).

The third type of mutation is that which is seen in SCA8, an untranslated CTG expansion, which is comparable to the genetic abnormality associated with myotonic dystrophy.

A persistent mystery about the ataxias has been why and how mutations in genes—many of which are expressed widely in the brain and elsewhere—primarily cause ataxia, and not, for example, epilepsy or dementia. SCA is genetically extremely heterogeneous, involving some genes with ubiquitous expression (discussed below). For example, why should a poly-glutamine stretch in TATA binding protein (which is important in all cells) particularly disrupt cerebellar coordination? Advances in the genetics of cerebellar ataxias provide enough insight into the mechanism of the disorder to suggest a rational hypothesis for how so many different genes lead to predominantly cerebellar defects. One unifying feature of many of the genes involved in cerebellar ataxias is their impact on the unusual mechanism of plasticity used in the spines of cerebellar Purkinje cells which is thought to underlie many forms of cerebellar learning and coordination. This mechanism is postulated by Schorge et al. (2009) to be a unifying pathogenic mechanism in the ataxias, and is attractive because it would extend from the SCAs to other inherited and acquired ataxias.

More than 390 entries in the Online Mendelian Inheritance in Man (OMIM) database refer to "cerebellar ataxia." Of these, the 27 that are associated with spinocerebellar ataxia and the two genes that are clearly linked to episodic ataxia can all be integrated into the Schorge model. However, there are several types of ataxia that do not involve directly targeting cerebellar plasticity. For example, six different mitochondrial genes are implicated in ataxia, and more than ten mutations in 'house

Table 2 Pathophysiological Mechanisms Common to Dominant Ataxias

Pathophysiological Mechanism	Ataxias	Other Disorders with Similar Genetics	Pathological Features	Proposed Cellular Mechanisms
CAG repeat	SCA1,2,3,7,12, DRPLA	Huntington's disease	Neuronal intranuclear inclusions	Toxic gain of function or loss of transcription factors
Channelopathy	EA1/SCA6, EA2		Purkinje cell dominant cortical cerebellar degeneration, lack of ubiquitin immunoreactive nuclear inclusions.	Impaired activity of ion channels
CTG (intronic) repeat	SCA8	Myotonic dystrophy	Cerebellar atrophy, depigmentation of the substantia nigra, severe loss of Purkinje cells replaced by fibrillary accumulations resembling afferent axons.	Consumption of transcription factors, other key proteins
CGG repeat expansion (permutation)	FXTAS	Fragile X (full mutation)	Intranuclear neuronal and astrocytic inclusions	Toxic gain of function (vs. loss of function in Fragile X)

DRPLA = dentatorubral pallidoluysian atrophy; EA = episodic ataxia; FXTAS = fragile X-associated tremor ataxia syndrome; SCA = spinocerebellar ataxia.

keeping' genes involved in DNA repair, RNA processing, or protein folding lead to cerebellar ataxias, which in some cases lead to a fairly pure cerebellar phenotype. Why loss of what are ubiquitously important proteins would cause ataxia (and not, say, muscle disease, dementia, other movement disorders, or even death) is not known. One can speculate that both mitochondrial and 'housekeeping' mutations may lead to ataxia because of the very large Purkinje cell size, extensive connectivity, and high metabolic demand.

Genetic Contribution(s) to Condition, as Known

There are over 30 currently identified causal genes for hereditary forms of ataxia. There are autosomal dominant (such as the spinocerebellar ataxias), autosomal recessive (such as Friedreich's ataxia and ataxia telangiectasia), X-linked recessive (fragile X tremor ataxia syndrome), and mitochondrial (neuropathy, ataxia, and retinitis pigmentosa, [NARP], mitochondrial encephalomyopathy, lactic acidosis with stroke-like episodes, [MELAS] and myoclonus epilepsy with ragged red fibers [MERRF]) conditions which all can be associated with ataxia. The SCAs and fragile X tremor ataxia syndrome (FXTAS) are the forms most likely to present in adulthood. Friedreich's ataxia (FA) and ataxia telangiectasia (AT) are more likely to occur in adolescents (FA) or children (AT). In addition to those ataxias listed in Table 2, there are many autosomal or X-linked recessive ataxias described in the literature. These are typically in a single family or small number of cases, and almost all are childhood onset, and so, will not be discussed further here.

Clinical Presentation(s)

Ataxia, a primary disorder of cerebellar function, causes a breakdown in the central motor program resulting in inaccuracy in range, force, timing, and direction of movements. Ataxic symptoms may be quite variable and can develop chronically or occur acutely, depending on the cause. Typically, the patient will complain of lack of coordination, hand tremor, slurring of speech, or difficulty with balance. In particular, patients may report one or a combination of the following symptoms: Unsteady walk and a tendency to stumble; difficulty with fine-motor tasks, such as eating, writing or buttoning a shirt due to incoordination or tremor; change in speech, including sounding "drunk"; difficulty swallowing; head or hand tremor or "shaking." While ataxia is a disorder of movement timing, rather than of weakness, a patient may come with a chief complaint of general

weakness as well, misinterpreting their symptoms as a problem with their muscles.

The clinical classification of Harding (1983) divides adult dominant cerebellar ataxias (ADCAs) into three different groups based on the presence or absence of associated findings. In ADCA I, cerebellar ataxia of gait and limbs is associated with supranuclear ophthalmoplegia, pyramidal or extrapyramidal signs, mild dementia, and peripheral neuropathy. ADCA I includes spinocerebellar ataxia type 1 (SCA1), SCA2, and SCA3 (Machado-Joseph disease). In ADCA II, macular and retinal degeneration are seen. ADCA III is a pure form of late-onset cerebellar ataxia. However, the variability within as well as across the different types of ataxia, even within a single family with the same genetic cause, has made the ADCA categorization less useful clinically. Many genetically caused types of ataxia have commercial genetic tests available, and those should be part of the diagnostic evaluation (see below).

Schols et al. (1997) compared clinical, electrophysiologic, and magnetic resonance imaging (MRI) findings to identify phenotypic characteristics of genetically defined SCA subtypes. Slow saccades, hyporeflexia, myoclonus, and action tremor suggested SCA2. SCA3 patients frequently developed diplopia, severe spasticity or pronounced peripheral neuropathy, and impaired temperature discrimination, apart from ataxia. SCA6 presented with a predominantly cerebellar syndrome, and patients often had onset after 55 years of age. SCA1 was characterized by markedly prolonged peripheral and central motor conduction times in motor evoked potentials. MRI scans showed pontine and cerebellar atrophy in SCA1 and SCA2. In SCA3, enlargement of the fourth ventricle was the main sequel of atrophy. SCA6 presented with pure cerebellar atrophy on MRI. Overlap between the 4 SCA subtypes studied was broad, however. Furthermore, these distinctions are somewhat academic, because commercial testing is available for all of these but SCA4.

In some Chinese and American Hispanic families a phenotype that is almost indistinguishable from Parkinson's disease (PD) clinically and on PET neuroimaging occurs. As repeat sizes increase, the phenotype more closely resembles ataxia. SCA2 is responsible for almost 10% of familial parkinsonism cases in the ethnic Chinese in some series. Like SCA2, in SCA3 (Machado Joseph disease) affected members of Caucasian families typically present with ataxia, although mixed ataxia-parkinsonism is also seen. In contrast, in people of African origin with SCA3, ataxia overlapped with parkinsonism in a given patient is common. It is notable that the PD phenotype for both SCA2 and 3 may be more common in those with intermediate-range repeat numbers; this narrow range requires precise determination of repeat size, which is not done by all

Table 3 Selected Hereditary Ataxias

Designation	Typical Onset	Frequent (but not invariable) Additional Clinical and Laboratory Features	Gene (locus)/OMIM #	Genetic Abnormality	Commercial Testing
Autosomal Dominant					
SCA1	4th decade	Bulbar, UMN signs, EPS. Olivopontocerebellar atrophy on imaging. May see peripheral nerve involvement.	ATXN1 (6p23)/#164400	CAG expansion in ataxin-1	Available
SCA2 (OPCA2)	4th–7th decade	Slow saccades (@100%), neuropathy, dementia, EPS (including typical PD). Olivopontocerebellar atrophy on imaging. May present as typical PD especially in Asian, Native American.	ATXN2/ (12q24)/#183090	CAG expansion in ataxin-2	Available
SCA3 (MJD)	4th–7th decade	EPS (including typical PD, especially African American), proptosis, facial fasciculations, gaze evoked nystagmus peripheral nerve involvement. Sparing of olives on imaging.	ATXN3/; MJD protein 1 (14q24.3-q31)	CAG expansion in ataxin-3	Available
SCA4	4th or 5th decade	Sensory axonal neuropathy	(16q22.1)/#600223	Unknown	N/A
SCA5	1st–6th decade	Downbeat nystagmus, very slow progression. "Lincoln ataxia."	SPTBN2/ (11q13)/ #600224	Spectrin beta chain, brain 2 mutation (involved in glutamate transporter stability)	N/A
SCA6	6th decade	Peripheral nerve involvement, gaze evoked nystagmus.	CACNA1A (19p13)/#183086	CAG expansion in the Voltage-dependent P/Q-type calcium channel alpha-1A subunit (or also missense mutation)	Available
SCA7	Birth through 5th decade	OPCA3. Ophthalmoplegia, retinopathy, UMN abnormalities, EPS, sensory loss, dementia.	ATXN7/ataxin-7 (3p21.1-p12)/#164500	CAG expansion in ataxin-7	Available
SCA8	2nd–7th decade	Spastic and ataxic dysarthria, nystagmus, UMN, diminished vibration	ATXN8OS (13q21)/#608768	CTG expansion in SCA8 gene	Available
SCA9		SCA 9 is reserved for disorders yet to be described in the literature			N/A
SCA10	2nd–4th decade	Isolated ataxia; or variably seizures, mood disorders, cognitive and psychiatric impairment, pyramidal tract signs, EEG abnormalities, and sensorimotor polyneuropathy. Mexican, Argentinean, Brazilian kindreds.	ATXN10/ataxin-10; E46L (22q13)/ #603516	Expanded 5-bp repeat (ATTCT) intronically in the ATXN10 gene	Available
SCA11	3rd decade	Isolated ataxia; or UMN	(15q14-q21.3)/ #604432	Tau tubulin kinase-2 mutation	N/A
SCA12	1st–6th decade	Head tremor	PPP2R2B/ (2A5q31-q33)/ #604326	CAG expansion in Brain-specific regulatory subunit of protein phosphatase	N/A
SCA13	1st–7th decade	Dysarthria, moderate mental retardation, mild developmental delay in motor acquisition	KCNC3 (19q13.3-q13.4)/ #605259	Voltage-gated potassium channel, Shaw-related subfamily, member-3 gene mutation	Available
SCA14	1st–6th decade	Isolated ataxia; or dysphagia, nystagmus, facial myokymia, chorea, decreased vibration sense	PRKCG (19q13.4)/ #605361	Protein kinase C, gamma subtype mutation	Available
SCA15	3rd–5th decade	Isolated ataxia	ITPR1 (3p26.1-p25.3)/ #606658	Inositol 1,4,5-triphosphate receptor deletion (related to Calcium release)	N/A
SCA16		Same as SCA15 (Miura et al. 2006)			
SCA17	4th decade	EPS, cognitive impairment dysarthria, and dysphagia, and most showed psychiatric symptoms, dementia, dystonia. May resemble HD.	TBP (6q27)/#607136	Expansion of a CAG/CAA in the TATA-box binding protein	Available
SCA18	2nd decade	Sensory motor neuropathy.	(7q22-q32)/#607458	Unknown	N/A
SCA19	3rd–4th decade	Cognitive impairment, myoclonus, postural tremor. (debated-same disorder as SCA22?)	(1p21-q21)/#607346	Unknown	N/A

(Continued)

Table 3 Continued

Designation	Typical Onset	Frequent (but not invariable) Additional Clinical and Laboratory Features	Gene (locus)/OMIM #	Genetic Abnormality	Commercial Testing
SCA20	5th decade	May be pure ataxia; or also spasmodic coughing, dysphonia, dentate calcifications.	(11p13-q11)/#608687	Unknown	N/A
SCA21	1st-4th decade	EPS, dysarthria, dysgraphia, hyporeflexia, postural tremor, cognitive impairment (single family)	(7p21.3-p15.1)/ #607454	Unknown	N/A
SCA22	3rd-4th	(debated-same disorder as SCA19?)	(1p21-q21)/#607346	Unknown	N/A
SCA23	5th-6th decade	UMN; pathologically neuronal loss in the cerebellar vermis, dentate nuclei, olives, but not pons (single family).	(20p13-p12.3)/ #610245	Unknown	N/A
Formerly SCA24 (now SCAR4)	3rd decade	No longer termed SCA24; is categorized as SCAR4. Saccadic instrusions, EPS, UMN, pes cavus, sensory neuropathy in all modalities.	(1p36)/#607317	Unknown	N/A
SCA25	2nd-4th decade	Areflexia, sensory neuropathy	(2p21-p13)/#608703	Unknown	N/A
SCA26	2nd-6th decade	Pure ataxia (single family)	(19p13.3)/#609306	Unknown	N/A
SCA27	2nd decade	Orofacial dyskinesias, aggression, cognitive difficulties.	FGF14/ (13q34)/ #609307	Fibroblast growth factor 14 mutation	
SCA28	1st-4th decade	Gaze-evoked nystagmus (shorter disease duration); dysmetric saccades, slow saccades, ophthalmoparesis, and ptosis (longer disease duration)	(18p11.22-q11.2)/ #610246	Unknown	N/A
SCA29	May be present at birth	Truncal ataxia, mild limb dysmetria, upbeating nystagmus, and gaze-provoked horizontal nystagmus. Episodes of vertigo and ataxia with vertical oscillopsia, similar to an episodic ataxia syndrome. Non-progressive in some.	(3p26)/#117360	Unknown	N/A
DRPLA	1st-4th decade	Myoclonic epilepsy, dementia, ataxia, chorea, myoclonus, clinically resembles HD in some families (especially African American, aka "Haw River syndrome").	ATN1/ (12p13.31)/ #125370	CAG expansion in atrophin1-related protein gene	Available
EA1	1st or 2nd decade	Episodic ataxia, myokymia. May be brought on by physical exertion, emotional stimulus. Ataxia may be mild or even absent. May respond to phenytoin.	KCNA1 (12p13)/ #160120	Potassium voltage-gated channel component mutation	Available
EA2	1st or 2nd decade	Episodic ataxia. Often induced emotional stimuli, carbohydrate rich meals, fever. Downbeating nystagmus, dystonia, isolated vermian atrophy. Responsive to acetazolamide.	CACNA1A (19p13)/ #108500	Voltage-dependent P/Q-type calcium channel alpha-1A subunit mutation	Available
Autosomal Recessive					
Friedreich's ataxia	1st or 2nd decade	Areflexia, pes cavus, cardiac manifestations. European, East Indian, and Middle Eastern origin people.	FRDA1 (9q13,); FRDA2 (9p23-p11) /#229300	Frataxin gene-CAA expansion (FRDA1); FRDA2=Unknown	Available (FRDA1)
Ataxia-Telangiectasia	1st or 2nd decade	Ataxia, telangiectases, immune defects, predisposition to malignancy.	ATM(11q22.3) /#208900	Phosphatidylinositol 3-kinase mutation (related to DNA repair)	Available
X-Linked					
FXTAS	5th-9th decade	Tremor, ataxia. Family history of MR (Fragile X syndrome); short-term memory loss, executive function deficits, cognitive decline, EPS, peripheral neuropathy, lower limb proximal muscle weakness, and autonomic dysfunction	FMR-1 (Xq27.3)/ #300623	Permutation (expanded CGG trinucleotide repeats) in FMR1	Available

AD = autosomal dominant; ADCA = autosomal dominant cerebellar ataxia (Harding criteria); AR = autosomal recessive; EPS = extrapyramidal syndrome; DRPLA = dentatorubral pallidoluysian atrophy; EA = episodic ataxia; FXTAS = fragile X-associated tremor ataxia syndrome; HD = Huntington's disease; PD = Parkinson's disease; MJD = Machado Joseph disease; MR = mental retardation; N/A = not available; OMIM = Online Mendelian Inheritance in Man; OPCA2 = olivopontocerebellar atrophy type 2; SCA=spinocerebellar ataxia; UMN-upper motor neuron.

diagnostic laboratories. Therefore, when ruling out SCA2 and SCA3 as a cause of PD, it is important that methods which accurately assess the repeats in this intermediate (a.k.a. borderline) range be used. Similarly, the DRPLA phenotype in Japanese and European populations, and Haw River syndrome in African Americans, was disparate enough to hide the fact these diseases were caused by the same gene mutation.

Diagnosis: History, Exam, Imaging, Laboratory Tests, Exclusionary Conditions

History

In taking the history of a person with suspected ataxia, it is essential to assess for the following:

♦ Onset of ataxia (acute vs. rapid vs. slow);

♦ Exposure to toxic substances, drugs, medications;

♦ History of alcohol use or abuse;

♦ History of viral illness;

♦ Family history of ataxia, parkinsonism or other movement disorders, dementia;

♦ Complete review of systems including symptoms consistent with thyroid problems, malabsorption syndromes;

♦ Neurological review of systems including cognitive difficulties, symptoms suggestive of peripheral neuropathy, past neurological problems "separated in time or space"; autonomic symptoms, including control of blood pressure (problems with the autonomic system may suggest a diagnosis of multiple system atrophy).

If the person has hand tremor, it is important to know whether the tremor is activation tremor (hands do not shake at rest, but do shake when the patient uses the hands in eating, writing, or other activities). Ataxic tremor will not typically occur at rest; however, many of the ataxic syndromes, especially, hereditary ataxias, have concurrent parkinsonism.

Ataxic patients may complain of head tremor or swaying of the body when seated. Abnormal speech is extremely common in most forms of ataxia. This may be pure ataxic speech and the patient may report that the voice "sounds like they are drunk" but can also be a combination of ataxic and spastic speech.

Examination

Ataxia may be the only neurologic finding, or, depending on the disorder, may be accompanied by dementia, seizures, myoclonus, dystonia, parkinsonism, and other signs including extrapyramidal features, upper motor neuron dysfunction (including spastic speech), and peripheral nerve dysfunction.

A mental status examination is essential, as many forms of ataxia, both secondary and hereditary, may have an associated cognitive abnormality.

On speech examination, vocal quality may be harsh. Patients with ataxic dysarthria tend to place equal and excessive stress on all syllables spoken. The term "scanning speech" has been used in the past to describe this prosodic pattern. A useful technique to evaluate prosody is to have the patient say the "pa-ta-ca" exercise, in which a patient says "pa pa pa pa, etc." followed by the other two sounds, and then combines them all together (pa-ta-ca, pa-ta-ca, etc.). It is important to have them repeat this at least twenty times each sound, as the ataxic quality of speech may not emerge initially. Because the volume of

speech often varies and requires increase, ataxic speech is sometimes described as explosive speech. Hypernasality is not common, but may occur.

Eye movement abnormalities are extremely common in ataxic disorders, and in fact, it would be quite unusual for an ataxic patient to have completely normal eye movements. Abnormalities may include abnormal pursuits, inaccurate saccades, and nystagmus. Square wave jerks (involuntary back and forth movements of the eyes, with equal movements in both directions, which occur when gazing upon a fixed target) are also seen. In addition to asking the patient to follow a moving finger (or hand-held object) with their eyes, which will reveal saccadic pursuits, it is valuable to ask the patient to fix their gaze directly on a non-moving target in order to solicit square wave jerks. Having a patient look from one fixed lateral target to another on the opposite side (i.e., saccades from side to side, with the examiner holding a finger at the edge of each peripheral visual field) is useful for assessing hyper- and hypodysmetria.

Some oculomotor abnormalities unrelated to cerebellar dysfunction but which may be seen include gaze palsy, ptosis, and blepharospasm. May patients have additional bulbar deficits such as facial atrophy and facial fasciculations.

Head tremor due to cerebellar disease is typically symmetric, regular, and not associated with pain. It is typically side to side, without any rotational component. An irregular, jerky, rotational, asymmetric, or painful head tremor is suggestive of cervical dystonia. Note however, that dystonia can also accompany some forms of ataxia.

Limb movements will typically show upper extremity intention tremor (tremor is most pronounced at the end of a movement). Examination will also demonstrate impaired alternating movements (during activities such as turning the hand over and back). Impaired movements to an intended position, such as reaching for an object, for example, on finger to nose to finger testing; the tremor will dramatically worsen as the target is neared. During lower extremity testing, a heel-knee-shin examination (sliding the heel up and down the front of the shin and back again) may show unsteadiness with difficulty keeping the heel on the shin.

The term "ataxia" classically refers to a gait disorder, as noted above, and all patients with ataxia will have an abnormal gait, even if subtle. The patient may complain of feeling unstable or having lack of balance. They may also say that people have told them, or that they have noticed that they "walk like they are drunk." On examination, the classic finding is a wide-based stance. Cadence of gait is irregular, and the rest of the body may sway from side to side as the patient struggles to right themselves. Often, the findings are more subtle than this, and wide-based stance may be the limit of the findings on gait examination. There may also be truncal swaying (this feature in the head or trunk is often referred to as titubation). It is essential to perform a Romberg test on each patient, as a sensory neuropathy may lead to an apparent ataxic gait. Because many patients have both sensory neuropathy and ataxia, a thorough examination for both is important.

Laboratory Tests

Broadly speaking, laboratory tests primarily are done to rule out secondary causes (Table 1), and to evaluate for genetic abnormalities (Table 2). Acute onset of ataxia should be considered a neurologic, and potentially a neurosurgical, emergency until structural, vascular, or toxic causes of acute ataxia are ruled out.

Imaging should be done to rule out space-occupying lesions, evidence of stroke, and demyelinating diseases. Blood tests, especially for vitamin B12 or E deficiencies, infection, metabolic syndromes, and Wilson's disease are appropriate, and are quite important as they may reveal reversible causes of ataxia. Imaging in most of the hereditary ataxias will reveal progressive atrophy of the cerebellum. There may also be atrophy of the pons, medulla, middle cerebellar peduncles, and upper cervical cord, the latter, especially, with the SCAs. CSF studies may be needed to evaluate for prion disease and to evaluate for malignant cells.

SCAs, vitamin E deficiency, and paraneoplastic syndromes can exhibit abnormalities on peripheral nerve testing and EMG; many ataxic disorders cause motor or sensory neuropathy. Autonomic testing, when multiple system atrophy (MSA) is suspected, may also be abnormal. An EEG may also be indicated, especially in episodic ataxias or where a family history of a seizure disorder is elicited.

Examination and laboratory studies other than genetic testing will not definitively differentiate between the various hereditary ataxias; these diagnoses require molecular evaluation. There is commercial testing available for many of the SCAs, as well other hereditary ataxic syndromes (Table 2). In patients with an identified genetic cause, testing of unaffected family members should be performed using the Huntington protocol.

Treatments Available, Recommended Prioritization of Treatments

There is no cure for the hereditary ataxias and symptomatic treatment is largely limited for most types of ataxia. The exception is EA2, as noted below. If the ataxia is caused by another condition, that underlying condition should be treated and the ataxia may stabilize, or even improve or resolve. For example, ataxia caused by a metabolic disorder may be treated with medications and a controlled diet. Vitamin deficiency is treated with vitamin therapy. A variety of drugs may be used to treat gait and swallowing disorders. Physical therapy can strengthen muscles, while special devices or appliances can assist in walking and other activities of daily life (see below).

Several agents have been inconsistently reported to improve ataxia. Amantadine, L-5-hydroxytryptophan, odansetron, physostigmine, branched-chain amino acid therapy, gabapentin, and piracetam all have been reported in case reports or open-label studies to be of benefit, but no well designed clinical trials have been successful to date. Surgical ablation or deep brain stimulation surgery of the ventral intermediate nucleus of the thalamus (VIM) may be effective in reducing cerebellar tremor, however, they often do not significantly lessen ataxia, although a few cases have been reported with benefit (e.g. SCAs).

Some patients with EA1 respond to phenytoin. Most patients with EA2 respond to acetazolamide.

Idebenone, a free-radical scavenger, has been explored as a possible therapy for Friedreich's ataxia (FA), based upon the rationale that the frataxin gene is involved in the regulation of mitochondrial iron content, which is abnormal in FA, and clinical trials are suggestive of benefit.

Natural Progression of Disease, Optimal Treatment Outcomes

The natural history of any form of ataxia depends, of course, on the underlying cause. Ataxias due to stroke and multiple sclerosis may plateau as any subsequent lesions may be in a different location and those responsible for the ataxia may stabilize. Ataxia due to space-occupying lesions likewise will have a course dependent upon the illness itself. Paraneoplastic ataxic disorders may resolve completely with treatment of the underlying cancer, or may result in residual ataxia symptoms.

The adult onset hereditary ataxias are typically inexorably, but often very slowly, progressive. Gait will worsen and most patients will ultimately be wheelchair bound, though the rate of progression varies not only between the different types of ataxia, but even within a given type and sometimes even varies a great deal within families all with the same genotype. Clearly there are modifying genetic factors at play that remain to be discovered.

The triplet repeat disorders are among the earliest discovered genetic causes of hereditary neurological disease, and yet remain among those for which almost no significant treatment inroads have been made. These disorders are ripe for translational research and therapeutics development because their molecular pathogenesis is increasingly well characterized.

Rehabilitative/Psychological Aspects as Pertinent

After correction of symptomatic causes, management typically includes physical, occupational, and speech therapy. Rehabilitation efforts begin with evaluation of motor strength, coordination, and with a skills assessment. Based on this assessment, devices may be recommended including neck supports, canes, walkers, and wheelchairs. Devices are also available to assist with writing, eating, and self care. Speech therapy may play an important role and devices to assist in communication may also be useful. Speech and swallowing therapy may assist in preventing problems with swallowing.

Gait rehabilitation includes using visual and somatosensory systems to provide feedback to enhance the gait pattern. For patients with concurrent sensory polyneuropathies, the latter approach may be difficult; auditory feedback devices may also be useful. Portable visual or auditory feedback apparati are the subject of clinical research currently and may become part of the treatment armamentarium in the future. Exercise regimens which may be of value include proprioceptive neuromuscular facilitation, rhythmic motor tasks and other coordination exercises, and aquatic therapy. Rehabilitation efforts ideally should remain lifelong for those suffering from ataxia to allow those with these disorders to maximize their function.

Future Directions

Many areas of research are needed in the field of ataxia for moving forward with improved diagnostic categorization and treatment strategies.

Epidemiological studies are needed. While ataxia is relatively rare, and each particular type of ataxia is quite rare (with SCA3, SCA2, SCA1, EA1, and EA2 being the most likely to be encountered), the actual burden of ataxic illness is great not only because it affects the individual, typically during the most productive era of their lives, but also because it affects the family of the patient significantly and creates significant caregiver psychological and financial burden. The first step in better understanding the burden of ataxia to patients and society is to have accurate information regarding the incidence and prevalence of both inherited and acquired ataxia.

Great leaps have been made in the ability to molecularly diagnose the hereditary ataxias. Commercial testing is now available for a large number of genetic disorders which can cause ataxia. However, until meaningful treatment is available, genetic testing will be useful only in helping to predict the natural history in extremely vague terms. The classical pathway of disease definition has been to clarify a constellation of symptoms and to categorize diseases accordingly, as was done to develop the Harding ADCA criteria. Future treatments for hereditary ataxias are likely to be based on molecular pathogenesis, not merely palliative measures, as they are currently. This will allow treatment to stem from the underlying biology of disease and hence, to tackle the disease at its root cause rather than a series of what might be common final pathways for a variety of biological processes, all leading to similar or the same phenotype. Patients with similar clinical phenotypes might need very different treatments, depending on genetic cause or risk factors. For example, based on the above discussed data, treatment decisions in ataxia will be relevant to a subset of ataxia patients, and the size of this subset will differ in differing populations. This is likely to be true for a variety of disorders. Inclusion/exclusion criteria for clinical studies may need to consider molecular characterizations as well, in order to refine diagnostic categories and allow more sophisticated treatment response analyses.

We need additional genetic, epidemiologic and pathologic investigations of neurodegenerative disease in different populations. In these investigations, it will be inappropriate to naively and uniformly apply consensus criteria derived from the analysis of Caucasian populations: Rather, criteria will have to be considered in many ethnic and racial groups. Such investigations, despite their challenges from a design standpoint, are essential if we are to achieve appropriate diagnosis and treatment for non-Caucasian and Caucasian populations alike.

Several studies have looked at a given disease, and within that diagnosis determined differences in genotype for differing manifestations. It is time to tackle this from the opposite angle: By using genetic factors to define the underlying biology, we can broaden our understanding of the possible phenotypes both clinically, and ultimately, pathologically, that might be manifest as a result of a given genetic variant. For example, a patient with ataxia may need to be in the same treatment trial as one with Huntington's disease, whereas another might be better off in a trial with a group of patients with a clinical diagnosis of, for example, epilepsy. Only when we open our minds to what we mean by the words "diagnosis" and "disease" in the context of what is currently the era of molecular diagnosis, will we be able to move forward to help these patients in a meaningful way.

Summary

Ataxia is not a single diagnostic category, but rather, a symptom which can accompany many different illnesses and syndromes. There are many causes of both acquired and hereditary ataxia. Molecular diagnosis of ataxia has advanced dramatically in the last decade. Understanding of some of the pathological processes of ataxia on a cellular level has engendered translational research which is essential if meaningful therapeutic interventions for ataxia can occur.

References

Blattner K. Friedreich's ataxia: A suggested physical therapy regimen. *Clinical Management* 1988;8(4)14–15.

Bower JH. Familial adult-onset spinocerebellar degenerations. In CH Adler, JE Ahlskog, eds. *Parkinson's disease and movement disorders: Diagnosis and treatment for the practicing physician.* Totowa, NJ: Humana Press, 2007;243–252.

Brusse E, Maat-Kievet JA, and van Swieten JC. Diagnosis and management of early- and late-onset cerebellar ataxia. *Clin Genet* 2007;71:12–24.

Burke JR, Ikeuchi T, Koide R, Tsuji S, Yamada M, Pericak-Vance MA, and Vance JM. Dentatorubral-pallidoluysian atrophy and Haw River syndrome. (Letter) *Lancet* 1994;344: 1711–1712.

Albin RL. Dominant ataxias and Friedreich ataxia: An update. *Mov Disord* 2000 Jul;15(4):604–12.

Evidente VG, Gwinn-Hardy KA, Caviness JN, and Gilman S. Hereditary ataxias. *Mayo Clin Proc* 2000 May;75(5):475–90.

Freidrich's Ataxia Research Alliance. *FA beginner's primer.* http://www. curefa.org/primer.html. Accessed July 17, 2009.

Gwinn-Hardy K, Chen JY, Liu H.-C, Liu TY, Boss M, Seltzer W, et al. Spinocerebellar ataxia type 2 with parkinsonism in ethnic Chinese. *Neurology* 2000;55:800–805.

Gwinn-Hardy K, Singleton A, O'Suilleabhain P, Boss M, Nicholl D, Adam A, et al. Spinocerebellar ataxia type 3 phenotypically resembling Parkinson disease in a black family. *Arch Neurol* 2001;58:296–299.

Gwinn-Hardy K. When is ataxia not ataxia? *Arch Neurol* 2004;61:25–26.

Harding AE. The clinical features and classification of the late onset autosomal dominant cerebellar ataxias. A study of 11 families including descendants of the "Drew family of Walworth." *Brain* 1982;105:1–28.

Harding, AE. Classification of the hereditary ataxias and paraplegias. *Lancet* 1983;321:1151–1155.

Hardy J and Gwinn-Hardy K. Neurodegenerative disease: A different view of diagnosis. *Mol Med Today* 1999; 5:514–7

Hardy J, Singleton A, and Gwinn-Hardy K. Ethnic differences and disease phenotypes. *Science* 2003 May 2;300(5620):739–40.

Holmes G. An attempt to classify cerebellar disease, with a note on Marie's hereditary cerebellar ataxia. *Brain* 1907;30:545–67.

Hussey J, Lockhart PJ, Seltzer W, Wszolek ZK, Payami H, Hanson M, et al. Accurate determination of ataxin-2 polyglutamine expansion in patients with intermediate-range repeats. *Genet Test* 2002;6(3): 217–220.

Jen JC, et al. Primary episodic ataxias: Diagnosis, pathogenesis and treatment. *Brain* 2007;130:2484.

Klockgether T, Wüllner U, Spauschus A, and Evert B. The molecular biology of the autosomal-dominant cerebellar ataxias (Review). *Mov Disorders* 2000(15);4:604–12.

Machkhas, H. et al., A mild case of Friedreich's ataxia: Lymphocyte and sural nerve analysis for GAA repeat length reveals somatic mosaicism. *Muscle & Nerve* 1998;21:390–393.

Margolis, R. L. Dominant spinocerebellar ataxias: A molecular approach to classification, diagnosis, pathogenesis and the future. *Expert Rev Molec Diag* 2003;3: 715–732.

Matsuura T, Achari M, Khajavi M, Bachinski LL, Zoghbi HY, and Ashizawa T. Mapping of the gene for a novel spinocerebellar ataxia with pure cerebellar signs and epilepsy. *Ann Neurol* 1999:45:407–411.

Miura S, Shibata H, Furuya H, Ohyagi Y, Osoegawa M, Miyoshi Y, et al. The contactin 4 gene locus at 3p26 is a candidate gene of SCA16. *Neurology* 2006;67(7):1236–41.

McKinnon WC, Baty BJ, Bennett RL, Magee M, Neufeld-Kaiser WA, Peters KF, et al. Predisposition genetic testing for late-onset disorders in adults: A position paper of the National Society of Genetic Counselors. *JAMA* 1997;278: 1217–1220.

National Cancer Institute. *Ataxia telangiectasia: Fact sheet.* http://www. cancer.gov/cancertopics/factsheet/ataxiaqa. Accessed July 17, 2009.

National Institute of Neurological Disorders and Stroke. NINDS Ataxia telangiectasia information page. http://www.ninds.nih.gov/disorders/ a_t/a-t.htm. Accessed Jan 29, 2009.

National Institute of Neurological Disorders and Stroke. NINDS ataxias and cerebellar or spinocerebellar degeneration information page. http://www.ninds.nih.gov/disorders/ataxia/ataxia.htm. Accessed Jan 29, 2009.

National Institute of Neurological Disorders and Stroke. NINDS Friedreich's ataxia information page. http://www.ninds.nih.gov/disorders/ friedreichs_ataxia/friedreichs_ataxia.htm. Accessed June 5, 2009.

National Institute of Neurological Disorders and Stroke. NINDS paraneoplastic syndromes information page. http://www.ninds.nih. gov/disorders/paraneoplastic/paraneoplastic.htm. Accessed June 5, 2009.

Online Mendelian Inheritance in Man (OMIM). http://www.ncbi.nlm.nih.gov/omim/. Accessed July 26, 2009.

Opal P and Zoghbi HY. The spinocerebellar ataxias. http://www.uptodate.com/home/index.html. Accessed Jan. 5, 2009.

Orr HT and Zoghbi HY. Toward understanding polyglutamine-induced neurological disease in spinocerebellar ataxia type 1. *Cold Spring Harbor Symp Quant Biol* 1996;61:649–657.

Ranum LPW, Schut LJ, Lundgren JK, Orr HT, and Livingston DM. Spinocerebellar ataxia type 5 in a family descended from the grandparents of President Lincoln maps to chromosome 11. *Nature Genet* 8:280–284, 1994.

Rustin P, von Kleist-Retzow JC, Chantrel-Groussard K, Sidi D, Munnich A, and Rötig A. Effect of idebenone on cardiomyopathy in Friedreich's ataxia: A preliminary study. *Lancet* 1999;354(9177):477–9.

Schoenberg BS. Epidemiology of the inherited ataxias. *Adv Neurol* 1978;21:15–32.

Schöls L, Amoiridis G, Büttner T, Przuntek H, Epplen JT, and Riess O. Autosomal dominant cerebellar ataxia: Phenotypic differences in genetically defined subtypes? *Ann Neurol* 1997;42(6):924–32.

Stephanie Schorge S, van de Leemput J, Houlden H, and Hardy J. Human ataxias provide a genetic dissection of cerebellar LTD. *Trends in Neuroscience*, in press.

Wood NW and Harding AE. Cerebellar and spinocerebellar disorders. In *Neurology in clinical practice*, 3rd ed., Vol II. W.G. Bradley et al., eds. 1931–1951. 2000. Boston: Butterworth-Heinemann.

Worldwide Education and Awareness for Movement Disorders. *Adult ataxia information for patients and caregivers*. http://www.wemove.org/ataxia/. Accessed July 17, 2009.

28 Dyskinetic Movement Disorders

Sarah Pirio Richardson and Mark Hallett

Introduction

With normal aging, slowing of movements is a commonly observed phenomenon. Hypokinetic movement disorders such as Parkinson disease are seen frequently in the aging population, but hyperkinetic or dyskinetic movement disorders can also arise. Examples are dystonia, chorea, myoclonus, tics, stereotypies and tardive dyskinesia, all of which can manifest at any point in the life cycle but may present as late-onset disorders. Hyperkinetic movement disorders may manifest in the elderly patient as an isolated symptom (e.g., blepharospasm) or as part of a neurodegenerative disease (e.g., Huntington disease). Polypharmacy in the elderly is also a potential etiology of hyperkinetic movement disorder as dystonia, chorea, myoclonus, and tardive dyskinesia have all been reported to be due to a variety of medications that may be used in the elderly population such as the neuroleptics. Both the etiology and the treatment of these hyperkinetic movement disorders deserve special attention in the elderly population. Older patients diagnosed with a genetic etiology of their movement disorder may well have children, grandchildren, and even great grandchildren, raising implications of testing for a large number of family members. The treatment of hyperkinetic movement disorders in the elderly should be focused on alleviating intrusive symptoms while carefully considering medication interactions and potential cognitive and sedating side effects.

Dystonia

Dystonia is characterized by abnormal posturing due to sustained muscle contractions which interfere with the normal performance of motor tasks (Hallett 2004). Dystonia can be classified by age at onset, by distribution, and by cause (Tarsy and Simon 2006). Generalized dystonia is a disease of childhood, and multiple types of focal dystonia are seen in adults and the elderly. Age of onset of symptoms varies across the focal dystonias and, for example, blepharospasm has the oldest average age of onset (O'Riordan et al. 2004). In O'Riordan et al. they report that the mean age of onset of blepharospasm (including cranial dystonia) was 55.7 years. The other focal dystonias had younger age of onset: writer's cramp at 38.4 years, cervical dystonia at 40.8 years, and spasmodic dysphonia at 43 years (see Figure 1). A genetic predisposition is likely to play a role in the development of the dystonia; however, the exact nature of the abnormality is not known currently but it is unlikely to be a simple Mendelian trait (Defazio, Aniello, Masi, Lucchese, De Candia, and Martino 2003; Defazio, Berardelli, and Hallett 2007). Currently, the pathophysiology of dystonia is characterized primarily by abnormal sensorimotor integration (Abbruzzese and Berardelli 2003), loss of plasticity (Quartarone et al. 2005; Weise et al. 2006) and loss of inhibition—both in the motor system (Hallett 2004) and in the somatosensory system (Tinazzi, Rosso, and Fiaschi 2003).

Which of these pathophysiologic hallmarks of dystonia are primary to the disease, secondary, or compensatory is not known (Quartarone, Rizzo, and Morgante 2008). There is growing evidence from animal studies that abnormal sensorimotor integration is a key feature that links the various physiologic findings together (Evinger 2005).

The typical presentation of dystonia in the elderly is focal in its manifestation. Blepharospasm manifests as involuntary eyelid closure. An important differential diagnosis in involuntary eyelid closure is failure of the levator palpebrae to contract appropriately, resulting in apraxia of eyelid opening (Hallett, Evinger, Jankovic, and Stacy 2008). Diagnosis of blepharospasm is made on clinical grounds. Interestingly, patients with blepharospasm have increased blink rates at rest and also show a reversal of the normal pattern that blinking increases during conversation (Bentivoglio, Daniele, Albanese, Tonali from PA, and Fasano 2006). This reversal of the normal pattern may account for blepharospasm patients' reports that talking acts as a "sensory trick" and improves their blepharospasm while in conversation. Photophobia is a common complaint of blepharospasm patients and light can precipitate eyelid spasm.

The natural history of the focal dystonias varies according to the body part involved. Blepharospasm may be more likely to spread to other body parts than the other focal dystonias. In a study of more than 600 patients, 31% of blepharospasm patients experienced spreading of their dystonia beyond the initial focal manifestation (Weiss et al. 2006). This is in contrast with 9% spread in cervical dystonia, 12% in laryngeal dystonia, and 16% in focal arm dystonia. In general the pattern of spread occurs in the first few years and then plateaus. This pattern has been verified in several reports (Abbruzzese et al. 2008; Svetel et al. 2007).

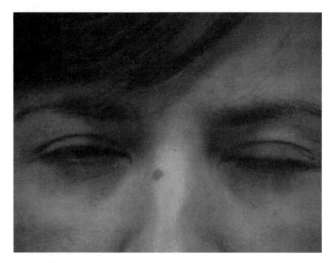

Figure 1 Patient with blepharospasm attempting eye opening and having persistent orbicularis oculi activation forcing eyes closed.

The mainstay of treatment of the focal dystonias is botulinum neurotoxin (BoNT) injections into the affected areas (e.g., for blepharospasm injections into orbicularis oculi) (Simpson et al. 2008). Medications that may be associated with some therapeutic benefit in the treatment of dystonia are the anticholinergics, particularly trihexyphenidyl. The data supporting trihexyphenidyl are from open label studies showing benefit in about 40% of patients (Greene, Shale, and Fahn 1986). Anticholinergic side effects can limit the usefulness of the drug, particularly in the elderly who tend to have more cognitive problems. There is limited data for the use of baclofen and benzodiazepines, but the available information suggests that a minority of patients may have some benefit with these drugs (Greene 1992). Patients who fail medical and BoNT therapy may be candidates for surgical therapy. In the past, the surgical treatments have focused on the end muscle/nerve structure. In blepharospasm and cervical dystonia, myectomy has been used (Patel and Anderson 1995). In cervical dystonia, myectomy and selective denervation have met with varied success. More recently, deep brain stimulation (DBS) surgery is being explored as a treatment option. Deep brain stimulation has shown success in cervical dystonia and in generalized dystonia. Several reports of success in cranial dystonia are emerging, but there are substantial side effects, and this therapy should be considered only experimental (Houser and Waltz 2005; Ostrem, Marks, Volz, Heath, and Starr 2007).

Chorea

Chorea, "to dance," is a hyperkinetic movement disorder characterized by involuntary, brief, non-rhythmic movements. The movements can occur in any part of the body and can flow from one body part to another without a predictable pattern. The clinical presentation of chorea ranges from subtle finger movements to disabling, flinging movements. When the movements are small, they can resemble fidgetiness and sometimes are incorporated in voluntary movements known as parakinesias. Slow, writhing movements of arms, legs, neck, or trunk can accompany chorea and is called choreoathetosis. The exact prevalence or incidence of chorea, especially late-onset chorea, is not known. There are several articles in the literature that explore the frequency of the diagnosis of chorea in the elderly population. A study set in the inpatient environment shows rare admissions for chorea in patients over the age of 55 of less than 0.3% (Piccolo, Sterzi, Thiella, Minazzi, and Caraceni 1999). Inpatient studies are likely to underestimate the prevalence of chorea due to the severity of symptoms that would be required for hospitalization. In the outpatient setting, one study looking at this question identified 12 patients with chorea from age 50 to 89, but did not detail the total number of patients seen during the three-year study period (Warren, Firgaira, Thompson, Kneebone, Blumbergs, and Thompson 1998). Another study from a tertiary outpatient referral center identified 0.7% of outpatients in an 11-year period had chorea with about half over the age of 55 (Dewey and Jankovic 1989).

The pathophysiology of chorea is not entirely clear but is likely a phenomenon produced by dysfunction of the basal ganglia and any corresponding outflow loops (Lorincz 2006). The basal ganglia are made up of the striatum, globus pallidus, subthalamic nuclei, and substantia nigra—all subcortical nuclei. The organization of the basal ganglia, in simple terms, is divided into direct and indirect pathways. Activity in the direct pathway results in increased output from the thalamus to the cortex; whereas the indirect pathway yields inhibition of cortical activity (Albin, Young, and Penney 1989). Dysfunction of the indirect pathway can disrupt the normal inhibitory input to the cortex and may be responsible for the abnormal, hyperkinetic movements seen in choreiform disorders.

Huntington disease (HD) is caused by excessive trinucleotide repeats in the HD gene (*IT15*) which results in a polyglutamine expansion in the huntingtin protein (Htt) (Roze, Saudou, and Caboche 2008). The medium spiny neurons in the striatum seem to be most vulnerable to the neurodegeneration seen in HD (Cepeda, Nanping, Veronique, Cummings, and Levine 2007). These same neurons originate in the indirect pathway and their demise disrupts the normal inhibitory flow to the cortex. The reason that these neurons are more at risk than the neurons participating in the direct pathway is not known. The neuronal structures that degenerate in this disease process are interconnected through long circuit loops such as corticostriatal connections, striatal outputs to globus pallidus and substantia nigra, substantia nigra/globus pallidus projections to thalamus, and then from the thalamus to the cortex. Given this complexity, there are multiple synaptic connections and alterations in any of these connections that could account for the various symptoms and signs seen in a disease like HD—including the chorea (Cepeda, Nanping, Veronique, Cummings, and Levine 2007).

The clinical presentation of late-onset chorea depends on the etiology (Table 1).

Although cerebrovascular disease may be the most common presentation of late-onset chorea, chorea as a stroke symptom is rare—about 0.4% in a study of 2500 patients with first stroke (Ghika-Schmid, Ghika, Regli, and Bogousslavsky 1997). The typical presentation is hemichorea affecting the hemibody contralateral to the ischemic lesion in the lenticular nuclei, thalamus, caudate, parieto-occipital junction, or white matter in internal capsule or subcortical areas. If severe, it is called hemiballismus, but in most cases the movements evolve to chorea. In the geriatric population, medications and toxins are the next most common etiology of chorea. Table 2 includes a list of medications reported to cause chorea. Of note, levodopa-induced dyskinesias in patients with Parkinson disease are likely to be the most common late-onset chorea in the geriatric population, but are covered elsewhere in this volume. Medication-induced chorea is characterized by development of the symptoms during treatment with the offending drug and resolution of the symptoms with discontinuation of the drug. Tardive dyskinesia where the movement disorder persists after discontinuation of the drug is discussed below.

Genetic causes of chorea can present in the elderly population, most notably, Huntington disease (HD). HD is a cytosine-adenine-guanine (CAG) repeat disorder which causes neurodegeneration. When the CAG repeat length is expanded greater than 36, symptomatic disease manifests with loss of saccadic eye movements, chorea, athetosis,

Table 1 Causes of Late-Onset Chorea

Cerebrovascular	Ischemic and hemorrhagic
Medications and toxins	See Table 2
Hereditary	Huntington's disease and neuroacanthosytosis
Autoimmune	SLE, lupus-like or probable SLE, primary antiphospholipid syndrome, and paraneoplastic
Metabolic	Hyperthyroidism, hyperglycemia, and hypocalcemia
Infectious	AIDS and CJD
Other	Polycythemia vera, senile chorea, and basal ganglion mineralization

Abbreviations: CJD, Creutzfeldt-Jakob disease; SLE, systemic lupus erythematosus. From Lorincz, 2006, used with permission from Elsevier.

Table 2 Medications and Toxins Reported to Cause Chorea

Antiparkinsonian medications	Levodopa, pramipexole, ropinirole, bromocriptine, pergolide, amantadine
Anticonvulsants	Phenytoin, carbamazepine, valproic acid, lamotragine, gabapentin
Simulants	Amphetamines, methyphenidate, methamphetamine, theophylline, caffeine
Psychiatric	Tricyclic antidepressants, fluoxetine, paroxetine, lithium, risperidone, phenothiazines, amoxapine
Steroids	Oral contraceptives, hormone replacement therapy, anabolic steroids
Opiates	Methadone
Other	Levofloxacin, ciprofloxacin, amoxapine, antihistamines, cimetidine, ranitidine, metoclopramide, digoxin, isoniazide, resirpine, triazolam, cyclosporine, propofol, sulfasalazine, cyproheptadine
Toxins	Ethanol/ethanol withdrawal, carbon monoxide, manganese, mercury, thallium, toluene, organophosphate poisoning

Data from Shoulson I. On chorea. *Clin Neuropharmacol* 1986;9(Suppl 2): S85–99; Cardoso F. Chorea: Non-genetic causes. *Curr Opin Neurol* 2004;17:433–6; Janavs JL and Aminoff MJ. Dystonia and chorea in acquired systemic disorders. *J Neurol Neurosurg Psychiatry* 1998;65:436–45. From Lorincz, 2006, used with permission from Elsevier.

dystonia, dyskinesia, bulbar symptoms of dysphagia and dysarthria, cognitive decline, psychiatric manifestations, and generalized wasting (Lorincz 2006). The CAG repeat size and the age of symptom onset are inversely correlated, making it possible for an affected individual to manifest symptoms in later life if they have a minimal number of abnormal repeats (e.g., 42 CAG repeats) (Langbehn, Brinkman, Falush, Paulsen, and Hayden 2004). In studies of patients with HD, 10% to 25% develop symptoms after 50 years of age and another 3% to 12% manifest after the age of 60 (Myers et al. 1985; Kremer et al. 1993). Typically in late-onset HD, patients present with cognitive decline and chorea jointly, but chorea can occasionally be the only symptom (Britton, Uitti, Ahlskog, Robinson, Kremer, and Hayden 1995). Dementia and chorea can also be seen in two other CAG repeat disorders, namely, spinocerebellar ataxia type 17 (SCA17) and dentatorubral-pallidoluysian atrophy (DRPLA). Both of these disorders can have heterogeneous presentations with chorea, dementia, ataxia, dystonia, and parkinsonism to variable degrees and can have onset of symptoms after the age of 50—although rarely (Bauer et al. 2004; Ikeuchi, Koide, Tanaka, et al. 1995). Other rare genetic causes of late-onset chorea include neuroacanthocytosis, a group of neurologic diseases with abnormal red blood cell morphology, namely acanthocytes (Walker et al. 2007). Among these disorders, autosomal-recessive chorea-acanthocytosis and X-linked Macleod syndrome can present over the age of 50. Typically these patients have other disease manifestations in addition to the chorea, such as axonal peripheral neuropathy.

Autoimmune disorders can cause chorea, but these disorders typically manifest in younger patients (e.g., Syndenham's chorea) (Marques-Dias, Mercadante, Tucker, and Lombroso 1997). Systemic lupus erythematosus (SLE) can present with chorea rarely, manifesting in 1% to 4% of SLE patients. (Jennekens and Kater 2002) This is particularly uncommon in patients over 60 years of age (Cervera et al. 1997). A paraneoplastic syndrome can present with chorea, often in the setting of limbic encephalitis (Rogemond and Honnorat 2000). Antibodies against collapsing response-mediating protein-5 (CRMP-5) (same

antibody as described in anti-CV-2) may be particularly associated with paraneoplastic chorea (Vernino et al. 2002). The presentation is typically after the age of 55 years and the chorea typically precedes the diagnosis of cancer. MRI may be abnormal (see Figure 2). Treatment of the cancer can resolve the chorea in about half of cases (Vernino et al. 2002). Finally, metabolic causes can very rarely present with chorea, namely, thyroid disease and nonketotic hyperglycemia (Shahar, Shapiro, and Shenkman 1988; Branca, Gervasio, Le Piane, Russo, and Aguglia 2005; Oh, Lee, Im, and Lee 2002). Nonketotic hyperglycemia should be considered in a diabetic with sudden onset of chorea.

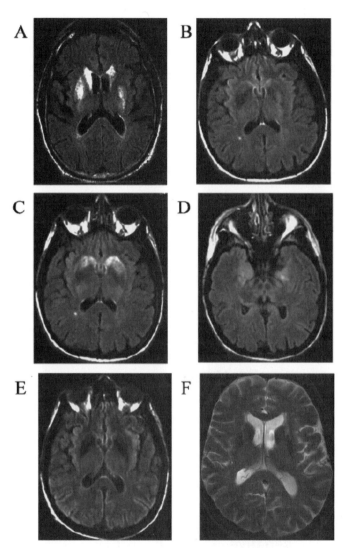

Figure 2 Magnetic resonance imaging (MRI) findings in patients with paraneoplastic chorea. (A) In Patient 1, one week after the onset of hemichorea, fluid-attenuated inverse recover (FLAIR) MRI revealed assymetric signal hyperintensity in the caudate and putamen. (B) In Patient 2, cranial MRI performed to evaluate forgetfulness (4 months before the onset of chorea) was normal except for minimal FLAIR hyperintensity of the caudate head and left putamen. (C, D) In Patient 2, one month after the onset of chorea, cranial MRI showed marked FLAIR hyperintensity in the caudate head and anterior putamen bilaterally as well as in the mesial temporal lobes. Chorea improved dramatically after chemotherapy for small-cell lung carcinoma. (E) In Patient 2, clinical improvement was accompanied by the resolution of FLAIR signal abnormalities in the basal ganglia. (F) In Patient 3, cranial MRI 9 months after the onset of chorea was unremarkable except for low T2 signals in the caudate and putamen. From Vernino S, et al. 2002, used with permission from John Wiley and Sons.

The workup of late-onset chorea can be extensive and of low yield, thus making necessary a staged diagnostic approach. First, contrast-enhanced MRI, a complete blood count with wet smear evaluation, erythrocyte sedimentation rate, and thyroid studies could be pursued. Depending on the normal or abnormal results of the first tests, HD gene testing, CRMP-5, and other paraneoplastic antibody testing with imaging of the chest, abdomen, and pelvis for a primary neoplasm, autoimmune workup (including antiphospholipid antibodies, lupus anticoagulant, β-2-glycoprotein I, antinuclear antibody, and extractable nuclear antigens), and metabolic profile to include calcium, phosphorous, and parathyroid hormone levels (Lorincz 2006).

Symptomatic treatment of chorea in general is aimed at depleting or antagonizing dopamine, but carries significant side effects. Tetrabenazine, a presynaptic dopamine depleter and D2 antagonist, has been recently approved for the treatment of HD chorea (Hayden, Leavitt, Yasothan, and Kirkpatrick 2009). The dosage of tetrabenazine begins at 25 mg/day for one day then increased to 25 mg twice daily. If tolerated, it can be increased by 25 mg/week to a recommended maximum of 50 mg twice daily. The major side effects are sedation, depression, suicidality, and parkinsonism. Other typical and atypical neuroleptics are used in the treatment of chorea and have similar associated side effects in terms of the parkinsonism as tetrabenazine, but also carry a risk of tardive dyskinesia, neuroleptic malignant syndrome, and weight gain. In sporadic chorea, it is reasonable to try withdrawing the anti-chorea medication after several months to see if sporadic chorea has resolved.

Myoclonus

Involuntary, brief, shock-like movements characterize myoclonus, which can be caused by muscle contractions (e.g., positive myoclonus) or by inhibition of muscle activity (e.g., negative myoclonus (Marsden, Hallett, and Fahn 1982) (see Figure 3). Myoclonus can present as an isolated symptom, in combination with epilepsy, or as symptomatic of a neurodegenerative illness, medication effect, or structural lesion

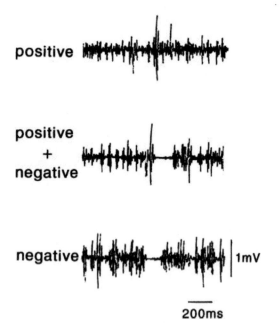

Figure 3 Electromyogram (EMG) correlates of cortical myoclonus, positive, negative, or combination of the two, recorded during sustained muscle contraction from a patient with progressive myoclonus epilepsy (PME). From Shibasaki and Hallett 2005, used with permission from John Wiley and Sons.

(Caviness and Brown 2004). The epidemiology of myoclonus depends on the population studied. One study looked at persistent myoclonus due to all causes in Olmsted County (Caviness, Alving, Maraganore, Black, McDonnell, and Rocca 1999). They found lifetime prevalence of persistent myoclonus was 8.6 cases per 100,000. The most common etiology was symptomatic myoclonus (72%)—a category that includes posthypoxia and neurodegenerative disease. The other etiologies found were epileptic myoclonus (17%) and essential myoclonus (11%). Other causes of myoclonus are toxic-metabolic and drug-induced, but are most often transient abnormalities and are unlikely to be captured in epidemiological studies (Caviness and Brown 2004). Although there is no epidemiologic study done directly in the older adult population, the prevalence would likely mimic that found above, namely, symptomatic myoclonus—including toxin-, metabolic-, and drug-induced—is likely to be most prevalent followed by epileptic myoclonus.

Myoclonus is classified depending on the neuroanatomical localization of the presumed generator of the abnormal movement: cortical, subcortical, and spinal (Shibasaki and Hallett 2005). Cortical myoclonus is subcategorized as spontaneous, cortical reflex myoclonus and epilepsia partialis (EPC). When cortical myoclonus is elicited by stimuli, it is called stimulus-sensitive and accounts for the most frequent presentation of cortical myoclonus—cortical reflex myoclonus (Shibasaki and Hallett 2005). Myoclonus from cortical generators is seen in a wide variety of diseases, including posthypoxic (Lance and Adams 1963), neurodegenerative disease (e.g., Alzheimer's disease, corticobasal degeneration) (Carella, Ciano, Panzica, and Scaioli 1997), prion disease (Creutzfeldt-Jacob disease (CJD)) (Maltête, Guyant-Maréchal, Mihout, and Hannequin 2006) and metabolic causes (e.g., uremia). There is a variety of inherited metabolic disorders that can present with cortical myoclonus, but would not be presenting in the older population. Progressive myoclonic epilepsy syndromes also have cortical generators of the myoclonus, but would be very unusual to present in the elderly population. Myoclonus generated by subcortical mechanisms is seen in essential myoclonus, dystonic myoclonus, reticular reflex myoclonus, startle syndromes, and in palatal tremor (previously called palatal myoclonus.) (Shibasaki and Hallett 2005) Spinal myoclonus usually presents as rhythmic myoclonus, which is often slightly irregular, affecting muscles within a spinal segment. A second type of spinal myoclonus, propriospinal myoclonus, is characterized by occasional axial jerks. The underlying basic mechanism of myoclonus is thought to be hyperexcitability of neuron groups. (Shibasaki and Hallett 2005)

The clinical presentation of myoclonus depends on the etiology and therefore on the neuroanatomical generator of the myoclonus. In general, cortical myoclonus tends to be of shortest duration and appears shock-like. It is usually present with posture and with movement. It is often irregular and is highly sensitive to stimuli. Subcortical myoclonus appears less shock-like than cortical myoclonus and tends to be present at rest. It is usually periodic and not stimulus-sensitive. Finally, spinal myoclonus can be shock-like and present at rest. It is often quasiperiodic or rhythmic and can have stimulus-sensitivity (Shibasaki and Hallett 2005). When assessing an older patient with new onset of myoclonus, the history should include mode of myoclonus onset, presence of additional neurologic symptoms, history of seizures, current and past medication and toxin exposures, concurrent medical problems and the family history. The physical exam should include the usual elements of the neurologic exam, but should focus attention on the distribution of the myoclonus, rhythmicity, activation pattern (e.g., present at rest, action, posture), and response of the myoclonus to stimulation (touch, sound, light, muscle stretch). At this point, differentiating the myoclonus into a major clinical syndrome category should be possible and can generally be distributed into four main categories: physiological myoclonus, essential myoclonus, epileptic myoclonus, and symptomatic myoclonus (Marsden, Hallett, and Fahn 1982).

Physiological myoclonus is present in healthy individuals, has no associated disability, and a normal physical exam (Marsden, Hallett, and Fahn 1982). Myoclonus at sleep transitions are the most common form of physiological myoclonus. This does not require any intervention except for reassurance. Essential myoclonus is characterized by the absence of associated neurologic symptoms and little or no progression (Marsden, Hallett, and Fahn 1982) Inherited forms of essential myoclonus present before the age of 20 and would not be encountered in the elderly population as a new symptom, this includes the myoclonus-dystonia syndrome (Asmus and Gasser 2004). Palatal myoclonus, which is also described as palatal tremor, either essential or symptomatic, could be encountered with an older age of onset (Pearce 2008). In essential palatal myoclonus, contractions of the tensor veli palatini cause ear clicks; the patient has an otherwise normal neurologic exam. For symptomatic palatal myoclonus, contraction of the levator veli palatini typically does not produce ear clicks and is a result of a disease within the triangle of Guillain and Mollaret, often with accompanying hypertrophy of the inferior olive nuclei (Pearce 2008).

Epileptic myoclonus is the next clinical category of myoclonus. In general the progressive myoclonic epilepsies and childhood myoclonic epilepsies would not be encountered in the geriatric age range. In older adults, it would be more common to encounter fragments of myoclonic epilepsy, including isolated epileptic myoclonic jerks, epilepsia partialis continua, idiopathic stimulus-sensitive myoclonus, and photosensitive myoclonus (Caviness and Brown 2004). The most frequent clinical presentation of myoclonus in the elderly would be symptomatic causes. Please see Table 3 for an edited list of symptomatic myoclonus etiologies that might present in the older adult (Caviness and Brown 2004; Marsden, Hallett, and Fahn 1982).

The initial workup could include electrolyte testing, thyroid function and antibody testing, glucose, renal and hepatic function tests, paraneoplastic antibodies in the appropriate clinical context, drug/toxin screening, MRI of the brain or spinal cord, and electroencephalography (Caviness and Brown 2004). If the neuroanatomical localization of the myoclonus generator is not apparent from the exam and initial workup, neurophysiologic testing can be done to determine the site of generation. This often includes surface electromyogram (EMG) recording, EEG, jerk-locked back-averaging of EEG, cortico-muscular coherence, transcranial magnetic stimulation, and evoked potentials (Shibasaki and Hallett 2005). If, based on the above investigations, an etiology is not determined and given the appropriate clinical context; advanced testing could include body imaging for an occult malignancy, cerebrospinal fluid examination, tests for malabsorption disorders, genetic testing, and mitrochondrial function studies.

The treatment strategy of myoclonus depends on the etiology. Toxin- and medication-induced myoclonus is often completely resolved by removal of the causative agent. In symptomatic myoclonus, treatment of the underlying disorder is indicated but may not be available. Furthermore, for many patients the complete resolution

Table 3 Symptomatic Myoclonus in the Aging Population

DEGENERATIVE	• Ramsay-Hunt syndrome • Friedreich's ataxia • Basal ganglia degenerations • Progressive supranuclear palsy • Huntington's disease • Parkinson disease	• Multisystem atrophy • Corticobasal degeneration • Creutzfeldt-Jakob disease • Alzheimer's disease • Dementia with Lewy bodies • Frontotemporal dementia
INFECTIOUS	• Encephalitis lethargic • Arbovirus encephalitis • Herpes simplex encephalitis • Human T-lymphotrophic virus I • HIV	• Post-infectious encephalitis • Lyme disease • Cryptococcus • Progressive multifocal leucoencephalopathy • Syphilis
METABOLIC	• Hyperthyroidism • Hepatic failure • Renal failure • Dialysis syndrome • Hyponatremia	• Hypoglycemia • Non-ketotic hyperglycemia • Hypoxia • Metabolic alkalosis • Vitamin E deficiency
TOXIN AND DRUG-INDUCED	• Psychiatric medications • Anti-infective agents • Narcotics • Anticonvulsants • Anesthetics	• Contrast media • Cardiac medications • Drug withdrawal • Other medications
PHYSICAL ENCEPHALOPATHY	• Post-hypoxic (Lance-Adams) • Post-traumatic • Heat stroke	• Electric shock • Decompression injury
FOCAL NERVOUS SYSTEM LESIONS	• Post-stroke • Post-thalamotomy • Tumor	• Inflammation • Trauma
MALABSORPTION	• Celiac disease	• Whipple's disease
PARANEOPLASTIC	• Encephalopathy	• Opsoclonus-myoclonus
UNKNOWN		

Adapted from Caviness and Brown, Myoclonus: Current concepts and recent advances, 2004, used with permission from Elsevier.

of symptomatic myoclonus with treatment is rarely achieved and the treatment is often found wanting. Cortical myoclonus treatment is aimed at decreasing any hyperexcitability. Sodium valproate is often used with doses between 1200–2000 mg daily. Other GABAergic medications used include clonazepam, primidone, and phenobarbital. Clonazepam seems to be the most of effective of these and large doses of this medication (up to 15 mg per day) are often needed (Caviness and Brown 2004). Levetiractem and piracetam have been noted to be useful. Other antiepileptic drugs have limited usefulness and some may worsen the myoclonus in certain conditions. Combination therapy is sometimes useful but sedation and gait disturbances can be limiting. Subcortical myoclonus does not respond to typical antiepileptic treatments. Partial response may be seen with clonazepam (Caviness and Brown 2004). Palatal myoclonus is quite difficult to treat. When the ear clicking is disabling, patients may undergo surgical treatments such as tensor veli palatine tenotomy and/or occlusion of the eustachian tube (Ensink, Vingerhoets, Schmidt, and Cremers 2003). Botulinum toxin injections have also been tried (Bryce and Morrison 1998). Spinal myoclonus may respond to clonazepam—especially if due to propriospinal or spinal segmental myoclonus. Rarely botulinum toxin has been reported to be a use in decreasing the movements associated with spinal segmental myoclonus (Lagueny, Tison, Burbaud, Le Masson, and Kien 1999).

Tic Disorders

Tics are defined as sudden, brief, stereotyped movements or sounds. They may be preceded by a premonitory urge and often are suppressible to some degree. In general tic disorders are typically considered childhood disorders and in fact, the diagnostic criteria for Tourette syndrome demands onset before the age of 18 or 21 years (American Psychiatric Association 1994; The Tourette Syndrome Classification Study Group 1993). A retrospective review of the clinical database of a tertiary care referral movement disorder clinic revealed that of 411 patients with tic disorders, 22 patients (5%) had onset of the tic after the age of 21 (Chouinard and Ford 2000). With careful questioning, nine of the 22 patients did reveal a transient history of tics in childhood, but the remaining 13 patients had clear onset in adulthood. About half (six patients) had secondary tics and half had idiopathic tic disorders. The mean age of tic onset was 40 years with a range between 24 and 63 years (Chouinard and Ford 2000). The secondary tics were in response to motor vehicle accident (two patients), neck strain (one patient), pharyngitis (one patient), and toxic/drug exposure (two patients).

Other reports of tic disorders beginning in adulthood have been in the form of case report or case series. Tic disorders in adults are generally described as a result of an acquired brain lesion (Krauss and Jankovic 1997) or peripheral injury (Factor and Molho 1997). The acquired brain lesions include trauma, neurologic/neuropsychiatric disease, and exposure to a variety of drugs (Kumar and Lang 1997). The latency to onset of tics after brain trauma ranges from within one day of injury to several months (Krauss and Jankovic 1997). The pathophysiological explanation for the development of the tics and the relationship to the trauma is unclear, as many of the case reports do not describe loss of consciousness or structural brain abnormalities (Kumar and Lang 1997). Herpes simplex (Northam and Singer 1991) and HIV-1 encephalitis (McDaniel and Summerville 1994) has been described in case reports to cause tics, in addition to other neurologic abnormalities.Tics rarely have been reported after stroke and the distribution of the tics has not necessarily corresponded to the location of the infarct, with the exception of a case report describing left body tics after a right middle cerebral artery distribution infarct

(Kumar and Lang 1997; Jankovic 1993). Adult-onset tics could rarely be a presentation of neurodegenerative disease, namely Huntington disease (HD), neuroacanthocytosis (NA) and, even more rarely, neurodegeneration with brain iron accumulation (NBIA) might also be considered. Patients with HD can present with chorea, as previously discussed, and rarely with motor and vocal tics. Interestingly, HD patients can also manifest obsessive-compulsive disorder similarly to patients with Tourette syndrome (Jankovic and Ashizawa 1995; Sacks 1982). Neuroacanthocytosis is a rare inherited disorder that presents with chorea, seizures, bulbar dysfunction, and axonal neuropathy. Lip and tongue self-mutilation through biting may be a manifestation of tics, but definitively differentiating this from chorea in these patients is challenging (Hardie et al. 1991). Even more rarely, neurodegeneration with brain iron accumulation (NBIA), formerly known as Hallervorden-Spatz disease, could present with tics as a manifestation of this rare progressive autosomal recessive disorder. This is typically a childhood disorder which presents with a variety of abnormal movements (dystonia, chorea, parkinsonism), pyramidal tract dysfunction, bulbar symptoms of dysarthria and dysphagia, behavioral and cognitive disturbances, and visual symptoms (Gregory, Polster, and Hayflick 2009). There is a case report in the literature presenting a patient with NBIA who had onset of motor symptoms after the age of 18 years and motor tics by the age of 37 years (Sacks, Aguilar, and Brown 1966).

Drug- or toxin-exposure has been reported in the literature to cause secondary tics in adults. The most common reports are for stimulant medications and cocaine use. The majority of these cases describe exacerbations of an underlying tic disorder (Price, Leckman, Pauls, Cohen, and Kidd 1986). There is a report of de novo tics in two patients who reported cocaine use, which lasted from weeks to months and then resolved (Pascual-Leone and Dhuna 1990). Tardive tourettism has also been described following chronic neuroleptic use (Bharucha and Sethi 1995). Many cases improved after cessation of the neuroleptic use or with trials of anti-tic medications (Kailan, Lerner, and Goldman 1993). There are questions on the clinical descriptions of the cases and whether these "tics" might better described as tardive akathisia (restlessness) (Kumar and Lang 1997). Other uncommon medications reported to cause tics include antihistamines and anticholinergic medications (Shafii 1986). Exacerbation of underlying Tourette syndrome or de novo tic onset in children has been reported with antidepressants and antiepileptics, but not in adults thus far.

In the study of tics in adulthood from a tertiary care referral center, of the patients who chose to have treatment for their tics, half had modest improvement with medications, including verapamil, botulinum toxin, clonazepam, and diazepam (Chouinard and Ford 2000). For the treatment of tics, medications that have class A evidence (good supportive evidence of safety and efficacy in at least two randomized, placebo-controlled trials) include haloperidol, pimozide, and risperidone (Swain, Scahill, Lombroso, King, and Leckman, 2007). Medications with class B evidence (fair supportive data with at least one positive placebo-controlled study) include clonidine, guanficine, pergolide, botulinum toxin type A, fluphenazine, tiapride, and zisprasidone (Swain, Scahill, Lombroso, King, and Leckman, 2007). In the older patient, consideration of medication side effects and medication interactions would have to be carefully weighed against the intrusiveness of the tic and the expected benefit of treatment.

Tardive Dyskinesia

Polypharmacy is an important issue in the elderly and with comorbid dementia and behavioral issues, older patients may be exposed to dopamine receptor blocking drugs. The dopamine receptor blocking drugs, whether phenothiazines or anti-emetic drugs, have the potential to produce tardive dyskinesia (TD), which can manifest as involuntary movement such as chorea, dystonia, akathisia, stereotypies, myoclonus, and tremor (Stacy and Jankovic 1991). Prevalence estimates of TD range from around 14% to more than 60% (Goetz 1997; Smith 1979). Interestingly, the higher prevalence estimate is found in patients over the age 70 with psychiatric illnesses (Smith 1979). Another study found that the incidence of TD in patients over the age of 55 years was six times that of younger patients (Saltz et al. 1991). Although the pathophysiology of TD is not known, there has been an association made with the development of TD and loss of D_2 receptors in the striatum—perhaps explaining the age-related risk (DeKosky and Palmer 1994).

Orofacial dyskinesia manifesting as rhythmic involuntary movements is a common tardive phenomenon (Stacy, Cardoso, and Jankovic 1993). In the report of Stacy et al., they found 61 out of 100 patients with tardive dyskinesia had orofacial movements. Spontaneous (i.e., not neuroleptic-induced) oral-lingual-buccal dyskinesias had an incidence of 6.8% in patients between the ages of 60 and 79 (Klawans and Barr 1982). A risk factor aside from age in the development of spontaneous orofacial dyskinesias is thought to be ill fitting or no dentures as seen in a study of Veterans Administration dental patients where 16% of edentulous patients had orofacial dyskinesias (Koller 1983). Typically, TD begins after at least a few months of neuroleptic treatment or up to years on the treatment. It can involve any part of the body but the orofacial dyskinesias are the most common. TD tends to worsen with excitement or anxiety and disappears with sleep. Although withdrawal of the offending drug may resolve the TD, it can be irreversible, necessitating attempts at treatment.

The first step in the management of TD is to discontinue neuroleptic therapy. Due to the underlying psychiatric symptoms if neuroleptic discontinuation is not possible, switching to another neuroleptic with less propensity for TD is indicated, such as quetiapine or clozapine (Haddad and Dursun 2008). In one study looking at clozapine, just under half of patients with TD (43%) converted to clozapine showed improvement in their TD symptoms (Lieberman, Salz, John, Pollak, Borenstein, and Kane 1991). Tetrabenazine, a D_2-antagonist and presynatic dopamine depleter, has been used to treat TD, but is associated with serious side effects of parkinsonism and depression (Kenney, Hunter, and Jankovic 2007). It is recently available in the United States as an FDA-approved therapy for chorea, associated with HD. Other medications with variable evidence for efficacy have been recommended for the treatment of TD. These include: vitamin E, sodium valproate, essential fatty acids, and benzodiazepines (Haddad and Dursun 2008). Reports in the literature and even a single-blinded trial suggest that botulinum toxin may be helpful in some cases for resistant TD (Tschopp, Salazar, and Micheli 2009; Slotema, van Harten, Bruggeman, and Hoek 2008). In severe cases with careful patient selection, deep brain stimulation of the globus pallidus interna may be an option (Kefalopoulou, Paschali, Markaki, Vassilakos, Ellul, and Constantoyannis 2009).

Summary

Late-onset hyperkinetic movement disorders can present with dystonia, chorea, myoclonus, tics, stereotypies, and tardive dyskinesia. These can be isolated symptoms or part of a symptom complex related to a neurodegenerative process or as a result of a cerebral insult. In addition, medication-related hyperkinetic movement disorders may present in the elderly and may be challenging to identify in the presence of polypharmacy. Treatment of these disorders is primarily pharmacologic, but careful consideration must be given to medication interactions and potential side effects in this population.

References

Abbruzzese, G. and Berardelli, A. (2003). Sensorimotor integration in movement disorders. *Mov Disord, 18* (3), 231–40.

Abbruzzese, G., Berardelli, A., Girlanda, P., Marchese, R., Martino, D., Morgante, F., et al. (2008). Long term assessment of the risk of spread in primary late-onset focal dystonia. *Journal of Neurology, Neurosurgery and Psychiatry, 79* (4), 392–396.

Albin, R., Young, A., and Penney, J. (1989). The functional anatomy of basal ganglia disorders. *Trends Neurosci, 12* (10), 366–375.

American Psychiatric Association. (1994). *Diagnostic and statistical manual of mental disorders.* 4th edition (DSM-IV). Washington DC: APA.

Asmus, F., and Gasser, T. (2004). Inherited myoclonus-dystonia. In S. Fahn, M. Hallett, and M. DeLong (Eds.), *Advances in Neurology, vol 94: Dystonia* 4 (pp. 113–119). Philadelphia: Lippincott Williams & Wilkins.

Bauer, P., Laccone, F., Rolfs, A., Wüllner, U., Bösch, S., Peters, H., et al. (2004). Trinucleotide repeat expansion in SCA17/TBP in white patients with Huntington's disease-like phenotype. *J Med Genet, 41* (3), 230–232.

Bentivoglio, A., Daniele, A., Albanese, A., Tonali, P.A., and Fasano, A. (2006). Analysis of blink rate in patients with blepharospasm. *Mov Disord* (21), 1225–1229.

Bharucha, K., and Sethi, K. (1995). Tardive tourettism after exposure to neuroleptic therapy. *Mov Disord, 10,* 791–793.

Branca, D., Gervasio, O., Le Piane, E., Russo, C., and Aguglia, U. (2005). Chorea induced by non-ketotic hyperglycaemia: A case report. *Neurol Sci, 26* (4), 275–277.

Britton, J., Uitti, R., Ahlskog, J., Robinson, R., Kremer, B., and Hayden, M. (1995). Hereditary late-onset chorea without significant dementia: Genetic evidence for substantial phenotypic variation in Huntington's disease. *Neurology, 45* (3 Pt 1), 443–447.

Bryce, G., and Morrison, M. (1998). Botulinum toxin treatment of essential palatal myoclonus tinnitus. *J Otolaryngol, 27,* 213–216.

Carella, F., Ciano, C., Panzica, F., and Scaioli, V. (1997). Myoclonus in corticobasal degeneration. *Mov Disord, 12,* 598–603.

Caviness, J. and Brown, P. (2004). Myoclonus: Current concepts and recent advances. *Lancet Neurol, 3,* 598–607.

Caviness, J., Alving, L., Maraganore, D., Black, R., McDonnell, S., and Rocca, W. (1999). The incidence and prevalence of myoclonus in Olmsted County. *Mayo Clin Proc, 74,* 565–569.

Cepeda, C., Nanping, W., Veronique, M., Cummings, D., and Levine, M. (2007). The corticostriatal pathway in Huntington's disease. *Progress in Neurobiology, 81* (5–6), 253–271.

Cervera, R., Asherson, R., Font, J., Tikly, M., Pallarés, L., Chamorro, A., et al. (1997). Chorea in the antiphospholipid syndrome. Clinical, radiologic, and immunologic characteristics of 50 patients from our clinics and the recent literature. *Medicine (Baltimore), 76* (3), 203–212.

Chouinard, S. and Ford, B. (2000). Adult onset tic disorders. *J Neurol Neurosurg Psychiatry, 68,* 738–743.

Defazio, G., Aniello, M., Masi, G., Lucchese, V., De Candia, D., and Martino, D. (2003). Frequency of familial aggregation in primary adult-onset cranial cervical dystonia. *Neurol Sci, 24* (3), 168–169.

Defazio, G., Berardelli, A., and Hallett, M. (2007). Do primary adult-onset focal dystonias share aetiological factors? *Brain, 130* (Pt 5), 1183–1193.

DeKosky, S. and Palmer, A. (1994). Neurochemistry of aging. In M. Albert, & J. Knoefel, *Clinical neurology of aging,* Ed. 2 (pp. 79-101). New York: Oxford University Press.

Dewey, R. J. and Jankovic, J. (1989). Hemiballism-hemichorea. Clinical and pharmacologic findings in 21 patients. *Arch Neurol, 46* (8), 862–867.

Ensink, R., Vingerhoets, H., Schmidt, C., and Cremers, C. (2003). Treatment for severe palatoclonus by occlusion of the eustachian tube. *Otol Neurotol, 24*, 714–716.

Evinger, C. (2005). Animal models of focal dystonia. *NeuroRx, 2* (3), 513–524.

Factor, S. and Molho, E. (1997). Adult-onset tics associated with peripheral injury. *Mov Disord, 12*, 1052-1055.

Ghika-Schmid, F., Ghika, J., Regli, F., and Bogousslavsky, J. (1997). Hyperkinetic movement disorders during and after acute stroke: The Lausanne Stroke Registry. *J Neurol Sci, 146* (2), 109–116.

Goetz, C. (1997). Tardive dyskinesia. In R. Watts, & W. Koller, *Movement disorders: Neurologic principles and practice* (pp. 519–526). New York: McGraw-Hill.

Greene, P. (1992). Baclofen in the treatment of dystonia. *Clin Neuropharm* (15), 276–288.

Greene, P., Shale, H., and Fahn, S. (1986). Analysis of open label trials in torsion dystonia using high dosages of trihexyphenidyl. *Mov Disord* (3), 46–60.

Gregory, A., Polster, B., and Hayflick, S. (2009). Clinical and genetic delineation of neurodegeneration with brain iron accumulation. *J Med Genet. 200, 46* (2), 73–80.

Haddad, P. and Dursun, S. (2008). Neurological complications of psychiatric drugs: Clinical features and management. *Hum Psychopharmacol, 23* (Suppl 1), 15–26.

Hallett, M. (2004). Dystonia: Abnormal movements result from loss of inhibition. *Adv Neurol* (94), 1–9.

Hallett, M., Evinger, C., Jankovic, J., and Stacy, M. (2008). Update on blepharospasm: Report from the BEBRF International Workshop. *Neurology, 71* (16), 1275–1282.

Hardie, R., Pullon, H., Harding, A., Owen, J., Pires, M., Daniels, G., et al. (1991). Neuroacanthocytosis. A clinical, haematological and pathological study of 19 cases. *Brain, 114*, 13–49.

Hayden, M., Leavitt, B., Yasothan, U., and Kirkpatrick, P. (2009). Tetrabenazine. *Nat Rev Drug Discov, 8* (1), 17–18.

Houser, M. and Waltz, T. (2005). Meige syndrome and pallidal deep brain stimulation. *Mov Disord* (20), 1203–1205.

Ikeuchi, T., Koide, R., Tanaka, H., et al. (1995). Dentatorubral-pallidoluysian atrophy: Clinical features are closely related to unstable expansions of trinucleotide (CAG) repeat. *Ann Neurol, 37* (6), 769–775.

Jankovic, J. (1993). Tics in other neurological disorders. In R. Kurlan (Ed.), *Handbook of Tourette's syndrome and related tic and behavioral disorders* (pp. 167–183). New York: Marcel Dekker.

Jankovic, J. and Ashizawa, T. (1995). Tourettism associated with Huntington's disease. *Mov Disord, 10*, 103–105.

Jennekens, F. and Kater, L. (2002). The central nervous system in systemic lupus erythematosus. Part 1. Clinical syndromes: A literature investigation. *Rheumatology (Oxford), 41* (6), 605–618.

Kailan, M., Lerner, V., and Goldman, M. (1993). Atypical variants of tardive dyskinesia, treated by a combination of clozapine with propanolol and clozapine with tetrabenazine. *J Nerv Ment Dis, 181*, 649–651.

Kefalopoulou, Z., Paschali, A., Markaki, E., Vassilakos, P., Ellul, J., and Constantoyannis, C. (2009). A double-blind study on a patient with tardive dyskinesia treated with pallidal deep brain stimulation. *Acta Neurol Scand, 119* (4), 269–273.

Kenney, C., Hunter, C., and Jankovic, J. (2007). Long-term tolerability of tetrabenazine in the treatment of hyperkinetic movement disorders. *Mov Disord, 22* (2), 193–197.

Klawans, H. and Barr, A. (1982). Prevalence of spontaneous lingual-facial-buccal dyskinesias in the elderly. *Neurology* (32), 558–559.

Koller, W. (1983). Edentulous orodyskinesia. *Annals of Neurology* (13), 97–99.

Krauss, J. and Jankovic, J. (1997). Tics secondary to craniocerebral trauma. *Mov Disord, 12* (5), 776–782.

Kremer, B., Squitieri, F., Telenius, H., Andrew, S., Theilmann, J., Spence, N., et al. (1993). Molecular analysis of late onset Huntington's disease. *J Med Genet, 30* (12), 991–995.

Kumar, R. and Lang, A. (1997). Secondary tic disorders. *Neurol Clin, 15* (2), 309–331.

Lagueny, A., Tison, G., Burbaud, P., Le Masson, G., and Kien, P. (1999). Stimulus-sensitive spinal segmental myoclonus improved with injections of botulinum toxin type A. *Mov Disord, 14*, 182–185.

Lance, J. and Adams, R. (1963). The syndrome of intention or action myoclonus: A sequel to hypoxic encephalopathy. *Brain, 86*, 111–136.

Langbehn, D., Brinkman, R., Falush, D., Paulsen, J., and Hayden, M. (2004). A new model for prediction of the age of onset and penetrance for Huntington's disease based on CAG length. *Clin Genet, 65* (4), 267–277.

Lieberman, J., Salz, B., John, C., Pollak, S., Borenstein, M., and Kane, J. (1991). The effect of clozapine in tardive dyskinesia. *Br J Psychiatry, 154*, 503–510.

Lorincz, M. (2006). Geriatric chorea. *Clin Geriatr Med, 22* (4), 879–897.

Maltête, D., Guyant-Maréchal, L., Mihout, B., and Hannequin, D. (2006). Movement disorders and Creutzfeldt-Jakob disease: A review. *Parkinsonism Relat Disord, 12* (2), 65–71.

Marques-Dias, M., Mercadante, M., Tucker, D., and Lombroso, P. (1997). Sydenham's chorea. *Psychiatr Clin North Am, 20* (4), 809–820.

Marsden, C., Hallett, M., and Fahn, S. (1982). The nosology and pathophysiology of myoclonus. In C. Marsden, and S. Fahn (Eds.), *Movement disorders* (pp. 196–248). London: Butterworth.

McDaniel, J. and Summerville, J. (1994). Tic disorder associated with encephalopathy in advanced HIV disease. *Gen Hosp Psychiatry, 125*, 298–300.

Myers, R., Sax, D., Schoenfeld, M., Bird, E., Wolf, P., Vonsattel, J., et al. (1985). Late onset of Huntington's disease. *J Neurol Neurosurg Psychiatry, 48* (6), 530–534.

Northam, R. and Singer, H. (1991). Postencephalitic acquired Tourette-like syndrome in a child. *Neurology, 41*, 592–593.

Oh, S., Lee, K., Im, J., and Lee, M. (2002). Chorea associated with non-ketotic hyperglycemia and hyperintensity basal ganglia lesion on T1-weighted brain MRI study: A meta-analysis of 53 cases including four present cases. *J Neurol Sci, 200* (1–2), 57–62.

O'Riordan, S., Raymond, D., Lynch, T., Saunders-Pullman, R., Bressman, S., Daly, L., et al. (2004). Age at onset as a factor in determining the phenotype of primary torsion dystonia. *Neurology, 63* (8), 1423–1426.

Ostrem, J., Marks, W. J., Volz, M., Heath, S., and Starr, P. (2007). Pallidal deep brain stimulation in patients with cranial-cervical dystonia (Meige syndrome). *Mov Disord* (22), 1885–1891.

Pascual-Leone, A. and Dhuna, A. (1990). Cocaine-associated multifocal tics. *Neurology, 40*, 999–1000.

Patel, B. and Anderson, R. (1995). Blepharospasm and related facial movement disorders. *Curr Opin Ophthalmol, 6* (5), 86–99.

Pearce, J. (2008). Palatal myoclonus (syn. palatal tremor). *Eur Neurol, 60* (6), 312–315.

Piccolo, I., Sterzi, R., Thiella, G., Minazzi, M., and Caraceni, T. (1999). Sporadic choreas: Analysis of a general hospital series. *Euro Neurol, 41* (3), 143–149.

Price, R., Leckman, J., Pauls, D., Cohen, D., and Kidd, K. (1986). Gilles de la Tourette's syndrome: Tics and central nervous system stimulants in twins and nontwins. *Neurology, 36* (2), 232–237.

Quartarone, A., Rizzo, V., and Morgante, F. (2008). Clinical features of dystonia: A pathophysiological revisitation. *Curr Opin Neurol, 21* (4), 484–490.

Quartarone, A., Rizzo, V., Bagnato, S., Morgante, F., Sant'Angelo, A., Romano, M., et al. (2005). Homeostatic-like plasticity of the primary motor hand area is impaired in focal hand dystonia. *Brain, 128* (Pt 8), 1943–1950.

Rogemond, V. and Honnorat, J. (2000). Anti-CV2 autoantibodies and paraneoplastic neurological syndromes. *Clin Rev Allergy Immunol, 19* (1), 51–59.

Roze, E., Saudou, F., and Caboche, J. (2008). Pathophysiology of Huntington's disease: From huntingtin functions to potential treatments. *Current Opinion in Neurology, 21,* 497–503.

Sacks, O. (1982). Acquired Tourettism in adult life. In A. Friedhoff, & T. Chase (Eds.), *Gilles de la Tourette Syndrome, advances in neurology* (pp. 89-92). New York: Raven Press.

Sacks, O., Aguilar, M., and Brown, W. (1966). Hallervorden Spatz disease: Its pathogenesis and place among the axonal dystrophies. *Acta Neuropath, 6,* 164–174.

Saltz, B., Woerner, M., Kane, J., Lieberman, J., Alvir, J., Bergmann, K., et al. (1991). Prospective study of tardive dyskinesia incidence in the elderly. *JAMA, 266* (17), 2402–2406.

Shafii, M. (1986). The effects of sympathomimetic and antihistaminic agents on chronic motor tics and Tourette's disorder. *N Engl J Med, 315,* 1228–1229.

Shahar, E., Shapiro, M., and Shenkman, L. (1988). Hyperthyroid-induced chorea. Case report and review of the literature. *Isr J Med Sci, 24* (4–5), 264–266.

Shibasaki, H. and Hallett, M. (2005). Electrophysiological studies of myoclonus. *Muscle Nerve, 31,* 157–174.

Simpson, D., Blitzer, A., Brashear, A., Comella, C., Dubinsky, R., Hallett, M., et al. (2008). Practice parameter: Botulinum neurotoxin for the treatment of movement disorders and spasticity: An evidence-based report of the therapeutics and technology assessment Subcommittee of the American Academy of Neurology. *Neurology, 70* (19), 1699–1706.

Slotema, C., van Harten, P., Bruggeman, R., and Hoek, H. (2008). Botulinum toxin in the treatment of orofacial tardive dyskinesia: A single blind study. *Prog Neuropsychopharmacol Biol Psychiatry, 32* (2), 507–509.

Smith, J. (1979). An assessment of tardive dyskinesia in schizophrenic outpatients. *Psychopharmacology, 64* (1), 99–104.

Stacy, M. and Jankovic, J. (1991). Tardive dyskinesia. *Current Opinion in Neurology and Neurosurgery* (4), 343–349.

Stacy, M., Cardoso, F., and Jankovic, J. (1993). Tardive stereotypy and other movement disorders in tardive dyskinesias. *Neurology* (43), 937–941.

Svetel, M., Pekmezovi , T., Jovi , J., Ivanovi , N., Dragasevi , N., Mari, J., et al. (2007). Spread of primary dystonia in relation to initially affected region. *J Neurol, 254* (7), 879–883.

Swain, J., Scahill, L., Lombroso, P., King, R., and Leckman, J. (2007). Tourette syndrome and tic disorders: A decade of progress. *J Am Acad Child Adolesc Psychiatry, 46* (8), 947–968.

Tarsy, D. and Simon, D. (2006). Dystonia. *N Engl J Med, 355* (8), 818–829.

The Tourette Syndrome Classification Study Group. (1993). Definitions and classification of tic disorders. *Arch Neurol, 50,* 1013–1016.

Tinazzi, M., Rosso, T., and Fiaschi, A. (2003). Role of the somatosensory system in primary dystonia. *Mov Disord, 18* (6), 605–622.

Tschopp, L., Salazar, Z., and Micheli, F. (2009). Botulinum toxin in painful tardive dyskinesia. *Clin Neuropharmacol, 32* (3), 165–6.

Vernino S.T.P., Adler, C., Meschia, J., Boeve, B., Boasberg, P., Parisi, J., et al. (2002). Paraneoplastic chorea associated with CRMP-5 neuronal antibody and lung carcinoma. *Ann Neurol, 51* (5), 625–630.

Walker, R., Jung, H., Dobson-Stone, C., Rampoldi, L., Sano, A., Tison, F., et al. (2007). Neurologic phenotypes associated with acanthocytosis. *Neurology, 68* (2), 92–98.

Warren, J., Firgaira, F., Thompson, E., Kneebone, C., Blumbergs, P., and Thompson, P. (1998). The causes of sporadic and 'senile' chorea. *Aust N Z J Med, 28* (4), 429–431.

Weise, D., Schramm, A., Stefan, K., Wolters, A., Reiners, K., Naumann, M., et al. (2006). The two sides of associative plasticity in writer's cramp. *Brain, 129* (Pt 10), 2709–2721.

Weiss, E., Hershey, T., Karimi, M., Racette, B., Tabbal, S., Mink, J., et al. (2006). Relative risk of spread of symptoms among the focal onset primary dystonias. *Mov Dis, 21* (8), 1175–1181.

29 Simple and Complex Sleep-related Movement Disorders in Older Adults

Madeleine Grigg-Damberger

When you are old and gray and full of sleep,
And nodding by the fire, take down this book,
And slowly read, and dream of the soft look
Your eyes had once, and of their shadows deep…

William Butler Yeats, from *The Rose*, 1893

Introduction

Sleep is an *active*, not passive, process characterized outwardly by a reversible behavior state of perceptual disengagement and relative insensitivity to the environment, typically accompanied by a recumbent posture, closed eyes, and absent or only slight mobility. Abrupt cessation of eye blinking soon then followed by slow eye movements (SEM) is the earliest sign of drowsiness (Santamaria and Chiappa 1987). SEM are binocular conjugate slow roving horizontal eye movements with an initial deflection lasting longer than 500 msec which progressively increase in amplitude and duration with deepening NREM 1 sleep, then decrease in amplitude or disappear with NREM 2 sleep (Iber, Ancoli-Israel et al. 2007; Silber, Ancoli-Israel et al. 2007).

We monitor submental electromyographic (EMG) skeletal axial muscle tone in a polysomnogram (PSG) because it exhibits sleep/wake state-specific changes. When awake, chin muscle activity is high and the tonically active chin EMG is interrupted by phasic muscle activity related to facial expression, chewing, talking, and tension. Even before sleep onset, the motor system reduces its level of activity. Chin EMG progressively decreases from lighter NREM 1 to deepest NREM 3 sleep. One to two body shifts per hour of NREM sleep and small flickering muscle twitches (called sleep myoclonus) normally interrupt the "pose of repose" of NREM sleep. A normal person brought to stand during NREM 3 sleep can walk because the axial skeletal motor systems are intact. However, skeletal muscle activity and tone are profoundly suppressed during REM sleep (except for extraocular movements and the diaphragm); this is known as "tonic" REM sleep. Superimposed upon tonic REM sleep are periods of "phasic" REM sleep when rapid eye movements and brief twitches of facial and limb muscles (periods of which are called "phasic" REM sleep) particularly occur (Figure 1). Rapid eye movements are conjugate, irregular, sharply peaked eye movements with an initial deflection usually lasting less than 500 msec (Iber, Ancoli-Israel et al. 2007).

Cells in the medial brainstem reticular formation are thought to control motor movements: active during wakefulness and REM sleep, reduced during NREM sleep. During REM sleep, the motor system is dominated by central activation and peripheral inhibition (Hening 2009). Loss of muscle tone and activity during tonic REM sleep is thought to be due to active inhibition of motor neuron at spinal level by GABA and glycine release onto the motorneurons (and decreased release of norepinephrine and serotonin). The central motor systems are highly active during REM sleep but motor neurons in the brainstem are tonically inhibited by hyperpolarization. Muscle twitches during phasic REM sleep are attributed to periodic bursts of excitatory activity breaking through the generalized tonic inhibitory state of REM sleep.

Effects of Age on Sleep and Sleep Architecture in Older Adults

Age is the strongest and most consistent factor affecting the patterns of sleep stages across the night. We need to appreciate the changes in the sleep architecture which occur with normal aging in order to understand the impact of excessive motor activity and different movement disorders upon sleep.

Sleep in older adults (even those who deny trouble sleeping) tends to become shorter (less total sleep time), shallower (a mild increase in NREM 1 with a marked decrease in NREM 3 sleep), more fragmented (increased numbers and duration of arousals and awakenings, more wake after sleep onset), and a longer time to fall asleep longer (Floyd, Medler et al. 2000; Espiritu 2008). Non-complaining elders typically get only 5.5–6.5 hours of sleep (total sleep time) per night compared to 7.5 hours in young adults (Tune 1969). Average nocturnal sleep time was 1.5 hours shorter in older compared with younger subjects (Klerman and Dijk 2008). Some argue that the total sleep time for a 24 hour period in elders may not decline, but sleep becomes more polyphasic and more time in bed is needed especially at night to obtain 7 to 8 hours of sleep (Bliwise 1993).

After adaptation to sleeping in the laboratory, healthy older adults spend only 5–10% of their total sleep time in NREM 3 sleep, compared to 25–35% in young adults (Hood, Bruck et al. 2004; Vitiello, Larsen et al. 2004). Their average sleep efficiency (time in bed spent sleeping) is typically 80–85% compared to 90% in younger adults. Compared to young adults who average 10 arousals per hour of sleep, older adults average 27 per hour (Boselli, Parrino et al. 1998). Healthy elders typically spend 18% of their sleep time in REM sleep compared to 20–25% in younger adults. REM sleep latency is often shorter in older adults (nearer to 50 minutes) perhaps because of the reduced amount (and amplitude) of NREM 3 sleep. A meta analysis examining age-related changes in sleep architecture among 65 studies of all-night PSG or actigraphy done on 3,577 healthy subjects, age 5 years to 102 years, has confirmed these age-related changes (Ohayon, Carskadon et al. 2004).

Aging also affects the EEG patterns of sleep. The amplitude and amount of sleep spindles (a marker of NREM 2 sleep) decreases, and their frequency slows to 12 Hz (cycles per second) (Dijk and Duffy 1999). The amplitude of NREM 3 slow wave activity (0.5–2.0 Hz) decreases with age, attributed to reduction of neuronal synchronization in the neocortex, increasing skull thickness, and/or changes in the subarachnoid space. REM density (mean number of eye movement bursts per minute of REM sleep) also decreases with advancing age (Ficca, Gori et al. 1999; Darchia, Campbell et al. 2003).

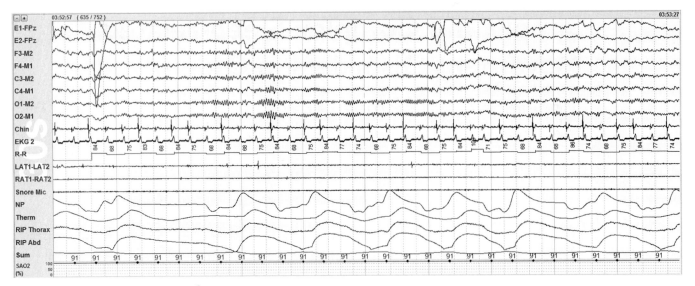

Figure 1 REM sleep. A 30-second epoch of stage REM sleep showing rapid eye movements, suppression of chin and limb EMG muscle activity, and an EEG background of low amplitude mixed frequencies in a 70-year-old man.

Effects of Age on Sleep-related Movement

Healthy adults change their body position in sleep between 3 to 36 times per night (Hobson, Spagna et al. 1978; De Koninck, Gagnon et al. 1983; De Koninck, Lorrain et al. 1992). Compared to younger controls, healthy older adults had significantly fewer body movements, which can emerge from any stage of sleep and are often followed by a shift from one stage of sleep to another (called a stage shift) or an awakening, whereas body movements in the younger subjects preferentially occurred during REM sleep and did not predict a stage shift or an arousal (Gori, Ficca et al. 2004). Another study found very old healthy subjects (ages 76–98 years) have even fewer body movements when sleeping than those 61 to 71 years of age (Giganti, Ficca et al. 2008). Another study found mean body shifts during sleep averaged 3.6, 2.7, and 2.1 per hour of sleep in healthy subjects ages 18–24, 35–45, and 65–80 years, respectively, and the oldest had longer periods of postural immobility often lasting 45 to 110 minutes (De Koninck, Lorrain et al. 1992).

The quantity of sleep-related movement is affected by the external environment of the sleeper. Progressively more intrusive environmental stimuli lead to recruitment of progressively more extensive motor sequences. Real words or calling a sleeper's name cause a differential responsiveness; the brain appears to perform a complex set of discriminations which can lead to movement, arousal, or waking when needed. How much a bed partner moves, depression, or sleeping in an insecure place result in greater numbers of movements when sleeping. The quality of sleep a subject reports was found to be inversely related to the motor activity: better sleep, less movement at night (Blagrove, Owens et al. 1998). Increased position shifts has been related to sleeping on an uncomfortable pillow or mattress, in unfamiliar surroundings or room temperature, bed partner movement, soft tissue compression, stress, noise, anxiety, and medical or musculoskeletal conditions (Martin-Du Pan, Benoit et al. 2004). A study of activity and sleep quality in 15 elders found greater motor activity during the day was associated with lower levels of motor activity at night and better sleep quality (Hashimoto and Kobayashi 1998).

Effects of Sleep Position Upon Sleep Quality, Health and Disease

By six years of age, individuals exhibit a preferred sleep position (Dunkell 1977) which often persists into young adulthood (Johns, Gay et al. 1971). Adults more often prefer to sleep in lateral decubitus position, especially on the right (Hobson, Spagna et al. 1978; De Koninck, Lorrain et al. 1992). Poor sleepers (who had more awakenings and more time awake) spent more time on their backs with their heads straight compared to good sleepers (De Koninck, Gagnon et al. 1983).

Sleeping in a left or right lateral decubitus position may impact upon health (Martin-Du Pan, Benoit et al. 2004). When sleeping on their left side, patients with congestive heart failure report more dyspnea, have greater awareness of an uncomfortable sensation of the enlarged heart beating against their left chest wall, lower vagal tone, and higher sympathetic nervous activity and plasma norepinephrine levels (Kuo, Chen et al. 2000; Miyamoto, Fujita et al. 2001; Miyamoto, Tambara et al. 2002; Leung, Bowman et al. 2003). Placing patients with severe coronary artery disease, CHF, or acute myocardial infarction without severe bradycardia in a right lateral body position is best because vagal tone was enhanced, sympathetic tone lowest, and arterial oxygen saturation higher when lying in this position (Kuo, Chen et al. 2000). However, sleeping in a right side position compared to the left predisposes to postprandial gastroesophageal reflux with more prolonged esophageal acid exposure (7% vs. 2%), higher number of reflux episodes (3.8/h vs. 0.9/h), more transient lower esophageal sphincter relaxations and higher number of these associated with reflux (6.5/h vs. 3.2/h, and 57% vs. 22% respectively) (van Herwaarden, Katzka et al. 2000). As always, choices must be made.

Diagnosing Simple Sleep-related Movement Disorders in Older Adults

A reasonable starting point when diagnosing abnormal movements during sleep is to determine whether they occur only in and around sleep, or also occur during wakefulness (Walters 2007). If the abnormal movements also occur awake, consider whether the patient has a movement disorder while awake. Contrary to older teachings, many diurnal movement disorders persist in sleep, though often then reduced in frequency and duration, and are discussed in Section 5. Next, determine whether the sleep-related movements are simple or complex. Complex sleep-related movement disorders are more often characterized by seemingly goal-directed, purposeful, but outside the awareness of patient, paroxysmal motor behaviors and vocalizations. Many are also classified as parasomnias and we discuss them in Section 4.

If the sleep-related movements are simple, determine if they preferentially affect the face, jaw, or legs (Walters 2007). If they involve only the jaw and face, consider sleep-related bruxism or faciomandibular myoclonus. If primarily leg movements, consider sleep-related leg cramps, restless legs, hypnagogic foot tremor, or periodic limb movements in sleep. Then ask whether almost all occur at sleep onset; if so, consider sleep starts. Next ask about the onset, duration, frequency, pattern, and description of the nocturnal movements and review the patient's past medical, medications, and family and social history. The physical examination should assess for a movement disorder awake, dementia, confusion, depression, anxiety, upper airway or body habitus at risk for obstructive sleep apnea, and underlying cardiac, pulmonary, neurodegenerative, or peripheral nerve disorders. A diagnostic nocturnal video-polysomnogram with expanded EEG and EMG channels may be needed to best characterize the motor behaviors and exclude other sleep disorders (e.g., sleep disordered breathing) contributing to their appearance. Figure 2 provides a flow chart for assessing sleep-related movement disorders in older adults.

Many sleep-related movement disorders may also represent impaired sleep state synchronization or "state dissociation" disorders. The transition between wakefulness, NREM, and REM sleep usually occurs amazingly smoothly and completely, but when the *transition* between two sleep states is more gradual (or rapidly oscillates), the physiological markers of one sleep state can linger or intrude into another. (Mahowald and Schenck 2005; Mahowald 2009) Narcolepsy with cataplexy is a prototypical "state dissociation" disorder because: 1) cataplexy (a sudden onset of REM sleep atonia while awake in response to an emotion-laden event); 2) sleep paralysis (an early or lingering

appearance of REM sleep atonia), and 3) hypnic hallucinations fragments of REM sleep dream mentation persisting into wakefulness.

Polysomnography is particularly warranted if the motor behaviors are frequent, have caused injury, or are potentially injurious to the patient (or bed partner). Techniques used to confirm the diagnosis of abnormal motor activities during sleep include in-laboratory overnight polysomnography with video (v-PSG) and adding additional surface EMG electrodes to the wrist extensors (Aldrich and Jahnke 1991; Chesson, Ferber et al. 1997; Kushida, Littner et al. 2005; Frauscher, Gschliesser et al. 2007). Many simple sleep-related movement disorders usually do not require, need, or have known treatment(s); others need to be remembered in order to differentiate them.

Simple Sleep-related Movement Disorders of Older Adults

Sleep Starts (Hypnic Jerks)

Sleep starts (also called hypnic jerks) occur in the transition from wakefulness to sleep, typically are one or two abrupt myoclonic flexion jerks (generalized or partial, often asymmetric), and are often accompanied by a feeling of falling, a sensory flash, and/or a bit of dream-like imagery. Seventy percent of people have experienced sleep starts at one time or another. They are thought to arise from sudden descending brainstem reticular formation volleys activated by the instability of the system in the wake/sleep transition. When captured on video-PSG, sleep starts are characterized by a single brief EMG burst which lasts less than 250 milliseconds (msec) in duration, which often occurs asymmetrically

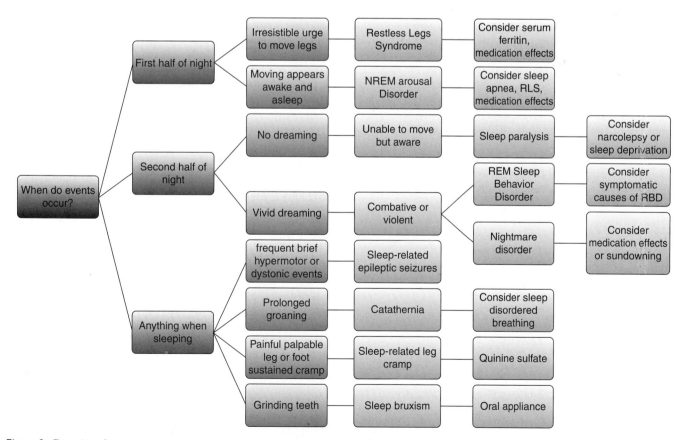

Figure 2 Flow chart for assessing sleep-related movement disorders in older adults.

and simultaneously, or sequentially in various muscles, and often causes a brief EEG arousal. Sleep starts are best treated by reassuring the patient (and bed partner) of their benign nature and by avoiding sleep deprivation or insufficient sleep which may contribute to their appearance.

Sleep-related Leg Cramps

Fifty percent of adults over 65 years of age complain of at least occasional sleep-related leg cramps (LC) (Haskell and Fiebach 1997; Pires, Benedito-Silva et al. 2007). Leg cramps occur nightly in 6% of adults 60 years or older (Abdulla, Jones et al. 1999) and are defined as forceful, painful involuntary muscle contractions of a leg or foot which cause intense pain and awaken the patient from any stage of sleep, occurring less often awake. The muscles of the posterior compartment of the leg and foot are most often affected, especially the triceps surae. The muscle cramp is palpable; the cramping muscles firm and tender while the cramp is present. The feet and toes are typically plantar flexed. Usually only one limb is affected at a time.

Leg cramps last from several seconds to minutes (a mean of 1.7 minutes) (Leung, Wong et al. 1999); their duration may be shortened by forceful stretching of the affected muscle (e.g., dorsal flexion of foot), or by standing or walking. Cramps may remit spontaneously but sometimes a residual tenderness may persist in the muscle for up to 30 minutes (Leung, Wong et al. 1999). EMG studies show LC are associated with a contraction of a slowly moving fraction of muscle fibers with extremely short potentials (Roeleveld, van Engelen et al. 2000). Repetitive stimulation of homonymous afferents of the nerve trunk has been shown to induce LC while cutaneous stimulation and Renshaw cell activation shorten them (Baldissera, Cavallari et al. 1994).

Predisposing factors for LC include: vigorous daytime exercise, arthritis, peripheral vascular disease, peripheral neuropathy, dehydration, hypothyroidism, hypoparathyroidism, diabetes mellitus type 2, hypomagnesemia, hypokalemia, hypcalcemia, uremia, overuse of diuretics, dehydration, spasticity, and rigidity. "Vespers curse" is a tetrad of painful nocturnal LC, pain, paresthesia, and fasciculations due to lumbar spinal stenosis with radiculopathy (LaBan, Viola et al. 1990). Medications associated with or exacerbating LC are listed in Table 1.

Quinine sulphate (200 to 325 mg by mouth before bed) remains the first line treatment for frequent LC. Several randomized double-blind, placebo controlled studies and a meta-analysis have shown that quinine reduces the frequency (but not the duration or severity) of LC (Connolly, Shirley et al. 1992; Man-Son-Hing, Wells et al. 1998; Diener, Dethlefsen et al. 2002). Four to six weeks of treatment with lowest dose of quinine is recommended (Butler, Mulkerrin et al. 2002). Quinine can worsen tinnitus and cause potentially fatal thrombocytopenia,

cutaneous photosensitivity, vasculitis, granulomatous hepatitis, and hypersensitivity reactions, and quinine overdose can cause epileptic seizures, confusion, blindness, coma, and even death, especially in older women (Brasic 2003; Townend, Sturm et al. 2004). Quinine acts by decreasing the excitability of the motor end plate, reducing muscle fiber contractility. The Food and Drug Administration has removed the pharmacological dose strength from the market due to the side effects discussed above.

Vitamin E (800 IU) was ineffective in comparison to placebo or quinine in reducing leg cramps (Connolly, Shirley et al. 1992). Quinine was significantly more effective than vitamin E in a double blind randomized control study (Sidorov 1993). However, one study found the combination of vitamins E and C was significantly effective in treating muscle cramps during hemodialysis (Khajehdehi, Mojerlou et al. 2001). Verapamil, gabapentin, carisoprodol, and orphenadrine have been tried with varying success to treat LC (Guay 2008; Young 2009). Calf-stretching exercises do not decrease the frequency or severity of LC (Coppin, Wicke et al. 2005).

Sleep Paralysis

Sleep paralysis (SP) is a transient inability to move despite being fully awake during a transition between sleep and wakefulness. It represents a brief persistence of the skeletal muscle motor suppression of REM sleep lingering into wakefulness. Sleep paralysis occurs most often and with greatest frequency in individuals who have narcolepsy with cataplexy, particularly in the transition from REM sleep to wakefulness (Overeem, Mignot et al. 2001).

Although the patient with SP often complains of difficulty breathing during an attack, breathing and eye movements are preserved. Sleep paralysis, when it sometimes appears in normal subjects, often causes anxiety especially the first time (Solomonova, Nielsen et al. 2008), often within the first two hours after sleep onset (Girard and Cheyne 2006) and is associated with partial sleep deprivation (Bell, Dixie-Bell et al. 1986; Fukuda, Miyasita et al. 1987; Takeuchi, Fukuda et al. 2002). Isolated SP without other features of narcolepsy has been reported to occur in families (Roth, Buuhova et al. 1968). Selective serotonin reuptake inhibitors can be effective in treating SP but is usually reserved for when it is frequent and bothersome.

Hypnagogic Foot Tremor and Alternating Leg Muscle Activation

Another benign simple sleep-related movement disorder is hypnagogic foot tremor (HFT). HFT is characterized by single short trains of *rhythmic* 1–2 per second oscillating movements of the toes or whole foot of one or both feet which occur most often during the transition from wakefulness to sleep, but often linger into stages NREM 1 or NREM 2 sleep, and may recur following sleep-related arousals (Wichniak, Tracik et al. 2001). A case-control study found HFT in 8% of 375 consecutive patients complaining of disturbed sleep and 5% of 20 healthy young controls (Wichniak, Tracik et al. 2001). When observed in the PSG, HFT is characterized by a series of single phasic EMG bursts lasting 300 to 700 msec recurring at 1 to 2 per second for 10 to 20 seconds (Wichniak, Tracik et al. 2001). Night-to-night variability in HFT has been reported (Wichniak, Tracik et al. 2001). When HFT alternates from one leg to another, it is called "alternating leg muscle activation" (ALMA). Alternating leg muscle activation was observed in 16 of 1500 patients who had overnight PSG for varying reasons (Chervin, Consens et al. 2003). The individual muscle bursts of HFT recorded from anterior tibialis surface EMG typically last 300 to 700 msec. Seventy percent of patients in one case series of ALMA were taking antidepressants (Chervin, Consens et al. 2003). HFT and ALMA usually do not disturb sleep, and do not require treatment.

Table 1 Drugs Associated with Sleep-related Leg Cramps

- Albuterol
- Asraloxifene
- Clofibrate
- Potassium-wasting diuretics
- Donepezil
- Prostigmine
- Nifedipine
- Statins
- Terbutaline
- Tolcapone
- Withdrawal from alcohol, barbiturates, narcotics, benzodiazepines

Propriospinal Myoclonus at Sleep Onset

Propriospinal myoclonus (PSM) is a rare, simple sleep-related movement disorder which can cause severe sleep-onset insomnia. Propirospinal myoclonus is a series of *involuntary* myoclonic jerks which begins in the upper rectus abdominus or lower intercostal muscles and *propagates* rostrally to the upper intercostals and caudally to the lower abdominus muscles. Propriospinal myoclonus occurs when the patient is relaxed and trying to fall asleep, usually disappears with the onset of NREM 2 sleep, but may recur following awakening and prevent sleep onset. EMG of PSM shows spontaneous intermittent rhythmic or arrhythmic brief myoclonic bursts which usually arise in the upper rectus abdominus or lower intercostal axial muscles followed by propagation rostrally to upper intercostal and caudally to the abdominal muscles at slow conduction velocities of 2 to 16 msec (Montagna, Provini et al. 2006). Propriospinal myoclonus is usually spontaneous but can sometimes be triggered by stimulus-sensitive flexion (or occasionally extension) movements of the axial trunk muscles (Chokroverty 1995); it can co-exist with symptoms of restless legs syndrome (RLS) and periodic limb movements (PLMS) (Vetrugno, Provini et al. 2005).

The neurological examination, brain and spinal MRI, somatosensory evoked potentials, and transmagnetic stimulation are usually normal (Vetrugno, Provini et al. 2001; Montagna, Provini et al. 2006). Myoclonic jerk time-locked to brain averaging has shown PSM does not originate in the cerebral cortex. PSG can develop within days or weeks of cervical trauma, suggesting it may represent a partial release of a spinal central pattern generator (Brown, Rothwell et al. 1994) propagated up and down the spinal cord by slow conducting pathways, such as propriospinal fibers (Chokroverty, Walters et al. 1992). Clonazepam (0.5–2 mg) before bed usually provides partial relief for patients with PSM who complain of inability to fall asleep because of the PSM (Montagna, Provini et al. 2006).

Excessive Fragmentary Myoclonus

If simple sleep-related movements are only minor ones of the fingers or toes, or twitches about the mouth, consider excessive fragmentary myoclonus (EFM); this is defined as small muscle twitches of the fingers, toes, or corners of the mouth or small muscle twitches which resemble muscle fasciculations because they cause *no* movement across a joint space (Broughton, Tolentino et al. 1985). Excessive fragmentary myoclonus occurs during all stages of sleep (most often REM sleep), does not occur in clusters or synchronously (as HFT or ALTA), or in wake/sleep transitions such as sleep starts (Lins, Castonguay et al. 1993). Excessive fragmentary myoclonus in a video-PSG appear as very brief (75–150 msec) EMG bursts in various muscles which occur asynchronously and asymmetrically in a sustained manner without clustering for at least 20 minutes of sleep (Medicine 2005). EEG-EMG back averaging has shown these are not generated by the cerebral cortex (Vetrugno, Plazzi et al. 2002). Excessive fragmentary myoclonus is most often an incidental finding in a PSG. Patients are not usually aware of the movements, nor do they affect sleep onset or sleep quality, or need treatment. Occasionally, a bed partner asks for an explanation for them.

Sleep-related Bruxism and Faciomandibular Myoclonus

Grinding or clenching of teeth during sleep, which often occurs with or following arousals, characterizes sleep-related bruxism (SB). The prevalence of SB decreases with age: reported in approximately 8% of young to middle-aged adults and 3% of older persons (Lavigne, Khoury et al. 2008). Sleep-related bruxism is diagnosed if a patient: 1) reports or is aware of tooth-grinding sounds or tooth clenching sleeping and complains of jaw muscle discomfort, fatigue, or pain and jaw lock; and 2) has on exam abnormal wear of the teeth with or without masseter muscle hypertrophy upon voluntary forceful jaw clenching. Sleep-related bruxism on video-PSG appears as recurring episodes of bruxing movements of masseter and temporalis muscles accompanied by the noise of grinding teeth which usually follow an arousal, and sometimes concludes with a swallow, and can occur in any stage of sleep but most often NREM 1 or NREM 2.

Sleep-related bruxism can lead to tooth destruction, temporomandibular joint pain, lock jaw, temporal headaches, cheek-biting, and mastication muscle hypertrophy. The noise of SB may disturb a sleeping bed partner. Major risk factors for SB include: tobacco, caffeine, heavy alcohol, type A personality, and other sleep disorders, especially sleep apnea or PLMS (Walters, Lavigne et al. 2007). Sleep-related bruxism is probably an extreme audible expression of rhythmic masticatory muscle activity (RMMA), occurs during sleep for most normal subjects (Lavigne, Kato et al. 2003), and probably represents another central pattern generator emerging during sleep. Sleep-related faciomandibular myoclonus (FM) at first glance resembles SB but is characterized on PSG by spontaneous myoclonic jerks of the facial, masticatory, and sometimes sternocleidomastoid muscles during NREM sleep without the tonic EMG masticatory activity typical of SB (Loi, Provini et al. 2007). Faciomandibular myoclonus may cause tongue biting and bleeding, and be mistaken for sleep-related epilepsy (Dylgjeri, Pincherle et al. 2009); SB, FM, and RMMA most likely represent sleep-related release of brainstem central pattern motor generators. Mouth guard or mandibular advance appliance worn when sleeping or clonazepam taken before bed are the most successive treatments for SB (Landry, Rompre et al. 2006; Huynh, Manzini et al. 2007; Landry-Schonbeck, de Grandmont et al. 2009).

Periodic Limb Movements in Sleep (PLMS)

Periodic limb movements in sleep (PLMS) are involuntary unilateral or bilateral stereotypic limb movements which occur periodically during sleep. PLMS usually involve the legs, occasionally the arms or trunk. Jerks are usually bilateral, but may shift, or predominate in one limb. PLMS may be first observed on a PSG immediately after sleep onset, are most frequent during stage NREM 2, tend to decrease in frequency during NREM 3 sleep, and are uncommon during REM sleep.

We record PLMS in a PSG from surface anterior tibialis muscle EMG (Zucconi, Ferri et al. 2006). PLMs are defined as a *periodic* sequence of four or more limb movements each lasting 0.5 to 10 seconds with 5 to 90 seconds from onset to onset of consecutive movements (Zucconi, Ferri et al. 2006; Iber, Ancoli-Israel et al. 2007; Walters, Lavigne et al. 2007). Most PLMs we see in a PSG last 1.5–2.5 seconds and usually recur at 20–40 second intervals (Figure 3).

Considerable debate continues as to the clinical significance of PLMS. PLMS occur during sleep in 4–10% of normal asymptomatic young adults and 30–86% of older adults when sleeping (Hornyak, Feige et al. 2006). Some argue that PLMS are "sufficiently distinct and common among RLS patients to be considered a motor sign of RLS" (Allen and Earley 2001), but 20% of patients with primary RLS had no PLMS on a first night PSG (Montplaisir, Boucher et al. 1997). An Iceland discovery sample searching for the PLM gene among patients with RLS found 35% who fulfilled all clinical criteria for RLS had no PLMS on their PSG and 50% with PLMS denied RLS (Stefansson, Rye et al. 2007). One-third of cardiac transplant patients had PLM-index $\geq$ 15/h but only 45% of them endorsed symptoms of RLS (Javaheri, Abraham et al. 2004).

A PLM-index (PLMI, mean number of PLMS per hour of sleep) of $\geq$ 10 per hour of sleep in an overnight PSG is considered abnormal in

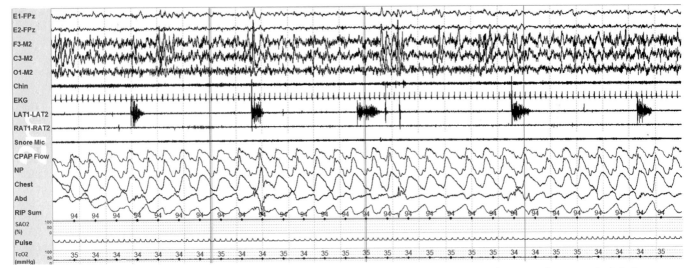

Figure 3 Periodic limb movements during sleep A two-minute epoch of PSG in NREM 2 sleep in a 63-year-old woman showing periodic limb movements recurring every 20 to 40 seconds.

an adult but often of uncertain clinical or diagnostic significance. PLMS and arousals seemingly related to PLMS occur with almost every other primary sleep disorder: 66% of patients with narcolepsy-cataplexy (Baumann 2007), 57–70% of patients with REM sleep behavior disorder (Olson, Boeve et al. 2000; Fantini, Michaud et al. 2002), and 39% of patients with obstructive sleep apnea (Haba-Rubio, Staner et al. 2005). PLMS in patients with other primary sleep disorders are usually older, and their PLMS usually do not cause arousals. A study of 1,124 adults who had overnight PSG for suspected or confirmed sleep disorders found the PLM-ArI was associated with *less* objective sleepiness but PLMS, which did not cause arousal, predicted nothing.

PLMS are especially common on PSG in patients treated with antidepressants. Yang et al. (2005) found 274 patients on antidepressants (except bupropion) had 10 to 14 PLMS per hour of sleep compared with 5 per hour among the 69 control subjects (Yang, White et al. 2005). Treatment with venlaxine or a selective serotonin reuptake inhibitor increased 5-fold the odds ratio of a PLMI >20/h; however, these leg movements usually did not cause arousals (PLM-ArI averaged only 3.2/h). Chervin argues that scoring PLMS in a PSG is of little diagnostic or clinical value unless the patient has a clinical history of PLMS, RLS, or a neurodegenerative disorder (Chervin 2001).

Complex Sleep-related Movement Disorders

REM Sleep Behavior Disorder

At the beginning of the 20th century, Freud suggested how fortunate we are to be paralyzed during sleep, so we cannot act our dreams (Freud 1958). Freud's early speculation was later proved true: Skeletal muscles (save those innervating eye muscles and the diaphragm) are paralyzed when we sleep, but normally *only* during REM sleep. However, patients with REM sleep behavior disorder (RBD) lose the skeletal atonia normally present during REM sleep, permitting them to "act out" their increasingly disturbing and violent dreams. RBD was first described in humans by Schenck and Mahowald in 1986 (Schenck, Bundlie et al. 1986).

Abnormal and often violent motor behaviors and vocalizations which emerge during recurring REM sleep periods characterize RBD. Once aroused, the patient is able to recount dreams which correspond to the observed behaviors (Schenck, Bundlie et al. 1986; Schenck,

Bundlie et al. 1987). RBD episodes usually appear in the first 90 minutes after sleep onset, typically last 1 to 5 minutes, and recur 3–5 times at 90 to 120 minute intervals across an entire night of sleep during recurring periods of REM sleep. Motor behaviors during RBD can be simple (talking, shouting, excessive jerking of limbs or body) or complex (arm flailing, slapping, kicking, sitting up, leaping from bed, running, crawling, gesturing, swearing) (AASM 2005). Speech can vary from mumbling to logical sentences; sometimes the dream enactment behavior is nonviolent (singing, dancing, clapping or snapping fingers) (Oudiette, De Cock et al. 2009). REM sleep behavior disorder is also a dream disorder: Dreams tend to involve frighteningly unfamiliar people or animals, confrontation, attacking, or chasing themes and the behaviors often depict the sleeper defending himself. Sleep-related injuries (bruises, abrasions, lacerations, fractures, choking episodes, and rarely subdural hematomas) to the patient or bed partner are the presenting complaint in 33% to 85% of patients.(Schenck, Milner et al. 1989; Schenck, Hurwitz et al. 1993; Olson, Boeve et al. 2000) The personality, temperament, and behavior of RBD patients awake are discordant with their nocturnal aggressive behaviors.

Video-PSG Used to Confirm REM Sleep Behavior Disorder

A clinical history of bizarre violent motor behaviors in an older adult which occur more than 90 minutes after sleep onset (especially if dream enactment is reported) warrants consideration of RBD. The clinical diagnosis of RBD requires confirmation by in-laboratory nocturnal video-PSG. Excessive amounts of phasic and/or tonic activity in the chin and/or limb muscles during REM sleep coupled with dream enactment behavior characterizes RBD in a PSG (Figure 4). The severity of the RBD motor and vocal behaviors during REM sleep vary in severity, often more severe at the end of the night when REM sleep is most plentiful (Iranzo, Santamaria et al. 2009). Motor behaviors are more frequent than vocal behaviors in RBD. Nonviolent behaviors may also occur (Oudiette, De Cock et al. 2009).

The clinical diagnosis of RBD requires video-PSG confirmation. Full criteria for the diagnosis of RBD include: 1) the presence of REM sleep without atonia (RSWA) (excessive amounts of sustained or intermittent elevation of submental EMG tone or excessive phasic submental or limb EMG twitching); 2) sleep-related injurious, potentially injurious, or disruptive behaviors by history and/or abnormal REM

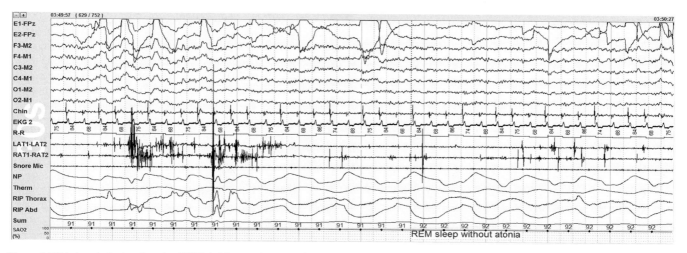

Figure 4 REM sleep behavior disorder (RBD) A 30-second epoch of a polysomnogram from a patient with REM sleep behavior disorder (RBD) showing loss of the normal skeletal atonia present during REM sleep. Loss of skeletal atonia during REM sleep permits patients with RBD to act out their increasing violent dreams. Compare the increased amounts of phasic and tonic muscle activity in the chin and limb channels to the normal amount seen in Figure 1.

sleep behaviors documented during video-PSG; and 3) exclusion of medication use, substance abuse, or another medical, neurological, psychiatric, or sleep disorder which better explains the sleep disturbance (Medicine 2005; Iber, Ancoli-Israel et al. 2007; Walters, Lavigne et al. 2007). However, there is no accepted methodology for which muscles should be sampled and measured (Burns, Consens et al. 2007; Frauscher, Gschliesser et al. 2007; Ferri, Manconi et al. 2008; Mayer, Kesper et al. 2008) or for classifying the behaviors (Sforza, Krieger et al. 1997; Fantini, Ferini-Strambi et al. 2005; Frauscher, Gschliesser et al. 2007).

Frauscher et al. (2007) found they were able to score greater amounts of excessive motor activity during REM sleep by simultaneously recording and analyzing EMG activity from the mentalis, flexor digitorum superficialis, and extensor digitorum brevis muscles (Frauscher, Gschliesser et al. 2007). Zhang et al. (2008) evaluated night-to-night variability in RSWA and clinical RBD (Zhang, Lam et al. 2008). They found: 1) they could diagnose RBD in 95% of patients by recording and carefully analyzing the amounts of REM-related EMG activity, RSWA, and motor events observed on video-PSG; 2) no significant difference in the amounts of phasic and tonic EMG activity during REM sleep between nights 1 and 2 but dream enactment motor events varied between nights; 3) inter-study agreement were lowest for video analysis (kappa coefficients of 0.64, 0.51, and 0.31 between nights 1 and 2 for REM sleep-related EMG activity, RSWA, and video analysis); and 4) they were able to diagnose RBD even in patients with concomitant obstructive sleep apnea treated with continuous positive airway pressure. Effective treatments for RBD (clonazepam, melatonin) may suppress the clinical behaviors but the excessive motor activity in REM sleep persists.

The most common expression of RBD is limb jerking. A case-control study found five PD patients with RBD had a mean of 54 ± 23 paroxysmal motor behaviors per 10 minutes of REM sleep compared 4 ± 2 per hour among age- and gender-matched controls; 75% of these lasted less than 2 seconds, 83% were simple, 14% complex, 11% vocalizations, and 4% violent (Frauscher, Gschliesser et al. 2007). Ninety-one percent of the motor events in the control group were simple. Manni et al. (2009) found paroxysmal motor RBD behaviors were more likely to occur in phasic rather than tonic REM sleep (Manni, Terzaghi et al. 2009). A fascinating video-PSG study found 38% of 53 PD patients moved much better and had louder more intelligible

speech during their RBD episodes than when awake (De Cock, Vidailhet et al. 2007).

REM Sleep Behavior Disorder Often Heralds a Neurodegenerative Disorder

REM sleep behavior disorder typically affects older men: 87% of 93 consecutive patients with RBD seen at the Mayo Clinic over a four-year period were male (Olson, Boeve et al. 2000); a male predominance is observed in most other large case series (Schenck, Hurwitz et al. 1993; Iranzo, Molinuevo et al. 2006; Postuma, Gagnon et al. 2009). The predilection for RBD to occur in men prompted speculation that testosterone contributed to its clinical expression in men but RBD was not associated with higher serum testosterone levels than in controls of patients with idiopathic RBD (Iranzo, Santamaria et al. 2007) or PD with RBD (Chou, Moro-De-Casillas et al. 2007).

REM sleep behavior disorder is often symptomatic of an undiagnosed neurological disorder (Table 2). More than half of older adults with RBD have or will develop a neurodegenerative disease, most often a synucleinopathy: dementia with Lewy bodies (DLB), multiple system atrophy (MSA), and Parkinson's disease (PD) (Boeve, Silber et al. 2001; Boeve, Silber et al. 2003; Boeve, Silber et al. 2004; Stiasny-Kolster, Doerr et al. 2005; Boeve and Saper 2006; Gagnon, Postuma et al. 2006; Iranzo, Molinuevo et al. 2006; Postuma, Lang et al. 2006; Weyer, Minnerop et al. 2006; Boeve, Silber et al. 2007). Boeve et al. (2007) found that 97% of 36 older patients with PSG-confirmed RBD and dementia and/or parkinsonism had an underlying α-synucleinopathy: 31 (92%) had DLB, four MSA, but one patient had progressive supranuclear palsy (PSP), which is a tauopathy (Boeve, Silber et al. 1998; Boeve, Silber et al. 2003; Boeve, Silber et al. 2007). RBD began at a mean age of 62 years, the mean age of cognitive decline six years later at age 68, and parkinsonism age 69 (Boeve, Silber et al. 1998).

REM sleep behavior disorder occurs in 50–80% of patients with DLB (Boeve, Silber et al. 2004). DLB is the second most common late-life dementia, and probably accounts for approximately 20% of all late-onset dementias, 10–15% at autopsy (McKeith, Dickson et al. 2005). The diagnosis of probable DLB is suggested by the presence of dementia and RBD with at least one of the three core features of visual hallucinations, fluctuating cognition, or parkinsonism (McKeith 2006). A diagnosis of possible DLB is suggested by dementia plus RBD

Table 2 Neurological Disorders and Medications Associated with REM Sleep Behavior Disorder

- ◆ Synucleinpathies:
  - ◆ Dementia with Lewy bodies;
  - ◆ Parkinson's disease;
  - ◆ Multiple system atrophy;
  - ◆ Pure autonomic failure);
- ◆ Non-synucleinopathies:
  - ◆ Parkinson's disease due to Parkin mutations;
  - ◆ Paraneoplastic limbic encephalitis with voltage-gated potassium channel antibodies;
  - ◆ Guadalupean Parkinsonism (sour sop ingestion);
  - ◆ Progressive supranuclear palsy (rare);
  - ◆ Huntington's disease (15%);
  - ◆ Spinocerebellar ataxia type 3 (Joseph-Machado disease);
- ◆ Structural lesions most often involving pontine tegmentum;
  - ◆ Ischemic infarction, multiple sclerosis;
  - ◆ Brain stem tumor, trauma, or surgery;
- ◆ Narcolepsy with cataplexy (including childhood onset);
  - ◆ Autism;
  - ◆ Medication-related:
    - ◆ Tricyclic antidepressants especially amitriptyline;
    - ◆ Selective serotonin reuptake inhibitors particularly mirtazapine (Remeron) and venlafaxine (Effexor);
    - ◆ Chocolate

alone (McKeith 2006). It is important to recognize LBD because patients with it often have a good response to cholinesterase inhibitors and an extreme sensitivity to the side effects of neuroleptics. DLB tends to have a more rapid progression than AD (mean survival 8 ± 3 years) and two-thirds are men (in contrast to the predominance of AD in women (McKeith, Dickson et al. 2005). DLB is often the cause of unexplained recurrent delirium or episodic disturbances of consciousness in elders. DLB patients may be unaware of their RBD symptoms: 18% of 17 consecutive DLB patients with video-PSG confirmed RBD could not recall unpleasant dreams and 59% were unaware of their RBD behaviors (Iranzo, Santamaria et al. 2009).

REM sleep behavior disorder occurs in approximately 15–50% of patients with PD (Comella, Nardine et al. 1998; Gagnon, Bedard et al. 2002; De Cock, Vidailhet et al. 2008; Lee, Kim et al. 2009). RBD may be even more common in patients with PD because 65% were unaware of their RBD symptoms and 24% did not recall violent dreams (Iranzo, Santamaria et al. 2005). Another third of PD patients have REM sleep without atonia (RSWA) on their PSG without any clinical history of RBD behaviors or symptoms (Gagnon, Bedard et al. 2002).

Recent studies suggest that PD patients with RBD may have a different neurodegenerative profile than those without RBD. RBD was less common in PD with tremor than those with rigid-akinetic PD (Kumru, Santamaria et al. 2007; Postuma, Gagnon et al. 2008). Another study found PD patients with RBD compared to those without RBD were older, had a longer duration of PD, were more disabled, and had a lower proportion of tremor (Lee, Kim et al. 2009). RBD was strongly associated with orthostatic hypotension in 36 PD patients (71% vs.

27%, p = .0076) (Postuma, Gagnon et al. 2008). PD patients with RBD were more likely to have slowed EEGs when awake (Gagnon, Fantini et al. 2004) and poorer performance in executive function, verbal memory, and visuospatial dysfunction on neuropsychological testing than PD without RBD (Vendette, Gagnon et al. 2007). However, RBD in PD was not associated with hypersomnia, sleep benefit, motor fluctuations, dyskinesias, or depression (Iranzo, Santamaria et al. 2009).

Almost all patients with multiple system atrophy (MSA) have RBD (or at least RSWA on their PSGs). Clinical RBD was reported in 69% of 39 consecutive cases of MSA, and 90% had RSWA on their video-PSG (Plazzi, Corsini et al. 1997). Many MSA patients are unaware of their RBD behaviors or bad dreams (Tachibana and Oka 2004). RBD is often the *initial* symptom of MSA (Tison, Wenning et al. 1995); RBD is a red flag for the diagnosis of MSA (Kollensperger, Geser et al. 2008). Consider MSA in a patient with an axial rigid syndrome (less often a jerky postural tremor) and RBD who have symptomatic orthostatic hypotension or urinary incontinence beginning less than one year after the onset of the parkinsonism, early postural instability and falls less than three years after onset; or rapid progression to wheelchair within less than five years despite dopaminergic therapy (Kollensperger, Geser et al. 2008). A longitudinal study found patients with MSA and RBD had a shorter duration of disease, a higher percentage of REM sleep without atonia, greater mean number of PLM per hour of sleep, and less total sleep time compared to those with PD and RBD (Iranzo, Santamaria et al. 2005). Consider MSA in an older woman with RBD because no gender predominance is observed in MSA (Iranzo, Santamaria et al. 2005; Plazzi, Corsini et al. 1997).

The onset of clinical RBD has been reported to occur with the introduction of tricyclic antidepressants, selective serotonin reuptake inhibitors, beta blockers and perhaps chocolate. RBD can occur in patients with other neurological or neurodegenerative disorders which are not synucleinopathies (Table 2). RBD in non-synucleinopathies tends to evolve in concert with or after the onset of parkinsonism, whereas RBD typically begins years after the onset of the cognitive and motor features in synucleinopathies (Boeve, Silber et al. 2007). Nine percent of patients with PD due to *parkin* gene mutations (which are not synucleinopathies) had symptoms suggestive of clinical RBD, 45% had RSWA on their PSG (Plazzi, Cortelli et al. 1998; Tachibana and Oka 2004; Iranzo, Santamaria et al. 2005; Limousin, Konofal et al. 2009). RBD rarely occurs in patients with tauopathies such as corticobasal degeneration or progressive supranuclear palsy (PSP) (Pareja, Caminero et al. 1996; Montplaisir, Petit et al. 1997; Arnulf, Merino-Andreu et al. 2005; Cooper and Josephs 2009), although some argue that these patients more often had mixed AD/DLB pathology upon autopsy (Boeve, Silber et al. 2007).

REM sleep behavior disorder has also been observed in 10–15% of patients with narcolepsy with cataplexy (Schenck and Mahowald 1992; Dauvilliers, Rompre et al. 2007; Billiard 2009) and others have RSWA without clinical RBD (Dauvilliers, Rompre et al. 2007). Medications prescribed to treat their cataplexy can induce or aggravate RBD (Schenck and Mahowald 1992; Abril, Carlander et al. 2007; Ahmed 2008). Video-PSG confirmed RBD was observed in five patients with limbic encephalitis associated with antibodies to voltage-gated potassium channels and their RBD resolved with immunosuppressive therapy (Iranzo, Munoz et al. 2003). RBD has been observed in 78% of patients with another tauopathy, Guadeloupean parkinsonism (and RBD preceded the symptoms in 43%) (De Cock, Lannuzel et al. 2007). Guadeloupean parkinsonism is characterized by levodopa-resistant parkinsonism, tremor, myoclonus, hallucinations, and a subcortical dementia with or without supranuclear palsy. RBD in these patients was intense, and all patients recalled their dream enactment behaviors (Iranzo, Santamaria et al. 2009). It appears to be caused by regular ingestion of sour sop (a tropical fruit available in the US). The fruit and leaves of sour sop contain acetogenins which are selective mitochondrial complex I inhibitors. Chronic administration of acetogenins to mice reproduced the characteristic midbrain lesions seen in humans (Lannuzel, Ruberg et al. 2008).

REM sleep behavior disorder has been observed in patients with spinocerebellar ataxias (Friedman, Fernandez et al. 2003; Iranzo, Munoz et al. 2003; Syed, Rye et al. 2003), especially Machado Joseph disease (type 3), an autosomal dominant disorder linked to CAG-triplet expansions in the ataxin-3 gene. We have single case reports of RBD developing after ischemic strokes, brainstem surgery, trauma, or associated with an exacerbation of multiple sclerosis with the brain MRI demonstrating lesions which most often involve the pons (Kimura, Tachibana et al. 2000; Plazzi and Montagna 2002; Tippmann-Peikert, Boeve et al. 2006).

What Is the Risk of a Patient with Chronic Idiopathic RBD Subsequently Developing a Neurodegenerative Disorder?

Patients who have the clinical and PSG findings of RBD but have no neurological condition or other particular cause for RBD when first diagnosed are regarded as having "idiopathic" RBD (iRBD). Recent case series and longitudinal studies suggest half to two-thirds of patients with iRBD will develop a neurodegenerative disorder, most often a synucleinopathy (DLB, PD, or MSA) within 5–10 years (Iranzo, Santamaria et al. 2009). Thirty-eight percent of 29 men developed parkinsonism, a mean of 12.7 years after the onset of RBD and 3.7 years after the diagnosis of RBD (Schenck, Bundlie et al. 1996); 65% seven years later (Schenck 2003). Another study found 45% of 44 iRBD patients (39 men, mean age 74 y) developed a neurological disorder a mean of 11.5 years after the RBD onset and 5.1 years after the diagnosis of iRBD (Iranzo, Molinuevo et al. 2006). Clinical diagnoses included: DLB in six, PD five, MSA one, and "mild cognitive impairment with prominent visuospatial dysfunction" in four. In 2009, Postuma et al. reports that six of 67 patients with iRBD they have followed prospectively since 2004 have developed PD, and 11 dementia (Postuma, Gagnon et al. 2009). They have found all tests of olfaction, color vision, autonomic function, depression, and quantitative measures of motor speed were similar in patients with PD and dementia. RBD was the initial manifestation of DLB, even before hallucinations or fluctuations in consciousness developed. Postuma et al. (2009), based upon their longitudinal study of 93 iRBD patients, estimated the 5-year risk of neurodegenerative disease with iRBD was 18%; the risk increased to 41% and 52% at 10- and 12-years, respectively (Postuma, Gagnon et al. 2009).

Are there diagnostic tests which can predict which patients with iRBD are at greater risk to develop a neurodegenerative disease? Many patients with iRBD exhibit subtle deficits also seen in patients with PD or DLB, including: subtle deficits in executive function (Massicotte-Marquez, Decary et al. 2008), color discrimination and olfactory dysfunction (Fantini, Postuma et al. 2006; Postuma, Lang et al. 2006; Stiasny-Kolster, Clever et al. 2007; Massicotte-Marquez, Decary et al. 2008; Miyamoto, Miyamoto et al. 2009), and prominent slow wave activity in their EEGs (Massicotte-Marquez, Carrier et al. 2005). A particularly promising diagnostic test identifying iRBD at risk for PD or DLB is early loss of cardiac sympathetic nerve terminals confirmed by ^{123}I-MIBG (metaiodobenzylguanidine) cardiac scintigraphy present in patients with iRBD, PD, or DLB but not those with MSA or PSP (Miyamoto, Miyamoto et al. 2006; Miyamoto, Miyamoto et al. 2008). Reduced cardiac MIBG uptake has been reported to be characteristic of patients with α-synucleinopathies such as PD and DLB (Wada-Isoe, Kitayama et al. 2007; Sawada, Oeda et al. 2009; Ishibashi, Saito et al. 2010).

Neuropathological Basis of REM Sleep Behavior Disorder

REM sleep without atonia (RSWA) was first induced experimentally by making bilateral lesions in the dorsolateral pontine tegmentum of cats (Jouvet 1965; Mahowald and Schenck 2004). Depending upon the size and extent of the brainstem lesions, the cats could stand, walk, attack, and "act out their dreams" (raised vertical and horizontal head movements as if watching something) during REM sleep, culminating in attack behaviors when they extended the lesions into midbrain, interrupting amygdalar pathways. Increased phasic locomotor tone and/or loss of REM sleep atonia are thought the likely mechanisms for clinical RBD (Boeve, Dickson et al. 2007; Mahowald, Schenck et al. 2007) in humans (Kimura, Tachibana et al. 2000), cats (Jouvet 1965; Hendricks, Lager et al. 1989), and rats (Lu, Sherman et al. 2006).

Skeletal atonia during REM sleep is regulated by neurons in the human equivalent of the pontine reticular formation sublaterodorsal nucleus (SLD) in the rat and the subcoeruleus region in cats (Saper, Cano et al. 2005; Lu, Sherman et al. 2006; Boeve, Silber et al. 2007). SLD neurons send direct projections (primarily glutaminergic and presumably excitatory) to nuclei in the reticularis magnocellularis of the medulla which in turn send direct inhibitory projections to inhibit α-motor neurons in the ventral spinal cord (causing hyperpolarization by glycinergic and GABAergic mechanisms) (Lu, Sherman et al. 2006).

Abnormalities in central dopamine function may underlie or contribute to RBD: SPECT studies have showed decreased numbers of striatal dopamine transporters in patients with RBD (Eisensehr, Linke et al. 2000; Eisensehr, Linke et al. 2003). Decreased striatal binding on PET scans in MSA patients with RBD correlated with increased amounts of RSWA on video-PSG (Gilman, Koeppe et al. 2003). Decreased striatal-binding RBD motor behaviors and frightening dreams may reflect brainstem and amygdalar dysfunction, respectively, but cortical areas must be activated in some patients because they sometimes sing, give long speeches, or exhibit elaborate motor sequences beyond what could be expected from central pattern generators. Many different anatomical and neurochemical brain lesions can individually or in combination lead to RBD, evident by multiple different classes of drugs, disorders, and diseases that can trigger it. Full understanding of this complex sleep-related movement disorder is still needed.

Differential Diagnosis of REM Sleep Behavior Disorder

Consider DLB in patients who have unexplained recurrent delirium, episodic disturbances of consciousness, syncope, and sleep disorders. RBD can be misdiagnosed as nocturnal panic attacks, agitated sleepwalking, sleep dissociation disorder, sleep-related epilepsy, nocturnal hallucinations, agitated delirium in intensive care units, and/or intentional spouse abuse. RSWA and even RBD-like behaviors can occur in patients with and without neurodegenerative disorders who are affected by obstructive sleep apnea, nocturnal epilepsy, hallucinations, sleep terrors, and delirium. Some patients with RBD additionally have sleep apnea, nocturnal epilepsy, confusional arousals, and sleepwalking. Suffice it to say, separating these out can be challenging.

Treating REM Sleep Behavior Disorder

Treating RBD begins with removing drugs which can cause or worsen RBD (Table 2). If a drug which is aggravating RBD cannot be discontinued (too often the case in patients with concomitant depression treated with venlafaxine or a selective serotonin reuptake inhibitor), try reducing the daily dose. Consider prescribing bupropion to treat depression in patients with RBD. Buproprion does not seem to worsen RBD, RLS or PLMs (Nofzinger, Fasiczka et al. 2000; Kim, Shin et al. 2005; Yang, White et al. 2005; Lee, Erdos et al. 2009).

REM sleep behavior disorder warrants treatment to: 1) prevent injuries in patients with violent dream enactment; 2) reduce the intensity of the unpleasant dreams; and 3) permit the bed partner to sleep comfortably and safely near the patient with RBD. The first step in treatment of RBD is to remove drugs that can precipitate or worsen it (Table 2). The next step is to secure the bedroom and protect the patient and bed partner from injury. No large randomized controlled trials of treatment for RBD have been published.

Small case series and case reports have found clonazepam effective in treating RBD in the majority (90%) of patients (Schenck, Bundlie et al. 1987; Schenck and Mahowald 1996; Comella, Nardine et al. 1998; Olson, Boeve et al. 2000; Massironi, Galluzzi et al. 2003; Nomura, Inoue et al. 2003; Fantini, Corona et al. 2005; Iranzo, Santamaria et al. 2005; Gagnon, Postuma et al. 2006; Iranzo, Santamaria et al. 2009). Clonazepam (0.25–4 mg before bed, mean dose 1 mg) usually decreases the frequency and severity of both dream enactment behaviors and unpleasant dream recall within the first week of treatment without loss of effectiveness or the development of tolerance over time. Clonazepam has an elimination half-life of 30–40 hours and maximum plasma concentrations occur within 1–4 hours after oral ingestion (Anderson and Shneerson 2009). Holding clonazepam for a single night in hospitalized RBD patients or periodic attempts to taper clonazepam resulted in almost immediate recurrence of their nocturnal behaviors (Schenck and Mahowald 1991; Schenck and Mahowald 1996). Even if the RBD behaviors are suppressed, RSWA usually remains on the video-PSG. Clonazepam suppresses the clinical RBD behaviors but does not improve RSWA or alter sleep architecture (Lapierre and Montplaisir 1992; Schenck and Mahowald 1990). The use of clonazepam to treat RBD is often limited early or late by side effects. The most common side effects are sedation especially upon awakening, early morning clumsiness, impotence, and confusion (Schenck and Mahowald 1990; Schenck and Mahowald 1996; Olson, Boeve et al. 2000). Clonazepam taken only at night can cause memory or word-finding difficulties, depression, disinhibition, and if the dose is too low may trigger SW/ST or confusional arousals, especially in older adults with or without dementia. Clonazepam is relatively contraindicated in patients with a history of substance or ethanol abuse, untreated sleep disordered breathing, cognitive or motor dysfunction, or a nocturnal dissociative disorder.

Clonazepam should be used with caution in patients with dementia, gait disorders, or concomitant obstructive sleep apnea, all of which develop in varying degrees over the clinical course of RBD (Ferman, Boeve et al. 1999).

Oral melatonin has been effectively used to treat RBD (Takeuchi, Uchimura et al. 2001; Boeve, Silber et al. 2003; Kunz, Mahlberg et al. 2004). We have begun to prescribe melatonin first in patients with RBD because it is often just as effective and has far fewer side effects than clonazepam. Melatonin alone can control RBD, usually in oral doses ranging from 3 to 12 mg before bed. If melatonin alone does not completely suppress RBD, it can be combined with small doses of oral clonazepam. Melatonin suppressed dream enactment behavior (Kunz, Mahlberg et al. 2004; Boeve, Silber et al. 2003; Takeuchi, Uchimura et al. 2001). Side effects of melatonin observed in some RBD patients include morning headache, morning sleepiness, delusions, or hallucinations (Boeve, Silber et al. 2003). PSG studies in RBD patients treated with melatonin showed a decrease in the number of REM sleep epochs without atonia and movement time during REM sleep (Kunz and Bes 1999; Kunz, Mahlberg et al. 2004; Takeuchi, Uchimura et al. 2001) and has few side effects.

RBD in some patients with PD or DLB may respond to treatment with either dopamine receptor agonists (pramipexole) or reversible acetylcholinesterase inhibitors (rivastigmine) (Fantini, Gagnon et al. 2003; Schmidt, Koshal et al. 2006; Kumru, Iranzo et al. 2008), although these medications can paradoxically activate RBD in others (Comella, Tanner et al. 1993; Tan, Salgado et al. 1996; Fantini, Gagnon et al. 2003; Schmidt, Koshal et al. 2006; Kumru, Iranzo et al. 2008). Doses of pramipexole which were effective in treating RBD in some PD patients ranged from 0.5 to 1.5 mg (Fantini, Gagnon et al. 2003; Schmidt, Koshal et al. 2006). Fantini et al. found pramipexole lessened the frequency and intensity of RBD motor behaviors and reduced the REM sleep time spent in RSWA in five of eight patients with iRBD (Fantini, Gagnon et al. 2003). Patients with RBD also have PLMS on their PSG and pramipexole did not lessen the number of these. Another video-PSG in 11 PD patients with RBD found pramipexole did not alter the RSWA, nor suppress or even lessen the RBD motor behaviors (Kumru, Iranzo et al. 2008). Pramipexole and levodopa may worsen RBD in some patients with PD, DLB, or iRBD.

Safety measures to protect the patient and bed partner from RBD behaviors include: padding bedrails, pillow or plastic screen barricades, pad sharp corner and move furniture away from the bed, remove dangerous objects from bedroom, locks on doors and windows, motion-detected alarms, and consider having the patient sleep on a mattress on the floor or in another bedroom (Olson, Boeve et al. 2000; Schenck and Mahowald 1991; Abad and Guilleminault 2004). Active restraints should not be used to restrain patients with RBD because sudden twisting movements during RBD events may lead to greater injury.

Sleepwalking and Sleep Terrors in Older Adults

NREM disorders of arousal (DOA) include sleepwalking (SW) (Hughes 2007), sleep terrors (ST), confusional arousals (Plazzi, Vetrugno et al. 2005; Hughes 2007), sleep-related eating (Vetrugno, Manconi et al. 2006), or sexual behaviors (Schenck, Arnulf et al. 2007). DOA usually occur 90 to 180 minutes after sleep onset, and emerge during NREM 3 sleep. Patients during DOA episodes appear confused, disoriented, and are slow to respond; exhibit automatic motor behaviors; have little or no responsiveness to their external environment; and misidentify objects and people. They are difficult to arouse from an episode, and if aroused, recall only fragmentary dream images (often of be trapped or attacked). They typically have retrograde amnesia for these events (although some adults can recall fragments of some events). Varying degrees of sympathetic nervous system activation accompany DOA: mild for "passive" SW, moderate in confusional arousals, marked for ST or "agitated" SW or ST (whereas heart rates do not increase during RBD episodes). Eyes are typically closed during RBD events. Whereas, eyes are open during DOA, visual inspection functions but objects are often misidentified (e.g. trying to use the bedside water glass as a telephone receiver). Patients when touched or held may recoil and their agitation increase.

Confusional arousals begin with a sudden arousal from NREM 3 sleep; the patient often sits up in the bed, may fumble with bedclothes, thrash, flail or kick, moan, whimper and/or utter often unintelligible words. "Passive" SW often begins as a confusional arousal but the patient leaves the bed, walking toward a sound, light, or a particular room. Central pattern motor generators released during DOA often lead them to the kitchen to eat (often foods they would not eat when awake) or to urinate (next to the toilet or in a closet), or outside (through a window or door). Patients respond inappropriately or not at all to voices; sometimes can follow calmly given orders to return to bed. Sympathetic activation is marked during ST and agitated SW. These often begin with a blood-curdling scream or cry; patients exhibit severe agitation, widely dilated pupils, tachycardia, and more vocalization. Agitated sleepwalkers flee their bed screaming or crying, run through the house, down the stairs, or out the front door. Agitated sleepwalkers are prone to injury (to themselves or others) but violent or aggressive behavior is rare, and not goal-directed. DOA usually last a few to 30 minutes, often followed by a calm return to their bed or sleep somewhere else in the house or outside.

Ohayon et al. found 2.0% of 4972 UK adults reported SW, 2.2% ST, and 4.2% CA (Ohayon, Guilleminault et al. 1999) but only 0.4% of adults sleepwalk nightly (Plazzi, Vetrugno et al. 2005). New onset or a late recurrence of SW/ST in adults warrants consideration of other primary sleep disorders (obstructive sleep disordered breathing, RLS, RBD, shift work, or jet lag), cumulative partial sleep deprivation, emotional stress, infections, extreme fatigue, or exercise (Ohayon, Guilleminault et al. 1999; Hughes 2007; Pressman 2007; Schenck, Arnulf et al. 2007). Drugs which may trigger DOA include alcohol or sedative-hypnotics (especially zalpedon, zolpidem, and zopiclone) (ADRAC 2007; Ferentinos and Paparrigopoulos 2009; Hoque and Chesson 2009). Stressful life events (changes in sleep environment, family or workplace conflicts) preceded SW in 56% of the adult subjects they studied (Lecendreux, Bassetti et al. 2003). Video-PSG is warranted in patients with atypical parasomnias, particularly when these: 1) onset or recurrence in an older adult; 2) occur more than 2–3 times per week; 3) are potentially injurious or caused injury to the patient or others. Treatment strategies for DOA in older adults are summarized in Table 3. Sleep specialists often prescribe clonazepam (0.5 mg–2 mg QHS) to suppress potentially injurious SW/ST in adults, although again there are no placebo-controlled trials have been done to confirm this. The effectiveness of clonazepam is more likely due to inhibition of arousals or locomotor activity rather than pharmacological suppression of NREM 3 sleep. Side effects and risks of clonazepam in older adults are summarized in section 4.1.6.

Sleep-related Epileptic Seizures in Older Adults

Sleep, particularly NREM, is a powerful activator of interictal epileptiform discharges, certain seizure types, and particular epilepsy syndromes. Sleep particularly activates partial seizures emanating from the frontal cerebral cortex (Bazil and Walczak 1997; Crespel, Coubes et al. 2000; Herman, Walczak et al. 2001). One study found 57% of partial seizures during sleep arose from the frontal, 44% lateral temporal, 40% mesial temporal, and 13% parieto-occipital regions (Herman,

Table 3 Treatment Strategies for NREM Sleep Disorders of Arousal (DOA) in Adults

---

- Avoid partial arousal, which can trigger a DOA event especially during the first third of the night, especially when the patient is sleep deprived

- Decrease noise, light, pain, nocturia, emotional stress, or dyspnea which may contribute to arousal

- Avoid cumulative partial sleep deprivation

- Optimize sleep/wake schedules, avoid jet lag, night shift and shift work

- Search for other primary sleep disorders: sleep apnea, restless legs, and narcolepsy

- Extreme exercise or fatigue

- Avoid antipsychotics, antidepressants, alcohol, antihistamines, sedative-hypnotics, benzodiazepines.

- Secure the bedroom; protect the patient and those nearby.

- Consideration clonazepam (0.5–2.0 mg QHS) for DOA when chronic and potential danger and sleep disturbance to self or others, or cause excessive daytime sleepiness, daytime stress, or weight gain.

Walczak et al. 2001). Skeletal motor inhibition and desynchronization of EEG during REM sleep are to explain why seizures rarely occur during REM sleep.

Typical features of nocturnal frontal seizures are: 1) abrupt, often explosive, awakening from NREM 2 sleep; 2) sustained asymmetric tonic posturing, and/or violent hyperkinetic motor behaviors (especially thrashing, pedaling, and kicking of the legs); 3) fairly stereotypical appearance for the individual patient; 4) brief, typically lasting 20–30 seconds, rarely longer than 1–2 minutes; 5) patients are often aware during the seizure, but say they cannot control their movements or vocalizations; 6) no post-ictal amnesia or confusion; and 7) often no scalp-recorded ictal EEG activity accompanying theseizures (Lugaresi, Cirignotta et al. 1986; Zucconi, Oldani et al. 1997; Provini, Plazzi et al. 1999). Luders et al. proposed the term "hypermotor" for this type of seizure (Luders, Acharya et al. 1998). Most nocturnal hypermotor seizures emanate from the frontal lobe, but one-third are temporal lobe in origin (Nobili, Cossu et al. 2004; Mai, Sartori et al. 2005) and a few from the insular cortex (Ryvlin, Minotti et al. 2006). Nocturnal frontal lobe seizures are often initially misdiagnosed as sleep terrors, nightmares, or a psychiatric problem (Guilleminault, Leger et al. 1998; Oldani, Zucconi et al. 1998; Silvestri and Bromfield 2004; Derry, Duncan et al. 2006; Hughes 2007; Nobili 2007). Longer lasting nocturnal frontal lobe seizures can lead to "episodic nocturnal wandering," easily misdiagnosed as sleepwalking (Plazzi, Vetrugno et al. 2005).

Diagnosing NLE can be challenging because these patients often have no interictal epileptiform discharges in their EEGs either awake or asleep. Worse yet, 20% of adults with nocturnal frontal lobe epilepsy (NFLE) have no ictal EEG activity recorded as scalp EEGs during a seizure. Interictal and ictal EEGs during prolonged inpatient video-EEG monitoring were normal in 26% of 40 adult NFLE patients (Oldani, Zucconi et al. 1998). The lack of scalp-recorded ictal EEG activity in patients with NFLE may be related to: 1) the brevity of the seizures, often then obscured by muscle artifact, with little or no post-ictal slowing; and/or 2) seizures which originate from the mesial frontal or inferior frontopolar regions are often undetected from scalp-recorded EEG.

A family history of sleep-related epilepsy is present in 30% of patients with NFLE; the pattern of inheritance autosomal dominant with a penetrance estimated at 70% (Scheffer, Bhatia et al. 1994; Oldani, Zucconi et al. 1998; Aridon, Marini et al. 2006; Marini and Guerrini 2007). Although more than 100 families with autosomal dominant NFLE (ADNFLE) have been identified, only a few of them have been linked to mutations in the genes coding for subunits of the neuronal nicotinic acetylcholine receptor located on three different chromosomes (8p12.3-8q12.3, 15q4 and 20q13.1-13.3) (Phillips, Scheffer et al. 1995; Aridon, Marini et al. 2006; Marini and Guerrini 2007). These gene mutations appear to confer a gain of function with increased sensitivity to acetylcholine (Hoda, Gu et al. 2008), which may be the basis for epileptogenesis (Marini and Guerrini 2007). The clinical features and video-EEG findings of ADNFLE do not differ from sporadic NFLE (Marini and Guerrini 2007). Patients with ADNFLE typically have normal neurological exam, intellect, and brain MRI; their epilepsy is typically lifelong, although their seizures often become less frequent and milder by middle age (Aridon, Marini et al. 2006).

The diagnosis is of sleep-related epilepsy in older adults is best confirmed by video-EEG, continuous prolonged inpatient recording if needed (Vignatelli, Bisulli et al. 2007). Overnight video-PSG is best reserved for patients in whom non-epileptic primary sleep disorders (sleep apnea, restless legs, DOA) are suspected. Older adults with epilepsy may *also* have obstructive sleep apnea exacerbating their epilepsy (Malow, Foldvary-Schaefer et al. 2008) and/or RBD (Manni, Terzaghi

Table 4 Adult Parasomnias Red Flags

Red Flag	Consider
Adult onset or late recurrence of "sleepwalking" or "sleep terrors"	Other sleep disorder triggering or other parasomnias
Episodes are potentially injurious or caused injury to themselves or others	Mandate for video-PSG
Spells occur just after sleep onset	Sleep-wake transition parasomnia or sleep-related epilepsy
Multiple episodes per night	REM sleep behavior disorder, sleep-related epilepsy
Acting out dreams, easy to awake from behaviors, particularly in second half of night	REM sleep behavior disorder
Spells are stereotyped	Sleep-related epilepsy
Daytime sleepiness, unrefreshing sleep, symptoms suggestive of sleep apnea, restless legs, panic attacks	Consider other primary sleep disorders such as sleep apnea or restless legs precipitating parasomnias.

et al. 2007). Undiagnosed or misdiagnosed episodes of idiopathic RBD co-existing with epilepsy was found in 13% of 80 older adults (mean age 71 years). RBD began before the epilepsy in four, after the epilepsy in six. Table 4 summarizes "red flags" in adults which warrant video-EEG or video-PSG monitoring.

Carbamazepine is an appropriate first drug for NFLE, often effective at low doses (Oldani, Zucconi et al. 1998; Provini, Plazzi et al. 1999). Carbamazepine completely controlled seizures in 20% of 100 consecutive adults with NFLE, and reduced seizure frequency by 50% or more in another 48% of 100 consecutive adults with NFLE (Provini, Plazzi et al. 1999). The particular effectiveness of carbamazepine in ADNFLE may be related to its particular ability to inhibit mutated nicotinic acetylcholine receptors (Picard, Bertrand et al. 1999; Hoda, Gu et al. 2008).

Nightmare and Post-Traumatic Stress Disorder in Older Adults

A nightmare is a long complicated frightening dream which usually awakens patient from REM sleep. Nightmares are often preceded by usually mild to moderate increase in heart rate, respiration, and increased numbers of rapid eye movements (REM density) on the PSG. Once aroused, patients are fully alert, report anxiety, fear, and/or disgust, and may have difficulty returning to sleep. Heart rates do not increase during RBD events, perhaps due in part to reduced heart rate variability often present. Older adults are less likely to complain of nightmares than younger adults (Salvio, Wood et al. 1992). Acute onset of nightmares in older adults warrants consideration whether these are secondary to medications such as beta-blockers, cholinergics, selective serotonin reuptake inhibitors, barbiturates, neuroleptics, and/or withdrawal of REM sleep-suppressing drugs including antidepressants, alcohol, or central nervous system stimulants.

Older adults are far from immune to post-traumatic stress disorder (PTSD), especially those with coronary artery disease (Cohen, Marmar et al. 2009). PSTD is associated with disturbed sleep and frequent, often recurring nightmares. Woodward et al. found patients with PTSD had significant reductions in sleep movement time compared to normal nightmare-free controls (Woodward, Leskin et al. 2002). They suggested that movement suppression in PTSD in these individuals with heightened anxiety was consistent with the suppression of movement ("freezing") exhibited by animals under conditions of perceived threat. Compared to age-matched controls, PTSD patients had faster respiratory and heart rates during both REM and NREM sleep, reflecting cardiac autonomic dysfunction (Woodward, Leskin et al. 2003; Woodward, Arsenault et al. 2009; Sheikh, Woodward et al. 2003). Using transmagnetic stimulation, Rossi et al. (2009) related heightened cortical excitability in patients with PTSD to decreased cerebral GABAergic tone which lateralized to the right cerebral hemisphere (Rossi, Capua et al. 2009). When nightmares are sufficiently frequent to be considered a sleep disorder, behavioral therapies such as dream reconstruction, imagery rehearsal, stress relaxation therapy, and systematic desensitization can be very effective (Leskin, Kaloupek et al. 1998).

Prazosin (5–10 mg QHS, mean dose 9.5 ± 0.5 mg) compared to placebo has been used with success to treat nightmares related to PTSD (Raskind, Peskind et al. 2003). Prazosin (a lipophilic alpha-1 adrenergic antagonist) is superior to placebo, significantly reducing: 1) recurrent distressing dreams; 2) difficulty falling or stay asleep; and 3) lessening PTSD severity and improving functional status (Raskind, Peskind et al. 2003). Prazosin (2–4 mg PO one hour before bedtime) was effective and well-tolerated in eight of nine older adults suffering from military or Holocaust-related nightmares (Peskind, Bonner et al. 2003).

Movement Disorders Often Persist or Recur During Sleep

Many were trained to believe only palatal myoclonus persists during sleep, but we now understand that the muscle fasciculations, tics, blepharospasm, oromandibular dystonia, chorea, athetosis, and hemiballismus often reappear during sleep, especially in transitions between wake and sleep, and between sleep stages (Silvestri, De Domenico et al. 1990). Fish et al. recorded video-EEG in 52 sleeping patients with Parkinson's disease (PD), Huntington's disease (HD), torsion dystonia, or Tourette syndrome and ten normal controls (Fish, Sawyers et al. 1991). Abnormal movements awake "occasionally" recurred during sleep in 50 of the 52 patients, most often after awakenings, during NREM 1 or in transitions to lighter stages of sleep, and rarely during NREM 3.

Restless Legs Syndrome

Restless legs syndrome (RLS) is a clinical diagnosis based upon the presence of an urge to move the legs at rest that is worse in the evening or night and relieved by movement (Allen, Picchietti et al. 2003). Unpleasant sensations (burning, tingling, creeping, crawling) are often, but not always, endorsed. RLS has a strong circadian rhythmicity with a peak of symptom severity between midnight and 3 AM and least between 9 to 11 AM (Hening, Walters et al. 1999; Trenkwalder, Hening et al. 1999), and patients more often seek treatment when restless legs disturb their sleep (Spiegelhalder and Hornyak 2008). Table 5 summarizes symptoms typical of RLS.

Even though the symptoms of RLS often begin before age 20, the majority of patients complaining of RLS are middle to older age (Desautels, Turecki et al. 2002; Tison, Crochard et al. 2005). Patients with moderate to severe RLS complain of tiredness, difficulty falling asleep, frequent nocturnal awakenings especially in the first half of the night when RLS are worse, reduced quality of life, cognitive

Table 5 Typical Restless Legs Symptoms

- RLS symptoms begin few to 60 min after lying or sitting; symptoms more intense longer rest period lasts.
- Patients emphasize symptoms cause them great discomfort.
- Vague discomfort deep within legs (not skin surface).
- Persistent stretching or movement needed for relief.
- Symptoms reduced by mental activity.
- Usually bilateral, can involve thighs, around knees, ankles, feet, less often arms or trunk.
- Excruciating when confined in theater, airplane, or hospital bed.
- Disturb their sleep, cause them insomnia.

dysfunction, and adverse effects upon their family and social lives (Allen, Walters et al. 2005; Pearson, Allen et al. 2006; Kushida, Martin et al. 2007). Unlike most diurnal movement disorders whose movements lessen in the sleep/wake transition, RLS is activated by relaxation. Benes et al. classify RLS as a "movement-responsive quiescegenic nocturnal focal akathisia usually with dysesthesias"(Benes, Walters et al. 2007).

The 12-month prevalence of RLS symptoms in the French adult population averaged 8.5% (10.8% women, 5.8% men), increasing from 5.2% ages 18 to 24 years to 11.3% in those 50 to 64 years (Tison, Crochard et al. 2005). A World Health Organization study found 9.8% of older adults met criteria for RLS (Rothdach, Trenkwalder et al. 2000). Another general population study found while 12% of 23,052 adults complained of RLS symptoms within a two-week period, only 3% reported these occurred at least twice weekly, interfered with their quality of life, and would prompt requests for medical therapy (Hening, Walters et al. 2004).

RLS appears to be twice as prevalent in women as men (Phillips, Young et al. 2000; Ohayon and Roth 2002; Berger, Luedemann et al. 2004; Tison, Crochard et al. 2005; Lee, Hening et al. 2006; Phillips, Hening et al. 2006; Celle, Roche et al. 2009). Thirty percent of 318 older French adults (mean age 68 years) complained of RLS compared with 12% men (Celle, Roche et al. 2009). Berger et al. found the number of childbirths may explain the increased prevalence of RLS in women: The prevalence of RLS in nulliparous women was similar to those among men up to age 64 years but the odds ratio for RLS was respectively 2, 3, and 3.6 for women with one, two, or three or more children (Berger, Luedemann et al. 2004). Desautels et al. found women with RLS were twice as likely to have a monoamine oxidase type A (MAO-A) gene with high transcription activity; an association not found among the male subjects in this study (Desautels, Turecki et al. 2002). MAO-A is one of the enzymes that breaks down dopamine. The investigators suggested the presence of a high transcription MAO-A allele in women may represent a modifying factor which contributes to greater severity of RLS in women (Desautels, Turecki et al. 2002).

RLS often runs in families. Walters et al. found that 81% of patients with onset of RLS symptoms before 20 years of age had a positive family history compared with 58% of patients with later-onset symptoms (Walters, Mandelbaum et al. 2000). Familial RLS appears to be a polygenetic disorder (Winkelmann and Ferini-Strambi 2006; Trotti, Bhadriraju et al. 2008; Winkelmann 2008; Winkelmann and Muller-Myhsok 2008; Xiong, Levchenko et al. 2008; Kemlink, Polo et al. 2009; Levchenko, Montplaisir et al. 2009; Trenkwalder, Hogl et al. 2009;

Young, Vilarino-Guell et al. 2009). To date, linkage studies have identified nine gene foci mapped to chromosomes 12q, 14q, 9p, 2q, and 20p (RLS1 through 5), 6p, 2p, 15 q and 16p (Lohmann-Hedrich, Neumann et al. 2008; Pichler, Hicks et al. 2008; Winkelmann 2008); all have an autosomal dominant pattern of inheritance save 12q (RLS1) which is inherited in an autosomal recessive pattern but with "pseudo-dominance" imitating autosomal dominance. Genome-wide association studies have identified common variants in genomic regions (MEIS1, BTBD9, and MAP2K5/LBXCOR1) on chromosomes 2p, 6p, and 15q (Stefansson, Rye et al. 2007; Winkelmann, Schormair et al. 2007; Schormair, Kemlink et al. 2008). Subjects carrying one of these alleles have a 50% increased risk of developing RLS. A recent study found BTBD9 was the only genomic regions found in cases of sporadic RLS (Kemlink, Polo et al. 2009).

Secondary (or symptomatic) causes of RLS in older adults include: anemia, iron and/or ferritin deficiency, renal failure, peripheral neuropathies, frequent blood donations, triggered or exacerbated by medications (Gigli, Adorati et al. 2004; Garcia-Borreguero, Egatz et al. 2006) and depression (Banno, Delaive et al. 2000; Picchietti and Winkelman 2005; Wesstrom, Nilsson et al. 2008; Szentkiralyi, Molnar et al. 2009). Medications can trigger or worsen RLS include antidepressants, antihistamines, and dopamine receptor blocking antipsychotics (Gigli, Adorati et al. 2004; Garcia-Borreguero, Egatz et al. 2006). Many patients with RLS have low ferritin (a sensitive marker of body iron stores) levels and iron deficiency, especially those with "late-onset" RLS (symptoms beginning after age 45 years). A prospective study by O'Keefe et al. found low serum ferritin level (<50 μg/L) in 39% of adults with the onset of RLS between ages 50 to 64 years and 58% of those whose RLS began after age 64 years (O'Keeffe 2005). Of note, 23% of the patients who reported the onset of RLS between ages 50 to 64 years had a family history of RLS, but only 8% whose RLS began after age 64 reported a family history. Frausher et al. found one-third of patients with RLS had low ferritin levels (<50 μg/L) and RLS symptoms correlated inversely with ferritin levels (Frauscher, Gschliesser et al. 2009). RLS is more common among frequent blood donors who suffer from iron deficiency (Ulfberg and Nystrom 2004). At least 20 to 30% of patients with end stage renal disease have RLS (Winkelman, Chertow et al. 1996; Murtagh, Addington-Hall et al. 2007). RLS in end stage renal disease is associated with an increased risk for the occurrence and progression of cardiovascular disease (Portaluppi, Cortelli et al. 2009) and chronic depression.

Most intriguing are studies which suggest moderate to severe RLS increases the risks for cardiovascular disease, especially among older adults. Winkelman et al. (2008) found the odds ratio were two-fold higher for both coronary artery and cardiovascular disease among the 3433 subjects (mean age 67.9 years) enrolled in the Sleep Heart Health Study who reported RLS symptoms at least 16 times per month (Winkelman, Shahar et al. 2008). Two earlier studies found cardiovascular disease was 2.5 times and hypertension 1.5 times more common in patients with RLS than in the general population (Ohayon and Roth 2002; Ulfberg, Nystrom et al. 2001). Cardiovascular disease was more common in postmenopausal women with RLS (Wesstrom, Nilsson et al. 2008). Pennestri et al. found systolic blood pressure rose an average of 22 mm Hg and diastolic blood pressure 11 mm Hg with PLMS (Pennestri, Montplaisir et al. 2007). Siddiqui et al. found systolic blood pressure rose a mean of 11 mm Hg with PLMS, even those without an EEG-associated arousal, compared to a rise of 3 mm Hg with a sham PLMS (Siddiqui, Strus et al. 2007). Whether repetitive rises in blood pressure and heart rate with PLMS in patients with RLS contribute to their increased risk of cardiovascular disease needs more study.

Table 6 Diagnostic Features of Restless Legs Syndrome in Cognitively Impaired Older Adults

- Signs of leg discomfort (rubbing their legs or groaning while holding their legs), move their legs excessively when sitting or resting in bed, and symptoms are worse in the evening or at night.

- Complaints of restless legs syndrome and symptoms in the past.

- A positive family history of restless legs syndrome.

- Periodic limb movements awake (and to a lesser extent when asleep).

- Better quality of daytime sleep than at night (because restless legs are typically worse in the evening or at night).

5.1.1. Diagnosing Restless Legs Syndrome in Older Adults, Including the Cognitively Challenged

Primary care physicians diagnose RLS in less than 10% of cases (Hening 2004). RLS is best diagnosed by obtaining the clinical history, searching for secondary causes, and assessing response of the symptoms to dopamine treatment. The diagnosis of RLS is supported by a positive family history of RLS (present in about half of all RLS patients), response to dopaminergic therapy (present in about 80%), and periodic limb movements (PLMS) on a PSG (in 70–80%). Consider ordering a complete blood count, iron indices, serum ferritin, hemoglobin A1C, and creatinine in older adults complaining of symptoms of RLS, screening for iron and/or ferritin deficiency, anemia, diabetes mellitus, or renal disease (Aul, Davis et al. 1998). Diagnosing RLS is particularly challenging in aphasic or cognitively impaired elders. Table 6 summarizes diagnostic criteria for RLS in cognitively impaired adults.

The neurological examination is usually normal in idiopathic or familial RLS. Signs of peripheral neuropathy (usually small fiber sensory in type) may be found in as many as 20% of older adults complaining of RLS (Gemignani, Brindani et al. 2007; Nineb, Rosso et al. 2007), particularly those who complain of burning feet (Szentkiralyi, Molnar et al. 2009). Patients with hereditary and predominantly motor neuropathies are at greater risk to develop RLS secondary to their neuropathy than those with acquired neuropathies (Hattan, Chalk et al. 2009; Lo Coco, Cannizzaro et al. 2009). Thirty-seven percent of patients with Charcot-Marie-Tooth type 2 complained of RLS but none of those with type 1 (Gemignani, Marbini et al. 1999).

Overnight PSG is initially indicated only if a co-existing sleep disorder such as obstructive sleep apnea is suspected. As discussed in section 3.8, PLMS are observed in overnight PSG of only 80% of patients with RLS (Montplaisir, Boucher et al. 1997), increasing to 90% with repeated studies because of night-to-night variability (Montplaisir, Boucher et al. 1997; Sforza and Haba-Rubio 2005; Haba-Rubio and Sforza 2006). Since PLMS are observed in overnight PSG in 40% of older adults *without* sleep complaints, their presence on a PSG is *not* specific for RLS (Montplaisir, Boucher et al. 1997). Ferri et al. argue that PLMS in an overnight PSG can confirm RLS when their periodicity and circadian distribution is analyzed (Ferri, Zucconi et al. 2005; Ferri, Zucconi et al. 2006; Ferri, Zucconi et al. 2006; Ferri, Manconi et al. 2008). Using computer analysis techniques, they found they could distinguish PLMS in RLS from those with narcolepsy with cataplexy, REM sleep behavior disorder, normal controls, and elders but PLMS occurring during the first half of the sleep period with an extraordinary periodicity only in patients with RLS (Ferri, Zucconi et al. 2005; Ferri, Zucconi et al. 2006; Ferri, Zucconi et al. 2006; Ferri, Manconi et al. 2008).

Montplaisir et al. argue that the presence of periodic limb movements awake (PLMW) define RLS with a high degree of sensitivity and specificity and better differentiate patients with RLS from age-matched controls than PLMS (Michaud 2006; Kohnen, Allen et al. 2007; Kume, Sato et al. 2009). Patients with RLS have excessive numbers of PLMW especially when encouraged to try not to move their legs while resting in bed (Montplaisir, Boucher et al. 1997). They developed and validated the Suggested Immobilization Test (SIT) to distinguish patients with RLS from age-matched controls. Subjects during the SIT are asked to sit in bed for 60 minutes before sleep onset (Michaud 2006; Kohnen, Allen et al. 2007; Kume, Sato et al. 2009). The investigators found patients with RLS had a mean of 100 PLMW per hour compared to 40 per hour in age-matched controls. Patients with RLS were especially distinguished from controls by the number of PLMW during the last 30 minutes of the test. Requesting that RLS patients not move often increases the number, severity, and periodicity of their PLMW. The differential diagnosis of conditions which mimic RLS is summarized in Table 7. A useful screening tool for RLS is the patient-completed Cambridge-Hopkins questionnaire (CH-RLSq) which helps distinguish RLS from positional discomfort or leg cramps (Allen, Burchell et al. 2009). Allen et al. (2009) validated the questionnaire, finding it had a sensitivity, specificity, and positive predictive value of 87%, 94%, and 86%, respectively (Allen, Burchell et al. 2009). The investigators found a definite diagnosis of RLS was confirmed by: 1) Recurrent uncomfortable feelings or sensations in the legs when sitting or lying down which were more likely to occur when resting than when physically active; and 2) These symptoms did not occur more often in the morning or equally at all times of day and night and were not associated with muscle cramps (Allen, Burchell et al. 2009).

Pathophysiology of RLS and PLMS

Dopaminergic systems are thought to play a central role in the pathophysiology of RLS. Cervenka et al. found significantly reduced D2-binding in the thalamus and anterior cingulate cortex on PET scans of RLS patients compared with controls and hypothesized that the sensory symptoms of RLS may be due to hypoactive central dopa dopaminergic transmission (Cervenka, Palhagen et al. 2006). A11 neurons in the diencephalon may be the anatomic site of dopamine dysfunction in RLS. These dopaminergic neurons project to the dorsal horns in the spinal cord (and the sensory cortex and limbic system). Destruction of A11 neurons in an animal model of RLS resulted in a long sleep latency, reduced sleep time, and excessive motor restlessness in rats, symptoms which were subsequently ameliorated by pramipexole (Ondo, He et al. 2000). The circadian pattern of RLS, worse in the evening or night, may be related to a fall in endogenous dopamine production at night (Garcia-Borreguero, Larrosa et al. 2004).

Decreased iron availability to the brain also appears to be involved in the pathogenesis of RLS (Connor 2008). Qu et al. (2007) further evaluated locomotor activity in normal mice, mice with A11 lesions, mice fed a low iron diet, and mice with A11 lesions deprived of iron (Qu, Le et al. 2007). They found locomotor activity was increased in both the A11-lesioned and iron-deprived mice compared with normal mice. A11-lesioned mice with iron deprivation showed even greater locomotor activity.

Serum and CSF ferritin levels are often low in patients with RLS (Earley, Connor et al. 2000; Mizuno, Mihara et al. 2005) and oral or intravenous iron therapy often ameliorates or resolves their RLS (Earley, Horska et al. 2009; Gorder, Kuntz et al. 2009; Wang, O'Reilly et al. 2009). Iron is an important cofactor in brain dopamine metabolism. RLS severity correlated with low iron levels in the substantia nigra on MRI (Allen, Barker et al. 2001) and low levels of intracellular iron in the substantia nigra were found at autopsy in patients with both primary and secondary RLS (Connor, Boyer et al. 2003). Patients with low peripheral iron stores (frequent blood donations,

Table 7 Restless Legs Mimics

Restless Legs Mimic	Clinical Features
Shaking leg(s)	Often unconscious
Positional discomfort	Usually occurs with sitting, fixed position, leg under tension, crossed, or bent in acute angle, relieved by position change. May be due to limb ischemia.
Local leg pathology	Usually worse sitting, feels worse at night, due to arthritis, vascular problems, fractures or torn ligaments
Painful legs and moving toes (Dressler, Thompson et al. 1994; Tan and Tan 1996)	Undulating movements of toes which are lessened by voluntary movements and most often triggered by pain (Dressler, Thompson et al. 1994; Tan and Tan 1996).
Leg muscle cramps (see Section "Sleep-related Leg Cramps")	Often unilateral, intensely painful, located precisely in muscle, felt as hard, tight muscle;
Neuroleptic-induced akathisia	Continuous urge to move legs which occurs independent of body position, often with a history of neuroleptic use; less often endorse sleep complaints; can be caused by anti-emetic or anti-vertigo medications
Hypotensive akathisia (Cheshire 2000)	Habitual voluntary irresistible leg movements which are transiently suppressible, occur only when sitting in patients with autonomic failure, strategies to avoid orthostatic hypotension.
Peripheral venous insufficiency	Usually accompanied by skin manifestations.

gastrointestinal bleeding, pregnancy) are at increased risk to develop or worsen RLS. Some patients with idiopathic RLS have been shown to have low brain iron stores even when they do not have iron deficiency anemia (Allen and Earley 2007).

Signs and symptoms of RLS respond to opiate therapy and may reflect altered central processing of pain in RLS (Walters, Ondo et al. 2009). The effects of opioids may be mediated indirectly through the dopaminergic system (Walters 2002). The dysesthesia of RLS may be modulated by central dopaminergic systems but since PLMS have been observed in patients with transected spinal cords, the motor programs for PLMS appear to exist at a spinal cord level (Lee, Choi et al. 1996). PLMS are thought to reflect disinhibition of the locomotor central pattern generator (Trenkwalder and Paulus 2004). Studies in humans have demonstrated that PLMS are associated with increased spinal cord excitability with lower thresholds and greater spatial spread of the spinal flexor reflexes (Bara-Jimenez, Aksu et al. 2000).

Treating Restless Legs Syndrome

Selective serotonin reuptake inhibitors, tricyclic antidepressants, lithium, and olanzapine can aggravate or unmask RLS. A retrospective case-control study found patients who were taking selective serotonin reuptake inhibitors or venflaxine had five-fold increased odds ratio of 20 or more PLMS per hour of sleep on their PSGs (Yang, White et al. 2005). Consider discontinuing these drugs to assess whether their use is contributing to the RLS. Bupropion usually does not worsen RLS, and may be tried as an alternative antidepressant in patients with RLS (Nofzinger, Fasiczka et al. 2000; Kim, Shin et al. 2005; Lee, Erdos et al. 2009).

Non-pharmacological treatment strategies for RLS include: 1) increase physical activity and mental alerting activities before bed to see if symptoms are lessened; 2) trial of abstinence from nicotine, alcohol, and/or caffeine which can worsen RLS in some and 3) iron supplementation if serum ferritin levels are low; and 4) sequential compression devices when in bed (Eliasson 2007).

Order serum ferritin levels in all patients with RLS and repeat them when RLS symptoms worsen (Trenkwalder, Hogl et al. 2008). A serum ferritin level less than 40–50 μg/L (and especially a level less than 25 μg/L) has been associated with increased severity of RLS (O'Keeffe, Gavin et al. 1994; Sun, Chen et al. 1998). If a patient with RLS has a low serum ferritin level, prescribe a three month course of oral ferric sulfate or ferric gluconate, 325 mg three times daily. Oral absorption of iron is enhanced by 100 to 300 mg of vitamin C with each dose of iron.

Oral iron absorption is further improved when it is taken on an empty stomach. Unfortunately, oral iron often causes constipation and abdominal discomfort, especially when taken on an empty stomach. Patients often cannot or will not take it more than once or twice a day, and tolerate it better when taken with food. Serum ferritin levels should be repeated three months after taking supplemental iron. Iron supplement can be discontinued if the serum ferritin level is greater than 50 μg/L, but serum ferritin levels should be rechecked three months after stopping iron to see if the levels again fall (Silber, Ehrenberg et al. 2004). Further diagnostic evaluation for the cause of iron deficiency anemia should be considered. If patient cannot tolerate oral iron, intravenous iron has been tried in patients with RLS with success (Earley, Heckler et al. 2004; Sloand, Shelly et al. 2004; Earley, Horska et al. 2009; Grote, Leissner et al. 2009).

Perhaps only 2–3% of adults have RLS symptoms of sufficient frequency and severity to warrant daily therapy. Classes of drugs used to treat RLS include: 1) dopamine receptor agonists (especially pramipexole or ropinirole); 2) carbidopa/levodopa; 3) opioids (codeine, tramadol); 4) antiepileptics (gabapentin, pregabalin); and 5) benzodiazepine agonists (clonazepam).

An effective treatment for *intermittent* RLS is carbidopa/levodopa. Prescribe one-half to one tablet of carbidopa/levodopa 25 mg/100 mg for intermittent symptoms of RLS which do not occur daily. The regular formulation of carbidopa/levodopa has an onset of action of 30 minutes, and usually effective for 3–4 hours, it can be effective in treating intermittent RLS symptoms which occur in the evening, at bedtime, upon awakening during the night, or when attending the theater, or riding for long distances in an airplane or car. The controlled release formula of carbidopa/levodopa 25 mg/100 mg can be dosed before bed in those patients who complain RLS awakens them in the night. A test dose of carbidopa/levodopa can be used to confirm a patient's complaints are RLS, initially effective in 80% or more of patients with RLS.

Alternative treatments for intermittent RLS include opioid and benzodiazepine agonists. Opioid receptor agonists (such as 30 to 60 mg of codeine or 50 to 100 mg of tramadol) before bed are effective, especially if a patient's RLS has a painful component. However, nausea and constipation may be intolerable side effects. Benzodiazepine agonists can be effective especially among those who also have chronic psychophysiological insomnia. Short-acting triazolam (0.125–0.5 mg), zolpidem (5–10 mg), or zalpedon (5–10 mg) may be helpful for those whose RLS prevents sleep onset. However, intermediate acting agents such as temazepam

(15–30 mg) or sustained release zolpidem (6.25–12.5 mg) may be a better choice if RLS awakens the patient in the middle of the night. Clonazepam (0.5 to 2 mg, mean dose 1 mg) one-half hour before bed can be effective for RLS, especially those with concomitant anxiety. Adverse effects already discussed in Section "Treating REM Sleep Behavior Disorder" may limit its use in older adults (Schenck and Mahowald 1996).

Unfortunately, chronic use of carbidopa/levodopa leads to RLS augmentation and rebound in 70% of RLS patients (Allen and Earley 1996), especially when taking 200 mg or more of levodopa a day (Earley and Allen 1996). RLS *augmentation* is characterized by increased severity of RLS symptoms including: 1) earlier onset of symptoms during the day; 2) faster onset of symptoms when at rest; 3) spreading of symptoms to the upper limbs and trunk; and 4) shorter duration of the treatment effect (Williams and Garcia-Borreguero 2009). RLS augmentation may initially be treated by adding an additional dose of the medication at an earlier hour but if the symptoms subsequently appear even earlier, the drug should be discontinued (Trenkwalder, Hening et al. 2008; Trenkwalder, Hogl et al. 2009; Williams and Garcia-Borreguero 2009). Substituting another dopaminergic drug is not beneficial; it is best to switch to either an opiate (codeine), or antiepileptic (gabapentin, pregabalin) and screen for a fall in serum ferritin levels. A recently published study found 31% of patients with RLS augmentation had serum ferritin levels < 50 μg/L (Trenkwalder, Hogl et al. 2008; Frauscher, Gschliesser et al. 2009). If ferritin levels are low, also prescribe iron supplementation.

The best strategy to prevent RLS augmentation is to keep the dose of dopaminergic medication as low as possible (Williams and Garcia-Borreguero 2009). A recently published multicenter prospective study found 60% of patients with idiopathic RLS developed augmentation within a median of 71 days, taking a mean maximum levodopa dose of 311± 105 mg per day and patients with augmentation compared to those without were significantly more likely to be on higher doses of levodopa (≥ 300 mg per day, 83% vs. 54%, P = 0.03) (Hogl, Garcia-Borreguero et al. 2009).

Dopamine receptor agonists are the drug of choice in most patients with *daily* moderate to severe RLS (Ferini-Strambi 2009; Trenkwalder, Hening et al. 2008). Onset of action of dopamine agonists is 90 to 120 minutes, reducing their value when treating intermittent and unpredictable RLS. The non-ergot agonists (pramipexole, ropinirole) are preferred because ergot agonists (pergolide, bromocriptine) have been associated with the rare development of cardiac valvular fibrosis (Worthington and Thomas 2008). Pramipexole is usually first prescribed as 0.125 mg taken 2 hours before the RLS symptoms start, increased by 0.125 mg every 2–3 days until relief is obtained (Silber, Ehrenberg et al. 2004). Most patients require 0.5 mg a day or less, but doses up to 2.0 mg may be needed. A starting dose for ropinirole is 0.25 mg 2 hours before RLS symptom onset, increased by 0.25 mg every 2–3 days; most patients need 2 mg or less a day, although some require up to 4 mg. Some patients do best with twice daily dosing of pramipexole or ropinirole, taking one half the dose in the late afternoon or early evening and a second dose before bed. Common side effects with dopamine agonists are: nausea, headache, and lightheadedness, but they often resolve within 10–14 days. Some patients report dopamine agonists cause them nasal stuffiness, constipation, insomnia, or leg edema. Daytime sleepiness and sleep attacks more often occur in patients with Parkinson's disease taking much larger doses of dopamine agonists during the day.

Even low doses of dopamine agonists can cause drug-related impulse disorders (compulsive gambling, uncontrolled spending, or hypersexuality) in 5–7% of patients with RLS who take them (Driver-Dunckley, Noble et al. 2007). The risk for developing these was increased among RLS patients complaining of mood and stress disorders (Pourcher, Remillard et al. 2009). Clinicians need to discuss the risks of impulse disorders with the patient (and family) before starting and when following patients treated with these agents (Quickfall and Suchowersky 2007; Tippmann-Peikert, Park et al. 2007; Leu-Semenescu, Karroum et al. 2009; Pourcher, Remillard et al. 2009). These impulse disorders are thought to reflect dopaminergic mesolimbic stimulation in the reinforcement process of rewarding behavioral sequences.

RLS augmentation developed in one-third of RLS patients taking pramipexole for two years (Silber, Girish et al. 2003). Rotigotine is a non-ergot dopamine agonist (not yet available in the U.S. formulated as a transdermal patch; it was found to be effective as long as three years in treating many patients with moderate to severe RLS (Baldwin and Keating 2008). Authors reported low incidence of RLS augmentation with transdermal rotigotine over three years of use, attributing this to continuous dopaminergic delivery. Patients with RLS often suffer from depressive or anxiety disorders. Consider using bupropion to treat depression in RLS patients. If a RLS patient also has an anxiety disorder, consider clonazepam to treat RLS and anxiety, prescribing the larger dose at bedtime (Schenck 2002). Screen RLS patients for depression and anxiety using the Beck Depression and Beck Anxiety inventories; referring patients with all but the mildest depression or anxiety to a psychiatrist or psychologist is usually beneficial and soliciting help from a clinical pharmacologist is warranted in patients on polytherapy (Schenck 2002).

Opiates are effective in RLS, but chronic use is best reserved for those with recurring RLS needing augmentation to dopaminergic agents. Still, some RLS can be treated with constant doses of 60 mg codeine nightly for years without developing tolerance or abuse (Walters, Winkelmann et al. 2001). Patients with RLS and sleep-related eating disorder respond well to dopaminergic therapy (especially levodopa) combined with opioids (usually codeine), and/or clonazepam (Schenck 2002). At least 20% of patients with end stage renal disease have RLS. Transplantation and erythropoietin may help treat their RLS, but dialysis does not (Winkelman, Chertow et al. 1996). Gabapentin (300 to 1200 mg) dosed only at night can be effective in some patients with RLS (Happe, Sauter et al. 2003; Micozkadioglu, Ozdemir et al. 2004; Tan, Derwa et al. 2006; Conti, Oliveira et al. 2008), particularly useful in mild to moderate RLS, RLS augmentation, or peripheral neuropathies. Several recent reviews cover treatment strategies for RLS in even greater detail (Silber, Ehrenberg et al. 2004; Trenkwalder, Kohnen et al. 2007; Trenkwalder, Hening et al. 2008; Trenkwalder, Hogl et al. 2009).

Parkinson's Disease

Patients with Parkinson's disease (PD) have many more sleep complaints than age-matched controls. Complaints of poor quality sleep (nighttime awakenings, difficulty returning to sleep, lying in bed awake, and early awakenings) are second only to locomotor disability in patients with PD (Tandberg, Larsen et al. 1998; Comella 2003). Poor sleep has a negative impact on quality of life not only for patients with PD (Scaravilli, Gasparoli et al. 2003), but also for their caregivers (Happe and Berger 2002). Higher dopaminergic medication doses, female sex, depression, and motor fluctuations were associated with nocturnal sleep complaints (Verbaan, van Rooden et al. 2008). Disease severity (Porter, Macfarlane et al. 2008), disease duration, depression, difficulty turning over in bed, nightmares, and female sex increase the likelihood of PD patients reporting poor quality sleep (Gjerstad, Wentzel-Larsen et al. 2007).

The rest tremor (and a myriad of other motor movements) of PD typically disappears with the onset of NREM 1 sleep, but brief bursts of tremor typically lasting <15 seconds often reappear in later NREM 1 or

NREM 2 sleep, during transitions to and from REM sleep; in phasic REM sleep, following arousal; and/or accompanying body movements in sleep (Fish, Sawyers et al. 1991; Autret, Lucas et al. 1994). The amplitude of the tremor is usually less than half that seen awake. Tremor is often absent (or reduced) in the first 1–2 hours after awakening from sleep in the morning (a so-called "sleep benefit" which can allow for delay in taking their daytime antiparkinsonian medications). Sleep benefit is reported by 10% to 55% of patients with PD. Sleep benefit lasts 30 minutes to more than three hours following morning awakening, and allows for postponing the morning dose of levodopa. Sleep benefit may be a result of improved dopaminergic function from increased pre-synaptic release during sleep. Table 8 summarizes the range of motor movements observed in PD patients when sleeping.

Progressive Supranuclear Palsy

Patients with progressive supranuclear palsy (PSP) compared to age-matched controls had significantly reduced sleep efficiency, a marked reduction in the percentage of time spent in REM sleep, and deceased numbers of sleep spindles and rapid eye movements (Laffont, Leger et al. 1988; Montplaisir, Petit et al. 1997; Arnulf, Merino-Andreu et al. 2005). Patients with PSP had greater amounts of WASO, twice as much NREM 1 sleep and sleep fragmentation, and lower percentages of time spent in REM sleep compared to those with PD and age- and gender-matched controls (Arnulf, Merino-Andreu et al. 2005). The percentage of epochs of REM sleep with RSWA were 33 ± 36% in the patients with PSP, 28 ± 35% in those with PD, and only 0.5 ± 1% among the age-matched controls. Clinical RBD was present in 13% of PSP compared with 20% of PD patients. The four PSP patients with EDS slept longer at night than the 11 patients who were alert during day, suggesting a central hypersomnia.

Palatal Myoclonus

Palatal myoclonus (PM) is continuous synchronous jerks of the soft palate which occur at a rate of 1 to 3 per second. The rate and amplitude of PM gradually decreases from NREM 1 to NREM 3 sleep (Kayed, Sjaastad et al. 1983; Yokota, Atsumi et al. 1990). PM recurred at variable intervals in brief clusters of 2–4 high amplitude movements in REM sleep (Kayed, Sjaastad et al. 1983; Yokota, Atsumi et al. 1990). In some patients, ocular myoclonus synchronized with PM is observed

Table 8 Range of Abnormal Motor Behaviors Seen in Patients with Parkinson's Disease During Sleep

- Excessive periodic and isolated leg jerks and twitches compared to age-matched controls
- Increased tonic muscle activity, episodic rigidity and dystonia in NREM and REM sleep
- Repeated eye blinking at sleep onset
- Inappropriate rapid eye movements during NREM sleep
- Blepharospasm at REM sleep onset
- Loss of REM sleep muscle atonia and REM sleep behavior disorder (RBD)
- Early morning dystonia prior to waking
- Episodic prolonged sustained extension or flexion of one or more limbs during NREM sleep
- Respiratory dyskinesias
- Myoclonus
- Sleep-related leg cramps

(Yokota, Atsumi et al. 1990). Ocular myoclonus may disappear during NREM sleep, recur, or appear only during REM sleep in some (Yokota, Atsumi et al. 1990).

Cells of the hypertrophied inferior olives can generate PM. PM can be idiopathic or secondary to acquired brainstem or cerebellar diseases (Deuschl, Mischke et al. 1990). Diagnostic tests in patients with PM should include: 1) a brain MRI with thin sections through the medulla and a T1-MRI of the posterior fossa with gadolinium; 2) video-ENT evaluation of palate and vocal cord. Unfortunately, PM is difficult to treat: only 20% respond to any treatment, including trials of botulinum toxin, radioablation of the palate, cutting of the levator palatini or tensor veli palatine muscles, lamotrigine, valproate, sumatriptan, or benzodiazepines (Scott, Evans et al. 1996; Jankovic, Scott et al. 1997; Nasr and Brown 2002; Srirompotong, Tiamkao et al. 2002; Aydin, Iseri et al. 2006; Krause, Leunig et al. 2006; Mondria, de Gier et al. 2007; Pal, Lakshmi et al. 2007).

Orofacial Dystonia (Meige Syndrome) and Torsion Dystonia

Patients with dystonia complain of disturbed sleep which worsens with progression of their disease. Blepharospasm (BS, involuntary eye closure or eye blinking) in patients with orofacial dystonias (Meige syndrome) tend to last an average of 25 seconds and recur twice a minute when awake (Silvestri, De Domenico et al. 1990; Sforza, Montagna et al. 1991). BS during sleep occurs least often in the first hours after sleep onset and during NREM 3 sleep. When BS recurs in sleep it typically lasts only 3–4 seconds and recurs once every five minutes (Silvestri, De Domenico et al. 1990; Sforza, Montagna et al. 1991). Treatments for orofacial movement disorders include local botulinum toxin injections, anticholinergics (trihexphenidyl, benztropine), less often by clonazepam, baclofen, or carbamazepine (Clark 2006; Clark and Ram 2007). Abnormal movements seen awake occasionally recur in patients with torsion dystonia when sleeping, again most often after awakenings, during NREM 1, or in transitions to lighter stages of sleep, and rarely during NREM 3 (Fish, Sawyers et al. 1991). Skeletal muscle atonia during REM sleep is preserved in patients with torsion dystonia (Fish, Sawyers et al. 1991).

Huntington's Disease

A case-control study found patients with mild to moderate Huntington's disease (HD) had significantly more movements when sleeping compared to age- and sex-matched controls (Hurelbrink, Lewis et al. 2005). Disturbed sleep is a frequent complaint in patients with HD: sleep complaints increase with progression of HD and correlate with atrophy of the caudate nuclei. Choreic or dystonic movements of HD are typically suppressed at sleep onset, but often recur during stages NREM 1, NREM 2, or with arousals, and can lead to arousals and sleep fragmentation (Fish, Sawyers et al. 1991; Wiegand, Moller et al. 1991; Silvestri, Raffaele et al. 1995).

A recently published study compared 25 patients with varying stages of HD to patients with narcolepsy and controls (Arnulf, Nielsen et al. 2008). Diagnostic evaluation included clinical interview, overnight video-PSG, and multiple sleep latency testing (MSLT). They found that HD patients had frequent insomnia, earlier sleep onset, lower sleep efficiency, increased N1 sleep, delayed and shortened REM sleep, and increased PLMs. Only three (12%) HD patients had RBD. The degree of sleep abnormality did not correlate with CAG triplet repeat length. Reduced REM sleep duration was present even in the two pre-manifest carriers and worsened with disease severity. Four HD patients had abnormally low mean sleep latencies on MSLT (< 8 minutes) but none had multiple sleep-onset REM periods.

Patients with HD compared to healthy controls exhibited increased sleep onset latency, reduced sleep efficiency, frequent nocturnal awakenings, more wake after sleep onset, and less NREM 3 sleep (Wiegand, Moller et al. 1991; Silvestri, Raffaele et al. 1995). Increased numbers of sleep spindles (termed spindle density) in NREM 2 sleep (Emser, Brenner et al. 1988; Wiegand, Moller et al. 1991; Silvestri, Raffaele et al. 1995) and reduced numbers of eye movements during REM sleep (decreased REM density) have been observed in patients with HD compared with controls (Starr 1967; Oepen, Clarenbach et al. 1981). Sleep-disordered breathing was not found in a small group of patients with HD (Bollen, Den Heijer et al. 1988).

Degenerative changes in the structures regulating sleep/wakefulness, medication effects, and depression may contribute to sleep disorders in patients with HD. Selective hypothalamic atrophy and loss of hypocretin-containing neurons occurs early in HD, and alterations in circadian rhythms common in these patients may be due to early selective loss of hypocretin neurons (Petersen and Bjorkqvist 2006). Alterations with sleep architecture and severity of sleep disruption in HD correlates with duration of the disease, severity of clinical symptoms, and degree of caudate atrophy on CT scan correlates with sleep disruption in patients with HD (Wiegand, Moller et al. 1991). An experimental model using transgenic mice with the HD gene mutation demonstrated selective impairment in endogenous circadian rhythms which correlated with cognitive decline; inducing sleep with aprazolam improved cognitive performance (Pallier, Maywood et al. 2007).

Conclusions

In conclusion, sleep modifies movement, and movement modifies sleep. Adequate (but not excessive) amounts of physical activity during the day lessen the quantity of movement when sleeping. Abnormal movements that present awake in patients with diurnal movement disorders recur when sleeping, usually briefer and of lesser amplitude more often in NREM 1, NREM 2, and REM sleep. Almost every diurnal movement disorder impairs the quality of nocturnal sleep and alters its architecture. Many simple sleep-related movement disorders require only identification and reassurance. Most complex sleep-related movement disorders are also regarded as parasomnias. New onset or late recurrence of sleepwalking or sleep terrors in older adults requires diagnostic evaluation. The majority of patients with REM sleep behavior disorder have or will develop a neurodegenerative disease, more often a synucleinopathy. Effective therapies are available for many but not all sleep-related movement disorders.

References

AASM (2005). REM sleep behavior disorder (including parasomnia overlap disorder and status dissociatus. *The International Classification of Sleep Disorders, Second Edition, diagnostic & coding manual*. M. J. Sateia. Westchester, IL, American Academy of Sleep Medicine: 148–152.

Abad, V. C. and C. Guilleminault (2004). Review of rapid eye movement behavior sleep disorders. *Curr Neurol Neurosci Rep* 4: 157–163.

Abdulla, A. J., P. W. Jones, et al. (1999). Leg cramps in the elderly: prevalence, drug and disease associations. *Int J Clin Pract* 53(7): 494–496.

Abril, B., B. Carlander, et al. (2007). Restless legs syndrome in narcolepsy: a side effect of sodium oxybate? *Sleep Med* 8(2): 181–183.

ADRAC (2007). Zolpidem and bizarre sleep related effects. *Aust Adv Drug React Bull* 26: 1.

Ahmed, Q. A. (2008). Effects of common medications used for sleep disorders. *Crit Care Clin* 24(3): 493–515, vi.

Aldrich, M. S. and B. Jahnke (1991). Diagnostic value of video-EEG polysomnography. *Neurology* 41(7): 1060–1066.

Allen, R. P., P. B. Barker, et al. (2001). MRI measurement of brain iron in patients with restless legs syndrome. *Neurology* 56(2): 263–265.

Allen, R. P., B. J. Burchell, et al. (2009). Validation of the self-completed Cambridge-Hopkins questionnaire (CH-RLSq) for ascertainment of restless legs syndrome (RLS) in a population survey. *Sleep Med*.

Allen, R. P. and C. J. Earley (1996). Augmentation of the restless legs syndrome with carbidopa/levodopa. *Sleep* 19(3): 205–213.

Allen, R. P. and C. J. Earley (2001). Restless legs syndrome: a review of clinical and pathophysiologic features. *J Clin Neurophysiol* 18(2): 128–147.

Allen, R. P. and C. J. Earley (2007). The role of iron in restless legs syndrome. *Mov Disord* 22 Suppl 18: S440–448.

Allen, R. P., D. Picchietti, et al. (2003). Restless legs syndrome: Diagnostic criteria, special considerations, and epidemiology. A report from the restless legs syndrome diagnosis and epidemiology workshop at the National Institutes of Health. *Sleep Med* 4(2): 101–119.

Allen, R. P., A. S. Walters, et al. (2005). Restless legs syndrome prevalence and impact: REST general population study. *Arch Intern Med* 165(11): 1286–1292.

Anderson, K. N. and J. M. Shneerson (2009). Drug treatment of REM sleep behavior disorder: the use of drug therapies other than clonazepam. *J Clin Sleep Med* 5(3): 235–239.

Aridon, P., C. Marini, et al. (2006). Increased sensitivity of the neuronal nicotinic receptor alpha 2 subunit causes familial epilepsy with nocturnal wandering and ictal fear. *Am J Hum Genet* 79(2): 342–350.

Arnulf, I., M. Merino-Andreu, et al. (2005). REM sleep behavior disorder and REM sleep without atonia in patients with progressive supranuclear palsy. *Sleep* 28(3): 349–354.

Arnulf, I., J. Nielsen, et al. (2008). Rapid eye movement sleep disturbances in Huntington disease. *Arch Neurol* 65(4): 482–488.

Aul, E. A., B. J. Davis, et al. (1998). The importance of formal serum iron studies in the assessment of restless legs syndrome. *Neurology* 51(3): 912.

Autret, A., B. Lucas, et al. (1994). [The influence of sleep on abnormal waking movements]. *Neurophysiol Clin* 24(3): 218–226.

Aydin, O., M. Iseri, et al. (2006). Radiofrequency ablation in the treatment of idiopathic bilateral palatal myoclonus: A new indication. *Ann Otol Rhinol Laryngol* 115(11): 824–826.

Baldissera, F., P. Cavallari, et al. (1994). Motor neuron 'bistability'. A pathogenetic mechanism for cramps and myokymia. *Brain* 117 (Pt 5): 929–939.

Baldwin, C. M. and G. M. Keating (2008). Rotigotine transdermal patch: in restless legs syndrome. *CNS Drugs* 22(10): 797–806.

Banno, K., K. Delaive, et al. (2000). Restless legs syndrome in 218 patients: associated disorders. *Sleep Med* 1(3): 221–229.

Bara-Jimenez, W., M. Aksu, et al. (2000). Periodic limb movements in sleep: state-dependent excitability of the spinal flexor reflex. *Neurology* 54(8): 1609–1616.

Baumann, A. (2007). Leg movements in narcolepsy patients. *Sleep Diagnosis and Therapy* 2(6): 36–39.

Bazil, C. W. and T. S. Walczak (1997). Effects of sleep and sleep stage on epileptic and nonepileptic seizures. *Epilepsia* 38(1): 56–62.

Bell, C. C., D. D. Dixie-Bell, et al. (1986). Further studies on the prevalence of isolated sleep paralysis in black subjects. *J Natl Med Assoc* 78(7): 649–659.

Benes, H., A. S. Walters, et al. (2007). Definition of restless legs syndrome, how to diagnose it, and how to differentiate it from RLS mimics. *Mov Disord* 22 Suppl 18: S401–408.

Berger, K., J. Luedemann, et al. (2004). Sex and the risk of restless legs syndrome in the general population. *Arch Intern Med* 164(2): 196–202.

Billiard, M. (2009). REM sleep behavior disorder and narcolepsy. *CNS Neurol Disord Drug Targets* 8(4): 264–270.

Blagrove, M., D. S. Owens, et al. (1998). Time of day effects in, and the relationship between, sleep quality and movement. *J Sleep Res* 7(4): 233–239.

Bliwise, D. L. (1993). Sleep in normal aging and dementia. *Sleep* 16(1): 40–81.

Boeve, B. F., D. W. Dickson, et al. (2007). Insights into REM sleep behavior disorder pathophysiology in brainstem-predominant Lewy body disease. *Sleep Med* 8(1): 60-64.

Boeve, B. F. and C. B. Saper (2006). REM sleep behavior disorder: A possible early marker for synucleinopathies. *Neurology* 66(6): 796–797.

Boeve, B. F., M. H. Silber, et al. (2003). Melatonin for treatment of REM sleep behavior disorder in neurologic disorders: Results in 14 patients. *Sleep Med* 4(4): 281–284.

Boeve, B. F., M. H. Silber, et al. (2004). REM sleep behavior disorder in Parkinson's disease and dementia with Lewy bodies. *J Geriatr Psychiatry Neurol* 17(3): 146–157.

Boeve, B. F., M. H. Silber, et al. (1998). REM sleep behavior disorder and degenerative dementia: an association likely reflecting Lewy body disease. *Neurology* 51(2): 363–370.

Boeve, B. F., M. H. Silber, et al. (2001). Association of REM sleep behavior disorder and neurodegenerative disease may reflect an underlying synucleinopathy. *Mov Disord* 16(4): 622–630.

Boeve, B. F., M. H. Silber, et al. (2003). Synucleinopathy pathology and REM sleep behavior disorder plus dementia or parkinsonism. *Neurology* 61(1): 40–45.

Boeve, B. F., M. H. Silber, et al. (2007). Pathophysiology of REM sleep behaviour disorder and relevance to neurodegenerative disease. *Brain* 130(Pt 11): 2770–2788.

Bollen, E. L., J. C. Den Heijer, et al. (1988). Respiration during sleep in Huntington's chorea. *J Neurol Sci* 84(1): 63–68.

Boselli, M., L. Parrino, et al. (1998). Effect of age on EEG arousals in normal sleep. *Sleep* 21(4): 351–357.

Brasic, J. R. (2003). Risks of the consumption of beverages containing quinine. *Psychol Rep* 93(3 Pt 2): 1022–1024.

Broughton, R., M. A. Tolentino, et al. (1985). Excessive fragmentary myoclonus in NREM sleep: a report of 38 cases. *Electroencephalogr Clin Neurophysiol* 61(2): 123–133.

Brown, P., J. C. Rothwell, et al. (1994). Propriospinal myoclonus: evidence for spinal "pattern" generators in humans. *Mov Disord* 9(5): 571–576.

Burns, J. W., F. B. Consens, et al. (2007). EMG variance during polysomnography as an assessment for REM sleep behavior disorder. *Sleep* 30(12): 1771–1778.

Butler, J. V., E. C. Mulkerrin, et al. (2002). Nocturnal leg cramps in older people. *Postgrad Med J* 78(924): 596–598.

Celle, S., F. Roche, et al. (2009). Prevalence and clinical correlates of restless legs syndrome in an elderly French population: The Synapse Study. *J Gerontol A Biol Sci Med Sci*.

Cervenka, S., S. E. Palhagen, et al. (2006). Support for dopaminergic hypoactivity in restless legs syndrome: a PET study on D2-receptor binding. *Brain* 129(Pt 8): 2017–2028.

Chervin, R. D. (2001). Periodic leg movements and sleepiness in patients evaluated for sleep-disordered breathing. *Am J Respir Crit Care Med* 164(8 Pt 1): 1454–1458.

Chervin, R. D., F. B. Consens, et al. (2003). Alternating leg muscle activation during sleep and arousals: a new sleep-related motor phenomenon? *Mov Disord* 18(5): 551–559.

Cheshire, W. P., Jr. (2000). Hypotensive akathisia: autonomic failure associated with leg fidgeting while sitting. *Neurology* 55(12): 1923–1926.

Chesson, A. L., Jr., R. A. Ferber, et al. (1997). The indications for polysomnography and related procedures. *Sleep* 20(6): 423–487.

Chokroverty, S. (1995). Propriospinal myoclonus. *Clin Neurosci* 3(4): 219–222.

Chokroverty, S., A. Walters, et al. (1992). Propriospinal myoclonus: A neurophysiologic analysis. *Neurology* 42(8): 1591–1595.

Chou, K. L., M. L. Moro-De-Casillas, et al. (2007). Testosterone not associated with violent dreams or REM sleep behavior disorder in men with Parkinson's. *Mov Disord* 22(3): 411–414.

Clark, G. T. (2006). Medical management of oral motor disorders: Dystonia, dyskinesia and drug-induced dystonic extrapyramidal reactions. *J Calif Dent Assoc* 34(8): 657–667.

Clark, G. T. and S. Ram (2007). Four oral motor disorders: Bruxism, dystonia, dyskinesia and drug-induced dystonic extrapyramidal reactions. *Dent Clin North Am* 51(1): 225–243, viii–ix.

Cohen, B. E., C. R. Marmar, et al. (2009). Posttraumatic stress disorder and health-related quality of life in patients with coronary heart disease: Findings from the Heart and Soul Study. *Arch Gen Psychiatry* 66(11): 1214–1220.

Comella, C. L. (2003). Sleep disturbances in Parkinson's disease. *Curr Neurol Neurosci Rep* 3(2): 173–180.

Comella, C. L., T. M. Nardine, et al. (1998). Sleep-related violence, injury, and REM sleep behavior disorder in Parkinson's disease. *Neurology* 51(2): 526–529.

Comella, C. L., C. M. Tanner, et al. (1993). Polysomnographic sleep measures in Parkinson's disease patients with treatment-induced hallucinations. *Ann Neurol* 34(5): 710–714.

Connolly, P. S., E. A. Shirley, et al. (1992). Treatment of nocturnal leg cramps. A crossover trial of quinine vs vitamin E. *Arch Intern Med* 152(9): 1877–1880.

Connor, J. R. (2008). Pathophysiology of restless legs syndrome: Evidence for iron involvement. *Curr Neurol Neurosci Rep* 8(2): 162–166.

Connor, J. R., P. J. Boyer, et al. (2003). Neuropathological examination suggests impaired brain iron acquisition in restless legs syndrome. *Neurology* 61(3): 304–309.

Conti, C. F., M. M. Oliveira, et al. (2008). "Anticonvulsants to treat idiopathic restless legs syndrome: systematic review." *Arq Neuropsiquiatr* 66(2B): 431–435.

Cooper, A. D. and K. A. Josephs (2009). Photophobia, visual hallucinations, and REM sleep behavior disorder in progressive supranuclear palsy and corticobasal degeneration: A prospective study. *Parkinsonism Relat Disord* 15(1): 59–61.

Coppin, R. J., D. M. Wicke, et al. (2005). Managing nocturnal leg cramps—calf-stretching exercises and cessation of quinine treatment: A factorial randomised controlled trial. *Br J Gen Pract* 55(512): 186–191.

Crespel, A., P. Coubes, et al. (2000). Sleep influence on seizures and epilepsy effects on sleep in partial frontal and temporal lobe epilepsies. *Clin Neurophysiol* 111 Suppl 2: S54–59.

Darchia, N., I. G. Campbell, et al. (2003). Rapid eye movement density is reduced in the normal elderly. *Sleep* 26(8): 973–977.

Dauvilliers, Y., S. Rompre, et al. (2007). REM sleep characteristics in narcolepsy and REM sleep behavior disorder. *Sleep* 30(7): 844–849.

De Cock, V. C., A. Lannuzel, et al. (2007). REM sleep behavior disorder in patients with Guadeloupean parkinsonism, a tauopathy. *Sleep* 30(8): 1026–1032.

De Cock, V. C., M. Vidailhet, et al. (2008). Sleep disturbances in patients with parkinsonism. *Nat Clin Pract Neurol* 4(5): 254–266.

De Cock, V. C., M. Vidailhet, et al. (2007). Restoration of normal motor control in Parkinson's disease during REM sleep. *Brain* 130(Pt 2): 450–456.

De Koninck, J., P. Gagnon, et al. (1983). Sleep positions in the young adult and their relationship with the subjective quality of sleep. *Sleep* 6(1): 52–59.

De Koninck, J., D. Lorrain, et al. (1992). Sleep positions and position shifts in five age groups: An ontogenetic picture. *Sleep* 15(2): 143–149.

Derry, C. P., J. S. Duncan, et al. (2006). Paroxysmal motor disorders of sleep: The clinical spectrum and differentiation from epilepsy. *Epilepsia* 47(11): 1775–1791.

Desautels, A., G. Turecki, et al. (2002). Evidence for a genetic association between monoamine oxidase A and restless legs syndrome. *Neurology* 59(2): 215–219.

Deuschl, G., G. Mischke, et al. (1990). Symptomatic and essential rhythmic palatal myoclonus. *Brain* 113 (Pt 6): 1645–1672.

Diener, H. C., U. Dethlefsen, et al. (2002). Effectiveness of quinine in treating muscle cramps: a double-blind, placebo-controlled, parallel-group, multicentre trial. *Int J Clin Pract* 56(4): 243–246.

Dijk, D. J. and J. F. Duffy (1999). Circadian regulation of human sleep and age-related changes in its timing, consolidation and EEG characteristics. *Ann Med* 31(2): 130–140.

Dressler, D., P. D. Thompson, et al. (1994). The syndrome of painful legs and moving toes. *Mov Disord* 9(1): 13–21.

Driver-Dunckley, E. D., B. N. Noble, et al. (2007). Gambling and increased sexual desire with dopaminergic medications in restless legs syndrome. *Clin Neuropharmacol* 30(5): 249–255.

Dunkell, S. (1977). *Sleep positions: The night language of the body.* London, Heinemann.

Dylgjeri, S., A. Pincherle, et al. (2009). Sleep-related tongue biting may not be a sign of epilepsy: a case of sleep-related faciomandibular myoclonus. *Epilepsia* 50(1): 157–159.

Earley, C. J. and R. P. Allen (1996). Pergolide and carbidopa/levodopa treatment of the restless legs syndrome and periodic leg movements in sleep in a consecutive series of patients. *Sleep* 19(10): 801–810.

Earley, C. J., J. R. Connor, et al. (2000). Abnormalities in CSF concentrations of ferritin and transferrin in restless legs syndrome. *Neurology* 54(8): 1698–1700.

Earley, C. J., D. Heckler, et al. (2004). The treatment of restless legs syndrome with intravenous iron dextran. *Sleep Med* 5(3): 231–235.

Earley, C. J., A. Horska, et al. (2009). A randomized, double-blind, placebo-controlled trial of intravenous iron sucrose in restless legs syndrome. *Sleep Med* 10(2): 206–211.

Eisensehr, I., R. Linke, et al. (2000). Reduced striatal dopamine transporters in idiopathic rapid eye movement sleep behaviour disorder. Comparison with Parkinson's disease and controls. *Brain* 123 (Pt 6): 1155–1160.

Eisensehr, I., R. Linke, et al. (2003). Increased muscle activity during rapid eye movement sleep correlates with decrease of striatal presynaptic dopamine transporters. IPT and IBZM SPECT imaging in subclinical and clinically manifest idiopathic REM sleep behavior disorder, Parkinson's disease, and controls. *Sleep* 26(5): 507–512.

Eliasson, A.H, Lettieri, C.J. (2007). Sequential compression devices for treatment of restless legs syndrome. Medicine (Baltimore) 86(6): 317–323.

Emser, W., M. Brenner, et al. (1988). Changes in nocturnal sleep in Huntington's and Parkinson's disease. *J Neurol* 235(3): 177–179.

Espiritu, J. R. (2008). Aging-related sleep changes. *Clin Geriatr Med* 24(1): 1–14, v.

Fantini, M. L., A. Corona, et al. (2005). Aggressive dream content without daytime aggressiveness in REM sleep behavior disorder. *Neurology* 65(7): 1010–1015.

Fantini, M. L., L. Ferini-Strambi, et al. (2005). Idiopathic REM sleep behavior disorder: toward a better nosologic definition. *Neurology* 64(5): 780–786.

Fantini, M. L., J. F. Gagnon, et al. (2003). The effects of pramipexole in REM sleep behavior disorder. *Neurology* 61(10): 1418–1420.

Fantini, M. L., M. Michaud, et al. (2002). Periodic leg movements in REM sleep behavior disorder and related autonomic and EEG activation. *Neurology* 59(12): 1889–1894.

Fantini, M. L., R. B. Postuma, et al. (2006). Olfactory deficit in idiopathic rapid eye movements sleep behavior disorder. *Brain Res Bull* 70(4-6): 386–390.

Ferentinos, P. and T. Paparrigopoulos (2009). Zopiclone and sleepwalking. *Int J Neuropsychopharmacol* 12(1): 141–142.

Ferini-Strambi, L. (2009). Treatment options for restless legs syndrome. *Expert Opin Pharmacother* 10(4): 545–554.

Ferman, T. J., B. F. Boeve, et al. (1999). REM sleep behavior disorder and dementia: cognitive differences when compared with AD. *Neurology* 52(5): 951–957.

Ferri, R., M. Manconi, et al. (2008). "Age-related changes in periodic leg movements during sleep in patients with restless legs syndrome." *Sleep Med* 9(7): 790–798.

Ferri, R., M. Manconi, et al. (2008). A quantitative statistical analysis of the submentalis muscle EMG amplitude during sleep in normal controls and patients with REM sleep behavior disorder. *J Sleep Res* 17(1): 89–100.

Ferri, R., M. Zucconi, et al. (2006). Different periodicity and time structure of leg movements during sleep in narcolepsy/cataplexy and restless legs syndrome. *Sleep* 29(12): 1587–1594.

Ferri, R., M. Zucconi, et al. (2005). Computer-assisted detection of nocturnal leg motor activity in patients with restless legs syndrome and periodic leg movements during sleep. *Sleep* 28(8): 998–1004.

Ferri, R., M. Zucconi, et al. (2006). New approaches to the study of periodic leg movements during sleep in restless legs syndrome. *Sleep* 29(6): 759–769.

Ficca, G., S. Gori, et al. (1999). The organization of rapid eye movement activity during rapid eye movement sleep is impaired in the elderly. *Neurosci Lett* 275(3): 219–221.

Fish, D. R., D. Sawyers, et al. (1991). The effect of sleep on the dyskinetic movements of Parkinson's disease, Gilles de la Tourette syndrome, Huntington's disease, and torsion dystonia. *Arch Neurol* 48(2): 210–214.

Fish, D. R., D. Sawyers, et al. (1991). Motor inhibition from the brainstem is normal in torsion dystonia during REM sleep. *J Neurol Neurosurg Psychiatry* 54(2): 140–144.

Floyd, J. A., S. M. Medler, et al. (2000). Age-related changes in initiation and maintenance of sleep: A meta-analysis. *Res Nurs Health* 23(2): 106–117.

Frauscher, B., V. Gschliesser, et al. (2009). The severity range of restless legs syndrome (RLS) and augmentation in a prospective patient cohort: Association with ferritin levels. *Sleep Med* 10(6): 611–615.

Frauscher, B., V. Gschliesser, et al. (2007). "Video analysis of motor events in REM sleep behavior disorder. *Mov Disord* 22(10): 14641470.

Freud, S. (1958). The intrepretation of dreams. *Standard edition of the complete psychological works of Sigmund Freud.* J. Strachey. London, Hogarth Press. 5: 567–568.

Friedman, J. H., H. H. Fernandez, et al. (2003). REM behavior disorder and excessive daytime somnolence in Machado-Joseph disease (SCA-3). *Mov Disord* 18(12): 1520–1522.

Fukuda, K., A. Miyasita, et al. (1987). High prevalence of isolated sleep paralysis: kanashibari phenomenon in Japan. *Sleep* 10(3): 279–286.

Gagnon, J. F., M. A. Bedard, et al. (2002). REM sleep behavior disorder and REM sleep without atonia in Parkinson's disease. *Neurology* 59(4): 585–589.

Gagnon, J. F., M. L. Fantini, et al. (2004). Association between waking EEG slowing and REM sleep behavior disorder in PD without dementia. *Neurology* 62(3): 401–406.

Gagnon, J. F., R. B. Postuma, et al. (2006). Rapid-eye-movement sleep behaviour disorder and neurodegenerative diseases. *Lancet Neurol* 5(5): 424–432.

Gagnon, J. F., R. B. Postuma, et al. (2006). Update on the pharmacology of REM sleep behavior disorder. *Neurology* 67(5): 742–747.

Garcia-Borreguero, D., R. Egatz, et al. (2006). Epidemiology of restless legs syndrome: the current status. *Sleep Med Rev* 10(3): 153–167.

Garcia-Borreguero, D., O. Larrosa, et al. (2004). Circadian variation in neuroendocrine response to L-dopa in patients with restless legs syndrome. *Sleep* 27(4): 669–673.

Gemignani, F., F. Brindani, et al. (2007). Restless legs syndrome in diabetic neuropathy: A frequent manifestation of small fiber neuropathy. *J Peripher Nerv Syst* 12(1): 50–53.

Gemignani, F., A. Marbini, et al. (1999). Charcot-Marie-Tooth disease type 2 with restless legs syndrome. *Neurology* 52(5): 1064–1066.

Giganti, F., G. Ficca, et al. (2008). Body movements during night sleep and their relationship with sleep stages are further modified in very old subjects. *Brain Res Bull* 75(1): 66–69.

Gigli, G. L., M. Adorati, et al. (2004). Restless legs syndrome in end-stage renal disease. *Sleep Med* 5(3): 309–315.

Gilman, S., R. A. Koeppe, et al. (2003). REM sleep behavior disorder is related to striatal monoaminergic deficit in MSA. *Neurology* 61(1): 29–34.

Girard, T. A. and J. A. Cheyne (2006). Timing of spontaneous sleep-paralysis episodes. *J Sleep Res* 15(2): 222–229.

Gjerstad, M. D., T. Wentzel-Larsen, et al. (2007). Insomnia in Parkinson's disease: Frequency and progression over time. *J Neurol Neurosurg Psychiatry* 78(5): 476–479.

Gorder, V., S. Kuntz, et al. (2009). Treatment of restless legs syndrome with iron infusion therapy. *JAAPA* 22(3): 29–32.

Gori, S., G. Ficca, et al. (2004). Body movements during night sleep in healthy elderly subjects and their relationships with sleep stages. *Brain Res Bull* 63(5): 393–397.

Grote, L., L. Leissner, et al. (2009). A randomized, double-blind, placebo controlled, multi-center study of intravenous iron sucrose and placebo in the treatment of restless legs syndrome. *Mov Disord* 24(10): 1445–1452.

Guay, D. R. (2008). Are there alternatives to the use of quinine to treat nocturnal leg cramps? *Consult Pharm* 23(2): 141–156.

Guilleminault, C., D. Leger, et al. (1998). Nocturnal wandering and violence: Review of a sleep clinic population. *J Forensic Sci* 43(1): 158–163.

Haba-Rubio, J. and E. Sforza (2006). Test-to-test variability in motor activity during the suggested immobilization test in restless legs patients. *Sleep Med* 7(7): 561–566.

Haba-Rubio, J., L. Staner, et al. (2005). Periodic limb movements and sleepiness in obstructive sleep apnea patients. *Sleep Med* 6(3): 225–229.

Happe, S. and K. Berger (2002). The association between caregiver burden and sleep disturbances in partners of patients with Parkinson's disease. *Age Ageing* 31(5): 349–354.

Happe, S., C. Sauter, et al. (2003). Gabapentin versus ropinirole in the treatment of idiopathic restless legs syndrome. *Neuropsychobiology* 48(2): 82–86.

Hashimoto, T. and T. Kobayashi (1998). Correlation between daytime activities and night sleep of aged individuals estimated by wrist activity and sleep log. *Psychiatry Clin Neurosci* 52(2): 187–189.

Haskell, S. G. and N. H. Fiebach (1997). Clinical epidemiology of nocturnal leg cramps in male veterans. *Am J Med Sci* 313(4): 210–214.

Hattan, E., C. Chalk, et al. (2009). Is there a higher risk of restless legs syndrome in peripheral neuropathy? *Neurology* 72(11): 955–960.

Hendricks, J. C., A. Lager, et al. (1989). Movement disorders during sleep in cats and dogs. *J Am Vet Med Assoc* 194(5): 686–689.

Hening, W., Allen, R.P., Walters, A.S., and Chokroverty, S. (2009). Motor functions and dysfunctions of sleep. *Sleep disorders medicine: Basic science, technical considerations and clinical aspects.* S. Chokroverty. Philadelphia, PA, Saunders Elsevier: 397–435.

Hening, W., A. S. Walters, et al. (2004). Impact, diagnosis and treatment of restless legs syndrome (RLS) in a primary care population: The REST (RLS epidemiology, symptoms, and treatment) primary care study. *Sleep Med* 5(3): 237–246.

Hening, W. A. (2004). Restless legs syndrome: The most common and least diagnosed sleep disorder. *Sleep Med* 5(5): 429–430.

Hening, W. A., A. S. Walters, et al. (1999). Circadian rhythm of motor restlessness and sensory symptoms in the idiopathic restless legs syndrome. *Sleep* 22(7): 901–912.

Herman, S. T., T. S. Walczak, et al. (2001). Distribution of partial seizures during the sleep–wake cycle: differences by seizure onset site. *Neurology* 56(11): 1453–1459.

Hobson, J. A., T. Spagna, et al. (1978). Ethology of sleep studied with time-lapse photography: Postural immobility and sleep-cycle phase in humans. *Science* 201(4362): 1251–1253.

Hoda, J. C., W. Gu, et al. (2008). Human nocturnal frontal lobe epilepsy: Pharmocogenomic profiles of pathogenic nAChR {beta}-subunit mutations outside the ion channel pore. *Mol Pharmacol.*

Högl, B., D. Garcia-Borreguero, et al. (2009). Progressive development of augmentation during long-term treatment with levodopa in restless legs syndrome: Results of a prospective multi-center study. *J Neurol.*;257(2): 230–237 (Epub 2009 Sep 11).

Hood, B., D. Bruck, et al. (2004). Determinants of sleep quality in the healthy aged: The role of physical, psychological, circadian and naturalistic light variables. *Age Ageing* 33(2): 159–165.

Hoque, R. and A. L. Chesson, Jr. (2009). Zolpidem-induced sleepwalking, sleep related eating disorder, and sleep-driving: Fluorine-18-flourodeoxyglucose positron emission tomography analysis, and a literature review of other unexpected clinical effects of zolpidem. *J Clin Sleep Med* 5(5): 471–476.

Hornyak, M., B. Feige, et al. (2006). Periodic leg movements in sleep and periodic limb movement disorder: Prevalence, clinical significance and treatment. *Sleep Med Rev* 10(3): 169–177.

Hughes, J. R. (2007). A review of sleepwalking (somnambulism): The enigma of neurophysiology and polysomnography with differential diagnosis of complex partial seizures. *Epilepsy Behav* 11(4): 483–491.

Hurelbrink, C. B., S. J. Lewis, et al. (2005). The use of the Actiwatch-Neurologica system to objectively assess the involuntary movements and sleep-wake activity in patients with mild-moderate Huntington's disease. *J Neurol* 252(6): 642–647.

Huynh, N., C. Manzini, et al. (2007). Weighing the potential effectiveness of various treatments for sleep bruxism. *J Can Dent Assoc* 73(8): 727–730.

Iber, C., S. Ancoli-Israel, et al. (2007). *The AASM manual for the scoring of sleep and associated events: Rules, terminology and technical specifications, 1st ed.* Westchester, IL, American Academy of Sleep Medicine.

Iranzo, A., J. L. Molinuevo, et al. (2006). Rapid-eye-movement sleep behaviour disorder as an early marker for a neurodegenerative disorder: A descriptive study. *Lancet Neurol* 5(7): 572–577.

Iranzo, A., E. Munoz, et al. (2003). REM sleep behavior disorder and vocal cord paralysis in Machado-Joseph disease. *Mov Disord* 18(10): 1179–1183.

Iranzo, A., J. Santamaria, et al. (2005). Characteristics of idiopathic REM sleep behavior disorder and that associated with MSA and PD. *Neurology* 65(2): 247–252.

Iranzo, A., J. Santamaria, et al. (2009). The clinical and pathophysiological relevance of REM sleep behavior disorder in neurodegenerative diseases. *Sleep Med Rev.*

Iranzo, A., J. Santamaria, et al. (2009). The clinical and pathophysiological relevance of REM sleep behavior disorder in neurodegenerative diseases. *Sleep Med Rev* 13(6): 385–401.

Iranzo, A., J. Santamaria, et al. (2007). Absence of alterations in serum sex hormone levels in idiopathic REM sleep behavior disorder. *Sleep* 30(6): 803–806.

Ishibashi, K., Y. Saito, et al. (2010). Validation of cardiac (123)I-MIBG scintigraphy in patients with Parkinson's disease who were diagnosed with dopamine PET. *Eur J Nucl Med Mol Imaging* 37(1): 3–11.

Jankovic, J., B. L. Scott, et al. (1997). Treatment of palatal myoclonus with sumatriptan. *Mov Disord* 12(5): 818.

Javaheri, S., W. T. Abraham, et al. (2004). Prevalence of obstructive sleep apnoea and periodic limb movement in 45 subjects with heart transplantation. *Eur Heart J* 25(3): 260–266.

Johns, M. W., T. J. Gay, et al. (1971). Sleep habits of healthy young adults: Use of a sleep questionnaire. *Br J Prev Soc Med* 25(4): 236–241.

Jouvet, M. (1965). Paradoxical sleep–a study of its nature and mechanisms. *Prog Brain Res* 18: 20–62.

Kayed, K., O. Sjaastad, et al. (1983). Palatal myoclonus during sleep. *Sleep* 6(2): 130–136.

Kemlink, D., O. Polo, et al. (2009). Replication of restless legs syndrome loci in three European populations. *J Med Genet* 46(5): 315–318.

Khajehdehi, P., M. Mojerlou, et al. (2001). A randomized, double-blind, placebo-controlled trial of supplementary vitamins E, C and their combination for treatment of haemodialysis cramps. *Nephrol Dial Transplant* 16(7): 1448–1451.

Kim, S. W., I. S. Shin, et al. (2005). Bupropion may improve restless legs syndrome: a report of three cases. *Clin Neuropharmacol* 28(6): 298–301.

Kimura, K., N. Tachibana, et al. (2000). A discrete pontine ischemic lesion could cause REM sleep behavior disorder. *Neurology* 55(6): 894–895.

Klerman, E. B. and D. J. Dijk (2008). Age-related reduction in the maximal capacity for sleep–implications for insomnia. *Curr Biol* 18(15): 1118–1123.

Kohnen, R., R. P. Allen, et al. (2007). Assessment of restless legs syndrome–methodological approaches for use in practice and clinical trials. *Mov Disord* 22 Suppl 18: S485–494.

Kollensperger, M., F. Geser, et al. (2008). Red flags for multiple system atrophy. *Mov Disord* 23(8): 1093–1099.

Krause, E., A. Leunig, et al. (2006). Treatment of essential palatal myoclonus in a 10-year-old girl with botulinum neurotoxin. *Otol Neurotol* 27(5): 672–675.

Kume, A., H. Sato, et al. (2009). An intradialysis diagnostic test for restless legs syndrome: A pilot study. *Am J Kidney Dis* 54(2): 318–326.

Kumru, H., A. Iranzo, et al. (2008). Lack of effects of pramipexole on REM sleep behavior disorder in Parkinson disease. *Sleep* 31(10): 1418–1421.

Kumru, H., J. Santamaria, et al. (2007). Relation between subtype of Parkinson's disease and REM sleep behavior disorder. *Sleep Med* 8(7–8): 779–783.

Kunz, D. and F. Bes (1999). Melatonin as a therapy in REM sleep behavior disorder patients: An open-labeled pilot study on the possible influence of melatonin on REM-sleep regulation. *Mov Disord* 14(3): 507–511.

Kunz, D., R. Mahlberg, et al. (2004). Melatonin in patients with reduced REM sleep duration: Two randomized controlled trials. *J Clin Endocrinol Metab* 89(1): 128–134.

Kuo, C. D., G. Y. Chen, et al. (2000). Effect of different recumbent positions on spectral indices of autonomic modulation of the heart during the acute phase of myocardial infarction. *Crit Care Med* 28(5): 1283–1289.

Kushida, C., M. Martin, et al. (2007). Burden of restless legs syndrome on health-related quality of life. *Qual Life Res* 16(4): 617–624.

Kushida, C. A., M. R. Littner, et al. (2005). Practice parameters for the indications for polysomnography and related procedures: An update for 2005. *Sleep* 28(4): 499–521.

LaBan, M. M., S. L. Viola, et al. (1990). Restless legs syndrome associated with diminished cardiopulmonary compliance and lumbar spinal stenosis–a motor concomitant of "Vesper's curse". *Arch Phys Med Rehabil* 71(6): 384–388.

Laffont, F., J. M. Leger, et al. (1988). [Sleep abnormalities and evoked potentials (VEP-BAER-SEP) in progressive supranuclear palsy]. *Neurophysiol Clin* 18(3): 255–269.

Landry-Schonbeck, A., P. de Grandmont, et al. (2009). Effect of an adjustable mandibular advancement appliance on sleep bruxism: A crossover sleep laboratory study. *Int J Prosthodont* 22(3): 251–259.

Landry, M. L., P. H. Rompre, et al. (2006). Reduction of sleep bruxism using a mandibular advancement device: an experimental controlled study. *Int J Prosthodont* 19(6): 549–556.

Lannuzel, A., M. Ruberg, et al. (2008). Atypical parkinsonism in the Caribbean island of Guadeloupe: Etiological role of the mitochondrial complex I inhibitor annonacin. *Movement Disorders* 23(15): 2122–2128.

Lapierre, O. and J. Montplaisir (1992). Polysomnographic features of REM sleep behavior disorder: Development of a scoring method. *Neurology* 42(7): 1371–1374.

Lavigne, G. J., T. Kato, et al. (2003). Neurobiological mechanisms involved in sleep bruxism. *Crit Rev Oral Biol Med* 14(1): 30–46.

Lavigne, G. J., S. Khoury, et al. (2008). Bruxism physiology and pathology: An overview for clinicians. *J Oral Rehabil* 35(7): 476–494.

Lecendreux, M., C. Bassetti, et al. (2003). HLA and genetic susceptibility to sleepwalking. *Mol Psychiatry* 8(1): 114–117.

Lee, H. B., W. A. Hening, et al. (2006). Race and restless legs syndrome symptoms in an adult community sample in east Baltimore. *Sleep Med* 7(8): 642–645.

Lee, J. E., K. S. Kim, et al. (2009). Factors related to clinically probable REM sleep behavior disorder in Parkinson disease. *Parkinsonism Relat Disord*.

Lee, J. J., J. Erdos, et al. (2009). Bupropion as a possible treatment option for restless legs syndrome" *Ann Pharmacother* 43(2): 370–374.

Lee, M. S., Y. C. Choi, et al. (1996). Sleep-related periodic leg movements associated with spinal cord lesions. *Mov Disord* 11(6): 719–722.

Leskin, G. A., D. G. Kaloupek, et al. (1998). Treatment for traumatic memories: Review and recommendations. *Clin Psychol Rev* 18(8): 983–1001.

Leu-Semenescu, S., E. Karroum, et al. (2009). Dopamine dysregulation syndrome in a patient with restless legs syndrome. *Sleep Med* 10(4): 494–496.

Leung, A. K., B. E. Wong, et al. (1999). Nocturnal leg cramps in children: incidence and clinical characteristics. *J Natl Med Assoc* 91(6): 329–332.

Leung, R. S., M. E. Bowman, et al. (2003). Avoidance of the left lateral decubitus position during sleep in patients with heart failure: Relationship to cardiac size and function. *J Am Coll Cardiol* 41(2): 227–230.

Levchenko, A., J. Y. Montplaisir, et al. (2009). Autosomal-dominant locus for restless legs syndrome in French-Canadians on chromosome 16p12.1. *Mov Disord* 24(1): 40–50.

Limousin, N., E. Konofal, et al. (2009). Restless legs syndrome, rapid eye movement sleep behavior disorder, and hypersomnia in patients with two parkin mutations. *Mov Disord*.

Lins, O., M. Castonguay, et al. (1993). Excessive fragmentary myoclonus: Time of night and sleep stage distributions. *Can J Neurol Sci* 20(2): 142–146.

Lo Coco, D., E. Cannizzaro, et al. (2009). Restless legs syndrome in a patient with multifocal motor neuropathy. *Neurol Sci*.

Lohmann-Hedrich, K., A. Neumann, et al. (2008). Evidence for linkage of restless legs syndrome to chromosome 9p: Are there two distinct loci? *Neurology* 70(9): 686–694.

Loi, D., F. Provini, et al. (2007). Sleep-related faciomandibular myoclonus: A sleep-related movement disorder different from bruxism. *Mov Disord* 22(12): 1819–1822.

Lu, J., D. Sherman, et al. (2006). A putative flip-flop switch for control of REM sleep. *Nature* 441(7093): 589–594.

Luders, H., J. Acharya, et al. (1998). Semiological seizure classification. *Epilepsia* 39(9): 1006–1013.

Lugaresi, E., F. Cirignotta, et al. (1986). Nocturnal paroxysmal dystonia. *J Neurol Neurosurg Psychiatry* 49(4): 375–380.

Mahowald, M. W. (2009). What state dissociation can teach us about consciousness and the function of sleep. *Sleep Med* 10(2): 159–160.

Mahowald, M. W. and C. H. Schenck (2004). REM sleep without atonia–from cats to humans. *Arch Ital Biol* 142(4): 469–478.

Mahowald, M. W. and C. H. Schenck (2005). Insights from studying human sleep disorders. Nature 437(7063): 1279–1285.

Mahowald, M. W., C. H. Schenck, et al. (2007). Pathophysiologic mechanisms in REM sleep behavior disorder. *Curr Neurol Neurosci Rep* 7(2): 167–172.

Mai, R., I. Sartori, et al. (2005). Sleep-related hyperkinetic seizures: Always a frontal onset? *Neurol Sci* 26 Suppl 3: s220–224.

Malow, B. A., N. Foldvary-Schaefer, et al. (2008). Treating obstructive sleep apnea in adults with epilepsy: A randomized pilot trial. *Neurology* 71(8): 572–577.

Man-Son-Hing, M., G. Wells, et al. (1998). Quinine for nocturnal leg cramps: A meta-analysis including unpublished data. *J Gen Intern Med* 13(9): 600–606.

Manni, R., M. Terzaghi, et al. (2009). Motor-behavioral episodes in REM sleep behavior disorder and phasic events during REM sleep. *Sleep* 32(2): 241–245.

Manni, R., M. Terzaghi, et al. (2007). REM sleep behaviour disorder in elderly subjects with epilepsy: Frequency and clinical aspects of the comorbidity. *Epilepsy Res* 77(2–3): 128–133.

Marini, C. and R. Guerrini (2007). The role of the nicotinic acetylcholine receptors in sleep-related epilepsy. *Biochem Pharmacol* 74(8): 1308–1314.

Martin-Du Pan, R. C., R. Benoit, et al. (2004). The role of body position and gravity in the symptoms and treatment of various medical diseases. *Swiss Med Wkly* 134(37–38): 543–551.

Massicotte-Marquez, J., J. Carrier, et al. (2005). Slow-wave sleep and delta power in rapid eye movement sleep behavior disorder. *Ann Neurol* 57(2): 277–282.

Massicotte-Marquez, J., A. Decary, et al. (2008). Executive dysfunction and memory impairment in idiopathic REM sleep behavior disorder. *Neurology* 70(15): 1250–1257.

Massironi, G., S. Galluzzi, et al. (2003). Drug treatment of REM sleep behavior disorders in dementia with Lewy bodies. *Int Psychogeriatr* 15(4): 377–383.

Mayer, G., K. Kesper, et al. (2008). Quantification of tonic and phasic muscle activity in REM sleep behavior disorder. *J Clin Neurophysiol* 25(1): 48–55.

McKeith, I. G. (2006). Consensus guidelines for the clinical and pathologic diagnosis of dementia with Lewy bodies (DLB): Report of the Consortium on DLB International Workshop. *J Alzheimers Dis* 9(3 Suppl): 417–423.

McKeith, I. G., D. W. Dickson, et al. (2005). Diagnosis and management of dementia with Lewy bodies: Third report of the DLB Consortium. *Neurology* 65(12): 1863–1872.

Medicine, A. A. o. S. (2005). *International classification of sleep disorders, 2nd edition: Diagnostic and coding manual (ICSD-2)*. Westchester, IL, American Academy of Sleep Medicine.

Michaud, M. (2006). Is the suggested immobilization test the "gold standard" to assess restless legs syndrome? *Sleep Med* 7(7): 541–543.

Micozkadioglu, H., F. N. Ozdemir, et al. (2004). Gabapentin versus levodopa for the treatment of restless legs syndrome in hemodialysis patients: An open-label study. *Ren Fail* 26(4): 393–397.

Miyamoto, S., M. Fujita, et al. (2001). Effects of posture on cardiac autonomic nervous activity in patients with congestive heart failure. *J Am Coll Cardiol* 37(7): 1788–1793.

Miyamoto, S., K. Tambara, et al. (2002). Effects of right lateral decubitus position on plasma norepinephrine and plasma atrial natriuretic peptide levels in patients with chronic congestive heart failure. *Am J Cardiol* 89(2): 240–242.

Miyamoto, T., M. Miyamoto, et al. (2006). Reduced cardiac 123I-MIBG scintigraphy in idiopathic REM sleep behavior disorder. *Neurology* 67(12): 2236–2238.

Miyamoto, T., M. Miyamoto, et al. (2009). Odor identification test as an indicator of idiopathic REM sleep behavior disorder. *Mov Disord* 24(2): 268–273.

Miyamoto, T., M. Miyamoto, et al. (2008). 123I-MIBG cardiac scintigraphy provides clues to the underlying neurodegenerative disorder in idiopathic REM sleep behavior disorder. *Sleep* 31(5): 717–723.

Mizuno, S., T. Mihara, et al. (2005). CSF iron, ferritin and transferrin levels in restless legs syndrome. *J Sleep Res* 14(1): 43–47.

Mondria, T., H. H. de Gier, et al. (2007). New device to control combined lingual and palatal myoclonus. *Mov Disord* 22(4): 573–576.

Montagna, P., F. Provini, et al. (2006). Propriospinal myoclonus at sleep onset. *Neurophysiol Clin* 36(5-6): 351–355.

Montplaisir, J., S. Boucher, et al. (1997). Clinical, polysomnographic, and genetic characteristics of restless legs syndrome: A study of 133 patients diagnosed with new standard criteria. *Mov Disord* 12(1): 61–65.

Montplaisir, J., D. Petit, et al. (1997). Sleep and quantitative EEG in patients with progressive supranuclear palsy. *Neurology* 49(4): 999–1003.

Murtagh, F. E., J. Addington-Hall, et al. (2007). The prevalence of symptoms in end-stage renal disease: a systematic review. *Adv Chronic Kidney Dis* 14(1): 82–99.

Nasr, A. and N. Brown (2002). Palatal myoclonus responding to lamotrigine. *Seizure* 11(2): 136–137.

Nineb, A., C. Rosso, et al. (2007). Restless legs syndrome is frequently overlooked in patients being evaluated for polyneuropathies. *Eur J Neurol* 14(7): 788–792.

Nobili, L. (2007). Nocturnal frontal lobe epilepsy and non-rapid eye movement sleep parasomnias: Differences and similarities. *Sleep Med Rev* 11(4): 251–254.

Nobili, L., M. Cossu, et al. (2004). Sleep-related hyperkinetic seizures of temporal lobe origin. *Neurology* 62(3): 482–485.

Nofzinger, E. A., A. Fasiczka, et al. (2000). Bupropion SR reduces periodic limb movements associated with arousals from sleep in depressed patients with periodic limb movement disorder. *J Clin Psychiatry* 61(11): 858–862.

Nomura, T., Y. Inoue, et al. (2003). Visual hallucinations as REM sleep behavior disorders in patients with Parkinson's disease. *Mov Disord* 18(7): 812–817.

O'Keeffe, S. T. (2005). Secondary causes of restless legs syndrome in older people. *Age Ageing* 34(4): 349–352.

O'Keeffe, S. T., K. Gavin, et al. (1994). Iron status and restless legs syndrome in the elderly. *Age Ageing* 23(3): 200–203.

Oepen, G., P. Clarenbach, et al. (1981). Disturbance of eye movements in Huntington's chorea. *Arch Psychiatr Nervenkr* 229(3): 205–213.

Ohayon, M. M., M. A. Carskadon, et al. (2004). Meta-analysis of quantitative sleep parameters from childhood to old age in healthy individuals: Developing normative sleep values across the human lifespan. *Sleep* 27(7): 1255–1273.

Ohayon, M. M., C. Guilleminault, et al. (1999). Night terrors, sleepwalking, and confusional arousals in the general population: Their frequency and relationship to other sleep and mental disorders. *J Clin Psychiatry* 60(4): 268–276; quiz 277.

Ohayon, M. M. and T. Roth (2002). Prevalence of restless legs syndrome and periodic limb movement disorder in the general population. *J Psychosom Res* 53(1): 547–554.

Oldani, A., M. Zucconi, et al. (1998). Autosomal dominant nocturnal frontal lobe epilepsy. A video-polysomnographic and genetic appraisal of 40 patients and delineation of the epileptic syndrome. *Brain* 121 (Pt 2): 205–223.

Olson, E. J., B. F. Boeve, et al. (2000). Rapid eye movement sleep behaviour disorder: demographic, clinical and laboratory findings in 93 cases. *Brain* 123 (Pt 2): 331–339.

Ondo, W. G., Y. He, et al. (2000). Clinical correlates of 6-hydroxydopamine injections into A11 dopaminergic neurons in rats: A possible model for restless legs syndrome. *Mov Disord* 15(1): 154–158.

Oudiette, D., V. C. De Cock, et al. (2009). Nonviolent elaborate behaviors may also occur in REM sleep behavior disorder. *Neurology* 72(6): 551–557.

Overeem, S., E. Mignot, et al. (2001). Narcolepsy: Clinical features, new pathophysiologic insights, and future perspectives. *J Clin Neurophysiol* 18(2): 78–105.

Pal, P. K., P. S. Lakshmi, et al. (2007). Efficacy and complication of botulinum toxin injection in palatal myoclonus: Experience from a patient. *Mov Disord* 22(10): 1484–1486.

Pallier, P. N., E. S. Maywood, et al. (2007). Pharmacological imposition of sleep slows cognitive decline and reverses dysregulation of circadian gene expression in a transgenic mouse model of Huntington's disease. *J Neurosci* 27(29): 7869–7878.

Pareja, J. A., A. B. Caminero, et al. (1996). A first case of progressive supranuclear palsy and pre-clinical REM sleep behavior disorder presenting as inhibition of speech during wakefulness and somniloquy with phasic muscle twitching during REM sleep. *Neurologia* 11(8): 304–306.

Pearson, V. E., R. P. Allen, et al. (2006). Cognitive deficits associated with restless legs syndrome (RLS). *Sleep Med* 7(1): 25–30.

Pennestri, M. H., J. Montplaisir, et al. (2007). Nocturnal blood pressure changes in patients with restless legs syndrome. *Neurology* 68(15): 1213–1218.

Peskind, E. R., L. T. Bonner, et al. (2003). Prazosin reduces trauma-related nightmares in older men with chronic posttraumatic stress disorder. *J Geriatr Psychiatry Neurol* 16(3): 165–171.

Petersen, A. and M. Bjorkqvist (2006). Hypothalamic-endocrine aspects in Huntington's disease. *Eur J Neurosci* 24(4): 961–967.

Phillips, B., W. Hening, et al. (2006). Prevalence and correlates of restless legs syndrome: Results from the 2005 National Sleep Foundation Poll. *Chest* 129(1): 76–80.

Phillips, B., T. Young, et al. (2000).Epidemiology of restless legs symptoms in adults. *Arch Intern Med* 160(14): 2137–2141.

Phillips, H. A., I. E. Scheffer, et al. (1995). Localization of a gene for autosomal dominant nocturnal frontal lobe epilepsy to chromosome 20q 13.2. *Nat Genet* 10(1): 117–118.

Picard, F., S. Bertrand, et al. (1999). Mutated nicotinic receptors responsible for autosomal dominant nocturnal frontal lobe epilepsy are more sensitive to carbamazepine. *Epilepsia* 40(9): 1198–1209.

Picchietti, D. and J. W. Winkelman (2005). Restless legs syndrome, periodic limb movements in sleep, and depression. *Sleep* 28(7): 891–898.

Pichler, I., A. A. Hicks, et al. (2008). Restless legs syndrome: An update on genetics and future perspectives. *Clin Genet* 73(4): 297–305.

Pires, M. L., A. A. Benedito-Silva, et al. (2007). Sleep habits and complaints of adults in the city of Sao Paulo, Brazil, in 1987 and 1995. *Braz J Med Biol Res* 40(11): 1505–1515.

Plazzi, G., R. Corsini, et al. (1997). REM sleep behavior disorders in multiple system atrophy. *Neurology* 48(4): 1094–1097.

Plazzi, G., P. Cortelli, et al. (1998). REM sleep behaviour disorder differentiates pure autonomic failure from multiple system atrophy with autonomic failure. *J Neurol Neurosurg Psychiatry* 64(5): 683–685.

Plazzi, G. and P. Montagna (2002). Remitting REM sleep behavior disorder as the initial sign of multiple sclerosis. *Sleep Med* 3(5): 437–439.

Plazzi, G., R. Vetrugno, et al. (2005). Sleepwalking and other ambulatory behaviours during sleep. *Neurol Sci* 26 Suppl 3: s193–198.

Portaluppi, F., P. Cortelli, et al. (2009). Do restless legs syndrome (RLS) and periodic limb movements of sleep (PLMS) play a role in nocturnal hypertension and increased cardiovascular risk of renally impaired patients? *Chronobiol Int* 26(6): 1206–1221.

Porter, B., R. Macfarlane, et al. (2008). The frequency and nature of sleep disorders in a community-based population of patients with Parkinson's disease. *Eur J Neurol* 15(1): 50–54.

Postuma, R. B., J. F. Gagnon, et al. (2008). Manifestations of Parkinson disease differ in association with REM sleep behavior disorder. *Mov Disord* 23(12): 1665–1672.

Postuma, R. B., J. F. Gagnon, et al. (2009). Quantifying the risk of neurodegenerative disease in idiopathic REM sleep behavior disorder. *Neurology* 72(15): 1296–1300.

Postuma, R. B., J. F. Gagnon, et al. (2009). Idiopathic REM sleep behavior disorder in the transition to degenerative disease. *Mov Disord.*

Postuma, R. B., A. E. Lang, et al. (2006). Potential early markers of Parkinson disease in idiopathic REM sleep behavior disorder. *Neurology* 66(6): 845–851.

Pourcher, E., S. Remillard, et al. (2009). Compulsive habits in restless legs syndrome patients under dopaminergic treatment. *J Neurol Sci.*

Pressman, M. R. (2007). Factors that predispose, prime and precipitate NREM parasomnias in adults: Clinical and forensic implications. *Sleep Med Rev* 11(1): 5–30; discussion 31–33.

Provini, F., G. Plazzi, et al. (1999). Nocturnal frontal lobe epilepsy. A clinical and polygraphic overview of 100 consecutive cases. *Brain* 122 (Pt 6): 1017–1031.

Qu, S., W. Le, et al. (2007). Locomotion is increased in a11-lesioned mice with iron deprivation: A possible animal model for restless legs syndrome. *J Neuropathol Exp Neurol* 66(5): 383–388.

Quickfall, J. and O. Suchowersky (2007). Pathological gambling associated with dopamine agonist use in restless legs syndrome. *Parkinsonism Relat Disord* 13(8): 535–536.

Raskind, M. A., E. R. Peskind, et al. (2003). Reduction of nightmares and other PTSD symptoms in combat veterans by prazosin: A placebo-controlled study. *Am J Psychiatry* 160(2): 371–373.

Roeleveld, K., B. G. van Engelen, et al. (2000). Possible mechanisms of muscle cramp from temporal and spatial surface EMG characteristics. *J Appl Physiol* 88(5): 1698–1706.

Rossi, S., A. D. Capua, et al. (2009). Dysfunctions of cortical excitability in drug-naïve posttraumatic stress disorder patients. *Biological Psychiatry* 66(1): 54–61.

Roth, B., S. Buuhova, et al. (1968). Familial sleep paralysis. *Schweiz Arch Neurol Neurochir Psychiatr* 102(2): 321–330.

Rothdach, A. J., C. Trenkwalder, et al. (2000). Prevalence and risk factors of RLS in an elderly population: the MEMO study. Memory and Morbidity in Augsburg Elderly. *Neurology* 54(5): 1064–1068.

Ryvlin, P., L. Minotti, et al. (2006). Nocturnal hypermotor seizures, suggesting frontal lobe epilepsy, can originate in the insula. *Epilepsia* 47(4): 755–765.

Salvio, M. A., J. M. Wood, et al. (1992). Nightmare prevalence in the healthy elderly. *Psychol Aging* 7(2): 324–325.

Santamaria, J. and K. H. Chiappa (1987). The EEG of drowsiness in normal adults. *J Clin Neurophysiol* 4(4): 327–382.

Saper, C. B., G. Cano, et al. (2005). Homeostatic, circadian, and emotional regulation of sleep. *J Comp Neurol* 493(1): 92–98.

Sawada, H., T. Oeda, et al. (2009). Diagnostic accuracy of cardiac metaiodobenzylguanidine scintigraphy in Parkinson disease. *Eur J Neurol* 16(2): 174–182.

Scaravilli, T., E. Gasparoli, et al. (2003). Health-related quality of life and sleep disorders in Parkinson's disease. *Neurol Sci* 24(3): 209–210.

Scheffer, I. E., K. P. Bhatia, et al. (1994). Autosomal dominant frontal epilepsy misdiagnosed as sleep disorder. *Lancet* 343(8896): 515–517.

Schenck, C. H. (2002). Restless legs syndrome and periodic limb movements of sleep: Global therapeutic considerations. *Sleep Med Rev* 6(4): 247–251.

Schenck, C. H., I. Arnulf, et al. (2007). Sleep and sex: what can go wrong? A review of the literature on sleep related disorders and abnormal sexual behaviors and experiences. *Sleep* 30(6): 683–702.

Schenck, C. H., S. R. Bundlie, et al. (1986). Chronic behavioral disorders of human REM sleep: A new category of parasomnia. *Sleep* 9(2): 293–308.

Schenck, C. H., S. R. Bundlie, et al. (1996). Delayed emergence of a parkinsonian disorder in 38% of 29 older men initially diagnosed with idiopathic rapid eye movement sleep behaviour disorder. *Neurology* 46(2): 388–393.

Schenck, C. H., S. R. Bundlie, et al. (1987). Rapid eye movement sleep behavior disorder. A treatable parasomnia affecting older adults. *JAMA* 257(13): 1786–1789.

Schenck, C. H., Bundlie, S.R., Mahowald, M.W. (2003). REM sleep behavior disorder (RBD) delayed emergence of parkinsonism and/or dementia in 65% of older men initially diagnosed with idiopathic RBD, and an analysis of the maximum and minium tonic and/or phasic electromyographic abnormalities found during REM sleep. *Sleep* 26 (Suppl.): A316.

Schenck, C. H., T. D. Hurwitz, et al. (1993). Symposium: Normal and abnormal REM sleep regulation: REM sleep behaviour disorder: an update on a series of 96 patients and a review of the world literature. *J Sleep Res* 2(4): 224231.

Schenck, C. H. and M. W. Mahowald (1990). A polysomnographic, neurologic, psychiatric, and clinical outcome report on 70 consecutive cases with REM sleep behavior disorder (RBD): sustained clonazepam efficacy in 89.5% of 57 treated patients. *Clev Clin J Med* 57(Suppl): S9–S23.

Schenck, C. H. and M. W. Mahowald (1991). Injurious sleep behavior disorders (parasomnias) affecting patients on intensive care units. *Intensive Care Med* 17(4): 219–224.

Schenck, C. H. and M. W. Mahowald (1992). Motor dyscontrol in narcolepsy: Rapid-eye-movement (REM) sleep without atonia and REM sleep behavior disorder. *Ann Neurol* 32(1): 3–10.

Schenck, C. H. and M. W. Mahowald (1996). Long-term, nightly benzodiazepine treatment of injurious parasomnias and other disorders of disrupted nocturnal sleep in 170 adults. *Am J Med* 100(3): 333–337.

Schenck, C. H., D. M. Milner, et al. (1989). A polysomnographic and clinical report on sleep-related injury in 100 adult patients. *Am J Psychiatry* 146(9): 1166–1173.

Schmidt, M. H., V. B. Koshal, et al. (2006). Use of pramipexole in REM sleep behavior disorder: Results from a case series. *Sleep Med* 7(5): 418–423.

Schormair, B., D. Kemlink, et al. (2008). PTPRD (protein tyrosine phosphatase receptor type delta) is associated with restless legs syndrome. *Nat Genet* 40(8): 946–948.

Scott, B. L., R. W. Evans, et al. (1996). Treatment of palatal myoclonus with sumatriptan. *Mov Disord* 11(6): 748–751.

Sforza, E. and J. Haba-Rubio (2005). Night-to-night variability in periodic leg movements in patients with restless legs syndrome. *Sleep Med* 6(3): 259–267.

Sforza, E., J. Krieger, et al. (1997). REM sleep behavior disorder: Clinical and physiopathological findings. *Sleep Med Rev* 1(1): 57–69.

Sforza, E., P. Montagna, et al. (1991). Sleep and cranial dystonia. *Electroencephalogr Clin Neurophysiol* 79(3): 166–169.

Sheikh, J. I., S. H. Woodward, et al. (2003). Sleep in post-traumatic stress disorder and panic: convergence and divergence. *Depress Anxiety* 18(4): 187–197.

Siddiqui, F., J. Strus, et al. (2007). Rise of blood pressure with periodic limb movements in sleep and wakefulness. *Clin Neurophysiol* 118(9): 1923–1930.

Sidorov, J. (1993). Quinine sulfate for leg cramps: Does it work? *J Am Geriatr Soc* 41(5): 498–500.

Silber, M. H., S. Ancoli-Israel, et al. (2007). The visual scoring of sleep in adults. *J Clin Sleep Med* 3(2): 121–131.

Silber, M. H., B. L. Ehrenberg, et al. (2004). An algorithm for the management of restless legs syndrome. *Mayo Clin Proc* 79(7): 916–922.

Silber, M. H., M. Girish, et al. (2003). Pramipexole in the management of restless legs syndrome: an extended study. *Sleep* 26(7): 819–821.

Silvestri, R. and E. Bromfield (2004). Recurrent nightmares and disorders of arousal in temporal lobe epilepsy. *Brain Res Bull* 63(5): 369–376.

Silvestri, R., P. De Domenico, et al. (1990). The effect of nocturnal physiological sleep on various movement disorders. *Mov Disord* 5(1): 8–14.

Silvestri, R., M. Raffaele, et al. (1995). Sleep features in Tourette's syndrome, neuroacanthocytosis and Huntington's chorea. *Neurophysiol Clin* 25(2): 66–77.

Sloand, J. A., M. A. Shelly, et al. (2004). A double-blind, placebo-controlled trial of intravenous iron dextran therapy in patients with ESRD and restless legs syndrome. *Am J Kidney Dis* 43(4): 663–670.

Solomonova, E., T. Nielsen, et al. (2008). Sensed presence as a correlate of sleep paralysis distress, social anxiety and waking state social imagery. *Conscious Cogn* 17(1): 49–63.

Spiegelhalder, K. and M. Hornyak (2008). Restless legs syndrome in older adults. *Clin Geriatr Med* 24(1): 167–180, ix.

Srirompotong, S., S. Tiamkao, et al. (2002). Botulinum toxin injection for objective tinnitus from palatal myoclonus: A case report. *J Med Assoc Thai* 85(3): 392–395.

Starr, A. (1967). A disorder of rapid eye movements in Huntington's chorea. *Brain* 90(3): 545–564.

Stefansson, H., D. B. Rye, et al. (2007). A genetic risk factor for periodic limb movements in sleep. *N Engl J Med* 357(7): 639–647.

Stiasny-Kolster, K., S. C. Clever, et al. (2007). Olfactory dysfunction in patients with narcolepsy with and without REM sleep behaviour disorder. *Brain* 130(Pt 2): 442–449.

Stiasny-Kolster, K., Y. Doerr, et al. (2005). Combination of 'idiopathic' REM sleep behaviour disorder and olfactory dysfunction as possible indicator for alpha-synucleinopathy demonstrated by dopamine transporter FP-CIT-SPECT. *Brain* 128(Pt 1): 126–137.

Sun, E. R., C. A. Chen, et al. (1998). "Iron and the restless legs syndrome." *Sleep* 21(4): 371–377.

Syed, B. H., D. B. Rye, et al. (2003). REM sleep behavior disorder and SCA-3 (Machado-Joseph disease). *Neurology* 60(1): 148.

Szentkiralyi, A., M. Z. Molnar, et al. (2009). Association between restless legs syndrome and depression in patients with chronic kidney disease. *J Psychosom Res* 67(2): 173–180.

Tachibana, N. and Y. Oka (2004). Longitudinal change in REM sleep components in a patient with multiple system atrophy associated with REM sleep behavior disorder: paradoxical improvement of nocturnal behaviors in a progressive neurodegenerative disease. *Sleep Med* 5(2): 155–158.

Takeuchi, N., N. Uchimura, et al. (2001). Melatonin therapy for REM sleep behavior disorder. *Psychiatry Clin Neurosci* 55(3): 267–269.

Takeuchi, T., K. Fukuda, et al. (2002). Factors related to the occurrence of isolated sleep paralysis elicited during a multi-phasic sleep-wake schedule. *Sleep* 25(1): 89–96.

Tan, A., M. Salgado, et al. (1996). Rapid eye movement sleep behavior disorder preceding Parkinson's disease with therapeutic response to levodopa. *Mov Disord* 11(2): 214–216.

Tan, A. K. and C. B. Tan (1996). "The syndrome of painful legs and moving toes—a case report." *Singapore Med J* 37(4): 446–447.

Tan, J., A. Derwa, et al. (2006). Gabapentin in treatment of restless legs syndrome in peritoneal dialysis patients. *Perit Dial Int* 26(2): 276–278.

Tandberg, E., J. P. Larsen, et al. (1998). A community-based study of sleep disorders in patients with Parkinson's disease. *Mov Disord* 13(6): 895–899.

Tippmann-Peikert, M., B. F. Boeve, et al. (2006). REM sleep behavior disorder initiated by acute brainstem multiple sclerosis. *Neurology* 66(8): 1277–1279.

Tippmann-Peikert, M., J. G. Park, et al. (2007). Pathologic gambling in patients with restless legs syndrome treated with dopaminergic agonists. *Neurology* 68(4): 301–303.

Tison, F., A. Crochard, et al. (2005). Epidemiology of restless legs syndrome in French adults: a nationwide survey: the INSTANT Study. *Neurology* 65(2): 239–246.

Tison, F., G. K. Wenning, et al. (1995). REM sleep behaviour disorder as the presenting symptom of multiple system atrophy. *J Neurol Neurosurg Psychiatry* 58(3): 379–380.

Townend, B. S., J. W. Sturm, et al. (2004). Quinine associated blindness. *Aust Fam Physician* 33(8): 627–628.

Trenkwalder, C., W. A. Hening, et al. (2008). Treatment of restless legs syndrome: an evidence-based review and implications for clinical practice. *Mov Disord* 23(16): 2267–2302.

Trenkwalder, C., W. A. Hening, et al. (1999). Circadian rhythm of periodic limb movements and sensory symptoms of restless legs syndrome. *Mov Disord* 14(1): 102–110.

Trenkwalder, C., B. Hogl, et al. (2008). Augmentation in restless legs syndrome is associated with low ferritin. *Sleep Med* 9(5): 572–574.

Trenkwalder, C., B. Hogl, et al. (2009). Recent advances in the diagnosis, genetics and treatment of restless legs syndrome. *J Neurol* 256(4): 539–553.

Trenkwalder, C., R. Kohnen, et al. (2007). Clinical trials in restless legs syndrome–recommendations of the European RLS Study Group (EURLSSG). *Mov Disord* 22 Suppl 18: S495–504.

Trenkwalder, C. and W. Paulus (2004). Why do restless legs occur at rest? Pathophysiology of neuronal structures in RLS. Neurophysiology of RLS (part 2). *Clin Neurophysiol* 115(9): 1975–1988.

Trotti, L. M., S. Bhadriraju, et al. (2008). An update on the pathophysiology and genetics of restless legs syndrome. *Curr Neurol Neurosci Rep* 8(4): 281–287.

Tune, G. S. (1969). The influence of age and temperament on the adult human sleep-wakefulness pattern. *Br J Psychol* 60(4): 431–441.

Ulfberg, J. and B. Nystrom (2004). Restless legs syndrome in blood donors. *Sleep Med* 5(2): 115–118.

Ulfberg, J., B. Nystrom, et al. (2001). Prevalence of restless legs syndrome among men aged 18 to 64 years: an association with somatic disease and neuropsychiatric symptoms. *Mov Disord* 16(6): 1159–1163.

van Herwaarden, M. A., D. A. Katzka, et al. (2000). Effect of different recumbent positions on postprandial gastroesophageal reflux in normal subjects. *Am J Gastroenterol* 95(10): 2731–2736.

Vendette, M., J. F. Gagnon, et al. (2007). REM sleep behavior disorder predicts cognitive impairment in Parkinson disease without dementia. *Neurology* 69(19): 1843–1849.

Verbaan, D., S. M. van Rooden, et al. (2008). Nighttime sleep problems and daytime sleepiness in Parkinson's disease. *Mov Disord* 23(1): 35–41.

Vetrugno, R., M. Manconi, et al. (2006). Nocturnal eating: Sleep-related eating disorder or night eating syndrome? A videopolysomnographic study. *Sleep* 29(7): 949–954.

Vetrugno, R., G. Plazzi, et al. (2002). Excessive fragmentary hypnic myoclonus: clinical and neurophysiological findings. *Sleep Med* 3(1): 73–76.

Vetrugno, R., F. Provini, et al. (2001). Propriospinal myoclonus at the sleep-wake transition: a new type of parasomnia. *Sleep* 24(7): 835–843.

Vetrugno, R., F. Provini, et al. (2005). Propriospinal myoclonus: A motor phenomenon found in restless legs syndrome different from periodic limb movements during sleep. *Mov Disord* 20(10): 1323–1329.

Vignatelli, L., F. Bisulli, et al. (2007). Interobserver reliability of video recording in the diagnosis of nocturnal frontal lobe seizures. *Epilepsia* 48(8): 1506–1511.

Vitiello, M. V., L. H. Larsen, et al. (2004). Age-related sleep change: Gender and estrogen effects on the subjective-objective sleep quality relationships of healthy, noncomplaining older men and women. *J Psychosom Res* 56(5): 503–510.

Wada-Isoe, K., M. Kitayama, et al. (2007). Diagnostic markers for diagnosing dementia with Lewy bodies: CSF and MIBG cardiac scintigraphy study. *J Neurol Sci* 260(1–2): 33–37.

Walters, A. S. (2002). Review of receptor agonist and antagonist studies relevant to the opiate system in restless legs syndrome. *Sleep Med* 3(4): 301–304.

Walters, A. S. (2007). Clinical identification of the simple sleep-related movement disorders. *Chest* 131(4): 1260–1266.

Walters, A. S., G. Lavigne, et al. (2007). The scoring of movements in sleep. *J Clin Sleep Med* 3(2): 155–167.

Walters, A. S., D. E. Mandelbaum, et al. (2000). Dopaminergic therapy in children with restless legs/periodic limb movements in sleep and ADHD. Dopaminergic Therapy Study Group. *Pediatr Neurol* 22(3): 182–186.

Walters, A. S., W. G. Ondo, et al. (2009). Does the endogenous opiate system play a role in the Restless Legs Syndrome? A pilot post-mortem study. *J Neurol Sci* 279(1-2): 62–65.

Walters, A. S., J. Winkelmann, et al. (2001). Long-term follow-up on restless legs syndrome patients treated with opioids. *Mov Disord* 16(6): 1105–1109.

Wang, J., B. O'Reilly, et al. (2009). Efficacy of oral iron in patients with restless legs syndrome and a low-normal ferritin: A randomized, double-blind, placebo-controlled study. *Sleep Med*.

Wesstrom, J., S. Nilsson, et al. (2008). Restless legs syndrome among women: Prevalence, co-morbidity and possible relationship to menopause. *Climacteric* 11(5): 422–428.

Weyer, A., M. Minnerop, et al. (2006). REM sleep behavioral disorder in pure autonomic failure (PAF). *Neurology* 66(4): 608–609.

Wichniak, A., F. Tracik, et al. (2001). Rhythmic feet movements while falling asleep. *Mov Disord* 16(6): 1164–1170.

Wiegand, M., A. A. Moller, et al. (1991). Nocturnal sleep in Huntington's disease. *J Neurol* 238(4): 203–208.

Wiegand, M., A. A. Moller, et al. (1991). Brain morphology and sleep EEG in patients with Huntington's disease. *Eur Arch Psychiatry Clin Neurosci* 240(3): 148–152.

Williams, A. M. and D. Garcia-Borreguero (2009). Management of restless legs syndrome augmentation. *Curr Treat Options Neurol* 11(5): 327–332.

Winkelman, J. W., G. M. Chertow, et al. (1996). Restless legs syndrome in end-stage renal disease. *Am J Kidney Dis* 28(3): 372–378.

Winkelman, J. W., E. Shahar, et al. (2008). Association of restless legs syndrome and cardiovascular disease in the Sleep Heart Health Study. *Neurology* 70(1): 35–42.

Winkelmann, J. (2008). Genetics of restless legs syndrome. *Curr Neurol Neurosci Rep* 8(3): 211–216.

Winkelmann, J. and L. Ferini-Strambi (2006). Genetics of restless legs syndrome. *Sleep Med Rev* 10(3): 179–183.

Winkelmann, J. and B. Muller-Myhsok (2008). Genetics of restless legs syndrome: A burning urge to move. Neurology 70(9): 664–665.

Winkelmann, J., B. Schormair, et al. (2007). Genome-wide association study of restless legs syndrome identifies common variants in three genomic regions. *Nat Genet* 39(8): 1000–1006.

Woodward, S. H., N. J. Arsenault, et al. (2009). Autonomic activation during sleep in posttraumatic stress disorder and panic: a mattress actigraphic study. *Biol Psychiatry* 66(1): 41–46.

Woodward, S. H., G. A. Leskin, et al. (2002). Movement during sleep: associations with posttraumatic stress disorder, nightmares, and comorbid panic disorder. *Sleep* 25(6): 681–688.

Woodward, S. H., G. A. Leskin, et al. (2003). Sleep respiratory concomitants of comorbid panic and nightmare complaint in post-traumatic stress disorder. *Depress Anxiety* 18(4): 198–204.

Worthington, A. and L. Thomas (2008). Valvular heart disease associated with taking low-dose pergolide for restless legs syndrome. *Eur J Echocardiogr* 9(6): 828–830.

Xiong, L., A. Levchenko, et al. (2008). Genetic association studies of neurotensin gene and restless legs syndrome in French Canadians. *Sleep Med* 9(3): 273–282.

Yang, C., D. P. White, et al. (2005). Antidepressants and periodic leg movements of sleep. *Biol Psychiatry* 58(6): 510–514.

Yokota, T., Y. Atsumi, et al. (1990). Electroencephalographic activity related to palatal myoclonus in REM sleep. *J Neurol* 237(5): 290–294.

Young, G. (2009). Leg cramps. *Clin Evid* (Online) 2009.

Young, J. E., C. Vilarino-Guell, et al. (2009). Clinical and genetic description of a family with a high prevalence of autosomal dominant restless legs syndrome. *Mayo Clin Proc* 84(2): 134–138.

Zhang, J., S. P. Lam, et al. (2008). Diagnosis of REM sleep behavior disorder by video-polysomnographic study: Is one night enough? *Sleep* 31(8): 1179–1185.

Zucconi, M., R. Ferri, et al. (2006). The official World Association of Sleep Medicine (WASM) standards for recording and scoring periodic leg movements in sleep (PLMS) and wakefulness (PLMW) developed in collaboration with a task force from the International Restless Legs Syndrome Study Group (IRLSSG). *Sleep Med* 7(2): 175–183.

Zucconi, M., A. Oldani, et al. (1997). Nocturnal paroxysmal arousals with motor behaviors during sleep: Frontal lobe epilepsy or parasomnia? *J Clin Neurophysiol* 14(6): 513–522.

5
Sensory Disturbance in Aging

30 Neuro-ophthalmology of the Afferent Visual System in Aging

Molly E. Gilbert and James Goodwin

This chapter focuses on neuro-ophthalmic disorders that have a propensity for occurring in elderly patients. However, a number of the diseases discussed can affect younger patients as well. This chapter will emphasize the history and physical findings that are keys to recognizing these disorders. In addition, typical diagnostic maneuvers and treatment plans will be discussed.

Temporal Arteritis

Temporal arteritis (giant cell, cranial, granulomatous, Horton's), a systemic vasculitis, is associated with a wide range of symptoms including fatigue, fever, headaches, jaw claudication, loss of vision, scalp tenderness, polymyalgia rheumatica, and aortic arch syndrome (Machado et al. 1988). The risk of blindness from giant cell arteritis (GCA) makes accurate diagnosis and prompt aggressive treatment critically important.

It is estimated that visual loss occurs in 7–60% of patients with GCA (Hayreh et al. 1997) typically from either anterior ischemic optic neuropathy, central retinal artery occlusion, or less frequently, occipital infarction (Chlemeski et al. 1992). The visual loss is typically profound with the majority of patients having acuities of 20/200 or less (Chlemeski et al. 1992; Danesh-Meyer, Savino, and Gamble 2005). Visual loss is frequently the symptom that brings patients to medical attention. The risk of progressive visual loss despite apparently adequate therapy is high. Two prospective studies have demonstrated that even with the early institution of high dose corticosteroids, 13–27% of patients experience progressive loss of vision within the first 5–6 days making presentation with visual loss an ophthalmic emergency (Danesh-Meyer, Savino, and Gamble 2005; Hayreh and Zimmerman 2003).

Pathology

Temporal arteritis involves large and mid-sized arteries which have an elastic lamina. The vasculitis preferentially targets the superficial temporal, vertebral, ophthalmic, and posterior ciliary arteries (Wilkinson and Russell 1992). This explains the frequency of blindness and neurologic findings seen in these patients. Less commonly involved vessels include the internal carotid, external carotid, and central retinal arteries. Dissection of the aorta and involvement of the coronary arteries have also been reported (Save-Soderbergh, Malmvall, and Andersson 1986).

Demographics

Temporal arteritis (TA) is more common in women than men (3:1) and affects patients of Northern European descent most frequently. However, patients in other ethnic groups are also be affected. The prevalence increases with increased age. The incidence of TA increased from 2.3 per 100,000 in the sixth decade to 44.7 per 100,000 in the ninth decade and older. It rarely occurs in patients under the age of 50 but there have been individual case reports in the ages from 30–50 years (Hunder 2001; Lie et al. 1975; Biller, Asconape, and Weinblatt 1982).

Ocular and Neuro-ophthalmologic Manifestations

Visual loss may be transient or permanent and may affect one or both eyes. Transient visual loss typically occurs a few days or hours before permanent loss of vision develops. This transient amaurosis is identical to the transient visual loss in patients with carotid artery disease or cardiac valvular disease, although it may alternate between the two eyes (Finelli 1997).

Unilateral or bilateral central retinal artery occlusion (CRAO) can occur in patients with TA; however, only 5–10% of patients with CRAO have TA (Appen, Wray, and Cogan 1975). These patients may have clinically silent choroidal ischemia that can be detected during the acute phase by fluorescein angiography. Branch retinal artery occlusion can also occur, but is less frequently seen than CRAO.

Anterior ischemic optic neuropathy (AION) is the most common cause of visual loss in patients with TA (Keltner 1982; Jonasson, Cullen, and Elton 1979). It is usually unilateral and the second eye may become involved. Involvement of the second eye most commonly occurs within the first 5–6 days after the first eye is involved (Danesh-Meyer, Savino, and Gamble 2005; Hayreh and Zimmerman 2003). However, it may occur weeks or months after the first eye is involved, particularly if treatment is tapered too rapidly. The loss of vision with AION in TA is profound, with over 80% of patients having visual acuity of hand motion or worse (Liu, Glaser, and Schatz 1994; Aiello, Trautmann, and McPhee 1993). The affected optic nerve shows pallid edema that may be associated with intraretinal hemorrhages and/or cotton wool spots (see Figure 1).

Posterior ischemic optic neuropathy (PION) can also occur in TA. It is much less common than AION. These patients have normal appearing fundi with sudden visual loss and afferent papillary defects (Isayama, Takahashi, and Inoue 1983). The visual loss may not be as profound as is seen in patients with AION secondary to TA.

Homonymous visual field defects can occur from damage to the retrochiasmal visual pathway. This usually indicates an occipital lobe infarction from inflammatory thrombosis in the vertebrobasilar arterial system. Cortical blindness can develop from involvement of both occipital lobes (Hollenhorst, Brown, and Wagener 1960).

Approximately 25% of patients with TA will present with diplopia. Most frequently, the ocular motor nerve is affected. However, the fourth and sixth cranial nerves can be involved. In addition, diplopia may be a result of brainstem ischemia and a resultant skew deviation or internuclear ophthalmoplegia (Barricks, Traviesa, and Glaser 1977).

Systemic Manifestations

Most patients with TA will have premonitory systemic symptoms prior to their visual symptoms. These may include; new onset headache (Goodwin 1979), jaw claudication, weight loss, malaise (Liu, Volpe, and Galetta 2001), polymyalgia rheumatica, fever, scalp tenderness

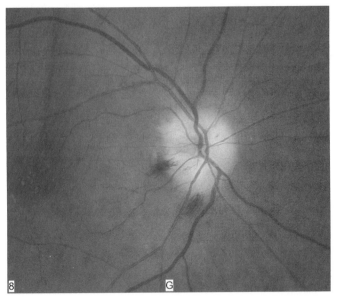

Figure 1 Pallid swelling and nerve fiber layer hemorrhages in a patient with giant cell arteritis.

(Hunder 2001), anemia, tongue claudication, tinnitus or vertigo. Jaw claudication is one the most specific systemic symptoms associated with TA (Hayreh, Podhajsky, and Raman 1997). It is important to differentiate jaw claudication from temporomandibular joint (TMJ) pain by history. Patients with jaw claudication will describe crescendo pain in the masseter muscles that begins after a period of chewing and abates when chewing ceases. Patients with TMJ report maximal pain when opening the jaw or immediately upon chewing.

Diagnosis

The American College of Rheumatology has published a list of diagnostic criteria. They specify that the diagnosis may be made when patients meet three of the five identified criteria including: age over 50, new onset headache, scalp tenderness or decreased temporal artery pulse, ESR greater than 50, or a positive temporal artery biopsy (TAB) (Hunder et al. 1993). Other authors have suggested that in the presence of AION or CRAO, any combination of age over 50, typical fundus appearance, typical systemic symptoms, high erythrocyte sedimentation rate (ESR), positive temporal artery biopsy (TAB), high C-reactive protein (CRP), and abnormal fluorescein angiography is sufficient to make the diagnosis (Liu, Volpe, and Galetta 2001). Some patients with TA may have no systemic symptoms, so called occult TA, but these patients will generally have elevated acute phase reactants.

Blood Tests

Normal ESRs include age divided by 2 for men and age +10/2 for women (Miller, Green, and Robinson 1983). However, elevated ESRs are nonspecific and furthermore, up to 22% of patients with TA can have normal ESRs.

Other's have shown that elevated CRP (>2.45 mg/dl) is more sensitive than ESR and that the combination of an elevated ESR and CRP is 97% specific for the diagnosis of TA (Hayreh, Podhajsky, and Raman 1997).

Another recent study has shown that thrombocytosis has a higher specificity, positive predictive value, and negative predictive value for TA than ESR alone (Foroozan et al. 2001). Thrombocytosis may increase the risk of subsequent visual or neurologic ischemic events (Krishna and Kosmorsky 1997).

Temporal Artery Biopsy

All patients suspected of having TA should undergo a temporal artery biopsy (TAB). It is 95% sensitive and 100% specific for TA. Although the American College of Rheumatology criteria do not mandate a TAB to make the diagnosis, it is prudent medicolegally given the side effects that can occur from treatment of TA.

There is very little risk from TAB, which include hematoma or brow droop from transecting a branch of the facial nerve (Slavin 1986). Since the risks are low and the complications of inappropriately treated disease are high, there should be a very low threshold for performing TAB.

Since the pathology of the vasculitis can include skip areas, it is important to ensure the biopsy specimen be of sufficient length to reduce the risk of missing the involved portion of the vessel. The recommended specimen length is at least two centimeters to take into account skip areas as well as artifactual shrinkage of the artery due to processing (Klein, Campbell, and Hunder 1986; Chambers, and Bernadoino 1988).

Biopsies should be embedded on end and serial sections should be stained with hematoxylin and eosin as well as elastin. Disruption of the internal elastic membrane is diagnostic of TA. Obliteration of the lumen and epithelioid giant cells may also be seen but are not necessary for diagnosis.

There is no need to withhold therapy while awaiting a TAB. Attempts should be made to undertake TAB within the first week of starting corticosteroid therapy. However, experienced pathologists can make the diagnosis of "healed arteritis," characterized by lymphocytic infiltration and scarring, even after several weeks of therapy with corticosteroids (McDonnell, Moore, and Miller 1986).

In patients for whom there is a high suspicion of TA but a negative TAB was performed, the diagnosis of TA is not eliminated. Therefore, a second TAB should be undertaken in these patients. The yield of a second TAB ranges from 5% to 13% (Klein, Campbell, and Hunder 1986).

Management

When patients present with vision loss, the goal of therapy is to prevent second eye involvement. The is evidence from retrospective studies is that corticosteroids retard the progression of visual loss, diminish the risk of fellow eye involvement, and may restore vision in some cases (up to 34%). Furthermore, IV steroids may be more effective than oral steroid in protecting the visual prognosis due to their higher bioavailability (Rosenfeld, Kosmorsky, and Klingele 1986; Matzkin, Slamovits, and Sachs 1992). Most neuro-ophthalmologists recommend immediate methylprednisolone 1 gram/day in patients presenting with visual loss who are suspected of TA. This must be given with ulcer prophylaxis for 3–5 days, after which it may be tapered to prednisone 1 mg/kg orally daily. The steroid dose is tapered after one month provided that the ESR remains normal and there is no reemergence of systemic symptoms. This taper is very slow and may last 6–12 months or longer.

Some cases of TA are refractory to corticosteroids. There have been some reports of heparinization being useful in these patients if flow-related ophthalmologic or neurologic phenomena are observed (Galetta, Balcer, and Liu 1997). In other refractory cases, or when steroids cannot be tolerated, steroid sparing immunomodulating therapy such as methotrexate or dapsone can be considered.

Nonarteritic Anterior Ischemic Optic Neuropathy

Nonarteritic ischemic optic neuropathy (NAION) is the most common cause of unilateral optic disc edema and optic neuropathy in patients over 50 years old (Johnson, and Arnold 1994). These patients describe a sudden onset of monocular visual loss, most commonly upon awakening. It is usually nonprogressive. There are no associated ocular symptoms or systemic symptoms. Typically, the patients describe a painless loss of vision; however, pain has been reported in up to 10% of patients (Swartz, Beck, and Savino 1995).

Demographics

Most patients are between 60–70 years old with a mean age of 66 +/− 8.7 years (Ischemic Optic Neuropathy Decompression Trial Study Group 1996). The annual incidence is 2.3 per 100,000 population per year (Johnson, and Arnold 1994). The rate is higher in Caucasians than in African Americans or Hispanic patients.

Pathogenesis

In order to discuss NAION, it is important to review the physiology of blood flow to the optic nerve. Blood flow to the optic nerve is determined by the perfusion pressure/resistance to flow (PP/RF). Perfusion pressure to the anterior optic nerve is expressed as mean arterial pressure (MAP) minus intraocular pressure (IOP) (MAP-IOP). Any variable that increases the RF or IOP or decreases the MAP can therefore compromise the perfusion of the optic nerve head (ONH) (Roth, and Pietrzyk 1994).

Furthermore, it has been shown that RF is autoregulated so that a constant rate of flow to the ONH is maintained when the MAP and IOP vary (Hayreh 1997). Autoregulation is maintained by endothelially derived vasoactive agents such as thromboxane A2 (vasoconstrictor) or nitric oxide and prostacyclin (vasodilators). However, there is a central range of perfusion pressure over which autoregulation works. Any vascular process which damages the endothelium can therefore lead to disruption of autoregulation (Hayreh 1999).

Patients with microvascular disease such as diabetes mellitus, hypertension, atherosclerosis, or smoking may have poor autoregulation of blood flow (Hayreh 1997), although some studies have questioned the role of these diseases in AION (Jacobson, Vierkant, and Belongia 1997). The Ischemic Optic Neuropathy Decompression Trial (IONDT), the largest source of the natural history of the disease, found that 47% of patients with NAION had systemic hypertension and 24% had diabetes (Ischemic Optic Neuropathy Decompression Trial Study Group 1996). Patients without these systemic risk factors did not have visual loss as severe as that seen in patients with systemic risk factors.

In addition it has been shown that autoregulation only acts over a certain range of perfusion pressure. Therefore, very elevated IOP or very low MAP may preclude the normal autoregulatory function of the endothelium. The role of nocturnal hypotension has therefore also been suggested as a separate risk factor that may explain the loss of vision upon awakening (Hayreh, Podhajsky, and Zimmerman 1997; Hayreh, Podhajsky, and Zimmerman 1999). In particular, patients who take antihypertensive medications before going to bed at night are at particular risk. The peak effectiveness of their medications tends to correspond to the normal dip in MAP that occurs in the very early morning hours. This potentiates the drop in MAP and compromises blood flow to the posterior ciliary vessels in these patients, increasing the risk of NAION.

Finally, up to 20% of healthy individuals have abnormal autoregulation of the perfusion pressure to part or all of their ONHs (Pillunat et al. 1997).

Another risk factor for development of NAION is the crowded optic nerve head or so called "disc at risk" (Doro and Lessell 1993). NAION occurs more often in patients with congenitally small discs. Therefore, the same number of nerve fibers must pass through a smaller lamina, leading to crowded nerves. Any insult that leads to swelling of the nerve fibers may then cause a compartment syndrome as the swollen fibers compress the blood supply to surrounding fibers (Hayreh 1997). Furthermore, the posterior ciliary arteries that supply the ONH have variable watershed zones in different individuals, making some people more likely to develop ION in the setting of predisposing or precipitating factors.

In addition to the atherosclerotic risk factors of diabetes and hypertension, patients with antiphospholipid antibodies have been reported to develop NAION (Galetta, Plock, and Kushner 1991; Bertram, Remky, and Arend 1995). Therefore, any patient who is younger than 50 should be investigated for this possibility. However, it is important to note that in general, prothrombotic states are not associated with NAION and therefore do not need to be investigated beyond this particular exception (Salomon, Huna-Baron, and Kurtz 1999).

Neuro-ophthalmic Signs

Patients present with decreased visual acuity at any range, although it is typically not as profound as that seen with TA. In the IONDT, 49% of patients had acuity better than 20/64 and 34% had acuity worse than 20/200. In addition, they have dyschromatopsia, an afferent papillary defect and visual field defects. The most common visual field defect is inferior altitudinal (Repka, Savino, and Schatz 1983). However, the visual field defect can be any "optic nerve" type defect, meaning it can be a central scotoma or anything that respects the horizontal meridian. The disc edema is sectoral in nature with splinter hemorrhages and dilated capillaries on the surface (see Figure 2). Over time as the edema resolves, the patients are left with sectoral pallor of the optic nerve head.

Diagnosis

In patients over the age of 50 years, an ESR and CRP should be checked to screen for TA. MRI is generally not necessary except in cases where there is concern for a compressive or infiltrative condition. MRI has been shown to have increased white matter ischemic changes that are reflective of the underlying presence of vasculopathic risk factors (Arnold, Hepler, and Hamilton 1995).

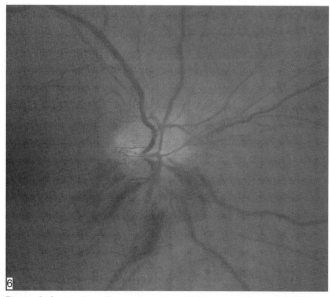

Figure 2 Sectoral swelling and capillary dilatation seen in nonarteritic anterior ischemic optic neuropathy.

Clinical Course

Most patients have a fixed deficit; however, certain subsets of patients were found to have progressive courses or spontaneous recovery in the IONDT. Forty-three percent of non-treated patients recovered three or more lines of vision; this has been supported by other studies as well (Arnold and Hepler 1994; Barrett, Glaser, and Schatz 1992). Approximately 10–15% of patients have a progressive loss of vision over the first month after diagnosis.

There is a lifetime risk of 30–40% of second eye involvement (Beri, Klugman, and Kohler 1989). The rates are higher in older patients and in patients with diabetes and hypertension. There is no demonstrated correlation that the visual outcome in one eye is predictive of the disease course in the second eye. Finally, there is no definitively established increased risk of cerebrovascular or cardiovascular disease in NAION patients.

Phosphodiesterase 5 (PDE 5) inhibitors merit a brief mention, if only to discuss the current thinking about how they may contribute to NAION. Transient visual symptoms such as altered color perception, a blue tinge to the environment, or changes in brightness perceptions are common with this class of drugs and related to the role of phosphodiesterase 6 and its effect on cGMP in the photoreceptors of the retina. As of October 2005, Pfizer reported that 23 million men worldwide had been written prescriptions for sildenafil; therefore over a billion doses had been taken. As of March 2006, the FDA's Adverse Event Reporting System had accumulated a total of 43 cases of PDE-5-associated NAION including those reported in the scientific literature. This rate of NAION is somewhat lower that the rates noted above in the general population. Therefore, PDE-5 inhibitors probably are such a rare cause of NAION, that it is impossible to make recommendations regarding its use. Neuro-ophthalmologists would recommend against the use of PDE-5 inhibitors in patients who have already experienced an episode of NAION in one eye. However, the risk of NAION is so small that no recommendations can be made regarding its use in the general population (Danesh-Meyer and Levin 2007).

Retinal Vascular Emboli

Retinal vascular insufficiency should be suspected in cases of transient or permanent monocular visual loss. Patients complain of a painless loss of vision that, if transient, lasts 1–5 minutes and involves darkening of the visual field in an altitudinal pattern (Volpe, Liu, and Galetta 1998).

Emboli

Retinal emboli prevalence increases with age and are more common in men. The prevalence is approximately 1% (Klein, Klein, and Jensen 1999). They are associated with hypertension, smoking, vascular disease, and previous surgery (Mitchell, Wang, and Li 1997; Bruno, Russell, and Jones 1992). The three types of emboli are cholesterol, calcific, and platelet-fibrin (Arruga and Sanders 1982; Howard and Russell 1987; Younge 1989). They are difficult to differentiate on ophthalmoscopy, but cholesterol emboli (Hollenhorst plaques) are the most common.

Events Associated With Retinal Vascular Insufficiency

Amaurosis Fugax

Fleeting transient monocular blindness that patients describe as a shade or curtain that obscures vision in one eye. The visual loss may be altitudinal peripheral or central. There are no photopsias or positive visual phenomena as may be seen with migraines. Emboli from the carotid vasculature are the most common cause. Patients with carotid artery disease may also describe a phenomenon of transient monocular blindness after exposure to sunlight or a white wall (bright light amaurosis) (Sempere, Duarte, and Coria 1992). The risk of stroke per year with amaurosis fugax is 2%, with a 1% risk of permanent visual loss (Poole and Russell 1985). This is significantly less than the stroke risk of 5–8% after a transient ischemic attack (TIA) (Streifler, Eliasziw, and Benaventer 1995).

Central Retinal Artery Occlusion (CRAO)

Acute CRAO is an ophthalmic emergency because the potential to restore vision may exist for the first 12 hours. The retina appears white with a cherry red spot in the fovea that results from the choroidal circulation showing through against the surrounding edematous retinal ganglion cells. Ten to 20% of patients with CRAO will have an associated visible embolus in the central retinal artery (see Figure 3). A number of heroic measures have been suggested to improve blood flow to the retina including anterior chamber paracentesis, inhalation of carbogen for vasodilation, lowering intraocular pressure with medications, and ocular massage. The efficacy of these measures has not been proven, however. These patients should be investigated for carotid or cardiac sources of emboli as well as TA.

Branch Retinal Artery Occlusion (BRAO)

These patients tend to maintain better visual acuity than patients with CRAO. BRAO is more commonly associated with visible retinal emboli (up to 70%). Ophthalmoscopy shows retinal whitening involving a section of the retina with partial cherry red spots. These patients should undergo the same work up for carotid and cardiac sources of emboli as patients with CRAO.

Patients with visible cholesterol or platelet fibrin retinal emboli, whether they are asymptomatic, or causes of CRAO or BRAO, have an increased risk of stroke or myocardial infarction (Klein, Klein, and Jensen 1991). One study has reported that the annual stroke rate for patients with retinal emboli was 8.5% versus 0.8% in control patients (Bruno, Jones, and Austin 1995). These factors lead to a reduced life expectancy, which underscores the importance of appropriate investigation and treatment of carotid disease.

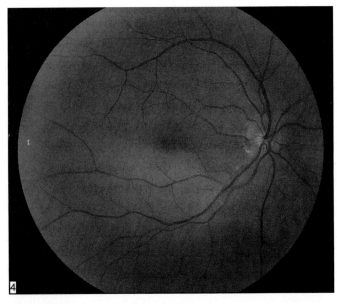

Figure 3 Central retinal artery occlusion showing retinal whitening and cherry red spot.

Ocular Ischemic Syndrome

Severe carotid disease may cause hypoperfusion and globe ischemia that produces a variety of signs involving the anterior and posterior segments of the eye (Mizener, Podhajsky, and Hayreh 1997; Costa, Kuzniec, and Molnar 1997; Brown and Magargal 1988). Patients may complain of amaurosis fugax, or gradual or sudden loss of vision. Ophthalmoscopy may show venous stasis retinopathy with dot blot hemorrhages in the fundus. Optic nerve edema may also be observed. Anteriorly, the eye may have injected conjunctiva or sclera, corneal swelling, anterior chamber cell and flare, and/or may be hypotonous. The vascular occlusion is located either in the ipsilateral internal carotid or in the ophthalmic arteries.

Carotid Artery Disease

Extracranial internal carotid artery disease is the most common cause of ischemic retinal visual loss (Adams, HP, Putnam, SF, Corbett 1983; Kollaritis, Lubow, and Hissong 1972). The origin of the internal carotid at its bifurcation may be narrowed by plaque formation, mural thrombi, plaque ulceration, or hemorrhage (Hayward, Davies, and Lamont 1995; Garcia and Khang-Loon 1996).

Diagnosis of carotid artery disease involves several modalities. In general, the presence or absence of a carotid bruit is not helpful. The incidence of carotid bruits increases with age, but the accuracy of this physical finding is low. Furthermore, in patients with high grade carotid stenosis, there may not be enough flow to produce an audible bruit (Levine, Crofts, and Lesser 1988). Carotid ultrasound is an effective screening tool for identification and estimation of extracranial internal carotid artery stenosis (el Asrar, Naddaf, and al Momen 1995). The limitation of this modality is the inability to differentiate between 99% stenosis and total occlusion. Magnetic resonance imaging angiography (MRA) is a noninvasive method of evaluating carotid disease that also provides a view of the intracranial circulation (Noble 1994). The limitation of this method is that it tends to overestimate stenoses. This is still useful however, because a normal MRA effectively rules out any carotid disease. Conventional angiography is the still the gold standard for quantifying carotid stenoses. The drawbacks to this method include the risk of stroke, which has been described at 1.2% (Mizener, Podhajsky, and Hayreh 1997).

Medical treatment of patients with mild, moderate or high grade stenosis, but other medical problems which preclude endarterectomy should start on treatment with aspirin. If symptoms of amaurosis fugax or transient ischemic attacks continue, larger doses of aspirin or clopidogrel, ticlopidine, or warfarin can be instituted.

The North American Symptomatic Carotid Endarterectomy Trial (NASCET) established the benefit of carotid surgery for stenosis greater than 70% in patients with retinal or hemispheric TIAs (North American Symptomatic Carotid Endarterectomy Trial Collaborators 1991; Barnett, Taylor, and Eliasziw 1998). This procedure can also be considered in patients without underlying medical conditions who are symptomatic but have only 50–70% stenosis. The surgical management of asymptomatic carotid stenosis is controversial. Meta analyses suggest that the risk of ipsilateral stroke is reduced but the benefit is small (Benavente, Moher, and Pham 1998). The NASCET study excluded patients greater than 80 years old who had significant intracranial disease, cardiac emboli, or life-threatening disease (North American Symptomatic Carotid Endarterectomy Trial (NASCET) Steering Committee 1991). Despite these exclusion criteria, the perioperative complication rate for major stroke and death was 2.1% (Barnett, Taylor, and Eliasziw 1998). Therefore, surgery on asymptomatic patients should take into account the age and health of the patients as well as the experience of the surgeon.

Cardiac Disease

Although less common than carotid emboli, cardiac emboli can also reach the retinal circulation. These emboli are calcific and lodge near the optic nerve head. Diagnosis of cardiac disease should include examination for irregular pulse rate, suggesting atrial fibrillation or a murmur suggestive of cardiac valvular disease. Laboratory evaluation including electrocardiography, 24-hour Holter monitoring, and transesophageal echocardiography should be undertaken. Transesophageal echocardiography has been shown to give a better view of the left atrial appendage, the aorta, the interatrial septum, and patent foramen ovales than traditional transthoracic echocardiography (Wisotsky and Engel 1993).

Retrochiasmal Disorders of the Visual Pathway

The retrochiasmal afferent visual pathways include the optic tract, lateral geniculate nucleus, optic radiations, and striate cortex. In adults, especially older adults, the most common cause of damage to this pathway is stroke or cerebrovascular disease. The most common neuro-ophthalmic presentation of damage to the afferent retrochiasmal pathway is a homonymous hemianopia.

This section will review the symptoms and signs associated with damage from stroke to each part of the retrochiasmal pathway, particularly the optic radiations and occipital lobe. We will also review the anatomy and blood supply of the retrochiasmal pathway.

Damage to the retrochiasmal pathway in adults is most commonly the result of ischemic stroke. Often these patients have cerebrovascular risk factors such as atrial fibrillation, hypertension, diabetes, smoking, and/or hypercholesterolemia (Dyken, Wolf, and Barnett 1984; Colditz, Bonita, and Stampfer 1988; Wolf, Agostino, and Kannel 1988; Iso, Jacobs, and Wentworth 1989). In any patient with new neurologic signs, neuroimaging is necessary. Computed tomography (CT) can be done in the emergency setting to differentiate between an ischemic and hemorrhagic stroke. However, MRI may be more effective at demonstrating small strokes, especially on T2-weighted imaging. Diffusion weighted imaging is useful for identifying ischemic areas in the first six hours after stroke (Bruno, Russell, and Jones 1992).

Optic Tract

The ganglion cell axons leave the optic chiasm and diverge to become the left and right optic tracts. Each optic tract carries the temporal retinal fibers from the ipsilateral eye and the contralateral nasal fibers. The majority of these fibers ultimately synapse in the ipsilateral lateral geniculate nucleus (LGN). However, some of the axons pass the LGN to synapse in the pretectal nuclei and from there connect bilaterally to the Edinger Westphal subnuclei of the oculomotor complex. The blood supply of the optic tract is from branches of the posterior communicating and anterior choroidal arteries (Kupersmith 1993).

Only 3% of hemianopias in adults result from optic tract lesions (Smith 1962). The majority of these lesions are due to strokes. The patients tend to have very incongruous homonymous hemianopia. The incongruity is due to the fact that the fibers are widely separated (Harrington and Drake 1990). Therefore, a partial tract lesion will affect the visual field in each eye asymmetrically (Figure 4). These hemianopias are associated with preserved acuity but there may be a relative afferent papillary defect noted in the contralateral eye. This is because more of the retinal ganglion cells cross in the chiasm to travel in the contralateral optic tract. Associated neurologic signs may include a hemiparesis ipsilateral to the hemianopia due to involvement of the cerebral peduncles, endocrine disturbances from involvement of the

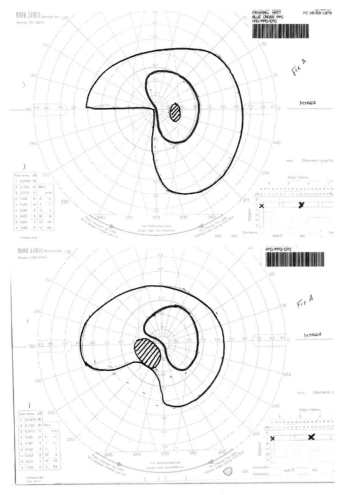

Figure 4 Noncongruous homonymous hemianopia in a patient with optic tract syndrome.

pituitary or hypothalamus, or visual hallucinations due to temporal lobe involvement (Bender, Bodis, and Wollner 1978).

Optic Radiations

Postsynaptic fibers from the LGN exit to become the optic radiations which travel in two major bundles. The superior bundle passes through the parietal lobe and carries visual information from the contralateral inferior quadrant. The inferior bundle travels through the temporal lobe (Meyer's loop) and contains visual information from the contralateral superior quadrant. Lesions of Meyer's loop will produce a contralateral incongruous homonymous hemianopia densest superiorly (Hughes, Abu-Khalil, and Lavin 1999). Lesions of the parietal lobe produce incongruous contralateral hemianopias densest inferiorly. In addition, lesions deep in the parietal lobe may have defective optokinetic responses in the direction ipsilateral to the lesion. Other cortical signs include complex partial seizures, memory deficits, fluent aphasia, or Kluver-Bucy syndrome if the temporal lobes are involved. If the dominant parietal lobe is involved, finger agnosia, agraphia, acalculia, and right-left disorientation may be observed. If the non dominant parietal lobe is involved, the patients may have left-sided neglect, memory loss, or dressing apraxias. As with optic tract lesions, the most common cause of damage to the optic tracts in adults is ischemic stroke in the middle cerebral artery distribution.

Occipital Lobe

The striate cortex has upper and lower banks above and below the calcarine fissure of the occipital lobe. Anterior to the striate cortex is the splenium of the corpus callosum. Fibers from the LGN that carry information from the superior retina project to the upper bank while those from the inferior retina project to the lower bank. Macular projections from the central 10 degrees of vision synapse in the occipital pole and occupy 60% of the striate cortex (Horton and Hoyt 1991). The occipital tip is devoted to foveal vision and the anterior-most striate cortex is monocularly innervated and subserves the most temporal 30 degrees of the visual field of the contralateral eye. The majority of the blood supply is from the branches of the posterior cerebral artery (PCA), especially the calcarine artery. There are minor contributions from the posterior temporal and parieto-occipital arteries (Smith and Richardson 1966). The occipital tip has dual blood supply from the PCA and the temporo-sylvian branch of the MCA.

Infarction of the PCA produces a hemianopia with macular sparing. Alternatively, if the occipital tip is affected, small homonymous hemianopic central scotomas may result. Lesions that do not affect the anterior most part of the calcarine cortex may spare the temporal crescent of the contralateral eye. Visual acuity is affected only if bilateral lesions are present. If the PCA is occluded proximally, an ipsilateral third nerve palsy, contralateral ataxia, or hemiparesis may also be present (Yamamoto, Georgiadis, and Chang 1999).

Neurophthalmological disease processes have many manifestations in the aging population. This chapter has covered the major diseases occurring in elderly patients that affect the afferent ophthalmologic pathways.

References

Adams, HP, Putnam, SF, and Corbett, JJ. Amaurosis fugax: The results of arteriography in 59 patients. *Stroke*. 1983;14:742–744.

Aiello, PD, Trautmann, JC, and McPhee, TJ. Visual prognosis in giant cell arteritis. *Ophthalmology*. 1993;100:550–555.

Appen, RE, Wray, SH, and Cogan, DG. Central retinal artery occlusion. *Am J Ophthalmology*. 1975; 79:374–381.

Arnold, AC and Hepler, RS. Natural history of nonarteritis ischemic optic neuropathy. *J Neurophthalmol*. 1994;14:66–69.

Arnold, AC, Hepler, RS, and Hamilton, DR. Magnetic resonance imaging of the brain in nonarteritic ischemic optic neuropathy. *J Neuro-ophthalmol*. 1995;15:158–60.

Arruga, J and Sanders, MD. Ophthalmologic findings in 70 patients with evidence of retinal embolism. *Ophthalmology*. 1982, 89;1336–1347.

Barnett, HJM, Taylor, DW, and Eliasziw, M. Benefit of carotid endartectomy in patients with symptomatic moderate or severe stenosis. *N Engl J Med*. 1998;339:1415–25.

Barrett, DA, Glaser, JS, and Schatz, NJ. Spontaneous recovery of vision in progressive anterior ischaemic optic neuropathy. *J Clin Neuro-ophthalmol*. 1992;12:219–225.

Barricks, ME, Traviesa, DB, and Glaser, JS. Ophthalmoplegia in cranial arteritis. *Brain*. 1977;100:209–221.

Benavente, O, Moher, D, and Pham, B. Carotid endarterectomy for asymptomatic carotid stenosis: A meta analysis. *BMJ*. 1998;317:1477–1480.

Bender, MB, Bodis, and Wollner, I. Visual dysfunction in optic tract lesions. *Ann Neurol*. 1978, 3:187–193.

Beri, M, Klugman, MR, and Kohler, JA. Anterior ischemic optic neuropathy VII. Incidence of bilateralitiy and various influencing factors. *Ophthalmology*. 1989;94:1020–1055.

Bertram, B, Remky, A, and Arend, O. Protein C, protein S, and antithrombin III in acute ocular occlusive diseases. *Ger J Ophthalmol*. 1995;4:332–5.

Biller, J, Asconape, J, and Weinblatt, ME. Temporal arteritis associated with a normal sedimentation rate. *JAMA*. 1982;247:486–487.

Brown, GC and Magargal, LE. The ocular ischemic syndrome. Clinical, fluorescein angiographic and carotid angiographic features. *Int Ophthalmol*. 1988;11:239–251.

Bruno, A, Jones, WL, and Austin, JK. Vascular outcome in men with asymptomatic retinal cholesterol emboli. A cohort study. *An Intern Med*. 1995;122:249–253.

Bruno, A, Russell, PW, and Jones, WL. Concomitants of asymptomatic retinal cholesterol emboli. *Stroke*. 1992;23:900–902.

Chambers, WA, and Bernadoino, VB. Specimen length in temporal artery biopsies. *J Clin Neuro-ophthalmol*. 1988;8:121–125.

Chlemeski, W, McKnight, K, Agudelo, C, and Wise, C. Presenting features and outcome in patients undergoing temporal artery biopsy: A review of 98 patients. *Arch Intern Med*. 1992;152:1690–1695.

Colditz, GA, Bonita, R, and Stampfer, MJ. Cigarette smoking and risk of stroke in middle aged women. *N Engl J Med*. 1988, 937–941.

Costa, VP, Kuzniec, S, and Molnar, LJ. Clinical findings and hemodynamic changes associated with severe occlusive carotid artery disease. *Ophthalmology*. 1997;104:1994–2002.

Danesh-Meyer, HV, and Levin, LA. Erectile dysfunction drugs and risk of anterior ischaemic optic neuropathy: Casual or causal association? *Br J Ophthalmol*. 2007;91: 1551–1555.

Danesh-Meyer, H, Savino, PJ, and Gamble, GG. Poor prognosis of visual outcome after visual loss from giant cell arteritis. *Ophthalmology*. 2005;112:1098–1103.

Doro, S and Lessell, S. Cup: Disc ration and ischemic optic neuropathy. *Arch Ophthalmol*. 1993;103:1143–1144.

Dyken, ML, Wolf, PA, and Barnett, HJM. Risk factors in stroke. *Stroke*. 1984;15:1105–1111.

El Asrar, AM, Naddaf, HO, and al Momen, AK. Systemic lupus erythematosus flare up manifesting as a cilioretinal artery occlusion. *Lupus*. 1995;4:158–160.

Finelli, PF. Alternating amaurosis fugax and temporal arteritis. *Am J Ophthalmol*. 1997;123: 850–851.

Foroozan, R, Danesh-Meyer, H, Savino, PS, Gamble, G, Mekari-Sabbagh, ON, and Sergott, RC. Thrombocytosis in patients with biopsy proven giant cell arteritis. *Ophthalmology*. 2002;109:1267–1271.

Galetta, SL, Balcer, LJ, and Liu, GT. Giant cell arteritis with unusual flow related neuro-ophthalmologic manifestations. *Neurology*. 1997:1483–1465.

Galetta, SL, Plock, GL, and Kushner, MJ. Ocular thrombosis associated with antiphospholipid antibodies. *Ann Ophthalmol*. 1991;23:207–212.

Garcia, JH, and Khang-Loon, H. Carotid atherosclerosis. Definition, pathogenesis, and clinical significance. *Neuroimag Clin North Am*. 1996:6:801–810.

Goodwin, BW Jr. Temporal arteritis. *Am J Med*, 1979;67:839–852.

Harrington, DO and Drake, MV. Postchiasmal visual pathway. In: *The visual fields. Text and atlas of clinical perimetry, 6th edition*. pp 311–361. St. Louis: CV, Mosby, 1990.

Hayreh, SS. Anterior ischemic optic neuropathy. *Clin Neurosci*. 1997; 4: 383–417.

Hayreh, SS. Factors influencing blood flow in the optic nerve head. *J Glaucoma*. 1997; 6:412–425.

Hayreh, SS. Retinal and optic nerve head ischemic disorders and atherosclerosis: Role of serotonin. *Progr Retin Eye Res*. 1999;18: 191–221.

Hayreh, SS, Podhajsky, PA, Raman, R, and Zimmerman, B. Giant cell arteritis: Validity and reliability of various diagnostic criteria. *Am J Ophthalmol*. 1997a;123:285–296.

Hayreh, SS, Podhajsky, PA, and Zimmerman, B. Nonarteritic anterior ischemic optic neuropathy: Time of onset of visual loss. *Am J Ophthalmol*. 1997b;124:641–647.

Hayreh, SS, Podhajsky, P, and Zimmerman, MB. Role of nocturnal arterial hypotension in optic nerve head ischemic disorders. *Ophthalmologica*. 1999;213:76–96.

Hayreh, SS and Zimmerman, B. Visual deterioration in giant cell arteritis patients while on high doses of corticosteroid therapy. *Ophthalmology*. 2003;110:1204–1215.

Hayward, JK, Davies, AH, and Lamont, PM. Carotid plaque morphology: A review. *Eur J Vasc Endovasc Surg*. 1995;9:368–374.

Hollenhorst, RW, Brown, JR, and Wagener, HP. Neurologic aspects of temporal arteritis. *Neurology*. 1960;10:490–498.

Horton, JC and Hoyt, WF. The representation of the visual field in human striate cortex. A revision of the classic Holmes map. *Arch Ophthalmol*. 1991;109:816–24.

Howard, RS and Russell, RW. Prognosis of patients with retinal embolism. *J Neurol Neurosurg Psychiatry*. 1987;50:1142–1147.

Hughes, TS, Abu-Khalil, B, and Lavin, PJM. Visual field defects after temporal lobe resection. A prospective quantitative analysis. *Neurology*. 1999;53:167–172.

Hunder, GG. Giant cell arteritis and polymyalgia rheumatica. In Ruddy, S, Harris, ED, and Sledge, CB eds. Kelley's *Textbook of rheumatology*, Ed 6. Philadelphia: WB Saunders, 2001:1155–1164.

Hunder, GG, Block, DA, Michel, BA, et al. The American College of Rheumatology 1990 criteria for the classification of giant cell arteritis. *Arthritis and Rheum*. August 1990;33:1122–1128.

Isayama Y, Takahashi, T, and Inoue, M. Posterior ischemic optic neuropathy. III: Clinical diagnosis. *Ophthalmologica*. 1983;187:141–147.

Ischemic optic neuropathy decompression trial study group. Characteristics of patients with nonarteritic anterior ischemic optic neuropathy eligible for the Ischmeic Optic Neuropathy Decompression Trial. *Arch Ophthalmol*. 1996;114:1366–74.

Iso, H, Jacobs, DR, and Wentworth, D. Serum cholesterol levels and six year mortality from stroke in 350,977 men screened for the multiple risk factor intervention trial. *N Engl J Med*. 1989; 320:904–910.

Jabs, DA. The rheumatic diseases. In Ryan, J, Schachat, AP, and Murphy, RP eds. *Retina. Vol 2*. St. Louis: CV Mosby, 2001:1410–1433.

Jacobson, DM, Vierkant, RA, and Belongia, EA. Nonarteritic anterior ischemic optic neuropathy: A case control study of potential risk factors. *Arch Ophthalmol*. 1997;115:1403–1407.

Jonasson, F, Cullen, JF, and Elton, PA. Temporal arteritis. *Scott Med* J. 1979;24:111–117.

Johnson, LN and Arnold, AC. Incidence of nonarteritic and arteritic anterior ischemic optic neuropathy. Population based study in the state of Missouri and Los Angeles County, California. *J Neuro-ophthalmol*. 1994;14:38–44.

Kachmaryk, MM, Trimble, SMN, and Gieser, RG. Cilioretinal artery occlusion in sickle cell trait and rheumatoid arthritis. *Retina*. 1995;15:501–504.

Keltner, JL. Giant cell arteritis. Signs and symptoms. *Ophthalmology*, 1982;89:1101–1110.

Klein, RG, Campbell, RJ, and Hunder, GG. Skip lesions in temporal arteritis. *Mayo Clin Proc*. 1976;51:504–510.

Klein, R, Klein, BE, and Jensen, SC. Retinal emboli and stroke. The Beaver Dam Eye Study. *Arch Ophthalmol*. 1999;117:1063–1068.

Kollaritis, CR, Lubow, M, and Hissong, SL. Retinal stroke: Incidence of carotid disease. *JAMA*. 1972;222:1273–1276.

Krishna, R and Kosmorsky, GS. Implications of thrombocytosis in giant cell arteritis. *Am J Ophthalmol*. 1997;124:103.

Kupersmith, MJ. Circulation of the eye, orbit, cranial nerves and brain. In: *Neurovascular neuro-ophthalmology*. pp. 1–67. Berlin: Springer-Verlag, 1993.

Levine, SR, Crofts, JW, and Lesser, GR. Visual symptoms associated with the presence of a lupus anticoagulant. *Ophthalmology*. 1988;95:686–692.

Lie, JT, Gordon, LP, and Titus, JL. Juvenile temporal arteritis: Biopsy study of four cases. *JAMA* 1975;234:572–577.

Liu, GT, Glaser, JS, and Schatz, NJ. Visual morbidity in giant cell arteritis: Clinical characteristics and prognosis for vision. *Ophthalmology*. 1994;101:1779–1785.

Liu, GT, Volpe, NJ, and Galetta, SL. Visual loss: Optic neuropathies. In *Neuro-Ophthalomology*. WB Saunders Company, 2001.

Lutsep, HL, Albers, GW, and DeCrespigny, A. Clinical utility of diffusion weighted magnetic resonance imaging in the assessment of ischemic stroke. *Ann Neurol*. 1997;41:574–580.

Machado, E, Michet, C, Ballard, D, et al. Trends in incidence and clinical presentation of temporal arteritis in Olmsted County, Minnesota, 1950-1985. *Arthritis Rheum*. 1988;31:745–749.

Matzkin, DC, Slamovits, TL, and Sachs, R. Visual recovery in two patients after intravenous methylprednisolone treatment of central retinal artery occlusion secondary to giant cell arteritis. *Ophthalmology*. 1992;99:68–71.

McDonnell, PJ, Moore, GW, and Miller, NR. Temporal arthritis: A clinicopathologic study. *Ophthalmology*. 1986;93:518–530.

McFadzean, R, Brosnahan, D, and Hadley, D. Representation of the visual field in the occipital striate cortex. *Br J Ophthalmol*. 1994;78:185–190.

Miller, A, Green, M, and Robinson, D. Simple rule for calculating normal erythrocyte sedimentation rate. *Br Med J*. 1983;286:266.

Mitchell, P, Wang, JJ, and Li, W. Prevalence of asymptomatic retinal emboli in an Australian urban community. *Stroke*. 1997;28:63–66.

Mizener, JB, Podhajsky, P, and Hayreh, SS. Ocular ischemic syndrome. *Ophthalmology*. 1997;104:859–64.

Noble, KG. Central retinal vein occlusion and cilioretinal artery infarction. *Am J Ophthalmol*. 1994;118:811–813.

North American Symptomatic Carotid Endarterectomy Trial (NASCET) Steering Committee. North American Symptomatic Carotid Endarterectomy Trial. Methods, patient characteristics, and progress. *Stroke*. 1991;22:711–720.

North American Symptomatic Carotid Endarterectomy Trial Collaborators. Beneficial effect of endareterectomy in symptomatic patients with high-grade carotid stenosis. *N Engl J Med*. 1991; 325:445–53.

Pillunat, LE, Anderson, DR, Knighton, RW, Joos, KM, and Feuer, WJ. Aurtoregulation of human optic nerve head circulation in response to increased intraocular pressure. *Exp Eye Res*. 1997; 64:737–744.

Poole, CJM and Russell, RWR. Mortality and stroke after amaurosis fugax. *J Neurol Neurosurg Psychiatr*. 1985;48:902–905.

Repka, MX, Savino, PJ, and Schatz, NJ. Clinical profile and long term implications of anterior ischemic optic neuropathy. *Am J Ophthalmol*. 1983;96:478–483.

Roth, S, and Pietrzyk, Z. Blood flow after retinal ischemia in cats. *Invest Ophthalmol Vis Sci*. 1994; 35: 209–217.

Salomon, O, Huna-Baron, R, and Kurtz, S. Analysis of prothrombotic and vascular risk factors in patients with nonarteritic anterior ischemic optic neuropathy. *Ophthalmology*. 1999;106:737–742.

Save-Soderbergh, J, Malmvall, BE, and Andersson, R. Giant cell arteritis as a case of death. *JAMA*. 1986;255:493–96.

Sempere, AP, Duarte, J, and Coria, F. Loss of vision induced by the color white: A sign of carotid occlusive disease. *Stroke*. 1992; 23:1179.

Slavin, ML. Brow droop after superficial temporal artery biopsy. *Arch Ophthalmol*. 1986;128:211–215.

Smith, CG and Richardson, WFG. The course and distribution of the arteries supplying the visual (striate) cortex. *Am J Ophthalmol*. 1966;61: 1391–96.

Smith, JL. Homonymous hemianopia. A review of 100 cases. *Am J Ophthalmol*. 1962, 54:616–622.

Streifler, JY, Eliasziw, B, and Benaventer, OR. The risk of stroke in patients with first ever retinal vs. hemispheric transient ischemic attacks and high grade carotid stenosis. *Arch Neurol*. 1995;52:246–249.

Volpe, NJ, Liu, GT, and Galetta, SL. Transient visual loss. *Curr Concepts Ophthalmol*. 1998;6:55–59.

Wilkinson, IMS and Russell, RWR. Arteries of the head and neck in giant cell arteritis. A pathological study to show the pattern of arterial involvement. *Arch Neurol*. 1972;27:378–391.

Wisotsky, BJ and Engel, HM. Transesophageal echocardiography in the diagnosis of branch retinal artery obstruction. *Am J Ophthalmol*. 1993;115:653–656.

Wolf, PA, D Agostino, RBM, and Kannel, WB. Cigarette smoking as a risk factor for stroke. The Framingham Study. *JAMA*. 1988;259:1025–1029.

Wong, AMF and Sharpe, JA. Presentation of the visual field in human occipital cortex. *Arch Ophthamol*. 1999;208–217.

Yamamoto, Y, Georgiadis, AL, and Chang, HM. Posterior cerebral artery territory infarcts in the New England Medical Center posterior circulation registry. *Arch Neurol*. 1999;56:824–832.

Younge, BR. The significance of retinal emboli. *J Clin Neuroophthalmol*. 1989;9:190–194.

31 The Aging Auditory System

Michael H. Flores, Gabrielle H. Saunders, and Bradley P. Pickett

"My misfortune is doubly painful to me because I am bound to be misunderstood; for me there can be no relaxation with my fellow men, no refined conversations, no mutual exchange of ideas. I must live almost alone, like one who has been banished; I can mix with society only as much as true necessity demands. If I approach near to people a hot terror seizes upon me, and I fear being exposed to the danger that my condition might be noticed."

Ludwig van Beethoven, 6 October 1802, in a letter to his brothers

An 85-year-old man presents for a routine medical evaluation accompanied by his spouse and daughter. The family is concerned that the patient is showing signs of Alzheimer's disease. For the past few years, his responses have become increasingly inappropriate, he has difficulty remembering instructions, appears frustrated at social gatherings, and has begun to isolate himself from others. During the evaluation, the gentleman speaks loudly and frequently misunderstands what is said; everything has to be repeated for him to understand. When asked, the patient acknowledges having progressive hearing difficulties for at least five years, especially in noisy listening environments. These problems have made it virtually impossible for him to interact with his wife, other family, and friends.

Medical providers who work with the elderly will recognize the above scenario. Although some adults maintain excellent hearing as they age, hearing loss is the third most common chronic complaint encountered within the geriatric population. Only hypertension and arthritis are more prevalent (National Health Interview 1994). While hearing loss is not life threatening, adults who do not receive adequate help for hearing impairment suffer greatly. Fear of failure when conversing with friends and family leads to withdrawal, social isolation, depression, and diminished functional and cognitive health. Given its prevalence and consequences, it's important that hearing loss not be overlooked or be unrecognized by health care providers.

Prevalence of Hearing Loss

With improved health care, nutrition, and hygiene, the average life span in the US has increased from 47 years in 1900 to 77 years today. According to the US Census Bureau, there will be 40 million people over age 65 years in 2010, with almost 6 million of these being over age 85 years. By 2050 these numbers are projected to rise to 88.5 million and 19 million respectively (US Census Bureau 2008). At least 31 million people in the US are thought to have some degree of hearing impairment (Kochkin 2005b), but as the baby boomer generation ages, this number will nearly double by the year 2030. Figure 1 shows the extent to which the prevalence of hearing loss increase with age. The percentage of 50–59 year olds with high frequency hearing impairment is 53%, but among the 60–69 year age group, this number is 77%. There do not appear to be any studies that have attempted to estimate the

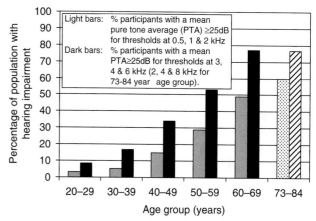

Figure 1 Data from the 1994–2004 National Health and Nutrition Examination survey of 5742 adults aged 20 to 69 and from the Health, Aging and Body Composition Study of 2052 adults aged 73–84 years. Data from: Agrawal, Y., Platz, E., & Niparko, J. (2008). Prevalence of hearing loss and differences by demographic characteristics among US adults. *Archives of Internal Medicine, 168*(14), 1522–1530. Helzner, E., Cauley, J., Pratt, S., Wisniewski, S., Zmuda, J., Talbott, E., et al. (2005). Race and sex differences in age-related hearing loss: the Health, Aging and Body Composition Study. *Journal of the American Geriatric Society, 53*(12), 2119–2127.

economic cost of presbycusis specifically, but as the prevalence of presbycusis increases, so will the economic and social burdens on society.

Anatomy and Physiology

It is necessary to have a basic knowledge about the anatomy and physiology of the auditory system in order to understand the changes that occur with age. The auditory system is sensitive to variations in sound pressure of less than one billionth of an atmosphere at frequencies between 20 Hz and 20 kHz. The healthy ear has a dynamic range (softest sound detectable to most intense sounds tolerated) of about 130 dB, made possible by the external, middle, and inner ear physiology, and central adaptation which intensifies low amplitude sounds but dampens high amplitude sounds to help to prevent acoustic trauma.

Figure 2 shows the anatomy of the outer, middle, and inner ear.

The outer ear consists of the pinna and the external auditory canal. The pinna helps to locate and amplify sound. The external auditory canal is a tube which protects the middle ear through its tortuous shape and cleansing properties and acts as a resonator which boosts the level of sounds between 2000 and 5500 Hz.

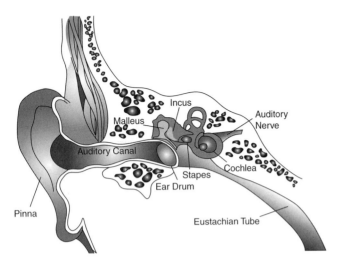

Figure 2 Diagram of the ear. Courtesy NIDCD; www.nidcd.nih.gov

The middle ear ossicles amplify the signal by about 30 dB by changing the sound energy into a mechanical vibration. This is necessary to compensate for the loss of intensity that occurs when the sound waves pass from air into the fluid medium of the inner ear (Yost 2007). The footplate of the stapes then transfers the mechanical energy to the cochlear fluids through the oval window of the cochlea by acting like a small piston.

The inner ear is located in the dense petrous portion of the temporal bone. It consists of a bony vestibular labyrinth for balance function and the cochlea. The cochlea converts the mechanical energy that arrived at the oval window, into electrical energy that is transmitted to the brain via the auditory nerve. The cochlea is divided into three radially spiraling fluid-filled compartments. The middle compartment, called the scala media, contains the organ of Corti. Hair cells in the organ of Corti are the microphone for the pressure impulses that are transmitted along the upper and lower compartments of the scala tympani and scala vestibuli when sound energy enters the oval window. The hair cells act as an electromechanical transducer that converts mechanical energy into electrical energy, a nerve impulse. These auditory signals are then transmitted from the cochlea to the auditory cortex in the brain through the primary auditory pathway, The primary auditory pathway is important for the initial decoding of the basic signal, including duration, intensity, and frequency and it is where sound localization occurs. Initial decoding of the signal duration, intensity, and frequency occurs in the primary auditory pathway. The auditory pathway synapses in the medial geniculate body within the thalamus before reaching the auditory cortex, at which time the content is recognized, memorized, and perhaps integrated into a voluntary response.

Auditory System Changes Associated with Aging

Age-related changes of the external ear include loss of cartilage, elasticity, atrophy of cerumen glands, and narrowing of the external auditory canal. These anatomical changes do not necessarily cause a change in hearing thresholds, although loss of ear canal tissue elasticity and cerumen accumulation do cause mechanical disruption of sound conduction, and in the case of collapse of the ear canal during testing with headphones, can cause factitious hearing loss. A study of 104 elderly nursing home residents found that 41% had collapsed ear canals

during audiometric testing (Schow and Goldbaum 1980). Canal collapse can be avoided by using insert earphones. Cerumen impaction is common in the geriatric population, with between 25% and 49% of elderly individuals having occluded ear canals due to impacted cerumen (Culbertson, Griggs, and Hudson 2004; Mahoney 1993). Cerumen impaction has measurable impacts on hearing thresholds and performance on the Folstein Mini-Mental Status Exam (Moore et al. 2002) and thus impacted cerumen should be removed before evaluation.

Middle ear changes associated with aging might include atrophy or thinning of the tympanic membrane. This has no effect on the conduction of sound to the middle or inner ear and or on hearing. Conversely, elderly patients with a life long history of chronic middle ear disease may have tympanosclerosis or thickening of the tympanic membrane which usually has minimal impact on hearing thresholds (Gates and Rees 2003). Otitis media in the elderly can result from obstruction of the eustachian tube that is associated with a viral or bacterial upper respiratory infection. However, when elderly patients who have no prior history of middle ear disease or chronic eustachian tube dysfunction develop middle ear effusions that fail to resolve, imaging of the nasopharynx and the skull base should be considered to evaluate for a neoplasm.

The primary cause of age-related hearing loss is associated with degeneration of hair cells in the cochlea and loss of peripheral auditory enervation. Schuknecht (1964) and Schuknecht and Gacek (1993) used histological sections of the cochlea to derive six distinct categories of presbycusis: sensory, neural, strial (metabolic), cochlear conductive, mixed, and indeterminate. In most cases, multiple sites within the cochlea and along the peripheral auditory nervous system are affected and reflect the summation of several disease processes.

Sensory presbycusis is caused by a loss of hair cells in the basal end of the cochlea, and is characterized by a downward sloping high frequency hearing loss. Because the inner hair cells are still intact and they continue to stimulate afferent auditory nerves which send information to the auditory cortex, word recognition in patients with sensory presbycusis tends to be very good. Sensory presbycusis accounts for only about 10% of elderly patients with hearing loss.

Neural presbycusis is characterized by loss or degeneration of the afferent auditory neurons. Because of neuronal redundancy, word recognition scores in patients with neural presbycusis may not be affected until more than 50% of the peripheral afferent nerves have been lost. Changes in audiometric thresholds may not be detectable until 90% of the neurons are lost. A sloping or flat audiometric configuration, with poorer than expected word recognition is the hallmark of neural presbycusis. Neural presbycusis accounts for 15% to 30% of all cases of presbycusis.

Strial presbycusis is associated with degeneration of the cochlear stria vascularis. The stria vascularis is responsible for helping to maintain electrolyte homeostasis of the endolymphatic fluid that surrounds hair cells. Losses of 30% to 40% of the stria vascularis may occur before audiometric thresholds are affected. Hearing loss from strial presbycusis tends to affect all areas along the cochlea equally, resulting in a flat audiometric configuration. Because of afferent nerve redundancy, inner hair cell connection to the auditory cortex remains intact, and word recognition is maintained. Strial presbycusis accounts for an estimated 20% to 35% of all cases of presbycusis.

Conductive/mechanical presbycusis is thought to account for about 15% to 20% of all cases. Schuknecht hypothesized that this presbycusis was a result of alterations in the mechanical functions of the basilar membrane and spiral ligament atrophy. Cochlear mechanical presbycusis is characterized by a sloping sensorineural hearing loss and poor word recognition scores.

Mixed and indeterminate presbycusis may account for up to 25% of all cases of presbycusis. Mixed presbycusis is a combination of two distinct types of degeneration—sensory and strial. The audiometric configuration and speech recognition scores will reflect the sum of the two types of presbycusis. When there is no correlation between cochlear histopathology, audiometric configuration and word recognition performance, hearing loss in geriatric patients is categorized as indeterminate presbycusis in the Schuknecht classification system.

Aging also affects the central auditory system. Central presbycusis is distinguished from peripheral presbycusis by the presence of normal or near normal hearing thresholds accompanied by poor speech discrimination abilities, especially in noise (Stach 1990; Frisina 2001). Reduction in speech understanding in elderly patients may correlate with global changes in the brain and atrophy of auditory pathways which results in decreased temporal fidelity and degradation of rapid processing of afferent signals from the cochlea. Global changes in the brain include loss of neurons, reduction of synaptic connections, changes in the neural transmission along the auditory pathway, changes in cognitive processing of the acoustic signal, and a loss of long-term memory (Willott 1996). While most of the research has centered on changes in the afferent auditory signal with aging, some studies suggest that there are also changes in efferent function (Jacobson et al. 2003). These studies propose that the efferent system aids in speech perception in noise by reducing outer hair cell amplification and a dampening of the noise signal. A loss or reduction of function of the efferent auditory system could explain why elderly patients have reduced speech discrimination in noise.

Pathophysiology

Clinically, presbycusis is characterized by a decline in auditory sensitivity that begins in the highest frequencies and progresses to include the lower frequencies. The rate of progression, age at onset, and ultimate severity of the hearing loss is quite variable. In fact, a significant fraction of the geriatric population has normal hearing. In other words, presbycusis is not inevitable for aging adults. There are extrinsic and intrinsic factors that are either the sole etiology for hearing loss, or work synergistically with the pathophysiology of presbycusis to cause hearing loss. Extrinsic factors include noise exposure, head trauma, exposure to ototoxic agents, and tobacco use. Intrinsic factors include hypertension, cardiovascular disease, diabetes, sequellae of neoplastic disease, and genetic predisposition. Thus, to some degree, hearing loss in elderly patients is preventable.

The National Institute on Deafness and Other Communication Disorders reports that more than 30 million Americans are exposed to hazardous sound levels on a regular basis, and of the 32 million Americans who have some degree of hearing loss, more than one-third have been affected by damaging noise. Noise exposure is thought to cause both mechanical and metabolic changes in hair cells that leads to cell death (Pujol and Puel 1999). Noise-induced hearing loss (NIHL) progresses most rapidly during the first 10–15 years of exposure and this hearing loss is permanent. Gates et al. (2000) reported that NIHL occurring before old age reduces the effects of aging at noise-associated frequencies, but hastens the decline of hearing in adjacent frequencies. These findings suggest that the effects of noise damage may continue long after the noise exposure has stopped. The rate of decline from noise exposure is also influenced by simultaneous exposure to ototoxic medications, solvents, heavy metals, and tobacco smoke which may act synergistically with noise to cause an increased severity of the hearing loss (Morata 1998). Currently it is impossible to predict in advance which individuals will have increased loss from aging as a result of

noise exposure but by preventing NIHL, patients can reduce the impact of age-related changes on their hearing. Physicians should educate and motivate patients of all ages to avoid potentially damaging noise, and to use hearing protection when necessary.

Ototoxicity is defined as a loss of cochlear or peripheral vestibular function that is caused by exposure to agents that damage the neuroepithelium of the inner ear. There are at least 130 medications, solvents, and heavy metals that have proven ototoxic (Palomar et al. 2001). The most common ototoxic medications include aminoglycoside antibiotics, platinum-based chemotherapeutic agents, loop diuretics, macrolide antibiotics, antimalarials, and salycilates (Roland et al. 2004). Organic solvents and exposure to heavy metals have also been shown to cause hearing loss in animals and humans. Typical solvent exposures involved mixtures of xylene, toluene and/or methyl ethyl ketone and heavy metals include lead, mercury, nickel, trimethyltin, and arsenic. Ototoxic hearing loss is typically bilateral and symmetrical with severity that ranges from asymptomatic high frequency sensorineural loss to total deafness. The geriatric population is highly susceptible to ototoxic damage because a history of noise exposure, renal impairment, dehydration, magnesium deficiency, preexisting hearing loss, dizziness, Meniere's disease, prior exposure to ototoxic agents, and tinnitus increase risk. The following website is recommended as a source of information on ototoxic drugs and chemicals: http://www.tchain.com.

James Watson, a Nobel Prize laureate and world-renowned genetics researcher, once said, "We used to think that our fate was in our stars, but now we know that, in large measure, our fate is in our genes." (Jaroff, 1989) There are approximately 100 genes that are necessary for normal auditory function (Morton 1991). The relationship between genetic make-up and susceptibility to presbycusis is under study, and while a "presbycusis gene" has not yet been identified, many believe that multiple genes determine the degree of hearing loss from presbycusis, the age at onset of the hearing loss, and the audiometric configuration.

Presbycusis has been identified in families and twins with heredity estimates of 35–55% being attributed to genetics (Karlsson, Harris, and Svartengren 1997; Wingfield et al. 2007; DeStefano 2003). A Framingham study looking at age-related hearing loss in parents, their offspring, and between siblings indicated a clear genetic link for presbycusis. The study showed a stronger correlation between a mother's hearing and her children's hearing, than between fathers and their children. This link implies that some forms of presbycusis may be due to mitochondrial genetic problems, since mitochondria have their own DNA that comes entirely from the mother's egg (Gates, Couropmitree, and Myers 1999). At present, our knowledge of the genetic factors that are responsible for NIHL is still limited, especially when compared with the relatively well-studied environmental factors. However, there is mounting evidence that several genetic mutations could determine an individual and intrinsic predisposition to noise damage (Bovo, Ciorba, and Martini 2007). The identification and isolation of these genetic factors could have important and practical outcomes. For example, workers genetically predisposed ought to be more rigorously protected against noise, in order to preserve their auditory function.

Research investigating the relationship between extrinsic and intrinsic factors impacting the severity and progression of presbycusis has shown cardiovascular disease to exacerbate presbycusis among women but not men. However, because men have a high incidence of NIHL the association might be hidden (Gates et al. 1993; Torre et al. 2005). A study of elderly men and women found a probable correlation between high systolic and diastolic blood pressure and hearing loss in the low and mid frequencies in women aged 79 years old and older.

No consistent associations were seen in men or in younger women (Rosenhall 2006). Diabetes mellitus is also likely to be associated with presbycusis. Diabetics were found to have poorer hearing at low frequencies, poorer speech reception thresholds, and poorer otoacoustic emissions than age-matched controls. These problems especially affected the right ear of diabetics. One interpretation is that the decline in right ear advantage that occurs with age, is accelerated by diabetes (Frisina et al. 2006). Hormonal changes also might be associated with presbycusis. Recent studies have found that women undergoing estrogen therapy have less rapid progression and slower development of presbycusis than those who did not receive treatment (Hederstierna et al. 2007). Similarly, menopausal women receiving combined estrogen and progestin were found to have significantly worse hearing than women taking estrogen alone or no hormones at all (Guimaraes et al. 2006). Smoking has been implicated as a risk factor for presbycusis. Smoking may reduce oxygen delivery to the cochlea resulting in hypoxia as well as mitochondrial mutations and injury. There is evidence that this significantly impacts hearing loss associated with aging. A study found that smokers were 1.69 times as likely to have a hearing loss as nonsmokers and that non-smoking participants who lived with a smoker were also more likely to have a hearing loss than those who were not exposed to a household member who smoked (Cruickshanks et al. 1998).

In summary, intrinsic and extrinsic factors play a role in the progression of presbycusis; therefore, primary care providers can play an important role in maintaining hearing health by maintaining the general health of their patients.

Rehabilitation

Impacts of Hearing Loss

As a result of retirement, mobility limitations, and bereavement, elderly individuals are susceptible to loneliness and isolation (Donaldson and Watson 1996). The addition of hearing impairment can result in even less motivation to participate in social situations, like family gatherings and meetings with friends, which are important for maintaining a good quality of life. Besides, or as a result of, impairing communication, untreated hearing loss has many negative social and emotional effects. Studies have found that the individuals who needed hearing aids but did not use them participated in significantly fewer social activities and reported significantly more anxiety, depression, emotional instability, and paranoia than did hearing-aid users. The non-users of hearing aids also had lower self-esteem and less warmth in their interpersonal relationships than the hearing-aid users. Further, as compared to the families of hearing-aid users, the family of the non-hearing-aid users more often reported that their relative showed anger and frustration, poor cognitive abilities, and had become introverted (Kochkin and Rogin 2000).

Benefits of Hearing Aids

On a positive note, acquisition of hearing aids has been shown to result in improvements in social, emotional, cognitive, and psychological well-being. As reported by (Kochkin and Rogin 2000), data from the National Council on the Aging study showed that acquisition of hearing aids led to improved relationships at home, better self-esteem, an increased sense of safety, and decreased dependence on others. These improvements were reported by both the hearing-impaired individual and his or her relatives. Results from a randomized clinical trial were similar. In this trial, half of the participants were fitted with hearing aids immediately, while the other half were put on a waiting list to receive hearing aids once the study was completed. After six weeks the individuals that had received hearing aids had improved social,

Table 1 Impacts of Hearing Loss and the Reported Improvements Following Use of Hearing Aids

Impacts of Hearing Loss	Changes Following Hearing Aid Acquisition
Depression, paranoia	Improved mental health
Loneliness	Life overall has improved
Isolation	Improved social life
Dependence on others	Increased independence
Lack of participation in social activities	Participate in more group activities
Anxiety	Increased sense of safety
Poor self-esteem	Better self-esteem
Lack of warmth in personal relationships	Improved relationships at home

emotional, and cognitive function, and were less depressed than those who were still waiting for hearing aids, even though there were no group differences at the start of the study (Mulrow et al. 1990). Table 1 below summarizes the impacts of hearing loss and the improvements in life reported following acquisition and use of hearing aids.

Barriers to Treatment

Given the negative consequences of hearing loss and the positive benefits of hearing aid use, it should be apparent that hearing aids are a highly effective intervention for hearing impairment. Yet, the National Council on Aging Study (Kochkin and Rogin 2000) reported that six out of seven middle-aged Americans with hearing loss, and three out of five elderly Americans with hearing loss don't use hearing aids. Why is this and why would someone with hearing loss not seek medical advice? The reasons are numerous and varied. Among the most common reasons cited are a belief on the part of the hearing-impaired person that he/she does not need hearing aids, the expense of the hearing aids, the belief that hearing aids do not work, and that his/her physician has not recommended them.

Awareness of Hearing Loss

It is not uncommon for older persons with hearing impairment to underestimate the impact their hearing loss has on their function. Many possible explanations for this have been put forward, the most probable of which is that because the onset of presbycusis is so gradual, older individuals are simply unaware of the extent to which their hearing has deteriorated. Physicians and other allied health professionals should encourage their elderly patients to seek appropriate screening, diagnosis, and treatment if they suspect a hearing loss. Unfortunately, identification of patients with hearing loss is not emphasized during routine physical examinations. A survey of almost 16,000 households revealed that currently only about 13% of physicians routinely screen for hearing loss (Kochkin 2005b) even though there are easy-to-administer screening tests available. The simplest screening tool is plainly asking the patient, Do you think you have a hearing problem? More sophisticated screening tools are also available such as a hand-held screening otoscope for screening thresholds, or a short screening questionnaire. If an elderly patient fails to hear 40 dB HL tones presented with the screening otoscope they should be referred to an audiologist for further evaluation. A commonly-used screening questionnaire is the 10-item version of the Hearing Handicap Inventory for the Elderly (Weinstein 1994). This questionnaire has good sensitivity and specificity to hearing loss (Bess 1995; Gates et al. 2003). Hearing screenings need not take more than five minutes and can provide important information to the physician about whether referral to an audiologist is necessary. It is important to remember that the elderly individual is unlikely to report hearing difficulties even though their communication might be substantially disrupted, so it is the responsibility of the physician and other members of a health care team to take the initiative to conduct hearing screenings of elderly patients.

High Cost

In a survey of seniors, 55% of respondents cited cost as their reason for not using hearing aids (Kochkin 2007) Hearing aids are indeed expensive, with the higher-end digital aids costing at least $2,500 per aid, and basic hearing aids ranging from $900 to $1500 per aid. Since most health insurance plans don't cover more than a few hundred dollars, the burden of payment is borne almost entirely by the elderly user. Most elderly individuals are on a fixed and minimal income, thus, when the individual has to choose between his/her basic needs and hearing aids, the choice is typically to forgo the hearing aids. Unfortunately, inexpensive hearing aids are available on the Internet; however, these devices are rarely fitted appropriately, and likely do not compensate for the individual's hearing configuration.

Solutions for seniors who cannot afford hearing aids can sometimes be found through programs run by a local chapter of the Lions Club or a United Way agency. These agencies collect, refurbish, and distribute donated hearing aids. In addition, many audiologists participate with hearing aid manufacturers to provide low or no cost amplification to the most needy. Physicians and caregivers should familiarize themselves with their local resources in order to assist their patients who may find financial obstacles preventing them pursuing assistance.

Belief that Hearing Aids Do Not Work

According to MarkeTrak VII data, less than half of the 65+ age group who could benefit from hearing aids actually purchase them (Kochkin 2005b). Further, market research has shown that almost 20% of older adults who do purchase hearing aids discontinue using them. Among hearing aid owners, only three out of four people said they wore their hearing aids more than four hours a day. The top three reasons given for abandoning hearing aids were (a) hearing aids do not work well in noise (48%), (b) hearing aids do not restore hearing to normal (47%), and (c) hearing aids pick up too much background noise (45%) (Kochkin 2005a). Unfortunately, some of these complaints are based on reality, although newer technology does provide some solutions.

Potential hearing aid users often are deterred from obtaining hearing aids by negative reports from others and by their own negative biases. Nineteen percent of non-hearing aid users reported that the experiences of others influenced their decision not to get hearing aids and about 50% of people with hearing loss choose not to try hearing aids because the perceived stigma associated with their use (Kochkin 2007). That is, use of a hearing aid is an admission of hearing loss, which is considered embarrassing and a reflection of being old.

No Recommendation from the Physician

Despite the fact that auditory prosthetics (hearing instruments and implants) are the most common treatment for hearing loss, medical professionals and hearing health care specialists often discourage hearing-impaired people from obtaining hearing aids. Table 2 shows data from a survey of over 2000 hearing-impaired non-hearing aid users from across the US and the recommendations these individuals received from various medical professionals and hearing health care specialists regarding their hearing. Hearing aids were recommended to just 11% of patients seen by family doctors, as compared to 33% of patients seen by audiologists and 56% seen by hearing instrument specialists. In fact, family doctors were more likely to recommend *against* getting a hearing aid (17%) than for doing so (11%). ENT physicians

Table 2 Recommendations Received by Patients Regarding Their Hearing from Various Professionals

Professional	Recommendation Received			
	Referral for Further Testing	Wait and Retest	Get Hearing Aids	Do Not Get Hearing Aids
Family doctor	48	25	11	17
ENT	29	28	25	25
Audiologist	13	34	33	25
Hearing instrument specialist	6	19	56	20

Data reprinted with permission from Kochkin, S. (2007) MarkeTrak VII: Obstacles to adult non-user adoption of hearing aids. *The Hearing Journal* 60(4) 24–50.

were equally likely to recommend against hearing aids as for them, and audiologists were slightly more likely to recommend for hearing aids than against (Kochkin 2007). This is despite the fact that today hearing aids are sufficiently flexible as to provide at least some benefit for all types of hearing loss.

Kochkin (2007) emphasized the importance of the physician's role in hearing loss identification and treatment when he reported that persons with hearing loss are eight times more likely to be positively inclined to purchase a hearing instrument if their physician has recommended one. Since an increase in referrals has the potential to positively impact the lives of so many people, offering education for primary care physicians by audiologists should be initiated when possible with the goal of improving physicians' knowledge of treatment alternatives available for hearing improvement.

Expectations

The reports that hearing aids do not work is in part a function of limitations in the technology and in our knowledge of the auditory system. However, some of the problems are associated with the fact that with age come auditory processing difficulties which exacerbate listening problems in noise. Back in 1972, Jerger showed that older hearing-impaired listeners performed more poorly on tests of speech in noise than the young listeners with the same degree of hearing impairment. Since that time, other studies have shown that age affects temporal processing ability (Gordon-Salant and Fitzgibbons 2001), processing of time-compressed speech (Vaughan, Storzbach, and Furukawa 2006), understanding of speech in noise (Plomp and Mimpen 1979), and higher level linguistic processing (Wingfield et al. 2006). The combination of hearing loss and age-related decline in auditory processing ability means the listener needs to expend more effort than previously to process incoming speech. Even mild-to-moderate hearing impairment affects memory, presumably because the extra effort required to decode incoming speech signals uses the brain's resources that otherwise would be allocated to encoding the information into memory (McCoy et al. 2005). The result is that speech might be heard but not understood or remembered as well and this is especially true in adverse listening situations. Counseling is needed from both the audiologist and physician regarding the abilities of the technology and the limitations of the auditory system to ensure expectations are realistic. A reminder that hearing aids are hearing *aids*, not hearing *restorers*, can help with this difficult barrier.

Technology and Hearing Loss

The advent of digital technology and digital signal processing (DSP) has truly improved the performance and usability of hearing aids. Complaints about earlier generations of hearing aids included sounds being uncomfortably loud, feedback (whistling), and poor function in noisy places. Now there are hearing aids with compression algorithms which adjust the level of the hearing aid output to an individual patient's hearing sensitivity. Specifically, low intensity signals are amplified more than high level ones and in this way, the output of the hearing aid stays within the user's dynamic range (comfortable range of listening levels).

Many hearing aids now have digital feedback reduction circuitry. This has virtually eliminated feedback in all but the most profound losses. Feedback reduction allows for increased amplification, and thus improved performance, without the annoyance and embarrassment of feedback that often occurred when the user moved his/her jaw or head, or when the hearing aid was in close proximity to an object such as a telephone handset or a hat.

Most hearing aids today have the option of "directional microphones." These microphones amplify sounds differently, depending on the direction the sound is coming from. Assuming the hearing aid user is facing the source of sound they want to hear (the signal), and that sounds from behind are unwanted 'noise,' the hearing aid essentially increases the gain of the signal relative to the noise—known as increasing the signal-to-noise ratio. Hearing-impaired persons have particular difficulty hearing in noise, therefore any increase in the signal-to-noise ratio is extremely beneficial. In fact, directional microphones are the only newer hearing aid technology that has been shown to successfully improve the ability of users to hearing in noise. Most hearing aids today have 'automatic directionality.' This means that the user does not need to make decisions about the best setting for a particular listening environment, something users found difficult to judge (Walden, Surr, and Cord 2003).

Noise reduction circuitry is now a standard feature on most hearing aids. Noise reduction is somewhat of a misnomer in that these hearing aids do not truly reduce the level of background noise, rather they reduce the amplification of low frequency according to an algorithm. No research has shown improved ability to understand speech in noise with a noise reduction hearing aid. However, noise reduction algorithms make the hearing aid output sound more pleasant, and thus users are more likely to wear their hearing aids.

Telephones are sometimes the only connection between an elderly individual and their family and friends. Feedback can be a problem when a telephone handset is brought up to the aided ear. To overcome this, hearing aids have a built in 'telecoil' which picks up and amplifies the magnetic current generated by the telephone. Hearing aids with automatic telecoils are now common. These hearing aids have a magnet built into them which automatically activates the telecoil when the handset of a telephone is brought close to the ear.

It should be apparent that the hearing aid industry has made considerable improvements in hearing aid technology. In fact, technology has changed so drastically over the last ten years that almost 80% of users with new hearing aids (less than one year old) are satisfied with their aids, as compared to about 50% of users with hearing aids that are ten or more years old (see Figure 3).

Beyond Technology: Formula for Successful Rehabilitation

Aside from the hearing aid processing, there are many other aspects of a hearing aid that need to be considered if someone is to be a successful hearing aid user. Clearly, providing a device the user can handle is essential. Fine motor control and vision are both necessary for successful upkeep and manipulation of a hearing aid. More specifically, hearing aid insertion, manipulation of the hearing aid controls, and handling the battery require fine motor skills, while cleaning the

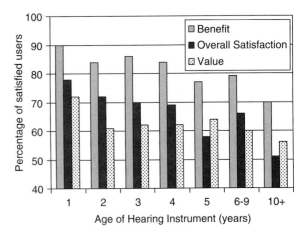

Figure 3 Data from MarkeTrak VII survey showing percentage of hearing aid users satisfied with their hearing aids by age of the instrument. Figure replotted with permission from The Hearing Journal. Kochkin, S. (2005) MarkeTrak VII: Customer satisfaction with hearing instruments in the digital age. *The Hearing Journal* 58(9) 30–44.

hearing aid and replacing the battery require adequate visual acuity. Indeed, several recent studies have shown that people with poor manual dexterity use their hearing aids less, and are less satisfied than those with better manual dexterity (Humes and Wilson 2003; Kumar, Hickey, and Shaw 2000; Wilson and Stephens 2002). Another study found that older people rated ease of handling to be the most important hearing aid attribute, after effectiveness for communicating in quiet and noisy environments (Meister et al. 2002). Usability is clearly an issue as demonstrated by a study that showed that 40% of people aged 90 and older could not use the volume control wheel, 36% could not change the hearing aid battery, and 34% could not clean the hearing aid ear mold due to manual and physical limitations (Parving and Philip 1991).

One way to quickly and informally evaluate an individual's dexterity and vision is to administer the 3-item Manual Dexterity and Vision scale of the Attitudes towards Loss of Hearing Questionnaire (Saunders et al. 2005) (Table 3 below). A patient who scores ten or more points will likely encounter difficulties handling a hearing aid. Due to cosmetic concerns, patients often want to select the smallest hearing aid available. It is hoped that once a patient has acknowledged dexterity and vision issues with the everyday tasks, he/she will be more accepting of a clinician's advice regarding selection of a hearing aid style.

Ease of Handling

It is the role of the physician and audiologist to advise and guide their patients towards selecting hearing aids with features that they can

Table 3 ALHQ Manual Dexterity and Vision Scale Items

	Strongly Disagree	Neither Agree nor Disagree			Strongly Agree
These days I find it hard to handle small things like push pins, buttons, or zippers.	a	b	c	d	e
I think I would have difficulty putting a small screw into a hole.	a	b	c	d	e
I find that I drop objects easily.	a	b	c	d	e

Table 4 Attributes of Different Styles of Hearing Aid

Attribute	Hearing Aid Style			
	BTE	ITE/ ITC	CIC	Open Canal
Power	+++	++	+	+
Feedback	–	+	++	+++
Battery size	Largest	Small	Tiny	Small
Ease of insertion	Harder	Easy	Hardest	Harder
Ease of handling	Easiest	Easy	Hardest	Easy
Visibility	++	+++	+	+

easily use and at the same time benefit from. There are five different styles of hearing aid commonly available for people with presbycusis: behind-the-ear (BTE), in-the-ear (ITE), in-the-canal (ITC), completely-in-the-canal (CIC) and mini-BTEs. They differ in their overall size and the way in which they sit in the ear. Each style has its pros and cons, depending on the needs and priorities of the user. Table 4 provides some information about each. The table can be used to help select the style of hearing aid most appropriate for the elderly.

For instance, BTE hearing aids would likely be a good choice for someone with a moderate-to-severe hearing loss and visual impairment, because BTEs can provide high amplification with little feedback, and their larger batteries and bigger controls are easier to use and see than those of other styles. On the other hand, an ITE or ITC hearing aid would be an appropriate choice for an individual with a milder hearing loss who has arthritic hands, because they are easier to insert than other styles and have a fairly large battery door and bigger controls.

In general, smaller hearing aids require smaller batteries. However, even the largest hearing aid batteries are only a few millimeters in diameter and thus are difficult for many older individuals to see and handle. At least two manufacturers of hearing aid batteries have come up with solutions to assist with battery insertion (the Duracell Easy Tab battery and the Energizer EZ-Change package), but even with these aids, battery insertion may not be possible for some individuals. Therefore, when dealing with an elderly individual who has visual impairments and/or peripheral neuropathy, this should be taken into account when selecting assistive devices.

Individuals often find it difficult to identify which hearing aid is for which ear. A simple solution is to color code the aids using nail polish. The typical convention is red for the right ear and blue for the left although obviously any identifying coding is fine. It is also advantageous to coordinate with a blind rehabilitation occupational specialist and low vision specialist when substantial visual loss is present. These services can substantially increase likelihood of successful auditory rehabilitation for the elderly individual with multi-sensory deficits.

Changes in Communication Needs

The communication needs of the aging population are at least as heterogeneous as those of the rest of society, and are largely dependent on the lifestyle the person is leading. A study of people over age 75 divided the lifestyles of the participants into 5 categories: Family-Oriented, Work-Oriented, Hobby-club Oriented, Quiet-life Living and Illness-Centered (Lähteenmäki and Kaikkonen 2008). Table 5 shows some likely communication needs associated with each and should illustrate that a 'one size fits all' approach to auditory rehabilitation is inappropriate. For instance, an individual living a 'Quiet-life Living' life-style, who primarily communicates with just one other person at home would likely be satisfied with a hearing aid that has omnidirectional microphones, an automatic telecoil, and no volume control. Someone living a 'Work-Oriented' or 'Hobby-club Oriented' life-style might want a hearing aid with a personal FM system with a wireless microphone to enhance communication during meetings and at restaurants. On the other hand, someone living an 'Illness-Centered' life-style, who does not want to deal with a hearing aid, might benefit most from an infrared personal television amplifier, an amplified telephone, and a wireless doorbell system.

In other words, when planning an auditory rehabilitation program, the needs and priorities of the patient should be taken into account. This can be done through an interview, or by having the patient complete a questionnaire like the Client Oriented Scale of Improvement (COSI; Dillon, James and Ginis 1997) or the Glasgow Hearing Aid Benefit Profile (GHABP; Gatehouse 1999). These questionnaires have the patient identify listening situations in which he/she specifically wants improved ability to hear (the COSI) or in which he/she considers it important to hear as well as possible (the GHABP). Once an individual's communication priorities have been established, the clinician can focus on designing auditory rehabilitation to optimize outcome for those particular listening situations.

Patient–Provider Communication

Cognitive aging will affect patient-provider communication, because as described above, elderly patients with even minimal peripheral hearing loss need longer time to process information, are likely to remember less of the information provided, and will fatigue sooner than younger patients with the same level of hearing. Further, if the patient is also visually impaired, he/she will be less able to use speech-reading and subtle non-verbal cues such as gestures, facial expressions, and body posture, than people with normal vision. Speech reading can improve sentence identification by up 60% over using auditory cues alone (Walden, Busacco, and Montgomery 1993). Non-verbal cues provide important metalinguistic information; specifically, facial expressions and posture can reveal the emotions of the speaker, gestures often provide information that supplement the verbal content, and eye contact provides an emotional link between the speaker and the listener. Another consequence of vision loss is an inability to clearly see written materials, such as informational brochures, prescription directions, referrals, and instructions on using medical devices. In fact,

Table 5 Five Life-styles of Elderly Individuals and Communication Situations Likely Encountered

Life-Styles	Likely Important Listening Situations			
Family-oriented	One-on-one in quiet	Young children	Dinner table	Telephone
Work-oriented	Group meetings	Telephone	Restaurants	
Hobby-club oriented	Group meetings	Noisy places	Restaurants	
Quiet-life living	One-on-One in quiet	TV	Telephone	Dinner table
Illness-centered lifestyle	One-on-one in quiet	TV	Telephone	

studies have shown that a major reason older people abandon assistive technology is that they don't know how to use it (Gitlin 1995). It should be the responsibility of the physician to ensure (a) the patient is following the content of all communication, (b) any written materials provided can be seen and understood by the patient, and (c) that they can troubleshoot and provide basic maintenance of a hearing aid. Short videos addressing this can be found online from, for example, Starkey: http://www.starkey.com/use_care/instrctional_videos.jsp.

Below are some simple guidelines for communicating with elderly patients, whether or not, but especially if, they have hearing impairment:

- Talk slowly, avoid redundancy, but include repetition.

- Light the office space with bright incandescent overhead lighting to avoid creating glare, but to optimize visibility (Kricos and Lesner 1995).

- Ensure your face can be clearly seen by making sure not to sit in front of a window or far from the patient across a large desk, to increase ease of lipreading.

- Provide written materials to reinforce verbal information. Encourage the patient to read them at home in a quiet non-stressful environment to ensure the information is understood and remembered.

- Have a magnifying glass and a portable personal listening device available for use in case the patient has forgotten, or does not have, eye glasses and/or hearing aids.

- Keep some hearing aid batteries of different sizes available in the office in case the patient's hearing aid batteries are dead.

In summary, patient-provider communication is a critical aspect of patient care, particularly as the older adult population has a higher prevalence of chronic disease than younger adults, and thus has the greatest need to engage in health-promoting behaviors. As pointed out by Kaplan (1996), "The goal of aural rehabilitation is to find the least expensive most versatile durable system that will address as many of the users communication needs as possible." Many of the recommendations in this chapter are applicable to anyone with hearing impairment, but are especially helpful to the older individuals whose limitations tend to go beyond the auditory system alone. It is essential that the physician to be aware of the potential for hearing impairment, to make the necessary referrals, and to ensure that communication with that patient is optimized.

Essential Points

- The prevalence of presbycusis rises with age, such that it affects about 50% of 50–59 year olds, about 75% of 60–69 year olds, and more than 80% of patients over age 85 years.

- Signs of presbycusis include gradual bilateral onset of hearing loss, difficulty understanding speech especially in noise, and problems hearing high-frequency sounds

- If not remediated, presbycusis can contribute to isolation and depression.

- Treatment of hearing loss with appropriately-fitted hearing aids and/or assistive listening devices, along with communication skills training, improves function and quality of life.

- When selecting hearing aids for older individuals it is important to consider: the nature and degree of hearing loss, the person's ability to manipulate the aid and adapt to its use, the persons

communication needs, and the social support and financial resources available to him or her.

- All elderly people should be screened at least annually for hearing loss.

- Physicians should take a role in the identification of hearing loss, and in making appropriate referrals for additional evaluation and treatment.

References

Bess, F. (1995). Applications of the Hearing Handicap Inventory for the Elderly—Screening Version (HHIE-S). *The Hearing Journal, 48*(6), 10, 51–57.

Bovo, R., Ciorba, A., and Martini, A. (2007). Genetic factors in noise-induced hearing loss. *Audiological Medicine, 5*(5), 25–32.

Cruickshanks, K., Klein, R., Klein, B., Wiley, T., Nondahl, D., and Tweed, T. (1998). Cigarette smoking and hearing loss: The epidemiology of hearing loss study. *The Journal of the American Medical Association, 279*(21), 1715–1719.

Culbertson, D., Griggs, M., and Hudson, S. (2004). Ear and hearing status in a multilevel retirement facility. *Geriatric Nursing, 25*(2), 93–98.

DeStefano, A., Gates, G., Heard-Costa, N., et al (2003). Genomewide linkage analysis to presbycusis in the Framingham Heart Study. *Archives of Otolaryngology Head Neck Surgery, 129*(3) 285–9.

Dillon, H., James, A., and Ginis, J. (1997). The Client Oriented Scale of Improvement (COSI) and its relationship to several other measures of benefit and satisfaction provided by hearing aids. *Journal of the American Academy of Audiology, 8*, 27–43.

Donaldson, J. and Watson, R. (1996). Loneliness in elderly people: An important area for nursing research. *Journal of Advanced Nursing, 24*(5), 952–959.

Frisina, R., (2001). Subcortical neural coding mechanisms for auditory temporal processing. *Hearing Research, 158*(1–2), 1–27

Frisina, S., Mapes, F., Kim, S., Frisina, D., and Frisina, R. (2006). Characterization of hearing loss in aged type II diabetics. *Hearing Research, 211*(1–2), 103–113.

Gatehouse, S. (1999). Glasgow Hearing Aid Benefit Profile: Derivation and validation of a client-centered outcome measure for hearing-aid services. *Journal of the American Academy of Audiology, 10*, 80–103.

Gates, G., Cobb, J., D'Agostino, R., and Wolf, P. (1993). The relation of hearing in the elderly to the presence of cardiovascular disease and cardiovascular risk factors. *Archives of Otolaryngology - Head and Neck Surgery, 119*(2), 156–161.

Gates, G., Couropmitree, N., and Myers, R. (1999). Genetic associations in age-related hearing thresholds. *Archives of Otolaryngology - Head and Neck Surgery, 125*(6), 654–659.

Gates, G., Murphy, M., Rees, T., and Fraher, A. (2003). Screening for handicapping hearing loss in the elderly. *Journal of Family Practice, 52*(1), 56–62.

Gates, G. and Rees, T. (2003). *Geriatric medicine: An evidence-based approach* (4th ed.). New York: Springer.

Gates, G., Schmid, P., Kujawa, S., Nam, B., and D'Agostino, R. (2000). Longitudinal threshold changes in older men with audiometric notches. *Hearing Research, 141*(1–2), 220–228.

Gitlin, L. (1995). Why older persons accept or reject assistive technology. *Generations, Spring*, 41–46.

Gordon-Salant, S. and Fitzgibbons, P. (2001). Source of age-related recognition difficulty for time-compressed speech. *Journal of Speech, Language and Hearing Research, 44*, 709–719.

Guimaraes, P., Frisina, S., Mapes, F., Tadros, S., Frisina, D., and Frisina, R. (2006). Progestin negatively affects hearing in aged women. *Proceedings of the National Academy of Sciences, 103*(38), 246–249.

Hederstierna, C., Hultcrantz, M., Collins, A., and Rosenhall, U. (2007). Prevalence of hearing loss, audiometric configuration and relation to hormone replacement therapy. *Acta Oto-Laryngologica, 127*(2), 149–155.

Humes, L. and Wilson, D. (2003). An examination of changes in hearing aid performance and benefit in the elderly over a 3-year period of hearing aid use. *Journal of Speech, Language and Hearing Research, 46*, 137–145.

Jacobson, M., Kim, S., Romney, J., Zhu, X., and Frisina, R. (2003). Contralateral suppression of distortion-product otoacoustic emissions declines with age: A comparison of findings in CBA mice with human listeners. *Laryngoscope, 113*(10), 1707–1713.

Jaroff, L. (1989). The Gene Hunt. Time Magazine 20 March: 62–67.

Jerger, J. (1972). Audiological findings in aging. *Advances in Otorhinolaryngology, 20*, 115–124.

Kaplan, H. (1996). Assistive devices for the elderly. *Journal of the American Academy of Audiology, 7*(3), 203–211.

Karlsson, K., Harris, J., and Svartengren, M. (1997). Description and primary results from an audiometric study of male twins. *Ear and Hearing, 18*(2), 114–120.

Kochkin, S. (2005a). Customer satisfaction with hearing instruments in the digital age. *The Hearing Journal, 58*(9), 30–44.

Kochkin, S. (2005b). MarkeTrak VII: Hearing loss population tops 31 million people. *The Hearing Review, 12*(7), 16–29.

Kochkin, S. (2007). MarkeTrak VII: Obstacles to adult non-user adoption of hearing aids. *The Hearing Journal, 60*(4), 24–46.

Kochkin, S. and Rogin, C. (2000). Quantifying the obvious: The impact of hearing instruments on the quality of life. *The Hearing Review, 7*, 6–34.

Kricos, P. and Lesner, S. (1995). *Audiologic rehabilitation for the elderly: A practical approach to rehabilitation.* Boston: Butterworth-Heinemann.

Kumar, M., Hickey, S., and Shaw, S. (2000). Manual dexterity and successful hearing aid use. *Journal of Laryngology and Otology, 114*, 593–597.

Lähteenmäki, M. and Kaikkonen, A. (2008). *Designing for aged people communications needs.* Retrieved 9/28/08, 2008, from http://www.dcs.gla.ac.uk/utopia/workshop/lahteenmaki.pdf

Mahoney, D. (1993). Cerumen impaction. Prevalence and detection in nursing homes. *Journal of Gerontological Nursing, 19*(4), 23–30.

McCoy, S., Tun, P., Cox, L., Colangelo, M., Stewart, R., and Wingfield, A. (2005). Hearing loss and perceptual effort: Downstream effects on older adults' memory for speech. *Quarterly Journal of Experimental Psychology. A: Human Experimental Psychology, 58*(1), 22–33.

Meister, H., Lausberg, I., Kiessling, J., von Wedel, H., and Walger, M. (2002). Identifying the needs of elderly, hearing-impaired persons: The importance and utility of hearing aid attributes. *European Archives of Otorhinolaryngology, 259*, 531–534.

Moore, A., Voytas, J., Kowalski, D., and Maddens, M. (2002). Cerumen, hearing, and cognition in the elderly. *Journal of the American Medical Directors Association, 3*(3), 136–139.

Morata, T. (1998). Assessing occupational hearing loss: Beyond noise exposures. *Scandinavian Audiology, Suppl. 48*(111–116).

Morton, N. (1991). Parameters of the human genome. *Proceedings of the National Academy of Sciences, 88*(7474–7476).

Mulrow, C., Aguilar, C., Endicott, J., Tuley, M., Velez, R., Charlip, W., et al. (1990). Quality-of-life changes and hearing impairment: A randomized trial. *Annals of Internal Medicine, 113*, 188–194.

National Health Interview. (1994). *National Health Interview Survey on Disability.* Retrieved 8/14/08, 2008, from http://www.cdc.gov/nchs/about/major/nhis_dis/nhis_dis.htm

Palomar, G., Abdulghani, M., Bodet, A., Andreu, M., and Palomar, A. (2001). Drug-induced ototoxicity: Current status. *Acta Oto-Laryngologica, 121*(5), 569–572.

Parving, A. and Philip, B. (1991). Use and benefit in the tenth decade—and beyond. *Audiology, 30*(2), 61–69.

Plomp, R. and Mimpen, A. (1979). Speech-reception threshold for sentences as a function of age and noise level. *Journal of the Acoustical Society of America, 66*(5), 1333–1342.

Pujol, R. and Puel, J. (1999). Excitotoxicity, synaptic repair, and functional recovery in the mammalian cochlea: A review of recent findings. *Annals of the New York Academy of Sciences, 884*(249–254).

Roland, P., Rybak, L., Hannley, M., Matz, G., Stewart, M., Manolidis, S., et al. (2004). Animal ototoxicity of topical antibiotics and the relevance to clinical treatment of human subjects. *Otolaryngology Head Neck Surgery, 130*(557–578).

Rosenhall, U. and Sundh, V. (2006). Age-related hearing loss and blood pressure. *Noise and Health, 8*(31), 88–94.

Saunders, G., Cienkowski, K., Forsline, A., and Fausti, S. (2005). Normative data for the Attitudes Towards Loss of Hearing Questionnaire. *Journal of the American Academy of Audiology, 16*, 637–652.

Schow, R. and Goldbaum, D. (1980). Collapsed ear canals in the elderly nursing home population. *Journal of Speech and Hearing Disorders, 45*(259–267).

Schuknecht, H. (1964). Further observations on the pathology of presbycusis. *Archives of Otolaryngology - Head and Neck Surgery, 80*(369–382).

Schuknecht, H. and Gacek, M. (1993). Cochlear pathology in presbycusis. *The Annals of Otology, Rhinology & Laryngology, 102*(2), 1–16.

Stach B.A, Jerger J., and Fleming K. (1985). Central presbycusis: A longitudinal case study. *Ear Hearing, 6*(6), 304–306.

Torre, P. R., Cruickshanks, K., Klein, B., Klein, R., & Nondahl, D. (2005). The association between cardiovascular disease and cochlear function in older adults. *Journal of Speech, Language and Hearing Research, 48*(2), 473–481.

US Census Bureau. (2008). *U.S. Population Projections.* Retrieved 9/25/2008, 2008, from http://www.census.gov/population/www/projections/files/nation/summary/np2008-t2.xls

Vaughan, N., Storzbach, D., and Furukawa, I. (2006). Sequencing versus nonsequencing working memory in understanding of rapid speech by older listeners. *Journal of the American Academy of Audiology, 17*(7), 506–518.

Walden, B., Busacco, D., and Montgomery, A. (1993). Benefit from visual cues in auditory-visual speech recognition by middle-aged and elderly persons. *Journal of Speech and Hearing Research, 36*(2), 431–436.

Walden, B., Surr, R., and Cord, M. (2003). Real-world performance of directional microphone hearing aids. *The Hearing Journal, 56*(11), 40–47.

Weinstein, B. (1994). Age-related hearing loss: How to screen for it, and when to intervene. *Geriatrics, 49*(8), 40–45.

Willott, J. (1996). Physiological plasticity in the auditory system and its possible relevance to hearing aid use, deprivation effects, and acclimatization. *Ear and Hearing, 17*(3), 66–77.

Wilson, C. and Stephens, D. (2002). Reasons for referral and attitudes toward hearing aids: Do they affect outcome? *Clinical Otolaryngology, 28*, 81–84.

Wingfield, A., McCoy, S., Peelle, J., Tun, A., and Cox, L. (2006). Effects of adult aging and hearing loss on comprehension of rapid speech varying in syntactic complexity. *Journal of the American Academy of Audiology, 17*(7), 487–497.

Wingfield, A., Panizzon, M., Grant, M., Toomey, R., Kremen, W., Franz, C., et al. (2007). A twin-study of genetic contributions to hearing acuity in late middle age. *The Journals of Gerontology Series A: Biological Sciences and Medical Sciences, 62*(11), 1294–1299.

Yost, W. (2007). *Fundamentals of hearing: An introduction* (5th ed.). Bedford MA: Academic Press.

32 Dizziness in the Elderly

Larry E. Davis

Introduction

Complaints of dizziness and vertigo are common in the elderly. Each year, dizziness sufficient enough to interfere with daily activities ranks as the third most common complaint for which elderly patients seek medical attention (Minor and Zee 2003). After the age of 75 years, dizziness becomes the most common complaint to primary care physicians (Baloh et al. 1992). One interview study of individuals at age 75 years found postural and balance disturbances in 40% of the women and 30% of the men (Sixt and Landahl 1987). Fifteen percent complained of intermittent vertigo. One-third described the problem as daily and one-fifth had fallen from the dizziness.

The evaluation of dizziness challenges the problem-solving ability of the clinician since the causes are many (Table 1). It is not uncommon that no diagnosis is made and no treatment is offered, which often leaves patients unsatisfied with the medical encounter. The consequences of dizziness can be serious as all forms of dizziness may lead to falls. It only takes a visit to the orthopedic floor of any hospital to observe the serious consequences of hip fractures that some elderly sustain after falling from being dizzy. This chapter discusses the components of normal balance, explores why the prevalence of dizziness increases with age, and covers the major causes of dizziness and their management options. The chapter assumes that the practitioner does not have a comprehensive vestibular clinical laboratory easily available.

Components of Normal Balance and Changes with Aging

Before discussing dizziness and vertigo, it is useful to understand the major components of normal balance. In simple terms, there are three major sensory inputs a person utilizes to maintain normal erect balance while standing and walking. The first sensory system starts with the peripheral position sensors located primarily in the joints of the feet that provide afferent sensory information about the position of the legs in space, characteristics of the floor, and movement of the feet. These position sensors send relevant afferent signals to the spinal cord via myelinated sensory nerves. Second order sensory nerves transmit the signal up the dorsal columns providing information to integrating centers in the medulla and pons and to consciousness in the cerebral cortex. It is common in the elderly to have impaired position sensors in the feet with peripheral neuropathies being the most common cause (Table 1). Loss of position sense in the feet can also occur following damage to the spinal cord dorsal columns as seen in vitamin B12 deficiency.

The second sensory system is the visual system that detects the horizon and deviation from it. Signals from the visual cortex are transmitted down to the same integrating centers in the medulla and pons. Vision provides important sensory input for keeping balance while in motion. As a person ages, visual acuity, dark adaptation, and accommodation diminish. Vision may also be impaired by cataracts, glaucoma, macular degeneration, or diabetic retinopathy (Table 1). Appropriate eye movements occur to allow optimal visual acuity with the target on the fovea as we move the head about. Control of the ocular muscles occurs via the vestibulo-ocular reflex for eye rotation and the visual system for vergence or accommodation to bring the target into best visual acuity by placing the target simultaneously on both fovea. Dysfunction of ocular muscles can produce diplopia or blurred vision and a sensation of dizziness.

The third sensory system is the inner ear vestibular system located bilaterally in the temporal bone adjacent to the cochlea. The vestibular system senses motion responding to changes in head or body spatial orientation to maintain body position and balance. It also holds visual

Table 1 Common Contributors to Dizziness and Vertigo in the Elderly by Anatomic Location

Vestibular System

    Benign positional vertigo

    Vestibular neuritis

    Meniere's disease

    Vestibular migraine

    Chronic vestibulopathy

Proprioceptive System

    Sensory peripheral neuropathy from

        Diabetes mellitus

        Alcoholism

        Vitamin B12 deficiency

    Spinal cord posterior column dysfunction

        Vitamin B12 deficiency

        Spinocerebellar atrophy

        Tabes dorsalis

Visual System

    Recent diplopia

    Mature cataracts bilaterally

    Glaucoma

    Macular degeneration

    Diabetic retinopathy

    Large refraction change in glasses, especially with plus lenses

Table 1 Continued

Brainstem and Cerebellum

Structural

Infarction (lateral medullary syndrome, cerebellar infarct)

Tumor (pontine glioma, cerebellar tumor)

Degenerative (multiinfarct dementia, multiple sclerosis)

Congenital (Chiari type 1)

Metabolic

Hypoglycemia, hyperglycemia

Hypothyroidism

Hyperventilation syndrome

Cardiovascular

Cardiac

Cardiac arrhythmia

Heart failure

Vascular

Orthostatic hypotension

Vasovagal syndrome

Hypoxia from chronic obstructive pulmonary disease, carbon monoxide, severe anemia

---

images steady on the retina during head rotation. Signals from the vestibular system travel to brainstem vestibular nuclei located at the junction of pons and medulla. Subsequent signals are sent to ocular and antigravity muscles and to the integrating center. The vestibular system is capable of remarkable neuroplasticity, enabling correcting adaptations to occur throughout life. However, after 40 years of age, histologic studies show vestibular primary afferent neurons and hair cells begin degenerating. This is reflected in a decline of vestibular function as determined by vestibular function tests. The speed and quality of adaptive changes slows with aging. Damage to one peripheral vestibular system in young patients results in transient vertigo for weeks that usually spontaneously resolves. Unfortunately, damage to the peripheral vestibular system in elderly patients may not always result in complete recovery, leaving them with permanent dizziness.

A fourth controversial sensory system is position sensors in the joints of the cervical vertebrae and posterior neck muscles. Its importance for normal balance in humans is uncertain but dysfunction of this system occasionally gives rise to dizziness upon turning the neck, particularly following a whiplash injury (Wrisley et al. 2000).

In summary, these sensory systems send critical information needed for normal balance to the brainstem integrating center where appropriate signals are sent to the ocular and antigravity muscles to maintain balance and prevent the world from spinning. Of importance, this sensory integration is sufficiently plastic and overlapping to maintain balance should one of the three sensory systems become impaired. The exception occurs in some elderly individuals who experience persistent dizziness because of preexisting dysfunction of multiple sensory systems.

Overview of Dizziness

The prevalence and types of dizziness in the elderly varies considerably because studies often have been performed in specialized neurotology clinics and reflect a bias towards the more severe and unusual forms of dizziness. However, one large epidemiological study explored dizziness in 1,622 community-dwelling adults 60 years and older in the southern U.S. (Sloane et al. 1989). They found the overall prevalence of dizziness to be 29% with a one-year incidence of 18% that was severe enough to seek a physician, take medication for dizziness, or interfere with daily activities. When compared to adults who denied dizziness, the authors found major predictors for dizziness to be: 1) neurosensory symptoms such as numbness in the legs, difficulty walking, poor vision, or neurologic disease, 2) cardiovascular disease or taking heart or blood pressure medication, and 3) psychiatric problems such as depression, anxiety, self perception as a nervous person, or taking psychoactive medication. The authors noted that patients tended to fall into two large groups—those with multisensory, cardiovascular, or high medication use and those with heightened self-awareness from depression, anxiety, or somatization. This study is similar to other reports (Belal and Glorig 1986; Davis 1994; Drachman and Hart 1972; Kroenke et al. 1992) that found dizziness did not predict death or institutionalization in the following 6–12 months, suggesting that for most the etiologies were chronic but not fatal.

History, Examination and Testing of a Dizzy Patient

Dizziness is a general term that most patients describe when they see a provider. It usually implies the patient experienced dysequilibrium, light headedness, or spinning. Careful questioning is necessary to further define the type of dizziness, which usually can be divided into four categories: vertigo, dysequilibrium, presyncope, and other.

To determine which category of dizziness best fits the patient's complaints, a careful history is the key. Almost all patients begin with the word dizziness. It is important to encourage the patient to amplify the description. Table 2 lists some characteristics of the history that are helpful. Side effects of medications are common in patients with

---

Table 2 Helpful Information in the History of a Dizzy Patient

1. Vertigo or Dizziness?

- Vertigo is the illusion that the room or person is spinning or tilting and implies dysfunction of the peripheral or central vestibular system

  - Information whether the vertigo is horizontal, vertical, rotary, or jumpy helps identify location of the vestibular dysfunction

- Dizziness has many descriptions but is not a spinning sensation

  - Implies dysfunction of one or more sensory systems (proprioception visual, vestibular) as well as brainstem or cerebellum

  - Cause may be structural, metabolic, or psychogenic

2. Loss of Consciousness or Feeling of Impending Faint?

- Syncope suggests cardiovascular cause such as orthostatic hypotension, vasovagal syncope, or cardiac arrhythmia

3. Duration of Vertigo Episode

- Seconds (less than a minute): Consider benign paroxysmal positional vertigo

- Hours: If recurrent and with unilateral hearing loss and tinnitus, consider Meniere's disease

---

Table 2 Continued

- Days: If only episode and without hearing changes, consider vestibular neuritis

- Continuous: Many causes but consider drug toxicity

4. Episode Triggers

- Head or body movements: If triggered by vertical head movement and is brief, consider benign paroxysmal positional vertigo

- Head position: If occurs with head hyperextended, consider vertebral artery stenosis at a cervical vertebrae

- Particular time of day: Many causes but consider hypoglycemia or adverse effect of medication taken within the hour

- When anxious: Consider panic or anxiety attack with hyperventilation

- If only when standing, consider orthostatic hypotension

- If only when coughing or urinating, consider post-tussive or micturation presyncope

5. Associated Symptoms or Signs

- Numbness or burning in feet—Consider proprioceptive dysfunction in feet

- Diplopia or new glasses—Consider visual dysfunction

- Recent unilateral hearing loss or tinnitus—Consider vestibular dysfunction

- Cranial nerve palsies—Consider brainstem dysfunction

- Chest pain, shortness of breath, leg edema—Consider cardiovascular or pulmonary problem

6. Medications (see Table 3 for common offenders)

- Always review all medications including over-the-counter and herbal medications

- Consider a medication if symptoms begin shortly after taking specific medications or began with a new medication

Note that elderly patients often have symptoms suggesting several causes.

Table 3 Common Drugs That Cause Dizziness

Vestibulo-Toxic Drugs (May cause permanent damage to the inner ear)

Aminoglycoside antibiotics (such as gentamycin, kanamycin, amikacin, vancomycin)

Cancer chemotherapeutic drugs (such as cisplatin, chlorambucil, vinblastine)

Loop diuretics (such as furosemide)

Central Nervous System Drugs

Sedatives (such as temazepam, lorazepam, diazepam, zolpidem)

Antipsychotic drugs (such as olanzapine, clozapine, haloperidol, quetiapine, risperidone)

Antidepressants (such as amitriptyline, SSRI, SNRI, lithium carbonate)

Anticonvulsants (such as carbamazepine, phenytoin, lamotrigine)

Circulatory Drugs

Vasodilators (such as isosorbide, nitroglycerin)

Ace inhibitors (such as lisinopril, captopril, enalapril)

Angiotensin receptor antagonists (such as losartan, candesartan, eprosartan)

Alpha blockers (such as prazosin, terazosin, tamsulosin)

Beta blockers (such as propanolol, labetalol, timolol, carvelidol)

Calcium channel blockers (amlodipine, nifedipine, nimodipine, verapamil)

Antiarrhythmics (such as amiodarone, mexiletine, flecainide)

Gastrointestinal Drugs

Anti-emetics (such as metoclopramide, ondansetron)

Anti-ulcer drugs (such as cimedtine, rantidine, omepraxole, lansoprazole)

Lipid-regulating drugs (such as simvastatin, atorvastatin, gemfibrozil)

Herbal Medicines and OTC Medications

Since the plant inside the bottle may not match the label, it is difficult to identify specific herbs.

Even excess aspirin can cause tinnitus and dizziness.

For a more extensive list of drugs that cause dizziness see Lee, et al. (2005)

dysequilibrium or presyncope and Table 3 lists some of the common medications that may cause dizziness.

The second step is to conduct a good general and neurological examination with appropriate laboratory tests to corroborate and better understand some of the patient's symptoms. Table 4 lists parts of the examination that are particularly helpful in determining which systems are involved. Table 5 lists several simple vestibular tests that can be conducted in the clinic that help clarify the type of vestibular dysfunction. If the patient complains of dizziness upon moving his head or body, the vestibular-ocular reflex (VOR) may be dysfunctional. One useful test is the head thrust test. Ask the patient to fixate on a target and observe the eyes after passive head thrusts horizontally and vertically. If after the head thrust an observed refixation saccade occurs, it indicates a decreased VOR. The test's sensitivity is moderate (33%) but the specificity is high (95%) (Tusa 2005). The head-shaking nystagmus test is also helpful. Ask the patient to close their eyes, tilt the head down 30 degrees, and then oscillate the head 20 times horizontally. Elicitation of nystagmus after head shaking indicates vestibular imbalance with a moderate sensitivity of 45% but a better specificity of 75% (Tusa 2005).

Laboratory Testing

For many types of dizziness, the history and examination are sufficient to establish the diagnosis, but occasionally laboratory tests are indicated. The MRI is helpful if the vertigo is suspected to be of central origin in the brainstem, cerebellum or cerebellopontine angle or from an infection or tumor of the middle or inner ear. CT is helpful when a fracture across the petrous bone or erosion of bones adjacent to the inner ear is suspected. An electronystagmogram (ENG) performs some of the above vestibular tests and is particularly helpful if the vestibular dysfunction is suspected to be bilateral, as bedside testing often does not determine whether one or both ears are involved. Examples of bilateral involvement include genetic causes and vestibulotoxicity from drugs. Elements of the ENG are described elsewhere in detail (Minor and Zee 2003). Of importance is that mild ENG abnormalities are frequently seen in normal elderly. Thus in general, the ENG

Table 4 Important Aspects in Examination of the Elderly Dizzy Patient

Vestibular System (see Table 5 for more information)

Eye exam for nystagmus

Hallpike maneuver for positional vertigo

Vestibulo-ocular reflex testing for movement induced vertigo

Fistula test for middle to inner ear fistula

Valsalva maneuver for rupture of round or oval window

External ear canal and tympanic membrane exam

Whisper test for hearing acuity

Proprioceptive System

Position sense testing of great toe and vibration testing with 128 cps tuning fork on toes, ankles and shins as necessary

Romberg test

Tandem gait test

Normal gait analysis

Visual System

Visual acuity to near and far vision

Visual field confrontation testing if suggested by history

Fundoscopic eye exam of lens and retina looking for cataracts, disk abnormalities, and retinal disease

Brainstem and Cerebellum

Cranial nerve exam, especially CN V and VII

Finger to nose testing and heel to shin testing

Simple speech evaluation for dysarthria

Cardiovascular System

Heart auscultation for murmurs and arrhythmias

Lying and standing blood pressure for orthostatic hypotension

Table 5 Simple Tests of Eye Movement and the Vestibular System

Eye and Eye Movements

- Observing for nystagmus when eyes are voluntarily moved 20–30 degrees from central gaze suggests gaze-evoked nystagmus. Minor nystagmus at the far end of eye gaze is often benign or due to drugs.

- Observing for head tilt that might suggest fourth cranial nerve palsy

- Extraocular eye movements looking for diplopia from third or sixth nerve palsy

- Ocular alignment using cover/uncover and cross cover tests

- Fundoscopic exam looking for cataracts, disk abnormalities, and retinal disease

Vestibulo-ocular System Tests

- Slow passive head rotation in horizontal or vertical plane with fixation on stationary target looking for catch-up saccadic eye movements.

- Rapid 15-degree head rotations or thrusts with fixation on stationary target looking for catch-up saccadic eye movements.

- Rapid horizontal head shaking for 15 seconds with eyes closed or with Frenzel goggles looking for nystagmus at end of maneuver when the eyes open.

- Looking for brief nystagmus with patient looking straight ahead.

- Vestibular nystagmus often can be suppressed by visual fixation and may be observed during fundoscopic exam of retina with the patient covering the opposite eye. One can often see nystagmus of the retinal blood vessels that disappears when the uncovered eye is opened.

- Dix-Hallpike maneuver looking for directional rotary nystagmus plus brief vertigo attack.

Vestibulo-spinal System Tests

- Tandem gait inability suggests many causes from poor position sense in the feet, orthopedic problems in the knees or hips, muscle weakness, poor vision, cerebellar dysfunction, and dysfunction of vestibulo

- Romberg test inability suggests poor position sense in the feet, cerebellar problems, and dysfunction of the vestibulo

Other Vestibular Tests

- Valsalva-induced nystagmus from closed glottis and pinched nostrils

- Dizziness or vertigo induced by hyperventilation with excessive deep breaths for 2–3 minutes

- Tragal compression-induced nystagmus from pressing the tragus of the ear pinna rapidly against the opening of the external ear canal. This changes the middle ear pressure and can detect a fistula between the middle and inner ear.

findings often support the clinical diagnosis determined by the history and examination but often do not provide additional definitive diagnostic information (Baloh et al. 1989). If syncope is considered, use of a Holter or continuous loop event monitor may detect intermittent cardiac arrhythmias. Examination of the patient on a tilt table may establish the diagnosis of orthostatic hypotension in a difficult patient.

The third step is to narrow down the list of possible diagnoses to the likely category.

Categories of Dizziness and Their Major Causes

The four categories presented below are common causes of dizziness and vertigo in the elderly. Of note, there are many less common etiologies and one is referred to several excellent books on dizziness for these conditions (Baloh 1997; Lustig et al. 2003).

Vertigo

Vertigo, from the Latin *vertere* (to turn), describes the illusion of the person or environment spinning or occasionally tilting and experiencing linear displacement. It results from an imbalance of the tonic vestibular inputs to the brainstem. Patients with vertigo have dysfunction of the vestibular system, which may be peripheral in the inner ear, along the vestibular nerve, central in the pons involving the vestibular nuclei or in the midline of the cerebellum. Patients typically describe a spinning sensation that is horizontal, like a "merry-go-round," vertical like a "Ferris wheel" or directional and rotary, which is often described as the world jumping about. The vertigo can be brief (seconds) or last hours to days and is commonly associated with nausea and vomiting. Peripheral vertigo is not a cause of syncope.

Benign Paroxysmal Positional Vertigo (BPPV)

BPPV is the most common cause of vertigo in the elderly and has a lifetime prevalence of 2.4% (Fife et al. 2008; Davis 1994). BPPV is a clinical syndrome characterized by brief recurrent episodes of vertigo triggered by changes in head position that occurs 85% of the time with movement in the vertical plane. This diagnosis is due to dysfunction of the peripheral labyrinth and excludes lesions in the CNS. Typical symptoms develop when the affected semicircular canal is moving in a vertical plane that is aligned with gravity. In practical terms, the vertigo usually follows vertical head movement. After a brief latency, the patient develops an abrupt whirling or jumping sensation that lasts less than a minute. Repeating the same head movement several times will fatigue the vertigo, often producing a period of hours of vertical head movements that do not trigger vertigo. The vertigo is so brief that the patient does not develop nausea, changes in hearing, tinnitus, or other neurologic symptoms. The patient is frustrated not by the severity of the vertigo but that it occurs unexpectedly. Many patients note that the BPPV often developed after minor head trauma. Current evidence finds that otoconia located in the macula of the utricle break free and fall by gravity usually into the posterior semicircular canal. Thus on vertical head movement, brief asymmetrical signals from the vestibular nerves leaving both posterior SCCs are sent to the brainstem and the mismatching signals produce the transient vertigo.

The clinical diagnosis is usually made (80% sensitivity and 75% specificity) by performing a Dix-Hallpike maneuver on the examining table that triggers a typical vertigo episode with directional-rotary nystagmus seen for several beats (Fife et al. 2008). This maneuver is performed by first turning the head 45 degrees to the right followed by rapidly moving the individual from a sitting position to lying with his head hanging below the examining table. Nystagmus is seen after a delay of a few seconds. If that maneuver does not trigger vertigo, it is repeated with the head turned to the left. Once the diagnosis is made, simple treatment with the canalith repositioning procedure (Epley maneuver) can be performed to often cure the patient (Fife et al. 2008). In essence, the patient is placed in the Dix-Hallpike maneuver position that triggered the attack and then with the head hanging down, the head is rotated slowly towards the opposite side of the body (Fife et al. 2008 has a nice video of the procedure). Most studies find that in about half the patients the BPPV is gone within a few days. If BPPV persists, having the patient repeat the maneuver twice a day at the foot of his bed may then result in a cure. With no treatment, BPPV usually spontaneously subsides over several weeks to a few months. Recurrences are not uncommon.

In 10% of patients the otoconia appear to lodge in one horizontal SCC instead of the posterior SCC. This results in the brief vertigo triggered by rapidly turning the head to the affected ear horizontally.

Vestibular Neuritis

Vestibular neuritis is considered the second most common cause of vertigo in the elderly. Although epidemiological figures are scarce, the incidence appears to be about 3–10/100,000/year. About half the patients describe an upper respiratory illness in the preceding two weeks. The onset is abrupt without warning and the vertigo is usually severe. Patients note a horizontal spinning sensation that causes severe ataxia sufficient to prevent walking without falling. Nausea and vomiting are common and often severe. There is no objective hearing loss

but some patients note fullness in one ear. On exam the patients typically have a horizontal nystagmus with the fast phase away from the involved ear. Falling and tilting are usually toward the side of the involved ear. Available histopathology is limited but has shown degeneration of the vestibular nerve branch going to the horizontal canal and sometimes the utricle (Schuknecht and Kitamura 1981). There may also be neuronal cell death in part of the vestibular ganglia. If caloric tests are performed in a vestibular laboratory, there usually is canal paresis or hypofunction on the involved side. The etiology is unclear but not thought to have a vascular basis. However, in elderly patients it is reasonable to obtain an MRI scan, as up to 15% of these patients have an infarction of the inferior midline cerebellum that mimics vestibular neuritis (Lee et al. 2006).

Management is first to reassure the patient of the benign nature of the symptom, followed by IV administration of anti-vertigo drugs such as promethazine at a dose of 10–25 mg every 4–6 hours as needed. Early administration of corticosteroids (methylprednisolone 100 mg tapered over 21 days or prednisone 1 mg/kg tapered over 21 days) shortens the duration of symptoms but not the extent of clinical recovery (Strupp et al. 2004; Shupak et al. 2008). Addition of acyclovir does not offer improvement in the clinical course over corticosteroids alone (Strupp et al. 2004).

The illness is self-limited as the severe vertigo ends in a few days and symptoms subside over 1–3 weeks. In general, patients should reduce and stop anti-vertigo medication as soon as they can tolerate the vertigo since these drugs may slow the rate of spontaneous recovery (Zee 1985). Recurrences are uncommon.

Meniere's Disease or Idiopathic Endolymphatic Hydrops

Meniere's disease is an inner ear disease characterized by spontaneous unprovoked attacks of vertigo, transient hearing loss during the attack, tinnitus, and aural fullness. Although Meniere's disease accounts for about 10% of patients in specialized neurotology clinics with 15% of the patients being over 65 years, it is far less common in the general population and often over diagnosed by primary care providers.

The frequency of attacks varies widely. Some patients have clusters of attacks while in others the attacks occur once or twice a month and occasionally less often. The attacks usually occur without a warning or recognized trigger and persist one to several hours. The vertigo intensity varies from moderate to severe. Patients describe the abrupt onset of a spinning or twirling motion, an up-and-down rotary sensation, or a dropping sensation (da Costa et al. 2002; Saffadi and Paparella 2008). Nausea and vomiting may develop. There is often a roaring tinnitus, muffled hearing, and a sensation of fullness in the involved ear. Early in the illness there is a loss of low frequency hearing in the involved ear but over time all frequencies are slowly lost until the patient becomes deaf. At that time, episodes of vertigo typically cease as all neurosensory elements of the inner ear are destroyed.

Inner ear pathology shows distention of the endolymphatic fluid-containing spaces (hydrops) of the cochlea and vestibular organs with degeneration of hair cells in the organ of Corti, macula, and ampulla (da Costa et al. 2002; Saffadi and Paparella 2008). Attacks are thought to result from rupture of an endolymphatic membrane, allowing rapid admixture of perilymphatic and endolymphatic fluid that produces electrolyte and ionic changes. The etiology is unknown but the theories suggest attacks may result from inadequate absorption or overproduction of endolymphatic fluid, causing ballooning of endolymphatic fluid compartments and rupture of an endolymphatic fluid membrane.

Treatment for the acute attack is symptomatic and aimed at reducing the vertigo and nausea by administering anticholinergics, antihistamines, benzodiazepines or phenothiazines (da Costa et al. 2002; Saffadi and Paparella 2008). Since the attacks are recurrent, use of promethazine suppositories (25–50 mg) are often beneficial, as nausea/vomiting often prevent use of oral medications. Patients should be warned that these medications may be sedating. There is no simple method to prevent attacks. Low sodium diets and diuretics are commonly administered but a recent Cochrane review did not find strong evidence for a benefit (Thirlwall and Kundu 2006). For patients with incapacitating frequent attacks, administration of small amounts of gentamycin can be injected into the middle ear through the tympanic membrane or directly into the inner ear through the oval or round window. The gentamycin destroys the vestibular sensory system, unilaterally stopping the vertigo attacks but gentamycin also destroys the organ of Corti, resulting in marked hearing loss (da Costa et al. 2002). Rarely in the elderly are surgical procedures performed such as cutting the vestibular nerve. Meniere's disease is usually unilateral but a few patients develop the disease on the opposite side.

Vestibular Migraine

Vestibular migraine is a relatively new category of vertigo that is included in the basilar-type migraine group of the International Headache Society classification system. One survey of migraine patients reported vertigo or dizziness was common and occurred in 52%, especially if they experienced migraine with aura (Vukovic et al. 2007). At the moment there is no clear set of diagnostic features that establish this diagnosis and it is often misdiagnosed as Meniere's disease without auditory findings.

Patients have a history of migraine headaches although a headache often does not develop with each episode of vertigo (Brantberg et al. 2005; Neushauser et al. 2001). Hearing loss or sudden tinnitus should not occur with the vertigo. The episodes last from seconds to hours and occur from once a month to over 40 times a month. Between episodes the balance is normal. Vestibular migraine occurs more commonly in women and younger individuals than in the elderly. There is often a family history of similar vertiginous episodes with migraine. Current criteria for diagnosis include: 1) episodic vestibular symptoms of at least moderate severity that include rotational vertigo, other illusory self or object motion, positional vertigo or head motion intolerance (sensation of imbalance or illusory motion provoked by head movements), 2) current or previous history of migraine, 3) one of the following migraine symptoms during at least two vertigo attacks of migraine headache: photophobia, phonophobia, or visual auras, and 4) no other known cause (Neuhauser et al. 2001).

There are no established treatment protocols or double blind treatment trials for vestibular migraine. Episodes that are infrequent or brief do not require treatment. For frequent episodes that interfere with daily functioning, verapamil (120–240 mg orally daily), nortriptyline (25–50 mg orally daily), or valproate (125–500 mg orally daily) has sometimes been helpful as a prophylaxis. Acute prolonged attacks may benefit from oral meclizine or promethazine (25 mg orally or by rectal suppository).

Cerebrovascular Disease and Vertigo

Brief vertigo as an isolated symptom is rarely caused by a transient ischemic attack or stroke (Kerber et al. 2006). However, vertigo as part of a compilation of other brainstem signs and symptoms is not uncommon in brainstem strokes and transient ischemic attacks. The most well recognized brainstem stroke causing severe vertigo is called a lateral medullary stroke or Wallenberg's syndrome (Mohr and Caplan

2004). These patients have a wedge infarction of the dorsolateral medulla just posterior to the olive that develops from occlusion of the ipsilateral vertebral artery or posterior inferior cerebellar artery. The infarction affects the vestibular nuclei beneath the floor of the fourth ventricle. Patients typically present with acute or subacute vertigo, nausea, vomiting, hiccups, diplopia, ataxia, dysphagia, and dysphonia. They commonly describe feelings of swaying, falling, feeling seasick, or being off-balance (Mohr and Caplan 2004). Others experience true vertigo with a whirling or rotational sensation or feel that they are being pulled by an external force towards the side of the lesion (lateropulsion). There is often a diminished sensation in the ipsilateral face, diminished pain and temperature sensation on the contralateral body, ipsilateral Horner's syndrome, horizontal and frequently rotary nystagmus, and ataxia. The vertigo slowly spontaneously improves over weeks to months.

In about 10% of patients with cerebellar infarctions, vertigo develops from occlusion of the medial branch of the posterior inferior cerebellar artery producing infarction of the nodulus and uvula, key components of the vestibulocerebellum. Patients experience prolonged vertigo and imbalance usually toward the side of the infarction that mimics the more common vestibular neuritis (Lee et al. 2006).

Other Vestibular Diagnoses and Chronic Vestibulopathy

Less common causes of vertigo in the elderly include middle ear infections with inflammatory toxins entering into the inner ear through the round or oval window, trauma to the inner ear, and perilymphatic fistulas from cholesteatomas eroding bone that opens into a perilymphatic space.

Unfortunately, in up to 50% of elderly patients with chronic vertigo, no specific diagnosis can be established and these patients are often coded as chronic vestibulopathy. Symptomatic treatment of these patients is often difficult, especially if the vertigo is intermittent.

Dysequilibrium

Patients complaining of dizziness commonly fall in this category (Fife and Baloh 1993). Dysequilibrium is mainly experienced when standing and often relieved upon sitting or lying down. The imbalance or unsteadiness usually develops from diminished sensory input from the vestibular, visual and proprioceptive systems or input from key motor centers, such as the basal ganglia and cerebellum (Baloh 1992). When there is a mismatch in brainstem input from one or more of the key sensory systems for balance, patients feel dysequilibrium. As an example, remember the odd sensations you felt when entering a "fun house" where the floor tilts downward but the hallway walls are built to give the visual perspective of going upwards. Described below are the more common causes of dysequilibrium.

Loss of Position Sense in the Feet

Patients with loss of position sense in their feet from a neuropathy or posterior column spinal cord disorder typically feel unsteady when standing or walking. Their unsteadiness is accentuated when walking at night as the ability to use vision to compensate is diminished. Sensory neuropathy from diabetes mellitus and chronic alcoholism are the most common but there are other less common etiologies (Table 1).

On exam, patients have diminished vibration appreciation from a 128 hertz tuning fork when placed on their great toe and difficulty in recognizing small movements of the great toe with their eyes closed. Other abnormalities include poor tandem gait (tested by walking a straight line with one foot in front of the other), and sway or falling on the Romberg test (tested by standing with feet together and eyes closed). The ability to improve balance and reduce dysequilibrium is difficult but improvement in glucose control in the diabetic patient or cessation of drinking alcohol may slow or stop the progression of the neuropathy. As such, management is mainly symptomatic aimed at improving balance with balance exercises (see end of chapter) and preventing falls with canes or walkers, placing bars in the shower or bath, and using strong night-lights.

Not to be overlooked in the elderly is B12 deficiency. Among the earliest clinical signs of low B12 serum levels is the slowly progressive loss of vibration and position sense in the feet that usually is out of proportion to loss of touch, temperature appreciation, and autonomic skin changes in the feet. Early diagnosis and treatment with B12 may improve balance.

Multiple Sensory Deficit Syndrome

This syndrome is common in the elderly. One study of elderly men found almost half had more than one sensory deficit to account for their complaint of dizziness (Davis 1994). These patients described being off balance and unsteady when standing or walking and were prone to falls. The classic dysequilibrium patient is the diabetic with loss of position sense in the feet from a peripheral neuropathy and visual impairment from cataracts and diabetic retinopathy. Should these individuals develop any dysfunction of the vestibular system or hypotension on standing, they experience severe dysequilibrium. Performing a physical examination as outlined in Table 4 helps identify the patient with multiple sensory deficits. Management is aimed toward minimizing the consequences of loss of sensory input. For example, if the patient has dense cataracts, surgical removal may improve vision to where dysequilibrium lessens and balance improves.

Bilateral Vestibular Hypofunction

Damage to one inner ear usually triggers vertigo, but damage to both vestibular systems often produces severe dysequilibrium without a sensation of vertigo. Patients are often incapacitated when standing and walking. The most common etiology in the elderly is exposure to vestibulotoxic drugs since genetic causes rarely first manifest in mature adults. While all aminoglycoside antibiotics can damage inner ear hair cells, gentamycin is the most common cause. Gentamycin kills vestibular hair cells more than hair cells in the organ of Corti so patients receiving the antibiotic may not experience marked hearing loss. Cisplatin and carboplatin (anticancer drugs), some macrolide antibiotics such as erythromycin, and loop diuretics can also be ototoxic (Lee 2005). Unfortunately, hair cell damage from gentamycin and cisplatin is irreversible so only symptomatic treatment with vestibular exercises is available. Other less common causes of bilateral vestibulopathy are reviewed elsewhere (Zingler et al. 2007).

Presyncope

Presyncope and syncope in the elderly are common. Presyncope is the feeling of light-headedness or of impending faint that may be associated with a feeling of unsteadiness. Some patients perspire, have palpations, and demonstrate pallor. The symptoms result from hypoperfusion or changes in blood chemical composition to the entire brain, especially the brainstem, and is rarely a symptom of focal cerebrovascular disease. Table 6 lists the more common causes of presyncope in the elderly.

If the cerebral hypoperfusion worsens, the presyncope symptoms are soon followed by syncope (fainting). Syncope is a transient loss of consciousness characterized by unresponsiveness and loss of postural muscle tone. The loss of consciousness is usually brief (less than one minute), followed by spontaneous recovery not requiring resuscitation interventions.

Syncope is in the elderly is estimated to develop at least once in 33% and the incidence increases for individuals over age 70 years (Soteriades et al. 2002). In a study of 822 patients with a mean age of 66 years, the causes of syncope included orthostatic or vasovagal in 31%, cardiac in 10%, medications in 7%, misdiagnosed seizure in 5%, stroke or TIA in 4%, other in 8%, and unknown in 37% (Soteriades et al. 2002). If preexisting cardiac disease was present, a cardiac cause for the syncope rose to 22% and these patients were at increased risk for death. A method to evaluate a patient with syncope is reviewed by Miller and Kruse (2005). Even simple faints can result in the bone fracture and some cardiac arrhythmias are life threatening.

In patients experiencing syncope, the episode may be difficult to distinguish from seizures. Useful clues include that the patient is usually standing and rarely supine and there is a warning feeling of light-headedness that often is followed by a graying and loss of vision. When fainting, patients lose muscle tone, become flaccid, and generally slump down to the floor. In contrast, patients with a generalized tonic clonic seizure become rigid and fall like a log, often hurting themselves. Syncopal patients usually are still for 10 to 60 seconds but may have a few simple muscle jerks. Patients with generalized seizures have a rhythmic shaking of their limbs for 30 seconds to 2 minutes. Post event syncopal patients usually become rapidly alert back to their baseline while seizure patients are confused up to an hour afterwards,

Table 6 Major Causes of Pre-Syncope and Syncope in the Elderly

1. Disorders of blood pressure
   a. Orthostatic hypotension
      i. Hypovolemia
      ii. Loss of blood vessel competence
      iii. Medications such as alcohol, antidepressants, antihypertensives, diuretics, narcotics, nitrates (also see Table 3)
   b. Vasovagal reactions
      i. Carotid sinus hypersensitivity
      ii. Situational syncope
         1. Post-tussive
         2. Micturition
         3. Postprandial
         4. Defecation
         5. Emotional crisis
         6. Visceral or vascular stimulation
2. Autonomic nervous system dysfunction
   a. Autonomic neuropathy from diabetes
   b. Amyloidosis
   c. Multisystem atrophy
   d. Myelopathy
   e. Tabes dorsalis

(Continued)

Table 6 Continued

3. Cardiac dysfunction

   a. Dysrrhythmias

      a. Tachydysrhythmias

      b. Bradydysrthmias

      c. Heart block

   b. Decreased pump function

      a. Myocardial infarction

      b. Cardiodepressive carotid sinus hypersensitivity

   c. Outflow obstruction

      a. Aortic stenosis

      b. Septal hypertrophy

      c. Atrial myxoma

4. Disorders of blood flow

   a. Vertebrobasilar artery insufficiency

   b. Subclavian steal syndrome

   c. Basilar artery migraine

   d. Hypovolemia

5. Metabolic/chemical/respiratory

   e. Hypoglycemia

   f. Hyperventilation

   g. Hypoxemia secondary to respiratory failure

6. Medications

   h. Cardioactive drugs including beta-blockers, calcium channel blockers, digoxin, oral antiarrhythmics

   i. Vasodilators including nitrates, alpha blockers, vasoselective calcium channel blockers

   j. Antihypertensives

   k. Antidepressants

   l. Psychoactive drugs such as atypical antipsychotics

   m. Antianxiety drugs

   n. Sedatives and narcotics

   o. Blood volume depleting drugs such as diuretics

   p. Herbal medications

For more extensive list of medications, see (Olsky and Murray 1990)

sometimes longer. It should be noted that if a syncopal patient cannot lie supine to allow blood to return to the brain, a brief generalized seizure might ensue. A full generalized seizure may develop if the patient has a prolonged cardiac arrhythmia.

Orthostatic Hypotension

Orthostatic hypotension is the most common cause of presyncope in the elderly. A study of 4,931 community living 75-year-old individuals found that asymptomatic orthostatic hypotension developed in 16% and dizziness from the orthostatic hypotension developed in 2% (Rutan et al. 1992). In institutionalized elderly patients, symptomatic postural hypotension was found in 20% (Linzer et al. 1997).

Symptomatic orthostatic hypotension is defined as a reduction in systolic blood pressure of at least 20 mm Hg or diastolic BP of at least 10 mm Hg within three minutes of standing that reproduces the patient's presyncopal symptoms. However, one study reported that orthostatic hypotension can develop in up to 40% of individuals after standing ten minutes (Gibbons and Freeman 2006). After a syncopal episode, the patient should lie down for at least ten minutes before standing.

There are several pathophysiologic causes of presyncope. Moving from the supine to upright position causes rapid pooling of up to 1 liter of blood in the dependent regions of the abdomen and legs. In healthy individuals, the redistribution of the circulating blood volume, cardiac output, and BP is countered by a baroreflex-mediated increase in sympathetic outflow and vagal inhibition leading to an increase in heart rate, cardiac output, and peripheral vascular resistance that maintains adequate blood pressure and cerebral perfusion. A variety of factors in the elderly can interfere with this complex reflex leading to a fall in BP. These include decreased sensitivity of the baroreflex, decline in increased heart rate to upright posture, and underlying cardiac disease with decreased cardiac filling (Lipsitz 1983). Factors predisposing to orthostatic hypotension include blood volume depletion (from vomiting, diarrhea, fluid restriction, or use of diuretic medication), carotid or vertebral artery stenosis, cardiac disease, adrenal insufficiency, diabetes mellitus, Parkinson's disease, myelopathy, peripheral neuropathies, autonomic neuropathies, varicose veins, and excessive antihypertensive medication. A few elderly patients may experience postprandial hypotension with dizziness or syncope during or following a large meal.

Often elderly patients arising from a lying posture note unsteadiness in their gait and a light-headed and dizzy sensation within a few seconds after standing. Stopping and standing may worsen the symptoms as leg muscles do not tighten to force blood upwards from legs. When the BP remains marginally low, the patient may not faint but a light-headed sensation may persist.

Treatment of the patient with presyncope consists of several simple maneuvers to alleviate symptoms. Upon noting symptoms, the patient can lie down or sit down and bend far forward bringing the heart and brain level (Weiling et al. 2004). Methods to prevent presyncope include having the patient sit for a minute before standing, using support hose, participating in exercise programs to improve muscle tone in the legs, and altering their antihypertensive medication. Patients often take several antihypertensive meds at the same time, which can predispose to hypotension for a few hours afterwards. Dividing the medications throughout the day may eliminate some orthostatic hypotension. Terazosin, a drug for benign prostatic hyperplasia, is an alpha-adrenergic blocking agent and may be a cause of orthostatic hypotension, particularly if taken with other antihypertensive agents. In severe cases, pharmacologic agents may be required to maintain blood pressure that include fludocortisone, midodrine, ibuprofen, caffeine, and increased salt intake (Gupta and Lipsitz 2007).

Reflex Mediated Blood Pressure Instability and Vasovagal Syncope

Presyncope and syncope following micturition, defecation, and coughing can occur (Lipsitz 1983). The hypotension comes from these events, creating a Valsalva maneuver (which produces elevated thorax pressure preventing venous return to the heart). Occasionally, difficulty in swallowing can produce presyncope from endobronchial, esophageal, or pharyngeal stimuli triggering afferent impulses carried by the vagus or glossopharyngeal nerves to the vasomotor center of the medulla. These individuals may develop reflex hypotension, bradycardia, or heart block (Hainsworth 2004; Lipsitz 1983). If the above maneuvers are done during monitoring, the BP falls and the heart rate slows.

Vasovagal or vasodepressor syncope is more common in the young patients but does occur in the elderly. The mechanism is incompletely understood but symptoms usually develop while standing. Premonitory signs include intense autonomic nervous system stimulation with weakness, sweating, pallor, nausea, blurred vision, hyperventilation, and a feeling of being unaware of the surroundings. When studied, the patients initially develop an increase in heart rate and blood pressure followed by abrupt peripheral vasodilatation, increased blood flow to muscles, and decrease in venous blood return to the heart (Lipsitz 1983).

Cardiac Arrhythmias

Cardiac arrhythmias are another common cause of presyncope or syncope, especially in the elderly (Table 6). Arrhythmias often cause palpitations with sensations of a rapid or irregular heartbeat. However, most patients with arrhythmias do not actually notice their palpations or may not report them to the doctor. Besides cardiac arrhythmias, other causes to consider for palpations include anxiety or panic attacks, hyperthyroidism, hypoglycemia, cardiac disease, and drugs such as caffeine, theophylline, digitalis, phenothiazines, cocaine, and tobacco (Abbott 2005).

An EKG is recommended in the presyncope workup and can give clues to preexisting cardiac disease or arrhythmias. If a cardiac arrhythmia is suspected, a referral to a cardiologist is recommended (Fogoros 1993). Often identification of the exact arrhythmia requires placement of an ambulatory EKG monitor such as a Holter monitor or event monitor (loop recorder) and sometimes a stress EKG test (Linzer et al. 1997).

Other Causes of Dizziness

This category covers a wide range of sensations that differ from the categories above. Patients complain of swimming, floating, drunkenness, wooziness, dissociation sensations, or visual distortions. The causes range from deconditioning, medication side effects to psychological causes such as anxiety or heightened self-awareness.

Deconditioning Associated Dizziness

Deconditioning in the elderly from bed rest occurs rapidly, often within a week. The changes include cardiovascular (decreased cardiac output and total blood volume), respiratory (atelectasis and hypoxemia), and muscular (loss of strength in legs can be as high as 5% per day) (Harper and Lyles 1988). These factors lead to a feeling of imbalance on getting out of chair, to swaying or falling while standing, walking, or turning. If a patient spends much of his day in bed or in a wheel chair, the deconditioning symptoms persist. Encouraging patients to participate in a physical therapy rehabilitation program helps lessen the symptoms.

Medication Induced Dizziness

Medications are common causes of complaints of dizziness. Well over a hundred drugs have been recognized to cause dizziness as a side effect (Lee et al. 2005). The more common offending medications tend to affect the central nervous or cardiovascular systems (Table 3). Clues that a medication may be the cause include dizziness persisting much of the day, becoming most intense an hour after taking the medication, and rarely producing vertigo. The disorientation and vague dizzy symptoms are often most intense when the drug is started, particularly if not started at low dosage.

Psychoactive drugs such as antidepressants, atypical antipsychotics, and antianxiety drugs are particularly common causes. Cardiovascular medications, such as antiarrhythmic drugs, may produce wooziness while drugs that cause coronary vasodilatation and many antihypertensives may produce presyncope sensations. Anticonvulsants (especially phenytoin and carbamazepine in high dosage) cause dizziness and ataxia. Sleeping pills and sedativesmay produce confusion and dysequilibrium in the morning or at night when the patient arises to void. Of note, some over-the-counter herbal medicines may cause dizziness.

Psychiatric Illnesses and Dizziness

Psychiatric illnesses characterized by chronic dizziness are commonly called phobic postural vertigo, psychogenic dizziness, and psychiatric dizziness. These disorders represent up to 20% of patients attending dizzy clinics (Brant 1996; Kroenke et al. 1992) but are considerably less common in the elderly. Predisposing psychiatric illnesses include chronic anxiety, panic disorders, major phobias such as agoraphobia, and somatization disorders. Symptoms of these patients include unsteadiness, rocking, swaying, fullness in the head, general anxiety, and hyperventilation. The dizzy episodes rarely cause fainting, vertigo, or oscillopsia and are often triggered by situations or environmental conditions that induce anxiety. Psychiatric dizziness occasionally may be the sole cause of the patient's complaints but often other minor causes of dizziness may be heightened by the underlying psychiatric condition (Staab 2006).

Conditions that induce hyperventilation produce dizziness by lowering the carbon dioxide content in blood and raising arterial pH. These arterial changes cause vasoconstriction of cerebral vasculature and biochemical changes in the brainstem. In some patients these biochemical changes can be maintained for prolonged periods without the patient appearing to hyperventilate. Having the patient breathe into a paper bag to increase the carbon dioxide content in their inhalation alleviates the dizziness. Before diagnosing hyperventilation syndrome in the elderly, always insure the patient does not have cardiac or pulmonary conditions that could trigger hyperventilation secondary to hypoxemia.

Traumatic Brain Injury

Mild traumatic brain injury (TBI) is fairly common in the elderly and is often secondary to falls. Studies of younger patients with mild TBI found that chronic dizziness affects about 20% of patients, ranks among the top five post-concussive symptoms, and can persist for months (Chamelian and Feinstein 2004). The symptoms may be from benign positional vertigo or may be non-specific often with spatial dysequilibrium (Hoffer et al. 2004). The symptoms are usually transient but vestibular exercises and rehabilitation are beneficial.

Rehabilitation Exercises for the Dizzy Patient

The above sections have focused on medical treatments for the dizzy patient. In addition, many patients also benefit from rehabilitation exercises aimed at improving balance and reducing their dysequilibrium. For many patients with acute severe vertigo, it is helpful to reassure them that most patients will undergo a natural recovery over several weeks.

The goal for vestibular rehabilitation is to improve the central compensation for a vestibular deficit through performing a series of vestibular exercises. These exercises are typically taught by a physical therapist and should be continued at home. Older individuals with a unilateral vestibular deficit improve slower than younger patients. Individuals with bilateral peripheral vestibular deficits never make a complete recovery but can be taught to strengthen the visual and proprioceptive reflexes to improve balance. Depending on the nature of the vestibular symptoms, several types of vestibular exercises are suggested (Baloh 2000). While these exercises were designed for patients recovering from vertigo, they are also helpful for patients with dysequilibrium.

If dizziness develops from moving the head, simple beneficial exercises include fixating on a target while moving the head. One exercise is to have the patient look at a target directly in front of him and slowly move his head from side to side trying to minimize the target moving or jumping as he turns. Repeat the exercise using up and down head motions. Over time, slowly move the head faster, keeping the target still. A second exercise is to select two targets far enough apart that that the patient has to move his head to look at them. The patient looks at one target and then turns to look at the other without closing his eyes. Slowly increase the rate of head turn speed. Both exercises can be done first sitting and later standing for at least two sessions each day until balance improves.

If the patient has dysequilibrium on walking, walking exercises are beneficial. Have the patient first walk down a long hall with his hand sliding against the wall for balance. Start slowly and then increase speed. The goal is to be able to walk down the middle of the hall in a straight line without using any canes or other assistive devices. Next have the patient start walking outside looking from side to side at the scenery. In the beginning the patient should carefully walk for 5 minutes and then as balance improves slowly increase speed and endurance to about a 30 minute walk. The patient may begin with a cane but should try to advance to where he does not need one. The third exercise is to practice turning by walking independently towards a spot on the wall and then slowly turning his body but not his head while keeping his eyes on the wall spot. During the turn, the patient should quickly close his eyes and move his head back into alignment with the body. He then opens his eyes and walks in a straight line away from the wall. The exercise then can be repeated with the eyes moving in the opposite direction. This exercise should be done several times a day.

Although the degree of balance recovery will depend on the etiology, one study reported after a mean of four sessions of vestibular rehabilitation therapy that two-thirds experience improvement in balance and one-fourth returned to normal (Cass et al. 1996). It is important to remember that some improvement may have been spontaneous from vestibular system neuroplasticity.

In summary, dizziness and dysequilibrium symptoms are very common in the elderly and have many causes and treatments. The condition can be diagnosed usually with clinical methods in the outpatient clinic setting, The majority of cases improve over time with treatment and exercises but symptoms often recur. It is important to address the problem aggressively since falling, injury and restriction of physical ctivity usually occur.

References

Abbott, A.V.: Diagnostic approach to palpitations. *Am Fam Physician* 71:743–750, 2005.

Baloh, R.W.: *Dizziness, hearing loss and tinnitus.* F.A. Davis, Philadelphia, 1997.

Baloh, R.W.: Vertigo in older people. *Curr Treat Option Neurol* 2:81–89, 2000.

Baloh, R.W.: Dizziness in older people. *J Am Geriatr Soc* 40:713–721, 1992.

Baloh, R.W., Sloane, P.D., and Honrubia, V.: Quantitative vestibular function testing in elderly patients with dizziness. *Ear Nose Throat J* 68:935–939, 1989.

Belal, A. and Glorig, A.: Disequilibrium of aging (presbyastasis). *J Laryngol Otol* 100:1037–1041, 1986.

Brandt, T.: Phobic postural vertigo. *Neurology* 46:1515–1519, 1996.

Brantberg, K., Trees, N., and Baloh, R.W.: Migraine-associated vertigo. *Acta Oto-Laryngol* 125:276–279, 2005.

Cass, S.P., Borello-France, D., and Furman, J.M.: Functional outcome of vestibular rehabilitation in patients with abnormal sensory-organization testing. *Am J Otol* 17:581–594, 1996.

Chamelian, L. and Feinstein, A.: Outcome after mild to moderate traumatic brain injury: The role of dizziness. *Arch Phys Med Rehabil* 85:1662–1666, 2004.

da Costa, S.S., de Sousa, L.C., and de Toledo Piza, M.R.: Meniere's disease: Overview, epidemiology, and natural history. *Otolaryngol Clin N Am* 35:455–495, 2002.

Davis, L.E.: Dizziness in elderly men. *J Am Geriatr Soc* 42:1184–1188, 1994.

Drachman, D.A. and Hart, C.W.: An approach to the dizzy patient. *Neurology* 22:323–334, 1972.

Fife, T.D. and Baloh, R.W.: Disequilibrium of unknown cause in older people. *Ann Neurol* 34:694–702, 1993.

Fife, T.D., Iverson, D.J., Lempert, T., et al.: Practice parameter: Therapies for benign paroxysmal positional vertigo (an evidence-based review). *Neurology* 70:2067–2074, 2008.

Fogoros, R.N.: Cardiac arrhythmias: Syncope and stroke. *Neurol Clin* 11:375–390, 1993.

Gibbons, C.H. and Freeman, R.: Delayed orthostatic hypotension. A frequent cause of orthostatic intolerance. *Neurology* 67:28–32, 2006.

Gupta, V. and Lipsitz, L.A.: Orthostatic hypotension in the elderly: Diagnosis and treatment. *Am J Med* 120:841–847, 2007.

Hainsworth, R.: Pathophysiology of syncope. *Clin Auton Res* 44 (suppl 1):I/18–I/24, 2004.

Harper, C.M. and Lyles, Y.M.: Physiology and complications of bed rest. *J Am Geriatr Soc* 36:1047–1054, 1988.

Hoffer, M.E., Gottshall, K.R., Moore, R., et al.: Characterizing and treating dizziness after mild head trauma. *Otol Neurotol* 25:135–138, 2004.

Kerber, K.A., Brown, D.L., Lisabeth, L.D., et al.: Stroke among patients with dizziness, vertigo, and imbalance in the emergency department. A population-based study. *Stroke* 37:2484–2487, 2006.

Kroenke, K., Lucas, C.A., Rosenberg, M.L., et al.: Causes of persistent dizziness. A prospective study of 100 patients in ambulatory care. *Ann Intern Med* 117:898–904, 1992.

Lee, C.A., Mistry, D., and Coatesworth, A.P.: Otologic side effects of drugs. *J Laryngol Otol* 119:267–271, 2005.

Lee, H., Sohn, S.I., Lee, S.R., et al.: Cerebellar infarction presenting isolated vertigo: Frequency and vascular topographical patterns. *Neurology* 67:1178–1183, 2006.

Linzer, M., Yang, E.H., Estes, M., et al.: Diagnosing syncope. Part 2: Unexplained syncope. *Ann Intern Med* 127:76–86, 1997.

Lipsitz, L.A.: Syncope in the elderly. *Ann Intern Med* 99:92–105, 1983.

Luslig, L.R., Niparko, J., Minor L.B., and Zee, D.S.: *Clinical neurotology: Diagnosing and managing disorders of hearing, balance, and the facial nerve.* Martin Dunitz, London, 2003.

Minor, L.B. and Zee D.S.: Clinical evaluation of the patient with dizziness. In *Clinical neurotology: Diagnosing and managing disorders of hearing, balance, and the facial nerve* (Lustig, L.R., Niparko, J. K., Eds). Martin Dunitz, Taylor & Francis Group, London, 2003, pp81–110.

Mohr, J.P. and Caplan, L.R.: Vertebrobasilar disease. In *Stroke pathophysiology, diagnosis, and management*, Ed. 4 (Mohr, J.R., Choi, D.W., Grotta, J.C., et al., Eds.). Churchill Livingston, Philadelphia, 2004, pp245–251.

Neuhauser, H., von Brevern, L.M., Arnold, G., and Lempert, T.: The interrelations of migraine, vertigo and migrainous vertigo. *Neurology* 56:436–441, 2001.

Olsky, M. and Murray, J.: Dizziness and fainting in the elderly. *Emerg Med Clin N Amer* 8:295–307, 1990.

Rutan, G.H., Hermanson, B., Bild, D.E., et al.: Orthostatic hypotension in older adults. The Cardiovascular Health Study. *Hypertension* 19:508–519, 1992.

Saffadi, H. and Paparella, M.M.: Meniere's disease. *Lancet* 372:406–414, 2008.

Schuknecht, H.F. and Kitamura, K.: Second Louis H. Clerf Lecture. Vestibular neuritis. *Ann Otol Rhinol Laryngol* Suppl 90(1 Pt 2):1–19, 1981.

Shupak, A., Issa, A., Golz, A. et al: Prednisone treatment for vestibular neuritis. *Otol Neurotol* 29:368–374, 2008.

Sixt, E. and Landahl, S.: Postural disturbances in a 75-year-old population: I. Prevalence and functional consequences. *Age Ageing* 16:393–398, 1987.

Sloane, P., Blazer, D., and George, L.K.: Dizziness in a community elderly population. *J Am Geriatr Soc* 37:101–108, 1989.

Soteriades, E.S., Evans, J.C., Larson, M.G., et al.: Incidence and prognosis of syncope. *N Engl J Med* 347:878–885, 2002.

Staab, J.P.: Chronic dizziness: The interface between psychiatry and neuro-otology. *Curr Opin Neurol* 19:41–48, 2006.

Strupp, M., Zingler, V.C., Arbusow, V., et al.: Methylprednisolone, valciclovir, or the combination for vestibular neuritis. *N Engl J Med* 351:354–361, 2004.

Thirlwall, A.S. and Kundu, S.: Diuretics for Meniere's disease or syndrome. *Cochrane Database Syst Rev* 3:CD003599, 2006.

Tusa, R.J.: Bedside assessment of the dizzy patient. *Neurol Clin* 23: 655–673, 2005.

Vukovic, V., Plavec, D., Galinovic, I., et al: Prevalence of vertigo, dizziness, and migrainous vertigo in patients with migraine. *Headache* 47:1427–1435, 2007.

Wieling, W., Colman, N., Krediet, C.T.P., and Freeman, R.: Nonpharmacological treatment of reflex syncope. *Clin Auton Res* 14(suppl 1):I62–I70, 2004.

Wrisley, D.M., Sparto, P.J., Whitney, S.L, and Furman, J.M.: Cervicogenic dizziness: A review of diagnosis and treatment. *J Orthoped Sports Phys Ther* 30:755–766, 2000.

Zee, D.S.: Perspectives on the pharmacotherapy of vertigo. *Arch Otolaryngol* 111:609–612, 1985.

Zingler, V.C., Cnyrim, C., Jahn, K., et al.: Causative factors and epidemiology of bilateral vestibulopathy in 255 patients. *Ann Neurol* 61:524–532, 2007.

33 Taste and Smell in Aging

Richard L. Doty

Introduction

Changes in the ability to taste and smell are common in later life and are not inconsequential. For example, in addition to being at greater risk from food poisoning, a disproportionate number of the elderly die from accidental gas poisonings and explosions (Chalke et al. 1958). In a study of 445 patients representing a range of ages, at least one hazardous event, such as failure to detect fire or leaking natural gas, was reported by 45.2% of those with anosmia, 34.1% of those with severe hyposmia, 32.8% of those with moderate hyposmia, 24.2% of those with mild hyposmia, and 19.0% of those with normal olfactory function (Santos et al. 2004).

Aside from safety issues is the fact that chemosensory loss impacts quality of life and can lead to decreased motivation to eat, as well as to nutritional deficiencies. In a study of 750 consecutive patients presenting to our center with complaints of taste or smell dysfunction, 68% experienced decreased quality of life, 46% changes in appetite or body weight, and 56% adverse influences on daily living or psychological well-being (Deems et al. 1991). Most of the cases of "taste" dysfunction reflected the loss of stimulation of the olfactory receptors via the retronasal route during deglutition (Burdach and Doty 1987). Sweet, sour, bitter, and salty perception is more resilient to major age-related changes, in part because of the redundancy of innervation of taste buds from several cranial nerves (i.e., CN VII, IX, & X). Nonetheless, such decrements in taste function do occur, particularly within circumscribed regions of the tongue and palate. Perhaps most debilitating are age-related distorted or phantom tastes, including persistent salty, sour, or bitter sensations.

This chapter has three main goals: first, to provide a brief overview of the anatomy and physiology of the senses of smell and taste; second, to review the age-related changes that occur in these sensory systems, including those associated with early Alzheimer's disease (AD); and third, to provide a synopsis of medications believed to influence chemosensation in the elderly.

Basic Anatomy and Physiology of the Olfactory System

To be perceived, odorants must first dissolve into the mucus that overlies the olfactory neuroepithelium, a pseudostratified columnar epithelium that lines sectors of the cribriform plate, superior septum, and the superior and middle turbinates. This mucus, which is mostly comprised of Bowman's gland secretions, consists of water, electrolytes, mucopolysaccharides, and proteins (Bradley and Beidler 2003). Some of its proteins degrade toxins and odorants, whereas others aid in transporting water insoluble odorants to the olfactory receptors (Ding and Dahl 2003; Getchell and Getchell 1990).

Once having traversed the mucus, odorants interact with olfactory receptors embedded in cilia that extend from dendritic knobs of bipolar receptor cells—cells that span the entire neuroepithelium (Menco 1997) (Figure 1). Other cell types within the olfactory epithelium include supporting cells, microvillar cells, and basal stem cells. Some of the latter cells differentiate to repopulate damaged or aged cells within the epithelium. Although it was previously believed that the olfactory receptor cells are automatically and continuously replaced over the course of a month or so (Moulton and Beidler 1967), we now know that long-lived receptor cells exist and that complex regulatory mechanisms alter the timing and extent of neurogenesis from the basal cell population (Mackay-Sim 2003). Unfortunately, receptor restoration following damage is often incomplete or nonexistent in both humans and animals.

The unmyelinated axons of the olfactory receptor cells coalesce into multiple bundles, termed the olfactory fila. Each filum contains fascicles ensheathed by glial cells with astrocyte- and Schwann cell mesaxon-like properties that play a role in axon guidance (Menco 1997). The axons of the receptor cells course within the fila through the cribriform plate, where they enter the olfactory bulb, an outgrowth of the forebrain made up of neurons, nerve fibers, microglia,

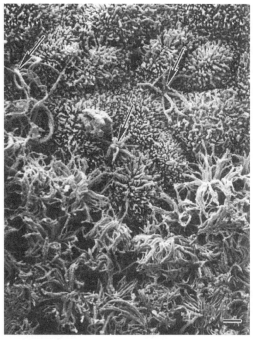

Figure 1 A surface transition region between the olfactory and respiratory epithelia. The bottom half displays olfactory epithelium, the top half respiratory epithelium. Arrows identify olfactory receptor cell dendritic endings with cilia. Bar = 5 μm. From Menco and Morrison (2003), with permission.

astrocytes, and blood vessels (Figure 2). The receptor cell axons synapse with dendrites of the major second-order neurons, the mitral and tufted cells. These synapses occur within the olfactory glomeruli, spherical structures that collectively make up a distinct layer of the bulb. The glomeruli are a major focal point of convergence, with many more neurons entering than leaving. The main transmitter of the olfactory receptor cells is the excitatory amino acid glutamate, which activates both NMDA and non-NMDA receptors on the dendrites of the second-order neurons (Berkowicz et al. 1994). Some cells intrinsic to the olfactory bulb, termed periglomerular cells, influence neural activity among glomeruli and are largely dopaminergic. During periods of intense odorant stimulation, these cells suppress olfactory nerve and mitral/tufted cell activity, in effect decreasing the volume of olfactory bulb output (Wilson and Sullivan 2003). GABAergic cells located in the core of the bulb, termed granule cells, extend processes into more peripheral bulbar layers and modulate olfactory bulb activity as a function of bodily needs such as hunger or arousal (Chen et al. 2000).

The axons of the mitral and tufted cell neurons exit the bulb via the olfactory tract to synapse ipsilaterally in the primary olfactory cortex. The primary components of this cortex are the anterior olfactory nucleus (AON), piriform cortex (the major recipient of the output neurons), anterior cortical nucleus of the amygdala, periamygdaloid cortex, and rostral entorhinal cortex (Figure 3). Some tertiary connections to the opposite hemisphere occur via the AON and anterior commissure.

Our understanding of how the complex machinery of the olfactory system recognizes thousands of odorants has greatly increased in recent years. Each of the estimated 6 to 10 million human olfactory receptor cells expresses one of 390 putative functional receptor genes and 465 pseudogenes (Olender et al. 2008). Olfactory receptor genes are found on all autosomes except chromosome 20, plus the X chromosome but not the Y chromosome (Olender et al. 2008). Axons of receptor cells expressing the same receptor protein project to the same glomeruli, making the glomeruli, in effect, functional units (Grosmaitre et al. 2006; Mombaerts et al. 1996). The receptor-dictated peripheral 'olfactory code' is embedded in the pattern of activity across the glomeruli—a pattern that becomes filtered in the olfactory bulb and ultimately matched to cell assembles largely dictated by experience and bodily state in higher brain structures (Wilson and Stevenson 2003).

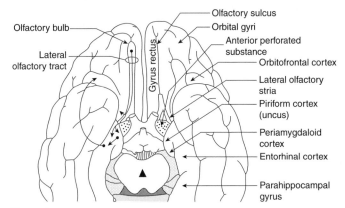

Figure 3 Cortical olfactory projections. From Alloway and Pritchard (2007), with permission.

Basic Anatomy and Physiology of the Taste System

Tastants are sensed by taste buds, goblet-shaped epithelial structures found on the tongue within fungiform, foliate, and circumvallate papillae, as well as on the soft palate, uvula, epiglottis, rostral esophagus, and the mucous membranes covering the laryngeal cartilages (Figure 4). Before entering the apical pore of a taste bud, a tastant must be solubilized into liquid form. Saliva aids in this process and dilutes, buffers, and alters the temperature of ingestants to protect the taste buds and other elements of the oral cavity from damage (Bradley and Beidler 2003). Aside from rinsing away foodstuffs, bacteria, and xenobiotics, saliva maintains taste buds via its trophic properties.

Anatomically, the taste buds contain receptor, supporting, and basal cells arranged in a grapefruit-like manner. As many as 200 taste buds are present in each circumvallate papilla, whereas far fewer buds are present on the other types of papilla. Indeed, many fungiform papillae contain only one or two taste buds. Some tastants, such as hot peppers,

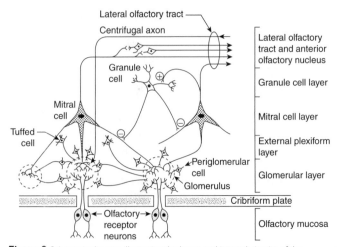

Figure 2 Schematic diagram illustrating the layers and internal circuits of the olfactory bulb. From Alloway and Pritchard (2007), with permission.

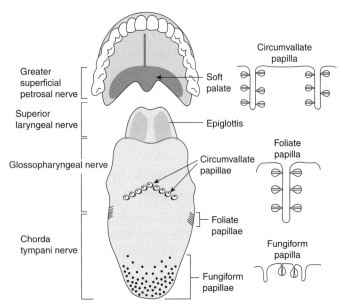

Figure 4 Distribution of taste buds. The distribution for the chorda tympani, glossopharyngeal, superior laryngeal, and superior petrosal nerves are shown on the left side. Cross sections of fungiform, foliate, and circumvallate papillae are shown on the right side. From Alloway and Pritchard (2007), with permission.

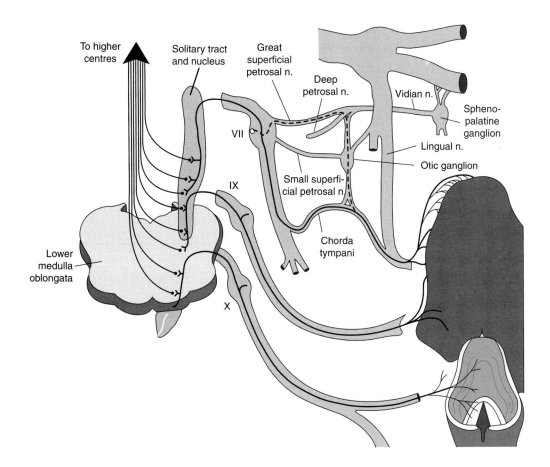

stimulate free nerve endings from CN V located within the oral mucosa, which mediate stinging, burning, and other somatosensory sensations.

The mechanisms of peripheral taste transduction differ according to taste modality (Alloway and Pritchard 2007; Gilbertson et al. 2000). *Salt taste perception* requires dissociation of NaCl into Na^+ and chloride (Cl^-) ions. Transduction begins by diffusion of Na^+ ions through amiloride-sensitive pores located on the surface of receptor cell microvilli. Positively charged Na^+ ions depolarize the receptor cell directly, resulting in the release of neurotransmitter into the synaptic cleft at the base of the cell. A similar process occurs for *sour taste perception*. Protons (H^+) donated by stimuli such as hydrochloric acid flow through amiloride-sensitive sodium channels. Such protons also block the potassium (K^+) channels located on the apical region of the cells, inhibiting the outward flux of K^+ that normally occurs. *Sweet and bitter taste* sensations depend upon specialized receptors located in the cell membrane, rather than on direct activation of ion channels (Chandrashekar et al. 2006). In the case of sweet perception, two separate transduction pathways have been identified, one which activates a G-protein associated adenylate cyclase–cAMP reaction that closes K^+ channels and another which uses an IP_3-mediated pathway to release Ca^{2+} from intracellular stores. The neurotransmitter used by taste buds, as well as by the primary taste nerves, is likely glutamate (Astback et al. 1995; Li and Smith 1997).

The neural projections of the human taste system are complex (Figure 5). The afferent fibers from the buds within the fungiform papillae enter the lingual nerve. There they join the chorda tympani branch of CN VII and merge with its main segment within the petrotympanic fissure of the temporal bone. The nerves that innervate the taste buds of the foliate and circumvallate papillae travel directly to the brainstem within the glossopharyngeal nerve (CN IX). The afferents from the taste buds on the palate travel with the greater superficial petrosal nerve which merges with the facial nerve at the geniculate ganglion. Taste buds of the larynx and esophagus send projections via the vagus nerve (CN X).

The gustatory nerve fibers enter the brain stem and project to the nucleus tractus solitarius (NTS), which extends from the rosterolateral medulla caudally along the ventral border of the vestibular nuclei. CN VII fibers synapse rostrally to the CN IX fibers (Figure 5) The axons of second-order neurons originating within the NTS then ascend ipsilaterally to the parvicellular division of the ventroposteromedial nucleus of the thalamus via the central tegmental tract (Pritchard 1991). From the thalamus, other neurons project to the primary taste cortex located at the junction of the anterior insula and the inner operculum. From this region, further projections are made to the orbitofrontal cortex, where visual, somatosensory, and olfactory information is known to converge.

Age-related Changes in Odor Perception

Major age-related decrements in the ability to smell are well documented (e.g., Choudhury et al. 2003; Deems and Doty 1987; Doty et al. 1984, 1989; Murphy et al. 2002; Rawson 2006; Schiffman 1991; Ship and Weiffenbach 1993; van Thriel et al. 2006;Wysocki and Pelchat 1993; Yousem et al. 1999). In addition, age-related declines are present in the responsiveness of the nasal mucosa to chemicals that produce irritation and other skin sensations via the free nerve endings of the trigeminal (CN V) nerve (Stevens et al. 1982). Large individual differences are present and men, on average, exhibit larger and earlier age-related declines in odor perception than women, Doty and Cameron (2009). An example of the age-related alterations in the ability to

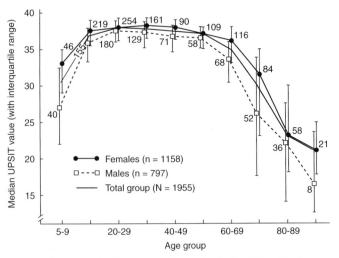

Figure 6 Scores on the University of Pennsylvania Smell Identification Test (UPSIT) as a function of age in a large heterogeneous group of subjects. Numbers by data points indicate sample sizes. From Doty et al. (1984b) with permission.

identify odors is shown in Figure 6 (Doty et al. 1984a). In general, individuals who exhibit comparatively low sensitivity to one odorant typically exhibit low sensitivity to others, whereas those who evidence comparatively high sensitivity to an odorant typically evidence high sensitivity to others. Such observations suggest that a "general olfactory acuity" factor exists, analogous to the general intelligence factor derived from items of intelligence tests (Doty et al. 1994; Yoshida 1984).

Causes of Age-related Losses of Olfactory Perception

The olfactory receptors are more or less directly exposed to the outside environment, making them susceptible to insult from bacteria, viruses, toxins, and other nosogenic agents. For this reason, environmentally induced damage to the receptor epithelium is the most common cause of age-related alterations in the ability to smell. Indeed, cumulative destruction of the olfactory neuroepithelium occurs throughout the entire life-span, with metaplasia from respiratory epithelium presenting as islands within the membrane (Nakashima et al. 1984). However, age-related physiological or structural changes may also directly damage or predispose the olfactory epithelium to damage from environmental insults. Such changes include reduced protein synthesis or metabolic insufficiency (as in hypothyroidism; Mackay-Sim and Beard 1987), loss of neurotrophic factors (Chuah et al. 1985), occlusion of cribriform plate foramina through which the olfactory nerve axons pass (Kalmey et al. 1998), decreased intramucosal blood flow (Hasegawa and Kern 1977), changes in the vascular elasticity of the epithelium (Somlyo and Somlyo 1968), altered airway patency (Frye 2003), increased nasal mucus viscosity (Koopmann 1989), atrophy of secretory glands and lymphatics (Koopmann 1989), and decreases in enzyme systems that deactivate xenobiotic materials within the olfactory mucosa (Ding and Dahl 2003). Importantly, pathology within more central pathways is also likely involved. For example, the olfactory bulbs of more than 40% of *non-demented* persons 50 years of age and older exhibit neurofibrillary tangles (NFTs) (Kishikawa et al. 1990). As described later in this chapter, considerable destruction of central olfactory structures has been noted in Alzheimer's disease and some other age-related diseases, such as Parkinson's disease.

Despite the fact that the olfactory receptor cells have the capacity to reconstitute themselves (Graziadei and Monti Graziadei 1979), this plasticity is altered by the aforementioned age-related processes, as demonstrated by studies of rodent and amphibian olfactory epithelia (Breipohl et al. 1986). For example, the ratio of dead or dying cells to the number of receptor cells increases in older animals, implying that receptor cells from older individuals have less mitotic activity than those from younger ones. Following chemical destruction of the olfactory receptors of mice with zinc sulfate or methyl-formimino-methylester, morphological repair is slower or nonexistent in older animals, unlike that in young animals (Matulionis 1982), indicating that the neurogenic process alters with age.

In general, destruction of the receptor elements of the olfactory neuroepithelium extends to the glomeruli of the olfactory bulb, where degeneration occurs. This fact was used by Smith (1942) to estimate age-related losses of human olfactory receptors. By assessing the number and form of glomeruli present in 205 olfactory bulbs of 121 individuals at autopsy, Smith concluded that loss of olfactory nerves begins soon after birth and continues to occur throughout life at approximately 1% per year. However, a reevaluation of Smith's data using medians rather than means leads one to the conclusion that there is no apparent average loss until the fifth decade of life. Although considerable variability among bulbs was seen at all ages examined, sex differences were not apparent in the data of this early study.

The widespread alterations in bulbar structures with age are perhaps best exemplified in a series of quantitative anatomical studies performed by Hinds and associates. Using the Sprague-Dawley rat strain, Hinds and McNelly (1977) examined the volume of main olfactory bulb components (including the glomerular, external plexiform, internal granular, and olfactory nerve layers) at 3, 12, 24, 27, and 30 months of age. In addition, the size and number of mitral cells were determined in both the main and accessory bulbs. Even though developmental increases in the layer volumes were noted during the first 24 months of age, decreases occurred after that time. Importantly, a sharp decrease in mitral cell number was noted, along with an increase in the volume of individual mitral cell dendritic trees and in the cell body and nucleus sizes.

Hinds and McNelly (1981) replicated these findings in the Charles River rat strain, although no loss in mitral cell number was apparent in the older animals. In this study, alterations within the olfactory neuroepithelium were assessed concurrently. A comparison of regression lines for changes in number of olfactory receptors on the septal epithelium with that of the size of mitral cell bodies suggested that the decline in receptor number began several months before the decline in mitral cell size, implying that the bulbar changes were secondary to the epithelial changes. A significant increase in the number of synapses per receptor was present in the oldest group evaluated, conceivably representing a compensatory increase in the relative numbers of synapses per receptor cell in the surviving receptor cell population.

Relative to the olfactory epithelium and bulb, the rat piriform cortex appears to exhibit little age-related change. Curcio et al. (1985), for example, examined the cells and synapses of the piriform cortices of rats ranging in age from 3 to 33 months and found no significant changes in the volumes of cortical laminae Ia and Ib or in the numerical and surface densities of the synaptic apposition zones in layer Ia (which are formed mainly by mitral cell axons). A modest (18%) decline in the proportion of layer Ia occupied by dendrites and spines was observed, although age-related changes in nuclear volume, soma volume, or numerical density of layer II neurons were not found. This decrease was accompanied by an increase in the proportion of glial processes, but not by an alteration in the proportion of axons and terminals.

Changes in Odor Perception Related to Alzheimer's Disease

Severe olfactory abnormalities are present in early stage Alzheimer's disease (for review, see Doty 2003). In a meta-analysis of studies on this topic, Mesholam et al. (1998) found that the AD-related deficits were relatively uniform across tests of odor identification, detection, and discrimination. Interestingly, no measure distinguished AD from PD, despite the likelihood of differing underlying olfactory pathology. Although some studies have reported that the AD-related olfactory deficit progresses over time (e.g., Nordin et al. 1997), the validity of psychophysical test results from more demented individuals is questionable. The majority (>90%) of AD patients seem unaware of their defective smell sense until formally tested (Doty et al. 1987), probably reflecting the fact that total anosmia is relatively rare. Such lack of awareness of less-than-total smell loss is a general phenomenon, since it is observed in non-demented patient groups as well (Nordin et al. 1995).

The olfactory loss in AD likely precedes the onset of dementia. In one prospective population-based study, 1,836 healthy people were tested at baseline using a 12-item odor identification test and a cognitive screening procedure (Graves et al. 1999). Reduced smell identification ability, particularly anosmia, was associated with an increased risk of cognitive dysfunction several years later. At baseline, anosmics who had at least one ApoE-4 allele had nearly five times the risk of developing subsequent cognitive decline. Similar observations of olfactory decline have been documented by others in longitudinal studies of older subjects with minimal or no cognitive defects on initial assessment (Bacon et al. 1998; Royall et al. 2002; Swan and Carmelli 2002; Wilson et al. 2007b), as well as in studies examining conversion from mild cognitive impairment to AD (Devanand et al. 2000, 2008).

Some close relatives of AD patients exhibit olfactory dysfunction, further implicating genetic determinants. For example, Serby et al. (1996) found 28 first-degree relatives of AD patients to have lower average scores on the University of Pennsylvania Smell Identification Test (UPSIT; Doty et al. 1984b) than 28 healthy controls, despite similar scores on the Mini-Mental State Exam (MMSE). Schiffman et al. (2002) reported that 33 at-risk relatives of AD patients had elevated phenyl ethanol detection thresholds relative to 32 controls, as well as decreased ability to remember smells, tastes, and narrative information. No association with ApoE-4 status was detectable. In contrast to these findings, Nee and Lippa (2001) found no association between UPSIT scores and subsequent development of clinical AD in a 10 year follow-up of 18 at-risk relatives of AD family members with the autosomal dominant presenilin-1 AD mutation. Two of the four family members who had AD upon retest 'converted' from normal smell function to abnormal function. This study suggests that, in this form of AD, either the olfactory dysfunction occurs less than 10 years before the expression of the clinical phenotype or olfactory dysfunction is not predictive of AD.

Causes of Losses of Olfactory Function in Alzheimer's Disease

Although AD-related olfactory dysfunction may reflect, to some degree, the physiological changes seemingly associated with normal aging, such changes are not the whole story. As noted above, even early-stage AD patients with mild dementia consistently score much more poorly on olfactory tests than age-matched controls—decrements not observed on visual tests designed to control for non-olfactory elements of the olfactory tests (Doty et al. 1987). Importantly, relatively high levels of NFTs and neuritic plaques (NPs) have been noted in brain structures involved in olfactory processing, including the anterior olfactory nucleus, olfactory bulb, hippocampal formation, periamygdaloid nucleus, piriform cortex, entorhinal cortex, orbitofrontal cortex, and dorsomedial thalamic nucleus (for review see Ferreyra-Moyano and Barragan 1989). Furthermore, changes within the olfactory epithelium and bulb have been reported, although their specificity to AD is questionable (Smutzer et al. 2003). Whether such damage is related to the transit of environmental toxins from the nasal cavity into the brain via the olfactory fila is unknown (the 'olfactory vector hypothesis') (Doty 2008). An alternative hypothesis is that damage to the olfactory system, per se, results in central brain changes that induce cognitive decline (the 'olfactory damage hypothesis'). This possibility is inferred from rat studies where rats that had been anosmic for some time have considerable difficulty learning an active avoidance learning task, unlike similarly aged and housed rats whose anosmia is of recent origin (Kurtz et al. 1989). Pearson et al. (1985) summarized the involvement of higher olfactory structures in AD as follows (p. 4534):

> The invariable finding of severe and even maximal involvement of the olfactory regions in Alzheimer's disease is in striking contrast to the minimal pathology in the visual and sensorimotor areas of the neocortex and cannot be without significance. In the olfactory system, the sites that are affected—the anterior olfactory nucleus, the uncus, and the medial group of amygdaloid nuclei—all receive fibers directly from the olfactory bulb. These observations at least raise the possibility that the olfactory pathway is the site of initial involvement of the disease.

More recently, Braak et al. (1998) proposed that the first AD-related pathological changes occur in the transentorhinal cortex, a bottleneck zone for cortical sensory afferents to the hippocampus. Abnormalities in this region are followed by changes in the adjacent entorhinal cortex—an area concerned with memory, emotion, and olfaction. However, Kovacs et al. (2001) reported that neurofibrillary tangles (NFTs) occurred in the anterior olfactory nucleus (AON) of some AD cases before any change was seen in the entorhinal cortex. The primary olfactory cortex was less severely affected than the medial orbitofrontal cortex (an olfactory association area) and there was a correlation between the pathology of the olfactory bulb and some non-olfactory areas. This led to the suggestion that NFT formation developed independently of synaptic connections, i.e., it was not a process that advanced along established fiber pathways as hypothesized by Braak et al. (1998).

In a recent study, Wilson et al. (2007a) found that odor identification test scores obtained prior to death were inversely related to entorhinal and hippocampal neurofibrillary tangle (NFT) numbers in elderly community dwelling subjects. This association remained after controlling for dementia or semantic memory, implying that the impaired olfaction of the elderly may be due, in part, to accumulation of NFTs in the primary olfactory cortex. Although two other postmortem-based studies reported no association between olfactory test scores and AD pathology (McShane et al. 2001; Olichney et al. 2005), smell impairment was associated with the presence of Lewy bodies (dementia with Lewy bodies or Lewy body variant).

Age-related Changes in Taste Perception

As in the case of the olfaction system, age-related decrements in taste threshold sensitivity are well documented. Such decrements occur regardless of whether the stimulus is electrical or chemical (Ahne et al. 2000; Baker et al. 1983; Drewnowski et al. 1999; Fikentscher et al. 1977; Gudziol and Hummel 2007; Kleinschmidt and Henning 1981; Koertvelyessy et al. 1982; Le Floch JP et al. 1990; Matsuda and Doty 1995; Mavi and Ceyhan 1999; Mojet et al. 2001; Murphy and Gilmore

1989; Nakazato et al. 2002; Nilsson 1979a,b; Weiffenbach 1984). Tests of small regions of the tongue show particularly large deficits (Matsuda and Doty 1995). Chemicals for which such decreases have been noted include caffeine, citric acid, hydrochloric acid, magnesium sulfate, phenyl thiocarbamide (PTC), propylthiouracil (PROP), quinine, sodium chloride, sucrose, tartaric acid, and a large number of amino acids. An example of the age-related decline in sensitivity to NaCl observed when small regions of the tongue are stimulated is shown in Figure 7.

Changes in suprathreshold taste perception to chemicals have also been observed. Thus, some studies have noted that functions relating tastant concentrations to perceived intensity are flatter for the elderly than for young adults, at least for some stimuli (Chauhan and Hawrysh 1988; Hyde and Feller 1981; Schiffman and Clark 1980). However, flatter functions need not be indicative of decreased sensitivity across the entire suprathreshold stimulus range. As pointed out by Bartoshuk et al. (1986), diminished slopes in log-log plots of stimulus concentration versus magnitude estimates often occur when decreased sensitivity is present for tastant concentrations only at the lower end of the stimulus continuum. Using a magnitude matching procedure, these authors had young and elderly subjects judge the relative intensity of tastants and interspersed sounds (white noise) during the same test session. Under the assumption that the intensity of low-pitch white noise is altered less by aging than is the intensity of the target tastants (sucrose, sodium chloride, citric acid, quinine), Bartoshuk et al. (1986) normalized the taste data across individuals by taking into account their different scaling strategies on the auditory continuum. With the exception of sodium chloride (where no differences between the young and the elderly were observed), the largest differences between the magnitude estimates of the two study groups were found at the lower stimulus concentrations for these tastants. However, very small but statistically significant decrements were observed at the highest concentration of citric acid and of quinine tested for both groups, suggesting that at least some decrement in taste sensitivity may be present for these two stimuli at high concentrations. Whether stimulus context effects (e.g., the tendency to rate stimuli as stronger in stimulus series containing a high proportion of weak stimuli) contribute to or are responsible for the latter phenomenon is not known.

As in the case of olfaction, a number of studies report that age-related alterations in taste function are not equivalent for men and women. Given that sex differences are present for a variety of taste tests in nonelderly populations (Doty 1978), there is no a priori reason to believe that such differences would not continue throughout life. In accord with this notion are reports of female superiority in taste perception within elderly populations, including superiority on detection threshold tests (Baker et al. 1983; Nilsson 1979b), recognition or identification threshold tests (Fikentscher et al. 1977; Lassila et al. 1988), suprathreshold scaling tests (Sorter et al. 2008; Weisfuse et al. 1986), and electrical taste threshold tests (Coates 1974). The magnitude of the age-related decline in taste sensitivity is greater for men than for women for some substances, a phenomenon also observed for the sense of smell (Doty et al., 1984a).

It should be emphasized that the age-related whole-mouth decrements in the ability to taste are not large, particularly in contrast to the magnitude of changes seen in olfaction, and are not consistently observed for all of the classic taste categories (i.e., sweet, sour, bitter, salty). For example, in a study of 81 healthy adults ranging in age from 23 to 88 years (including healthy elderly participants enrolled in the National Institute on Aging's Baltimore Longitudinal Study), Weiffenbach et al. (1982) found that sensitivity to sodium chloride and quinine sulfate decreased slightly with age, whereas that to sucrose and citric acid did not. Presumably such factors as the relative health of the subjects, study sample sizes, gender distributions, proportions of smokers and non-smokers within the tested groups, and specifics of the testing procedures contribute to the variance in findings among studies.

Causes of Age-related Losses of Taste Function

As in the case of other sensory modalities, a relationship exists between the number of functioning receptor elements and the taste system's

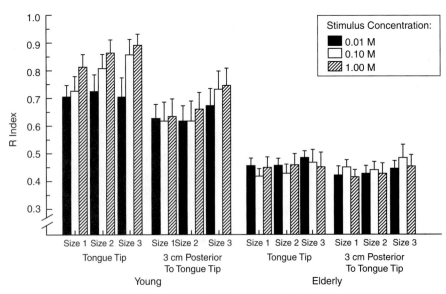

Figure 7 Mean (±SEM) sensitivity values obtained from 12 young and 12 elderly subjects for NaCl presented to two tongue regions for three stimulus areas (12.5, 25, and 50 mm²) and three stimulus concentrations. Note that the sensitivity of the older subjects was essentially at chance in all tongue regions and stimulus areas that were assessed. Unlike the young subjects, greater sensitivity was not seen on the tongue tip than on a more posterior tongue region. From Matsuda and Doty (1995), with permission. Copyright © 1995 Oxford University Press.

relative sensitivity. Thus, detection thresholds and the perceived intensity of tastants presented to small areas of the anterior tongue are proportional to the number and density of fungiform papillae and taste buds located in the stimulated regions (Doty et al. 2001; Miller and Reedy, Jr. 1990; Miller et al. 2002; Segovia et al. 2002; Smith 1971; Zuniga et al. 1993). The number of stimulus sensations derived from stimulation of individual papillae correlates with the number of taste buds present in the papillae, as determined from subsequent biopsy (Arvidson and Friberg 1980).

Given such associations, one might expect that age-related declines in taste function would reflect decreasing numbers of taste buds. However, the question as to whether human taste buds decrease in the later years is controversial. Some studies have reported age-related declines in human taste bud numbers, particularly in taste buds within the posteriorly located circumvallate papilla. Arey et al. (1935), for example, reported that the mean number of buds per circumvallate papilla was as follows: from 0 to 20 years of age, 248; from 20 to 70 years, 206; and from 74 to 85 years, 88. Mochizuki (1939) reported the following figures: from 0 to 20 years, 242; from 21 to 60 years, 196; and from 61 to 90 years, 116. Recently, Kano et al. (2007) reported statistically significant age-related decrements in taste bud numbers within the epiglottis. In contrast, Arvidson (1979) found no age or sex differences in taste bud numbers in 182 *fungiform* papillae collected, at autopsy, from 22 persons ranging in age from 2 to 90 years. Although the number of taste buds in a single papilla varied from 0 to 27, 63% of the papillae had no taste buds at all, 26% had 1–3 buds, and the remainder had 4 or more buds. The mean number of taste buds per papilla varied from 0 to 9 between individuals. Miller (1988) found no statistically meaningful relation between age and taste bud densities on either the tip or the midregion of tongues from young adults (22–36 years, $n = 5$), middle-aged adults (50–63 years, $n = 7$), and old adults (70–90 years, $n = 6$). This author noted that the marked variability in the number of taste buds at all ages is much more apparent than any age-related alterations. Mistretta and Oakley (1986) found the average percentage of *fungiform* papillae containing taste buds in Fischer 344 rats aged 4 to 6 months, 20 to 24 months, and 30 to 37 months to be 99.6%, 99.3%, and 94.7%, respectively.

Interestingly, neurophysiological recordings from the chorda tympani nerve (which innervates the taste buds on the anterior tongue) of older rats exhibited decreased neural responses to some salts, acids, and sugars (McBride and Mistretta 1986), despite the evidence that taste bud numbers are not meaningfully decreased (Mistretta and Oakley 1986). The reason for this decrease in responsiveness is unknown, but possibilities include decreased intrinsic reactivity of taste buds to taste solutions, decreased multiple neural innervation of taste buds by some taste fibers, alterations in the general structure of the epithelium (which, for example, might impair the movement of stimulus solution into the taste bud pore), and decreased taste nerve responsiveness per se. It is conceivable that although the full complement of taste buds is present, some buds are not fully functional. It should be kept in mind that taste buds function in a complex ionic milieu and that they are bathed with saliva and other secretory products, such as the secretions from von Ebner's glands near the foliate papillae, which themselves may undergo age-related changes.

Overall, the aforementioned studies suggest that the number of taste buds observed in histological preparations may not be the defining element responsible for age-related decrements in taste function. Nonetheless, however, it should be noted that studies which fail to find age-related taste bud decrements have sampled fungiform papillae, whereas those observing such decrements have sampled circumvallate

papillae. Moreover, studies reporting age-related effects have generally had much larger sample sizes than those reporting no such effects. It would seem that larger studies which assess fungiform, foliate, and circumvallate papillae from autopsy cases free of general pathology are needed before the question of age-related taste bud decrements will be fully resolved.

Changes in Taste Perception and Taste System Morphology in Alzheimer's Disease

Unlike olfaction, little research has been done on gustatory function in AD patients. Although one author has reported that patients with AD suffer no age-related taste deficits (Murphy et al. 1990), most studies find such deficits (Broggio et al. 2001; Lang et al. 2006; Schiffman et al. 1990; Waldton 1974). For example, Schiffman et al. (1990) found that patients with AD exhibit significant losses in the ability to detect the taste of glutamic acid. This decrement was not specific to AD, however, as it was also present in patients with other types of dementia. Whether this finding parallels the observation that several dementia-related disorders (e.g., multi-infarct dementia) are associated with varying degrees of olfactory dysfunction is a question that requires further study.

Influences of Medications on Taste and Smell Perception in Later Life

Chemosensory related complaints occur disproportionately in the elderly. Most such complaints relate specifically to taste, rather than to smell. Distorted or phantom taste sensations are very common and often stem from medication usage. According to the Physician's Desk Reference (PDR; Physician's Desk Reference 2009), hundreds of medications are associated with taste-related side effects. Terms used in the PDR to describe such side effects include "loss of taste," "altered taste," "ageusia," "taste loss," "dysgeusia," "bad taste," "hypogeusia;" "bitter taste," "metallic taste," "unpleasant taste," and "salty taste."

Among the major offending medications are antimicrobials, antifungals, antihypertensives, antihyperlipidemics, and antidepressants (Doty et al. 2008). Adverse chemosensory side effects are noted for 70 percent of the antihyperlipidemic drugs listed in the PDR. In a placebo-controlled study of Lipitor (atorvastatin calcium), side effects of altered taste and loss of taste were not uncommon (Physician's Desk Reference 2009). Similar side effects were found in clinical trials of Baycol, Lescol (fluvastatin), Provachol (pravastatin), Mevacor (lovastatin), and Zocor (simvastatin). Over a third of the antihypertensive drugs listed in the PDR reportedly have adverse taste side effects, including calcium channel blockers, diuretics (e.g., amiloride), and angiotensin-converting enzyme (ACE) inhibitors. ACE inhibitors block the enzyme that converts angiotensin I to angiotensin II, a potent vasoconstrictor that raises blood pressure and increases activation of bradykinin, a potent vasodilator. Captopril, the first orally active ACE inhibitor, is more frequently associated than any other ACE inhibitor with complaints of ageusia, metallic taste, and taste distortion (Grosskopf et al. 1984; McNeill et al. 1979). This drug can make sweet-tasting foods taste salty, and can produce chronic bitter or salty sensations, presumably by directly altering ion channels (Zervakis et al. 2000). Drug discontinuance usually reverses the taste disturbance within a few months, although in rare instances dysgeusias fail to resolve even after many months. A number of dysgeusias spontaneously remit over the course of several years (Deems et al. 1996).

Summary and Conclusions

The senses of taste and smell monitor the intake of all environmental nutrients and airborne chemicals required for life and largely determine the flavor and palatability of foods and beverages. In addition to purveying pleasure and displeasure, these senses alert us to spoiled foods, leaking natural gas, polluted air, and smoke.

It is clear from the studies reviewed in this chapter that chemosensory dysfunction is common in the older population. Such disturbances can be profound, significantly decreasing quality of life and increasing the risk of malnutrition, depression, and toxic poisoning. Olfactory dysfunction is easily detectable by a variety of sensory tests and is exaggerated in persons with early-stage AD. In fact, smell loss may precede the other clinical signs of AD. Medication-related dysgeusias or phantogeusias are present in some elderly that resolve only after long periods of drug discontinuance. Although damage to peripheral receptor cells and associated structures may explain some such changes, alterations within higher nervous system structures must also be considered, and it is likely that the structural and functional bases of many age-related chemosensory changes are multiple, interacting, and complex.

References

Ahne G, Erras A, Hummel T, and Kobal G (2000) Assessment of gustatory function by means of tasting tablets. *Laryngoscope* 110:1396–1401.

Alloway KD and Pritchard TC (2007) *Medical neuroscience*, 2nd ed. Hayes Barton, Raleigh NC.

Arey LB, Tremaine MJ, and Monzingo FL (1935) The numerical and topographical relations of taste buds to human circumvallate papillae throughout the life span. *Anat Rec* 64:9–25.

Arvidson K (1979) Location and variation in number of taste buds in human fungiform papillae. *Scand J Dent Res* 87:435–442.

Arvidson K and Friberg U (1980) Human taste: Response and taste bud number in fungiform papillae. *Science* 209:807–808.

Astback J, Arvidson K, and Johansson O (1995) Neurochemical markers of human fungiform papillae and taste buds. *Regulatory Peptides* 59:389–398.

Bacon AW, Bondi MW, Salmon DP, and Murphy C (1998) Very early changes in olfactory functioning due to Alzheimer's disease and the role of apolipoprotein E in olfaction. *Ann NY Acad Sci* 855:723–731.

Baker KA, Didcock EA, Kemm JR, and Patrick JM (1983) Effect of age, sex and illness on salt taste detection thresholds. *Age & Ageing* 12:159–165.

Bartoshuk LM, Rifkin B, Marks LE, and Bars P (1986) Taste and aging. *J Gerontol* 41:51–57.

Berkowicz DA, Trombley PQ, and Shepherd GM (1994) Evidence for glutamate as the olfactory receptor cell neurotransmitter. *J Neurophysiol* 71:2557–2561.

Braak H, Braak E, Bohl J, and Bratzke H (1998) Evolution of Alzheimer's disease related cortical lesions. *J Neural Trans Supplementum.* 54:97–106.

Bradley RM and Beidler LM (2003) Saliva: Its role in taste function. In: Doty, R. L. (ed) *Handbook of olfaction and gustation*, 2nd edn. Marcel Dekker, New York, pp 639–650.

Bradley RM, Stedman HM, and Mistretta CM (1985) Age does not affect numbers of taste buds and papillae in adult rhesus monkeys. *Anat Rec* 212:246–249.

Breipohl W, Mackay-Sim A, Grandt D, Rehn B, and Darrelmann C (1986) Neurogenesis in the vertebrate main olfactory epithelium. In: Breipohl, W. (ed) *Ontogeny of olfaction*. Springer-Verlag, Berlin, pp 21–33.

Broggio E, Pluchon C, Ingrand P, and Gil R (2001) [Taste impairment in Alzheimer's disease]. *Rev Neurol* (Paris) 157:409–413.

Burdach KJ and Doty RL (1987) The effects of mouth movements, swallowing, and spitting on retronasal odor perception. *Physiol Behav* 41:353–356.

Chalke HD, Dewhurst JR, and Ward CW (1958) Loss of smell in old people. *Pub Health* 72:223–230.

Chandrashekar J, Hoon MA, Ryba NJ, and Zuker CS (2006) The receptors and cells for mammalian taste. *Nature* 444:288–294.

Chauhan J and Hawrysh ZJ (1988) Suprathreshold sour taste intensity and pleasantness perception with age. *Physiol Behav* 43:601–607.

Chen WR, Xiong W, and Shepherd GM (2000) Analysis of relations between NMDA receptors and GABA release at olfactory bulb reciprocal synapses. *Neuron* 25:625–633.

Choudhury ES, Moberg P, and Doty RL (2003) Influences of age and sex on a microencapsulated odor memory test. *Chem Senses* 28:799–805.

Chuah MI, Farbman AI, and Menco BP (1985) Influence of olfactory bulb on dendritic knob density of rat olfactory receptor neurons in vitro. *Brain Res* 338:259–266.

Coates AC (1974) Effects of age, sex, and smoking on electrical taste threshold. *Ann Otol Rhinol Laryngol* 83:365–369.

Curcio CA, McNelly NA, and Hinds JW (1985) Aging in the rat olfactory system: Relative stability of piriform cortex contrasts with changes in olfactory bulb and olfactory epithelium. *J Comp Neurol* 235:519–528.

Deems DA and Doty RL (1987) Age-related changes in the phenyl ethyl alcohol odor detection threshold. *Trans Penn Acad Ophthalmol Otolaryngol* 39:646–650.

Deems DA, Doty RL, Settle RG, Moore-Gillon V, Shaman P, Mester AF, et al (1991) Smell and taste disorders, a study of 750 patients from the University of Pennsylvania Smell and Taste Center. *Arch Otolaryngol Head Neck Surg* 117:519–528.

Deems DA, Yen DM, Kreshak A, and Doty RL (1996) Spontaneous resolution of dysgeusia. *Arch Otolaryngol Head Neck Surg* 122:961–963.

Devanand DP, Liu XH, Tabert MH, Pradhaban G, Cuasay K, Bell K, de Leon MJ, Doty RL, Stern Y, and Pelton GH (2008) Combining early markers strongly predicts conversion from mild cognitive impairment to Alzheimer's disease. *Biol Psychiat* 64:871–879.

Devanand DP, Michaels-Marston KS, Liu X, Pelton GH, Padilla M, Marder K, et al (2000) Olfactory deficits in patients with mild cognitive impairment predict Alzheimer's disease at follow-up. *Amer J Psychiat* 157:1399–1405.

Ding X and Dahl AR (2003) Olfactory mucosa: Composition, enzymatic localization, and metabolism. In: Doty, R. L. (ed) *Handbook of olfaction and gustation*, 2nd edn. Marcel Dekker, New York, pp 51–73.

Doty RL (1989) Influence of age and age-related diseases on olfactory function. *Ann NY Acad Sci* 561:76–86.

Doty RL (1978) Gender and reproductive state correlates of taste perception in humans. In: McGill, T. E., Dewsbury, D. A., Sachs, B. D. (eds) *Sex and behavior: Status and prospectus*. Plenum Press, New York, pp 337–362.

Doty RL (2003) Odor perception in neurodegenerative diseases. In: Doty, R. L. (ed) *Handbook of olfaction and gustation*, 2nd edn. Marcel Dekker, New York, pp 479–502.

Doty RL (2008) The olfactory vector hypothesis of neurodegenerative disease: Is it viable? *Ann Neurol* 63:7–15.

Doty RL, Bagla R, Morgenson M, and Mirza N (2001) NaCl thresholds: Relationship to anterior tongue locus, area of stimulation, and number of fungiform papillae. *Physiol Behav* 72:373–378.

Doty RL and Cameron L (2009) Sex differences and reproductive hormone influences on human odor perception. *Physiology & Behavior* 97:213–228.

Doty RL, Reyes PF, and Gregor T (1987) Presence of both odor identification and detection deficits in Alzheimer's disease. *Brain Res Bull* 18:597–600.

Doty RL, Shah M, and Bromley SM (2008) Drug-induced taste disorders. *Drug Safety* 31:199–215.

Doty RL, Shaman P, Applebaum SL, Giberson R, Siksorski L, and Rosenberg L (1984a) Smell identification ability: Changes with age. *Science* 226:1441–1443.

Doty RL, Shaman P, and Dann M (1984b) Development of the University of Pennsylvania Smell Identification Test: A standardized microencapsulated test of olfactory function. *Physiol Behav* 32:489–502.

Doty RL, Smith R, McKeown DA, and Raj J (1994) Tests of human olfactory function: Principal components analysis suggests that most measure a common source of variance. *Percept Psychophys* 56:701–707.

Drewnowski A, Henderson SA, Hann CS, Barratt-Fornell A, and Ruffin M (1999) Age and food preferences influence dietary intakes of breast care patients. *Health Psychol* 18:570–578.

Ferreyra-Moyano H and Barragan E (1989) The olfactory system and Alzheimer's disease. *Intl J Neurosci* 49:157–197.

Fikentscher R, Roseburg B, Spinar H, and Bruchmuller W (1977) Loss of taste in the elderly: Sex differences. *Clin Otolaryngol Allied Sci* 2:183–189.

Frye RE (2003) Nasal patency and the aerodynamics of nasal airflow: Measurement by rhinomanometry and acoustic rhinometry, and the influence of pharmacological agents. In: Doty, R. L. (ed) *Handbook of olfaction and gustation*, 2nd edn. Marcel Dekker, New York, pp 439–460.

Getchell ML and Getchell TV (1990) Regulatory factors in the vetebrate olfactory mucosa. *Chem Senses* 15:223–231.

Gilbertson TA, Damak S, and Margolskee RF (2000) The molecular physiology of taste transduction. *Curr Opinion Neurobiol* 10:519–527.

Graves AB, Bowen JD, Rajaram L, McCormick WC, McCurry SM, Schellenberg GD, et al (1999) Impaired olfaction as a marker for cognitive decline: Interaction with apolipoprotein E epsilon4 status. *Neurology* 53:1480–1487.

Graziadei PPC and Monti Graziadei AG (1979) Neurogenesis and neuron regeneration in the olfactory system of mammals. I. Morphological aspects of differentiation and structural organization of the olfactory sensory neurons. *J Neurocytol* 8:1–18.

Grosmaitre X, Vassalli A, Mombaerts P, Shepherd GM, and Ma M (2006) Odorant responses of olfactory sensory neurons expressing the odorant receptor MOR23: A patch clamp analysis in gene-targeted mice. *Proc Nat Acad Sci USA* 103:1970–1975.

Grosskopf I, Rabinovitz M, Garty M, and Rosenfeld JB (1984) Persistent captopril-associated taste alteration. *Clin Pharm* 3:235.

Gudziol H and Hummel T (2007) Normative values for the assessment of gustatory function using liquid tastants. *Acta Otolaryngol (Stockh)* 127:658–661.

Hasegawa M and Kern EB (1977) The human nasal cycle. *Mayo Clin Proc* 52:28–34.

Hinds JW and McNelly NA (1977) Aging of the rat olfactory bulb: Growth and atrophy of constituent layers and changes in size and number of mitral cells. *J Comp Neurol* 72:345–367.

Hinds JW and McNelly NA (1981) Aging in the rat olfactory system: Correlation of changes in the olfactory epithelium and olfactory bulb. *J Comp Neurol* 203:441–453.

Hyde RJ and Feller RP (1981) Age and sex effects on taste of sucrose, NaCl, citric acid and caffeine. *Neurobiol Aging* 2:315–318.

Kalmey JK, Thewissen JG, and Dluzen DE (1998) Age-related size reduction of foramina in the cribriform plate. *Anat Rec* 251:326–329.

Kano M, Shimizu Y, Okayama K, and Kikuchi M (2007) Quantitative study of ageing epiglottal taste buds in humans. *Gerodontology* 24:169–172.

Kishikawa M, Iseki M, Nishimura M, Sekine I, and Fujii H (1990) A histopathological study on senile changes in the human olfactory bulb. *Acta Pathologica Japonica* 40:255-260.

Kleinschmidt EG and Henning L (1981) [Threshold for electric stimulation of taste in diabetes mellitus]. [German]. *Zeitschrift fur die Gesamte Innere Medizin und Ihre Grenzgebiete* 36:407–411.

Koertvelyessy TA, Crawford MH, and Hutchinson J (1982) PTC taste threshold distributions and age in Mennonite populations. *Hum Biol* 54:635–646.

Koopmann CF (1989) Effects of aging on nasal structure and function. *Amer J Rhinol* 3:59–62.

Kovacs T, Cairns NJ, and Lantos PL (2001) Olfactory centres in Alzheimer's disease: Olfactory bulb is involved in early Braak's stages. *Neuroreport* 12:285–288.

Kurtz P, Schuurman T, and Prinz H (1989) Loss of smell leads to dementia in mice: Is Alzheimer's disease a degenerative disorder of the olfactory system? *J Protein Chem* 8:448–451.

Lang CJG, Leuschner T, Ulrich K, Stößel C, Heckmann JG, and Hummel T (2006) Taste in dementing diseases and Parkinsonism. *J Neurol Sci* 248:177–184.

Lassila V, Sointu M, Raiha I, and Lehtonen A (1988) Taste thresholds in the elderly. *Proc Finn Dent Soc* 84:305–310.

Le Floch JP, Le Lievre G., Verroust J, Philippon C, Peynegre R, and Perlemuter L (1990) Factors related to the electric taste threshold in type 1 diabetic patients. *Diabet Med* 7:526–531.

Li CS and Smith DV (1997) Glutamate receptor antagonists block gustatory afferent input to the nucleus of the solitary tract. *J Neurophysiol* 77:1514–1525.

Mackay-Sim A (2003) Neurogenesis in the adult olfactory neuroepithelium. In: Doty, R. L. (ed) *Handbook of olfaction and gustation*, 2nd edn. Marcel Dekker, New York, pp 93–113.

Mackay-Sim A and Beard MD (1987) Hypothyroidism disrupts neural development in the olfactory epithelium of adult mice. *Brain Res* 433:190–198.

Matsuda T and Doty RL (1995) Regional taste sensitivity to NaCl: Relationship to subject age, tongue locus and area of stimulation. *Chem Senses* 20:283–290.

Matulionis DH (1982) Effects of the aging process on olfactory neuron plasticity. In: Breipohl, W. (ed) *Olfaction and endocrine regulation*. IRL Press, London, pp 299–308.

Mavi A and Ceyhan O (1999) Bitter taste thresholds, numbers and diameters of circumvallate papillae and their relation with age in a Turkish population. *Gerodontology* 16:119–122.

McBride MR and Mistretta CM (1986) Taste responses from the chorda tympani nerve in young and old Fischer rats. *J Gerontol* 41:306–314.

McNeill JJ, Anderson A, Christophidis N, Jarrott B, and Louis WJ (1979) Taste loss associated with oral captopril treatment. *BMJ* 2:1555–1556.

McShane RH, Nagy Z, Esiri MM, King E, Joachim C, Sullivan N, et al (2001) Anosmia in dementia is associated with Lewy bodies rather than Alzheimer's pathology. *J Neurol Neurosurg Psychiat* 70:739–743.

Menco BP (1997) Ultrastructural aspects of olfactory signaling. *Chem Senses* 22:295–311.

Menco BP and Morrison EE (2003). Morphology of the mammalian olfactory epithelium: Form, fine structure, function, and pathology. In: Doty, R. L. (ed) *Handbook of olfaction and gustation*, 2nd edn. Marcel Dekker, New York, pp 17–49.

Mesholam RI, Moberg PJ, Mahr RN, and Doty RL (1998) Olfaction in neurodegenerative disease: A meta-analysis of olfactory functioning in Alzheimer's and Parkinson's diseases. *Arch Neurol* 55:84–90.

Miller IJ (1988) Human taste bud density across adult age groups. *J Gerontol* 43:826–830.

Miller IJ, and Reedy FE, Jr. (1990) Variations in human taste bud density and taste intensity perception. *Physiol Behav* 47:1213–1219.

Miller SL, Mirza N, and Doty RL (2002) Electrogustometric thresholds: Relationship to anterior tongue locus, area of stimulation, and number of fungiform papillae. *Physiol Behav* 75:753–757.

Mistretta CM and Baum BJ (1984) Quantitative study of taste buds in fungiform and circumvallate papillae of young and aged rats. *J Anat* 138:323–332.

Mistretta CM and Oakley IA (1986) Quantitative anatomical study of taste buds in fungiform papillae of young and old Fischer rats. *J Gerontol* 41:315–318.

Mochizuki Y (1939) Studies on the papilla foliate of Japanese. 2. The number of taste buds. *Okajimas Folia Anatomica Japonica* 18:369.

Mojet J, Christ-Hazelhof E, and Heidema J (2001) Taste perception with age: Generic or specific losses in threshold sensitivity to the five basic tastes? *Chem Senses* 26:845–860.

Mombaerts P, Wang F, Dulac C, Chao SK, Nemes A, Mendelsohn M, et al (1996) Visualizing an olfactory sensory map. *Cell* 87: 675–686.

Moulton DG and Beidler LM (1967) Structure and function in the peripheral olfactory system. *Physiol Rev* 47:1–52.

Murphy C and Gilmore MM (1989) Quality-specific effects of aging on the human taste system. *Percept Psychophys* 45:121–128.

Murphy C, Gilmore MM, Seery CS, Salmon DP, and Lasker BR (1990) Olfactory thresholds are associated with degree of dementia in Alzheimer's disease. *Neurobiol Aging* 11:465–469.

Murphy C, Schubert CR, Cruickshanks KJ, Klein BE, Klein R, and Nondahl DM (2002) Prevalence of olfactory impairment in older adults. *JAMA* 288:2307–2312.

Nakashima T, Kimmelman CP, and Snow JB, Jr. (1984) Structure of human fetal and adult olfactory neuroepithelium. *Arch Otolaryngol* 110:641–646.

Nakazato M, Endo S, Yoshimura I, and Tomita H (2002) Influence of aging on electrogustometry thresholds. *Acta Otolaryngol (Stockh)* 122:16–26.

Nee LE and Lippa CF (2001) Inherited Alzheimer's disease PS-1 olfactory function: A 10-year follow-up study. *Amer J Alz Dis Other Dementias* 16:83–84.

Nilsson B (1979a) Taste acuity of the human palate. II. Studies with electrogustometry on subjects in different age groups. *Acta Odontol Scand* 37:217–234.

Nilsson B (1979b) Taste acuity of the human palate. III. Studies with taste solutions on subjects in different age groups. *Acta Odontol Scand* 37:235–252.

Nordin S, Almkvist O, Berglund B, and Wahlund LO (1997) Olfactory dysfunction for pyridine and dementia progression in Alzheimer disease. *Arch Neurol* 54:993–998.

Nordin S, Monsch AU, and Murphy C (1995) Unawareness of smell loss in normal aging and Alzheimer's disease: Discrepancy between self-reported and diagnosed smell sensitivity. *Journals of Gerontology* 50:187–192.

Olender T, Lancet D, Nebert DW (2008) Update on the olfactory receptor (OR) gene superfamily. *Hum Genomics* 3:87–97.

Olichney JM, Murphy C, Hofstetter CR, Foster K, Hansen LA, Thal LJ, and Katzman R (2005) Anosmia is very common in the Lewy body variant of Alzheimer's disease. *J Neurol Neurosurg Psychiat* 76: 1342–1347.

Pearson RCA, Esiri MM, Hiornes RW, Wilcock GK, and Powell TPS (1985) Anatomical correlates of the distribution of the pathological changes in the neocortex in Alzheimer's disease. *Proc Nat Acad Sci USA* 82:4531–4534.

Physician's Desk Reference (2009) 63rd edn. Thomson Reuters, Philadephia.

Pritchard TC (1991) The primate gustatory system. In: Getchell, T. V., Doty, R. L., Bartoshuk, L. M., and Snow, J. B., Jr. (eds) *Smell and taste in health and disease*. Raven Press, New York, pp 109–125.

Rawson NE (2006) Olfactory loss in aging. *Sci Aging Knowledge Environ* 2006:e6.

Royall DR, Chiodo LK, Polk MS, and Jaramillo CJ (2002) Severe dysosmia is specifically associated with Alzheimer-like memory deficits in nondemented elderly retirees. *Neuroepidemiology* 21:68–73.

Santos DV, Reiter ER, DiNardo LJ, and Costanzo RM (2004) Hazardous events associated with impaired olfactory function. *Arch Otolaryngol Head Neck Surg* 130:317–319.

Schiffman SS, Frey AE, Luboski JA, Foster MA, and Erickson RP (1991) Taste of glutamate salts in young and elderly subjects: Role of inosine 5'-monophosphate and ions. *Physiol Behav* 49:843–854.

Schiffman SS, Clark CM, and Warwick ZS (1990) Gustatory and olfactory dysfunction in dementia: Not specific to Alzheimer's disease. *Neurobiol Aging* 11:597–600.

Schiffman SS and Clark TB (1980) Magnitude estimates of amino acids for young and elderly subjects. *Neurobiol Aging* 1:81–91.

Schiffman SS, Graham BG, Sattely-Miller EA, Zervakis J, and Welsh-Bohmer K (2002) Taste, smell and neuropsychological performance of individuals at familial risk for Alzheimer's disease. *Neurobiol Aging* 23:397–404.

Segovia C, Hutchinson I, Laing DG, and Jinks AL (2002) A quantitative study of fungiform papillae and taste pore density in adults and children. *Brain Res Dev Brain Res* 20;138:135–146.

Serby M, Mohan C, Aryan M, Williams L, Mohs RC, and Davis KL (1996) Olfactory identification deficits in relatives of Alzheimer's disease patients. Biological Psychiatry 39:375–377.

Ship JA and Weiffenbach JM (1993) Age, gender, medical treatment, and medication effects on smell identification. *J Gerontol* 48:M26–M32.

Smith CG (1942) Age incident of atrophy of olfactory nerves in man. *J Comp Neurol* 77:589–594.

Smith DV (1971) Taste intensity as a function of area and concentration: Differentiation between compounds. *Journal of Experimental Psychology* 87:163–171.

Smutzer GS, Doty RL, Arnold SE, and Trojanowski JQ (2003) Olfactory system neuropathology in Alzheimer's disease, Parkinson's disease, and schizophrenia. In: Doty, R. L. (ed) *Handbook of olfaction and gustation*, 2nd edn. Marcel Dekker, New York, pp 503–523.

Somlyo AP and Somlyo AV (1968) Vascular smooth muscle. I. Normal structure, pathology, biochemistry, and biophysics. *Pharmacological Reviews* 20:197–272.

Sorter A, Kim J, Jackman AH, Tourbier I, Kahl A, and Doty RL (2008) Accuracy of self-report in detecting taste dysfunction. *Laryngoscope* 118:611–617;.

Stevens JC, Plantinga A, and Cain WS (1982) Reduction of odor and nasal pungency associated with aging. *Neurobiol Aging* 3:125–132.

Swan GE and Carmelli D (2002) Impaired olfaction predicts cognitive decline in nondemented older adults. *Neuroepidemiology* 21:58–67.

van Thriel TC, Schaper M, Kiesswetter E, Kleinbeck S, Juran S, Blaszkewicz M, et al (2006) From chemosensory thresholds to whole body exposures-experimental approaches evaluating chemosensory effects of chemicals. *Int Arch Occup Environ Health* 79:308–321.

Waldton S (1974) Clinical observations of impaired cranial nerve function in senile dementia. *Acta Psychiatr Scand* 50:539–547.

Warwick R and Williams PL (1973) *Gray's anatomy*. W.B. Saunders, Philadelphia.

Weiffenbach JM (1984) Taste and smell perception in aging. *Gerodontology* 3:137–146.

Weiffenbach JM, Baum BJ, and Burghauser R (1982) Taste thresholds: Quality specific variation with human aging. *J Gerontol* 37:372–377.

Weisfuse D, Catalanotto FA, and Kamen S (1986) Gender differences in suprathreshold taste scaling ability in an older population. *Special Care in Dentistry* 6:25–28.

Wilson DA and Stevenson RJ (2003) The fundamental role of memory in olfactory perception. *Trends in Neurosciences* 26:243–247.

Wilson DA and Sullivan RM (2003) Sensory physiology of central olfactory pathways. In: Doty, R. L. (ed) *Handbook of olfaction and gustation*. Marcel Dekker, New York, pp 181–201.

Wilson RS, Arnold SE, Schneider JA, Tang Y, and Bennett DA (2007a) The relationship between cerebral Alzheimer's disease pathology and odour identification in old age. *J Neurol Neurosurg Psychiat* 78:30–35.

Wilson RS, Schneider JA, Arnold SE, Tang Y, Boyle PA, and Bennett DA (2007b) Olfactory identification and incidence of mild cognitive impairment in older age. *Arch Gen Psychiat* 64:802–808.

Wysocki CJ and Pelchat ML (1993) The effects of aging on the human sense of smell and its relationship to food choice. *Critical Reviews in Food Science & Nutrition* 33:63–82.

Yoshida M (1984) Correlation analysis of detection threshold data for "standard test" odors. *Bull Fac Sci Eng Cho Univ* 27: 343–353.

Yousem DM, Maldjian JA, Hummel T, Alsop DC, Geckle RJ, Kraut MA, and Doty RL (1999) The effect of age on odor-stimulated functional MR imaging. *Amer J Neuroradiol* 20:600–608.

Zervakis J, Graham BG, and Schiffman SS (2000) Taste effects of lingual application of cardiovascular medications. *Physiology & Behavior* 2000 Jan;68:405–413.

Zuniga JR, Davis SH, Englehardt RA, Miller IJ, Jr., Schiffman SS, and Phillips C (1993) Taste performance on the anterior human tongue varies with fungiform taste bud density. *Chem Senses* 18:449–460.

34 Autonomic Dysfunction in the Elderly
William P. Cheshire, Jr.

Introduction

Disorders of the autonomic nervous system commonly occur with advancing age. As life expectancies increase in populations throughout the industrialized world, disturbances in autonomic function are becoming increasingly relevant to medical practice and have important implications for health and quality of life.

The autonomic nervous system maintains homeostasis in response to physiologic stress. Its sympathetic, parasympathetic, and enteric divisions provide integrative and adaptive functions to sustain the life and health of the body. Among its responsibilities are control of body temperature, heart rate, blood pressure, regional blood flow, pupillary size, lacrimation, salivation, gastrointestinal transit, urinary bladder emptying, and sexual function. The autonomic nervous system orchestrates a finely balanced repertoire of responses, adapting to environmental and internal changes with moment-by-moment adjustments in neural outflow. Within the brain, the central autonomic network receives signals from numerous peripheral and visceral sensors and sends delicately coordinated and graded responses through autonomic ganglia and peripheral autonomic nerves to reach every organ system. Autonomic reflexes lie beyond conscious control. Many, but not all, autonomic functions escape awareness unless age or disease causes them to falter or fail.

Aging may lead to symptoms of autonomic dysfunction in several ways. Normal human aging itself leads to structural and functional changes in neurons underlying autonomic responses. Age also increases the risk of developing systemic and neurological diseases that may impair autonomic function. Additionally, the elderly are more likely to be taking drugs that modify autonomic reflexes.

Epidemiology and Impact

Blood Pressure Regulation

One of the most important functions of the autonomic nervous system is to maintain an adequate blood pressure to supply oxygen to the brain and other metabolically active tissues. Consequently, one of the most debilitating forms of autonomic dysfunction is orthostatic hypotension, which is defined as a systolic blood pressure decrease of at least 20 mm Hg or a diastolic blood pressure decrease of at least 10 mm Hg within 3 minutes of standing (Consensus 1993). Community-based studies have found the prevalence of orthostatic hypotension in ambulatory elderly persons to be 6–30% (Ensrud et al. 1992; Matsubayashi et al. 1997; Rutan et al. 1992; Tilvis et al. 1996; Wu et al. 2008). Orthostatic hypotension is associated with increased risks of falling, difficulty walking, transient ischemic attacks, osteoporotic fractures, myocardial infarction, and all-cause mortality (Rutan et al. 1992; Ensrud et al. 1992; Verwoert et al. 2008).

Some elderly patients develop marked, symptomatic reductions in blood pressure following a carbohydrate meal, which may present as postprandial fatigue or orthostatic syncope (Mathias 1991; Jansen and Lipsitz 1995). In a Dutch study of hospitalized patients aged 60–98 years, 67% were found to have postprandial and 52% orthostatic hypotension (Vloet et al. 2005). In a prospective cohort study of semi-independent, low-level care residents aged 65 years and older, postprandial hypotension was the only blood pressure parameter that significantly and independently explained all-cause mortality (relative risk 1.79, p = 0.005), with no added predictive value explained by orthostatic hypotension (Fisher et al. 2005).

Thermoregulation

Thermoregulation is frequently impaired in elderly persons and may result from autonomic dysfunction, physical deconditioning, or diseases or medications that impair the behavioral and physiologic responses to changes in ambient temperature (Wongsurawat et al. 1990). The elderly are especially vulnerable during summer heat waves to developing hyperthermia, defined as a core body temperature >38 °C (>100.4 °F). Hyperthermia leads to dehydration, encephalopathy, muscle cramps, cardiac and renal failure (Cheshire and Low 2007). In the United States from 1979 to 1997, there were 7000 deaths attributable to excessive heat (Bouchama and Knochel 2002).

The elderly are also vulnerable to hypothermia, defined as a core body temperature <35 °C (<95 °F), from exposure in temperate as well as cold climates. Hypothermia leads to potentially fatal central nervous system depression, cardiac arrhythmias, and renal failure. In the United States from 1999 to 2002, there were 4607 deaths related to hypothermia, and of them 49% were >65 years of age (CDC 2006).

Autonomic Neuropathy

Increasing obesity and decreased physical activity are contributing to a rising prevalence of diabetes mellitus in the elderly (Marquess 2008). Autonomic dysfunction is common in diabetes mellitus. A population-based study found symptoms of autonomic dysfunction in 54% of type I and 73% of type II diabetic subjects. The severity of autonomic neuropathy was mild overall, but 14% had moderate to severe generalized autonomic failure, and orthostatic hypotension was detected in 8.4 and 7.4% of type I and II diabetic subjects, respectively (Low et al. 2004). Meta-analyses of published data suggest that the presence of cardiovascular autonomic neuropathy in diabetics is associated with an approximately doubled risk of silent myocardial ischemia and mortality (Vinik et al. 2003).

Bladder Dysfunction

The prevalence of urinary bladder dysfunction increases with advancing age. Overactive bladder affects more than 17 million people in the United States (Appell et al. 2001). Estimates of the prevalence of urinary incontinence vary from 5-15% in men to 14–41% in women (Tyagi et al. 2006). Overactive bladder symptoms are associated with an increased risk of falling and fractures (Tyagi et al. 2006). Stratified by age, the prevalence of overactive bladder for men and women, respectively, is approximately 3% and 9% in the fifth decade, 10% and 12% in the sixth decade, 19% and 17% in the seventh decade, 22% and 22% in the eighth decade, and 42% and 31% for ages greater than 75 years (Tyagi et al. 2006). Women with weekly urge incontinence have 26% and 34% greater risks of sustaining a fall or fracture, respectively, whereas daily urge incontinence carries a 35% and 45% increased risk (Tyagi et al. 2006).

Gastrointestinal Dysfunction

Enteric neurodegeneration contributes to the age-related decline in esophageal, gastric, and intestinal motility. Population studies have estimated the prevalence of chronic constipation in the elderly at 24% (Camilleri et al. 2008). Fecal soiling affects as many as 28% of the elderly (McCrea et al. 2008).

Urinary incontinence, constipation, and sexual dysfunction in the elderly are typically multifactorial and more often the result of medications and intercurrent disease than primary autonomic dysfunction (Lipsitz and Novak 2008; Spinzi 2007).

Pathophysiology

The precise mechanisms of aging of the autonomic nervous system remain to be fully elucidated. However, a number of changes in neuronal structures are known to occur with aging. Morphometric studies of the human hypothalamus have shown a decreased number of vasoactive intestinal polypeptide neurons in the suprachiasmatic nucleus in middle-aged males, hypertrophic neurokinin B neurons in postmenopausal women, and increased numbers of arginine vasopressin and corticotrophin-releasing hormone neurons in the paraventricular nucleus in both genders (Zhou and Swaab 1999). Progressive loss of catecholaminergic neurons occurs in the locus ceruleus during normal aging as assessed by histologic studies (Mann et al. 1983; Manaye et al. 1995) and magnetic resonance imaging (Shibata et al. 2006).

Morphometric studies of the human intermediolateral cell column have shown a progressive reduction in preganglionic sympathetic neurons of 5–8% per decade beginning in adult life (Low et al. 1977). With aging, lipofuscin pigment accumulates progressively in sympathetic ganglia (Pick et al. 1964). In the superior cervical ganglion, there is attrition of postganglionic neurons and marked reduction in nerve growth factor receptor p75 in older human subjects (Takahashi 1966; Liutkiene et al. 2007). In the superior mesenteric and celiac ganglia, but to a much lesser degree in the superior cervical ganglion, swollen argyrophilic dystrophic axon terminals develop with aging as well as in diabetic autonomic neuropathy (Schmidt 2002).

Morphometric studies of the human sural nerve, which contains a small proportion of unmyelinated sympathetic postganglionic nerve fibers, have shown axonal degeneration and decreased fiber density with aging (Jacobs and Love 1985; Ochoa and Mair 1969). Epidermal skin biopsies, although showing preserved intraepidermal total nerve fiber density (McArthur et al. 1998), have demonstrated decreased density of sympathetic nerve endings innervating sweat glands in the elderly (Abdel-Rahman et al. 1992). Age-related deterioration in autonomic nerves may be explained by a reduction in the expression and axonal transport of cytoskeletal proteins, diminished myelin regeneration, decline in trophic factors, and decreased rate of axonal regeneration and sprouting (Verdú et al. 2000).

There are two main categories of theories that attempt to explain cellular aging. Genetic programming theories account for aging as an intrinsic program in which lifespan is demarcated by the genome's internal clock (Hayflick 2007). Damage accumulation theories are based on the loss of molecular fidelity resulting from cumulative cellular damage by extrinsic factors resulting in free oxygen radicals, protein glycosylation, macromolecule error catastrophe, or increasing genomic informational entropy (Valko et al. 2006; Knight 2001).

Considerable evidence supports the free radical theory of aging to explain the complex intracellular events leading to the progressive decline in autonomic and other neurologic functions. The free radical theory is based on the fact that oxidative stress is deleterious to intracellular structures. Excessive superoxide radicals are formed by stimulation of nicotine adenine dinucleotide phosphate oxidase, which reduces molecular oxygen, and nonenzymatically by oxygen leakage from the mitochondrial electron transport chain. Excessive superoxide radicals result in cumulative damage to mitochondrial DNA (mtDNA) and proteins. The elevated mutation load in injured mtDNA, which encodes genes essential for energy production, progressively impairs mitochondrial respiration, leading to a vicious cycle of further free radical leakage, oxidative stress, mtDNA damage, disruption of cellular calcium homeostasis, endoplasmic reticulum stress, and ultimately cell death (Valko et al. 2006; Manczak et al. 2005; Cowen 2002).

Decreased levels of endogenous neurotrophic factors may also contribute to the impaired capacity of autonomic neurons to resist the degeneration wrought by free radicals that accumulates with age. The survival of adult sympathetic neurons requires both nerve growth factor and neurotrophin 3, which are derived from effector tissues and retrogradely transported by post-ganglionic neurons (Zhou and Rush 1996).

Additionally, molecular studies of cellular dysfunction in normal aging and disease are unraveling the complex molecular events leading to apoptosis, or programmed neuronal death. Apoptosis is a normal process whereby unnecessary cells are eliminated during embryogenesis and development. The number of apoptotic neurons increases with normal aging. Accelerated neuronal loss in some neurodegenerative disorders may reflect aberrant modulation of apoptosis. Numerous mediators influence the biochemical apoptotic cascade. These include upstream effectors such as Par-4, p53 and proapoptotic Bcl-2 family members, which mediate mitochondrial dysfunction and subsequent release of proapoptotic proteins, such as cytochrome c and apoptosis inducing factor, as well as caspase-dependent and caspase-independent pathways which degrade proteins and nuclear DNA (nDNA) (Culmsee and Landshamer 2006).

Genetic Contributions

Genes encoding the natural protective mechanisms that neutralize reactive oxygen species, such as superoxide dismutase, glutathione and catalase, may influence the aging process (Knight 2001). Moreover, it is plausible that individual variations in the autonomic dysfunction that accompanies aging may relate to nDNA or mtDNA polymorphisms encoding or regulating natural antioxidant pathways. A wide variety of mutations in mtDNA have been identified in organs that are greatly dependent on oxidative metabolism, which may partly explain why the brain has a selective vulnerability for degenerative disorders (Wallace 2005; Suen et al. 2008). These relationships suggest a fundamental link between free radical and genomic theories of neuronal aging.

Correlations of genes encoding components of the sympathetic nervous system to age-related autonomic dysfunction are emerging. Polymorphisms of the Gs protein α-subunit (GNAS1 T131C) and the β3-subunit (GNB3 C825T), for example, were strongly correlated with orthostatic hypotension in a study of community-dwelling elderly subjects (Tabara et al. 2002). Additionally, the arginine-for-tryptophan substitution at codon 64 (Trp64Arg) polymorphism for the β_3-adrenergic receptor has been associated with decreased resting autonomic nervous system activity as assessed by R-R power spectral analysis

(Shihara et al. 1999). As the β_3-adrenergic receptor influences lipolysis and thermogenesis in adipocytes, such polymorphisms may modulate basal metabolic rate, which has implications for aging.

Genetic polymorphisms have also been shown to contribute to the variation in autonomic dysfunction among individuals affected by disease. For example, cardiac autonomic function is more severely impaired in the 1% of type II diabetes associated with the mitochondrial tRNA mutation at base pair 3243 (Mt3243) as compared to ordinary diabetic patients (Momiyama et al. 2002; Majamaa-Voltti et al. 2004).

The genetically-determined accelerated aging syndromes may impair autonomic function. In Down syndrome, for example, baroreflex sensitivity and the heart rate and blood pressure responses to exercise are attenuated (Heffernan et al. 2005; Figueroa et al. 2005). Cardiac conduction defects may occur in Hutchinson-Gilford progeria syndrome, Emery-Dreifuss muscular dystrophy and Werner syndrome, all of which cause premature cardiovascular disease (Capell et al. 2007). Tachycardia, diaphoresis, flushing, and dry eyes have been described in Hutchinson-Gilford progeria syndrome (Merideth et al. 2008).

Clinical Presentations

The type and severity of autonomic phenotypes associated with advanced age differ markedly among individuals. Common patterns of autonomic dysfunction are summarized in Table 1. Among these, cardiovascular changes have been the most extensively studied.

Blood Pressure Regulation

Upon assuming the erect posture, the force of gravity displaces approximately 500–1000 ml of blood to the splanchnic and lower extremity vascular beds. This leads to decreased venous return to the heart, decreased ventricular filling, and a transient decrease in cardiac output and arterial blood pressure. In response, carotid and aortic baroreceptors signal the nucleus of the tractus solitarius in the brain stem to increase sympathetic outflow and decrease parasympathetic outflow. The resulting increase in peripheral vascular resistance and cardiac output restores and maintains blood pressure.

Age-related changes in cardiovascular and cerebrovascular blood flow regulation may predispose the elderly to orthostatic hypotension.

Table 1 Patterns of Autonomic Dysfunction in the Elderly

Orthostatic hypotension

Postprandial hypotension

Loss of heart rate variability

Hypothermia

Hyperthermia

Hyperhidrosis

Anhidrosis

Gastroparesis

Constipation

Loss of appetite

Overactive bladder

Atonic bladder

Incontinence

Sexual impotency

Dry mouth

Dry eyes

Orthostatic hypotension may be symptomatic or asymptomatic, and thus diagnosis should be based on supine and standing blood pressure measurements. Symptoms upon standing may include lightheadedness, dizziness, fatigue, impaired cognition, syncope, or, less frequently, dyspnea, occipitonuchal pain, chest pain, or nausea (Gupta and Lipsitz 2007; Gibbons and Freeman 2005). Even when asymptomatic, orthostatic hypotension poses a risk of falling. For many older patients, orthostatic hypotension is an inconsistent finding (Weiss et al. 2002) and may become symptomatic only under conditions of stress or illness. Prolonged bedrest, for example, deconditions vascular reflexes. Other stresses may include volume depletion from decreased fluid intake, diuresis or diarrhea; anemia; hypotensive side effects of diuretic or antihypertensive drugs; or intercurrent febrile illness. Some healthy older individuals may experience orthostatic hypotension following meal ingestion (Oberman et al. 2000).

A number of age-related changes in the autonomic nervous system combine to cause orthostatic hypotension. Normal aging is associated with an increase in sympathetic outflow combined with a decrease in sympathetic effector responsiveness. The increase in sympathetic outflow is evident in the tonic increases in muscle sympathetic nerve activity assessed by microneurographic recordings (Grassi et al. 1997; Sundlöf and Wallin 1978), as well as by increased circulating plasma catecholamine spillover (Ziegler et al. 1976; Esler et al. 1995). The decrease in sympathetic responsiveness is evident in the age-related decrease in baroreflex sensitivity which regulates the cardiovascular response to reduced venous return to the heart upon standing (Monahan 2007; Huang et al. 2007; Kornet et al. 2005; Jones et al. 2003; Shi et al. 1996). With age, the cardioacceleratory response to β_1-adrenergic stimulation is blunted (Bühler et al. 1980; Vestal et al. 1979). Additionally, α_1-adrenergic vasoconstrictor responsiveness decreases in healthy elderly subjects (Dinenno et al. 2002; Hogikyan and Supiano 1994). The observation that this decreased adrenoceptor responsiveness can be reversed by pharmacologic suppression of sympathetic nervous system activity suggests that it may result from receptor desensitization in response to the age-related increase in basal sympathetic nerve activity (Lipsitz and Novak 2008; Seals and Esler 2000).

The increase in supine blood pressure with age is also an important determinant in the postural drop in pressure (van Dijk et al. 1994). The age-related decline in parasympathetic tone results in less cardioacceleration from vagal withdrawal (De Meersman and Stein 2007; Lipsitz et al. 1990). Orthostatic hypotension in the elderly is also partly due to impaired diastolic filling from loss of cardiac compliance and the impaired muscle pump that occurs with declining lower extremity muscle mass (Rogers and Evans 1993). Aging entails progressive reduction in skeletal muscle mass due to decreased protein synthesis, increased muscle protein degradation, and decreased capacity for muscle regentation (Di Iorio et al. 2006). Finally, decreased levels of renin, angiotensin, and aldosterone with aging reduce the renal capacity to conserve sodium during conditions of fluid restriction or volume loss (Gupta and Lipsitz 2007).

Heart rate variability, which is closely linked with parasympathetic cardiovagal modulation, declines with age and may lessen the ability of the heart to respond to environmental stress (Sloan et al. 2008). Normal aging is associated with decreased R-R intervals during respiration, coughing, and the Valsalva maneuver. Decreased heart rate variability is also seen during sleep, especially since the proportion of deep sleep decreases with aging (Brandenberger et al. 2003; Crasset et al. 2001). A higher risk of myocardial postinfarction mortality with reduced heart rate variability is well-recognized (Wolf et al. 1978; De Meersman and Stein 2007; Kaye and Esler 2008).

Cerebrovascular Regulation

Orthostatic hypotension may occasionally present with focal neurologic symptoms in patients with hemodynamically precarious tandem carotid stenosis (Cheshire and Meschia 2006). Transcranial Doppler sonography evidence indicates that dynamic autoregulation of cerebral blood flow is preserved in the elderly at rest and during orthostatic challenge (van Beek et al. 2008; Carey et al. 2003), although cerebral vasomotor reserve as a function of cardiovagal function is decreased (Fu et al. 2006).

Exercise Capacity

An age-related decrease in maximal exercise heart rate limits aerobic exercise capacity in advanced age. Although due in part to loss of cardiac β-adrenergic sensitivity, the dominant factor is a decline in intrinsic heart rate (Christou and Seals 2008). Age also impairs both vasodilator and vasoconstrictor responses in resistance arteries and arterioles in skeletal muscle (Payne and Bearden 2006). Older subjects demonstrate greater vasoconstrictor tone and reduced blood flow in exercising muscles due to impaired ability of contracting muscle to blunt α-adrenergic vasoconstriction (Koch et al. 2003; Dinenno et al. 2005). In advanced age there is also a decline in endothelium-dependent vasodilation, which occurs more readily in resistance vessels in oxidative as compared to glycolytic muscle (Muller-Delp 2006).

Thermoregulation

Aging is characterized by impairment in the autonomic response to thermal challenge (Cheshire and Low 2007). Heat acclimatization, which results in a lowered sweating threshold and increased sweat quantity for a given rise in temperature, may be limited in older subjects (Wagner et al. 1972), although some of these changes may be reversible with fitness training (Robinson et al. 1965). The liability of older subjects to heat stress and heat stroke is partly due to age-related decline in the sensitivity of peripheral thermoreceptors (Inoue et al. 1999). There is, however, considerable variation among individuals which may be explained by differences in physical fitness, acclimatization, and medications (Foster et al. 1976; Ogawa 1988).

Whereas muscle sympathetic nerve activity progressively increases with age, by contrast, skin sympathetic nerve activity, which plays a key role in thermoregulation, undergoes a progressive and marked reduction in responsiveness to both heat and cold stimuli (Grassi et al. 2003).

Bladder Dysfunction

Overactive bladder syndrome presents with symptoms of urgency with frequency or urge incontinence. By contrast, the atonic or neurogenic bladder is typically due to parasympathetic failure and presents initially with infrequent micturition followed by delayed and incomplete emptying and overflow incontinence.

Gastrointestinal Dysfunction

Esophageal manometry studies in healthy elderly subjects have shown a small decrease in the amplitude of esophageal contractions, an increase in the frequency of simultaneous contractions of the upper and lower esophagus, and a decrease in the periodicity of peristaltic waves after swallowing (Ferriolli et al. 1998). Episodes of gastroesophageal reflux were found to be as frequent, but longer in duration, in older as compared to younger subjects (Ferriolli et al. 1998).

Gastroparesis may present with symptoms of anorexia, early satiety, bloating, nausea, or vomiting of undigested food.

Bowel dysfunction in the elderly significantly impacts functional status, independence, and quality of life. Constipation may consist of hard stools, infrequent stools, the need for straining, or incomplete or unsuccessful evacuation. Because of the subjective nature of constipation, no consensus definition exists. In general, stool frequency of less than three times per week may be considered abnormal (McCrea et al. 2008). Constipation is often the result of inactivity, low fiber diet, depression, medications that slow intestinal transit, neurological disorders that restrict mobility, and poor rectal sensation and evacuation dynamics (Camilleri et al. 2008). Age-related reductions in internal anal sphincter pressure, pelvic muscle strength, rectal sensitivity, and anal function contribute to the potential for constipation (McCrea et al. 2008).

Neurologic conditions that predispose to constipation include Parkinson's disease, stroke, spinal cord injury, multiple sclerosis, autoimmune autonomic ganglionopathy and autonomic neuropathies.

Constipation results also from neurodegeneration in the enteric nervous system. There is evidence of age-related loss of excitatory enteric neurons and interstitial cells of Cajal, resulting in a decrease in colonic propulsive activity, whereas inhibitory neurons appear to be retained (Camilleri et al. 2008). The number of neurons in the myenteric ganglia of colons of subjects older than 65 years is decreased as compared to those aged 20–35 years (Gomes et al. 1997).

The attenuation in thirst that occurs with aging (Farrell et al. 2008) may contribute to constipation as well as orthostatic hypotension.

Sexual Dysfunction

Male sexual dysfunction is characterized by infrequent or poorly sustained erections which may progress to complete erectile failure.

Pupillary Dysfunction

With age, dark-adapted pupil size declines, and latency of the light response is prolonged due to decreased iris sympathetic and parasympathetic activity, respectively. The time to achieve maximum dilation, however, does not decline with age (Pfeifer et al., 1983).

The physiologic changes which underlie the autonomic signs and symptoms associated with aging are summarized in Table 2.

Diagnosis

Beginning with a neurological history, a detailed system review is of paramount importance toward recognizing the presence, distribution, and severity of autonomic dysfunction. The patient with intermittent

Table 2 Age-related Physiologic Changes in the Autonomic Nervous System

Decreased	Increased
Baroreflex sensitivity	Muscle sympathetic nerve activity
Maximum heart rate with exercise	Plasma catecholamine spillover
α-adrenergic vasoconstrictor response to sympathetic activation	α$_1$-adrenergic vasoconstriction in exercising muscles
β$_1$-adrenoreceptor-mediated cardioacceleration and inotropic response	
β$_2$-adrenoreceptor-mediated vasodilatation	
Parasympathetic tone and heart rate variability	
Preganglionic sympathetic neurons	
Thirst when deprived of water	

autonomic dysfunction should be questioned regarding symptom timing and aggravating circumstances.

The history should also explore potential drug effects that can mimic autonomic disorders. Anhidrotic medications, for example, anticholinergics and carbonic anhydrase inhibitors can impair thermoregulatory sweating and contribute to hyperthermia (Cheshire and Fealey 2008). Neuroleptic malignant syndrome is a rare idiosyncratic reaction to dopamine antagonists characterized by hyperthermia, rigidity, hemodynamic instability, delirium, and elevated creatine kinase. In the patient with orthostatic hypotension, it is important to note medications such as diuretics, tricyclic antidepressants, or levodopa, all of which can lower orthostatic blood pressure.

A systematized Composite Autonomic Symptom Scale (COMPASS) has been developed and validated against clinical autonomic test scores (Suarez et al. 1999). This profile consists of 169 items directed at 7 domains of autonomic symptoms with weighted scores. The categories comprise orthostatic intolerance, sexual failure, bladder dysfunction, diarrhea, gastroparesis, secretomotor dysfunction, constipation, vasomotor dysfunction, and pupillomotor impairment. The questionnaire scores the presence and severity of each symptom and has a sensitivity and specificity of 76% and 87%, respectively, in detecting autonomic failure.

At the bedside, autonomic evaluation proceeds from a careful history to a general and neurological examination (Cheshire and Kuntz 2008). A number of features are of particular importance to the assessment of autonomic function and dysfunction. Assessment of hypothermia or hyperthermia should rely on measurements of core body temperature. The skin should be examined for signs of dryness, excessive or asymmetric sweating, unusual coolness or warmth, and distal or regional vasomotor color changes. Eyelid asymmetry or ptosis should be noted. Pupillary size, shape, and responsiveness to a light stimulus and to accommodation should be assessed. The amplitude and regularity of the pulse is palpated. Blood pressure and heart rate should be checked supine and after one to three minutes of standing. The finding of orthostatic hypotension (Consensus 1996) without reflex tachycardia is good evidence of generalized sympathetic adrenergic and cardiovagal failure, provided the patient is not taking a β-blocker. If reflex tachycardia is present, then hypovolemia should be considered.

Plasma volume may be estimated by measuring 24-hour urine sodium excretion. More accurate, and more cumbersome, methods of assessing hydration status include isotope dilution, bioelectrical impedance, and body mass change (Armstrong 2005).

Laboratory testing of autonomic function commonly consists of tests of adrenergic, cardiovagal, and sudomotor function. The Composite Autonomic Severity Score (CASS) grades the combined severity of autonomic failure in each of these domains, adjusted for age and gender (Low 1993).

Adrenergic function is assessed by the beat-to-beat blood pressure response to the Valsalva maneuver and to head-up tilt. One minute of upright tilt will detect orthostatic hypotension due to adrenergic failure in 88% of patients and three minutes will detect the remainder (Gehrking et al. 2005). A small minority of patients will manifest a delayed form of orthostatic hypotension (Gibbons and Freeman 2006). Baroreflex sensitivity is assessed by plotting the relationship between increasing or decreasing blood pressure and corresponding changes in R-R interval (La Rovere et al. 2008).

Cardiovagal function is assessed by the difference in R-R intervals during deep breathing at 5–6 breaths per minute (respiratory sinus arrhythmia), the Valsalva ratio, or spectral analysis of heart rate variability (Low 2003).

Sudomotor function is assessed by the quantitative sudomotor axon reflex test (QSART), which evaluates postganglionic sweating in response to transdermal iontophoresis of acetylcholine (Cheshire and Low 2007). A modified quantitative direct and indirect test (QDIRT) analyzes high-resolution digital photography of silicone impressions of sweat droplets (Gibbons et al. 2008). The thermoregulatory sweating test utilizes the colorimetric change of alizarin red or starch iodine to demarcate areas of sweating from areas of anhidrosis over the anterior body surface in response to raising the core temperature (Fealey et al. 1989).

Gastric emptying is assessed by scintigraphy and stable isotope breath tests (Haans and Masclee 2007). Postprandial hypotension is assessed by measuring blood pressure before and one hour after a large carbohydrate meal (Cheshire and Meschia 2006).

Erectile dysfunction may be evaluated by nocturnal penile tumescence studies, penile electromyography, penile plethysmography, penile blood pressures, selective internal pudendal pharmacoangiography, Doppler sonography, dynamic infusion cavernosometry, or nuclear washout radiography (Broderick 1998).

Treatments Available, Recommended Prioritization of Treatments

The management of autonomic dysfunction is best individualized to the type and severity of the patient's condition, taking into account medical comorbidity and potential adverse effects of the recommended treatment.

Orthostatic Hypotension

Mild forms of orthostatic hypotension can often be successfully managed by nonpharmacologic measures. The goals of treatment are to reduce orthostatic symptoms such as tiredness, dizziness, or cognitive impairment, decrease the risk of falling, and maximize the patient's level of function, rather than to achieve arbitrarily set blood pressure goals.

Plasma volume expansion with liberalization of oral fluids and salt is essential. In general, unless contraindicated by cardiac or renal disease, patients should consume from 2 to 2.5 L of fluid and approximately 10 g of sodium daily. Potentially hypotensive medications such as diuretics, tricyclic antidepressants, or adrenoreceptor antagonists should be tapered if possible. The patient with neurogenic orthostatic hypotension may be advised to anticipate the potential for a postural fall in blood pressure when exposed to a warm environment, after a hot bath, after a meal, after taking nitroglycerin for chest pain, or when straining during micturition or defecation. Orthostatic blood pressure is also lower in the morning hours and after prolonged recumbency because of a larger fall in stroke volume and cardiac output (Omboni et al. 2001). Thus, the patient may lessen orthostatic symptoms by moving from supine to standing in gradual stages and minimizing straining. Once the patient learns to recognize symptoms of hypotension, physical countermaneuvers such as leg-crossing, squatting, bending forward, or placing one foot on a chair, can be easily performed at the time of symptoms (Wieling et al. 1993). These maneuvers compress venous capacitance vessels and assist the return of blood to the heart.

Another useful measure is the use of head-up tilt during sleep. This procedure reduces renal arterial pressure and thereby also nocturnal natriuresis, with the result of increasing blood volume, as well as reducing the cerebrovascular load in patients with nocturnal supine hypertension (Bannister and Mathias 1992).

Custom-fitted, waist-high compressive stockings, alone or in combination with an abdominal binder, are often safe and effective for the nonpharmacologic treatment of neurogenic orthostatic hypotension. Compressive stockings may, however, be very difficult for the patient with limited hand function to apply and remove. Compressive stockings tend to be poorly tolerated in hot and humid climates and should be used cautiously in patients with limited cardiac reserve (McCardell et al. 1999).

Pharmacologic measures should be considered for the treatment of neurogenic orthostatic hypotension that is severe, unresponsive to conservative measures, or results in falling (Gupta and Lipsitz 2007). Fludrocortisone expands body fluid (either blood volume or fluid volume at the perivascular space) and enhances the sensitivity of blood vessels to circulating catecholamines (Freeman 2008; van Lieshout et al. 2000). Midodrine is an α_1-adrenoreceptor agonist that causes venous and arterial vasoconstriction, thus decreasing venous pooling and increasing peripheral vascular resistance.

A frequent clinical dilemma is the patient with adrenergic failure who has both orthostatic hypotension and supine hypertension, since treatment of either condition can worsen the other. Nocturnal supine hypertension, which is due to residual sympathetic tone, may be managed by elevating the head of the bed and avoiding taking midodrine within five hours of bedtime. A bedtime dose of clonidine or transdermal nitroglycerin may be beneficial (Shibao et al. 2006). Twenty-four hour ambulatory blood pressure testing is a useful method for diagnosing and monitoring both nocturnal hypertension and postprandial hypotension.

For the patient with severe supine hypertension, pyridostigmine, which enhances ganglionic transmission, has been shown to be effective in the management of orthostatic hypotension (Singer et al. 2006). Unlike midodrine, and to some degree fludrocortisone, which exacerbate supine hypertension, pyridostigmine significantly improves standing BP in patients with OH without worsening supine hypertension. The greatest effect is on diastolic BP, suggesting that the improvement is due to increased total peripheral resistance (Singer et al. 2006).

Droxidopa is an orally active synthetic precursor of norepinephrine that is currently approved and available in Japan for the treatment of neurogenic orthostatic hypotension and is undergoing clinical trials in Europe and North America (Mathias 2008).

Postprandial Hypotension

Avoiding large carbohydrate loads, including alcohol, is often sufficient to prevent or minimize postprandial hypotension. Caffeine, midodrine, acarbose, and octreotide with meals have been reported to be helpful (Mathias 1991; Jansen and Lipsitz 1995).

Hyperthermia

Vulnerability to the stress of heat or cold should be anticipated in the elderly patient. Hyperthermia can be prevented by seeking shade in hot weather, maintaining hydration, and avoiding overdressing. Symptoms of heat exhaustion, such as dizziness, malaise, nausea, or fatigue associated with elevated temperature can be managed by exposing the skin to fans and as necessary dampening the skin with water (Cheshire and Low 2007).

Hypothermia

Hypothermia can be prevented by dressing warmly, staying dry in cold weather, modifying activity level, making shelter available, and avoiding alcohol and dehydration (Cheshire and Low 2007).

Bladder Dysfunction

Muscarinic receptor antagonists are commonly used for overactive bladder symptoms. These anticholinergic drugs suppress involuntary bladder contractions. Dry mouth is the most frequent side effect. Anhidrosis may also occur (Cheshire and Fealey 2008). Tolterodine

and oxybutynin are comparable in efficacy, whereas tolterodine has less incidence of dry mouth (Hay-Smith et al. 2005). Extended-release preparations may afford additional tolerability (Appell et al. 2001). Intramural injections of botulinum toxin have shown initial promise in the treatment of refractory detrusor overactivity (Drake 2008).

Gastroparesis

Several dietary measures may reduce the symptoms of gastroparesis. Advice should include avoiding fatty foods and late evening meals, eating smaller portions, and dividing portions more frequently during the day, remaining upright after a meal, and limiting fiber intake. More severe symptoms may require prokinetic drugs such as metoclopramide or domperidone, both of which occasionally induce extrapyramidal reactions in susceptible patients. Erythromycin may be helpful in the short term but is less effective chronically. Intrapyloric botulinum toxin has been reported as helpful in select patients with severe gastroparesis and pyloric dysfunction (Haans and Masclee 2007).

Constipation

Constipation may be amenable to simple measures such as increasing oral fluid intake, dietary fiber, and physical activity. For resistant constipation, laxatives may be recommended, and the medication profile should be scrutinized for any constipating drugs that can be tapered or discontinued (Spinzi 2007).

Natural Progression of Disease, Optimal Treatment Outcomes

Autonomic dysfunction in the elderly may continue slowly to worsen with advancing years or, once detected, it may remain stable over time. Apparent worsening or improvement in autonomic dysfunction is frequently due to concurrent factors that shift autonomic physiology past the symptomatic threshold. Medical treatment aims to optimize the patient's ability to ambulate without falling, to function as independently as possible and with a satisfactory quality of life.

The time that the patient is able to remain standing without developing symptoms can be a useful index of the symptom severity of orthostatic hypotension. A treatment that allows the patient to stand as long as 5 or 10 minutes can restore the patient's ability to engage in most activities of ordinary daily living.

Rehabilitative Aspects

Regular physical activity has consistently been shown to reduce or prevent a number of functional and health-associated declines related to advancing age. The benefits of aerobic fitness and strength resistance training include lower rates of myocardial infarction, stroke, hypertension, obesity, osteoporosis, depression, falls, fractures, and overall mortality (Hollman et al. 2007; Mazzeo and Tanaka 2001).

The benefits of regular exercise extend to the autonomic nervous system. There is considerable evidence associating daily physical exercise with preserved respiratory heart rate variability in elderly men and women (Melo et al. 2005; Buchheit et al. 2004; Reland et al. 2004; Perini et al. 2000). Moreover, exercise training has been shown to enhance vagal modulation of heart rate variability in elderly subjects (Leicht et al. 2003; Stein et al. 1999). Since a low level of heart rate variability is an established risk factor for cardiac mortality (Laitio et al. 2007; Filipovic et al. 2003; Tsuji et al. 1994), some investigators have speculated that lessening the age-related decline in parasympathetic modulation of heart rate might be one of the ways in which a physically active lifestyle confers protection against cardiac events (De Meersman and Stein 2007).

Maintenance of an athletic lifestyle has also been shown to improve orthostatic tolerance in the elderly (Fortney et al. 1992). The mechanism involves increased blood volume, enhanced left ventricular performance and improved venous return (Hagberg et al. 1998; Seals et al. 1994; Petrella et al. 1989).

Age-related mitochondrial dysfunction partly normalizes with regular endurance exercise (Lanza et al. 2008). Additionally, the age-related decline in thermoregulatory sweating may be partly negated by physical fitness and acclimatization (Pandolf 1994; Ogawa 1988).

Future Directions

Further progress in preserving autonomic function and managing autonomic dysfunction in advanced age will require a union of science, clinical implementation, and education.

In the realm of science, clinical autonomic testing, now a standard part of the tertiary evaluation of the patient with autonomic symptoms, will likely become more routinely implemented to detect, quantify, and follow objective signs of autonomic dysfunction. With advances in pharmacogenomics, the physician increasingly will have the ability to predict individual differences in disease susceptibility, prognosis, and response to medications. New and affordable methods of genetic testing will make it possible to identify individual variations in metabolism, neurotransmitter transport, and receptor function that influence age-related autonomic dysfunction. Continued drug development will yield more effective and safer drugs to treat orthostatic hypotension, urinary bladder dysfunction, gastroparesis, constipation, and sexual dysfunction.

Further into the future, sophisticated autonomic prostheses may become possible. Implanted nanoscale devices, for example, may one day monitor beat-to-beat blood pressure to detect and respond to orthostatic hypotension, or other sensors may similarly monitor core body temperature, plasma glucose, or catecholamine levels (Cheshire 2007). Cellular regenerative therapies derived from ethical sources may also find applications in restoring lost autonomic functions (Cheshire et al. 2003).

Education will be essential to the realization of these benefits of clinical science. Medical school and residency curricula must remain current with advances in molecular biology, genomics, and neurophysiology. Continuing medical education must keep practicing physicians abreast of new developments and evidence-based therapies. Educational efforts are also needed at the bedside and beyond, so that patients are equipped to recognize indications of autonomic dysfunction and empowered to manage their symptoms effectively. Education should also be aimed at helping all who live a long life to adopt a lifestyle that averts and delays the loss of autonomic function that comes with advancing age.

Summary

Decline in autononomic function is inevitable in old age, whether due to neuronal degeneration, illness, or physical passivity. Orthostatic and postprandial hypotensions are among the most incapacitating manifestations. Other aspects of autonomic dysfunction include loss of heart rate variability, inadequate thermoregulation, and gastric, bowel, bladder, and sexual dysfunction. These problems impact mortality, morbidity, and quality of life. A directed autonomic neurological evaluation can detect and characterize autonomic dysfunction in the elderly and lead to specific treatments, which should be individualized to the particular patient.

References

Abdel-Rahman, T.A., Collins, K.J., Cowen, T., and Rustin, M.: Immunohistochemical, morphological and functional changes in the peripheral sudomotor neuro-effector system in elderly people. *J Auton Nerv Syst* 37:187–197, 1992.

Armstrong, L.E.: Hydration assessment techniques. *Nutr Rev* 63:S40–S54, 2005.

Appell, R.A., Sand, P., Dmochowski, R., et al.: Prospective randomized controlled trial of extended-release oxybutynin chloride and tolterodine tartrate in the treatment of overactive bladder: Results of the OBJECT study. *Mayo Clin Proc* 76:358–363, 2001.

Bannister, R. and Mathias, C.J.: Management of postural hypotension. In *Autonomic failure: A textbook of clinical disorders of the autonomic nervous system*, Ed. 3. (Bannister, R., Mathias, C.J., Eds.) Oxford University Press, Oxford, 1992, pp. 622–645.

Bouchama, A. and Knochel, J.P.: Heat stroke. *N Engl J Med* 346:1978–1988, 2002.

Brandenberger, G., Viola, A.U., Ehrhart, J., et al.: Age-related changes in cardiac autonomic control during sleep. *J Sleep Res* 12:173–180, 2003.

Broderick, G.A.: Evidence based assessment of erectile dysfunction. *Int J Impot Res* 10 Suppl 2:S64–S73, 1998.

Buchheit, M., Simon, C., Viola, A.U., et al.: Heart rate variability in sportive elderly: Relationship with daily physical activity. *Med Sci Sports Exerc* 36:601–605, 2004.

Bühler, F.R., Kiowski, W., van Brummelen, P., et al.: Plasma catecholamines and cardiac, renal and peripheral vascular adrenoceptor-mediated responses in different age groups of normal and hypertensive subjects. *Clin Exp Hypertens* 2:409–426, 1980.

Camilleri, M., Cowen, T., and Koch, T.R.: Enteric neurodegeneration in ageing. *Neurogastroenterol Motil* 20:418–429, 2008.

Capell, B.C., Collins, F.S., and Nabel, E.G.: Mechanisms of cardiovascular disease in accelerated aging syndromes. *Circ Res* 101:13–26, 2007.

Carey, B.J., Panerai, R.B., and Potter, J.F.: Effect of aging on dynamic cerebral autoregulation during head-up tilt. *Stroke* 34:1871–1875, 2003.

Centers for Disease Control and Prevention (CDC): Hypothermia-related deaths—United States, 1999–2002 and 2005. *MMWR Morb Mortal Wkly Rep* 55:282–284, 2006.

Cheshire, W.P.: Doing small things well: Translating nanotechnology into nanomedicine. In *Nanoscale: Issues and Perspectives for the Nano Century.* (Cameron, N.M.deS., Mitchell, M.E., Eds.) John Wiley and Sons, Inc.: Hoboken, N.J., 2007, pp. 315–336.

Cheshire, W.P. and Fealey, R.D.: Drug-induced hyperhidrosis and hypohidrosis: Incidence, prevention and management. *Drug Saf* 31:109–126, 2008.

Cheshire, W.P. and Kuntz, N.L.: Clinical evaluation of the patient with an autonomic disorder. In *Clinical autonomic disorders*, Ed. 3 (Low, P.A., Benarroch, E.E., Eds.). Lippincott Williams & Wilkins, Philadelphia, 2008, pp. 121–140.

Cheshire, W.P. and Low, P.A.: Disorders of sweating and thermoregulation. *Continuum Lifelong Learning Neurol* 13:143–164, 2007.

Cheshire, W.P. and Meschia, J.F.: Postprandial limb-shaking: An unusual presentation of transient cerebral ischemia. *Clin Auton Res* 16:243–246, 2006.

Cheshire, W.P., Pellegrino, E.D., Bevington, L.K., et al.: Stem cell research: Why medicine should reject human cloning. *Mayo Clin Proc* 78:1010–1018, 2003.

Christou, D.D. and Seals, R.: Decreased maximal heart rate with aging is related to reduced β-adrenergic responsiveness but is largely explained by a reduction in intrinsic heart rate. *J Appl Physiol* 105:24–29, 2008.

Consensus Committee of the American Autonomic Society and the American Academy of Neurology: Consensus statement on the definition of orthostatic hypotension, pure autonomic failure, and multiple system atrophy. *Neurology* 46:1470, 1996.

Cowen, T.: Selective vulnerability in adult and ageing mammalian neurons. *Auton Neurosci* 96:20–24, 2002.

Crasset, V., Mezzetti, S., Antoine, M., et al.: Effects of aging and cardiac denervation on heart rate variability during sleep. *Circulation* 103:84–88, 2001.

Culmsee, C. and Landshamer, S.: Molecular insights into mechanisms of the cell death program: Role in the progression of neurodegenerative disorders. *Curr Alzheimer Res* 3:269–283, 2006.

De Meersman, R.E. and Stein, P.K.: Vagal modulation and aging. *Biol Psychol* 74:165–173, 2007.

Dinenno, F.A., Masuki, S., and Joyner, M.J.: Impaired modulation of sympathetic α-adrenergic vasoconstriction in contracting forearm muscle of ageing men. *J Physiol* 567:311–331, 2005.

Dinenno, F.A., Dietz, N.M., and Joyner, M.J.: Aging and forearm postjunctional alpha-adrenergic vasoconstriction in healthy men. *Circulation* 106:1349–1354, 2002.

Di Iorio, A., Abate, M., Di Renzo, D., et al.: Sarcopenia: Age-related skeletal muscle changes from determinants to physical disability. *Int J Immunopathol Pharmacol* 19:703–719, 2006.

Drake, M.J.: Mechanisms of action of intravesical botulinum treatment in refractory detrusor overactivity. *BJU Int* 102 Suppl 1:11–16, 2008.

Esler, M.D., Turner, A.G., Kaye, D.M., et al.: Aging effects on human sympathetic neuronal function. *Am J Physiol* 268:R278–R285, 1995.

Ensrud, K.E., Nevitt, M.C., Yunis, C., et al.: Postural hypotension and postural dizziness in elderly women. The study of osteoporotic fractures. *Arch Intern Med* 152:1058–1064, 1992.

Farrell, M.J., Zamarripa, F., Shade, R., et al.: Effect of aging on regional cerebral blood flow responses associated with osmotic thirst and its satiation by water drinking: A PET study. *Proc Natl Acad Sci USA* 105:382–387, 2008.

Fealey, R.D., Low, P.A., and Thomas, J.E.: Thermoregulatory sweating abnormalities in diabetes mellitus. *Mayo Clin Proc* 64:617–628, 1989.

Ferriolli, E., Oliveira, R.B., Matsuda, N.M., et al.: Aging, esophageal motility, and gastroesophageal reflux. *J Am Geriatr Soc* 46:1534–1537, 1998.

Figueroa, A., Collier, S.R., Baynard, T., et al.: Impaired vagal modulation of heart rate in individuals with Down syndrome. *Clin Auton Res* 15:45–5, 2005.

Filipovic, M., Jeger, R., Probst, C., et al.: Heart rate variability and cardiac troponin I are incremental and independent predictors of one-year all-cause mortality after major noncardiac surgery in patients at risk of coronary artery disease. *J Am Coll Cardiol* 42:1767–1776, 2003.

Fisher, A.A., Davis, M.W., Srikusalanukul, W., and Budge, M.M.: Postprandial hypotension predicts all-cause mortality in older, low-level care residents. *J Am Geriatr Soc* 53:1313–1320, 2005.

Fortney, S., Tankersley, C., Lightfoot, J.T., et al.: Cardiovascular responses to lower body negative pressure in trained and untrained older men. *J Appl Physiol* 73:2693–2700, 1992.

Foster, K.G., Ellis, F.P., Doré, C., et al.: Sweat responses in the aged. *Age Ageing* 5:91–101, 1976.

Freeman, R.: Current pharmacologic treatment for orthostatic hypotension. *Clin Auton Res* 18 (Suppl 1):14–18, 2008.

Fu, C.-H., Yang, C.C.H., and Kuo, T.B.J.: Age-related changes in cerebral hemodynamics and their correlations with cardiac autonomic functions. *Neurol Res* 28:871–876, 2006.

Garland, E.M. and Biaggioni, I.: Genetic polymorphisms of adrenergic receptors. *Clin Auton Res* 11:67–78, 2001.

Gehrking, J.A., Hines, S.M., Benrud-Larson, L.M., et al.: What is the minimum duration of head-up tilt necessary to detect orthostatic hypotension? *Clin Auton Res* 15:71–75, 2005.

Gibbons, C.H. and Freeman, R.: Orthostatic dyspnea: A neglected symptom of orthostatic hypotension. *Clin Auton Res* 15:40–44, 2005.

Gibbons, C.H., Illigens, B.M., Centi, J., and Freeman, R.: QDIRT: Quantitative direct and indirect test of sudomotor function. *Neurology* 70:2299–2304, 2008.

Gibbons, C.H. and Freeman, R.: Delayed orthostatic hypotension: A frequent cause of orthostatic intolerance. *Neurology* 67:28–32, 2006.

Gomes, O.A., de Souza, R.R., and Liberti, E.A.: A preliminary investigation of the effects of aging on the nerve cell number of the myenteric ganglia of the human colon. *Gerontology* 43:210–217, 1997.

Grassi, G., Bolla, G., Seravalle, G., et al.: Comparison between reproducibility and sensitivity of muscle sympathetic nerve traffic and plasma noradrenaline in man. *Clin Sci (Lond)* 92:285–289, 1997.

Grassi, G., Seravalle, G., Turri, C., et al.: Impairment of thermoregulatory control of skin sympathetic nerve traffic in the elderly. *Circulation* 108:729–735, 2003.

Gupta, V. and Lipsitz, L.A.: Orthostatic hypotension in the elderly: Diagnosis and treatment. *Am J Med* 120:841–847, 2007.

Haans, J.J. and Masclee, A.A.: Review article: The diagnosis and management of gastroparesis. *Aliment Pharmacol Ther* 26 Suppl 2:37–46, 2007.

Hagberg, J.M., Goldberg, A.P., Lakatta, L., et al.: Expanded blood volumes contribute to the increased cardiovascular performance of endurance-trained older men. *J Appl Physiol* 85:484–489, 1998.

Hayflick, L.: Biological aging is no longer an unsolved problem. *Ann N Y Acad Sci* 1100:1–13, 2007.

Hay-Smith, J., Herbison, P., Ellis, G., and Morris, A.: Which anticholinergic drug for overactive bladder symptoms in adults. *Cochrane Database Syst Rev* 20:CD005429, 2005.

Heffernan, K.S., Baynard, T., Goulopoulou, S., et al.: Baroreflex sensitivity during static exercise in individuals with Down syndrome. *Med Sci Sports Exerc* 37:2026–2031, 2005.

Hogikyan, R.V. and Supiano, M.A.: Arterial alpha-adrenergic responsiveness is decreased and SNS activity is increased in older humans. *Am J Physiol* 26:E717–E724, 1994.

Hollmann, W., Strüder, H.K., Tagarakis, C.V.M., and King, G.: Physical activity and the elderly. *Eur J Cardiovasc Prev Rehabil* 14:730–739, 2007.

Huang, C.-C., Sandroni, P., Sletten, D.M., et al.: Effect of age on adrenergic and vagal baroreflex sensitivity in normal subjects. *Muscle Nerve* 36:637–642, 2007.

Inoue, Y., Shibasaki, M., Ueda, H., and Ishizashi, H.: Mechanisms underlying the age-related decrement in the human sweating response. *Eur J Appl Physiol Occup Physiol* 79:121–126, 1999.

Jacobs, J.M. and Love, S.: Qualitative and quantitative morphology of human sural nerve at different ages. *Brain* 108:897–924, 1985.

Jansen, R.W. and Lipsitz, L.A.: Postprandial hypotension: Epidemiology, pathophysiology, and clinical management. *Ann Intern Med* 122:286–295, 1995.

Jones, P.P., Christou, D.D., Jordan, J., and Seals, D.R: Baroreflex buffering is reduced with age in healthy men. *Circulation* 107:1770–1774, 2003.

Kaye, D.M. and Esler, M.D.: Autonomic control of the aging heart. *Neuromolecular Med* 10:179–186, 2008.

Kirstein, S.L. and Insel, P.A.: Autonomic nervous system pharmacogenomics: A progress report. *Pharmacol Rev* 56:31–52, 2004.

Knight, J.A.: The biochemistry of aging. *Adv Clin Chem* 35:1–62, 2001.

Koch, D.W., Leuenberger, U.A., and Proctor, D.N.: Augmented leg vasoconstriction in dynamically exercising older men during acute sympathetic stimulation. *J Physiol* 551:337–344, 2003.

Kornet, L., Hoeks, A.P.G., Janssen, B.J.A., et al.: Neural activity of the cardiac baroreflex decreases with age in normotensive and hypertensive subjects. *J Hypertens* 23:815–823, 2005.

Laitio, T., Jalonen, J., Kuusela, T., and Scheinin, H.: The role of heart rate variability in risk stratification for adverse postoperative cardiac events. *Anesth Analg* 105:1548–1560, 2007.

Lanza, I.R., Short, D.K., Short, K.R., et al.: Endurance exercise as a countermeasure for aging. *Diabetes* 57:2933–2942, 2008.

La Rovere, M.T., Pinna, G.D., and Raczak, G.: Baroreflex sensitivity: Measurement and clinical implications. *Ann Noninvasive Electrocariol* 13:191–207, 2008.

Leicht, A.S., Allen, G.D., and Hoey, A.J.: Influence of age and moderate-intensity exercise training on heart rate variability in young and mature adults. *Can J Appl Physiol* 28:446–461, 2003.

Lipsitz, L.A., Mietus, J., Moody, G.B., Goldberger, A.L.: Spectral characteristics of heart rate variability before and during postural tilt. Relations to aging and risk of syncope. *Circulation* 81:1803–1810, 1990.

Lipsitz, L.A. and Novak, V.: Aging and autonomic function. In *Clinical autonomic disorders,* Ed. 3 (Low, P.A., Benarroch, E.E., Eds.). Lippincott Williams & Wilkins, Philadelphia, 2008, pp. 164–178.

Liutkiene, G., Stropus, R., Pilmane, M., and Dabuzinskiene, A.: Age-related structural and neurochemical changes of the human superior cervical ganglion. *Ann Anat* 189:499–509, 2007.

Low, P.A.: Testing the autonomic nervous system. *Semin Neurol* 23:407–421, 2003.

Low, P.A.: Composite autonomic scoring scale for laboratory quantification of generalized autonomic failure. *Mayo Clin Proc* 68:748–752, 1993.

Low, P.A., Benrud-Larson, L.M., Sletten, D.M., et al.: Autonomic symptoms and diabetic neuropathy: A population-based study. *Diabetes Care* 27:2942–2947, 2004.

Low, P.A., Okazaki, H., and Dyck, P.J.: Splanchnic preganglionic neurons in man. I. Morphometry of preganglionic cytons. *Acta Neuropathol* 40:55–61, 1997.

Majamaa-Voltti, K., Majamaa, K., Peuhkurinen, K., et al.: Cardiovascular autonomic regulation in patients with 3243 A>G mitochondrial DNA mutation. *Ann Med* 36:225–231, 2004.

Manaya, K.F., McIntire, D.D., Mann, D.M., and German, D.C.: Locus coeruleus cell loss in the aging human brain: A non-random process. *J Comp Neurol* 358:79–87, 1995.

Manczak, M., Jung, Y., Park, B.S., et al.: Time-course of mitochondrial gene expressions in mice brains: Implications for mitochondrial dysfunction, oxidative damage, and cytochrome c in ageing. *J Neurochem* 92:494–504, 2005.

Mann, D.M., Yates, P.O., and Yawkes, J.: The pathology of the human locus ceruleus. *Clin Neuropathol* 2:1–7, 1983.

Marquess, J.G.: The elderly and diabetes: An age trend and an epidemic converging. *Consult Pharm* 23 Suppl B: 5–11, 2008.

Maser, R.E. and Lenhard, M.J.: Cardiovascular autonomic neuropathy due to diabetes mellitus: Clinical manifestations, consequences, and treatment. *J Clin Endocrinol* Metab 90:5896–5903, 2005.

Mathias, C.J.: L-dihydroxyphenylserine (Droxidopa) in the treatment of orthostatic hypotension: The European experience. *Clin Auton Res* Suppl 1:25–29, 2008.

Mathias, C.J.: Postprandial hypotension. Pathophysiological mechanisms and clinical implications in different disorders. *Hypertension* 18:694–704, 1991.

Matsubayashi, K., Okumiya, K., Wada, T., et al.: Postural dysregulation in systolic blood pressure is associated with worsened scoring on neurobehavioral function tests and leurkoaraiosis in the older elderly living in a community. *Stroke* 28:2169–2173, 1997.

Mazzeo, R.S. and Tanaka, H.: Exercise prescription for the elderly: Current recommendations. *Sports Med* 31:809–818, 2001.

McArthur, J.C., Stocks, E.A., Hauer, P., et al.: Epidermal nerve fiber density: Normative reference range and diagnostic efficiency. *Arch Neurol* 55:1513–1520, 1998.

McCardell, C.S., Berge, K.H., Ijaz, M., and Lanier, W.L.: Acute pulmonary edema associated with placement of waist-high, custom-fit compressive stockings. *Mayo Clin Proc* 74:478–480, 1999.

McCrea, G.L., Miaskowski, C., Stotts, N.A., et al.: Pathophysiology of constipation in the older adult. *World J Gastroenterol* 14:2631–2638, 2007.

Melo, R.C., Santos, M.D.B., Silva, E., et al.: Effects of age and physical activity on the autonomic control of heart rate in healthy men. Braz J Med Biol Res 38:1331–1338, 2005.

Merideth, M.A., Gordon, L.B., Clauss, S., et al.: Phenotype and course of Hutchinson-Giford progeria syndrome. *N Engl J Med* 358: 592–604, 2008.

Momiyama, Y., Suzuki, Y., Ohtomo, M., et al.: Cardiac autonomic nervous dysfunction in diabetic patients with a mitochondrial DNA mutation: Assessment by heart rate variability. *Diabetes Care* 25:2308–2313, 2002.

Monahan, K.D.: Effect of aging on baroreflex function in humans. *Am J Physiol Regul Integr Comp Physiol* 293:R3–R12, 2007.

Muller-Delp, J.M.: Aging-induced adaptations of microvascular reactivity. *Microcirculation* 13:339–352, 2006.

Oberman, A.S., Gagnon, M.M., Kiely, D.K., et al.: Autonomic and neurohumoral control of postprandial blood pressure in healthy aging. *J Gerontol A Biol Sci Med Sci* 55:477–483, 2000.

Ochoa, J., and Mair, W.G.P.: The normal sural nerve in man. II. Changes in the axons and Schwann cells due to aging. *Acta Neuropathol (Berl)* 13:217–239, 1969.

Ogawa, T.: Influence of aging on sweating activity. In *Cutaneous aging.* (Kligman, A.M., Takase, Y., Eds.). University of Tokyo, Tokyo, 1988, pp. 111–125.

Omboni, S., Smitt, A.A., van Lieshout, J.J., et al.: Mechanisms underlying the impairment in orthostaitc tolerance after nocturnal recumbency in patients with autonomic failure. *Clin Sci (Lond)* 101:609–618, 2001.

Pandolf, K.B.: Heat tolerance and aging. *Exp Aging Res* 20:275–284, 1994.

Payne, G.W., and Bearden, S.E.: The microcirculation of skeletal muscle in aging. *Microcirculation* 13:275–277, 2006.

Perini, R., Milesi, S., Fisher, N.M., et al.: Heart rate variability during dynamic exercise in elderly males and females. *Eur J Appl Physiol* 82:8–15, 2000.

Petrella, R.J., Cunningham, D.A., and Smith, J.J.: Influence of age and physical training on postural adaptation. *Can J Sport Sci* 14:4–9, 1989.

Pfeifer, M.A., Weinberg, C.R., Cook, D., et al.: Differential changes of autonomic nervous system function with age in man. *Am J Med* 75:249–258, 1983.

Pick, J., De Lemos, C., and Gerdin, C.: The fine structure of sympathetic neurons in man. *J Comp Neurol* 122:19–67, 1964.

Reland, S., Ville, N.S., Wong, S., et al.: Does the level of chronic physical activity alter heart rate variability in healthy older women? *Clin Sci* 107:29–35, 2004.

Robinson, S., Belding, H.S., Consolazio, F.C., et al.: Acclimatization of older men to work in heat. *J Appl Physiol* 20:583–586, 1965.

Rogers, M.A. and Evans, W.J.: Changes in skeletal muscle with aging: Effects of exercise training. *Exerc Sport Sci Rev* 21:65–102, 1993.

Rutan, G.H., Hermanson, B., Bild, D.E., et al.: Orthostatic hypotension in older adults: The cardiovascular health study. *Hypertension* 19:508–519, 1992.

Schmidt, R.E.: Age-related sympathetic ganglionic neuropathology: Human pathology and animal models. *Auton Neurosci* 96:63–72, 2002.

Seals, D.R. and Esler, M.D.: Human ageing and the sympathoadrenal system. *J Physiol* 528:407–417, 2000.

Seals, D.R., Hagberg, J.M., Spina, R.J., et al.: Enhanced left ventricular performance in endurance trained older men. *Circulation* 89:198–205, 1994.

Shi, X., Gallagher, K.M., Welch-O'Connor, R.M., and Foresman, B.H.: Arterial and cardiopulmonary baroreflexes in 60- to 69- vs. 18- to 36-yr-old humans. *J Appl Physiol* 80:1903–1910, 1996.

Shibao, C., Gamboa, A., Abraham, R., et al.: Clonidine for the treatment of supine hypertension and pressure natriuresis in autonomic failure. *Hypertension* 47:522–526, 2006.

Shibata, E., Sasaki, M., Tohyama, K., et al.: Age-related changes in locus ceruleus on neuromelanin magnetic resonance imaging at 3 Tesla. *Magn Reson Med Sci* 5:197–200, 2006.

Shihara, N., Yasuda, K., Moritani, T., et al.: The association between Trp[64]Arg polymorphism of the β_3-adrenergic receptor and autonomic nervous system activity. *J Clin Endocrinol Metab* 84:1623–1627, 1999.

Singer, W., Sandroni, P., Opfer-Gehrking, T.L., et al.: Pyridostigmine treatment trial in neurogenic orthostatic hypotension. *Arch Neurol* 63:513–518, 2006.

Sloan, R.P., Huang, M.-H., McCreath, H., et al.: Cardiac autonomic control and the effects of age, race, and sex: The CARDIA study. *Auton Neurosci* 139:78–85, 2008.

Spinzi, G.C.: Bowel care in the elderly. *Dig Dis* 25:160–165, 2007.

Stein, P.K., Ehsani, A.A., Domitrovich, P.P., et al.: Effect of exercise training on heart rate variability in healthy older adults. *Am Heart J* 138:567–576, 1999.

Suarez, G.A., Opfer-Gehrking, T.L., Offord, K.P., et al.: The Autonomic Symptom Profile: A new instrument to assess autonomic symptoms. *Neurology* 52:523–528, 1999.

Suen, D.-F., Norris, K.L., and Youle, R.J.: Mitochondrial dynamics and apoptosis. *Genes & Dev* 22:1577–1590, 2008.

Sundlöf, G. and Wallin, B.G.: Human muscle nerve sympathetic activity at rest. Relationship to blood pressure and age. *J Physiol* 274:621–637, 1978.

Tabara, Y., Kohara, K., and Miki, T.: Polymorphisms of genes encoding components of the sympathetic nervous system but not the renin-angiotensin system as risk factors for orthostatic hypotension. *J Hypertens* 20:651–656, 2002.

Takahashi, K.: A clinicopathologic study on the peripheral nervous system of the aged. Sciatic nerve and autonomic nervous system. *Geriatrics* 21:123–133, 1966.

van Lieshout, J.J., ten Harkel, A.D.J., and Wieling, W.: Fludrocortisone and sleeping in the head-up position limit the postural decrease in cardiac output in autonomic failiure. *Clin Auton Res* 10:35–42, 2000.

Tilvis, R.S., Hakala, S.M., Valvanne, J., and Erkinjuntti, T.: Postural hypotension and dizziness in a general aged population: A four-year follow-up study of the Helsinki Aging Study. *J Am Geriatr Soc* 44:809–814, 1996.

Tsuji, H., Venditti, F.J.Jr., Manders, E.S., et al.: Reduced heart rate variability and mortality risk in an elderly cohort. The Framingham Heart Study. *Circulation* 90:878–883, 1994.

Tyagi, S., Thomas, C.A., Hayashi, Y., and Chancellor, M.B.: The overactive bladder: Epidemiology and morbidity. *Urol Clin N Am* 33:433–438, 2006.

Valko, M., Liebfritz, D., Moncol, J., et al.: Free radicals and antioxidants in normal physiological functions and human disease. *Int J Biochem Cell Biol* 39:44–84, 2006.

van Beek, A.H., Claassen, J.A., Rikkert, M.G., and Jansen, R.W.: Cerebral autoregulation: An overview of current concepts and methodology with special focus on the elderly. *J Cerebr Blood Flow Metab* 28:1071–1085, 2008.

van Dijk, J.G., Tjon-A-Tsien, A.M., Kamzoul, B.A., et al.: Effects of supine blood pressure on interpretation of standing up test in 500 patients with diabetes mellitus. *J Auton Nerv Syst* 47:23–31, 1994.

van Lieshout, J.J., ten Harkel, A.D., and Wieling, W.: Fludrocortisone and sleeping in the head-up position limit the postural decrease in cardiac output in autonomic failure. *Clin Auton Res* 10:35–42, 2000.

Verdú, E., Ceballos, D., Vilches, J.J., and Navarro, X.: Influence of aging on peripheral nerve function and regeneration. *J Peripher Nerv Syst* 5:191–208, 2000.

Verwoert, G., Mattace-Raso, F.U.S., Hofman, A., et al.: Orthostatic hypotension and the risk of cardiovascular disease in elderly people: The Rotterdam Study. *J Am Geriat Soc* 56:1816–1820, 2008.

Vestal, R.E., Wood, A.J., and Shand, D.G.: Reduced beta-adrenoceptor sensitivity in the elderly. *Clin Pharmacol Ther* 26:181–186, 1979.

Vinik, A.I., Maser, R.E., Mitchell, B.D., and Freeman, R.: Diabetic autonomic neuropathy. *Diabetes Care* 26:1553–1579, 2003.

Vloet, L.C., Pel-Little, R.E., Jansen, P.A., et al.: High prevalence of postprandial and orthostatic hypotension among geriatric patients admitted to Dutch hospitals. *J Gerontol A Biol Sci Med Sci* 60:1271–1277, 2005.

Wagner, J.A., Robinson, S., Tzankoff, S.P., and Marino, R.P.: Heat tolerance and acclimatization to work in the head in relation to age. *J Appl Physiol* 33:616–622, 1972.

Wallace, D.C.: A mitochondrial paradigm of metabolic and degenerative diseases, aging, and cancer: A dawn for evolutionary medicine. *Annu Rev Genet* 39:359–407, 2005.

Weiss, A., Grossman, E., Beloosesky, Y., and Grinblat, J.: Orthostatic hypotension in acute geriatric ward: Is it a consistent finding? *Arch Intern Med* 162:2369–2374, 2002.

Wieling, W., Van Lieshout, J.J., and Van Leeuwen, A.M.: Physical maneuvers that reduce postural hypotension in autonomic failure. *Clin Autonom Res* 3:57–65, 1993.

Wolf, M.M., Varigos, G.A., Hunt, D., and Sloman, J.G.: Sinus arrhythmia in acute myocardial infarction. *Med J Australia* 2:52–53, 1978.

Wongsurawat, N., Davis, B.B., and Morley, J.E.: Thermoregulatory failure in the elderly. *J Am Geriat Soc* 38:899–906, 1990.

Wu, J.-S., Yang, Y.-C., Lu, F.-H., et al.: Population-based study on the prevalence and correlates of orthostatic hypotension/hypertension and orthostatic dizziness. *Hypertens Res* 31:897–904, 2008.

Zhou, J.N. and Swaab, D.F.: Activation and degeneration during aging: A morphometric study of the human hypothalamus. *Microsc Res Tech* 44:36–48, 1999.

Zhou, X.F. and Rush, R.A.: Functional roles of neurotrophin 3 in the developing and mature sympathetic nervous system. *Mol Neurobiol* 13:185–197, 1996.

Ziegler, M.G., Lake, C.R., and Kopin, I.J.: Plasma noradrenaline increases with age. *Nature* 261:333–335, 1976.

6
Peripheral Neurology in Aging

35 Spinal Disorders in the Elderly

Stephen M. Selkirk and Robert L. Ruff

Introduction

The geriatric population will increase due to increases in life expectancies and the aging of the baby boom generation. Treatment of spinal disorders in the elderly is a difficult challenge that involves numerous medical, surgical, and social issues. This chapter provides an overview of spinal disorders in the elderly. Multiple factors, such as immobilization, medical comorbidities, polypharmacy associated with multiple medical disorders, and skeletal degeneration, that vary among the elderly make it difficult to develop generalized treatment strategies. Care needs to consider the specific challenges of each patient. Treatment plans should emphasize early mobilization and functional rehabilitation. The treatment goals and surgical indications will differ from those for younger patients without comorbidities.

Geriatric-related spinal disorders can be divided into osteoarthritis and degenerative disk disease, degenerative deformities, traumatic disorders (covered in a separate chapter), spinal tumors, infections, and inflammatory disorders. Spinal disorders can produce pain and may be associated with myelopathy and radiculopathy. Non-traumatic myelopathy may develop subacutely and be related to ongoing systemic medical conditions such as spinal degenerative arthritis, disk disease, or metastatic cancer. It is critical to recognize myelopathy early to prevent permanent loss of motor function and bladder and bowel control. Nonoperative techniques such as adequate pain management and physical therapy can promote early mobilization and enhance functional recovery.

The Spine of Elderly Patients

Several factors contribute to the pathophysiology of spinal disorder in the elderly. Spondylosis, osteoporosis, and malignancy are more common in the elderly. Spondylosis is a degenerative local process specifically affecting the spine, whereas osteoporosis and other metabolic bone diseases are systemic processes that preferentially affect the spine. Malignant neoplasms affecting the spinal column and cord are most commonly metastatic.

Spondylosis

Degenerative changes of the spinal column usually begin in the third to fourth decade of life. The degenerative cascade is hypothesized to begin at the disk level where the water content of the nucleus pulposus begins to diminish and the collagen content increases. Radial and circumferential tears then are seen in the annulus fibrosis as the nucleus pulposus is less capable of load sharing. Biochemical alterations of the disk lead to mechanical insufficiency with reduction in disk height. As the intervertebral disks collapse, bulging of the annulus leads to lateral protrusion producing buckling of the ligamentum flavum into the spinal canal that may produce cord compression in the cervical and thoracic spine or thecal sac compression in the lumbar spine. Disk collapse decreases the size of the neural foramina and can produce radiculopathy. Spinal disk degeneration changes the mechanical loading of the vertebral endplates and posterior facet joints which triggers the genesis of vertebral body and facet osteophytes. Osteophytes can compress the spinal cord or nerve roots. The degenerative process may affect adjacent sites of spinal column motion leading to either stiffness or instability. Stiffened levels often are characterized by diminished disk height, ligament calcification, and bridging osteophyte formation. Hypermobile or unstable segments are characterized by spinal deformity such as degenerative spondylolisthesis or degenerative scoliosis. Compression of the spinal cord or roots can result from either static deformity or dynamic instability as seen in the positional dependent compression of the thecal sac in degenerative spondylolisthesis.

Osteoporosis

Osteoporosis is a systemic, age-related metabolic disorder. Osteoporosis is characterized by a decrease in bone mass and increased susceptibility to fractures. Two types of primary osteoporosis are Type I (postmenopausal and osteoclast-mediated) and Type II (senile and osteoblast-mediated). Both forms affect women more than men.

Osteoporosis and other metabolic bone diseases involve the spine because it contains the largest quantity of metabolically active trabecular bone. The preferential decrease in the horizontal trabeculae of the vertebral bodies in osteoporosis reduces the ability of the spinal column to withstand compressive loads. Therefore, vertebral compression can occur in the setting of minor, incidental trauma. The impaired mechanical integrity of vertebrae demands that special considerations be given when spinal procedures and instrumentation are considered.

Miscellaneous Conditions

The incidence of malignant spinal tumors is much higher in elderly patients. Other conditions such as ankylosing spondylitis and Paget's disease also have a greater prevalence in the elderly and also must be considered in the differential diagnosis of any elderly patient with recalcitrant spinal pain.

Special Considerations in the Elderly

Treatment goals and expectations may be different for the elderly. The realization that complete pain relief and cure may not be possible can be frustrating for the patient and the physician. However, appreciating the challenges of treating spinal disorders in the elderly may prevent potential complications and maximize the likelihood of a successful, though imperfect, result.

Nonoperative Treatment

Treatments of spine disorders in the elderly are complicated by medical comorbidities associated with numerous chronic medications to address the comorbidities. Caution must be exercised to avoid having the treatment be worse than the spinal disorder. Medical disorders such as chronic liver disease may preclude the use of acetaminophen. Likewise, nonsteroidal anti-inflammatory drugs (NSAIDs) should be used cautiously in elderly patients with a history of renal insufficiency, gastritis, or peptic ulcer disease. Glucocorticoid treatment will complicate diabetes mellitus. Medications that produce minimal drug interactions and provide a safer side-effect profile should be considered.

Adequate pain management is imperative. While elderly may be more prone to cognitive side effects of opioid medication, narcotic addiction is less frequent in this population. The elderly patient is more susceptible to muscle deconditioning and disuse osteopenia, which can occur when analgesia is not adequate and physical therapy is not implemented. A well-organized physical therapy program not only provides symptomatic relief, it also encourages overall fitness and general health.

Considerations in Operative Treatment

When surgery is considered, a thorough assessment of the risks and benefits of nonoperative and operative treatments is mandatory and frequently requires consultation from various specialists. The medical state must be optimized preoperatively. Poor nutritional status can complicate the surgical outcome. It is associated with poor wound healing and infection. Serologic markers of nutritional status including a prealbumin level should be done in any geriatric patient suspected to have nutritional compromise. The altered anatomy of diseased spinal elements can complicate surgery. For example, hypertrophic facet joints can obscure surgical landmarks for pedicle screw placement. Another important intraoperative consideration in the elderly is impaired bone mechanical integrity, which decreases the likelihood of a successful bone graft and adversely affects the quality of implant fixation.

Degenerative Disorders

Spinal degenerative disorders typically involve the cervical and lumbar spine. Degenerative lumbar disorders can cause axial symptoms (back pain) resulting from lumbar spondylosis, segmental instability, and spinal deformity, or can cause lower extremity symptoms (neurogenic claudication in central stenosis or radiculopathy in lateral stenosis) resulting from lumbar spinal canal stenosis. Similarly, degenerative cervical disorders can cause axial symptoms (neck pain) and/or can cause myelopathy in central stenosis or radiculopathy in lateral stenosis.

Lumbar Degenerative Disease
Pathophysiology

Degenerative disk disease, lumbar spondylosis, and lumbar spinal stenosis are common findings in the elderly. It is critical to distinguish axial symptoms from appendicular symptoms. In the evaluation of the elderly patient with lower extremity symptoms, neurogenic claudication resulting from lumbar spinal stenosis is among the most common causes. Neurogenic claudication is caused by significant central spinal stenosis. Appendicular symptoms such as pain or paresthesias radiating to the lower extremities can occur but usually are not reported below the knee, in contradistinction to lumbar radiculopathy caused by a herniated nucleus pulposus. Neurogenic claudication is usually characterized by a deep, aching pain beginning in the buttocks and radiating down the thighs, which is exacerbated during ambulation. Often pain is relieved by positions of lumbar flexion. Because comorbidities such as peripheral vascular disease and diabetic neuropathy are seen commonly in the elderly, it is important that neurogenic claudication be distinguished from vascular claudication and peripheral neuropathy.

Clinical Presentation and Diagnosis

The examination of the patient often reveals a normal neurologic examination. Diminished motor strength and atrophy usually are seen only in patients with severe or long-standing disease. Lower exercise may elicit weakness or loss of deep tendon reflexes. Plain radiographs taken with the patient standing often show nonspecific degenerative changes, but are important in ruling out any deformity or any instability. Magnetic resonance imaging (MRI) provides additional information and anatomic detail. It is important to correlate the findings on MRI with the clinical presentation.

Treatment and Natural History

Most patients with degenerative lumbar disease can be treated successfully by nonoperative modalities, which include oral NSAIDs, pain treatment, and physical therapy. Fluoroscopically assisted local injections can be used diagnostically and therapeutically. Diagnostic nerve root blocks often help to localize the source of leg pain. Therapeutic epidural steroid injections often can provide transient relief.

Surgical treatment is indicated in only a small percentage of patients with lumbar degenerative disease. The goals of surgical treatment are to provide pain relief, to halt or reverse any neurologic deficit, and ultimately, to restore function. Posterior lumbar decompression (laminectomy, laminotomy, or laminoplasty) is done for any neural compression-producing disabling appendicular symptoms. Good-to-acceptable results after posterior lumbar decompression have been reported in 85% of patients 80 years or older (Devo et al. 1992). Spinal stabilization with anterior fusion, posterior fusion, or both is done for severe degenerative disk disease producing incapacitating axial symptoms, spinal instability, or spinal deformity (Devo et al. 1992).

Cervical Spondylosis

Degenerative disease of the cervical spine, or cervical spondylosis (CS), is the most common cause of spinal cord pathology in the elderly (Young 2000). It is the most common cause of nontraumatic spinal cord injury, estimated to be the main contributing factor in a quarter of these cases (Moore and Blumhardt 1997). Furthermore, CS is a contributing factor to spinal cord injury after minor falls as described earlier. It has been defined as non-inflammatory vertebral osteophytosis secondary to degenerative disk disease. This is distinctly different from inflammatory arthritis which classically involves the synovial membranes of diarthrodial joints. Spondylosis is thought to be part of the natural aging process as by the age of 65 it can be identified in 95% of individuals (Fehlings and Skaf 1998).

Pathophysiology

CS occurs as spinal elements degenerate over time, ultimately resulting in compromise of the vascular supply to the spinal cord which actually causes irreversible damage. The degenerative process, which can be identified in up to 10% of individuals by age 25, begins with disk desiccation (Ferguson and Caplan 1985). This loss of water content results in changes in the biochemical composition of the disk including an increase in the keratin sulfate to chondroitin sulfate ratio (Benzel 2001) and a decrease in the protein and mucopolysaccharide content. The result is a nucleus pulposus that is less elastic, smaller, and fibrotic, causing a shift in weight bearing to the annulus fibrosis resulting in increased likelihood of disk bulging into the spinal canal (Benzel 2001). There is also a significant loss of disk space height ventrally. Loss of disk space results in a greater load on uncovertebral joints resulting in ventral redirection of the vertebral bodies and degeneration (Ferguson and Caplan 1985). The alterations in the biochemical composition of the vertebral body producing changes in biomechanical forces cause Sharpey's fibers to dissect away from the edges of vertebral bodies and the posterior ligament to buckle and peel away from the endplates (Verbiest 1973). These bare edges of the vertebral body are the focal point of reactive bone formation and subsequently spondylotic spurs form. Spondylotic spur (osteophyte) formation is accelerated by motion, promoting a greater degree of pathology at C5–C6, C6–C7.

Over time, a combination of these changes (osteophyte formation, degeneration uncovertebral joints, herniated disk and facet joint disease) results in a reduction in the diameter of the cervical spinal canal and subsequent symptomatology (Benzel 1996; Epstein 1978). The normal sagittal diameter of the cervical spinal cord in adults is about 17 mm (Bohlman and Emery 1988). In order to make the diagnosis of cervical spondylosis, Ferguson and Caplan (1985) suggest that the diameter must be less than 13 mm, while White and Panjabi (1988) report that patients with less than 14.8 mm were at high risk of developing myelopathy. The precise reduction in sagittal diameter required to cause myelopathy is debatable, but generally speaking most patients with a diagnosis of cervical spondylosis have a diameter at least 3 mm smaller than normal. Dynamic flexion and extension of the spinal cord can worsen the degenerative changes described above. Flexion lengthens the cord, stretching it over developing osteophytes and extension can result in pinching of the cord between weakened ligamentum flavum and ventral osteophytes (Fehlings and Skaf 1998). In the presence of spondylytic changes resulting in narrowing of the diameter of the spinal cord, repeated hyperextension of the cervical spine results in transient acute compression and shear stress analogous to that inflicted during an acute spinal cord injury.

Gross pathology findings including indentation of the spinal cord by osteophytic processes and diffuse flattening due to widespread mechanical changes. Histological changes are most evident in the dorsal and lateral column of the cord and demonstrate prominent demyelination over osteophytic areas. Interestingly, necrosis and cavitation of the central gray and medial white matter is readily identified in chronic cases and is suggestive of ischemic insult. Ischemia may also account for the prominent demyelination/dysmyelination as oligodendrocytes are particularly sensitive to ischemia (Fehlings and Skaf 1998). Animal models utilizing a combination of ischemic and compressive injury recapitulate these pathological changes as do studies measuring perfusion pressures (Fehling and Skar 1998). Evidence also suggests that micro-arterial circulation is likely responsible for ischemic changes (Al-Mefty et al. 1993) but venous congestion and/or compression of large arteries may also play a role in slow developing, chronic disease (McCormick et al. 2003). Less well defined, the role of apoptosis, free-radical damage, and cation-mediated cell death may also be significant contributors to the pathology of CS (Fehlings and Skar 1998).

Clinical Presentation

Patients with CS can present with the complaint of neck pain or stiffness prior to the onset of detectable neurological signs and symptoms. Signs and symptoms can be divided into radicular, occurring from compression of the nerve roots without spinal cord compression, and myelopathic, secondary to spinal cord compression, or a combination of both. Radicular signs and symptoms include pain radiating from the spinal cord into the affected limb and diminished or absent deep tendon reflexes (DTRs) with variable loss of strength and/or sensation. The most common site of radiculopathy with spondylosis is at C6

(Crandall and Batzdorf 1966). The C6 nerve is the only nerve innervating the extensor carpi radialis muscle and therefore weakness of wrist extension in combination with weakness of the biceps and diminished biceps or brachioradialis reflexes are consistent with a C6 radiculopathy.

Classical symptoms of myelopathy from CS are subacute, subtle gait disturbance and/or weakness and/or stiffness of the bilateral lower extremities in conjunction with a loss of dexterity in the bilateral upper extremities. Loss of dexterity can manifest as complaints about changes in hand writing or difficulty with buttons or zippers. Loss of sphincter control and urinary incontinence is uncommon; however, a significant number of patients may complain of urgency (McCormack 1996). Patients will have a typical upper motor neuron (UMN) pattern of injury including exaggerated DTRs, spasticity, clonus, and an extensor plantar response. The jaw jerk reflex can be particularly useful in localizing signs of UMN dysfunction as an absent jaw jerk suggests the lesion location is below the foramen magnum, while the converse is true if the jaw jerk is exaggerated. Similarly useful, the presence of an exaggerated pectoralis muscle reflex suggests high cervical cord compression. Muscle atrophy and fasiculations are considered late signs of myelopathic changes secondary to spondylosis and their presences early should initiate further evaluation to exclude amyotrophic lateral sclerosis. Later in the course, wasting of the intrinsic hand muscles is a classical finding (Goodridge et al. 1987).

Elderly patients with CS are at high risk for acute spinal cord injury due to loss of proprioception and gait disturbances predisposing to falls. The progressive bio-mechanical changes associated with CS can make apparent trivial falls life-altering events. Most commonly a fall, particularly if one strikes the forehead, will result in hyperextension of the already compromised cord resulting in acute compression (Maroon 1977) and central cord syndrome.

Diagnosis

MR-imaging is the *sine qua non* for the diagnosis of CS in patients presenting with cervical pain, decreased neck mobility, or signs and symptoms of cervical myelopathy or radiculopathy (Al-Mefty et al. 1988). CT scan is an additional important element for the diagnosis of CS, often complimenting the information generated from MR-imaging. It is superior for the identification of osteophyte formation, defining bony elements and the neural foramina (Freeman and Martinez 1992). Other modalities are much less useful. Myelography remains useful in patients who cannot undergo MRI, while plain films will be interpreted as demonstrating spondylotic changes in nearly all elderly patients (Alexander 1996) and therefore are of limited utility as a screening or diagnostic mechanism. Similarly, electromyography is not useful for the diagnosis of CS but should be employed to rule out ALS if there is concern for this diagnosis. Other possible diagnoses not eliminated by MRI imagining can be eliminated by laboratory studies including HIV, B12 deficiency, and a comprehensive family history.

Treatment

The value of surgical intervention for patients compared to medical management and close clinical follow-up is widely debated. The high risk for minor trauma resulting in acute SCI suggests that early surgical intervention in patients with deteriorating gait in the elderly would be a valid intercession. Having said this, the data on surgical outcomes does not necessarily support this conclusion and is confounded by a poorly defined natural history and a lack of solid prognostic indicator in patients with CS. Treatment of symptomatic patients with surgical intervention versus medical management has been compared in only two well designed studies (of 13209 citations) and reviewed by Fouyas et al. (2002) in a Cochrane review. The most efficacious surgical intervention is also not defined; however, the aim is to decompress the affected cord and/or nerve root. The two studies reviewed by Fouyas et al. (2002) utilized either an anterior approach using an allograft or autograft while the remainder underwent posterior decompression with laminectomy or laminoplasty. The medical management groups in these studies received a variety of interventions including physical therapy, hard collar, soft collar, anti-inflammatory agents, bed rest, and avoidance of strenuous activity. These studies failed to show a significant benefit from surgery at more extensive time points using measures of pain or function in patients with either radiculopathy or myelopathy from CS (Bednarik et al. 1999).

The main point of these data is that patients with CS need to be carefully selected for surgery, albeit with little or no principles to guide this selection. This fact is underscored by Glaser et al. (1998) who did a study asking academic neurosurgeons presented with clinical cases to recommend treatment. He concluded: "that there is a wide range of surgical opinion regarding the appropriate type of management of cervical spine injuries, even among a relatively small sample of mostly academic surgeons…" Clearly untreated patients with CS do not all develop progressive neurological deterioration over time and some patients with progressive disease stabilize for long time periods without intervention. Perhaps the most vulnerable population is elderly individuals with myelopathy-induced gait dysfunction predisposing them to recurrent minor falls and ultimately devastating acute SCI.

Natural History

The natural history of CS is variable. For the majority of cases there appears to be a slowly progressive deterioration with a subsequent prolonged static phase during which disability level is not altered (Lee and Turner 1963). This static phase is hypothesized to develop through fusion of ventral osteophytes in contiguous vertebrae resulting in stabilization of the cervical spine with diminished mobility. There is no evidence that patients with radiculopathy will eventually develop myelopathy. Subgroup analysis suggests that patients with moderate disability, progressive disability, or patients older than 60 with progressive disease were noted to deteriorate more frequently and therefore it is recommended that surgical intervention be reserved for this subgroup of patients. Overlying this data is the increased risk of acute SCI after minor trauma in patients with CS (Firooznia et al. 1985). This factor argues for early surgical intervention and is particularly germane to elderly individuals who are at increased risk for repeated trauma from falls. Multiple publications have documented the nefarious outcome in elderly patients following acute cervical SCI. Alander et al. (1994) reported a rather dramatic association between mortality and age: 23% of patients over age 50 did not survive an acute cervical spinal cord injury and mortality of patients over 65 years of age was 100% at early time points. Other data supports this with two year data post injury demonstrating 50% mortality in the 50–84 year age range (Foo 1986) and a separate report showing one year post injury mortality of 75% in patients older than 45 years of age and 20% in patients younger than 45 years of age (Sneddon and Bedbrook 1982). Further complicating the issue is the concept that the elderly population has worse outcomes after surgical decompression and stabilization after spinal cord injury, resulting in a less aggressive approach to treatment based on age.

Spinal Canal Deformity

Spinal deformity in the elderly population typically results from late-stage, advanced degenerative disk disease and should be differentiated from other causes (congenital, posttraumatic, idiopathic) of deformity seen in younger patients. Two of the more common deformities in adults are degenerative spondylolisthesis and degenerative scoliosis and predominantly are seen in the lumbar spine.

Degenerative Spondylolisthesis

Pathophysiology

Degenerative spondylolisthesis is one of the most common spinal deformities in the elderly population. It typically involves the L4–L5 level, in contrast to congenital spondylolisthesis which involves the L5–S1 level. Progressive disk and facet degeneration from spondylosis coupled with the sagittal orientation of the lumbar facet joints in insufficiency of the posterior elements to resist the anteriorly directed force of the body's center of gravity. Consequently, anterolisthesis of the superior vertebra on the inferior vertebra occurs. Unlike congenital or dysplastic spondylolistheses, the posterior elements in degenerative spondylolisthesis remain relatively intact, and slippage is mild, usually less than 33%.

Clinical Presentation

Patients with degenerative spondylolisthesis frequently have advanced degenerative disk disease and will report back pain, buttock and leg pain, or both. An important component in patient evaluation is to assess whether back pain or leg pain is the predominant symptom. Dynamic instability may exacerbate neurologic symptoms, and positions that relieve symptoms such as lumbar flexion, which increase the spinal canal and foraminal dimensions, should be elucidated.

Diagnosis

Plain radiographs and dynamic flexion and extension radiographs are mandatory in any patient with spondylolisthesis. MRI is indicated for patients with significant neurologic symptoms; additionally, dynamic flexion and extension MRI may help to visualize neural compression.

Treatment

Most patients with degenerative spondylolisthesis benefit from nonoperative treatment using a combination of NSAIDs, physical therapy, and if needed, epidural glucocorticoid injections. Surgical treatment is reserved for elderly patients with neurologic deterioration and/or patients who are unresponsive to a lengthy course of nonsurgical treatment.

When the clinical symptoms correspond to the findings on imaging studies and are refractory to nonoperative treatment, a posterior lumbar decompression and in situ posterolateral fusion can benefit patients. Posterior decompression alone will increase the instability at the level of the spondylolisthesis. In situ posterolateral fusion relieves preoperative axial symptoms and will stabilize the spine. Reduction usually is not necessary in degenerative spondylolisthesis because the deformity generally is mild. The benefits of instrumentation to provide immediate stability and to permit early mobilization without bracing outweigh the risks in most healthy older patients.

Degenerative Scoliosis

Pathophysiology

Degenerative scoliosis, often termed de novo scoliosis, is secondary to long-standing spondylotic disease and as a result, often is painful. It is differentiated from an adult with adolescent idiopathic scoliosis by the age of onset of the spinal deformity. It occurs predominantly in the lumbar spine as opposed to idiopathic scoliosis, which usually occurs in the thoracic spine. Also, degenerative curves generally involve fewer levels and are smaller in magnitude than idiopathic curves.

Clinical Presentation

Patients commonly will report neurogenic claudication or radicular symptoms, which often will outweigh the chronic back pain. Patients usually have radiculopathies on the concave side of the lumbar curve. Truncal balance is impaired with coronal or sagittal decompensation.

Diagnosis

Full-length scoliosis series radiographs should be taken with the patient standing to evaluate any compensatory curves above the usual lumbar curve and to assess coronal and sagittal alignment. Lateral radiographs often show a loss of lordosis or kyphotic thoracolumbar junctions. Most degenerative curves are mild. Hence, often MRI is adequate to observe spinal column elements and spinal cord. Bending and flexion and extension radiographs taken with the patient supine can assess the flexibility of the spine in the coronal and sagittal planes and identifies fusion levels in patients being considered for surgical intervention. Most degenerative curves are rigid and stiff.

Treatment

The standard nonoperative treatment including NSAIDs, opioid analgesics, physical therapy, and perhaps epidural steroid injections, may provide some symptomatic relief. Accommodative, not corrective, flexion bracing also may help alleviate symptoms. Unlike idiopathic scoliosis, the surgical indication for degenerative scoliosis is upon symptoms rather than the magnitude of the scoliosis. The main indications for surgical intervention are incapacitating back or leg pain or progressive neurologic deficits that are refractory to nonoperative treatment. The goals of surgical treatment are neural decompression, spinal balance, and spinal stabilization.

With degenerative scoliosis, any posterior decompression usually requires additional spinal canal stabilization. A posterolateral arthrodesis is sufficient in most patients. Additional interbody fusion enhances the correction of the sagittal alignment and improves the likelihood of fusion. Similar to degenerative spondylolisthesis, interbody fusion is indicated in patients in whom there is significant sagittal plane deformity, severe disk collapse with foraminal compromise, deficient posterior bone stock, or previous posterior decompressive surgery. When long fusions are done to the sacrum, interbody fusion also is recommended to augment posterior fixation and reduce the stress on instrumentation at the lumbosacral junction. Infrequently, patients present with large, rigid, stiff curves and with severe truncal decompensation that cannot be corrected with standard anterior and posterior techniques. In these patients, osteotomies and vertebral column resections are indicated to obtain appropriate correction.

Spinal Cord Compression in Metastatic Cancer

It is estimated that between 12,700 and 25,000 patients per year with a diagnosis of cancer in the U.S. will develop spinal cord compression. Of the estimated 500,000 patients dying of cancer annually, likely 1 in 20 of these patients will be diagnosed with spinal cord compression (Loblaw et al. 2003). The risk for spinal cord involvement is dependent upon the primary source and is highest for breast, prostate, and lung cancer. Together these three sources account for 50% to 60% of all cases involving spinal cord compression, with renal cell carcinoma, myeloma, non-Hodgkin lymphoma and colon cancer accounting for most of the remaining cases (Schiff 2003). However, nearly all forms of systemic cancer have been reported to seed the epidural space and a measureable percentage of cases are of unknown primary origin. Spinal cord compression usually manifests in patients with a pre-existing cancer diagnosis, however in 20% of patients it is the presenting symptom of cancer and 30% of these patients will eventually be diagnosed with lung cancer (Schiff et al. 1997). The focus of the following

will be epidural spinal cord metastases as intramedullary spinal cord metastases are considered to be extremely rare, found in only approximately 2% of cases at autopsy (Schiff et al. 1997).

Pathophysiology

Spinal cord dysfunction occurs when malignant cells seed and then expand within the spinal epidural space resulting in epidural spinal cord compression (ESCC). Malignant cells can enter the epidural space via expansion of a paravertebral tumor through an intervertebral foramen and into the spinal canal compressing the cord (Gilbert et al. 1978). More commonly, cells reach the vertebral bodies via hematogenous spread, followed by proliferation in the bone and spread into the epidural space. Acute symptomatology presumably results when bony destruction is sufficient to cause collapse and displacement into the epidural space. Direct compression of the cord by either mechanism results in acute oligodendrocyte and myelin loss followed by secondary axonal transection and glial scar formation. Anterior invasion compresses and eventually occludes venous drainage, resulting in loss of the blood-spinal cord barrier and edema. As compression continues, arterial supply is eventually compromised and infarction ensues resulting in irreversible damage (Kato et al. 1985). Thus ischemia secondary to compression rather than compression itself leads to spinal cord dysfunction and irreversible neurological damage.

Hematogenous dissemination of malignant cells to the vertebral column was thought to occur via Batson's vertebral venous plexus since Batson proposed the theory in 1940. More recent theories center on arterial dissemination and rely primarily on experimental animal data (Arguello et al. 1990).

Clinical Presentation

Pain is a nearly ubiquitous symptom in patients with ESCC with some studies demonstrating up to 95% of patients noting back pain prior to diagnosis (Schiff 2003). It is the presenting symptom of cancer in 20% of cases and the median time from pain onset to diagnosis is as long as eight weeks in some series (Gilbert et al. 1978). Pain can be caused by damage to bony vertebral structure causing localized pain or by nerve compression causing radicular pain. Often, pain may be referred and present as hip pain (girdle discomfort) or scapular pain with thoracic level or cervical level involvement respectively (Levack et al. 2002). Localized pain develops as cells extend into the soft tissue structures or stretches the periosteum. It usually develops first and is concomitant with the level of spinal cord involvement which is directly related to the volume of bone and the extent of blood flow to various segments of the cord. The majority of ESCC occur in the thoracic cord (60%), followed by lumbosacral (30%), and 10% are cervical (Schiff 2003). As the mass expands, nerve roots are compressed resulting in a radicular pain quality with increasing intensity. Radicular pain is usually unilateral in the cervical and lumbar nerve compression but bilateral with thoracic invasion. Radicular pain is characteristically worsened by movement and Valsalva and usually worse at night as the recumbent position lengthens the spine and distends the epidural venous plexus. Finally, mechanical pain, characterized by worsening with movement and improvement with lying still, is caused by vertebral body collapse and in general is a foreboding symptom associated with extensive bony invasion by cancer cells.

Weakness is the second most common presenting sign in patients diagnosed with ESCC; present in up to 75% of patients at diagnosis (Bach et al. 1990). Remarkably, in one series 68% of patients were non-ambulatory at the time of diagnosis (Gilbert et al. 1978). Weakness from ESCC is more often asymmetrical when presenting in an upper motor neuron (UMN) pattern and symmetrical with a lower motor neuron pattern (LMN). Other symptoms of spinal cord compression are highly variable and more dependant upon location and extent of involvement at the time of presentation. A pattern of distal sensory loss progressing proximally is common and sensory symptoms are present in at least one-half of patients at the time of diagnosis, but rarely precede motor dysfunction (Helweg-Larson 1996; Gilbert et al. 1978). Isolated ataxia has been reported with early isolated involvement of the spinocerebellar tract but this is uncommon (Gilbert et al. 1978). Equally uncommon is isolated autonomic dysfunction; however, bowel and bladder dysfunction is reported as being present in about 50% of patients at diagnosis (Bach et al. 1990).

Diagnosis

Although a thorough history and complete neurological evaluation are important, any patient presenting with new onset back pain and a pre-existing diagnosis of cancer should have diagnostics studies to exclude ESCC. Studies in the Netherlands, where access to MRI is limited secondary to economic constraints on the health care system, have demonstrated that no sign or symptom in a patient with cancer presenting with back pain can preclude the need for the definitive radiological study-MRI (Kienstra et al. 2000). The sensitivity and specificity of MRI for the diagnosis of ESCC is 93% and 97% respectively (Li and Poon 1988). It is superior to CT in terms of defining surrounding anatomy and its routine use adds information beyond a CT scan changing the parameters used in radiation therapies in 40%–53% of cases (Colletti et al. 1996). MRI also allows for evaluation of the entire spine in a short time window which is important as one-third of patients will have compression at multiple sites along the cord. These findings always affect surgical decision making and therefore imaging of the entire spine should be routine (Portenoy et al. 1987; Ruff and Lanska 1989).

Other imaging techniques are limited in diagnostic potential. Plain film studies have a 15% false negative rate and require extensive bony erosion before a compressive lesion can be identified (Bach et al. 1990). Classical findings include pedicle thinning, increased size of the neural foramina, altered osseous density, compression fractures and paravertebral masses (Portenoy et al. 1989). However, these are late findings. Radionuclide bone scans offer increased sensitivity compared to plain films but are unable to identify whether epidural tumor if present (Gosfield et al. 1993). Positron emission tomography (PET) using fluorodeoxyglucose (FDG) is superior to radionuclide bone scans as it is reliant upon metabolic activity rather than indirectly identifying metastasis through increased bone turnover. However, PET scans lack the appropriate resolution for diagnosis. Finally, CT scan with myelography, which was the radiologic study of choice prior to MRI for the diagnosis of ECSS, is now reserved for patients that cannot undergo MRI because of implanted devices but is preferred for the guidance of percutaneous needle biopsies.

Treatment

Given the poor median survival of patients diagnosed with ESCC, the definitive treatment is defined in terms of ameliorating symptoms rather than complete eradication of tumor cells in the spine. Early studies demonstrating the efficacy of corticosteroids in reducing neurological deficits in patients with CNS lesions were performed in the early 1960s (Cantu 1968). For patients with ESCC, steroids are the first line treatment and result in a rapid reduction in edema and inflammation resulting in an equally expeditious improvement of neurological deficits. The only randomized study demonstrating the efficacy of corticosteroid administration was reported in 1994 and tested steroid plus radiotherapy versus radiation therapy alone. Results showed a significant increase in the ability to ambulate at three (81% versus 63%) and six months (59% and 33%) post-treatment in the

steroid plus radiotherapy group (Sorenson et al. 1994). This study solidified the use steroids as first line treatment; however, controversy persists regarding the precise steroid regimen which optimizes relief of symptoms and minimizes side-effects. Complicating the issue are animal studies which demonstrate a dose-dependent effect (Delattre et al. 1989) while human studies failed to recapitulate an association between dose and relief of pain, maintaining ambulation or bladder function (Vecht et al. 1989). Spinal cord damage becomes irreversible soon after clinical onset, producing a justified sense of urgency by practitioners, resulting in a tendency to use steroids at the high-end of the dosing spectrum. This is particularly justified in patients who are not ambulatory at presentation or have rapidly progressive neurological deterioration. In these patients, a loading dose of 96 mg of dexamethasone intravenous followed by 96 mg per day for three days and then a 10-day taper is justified. For patients ambulating and with less progressive signs or symptoms a 10 mg loading dose followed by a 16 mg oral dose and then a taper may be acceptable.

Radiation therapy directed against the compressive lesion has been the standard treatment for ESCC for over 60 years, but efficacy has never been tested in a randomized controlled study. All evidence of efficacy versus supportive care is derived from retrospective analysis which has demonstrated a clear benefit to patients from radiotherapy (Barron et al. 1959). Similar to the use of corticosteroids, the most efficacious dose and treatment course has not been established, but the use of the modality itself is widely agreed upon. Clinical trials have been performed comparing different dosing and radiation schedules however interpretation of these studies are complicated by the variation in radio-sensitivity of different primary tumors and comparison to non-standard treatments. In general, patients with a poor prognosis for survival due to extensive systemic tumor burden should be treated with a short course of high dose radiotherapy ranging from 8 Gy in one fraction to 20 Gy in five fractions. Patients with controlled systemic disease and minimal to moderate neurological dysfunction should receive a more protracted course of 40 Gy in 20 fractions as this regimen results in less local recurrence of symptoms.

Prior to the widespread use of radiation therapy, laminectomy was the only available treatment. Later retrospective trials and one randomized prospective trial failed to demonstrate the efficacious of laminectomy either alone or in conjunction with radiotherapy and therefore it is no longer part of a treatment strategy for patients with ECSS. More recently, direct decompressive surgery, utilizing an anterior approach, immediate circumferential decompression, and spinal cord stabilization, has been shown to benefit patients beyond radiation therapy alone. In fact, the initial randomized trial comparing direct decompressive surgery and postoperative radiotherapy with only radiotherapy was halted prematurely after demonstrating statistical significance at only 50% of its target recruitment goal (Patchell et al. 2005). The combination therapy resulted in more patients able to walk after treatment, decreased need for pain medication and steroids, more patients maintaining ambulation for longer times, and more patients unable to walk at study start were able to walk after treatment. One caveat to this study was the recruitment of patients was limited to those with less radiosensitive tumor types. Current indications for surgery include: relapse after radiotherapy or progression during radiotherapy, unknown primary tumor, and evidence of instability of the spine or fractures. Particularly salient here, the complication rates from surgical management of ESCC was nearly double (Chen et al. 2007) for patients 65 years of age and older (71% versus 43%).

Finally, the use of chemotherapy is limited to patients with recurrence who cannot undergo surgery or radiotherapy. Tumor responsiveness and the prolonged time to obtain decompression of the spinal cord make this modality less useful.

Natural Progression

Untreated ESCC results in progressive incapacitating pain, weakness leading to paraplegia, and bowel and bladder dysfunction. Median survival of patients with ESCC is dependent upon the primary tumor type as well as the extent of metastatic disease and ambulatory ability at presentation. As stated previously, the goal of treatment is to alleviate symptoms and prevent further neurological decline as the median survival for patients even with radiosensitive tumors is at best 5 to 7 months while patients with lung cancer have a median survival of only 1.5 months (Loblaw et al. 2003). Patients ambulating after therapy had a median survival of 9 months while those nonambulatory only 1 to 2 months (Maranzano et al. 2005). More relevant to the proceeding section, patients with ESCC spend two times as many days hospitalized in the last year of life compared to cancer patients without ESCC (Loblaw et al. 2003), underlying the complexity of this diagnosis in terms of ongoing medical management and a need for an early and comprehensive rehabilitation program.

Patients who do survive for relatively extended periods are at high risk for recurrent ESCC. In fact, patients surviving 3-years post treatment of ESCC universally redeveloped compression from metastatic cells (Gilbert et al. 1978). Taken together, somewhere between 8% and 20% of patients with a diagnosis of ESCC will develop recurrent compression with one-half developing them at the identical spinal cord level and half at a different level (van der Sande et al. 1999). Although there is some controversy regarding how to best treat recurrent disease, current treatment paradigms recommend a second dose of radiotherapy for initial recurrence and then chemotherapy and surgery for future recurrences with the goal of maintaining ambulation as long as possible.

Rehabilitation

Given the short median survival of patients with ESCC, an early referral to a multi-disciplinary rehabilitation center is vital. The appropriate rehabilitation program should be short in duration and focus on improvements in mobility, transfer techniques, and self-care. The efficacy of rehabilitation in patients with a poor prognosis and with ESCC has been documented repeatedly. McKinley et al. (1996) reported on 32 patients with a median expected survival of three months who underwent rehabilitation and achieved functional improvements in mobility and self-care and maintained these improvements for at least three months after being discharged. Furthermore, 84% of these patients achieved discharge to home rather than a nursing facility. Two other reports demonstrated the benefits of a 2-week directed rehabilitation program focusing on transfers, skin care, and bladder/bowel management in nonambulatory patients with ECSS. Median survival was 26 weeks in patients undergoing rehabilitation versus six weeks in the control group. Lower pain levels, less depression, and improved quality of life were also associated with the rehabilitation program. These gains were durable and maintained until time of death (Ruff et al. 2007).

Future Directions

Emerging forms of highly directed radiotherapy hold promise for the treatment of ECSS. These spinal stereotactic radiosurgery (SRS) systems allow for accurate delivery of higher dose radiation to tumor cells while minimizing exposure of normal, uninvolved tissues. SRS systems are considered experimental as large randomized trials have yet to demonstrate efficacy versus standard radiotherapy regimens. But, published reports using CyberKnife® (Accuray Incorporated, Sunnyvale, CA) have shown a decrease in pain in treated patients, improvement in neurological deficits, or lack of progression in nearly 80% of patients treated with minimal adverse effects (Degen et al. 2005).

Infection

Pathophysiology

Elderly patients with vertebral osteomyelitis are challenging to treat. Elderly patients are not only at increased risk of failure of nonoperative treatment, but also at increased risk of neurologic deterioration. Spinal infections can be categorized in many ways: acute versus chronic, pyogenic versus granulomatous (tuberculous, fungal), or primary versus postsurgical. The most common location for pyogenic vertebral osteomyelitis is in the lumbar spine, whereas the most common location for tuberculous vertebral osteomyelitis is in the thoracic spine. (Feldenzer et al., 1988). Vertebral osteomyelitis usually is a secondary process from another focus of infection such as urinary tract infection, pneumonia, or skin infection and is the result of hematogenous seeding from arterial septic emboli or from retrograde flow from engorged venous channels of Batson's plexus. *Staphylococcus aureus* is the most common microorganism infecting the vertebral column. Gram negative infections such as *Escherichia coli* and *Pseudomonas* are characteristic of spinal osteomyelitis arising from a genitourinary tract infection. Atypical fungal and tuberculous infections are characteristic in immunocompromised patients because of HIV, cancer, or organ transplantation (Feldenzer et al. 1988).

Clinical Presentation

The clinical manifestation of spinal osteomyelitis is highly variable and dependent on host resistance and organism virulence. Because of the variability of presentation, spinal infection and spinal neoplasm should be considered in the differential diagnosis of any elderly patient with relentless, unremitting back pain. It usually is associated with a significant delay in diagnosis (sometimes greater than three months) and therefore, requires a high index of suspicion. Elderly patients especially are susceptible to complications from vertebral osteomyelitis. Risk factors for poor outcome include: advanced age, diabetes mellitus, rheumatoid arthritis (RA), *Staphylococcus aureus* infection, and epidural abscess in the cervical spine. The typical presentation of spinal osteomyelitis in an elderly patient is an insidious onset of unremitting back pain that is constant, awakens the patient from sleep, and is not related to activity. Constitutional symptoms such as fever, chills, and weight loss frequently are until late in the course of infection. Patients with acute infections are more likely to have the classic signs of infection than patients with more indolent infections. Physical examination is often nonspecific. Paravertebral spasm and tenderness may be elicited especially in patients with the acute stage of infection.

Diagnosis

Laboratory studies, including a leukocyte count with differential, erythrocyte sedimentation rate (ESR), C-reactive protein (CRP), and blood cultures, comprise the initial diagnostic workup. Plain radiographs often will show relatively normal findings at the acute phase of the infection (Hlavin et al. 1990). Disk space narrowing may be evident when there is advanced disk space infection. Rarefaction of bone may be present at six weeks, and new bone formation may be evident at 12 weeks from the onset of infection. Technetium-99 bone scanning when used in conjunction with gallium scanning is a sensitive and specific study that will show an infectious process long before any radiographic findings. Magnetic resonance imaging is the diagnostic modality of choice to observe the inflammatory process. It provides excellent soft tissue detail and permits observation of disk involvement, abscess formation, or neural compression. Magnetic resonance imaging can distinguish a pyogenic infection from a tuberculous infection or a spinal neoplasm. In pyogenic vertebral osteomyelitis, the vertebral body and affected disk will produce a dark signal on the

Tl-weighted sequence and a bright signal on the T2-weighted sequence. In a tuberculous infection and in a spinal tumor, the disk is usually relatively unaffected (An et al. 1991).

Treatment

The initial treatment is intravenous antibiotics and spinal column immobilization with an orthosis. Immobilization is a precautionary maneuver against vertebral body collapse or fracture that can produce spinal cord compression. Consultation with an infectious disease specialist is recommended for appropriate antibiotic selection after the microorganism has been isolated from blood cultures, biopsy specimens, or both. ESR and CRP can be used to monitor the response to antibiotic therapy.

Surgical intervention is indicated when: (1) a diagnosis cannot be made through blood culture or percutaneous biopsy; (2) systemic signs remain despite antibiotic therapy; (3) abscess formation is present; (4) there are progressive or evolving neurologic signs; or (5) there is evidence of spinal instability in the form of vertebral collapse or deformity. An anterior decompression generally is done because the underlying disease usually originates from the vertebral body. Reconstruction is done using autograft or allograft. Stabilization with the use of instrumentation is controversial and this treatment intervention is evolving.

Inflammatory Disorders

Two inflammatory disorders, rheumatoid arthritis (RA) and ankylosing spondylitis, are issues for the elderly. The treatment of RA considers its predisposition toward spinal instability, whereas the treatment of ankylosing spondylitis considers its predisposition toward spinal rigidity. In the geriatric population, RA and ankylosing spondylitis are challenging to treat because both often present as severe, advanced, late-stage disease.

Rheumatoid Arthritis

Pathophysiology

RA is a progressive seropositive polyarthropathy, predominantly affecting women. For reasons not completely understood, spinal RA is almost always restricted to the cervical spine.

Clinical Presentation

Three clinical manifestations of rheumatoid disease are evident in the cervical spine: atlantoaxial instability, basilar invagination, and subaxial instability. Usually, there is a sequential progression of cervical involvement beginning with atlantoaxial instability progressing to basilar invagination and then to subaxial subluxation. Most patients present with advanced disease, when all three findings are commonly present.

Presenting complaints of axial or appendicular pain or subtle findings of myelopathy often are masked by the peripheral deformities from late-stage rheumatoid disease. Overlooking subtle symptoms and missing cervical spinal disease in the patient with RA can lead to disastrous complications such as quadriparesis and sudden death. Therefore, every elderly patient with RA should be considered at risk for spinal RA until proven otherwise.

Diagnosis

Radiographic evaluation of atlantoaxial instability is determined with radiographs by measuring the posterior atlanto-odontoid process interval (PAOI), which should be greater than 14 mm in healthy subjects. Reduced PAOI often is observed on the lateral film taken with the spine in flexion. Measurement of the atlanto-odontoid interval

(AOI) (normal < 3.5 mm) is less reliable because accompanying basilar invagination may produce a falsely normal AOI. Numerous radiographic measurements to evaluate basilar invagination have been introduced.

The radiographic evaluation of subaxial instability is determined by measuring the space available for the cord, which is greater than 14 mm in healthy subjects, and by measuring translation and angulation of motion segments on the lateral radiographs taken with the spine in flexion and extension. An increase of greater than 3.5 mm translation or 10° angulation between motion segments is a radiographic sign of subaxial instability.

Treatment

The natural history of the rheumatoid cervical spine is a steadily progressive disability and loss of ambulation caused by myelopathy with sudden death in approximately 10% of patients. Goals of surgical treatment are neural decompression if needed, spinal stabilization, and early mobilization. Early aggressive surgical decompression and stabilization before permanent neurologic deficit are crucial to improve the functional recovery in these patients. Surgical stabilization with or without decompression is indicated for patients with any clinical evidence of myelopathy. Indications for surgical stabilization irrespective of the presence of neurologic deficit include patients who have atlantoaxial instability with a PAOI less than 14 mm, patients who have atlantoaxial instability and greater than 5 mm basilar invagination, and patients who have subaxial subluxation and less than 14 mm available for the spinal cord (Boden et al. 1993).

The surgical treatment chosen must address the underlying disease. C1–C2 fusion is indicated for patients with isolated atlantoaxial instability. The fusion should be extended to the occiput if there is any evidence of accompanying basilar invagination. The fusion should be extend caudad (an occiput-to-upper thoracic fusion) in patients with advanced disease in whom there also is additional subaxial subluxation or instability.

Natural History

The natural history of untreated cervical spine RA is a steadily progressive disability and loss of ambulation caused by myelopathy with sudden death in approximately 10% of patients.

Ankylosing Spondylitis

Although the typical age at onset of ankylosing spondylitis is approximately 40 years, it is a slowly progressive deformity with late-stage disease being difficult to treat. Because ankylosing spondylitis affects the elderly most severely, it deserves special consideration.

Clinical Presentation

Ankylosing spondylitis is an HLA-B27 seronegative spondyloarthropathy more commonly affecting males. It often begins at the sacroiliac joints and as the disease progresses ossification and ankylosis occur in an ascending manner. Multisystem involvement does occur, and associated conditions include uveitis, prostatitis, carditis, and pneumonitis. As the fusion progresses cephalad, it results in the development of a long rigid spinal column making it vulnerable to fracture, even in the setting of minor or incidental trauma. A high suspicion for acute fracture should be present for any patient with ankylosing spondylitis complaining of neck or back pain even with the history of minor or no trauma. Manifestations include loss of lordosis in the lumbar spine; progressive kyphotic deformities especially are seen in the thoracic and cervical spine. The thoracic and cervical deformity can progress to the point that the chin abuts the chest, making it difficult for the patient to look forward or eat.

Treatment

Extension osteotomies are reserved for progressive and severe kyphotic deformities that interfere with vision and eating. The procedure is technically demanding, and carries an appreciable risk due to the potential for spinal cord damage. Spinal cord monitoring is essential during spine surgery.

Because spinal ankylosis results in high torque of the rigid spinal column, mechanical stresses can produce fractures that lead to pseudarthrosis. When a fracture develops, particularly in the cervical spinal cord, prompt rigid immobilization by halo immobilization, surgical instrumentation, or both must be used to prevent additional fracture displacement, which could lead to epidural hematoma or mechanical spinal cord compression (Broom and Raycroft, 1988).

Natural History

Due to extensive ankylosis and kyphotic deformity, acute spinal fractures in patients with ankylosing spondylitis are associated with a high risk of profound neurologic deficit. There are also risks of spontaneous epidural hemorrhage, ascending paralysis, and death.

In summary, diagnosis and treatment of spinal disorders in the elderly is a difficult challenge that involves numerous medical and surgical issues and consideration of multiple co-morbid conditions and functional limitation in the elderly. A high index of suspicion and early diagnosis and imaging add to a favorable outcome in these conditions that represent a serious threat to health and independence in the elderly.

References

Al-Mefty O, Harkey HL, Marawi I, Haines DE, Peeler DF, Wilner HI, et al. Experimental chronic compressive cervical myelopathy. *Journal of Neurosurgery* 1993; 79: 550–561.

Al-Mefty O, Harkey LH, Middleton TH, Smith RR, and Fox JL. Myelopathic cervical spondylotic lesions demonstrated by magnetic resonance imaging. *Journal of Neurosurgery* 1988; 68: 217–222.

Alander DH, Andreychik DA, and Stauffer ES. Early outcome in cervical spinal cord injured patients older than 50 years of age. *Spine* 1994; 19: 2299–2301.

Alexander JT. Natural history and nonoperative management of cervical spon3dylosis. In Menezes AH, Sonntag VKH, Venzel EC, McCormick PC, Cahill DW, and Papadopoulos SM (eds): *Principles of spinal surgery*, New York: McGraw-Hill 1996, pp 547–557.

An HS, Vaccaro AR, and Dolinskas CA. Differentiation between spinal tumors and infections with magnetic resonance imagina. *Spine* 16(8 Suppl):S334–S338. 1991.

Arguello F, Baggs RB, Duerst RE, Johnstone, et al. Pathogenesis of vertebral metastasis and epidural spinal cord compression. *Cancer* 1990; 65: 98–106.

Bach F, Larsen B, Rhode K, et al. Metastatic spinal cord compression: Occurrence, symptoms, clinical presentations and prognosis in 398 patients with spinal cord compression. *Acta Neurochir (Wien)* 1990; 107: 37–43.

Barron K, Hirano A, Sraski S, et al. Experiences with metastatic neoplasm involving the spinal cord. *Neurology* 1959; 9: 91–106.

Bednarik J, Kadanka Z, Vohanka S, Stejskal L, Vlach O, and Schroder R. The value of somatosensory and motor-evoked potentials in predicting and monitoring the effect of therapy in spondylotic cervical myelopathy. Prospective randomized study. *Spine* 1999; 24: 1593–1598.

Benzel EC. *Biomechanics of spine stabilization.* Rolling Meadows: American Association of Neurological Surgeons Publications, 2001.

Benzel EC. Cervical spondylotic myelopathy: Posterior surgical approaches. In Menezes AH and Sonntag VKH (eds): *Principles of spinal surgery.* New York: McGraw-Hill, 1996, pp 571–580.

Boden SD, Dodge LD, Bohlman HH, and Rechtine GR: Rheumatoid arthritis of the cervical spine: A long-term analysis with predictors of paralysis and recovery. *J Bone Joint Surg* 75A: 1282–1297, 1993.

Bohlman HH and Emery SE. The pathophysiology of cervical spondylosis and myelopathy. *Spine* 1988; 13: 843–846

Broom MJ and Raycroft JF: Complications of fractures of the cervical spine in ankylosing spondylitis. *Spine* 1988; 13: 763–766,.

Cantu RC. Corticosteroids for spinal metastases. *Lancet* 1968; 2: 912.

Chen YJ, Chang G, Chen H, et al. Surgical results of metastatic spinal cord compression secondary to non-small cell lung cancer. *Spine* 2007; 32: E413–418.

Colletti PM, Siegal HJ, Woo MY, et al. The impact on treatment planning of MRI of the spine in patients suspected of vertebral metastasis: An efficacy study. *Comput Med Imaging Graph* 1996; 20: 159–162.

Crandall PH and Batzdorf U. Cervical spondylitic myelopathy. *Journal of Neurosurgery* 1966; 25: 57–66.

Degen JW, Gagnon GJ, Voyadzis J, et al. Cyberknife sterotactic radiosurgical treatment of spinal tumors for pain control and quality of life. *Journal of Neurosurgery Spine* 2005; 2: 540–549.

Delattre J, Arbit E, Thaler H, et al. A dose-response study of dexamethasone in a model of spinal cord compression caused by epidural tumor. *Journal of Neurosurgery* 1989; 70: 920–925.

Deyo RA, Gherkin DC, Loeser JD, Bigos SJ, and ClolMA: Morbidity and mortality in association with operations on the lumbar spine: The influence of age, diagnosis, and procedure. *J Bone Joint Surg* 1992; 74A: 536–543.

Epstein JA, Epstein BS, Lavine LS, Carras R, and Rosenthal AD. Cervical myelo-radiculopathy caused by arthritic hypertrophy of the posterior facets and laminae. *Journal of Neurosurgery* 1978; 49: 387–392.

Fehlings MG and Skaf G. A review of the pathophysiology of cervical spondylotic myelopathy with insights for potential novel mechanisms drawn from traumatic spinal cord injury. *Spine* 1998; 23: 2730–2737.

Feldenzer JA, McKeever PE, and Schaberg DR. The pathogenesis of spinal epidural abscess: Microangiographic studies in an experimental model. *J Neurosurg* 1988; 69: 110–14

Ferfuson RJ and Caplan LR. Cervical spondylosis myelopathy. *Neurologic clinics* 1985; 3: 373–382.

Firooznia H, Ahn JH, Rafii M, and Ragnarsson KT. Sudden quadriplegia after a minor trauma: The role of preexisting spinal stenosis. *Surgical Neurology* 1985; 23: 165–168.

Foo D. Spinal cord injury in forty-four patients with cervical spondylosis. *Paraplegia* 1986; 24: 301–306.

Fouyas IP, Statham PF, and Sandercock PA. Cochrane review on the role of surgery in cervical spondylotic radiculomyelopathy. *Spine* 2002; 27: 736–747.

Freeman TB and Martinez CR. Radiological evaluation of cervical spondylotic disease: Limitation of magnetic resonance imaging for diagnosis and preoperative assessment. *Perspectives Neurological Surgery* 1992; 3: 34–36.

Gilbert R and Posner J. Epidural spinal cord compression from metastatic tumor: Diagnosis and treatment. *Annals of Neurology* 1978; 3: 40–51.

Glaser JA, Jaworski BA, Cuddy BG, et al. Variation in surgical opinion regarding management of selected cervical spine injuries. A preliminary study. *Spine* 1998; 23: 975–982.

Goodridge AE, Feasby TE, Ebers GC, Brown WF, and Rice GP. Hand wasting due to mid-cervical spinal cord compression. *Canadian Journal Neurological Science* 1987; 14: 309–311.

Gosfield E, Alavi A, and Kneeland B. Comparison of radionuclide bone scans and magnetic resonance imaging in detecting spinal metastases. *Journal of Nuclear Medicine* 1993; 34: 2191–2200.

Helweg-Larsen S and Sorensen P. Symptoms and signs in metastatic spinal cord compression: A study from first symptom until diagnosis in 153 patients. *European Journal of Cancer* 1994; 30A: 396–398.

Hlavin ML, Kaminski HJ, Ross JS and Ganz E. Spinal epidural abcess: a ten year perspective. *Neurosurgery* 1990; 27: 177–184.

Kato A, Ushio Y, Hayakawa T, Yamada K, Ikeda H, et al. Circulatory disturbance of the spinal cord with epidural neoplasm in rats. *Journal of Neurosurgery* 1985; 63: 260–265.

Kienstra GEM, Terwee CB, Dekker FW, et al. Prediction of spinal epidural metastases. *Archives of Neurology* 2000; 57: 690–695.

Lees F and Turner J. Natural history and prognosis of cervical spondylosis. *British Medical Journal* 1963; 2: 1607–1610.

Li KC and Poon PY. Sensitivity and specificity of MRI in detecting malignant spinal cord compression and in distinguishing malignant from benign compression fractures of vertebrae. *Magn Reson Imaging* 1988; 6: 547–556.

Loblaw DA, Laperriere NJ, and Mackillop WJ. A population based study of malignant spinal cord compression in Ontario. *Clinical Oncology* 2003; 15: 211–217.

Maranzano E, Bellavita R, Rossi R, et al. Short-course versus split-course radiotherapy in metastatic spinal cord compression: Results of a phase III randomized, multicenter trial. *Journal Clinical Oncology* 2005; 23: 3358–3365.

Maranzano E, Latini P, Beneventi S, et al. Radiotherapy without steroids in selected metastic spinal cord copression patients: A phase II trial. *American Journal of Clinical Oncology* 1996; 19: 179–183.

Maroon JC. "Burning hands" in football spinal cord injuries. *Journal of the American Medical Association* 1977; 238: 2049–2051.

McCormack BM and Weinstein PR. Cervical spondylosis: An update. *Western Journal of Medicine* 1996; 165: 43–51.

McCormick WE, Steinmetz MP, and Benzel EC. Cervical spondylotic myelopathy: Make the difficult diagnosis, then refer for surgery. *Cleveland Clinic Journal of Medicine* 2003; 70: 899–904.

McKinley WO, Conti-Wyneken AR, and Vokac CW. Rehabilitative functional outcome of patients with neoplastic spinal cord compression. *Archives of Physical Medicine and Rehabilitation* 1996; 77: 892–895.

Moore AP and Blumhardt LD. A prospective survey of the causes of nontraumatic spastic paraparesis and tetraparesis in 585 patients. *Spinal Cord* 1997; 35: 361–367.

Patchell RA, Tibbs PA, Regine WF, et al. Direct decompressive surgical resection in the treatment of spinal cord compression caused by metastatic cancer: Randomized trial. *Lancet* 2005; 366: 643–648.

Portenoy R, Galer B, Salamon O, et al. Identification of epidural neoplasm: Radiography and bone scintigraphy in the symptomatic and asymptomatic spine. *Cancer* 1989; 64: 2207–2213.

Portenoy R, Lipton R, and Foley K. Back pain in the cancer patient: An algorithm for evaluation and management. *Neurology* 1987; 37: 134–138.

Ruff R and Lanska D. Epidural metastases in prospectively evaluated veterans with cancer and back pain. *Cancer* 1989; 63: 2234–2241.

Ruff RL, Adamson VW, Ruff SS, and Wang X. Directed rehabilitation reduces pain and depression while increasing independence and satisfaction with life for patients with paraplegia due to epidural metastatic spinal cord compression. *Journal of Rehabilitation Research and Development* 2007; 44: 1–10.

Schiff D, O'Neill B, and Suman V. Spinal epidural metastasis as the initial manifestation of malignancy: Clinical features and diagnostic approach. *Neurology* 1997; 49: 452–456.

Schiff D. Spinal cord compression. *Neurology Clinics* 2003; 21: 1–14.

Schneider RC, Cherry G, and Pantek H. The syndrome of acute central cervical spinal cord injury, with special reference to the mechanisms involved in hyperextension injuries of cervical spine. *J Neurosurgery* 1954; 11: 546–577.

Schneider RC and Schemm GW. Vertebral artery insufficiency in acute and chronic spinal trauma. *Journal of Neurosurgery* 1961; 18: 348–360.

Sneddon DG and Bedbrook G. Survival following traumatic tetraplegia. *Paraplegia* 1982; 20: 201–207.

Sorenson PS, Helweg-Larsen S, Mouridsen H, and Hansen HH. Effect of high-dose dexamethasone in carcinomatous metastatic spinal cord compression treated with radiotherapy: A randomized trial. *European Journal of Cancer* 1994; 30A: 22–27.

van der Sande J, Kroger R, and Boogerd W. Multiple spinal epidural metastases: An unexpectedly frequent finding. *Journal of Neurology, Neurosurgery and Psychiatry* 1990; 53: 1001–1003.

Vecht C, Haaxma-Reiche H, van Putten W, et al. Initial bolus of conventional versus high dose dexamethasone in metastatic spinal cord compression. *Neurology* 1989; 39: 1255–1257.

Verbiest H. Chapter 23. The management of cervical spondylosis. *Clinical Neurosurgery* 1973; 20: 262–294.

White AA 3rd and Panjabi MM. Biomechanical considerations in the surgical management of cervical spondylotic myelopathy. *Spine* 1988; 13: 856–860.

Young R, Post E, and King G. Treatment of spinal epidural metastases. Randomized prospective comparison of laminectomy and radiotherapy. *Journal of Neurosurgery* 1980; 53: 741–748.

36 Motor Neuron Disease

Yvonne D. Rollins and Steven P. Ringel

Motor Neuron Disease

Motor neuron disease includes a spectrum of neurodegenerative disorders. Amyotrophic lateral sclerosis is the most common and involves both upper and lower motor neurons. Progressive muscular atrophy, X-linked spinobulbar atrophy, and post-polio syndrome involve the lower motor neurons only, while primary lateral sclerosis involves the upper motor neurons.

Amyotrophic Lateral Sclerosis

Introduction

Amyotrophic lateral sclerosis (ALS) is a fatal neurodegenerative disease affecting the motor neurons in the motor cortex, brainstem, and spinal cord, characterized by progressive limb weakness, respiratory insufficiency, spasticity, dysphagia, and dysarthria. ALS is the most common disease of motor neurons, with an incidence ranging from 0.6 to 2.4 per 100,000 per year in several European and North American studies. (Tysnes et al. 1991; Cronin et al. 2007) Incidence may vary with ethnicity, as African, Asian, and Hispanics populations seem to have a lower incidence (reviewed in Cronin et al. 2007). The prevalence is 6 per 100,000 due to the relatively short mean survival time (3–5 years) after diagnosis. Approximately 25% of individuals with ALS are alive five years after diagnosis. The peak age of incidence is the seventh decade after which it appears to decline rapidly (reviewed in Logroscino et al. 2008). Outcome studies have repeatedly shown worse prognosis including more rapid decline to death with increasing age. The age of onset of the bulbar form of ALS is higher than the limb onset forms and correlates with a poorer prognosis (Piao et al. 2003). Men have a slightly higher rate than females at premenopausal ages that equalizes by the 8th decade. No clear environmental risk factors have been identified. Elevated occupational risk has been reported in military personnel and Italian soccer players. (Chió et al. 2005; Weisskopf et al. 2005). Forms associated with dementia, mainly frontotemporal, have been described. (Mitsuyama 1984; Neary et al. 2000), including in certain areas of the Western Pacific where it is associated with the Parkinson-dementia complex.

Pathophysiology

The pathophysiology of ALS is unknown. Degeneration of cortical spinal tracts, loss of the upper and lower motor neurons, and the presence of both Bunina bodies and ubiquinated TAR DNA-binding protein (TDP-43) positive skein-like inclusions are reported. Typically, there is sparing of the extra-ocular motor neurons and the motor neurons in the nucleus of Onufrowicz to the urethral and rectal sphincters. Onset of clinical symptoms does not occur until most of the motor neurons have degenerated. The neurodegeneration can affect more than the motor system. TDP-43 positive ubiquinated inclusions have also been reported in frontal temporal dementia (Neumann et al. 2006). Many theories of disease have been proposed including excitotoxicity, mitochondrial disturbance, impaired axonal transport, and calcium handling (reviewed in Brown and Robberecht 2001), although no clear mechanism has been elucidated to date.

Transgenic animal models made with mutated superoxide dismutase 1 (SOD1) genes modeled from patients with familial ALS have been instrumental in evaluating possible mechanisms of disease. Abnormal protein aggregates are seen both in human tissue and mouse models although there may be disparity between their compositions as the aggregates in transgenic mice and humans with SOD1 mutations are not TDP-43 positive. Theories of how aggregates of abnormally folded proteins cause disease include inhibition of proteosome activity, loss of protein function through co-aggregation, depletion of chaperone proteins, interference with mitochondrial or other organelle function, and programmed cell death from endoplasmic reticulum triggered stress (Nishotoh et al. 2008). It has been shown that mutations in both motor neurons and their supporting astroglia are required for motor neuron degeneration in cell culture (reviewed in Boillee et al. 2006).

Genetic Contributions

Approximately 90% of ALS is sporadic and 10% familial. In familial forms, autosomal dominant inheritance is most common, although recessive and X-linked forms have been described especially within highly consanguineous populations (Mulder et al. 1986; Figlewicz and Orrell 2003). A SOD1 mutation is associated with 10% to 20% of familial cases or approximately 2% of all ALS cases (Rosen et al. 1993). Clinically, familial and sporadic forms are indistinguishable except that familial cases tend to have an earlier age of onset. Over 100 mutations in SOD1 have been identified without particular clustering into functional regions. In transgenic mice models, mutant SOD1 has been shown to cause a toxic gain of function as opposed to a loss of function. Unfortunately, there has been poor correlation between effective pharmacologic therapies in the transgenic mice models with expanded numbers of mutated SOD1 and human responses to these same agents.

Clinical Presentations

Muscle weakness and atrophy can start in any region with an approximate distribution of 20% bulbar, 40% cervical, and 40% lumbar. There is evidence that motor neuron loss starts focally and progresses radially from the sight of onset (Brooks 1991; Ravits et al. 2007). With bulbar onset, patients develop slurring of speech (dysarthria) and difficulty swallowing (dysphagia). Emotional lability with inappropriate laughing and/or crying spells can occur and is referred to as pseudobulbar affect or inappropriate emotion expression disorder (IEED). With unilateral limb onset, weakness in one limb often is followed by weakness in the contralateral limb. Limb symptoms may present either distally or proximally and are usually asymmetric. In the cervical regions, loss of hand dexterity is a common presenting complaint. Symptoms of cervical weakness include difficulty holding arms overhead, gripping objects, or dressing. Lumbar weakness results in tripping or difficulty climbing stairs.

Diagnosis

The El Escorial Revisited diagnostic criteria are summarized in Table 1 (Brooks et al. 2000). These have become the standard criteria for inclusion in clinical research trials.

History

Patients present with progressive weakness, muscle atrophy, fasiculations, stiffness, and generalized fatigue. They frequently complain of muscle cramping, particularly at night. Pain is usually not prominent. Shortness of breath may be noticed with bulbar and thoracic involvement. Bulbar onset is more frequently seen in the elderly with prominent dysarthria and dysphagia.

Exam

A mixture of upper motor neuron (UMN) and lower motor neuron (LMN) signs are typically present. The LMN signs include asymmetric limb and/or bulbar weakness, muscle atrophy, fasiculations, and cramps. The UMN signs include increased tone, spasticity, slowed movement, weakness, and hyperreflexia including pathologic reflexes such as a snout reflex, hyperactive jaw jerk, positive Hoffman's sign, and Babinski response. Originally thought to spare cognition, deficits in verbal fluency, attention, and working memory can be demonstrated in at least 50% of patients using formal neuropsychiatric testing. Frank frontotemporal dementia is evident in only 5%.

Imaging

Brain MRI is unremarkable. Cervical and lumbosacral MRI in elderly individuals frequently show degenerative changes that are falsely attributed to cause weakness. Unfortunately, decompressive surgery is unhelpful. There are reported cases with rapid progression where acute spinal tract degeneration has been noted by T2 hyperintensity.

Laboratory Tests

Electromyography and nerve conduction studies (EMG/NCS) assist in diagnosis and are essential to exclude motor neuropathy such as multifocal motor neuropathy (MMN). On nerve conduction studies, a decrease in compound muscle action potential amplitudes and prolonged late responses without slowed conduction velocities are typically observed. If significant sensory involvement is found, either the patient has a superimposed sensorimotor neuropathy, commonly found in the elderly, or another diagnosis should be considered. On needle electromyography, large motor unit potentials characteristic of chronic denervation caused by loss of LMNs and subsequent reinnervation are seen. Abnormal spontaneous activity including fibrillations, positive sharp waves, and fasiculations reflect acute denervation.

The forced vital capacity (FVC) is frequently impaired and has been shown to be the best prognostic indicator of survival (Fallat et al. 1979; Ringel et al. 1993; Stambler et al. 1998). It is followed serially to gauge progression and timing for noninvasive positive pressure ventilation and percutaneous gastrostomy tube placement.

Exclusionary Conditions

Sensory loss in addition to weakness makes motor neuron disease less likely. In older individuals, the most commonly confused diagnoses are cervical and lumbosacral radiculopathies. Other mimics of ALS include X-linked spinal and bulbar atrophy (see below), multifocal motor neuropathy (MMN), and inclusion body myositis. MMN is important to identify, as it is potentially treatable. It typically begins with hand and arm weakness. EMG/NCS show conduction block and conduction velocity slowing in motor nerves. Positive IgM anti-GM1 antibodies are present in approximately 80% of patients with MMN.

Treatment

The only available FDA-approved drug therapy is riluzole, a glutamate inhibitor that was shown to prolong life for 2–3 months in clinical trials. The rate of progressive muscle weakness is not altered. No other disease-modifying pharmacologic agents are available.

Standard supportive therapy includes non-invasive positive pressure ventilation (NIPPV) for respiratory muscle weakness and percutaneous endoscopic gastrostomy (PEG) tube for dysphagia Initiation of NIPPV is recommended when the FVC drops below 50% or a sleep study is consistent with sleep disordered breathing from chest wall weakness. Advanced age and airway mucus accumulation are poor prognostic factors for survival despite treatment with NIPPV (Peysson et al. 2008). NIPPV is most effective if tolerated for more than four hours at night (Kleopa et al. 1999). Dyspnea can be managed with a low dose benzodiazepine or morphine titrated to symptom relief without inhibition of respiratory drive. Secretions are common and can be difficult to effectively treat. Cough assist machines are frequently helpful. The American Academy of Neurology practice parameters recommend metoprolol or propranolol for thick secretions; N-acetylcysteine can also be tried (Miller et al. 1999). Thin secretions leading to sialorrhea usually respond at least partially to amitriptyline or other medications with anticholinergic properties such as scopolamine transdermal patches. These drugs must be used with caution in the elderly because of an increased incidence of confusion and delirium. Botolinum toxin injected into parotid and/or submandibular glands or salivary gland radiotherapy may reduce secretions. Toxin injection and radiotherapy should only be considered in patients who derive their nutritional needs solely through a gastrostomy tube (Tysnes 2008).

Dysphagia is first ameliorated with changes in diet consistency and safe swallowing techniques. Gastrostomy is recommended before the FVC drops below 50% because of safety concerns regarding protecting the airway during the procedure. A feeding tube may be placed endoscopically or via direct puncture using interventional radiology if airway compromise is a concern. Alternative communication devices are recommended when speech becomes unintelligible. Options include point boards and speech synthesizers. Tracheotomy and long term mechanical ventilation needs to be fully discussed with the patient and family and finalized in advance directives. Physicians should review the advance directives periodically as patient preferences may change over time.

Table 1 El Escorial Criteria Revisited

Clinically Definite ALS	UMN and LMN signs in three regions
Clinically Probable ALS	UMN and LMN signs in two regions with UMN signs rostral to the LMN signs
Clinically Probable Laboratory-Supported ALS	UMN and LMN signs in one region or UMN signs alone in one region and LMN EMG findings in two regions
Clinically Possible ALS	UMN and LMN signs in one region or UMN alone in two or more regions + Other diagnoses excluded

Natural Progression

ALS is relentlessly progressive with mean survival of 3–5 years from date of diagnosis, although a minority of patients live for many years. Age at onset is one of the strongest predictors of survival. Increased age at onset, low FVC, bulbar onset, and short time from first symptom onset to diagnosis have been identified as poor prognostic factors (Ringel et al. 1993; Haverkamp et al. 1995). Respiratory function, as measured by FVC, decreases in a linear manner and is also a strong prognostic factor.

Rehabilitation/Psychological Aspects

Physical, occupational, and speech therapists can assist with issues of energy conservation, mobility assistance, retention of range of motion, specialized utensils, bracing, augmentative communication, and safe swallowing techniques. Depression is common and responds to anti-depressant agents (Rabkin et al. 2005). A major role of the neurologist is to facilitate the patient's self-determination and autonomy with regard to treatment and end-of-life decisions (Miller et al. 1999).

Future Directions

The discovery of biomarkers of ALS could facilitate earlier diagnosis and treatment. Radiologic, genomic, and proteomic profiling have been attempted although no clear biomarkers have emerged. The pathogenesis of ALS remains unknown. Transgenic mouse models constructed with mutations in SOD1 and TDP-43 continue to be used to elucidate disease mechanisms. Mutant SOD1 was recently shown to interact with an endoplasmic reticulum protein to cause both defective endoplasmic reticulum functioning and activation of a protein kinase involved in programmed cell death (Nishitoh et al. 2008).

Summary

ALS is a progressive form of motor neuron disease leading to paralysis and death from respiratory compromise. Advanced age and bulbar symptoms at the time of diagnosis are poor prognostic factors. Treatment remains mainly supportive.

Lower Motor Neuron Disorders

The lower motor neuron (LMN) disorders of the elderly include progressive muscular atrophy (PMA), X-linked spinal and bulbar atrophy (SBMA; Kennedy's disease), and post poliomyelitis syndrome (PPS).

Progressive Muscular Atrophy

Introduction

Aran in 1850 described eleven patients with LMN-only symptoms which he named progressive muscular atrophy (PMA). Epidemiologic studies to determine the specific incidence of LMN disease have proved to be difficult to perform, as patients must be followed for long time periods to exclude spinal onset ALS. Large studies of motor neuron disease have shown approximately 10% present with isolated LMN signs. A five-year prospective follow up study showed an average age of onset of 57 years, similar to that seen in ALS (Visser et al. 2007). In another prospective study, 70% of patients with LMN signs thought to be consistent with PMA developed UMN and bulbar signs characteristic of ALS after six years (Traynor et al. 2000).

Pathophysiology

The underlying pathophysiology of PMA is unknown, as is its relationship to the pathophysiology of ALS. Pathological examination demonstrates corticospinal tract involvement in 50% of cases in addition to ubiquinated inclusions similar to those seen in ALS (Ince et al. 2003).

Genetic Contributions

No genetic cause of PMA has been identified, although a subset of adult-onset lower motor neuron disease has been shown to be related to deletions in the survival motor neuron (SMN) gene, which is then designated spinal muscular atrophy type IV (Moulard et al. 1998).

Clinical Presentations

In PMA, patients present with slowly progressive weakness and atrophy. Clinically, it is difficult to distinguish progressive muscular atrophy from spinal onset ALS, as the majority of motor neuron disease patients that present with primarily LMN symptoms ultimately develop UMN symptoms and progress to ALS.

Diagnosis
History

Based on a cross sectional study of 49 sporadic adult-onset LMN disease patients with greater than four years of only LMN symptoms, four patterns of progressive weakness and wasting were present: a generalized pattern, a symmetric distal pattern, an asymmetric distal arm predominant, or asymmetric proximal arm predominant. Age of onset is significantly older with the generalized pattern of weakness with mean of 58 years (Van den Berg-Vos et al. 2003).

Exam

LMN signs of muscle weakness, muscle atrophy, and decreased or absent reflexes with a normal sensory exam are seen.

Imaging

MRI imaging is usually unremarkable although atrophy of the cervical or thoracic cord has been reported.

Laboratory Tests

FVC should be followed serially in PMA as patients do develop compromised respiratory function. EMG/NCS shows chronic denervation on needle EMG and can show decrease or absence of compound muscle action potentials.

Exclusionary Conditions

PMA must be distinguished from multifocal motor neuropathy (MMN), a treatable form of motor neuropathy. In MMN, persistent conduction block of motor nerve conduction on electrophysiologic exam is characteristic.

Treatment

There is currently no pharmacologic therapy to slow the progression of weakness in PMA. As in ALS, treatment is mainly supportive.

Natural Progression

Controversy remains with regard to PMA as a separate entity from ALS. A recent study of 37 PMA subjects followed prospectively for 18 months showed a similar progressive disease course to ALS with 70% mortality at 5 years (Visser et al. 2007).

X-Linked Spinobulbar Muscular Atrophy

Introduction

X-linked spinobulbar muscular atrophy (SBMA), also known as Kennedy's disease, is a progressive degenerative disorder of the lower motor neurons seen with late onset in men (Kennedy et al. 1968). It is one of the polyglutamine repeat expansion diseases and has an estimated prevalence of 1 in 40,000. A recent epidemiologic study from Italy determined an age-adjusted prevalence for males of 2.8/100,000. Average age of onset was 44.8 +/- 10.1 and average age at death was 71.3 +/- 4.7 years (Guidetti et al. 2001).

Pathophysiology

An expanded CAG repeat in the androgen receptor, a ligand-dependent nuclear transcription factor essential for the development of the male phenotype, results in a toxic gain of function. The normal number of repeats is 10 to 36, while disease is seen in the 40 to 62 range (La Spada et al. 1991). Age of onset tends to be lower with increasing number of repeats (La Spada et al. 1992). An attenuated phenotype can be seen in female carriers even if homozygous for the expanded repeat. Animal models have shown that male levels of testosterone are required for full manifestation of disease (Katsuno et al. 2002). Pathological evaluation shows progressive atrophy of all types of muscle fibers with replacement by fibrous tissue corresponding to loss of lower motor neurons in the spinal cord and brainstem. Nuclear inclusions containing mutant and truncated androgen receptors are found in motor neurons of the brain stem and spinal cord, as well as in the skin and testes (Li et al. 1998; Adachi et al. 2005). The pathogenic process by which CAG repeats cause disease is not known. It is thought that polyglutamine expansions lead to misfolding of proteins possibly through sequestration of folding proteins and interrupting proteolytic pathways that require molecular chaperones. Transcription factors in protein aggregates may lead to compromise of transcriptional regulation and gene expression.

Genetic Contributions

SBMA is a known X-linked disorder that was the first pathogenic CAG DNA triplet repeats described (La Spada et al. 1991). The triplet repeat occurs in the open reading frame of a coding exon leading to a polyglutamine expansion in the androgen receptor. Individuals with longer CAG repeats tend to develop disease at an earlier age, although disease onset can vary by greater than a decade within a single family (LaSpada et al. 1991; Mariotti et al. 2000).

Clinical Presentations

Older men present with slowly progressive muscle weakness, muscle atrophy, and fasiculations in bulbar and limb muscles. Symptom onset is between 30–50 years old, although may be so mild at onset that no intervention is sought. Characteristic perioral coarse fasciculations, hand tremor, and gynecomastia may be seen. Bulbar involvement includes dysphagia and dysarthria from facial, masseter, palatal, and tongue weakness. Aspiration pneumonia is common in the late stage of disease. Mild sensory impairment may be present.

Diagnosis

History

Postural hand tremor may be the earliest sign with subsequent development of muscle twitching, cramping, weakness, and wasting with difficulty climbing stairs, walking, and lifting. Most affected men develop problems with chewing and swallowing and/or difficulty speaking. Many complain of tremor and endocrine abnormalities including gynecomastia, infertility, and testicular atrophy.

Exam

Bulbar signs including weakness and atrophy of the tongue, jaw, and oropharynx are common. Sensory modalities may be decreased. No cerebellar or cognitive impairment should be present. Signs of androgen insensitivity include gynecomastia, and testicular atrophy may be present.

Imaging

MRI of the brain and cervical spine is obtained to exclude mass or demyelination as the cause of bulbar and spinal weakness.

Laboratory Tests

Gene testing is available in SBMA for both affected males and female carriers. The sizing of the CAG repeat is based on amplification of the region by polymerase chain reaction (PCR). Genetic testing should be considered if there is a known family history or a male presents with bulbar symptoms, gynecomastia, and sensory symptoms. Serum creatinine kinase may be elevated secondary to muscle wasting. Testosterone has been reported to be decreased, normal, and elevated. EMG shows chronic denervation with prolonged distal motor latencies found on NCS. Sensory nerve responses may be reduced or absent.

Treatment

Testosterone replacement was initially considered until animal models showed exacerbation of disease characteristics with testosterone supplementation. Rescue of the disease phenotype in a transgenic mouse model was achieved with chemical and surgical castration and small clinical trials have been performed with chemical blockade of testosterone with leuprorelin with minimal improvement (Katsuno et al. 2003). Because of the slow progression, clinical trials must be long term to demonstrate significant effects.

Natural Progression

SBMA patients have a slowly progressive clinical course and remain relatively active. A recent retrospective study of 25 patients followed for mean duration of 13 years showed a minimally reduced survival of patients with SBMA compared to age- and gender-matched controls (Chahin et al. 2008).

Future Directions

Long-term clinical trials testing chemical blockade of testosterone are in progress, which may provide therapeutic benefit in SBMA.

Post-polio Syndrome
Introduction

The poliomyelitis virus causes a paralytic syndrome by infecting the motor neurons of the brainstem and spinal cord. Large epidemics in Western countries occurred in the 1940s and 1950s that abated with the development of effective vaccines. Years after initial recovery, new neuromuscular symptoms including new muscle weakness, myalgias, arthralgias, and fatigue occur in 20–60% of polio survivors (Halstead and Rossi 1987; reviewed in Trojan and Cashman 2005). These late sequelae have been designated post-poliomyelitis syndrome (PPS).

Pathophysiology

The main theory of PPS pathophysiology is that continuous motor unit remodeling including denervation and renervation associated with loss of motor neurons from aging leads to motor neuron junction instability, causing weakness and fatigue (Wiechers and Hubbell 1981). Motor unit size can increase to eight times larger than normal during recovery from the initial infection. Based on findings on muscle biopsy after development of PPS symptoms, degeneration of a subset of the axons of one motor unit as opposed to death of an entire motor unit occurs, causing fatigability related to instability at the neuromuscular junction.

Clinical Presentations

With PPS, patients with a remote history of poliomyelitis present 8 to 71 years (mean interval 36 years) after the initial infection with new weakness, fatigue, and pain. The fatigue is described as a flu-like exhaustion that worsens over the course of the day and with physical activity. The weakness usually involves the originally involved muscles although does occur in those not originally involved. Muscle pain occurs in 38–86% and joint pain in 42–80%. Less commonly, patients complain of new muscular atrophy, respiratory insufficiency, sleep abnormalities, dysarthria, dysphagia, muscle cramps, cold intolerance, fasciculations, and joint deformities.

Diagnosis
History
To consider a diagnosis of PPS, a history of prior poliomyelitis needs to be confirmed, if necessary, by EMG/NCS examination. Slowly progressive weakness, fatigue, myalgias, and arthralgias are the most common complaints.

Exam
LMN signs of muscle weakness, muscle atrophy, and decreased or absent reflexes are present.

Imaging
Spinal MRIs are usually ordered to exclude compressive lesions.

Laboratory Tests
EMG and single fiber EMG are unable to distinguish between stable post-polio and patients with new weakness but can establish the prior poliomyelitis infection and exclude other neurologic disorders. FVC should be followed in PPS; some patients develop compromised respiratory function.

Treatment
Weakness is managed with exercise, avoidance of overuse, weight loss, orthoses, and assistive devices. Fatigue management includes energy conservation, pacing, regular rest intervals, and optimal sleep hygiene. Some patients have found improvement with changing to more sedentary jobs or working at home. Management of muscle pain includes reduction of activity, pacing, stretching, use of assistive devices, and lifestyle modifications. Symptomatic management of chronic muscle complaints can include amitriptyline, muscle relaxants, or other antidepressants which may be beneficial on an individual basis.

Natural Progression
One prospective study found no progressive weakness in post polio patients followed over five years (Windebank et al. 1996) and controversy remains with regard to progression of muscle weakness. It is rarely fatal although respiratory compromise and dysphagia can develop. Pain and fatigue remain fairly stable over time. A meta analysis of late-onset sequelae determined that the data was too limited to evaluate functional status over time and detectable decrease in muscle strength was only found if patients were followed for greater than four years (Stolwijk-Swuste et al. 2005).

Rehabilitation/psychological Aspects
Rehabilitation efforts are focused on supportive equipment and energy conservation. Patients with PPS may have difficulty adjusting to worsening of disability. It is unclear whether the rate of depression is higher than the general population.

Summary
The LMN forms of motor neuron disease create a heterogeneous group of disorders that require individualized courses of treatment. They tend to have a longer course and milder symptoms than in ALS.

Primary Lateral Sclerosis
Introduction
Primary lateral sclerosis (PLS) is an upper motor neuron (UMN) disorder accounting for approximately 3–5% of all motor neuron disease. Although PLS has a younger mean age of onset compared to ALS (Tartaglia et al. 2007), the known survival advantage of UMN predominance means a person with this disorder may live to be elderly. PLS can "convert" to ALS with the development of LMN involvement raising questions of whether it has a separate pathophysiologic cause from ALS. Development of LMN involvement has been recorded up to 27 years after onset of UMN symptoms (Bruyn et al. 1995). Only limited epidemiological data is available for PLS; no familial cases are known in adults.

Pathophysiology
As in ALS, the pathogenesis of PLS is unknown. Pathologic tissue examination in PLS consistently reports loss of Betz cells in layer 5 of the motor cortex along with atrophy in the corticospinal tracts and sparing of spinal anterior horn cells (Younger et al. 1988; Pringle et al. 1992; Hudson et al. 1995). The typical pathologic features of ALS, including Bunina bodies and ubiquinated inclusions, have been described in autopsy cases of PLS; unfortunately, most of the autopsied cases had evidence of mild LMN involvement either by denervation on muscle biopsy, development of LMN signs, or denervation by EMG examination, so that technically these cases may not be pure PLS.

Genetic Contributions
Patients reporting a family history are generally diagnosed with hereditary spastic paraplegia.

Clinical Presentations
Progressive lower extremity spasticity without significant loss of strength or limb wasting is the classic initial symptom. Dysarthria frequently develops. Bladder dysfunction is rare and usually occurs late in the course. Emotional lability is present approximately 50% of the time. Pringle (1992) proposed clinical diagnostic criteria based on eight patients: insidious onset of spastic paresis, adult onset in the fifth decade or later, absence of family history, gradually progressive without steep loss of function, duration greater than three years, and a symmetric distribution.

The usefulness of these criteria has been debated. Gordon et al. (2006) argued for a pure PLS syndrome distinct from an UMN-dominant ALS based on a cohort of 29 patients with only UMN signs and a normal EMG on initial evaluation. Thirteen of 29 patients developed evidence of denervation by EMG or clinical examination within four years of follow up. Disability rating, respiratory function, and life expectancy were superior in the pure PLS syndrome while the UMN dominant ALS group retained a better life expectancy compared to an ALS control group.

Diagnosis
PLS is a diagnosis of exclusion and must be distinguished from ALS and hereditary spastic paraplegia.

History
Patients usually complain of gradually increasing leg stiffness with or without mild weakness. Occasionally, the arms or speech is the site of symptom onset. Stiffness or spasticity is a significantly more common complaint in PLS than ALS (Tartaglia et al. 2007). Dysarthria develops

insidiously. The development of urinary complaints is more variable as is emotional lability.

Exam

Increased tone with a spastic gait, hyperreflexia, spastic dysarthria, and extensor plantar reflexes with relative sparing of strength, coordination, and sensation are found. Maintained muscle bulk is a distinguishing feature of PLS that is not found in ALS. The patient may also exhibit spells of inappropriate laughing or crying.

Imaging

Brain and spinal MRIs are obtained to exclude compression or other lesions that can cause an UMN pattern of deficit. With brain MRI, atrophy of the frontoparietal (mainly precentral) region of the brain with degeneration of the underlying white matter and selective T2 hyperintensity of the pyramidal tract may be seen (Kuipers-Upmeijer et al. 2001).

Laboratory Tests

To exclude other causes of UMN predominant signs, vitamin B12, RPR, Borrelia anitbodies, HTLV-1 antibodies, and very long-chain fatty acids should be obtained. CSF analysis is usually unremarkable although mildly increased protein has been reported. Electromyography (EMG) is useful to distinguish PLS from ALS based on the absence of diffuse chronic denervation, although mild denervation in patients with PLS has been reported. Cortically evoked motor potentials are often absent or significantly prolonged in patients with PLS, whereas in ALS they are often normal or mildly delayed (Kuipers-Upmeijer et al. 2001).

Exclusionary Conditions

It is difficult to distinguish PLS from hereditary spastic paraparesis (HSP) and is usually based on family history. In HSP, an autosomal dominant family history is usually present. HSP tends to present at a younger age (mean onset of 39) and is not associated with spastic dysarthria or pseudobulbar affect.

Treatment

No curative treatment is available for PLS. Treatment is symptomatic and includes baclofen, tizanadine, or dantrolene for spasticity; augmentive speech devices for severe dysarthria; PEG tube for dysphagia; and walker or wheelchair for gait impairment.

Natural Progression

PLS is a disease with very slowly progressive increasing spasticity and dysarthria that rarely result in death from the disease.

Rehabilitation/psychological Aspects

Rehabilitation focuses on retention of mobility and communication through assistive devices.

Future Directions

Further epidemiologic studies are needed to determine which proportion of patients with initially pure UMN signs and symptoms develop signs and symptoms of ALS. A biomarker may help to distinguish between these two disorders or determine if they have the same pathogenesis.

Summary

PLS is an UMN disease of unknown etiology that results in very slowly progressive spasticity and dysarthria. It is a diagnosis of exclusion with a subset of individuals progressing to develop LMN signs and therefore clinical ALS. Treatment is supportive.

References

Adachi, H., Katsuno, M., Minamiyama, M., et al.: Widespread nuclear and cytoplasmic accumulation of mutant androgen receptor in SBMA patients. *Brain* 128(Pt 3):659–670, 2005.

Aran, F.A.: Recherches sur une maladie non encore décrite du système musculaire (atrophie musculaire progressive). *Arch Gen Med* 24:5-35, 172–214, 1850.

Boillée, S., Vande Velde, C., and Cleveland, D.W.: ALS: A disease of motor neurons and their nonneuronal neighbors. *Neuron* 52(1):39–59, 2006.

Brooks, B.R.: The role of axonal transport in neurodegenerative disease spread: A meta-analysis of experimental and clinical poliomyelitis compares with amyotrophic lateral sclerosis. *Can J Neurol Sci* 18(3 Suppl):435–438, 1991.

Brooks, B.R., Miller . R.G., Swash, M., Munsat, T.L., for the World Federation of Neurology Reaseach Group on Motor Neuron Diseases: El Escorial revisited: Revised criteria for the diagnosis of amyotrophic lateral sclerosis. *ALS and other motor neuron disorders* 1:293–299, 2000.

Brown, R.H. Jr, and Robberecht W.: Amyotrophic lateral sclerosis: Pathogenesis. *Semin Neurol* 21(2):131–139, 2001.

Bruyn, R.P., Koelman, J.H., Troost, D., and de Jong, J.M.: Motor neuron disease (amyotrophic lateral sclerosis) arising from longstanding primary lateral sclerosis. *J Neurol Neurosurg Psychiatry* 58(6):742–744, 1995.

Chahin, N., Klein, C., Mandrekar, J., and Sorenson, E.: Natural history of spinal-bulbar muscular atrophy. *Neurology* 70(21):1967–1971, 2008.

Chió, A., Benzi, G., Dessena, M., et al.: Severely increased risk of amyotrophic lateral sclerosis among Italian professional football players. *Brain* 128(Pt 3):472–476, 2005.

Cronin, S., Hardiman, O., and Traynor, J.: Ethnic variation in the incidence of ALS: A systematic review. *Neurology* 68(13):1002–1007, 2007.

Fallat, R.J., Jewitt, B., Bass, M., Kamm, B., and Norris, F.H. Jr.: Spirometry in amyotrophic lateral sclerosis. *Arch Neurol* 36(2):74–80, 1979.

Figlewicz, D.A. and Orrell, R.W.: The genetics of motor neuron diseases. *Amyotrophic Lateral Scler Other Motor Neuron Disord* 4(4):225–231, 2003.

Gordon, P.H., Cheng, B., Katz, I.B., et al.: The natural history of primary lateral sclerosis. *Neurology* 66(5):647–653, 2006.

Guidetti, D., Sabadini, R., Ferlini, A., and Torrente, I.: Epidemiological survey of X-linked bulbar and spinal muscular atrophy, or Kennedy disease, in the province of Reggio Emilia, Italy. *Eur J Epidemiol* 17(6):587–591, 2001.

Halstead, L.S. and Rossi C.D.: Post-polio syndrome: Clinical experience with 132 consecutive outpatients. In *Research and clinical aspects of the late effects of polio-myelitis.* (Halstead, L.S. and Wiechers, D.O., Eds.). March of Dimes Birth Defects Foundation, White Plains, 1987, pp 13–26.

Haverkamp, L.J., Appel, V., and Appel, S.H.: Natural history of amyotrophic lateral sclerosis in a database population. Validation of a scoring system and a model for survival prediction. *Brain* 118(Pt 3): 707–719, 1995.

Hudson, A.J., Kiernan, J.A., Munoz, D.G., et al.: Clinicopathological features of primary lateral sclerosis are different from amyotrophic lateral sclerosis. *Brain Res Bull* 30(3–4):359–364, 1993.

Ince, P.G., Evans, J., Knopp, M., et al. Corticospinal tract degeneration in the progressive muscular atrophy variant of ALS. *Neurology* 60(8):1252–1258, 1993.

Katsuno, M., Adachi, H., Kume, A., et al. : Testosterone reduction prevents phenotypic expression in a transgenic mouse model of spinal and bulbar muscular atrophy. *Neuron* 35(5):843–854, 2002.

Katsuno, M., Adachi, H., Doyu, M., et al.: Leuprorelin rescues polyglutamine-dependent phenotypes in a transgenic mouse model of spinal and bulbar muscular atrophy. *Nat Med* 9(6):768–773, 2003.

Kennedy, W.R., Alter, M., and Sung, J.H.: Progressive proximal spinal and bulbar muscular atrophy of late onset. A sex-linked recessive trait. *Neurology* 18(7):671–680, 1968.

Kleopa, K.A., Sherman, M., Neal, B., et al.: Bipap improves survival and rate of pulmonary function decline in patients with ALS. *J Neurol Sci* 164(1):82–88, 1999.

Kuipers-Upmeijer, J., de Jager, A.E., Hew, J.M., et al. Primary lateral sclerosis: Clinical, neurophysiological, and magnetic resonance findings. *J Neurol Neurosurg Psychiatry* 71(5):615–620, 2001.

La Spada, A.R., Wilson, E.M., Lubahn, D.B., et al.: Androgen receptor gene mutations in X-linked spinal and bulbar muscular atrophy. *Nature* 352(6330):77–79, 1991.

La Spada, A.R., Roling, D.B., Harding, A.E., et al.: Meiotic stability and genotype-phenotype correlation of the trinucleotide repeat in X-linked spinal and bulbar muscular atrophy. *Nat Genet* 2(4):302–304, 1992.

Li, M., Miwa, S., Kobayashi, Y., et al. Nuclear inclusions of the androgen receptor protein in spinal and bulbar muscular atrophy. *Ann Neurol* 44(2):249–254, 1998.

Logroscino, G., Traynor, B.J., Hardiman, O., et al.: Descriptive epidemiology of amyotrophic lateral sclerosis: New evidence and unsolved issues. *J Neurol Neurosurg Psychiatry* 79(1):6–11, 2008.

Mariotti, C., Castellotti, B., Pareyson, D., et al.: Phenotypic manifestations associated with CAG-repeat expansion in the androgen receptor gene in male patients and heterozygous females: A clinical and molecular study of 30 families. *Neuromuscul Disord* 10(6):391–397, 2000.

Miller, R.G., Rosenberg, J.A,. Gelinas, D.F., et al.: Practice parameter: The care of the patient with amyotrophic lateral sclerosis (an evidence-based review): Report of the Quality Standards Subcommittee of the American Academy of Neurology; ALS Practice Parameters Task Force. *Neurology* 52(7):1311–1323, 1999.

Mitsuyama, Y.: Presenile dementia with motor neuron disease in Japan: Clinico-pathological review of 26 cases. *J Neurol Neurosurg Psychiatry* 47(9):953–959, 1984.

Moulard, B., Salachas, F., Chassande, B., et al.: Association between centromeric deletions of the SMN gene and sporadic adult-onset lower motor neuron disease. *Ann Neurol* 43(5):640–644, 1998.

Mulder, D.W., Kurland, L.T., Offord, K.P., and Beard, C.M.: Familial adult motor neuron disease: Amyotrophic lateral sclerosis. *Neurology* 36:511–517, 1986.

Neary, D., Snowden, J.S., and Mann, D.M.: Cognitive change in motor neurone disease/amyotrophic lateral sclerosis (MND/ALS). *J Neurol Sci* 180(1–2):15–20, 2000.

Neumann, M., Sampathu, D., Kwong, L.K., et al.: Ubiquinated TDP-43 in frontotemporal lobar degeneration and amyotrophic lateral sclerosis. *Science* 314(5796):130–133, 2006.

Nishitoh, H., Kadowaki, H., Nagai, A., et al.: ALS-linked mutant SOD1 induces ER stress- and ASK1-dependent motor neuron death by targeting Derlin-1. *Genes Dev* 22(11):1451–1464, 2008.

Peysson, S., Vandenberghe, N., Philit, F., et al.: Factors predicting survival following noninvasive ventilation in amyotrophic lateral sclerosis. *Eur Neurol* 59(3–4):164–171, 2008.

Piao, Y-S., Wakabayashi, K., Kakita, A., et al.: Neuropathology with clinical correlations of sporadic amyotrophic lateral sclerosis: 102 autopsy cases examined between 1962 and 2000. *Brain Pathol* 13(1):10–22, 2003.

Pringle, C.E., Hudson, A.J., Munoz, D.G., et al.: Primary lateral sclerosis. Clinical features, neuropathology, and diagnostic criteria. *Brain* 115(Pt 2):495–520, 1992.

Rabkin, J.G., Albert, S.M., Del Bene, M.L. et al.: Prevalence of depressive disorders and change over time in late-stage ALS. *Neurology* 65(1):62–66, 2005.

Ravits, J., Laurie, P., Fan, Y., and Moore, D.H. Implications of ALS focality: Rostral-caudal distribution of lower motor neuron loss postmortem. *Neurology* 68(19):1576–1582, 2007.

Ringel, S.P., Murphy, J.R., Alderson, M.K., et al.: The natural history of amyotrophic lateral sclerosis. *Neurology* 43(7):1316–1322, 1993.

Rosen, D.R., Siddique, T., Patterson, D., et al.: Mutations in Cu/Zn superoxide dismutase gene are associated with familial amyotrophic lateral sclerosis. *Nature* 362(6415):59–62, 1993.

Stambler, N., Charatan, M., and Cedarbaum, J.M.: Prognostic indicators of survival in ALS. ALS CNTF Treatment Study Group. *Neurology* 50(1):66–72, 1998.

Stolwijk-Swuste, J.M., Beelen, A., Lankhorst, G.J. et al.: The course of functional status and muscle strength in patients with late-onset sequelae of poliomyelitis: A systematic review. *Arch Phys Med Rehabil* 86(8):1693–1701, 2005.

Tartaglia, M.C., Rowe, A., Findlater, K., et al.: Differentiation between primary lateral sclerosis and amyotrophic lateral sclerosis: Examination of symptoms and signs at disease onset and during follow-up. *Arch Neurol* 64(2):232–236, 2007.

Traynor, B.J., Codd, M.B., Corr, B., et al.: Clinical features of amyotrophic lateral sclerosis according to the El Escorial and Arlie House diagnostic criteria. *Arch Neurol* 57(8):1171–1176, 2000.

Trojan, D.A. and Cashman, N.R.: Post-poliomyelitis syndrome. *Muscle Nerve* 31(1):6–19, 2005.

Tysnes, O-B., Vollset, S.E., and Aarli, J.A.: Epidemiology of amyotrophic lateral sclerosis in Hordaland county, western Norway. *Acta Neurol Scand* 83(5):280–285, 1991.

Tysnes, O.B.: Treatment of sialorrhea in amyotrophic lateral sclerosis. *Acta Neurol Scand Suppl* 188:77–81, 2008.

Van den Berg-Vos, R.M., Visser, J., Franssen, H., et al.: Sporadic lower motor neuron disease with adult onset: Classification of subtypes. *Brain* 126:1036–1047, 2003.

Visser, J., van den Berg-Vos, R.M., Franssen, H., et al.: Disease course and prognostic factors of progressive muscular atrophy. *Arch Neurol* 64(4):522–528, 2007.

Weisskopf, M.G., O'Reilly, E.J., McCullough, M.L., et al.: Prospective study of military service and mortality from ALS. *Neurology* 64(1):32–37, 2005.

Wiechers, D.O. and Hubbell, S.L.: Late changes in the motor unit after acute poliomyelitis. *Muscle Nerve* 4(6):524–528, 1981.

Windebank, A.J., Litchy, W.J., Daube, J.R., and Iverson, R.A. Lack of progression of neurologic deficit in survivors of paralytic polio: A 5-year prospective population-based study. *Neurology* 46(1):80–84, 1996.

Younger, D.S., Chou, S., Hays, A.P., Lange et al.: Primary lateral sclerosis. A clinical diagnosis reemerges. *Arch Neurol* 45(12):1304–1307, 1988.

37 Primary and Inflammatory Muscle Disorders in the Elderly

Mazen M. Dimachkie, Faisal Raja, and Richard J. Barohn

Muscle weakness in the elderly is a complex and not uncommon phenomenon. Muscle effort is regulated by several structures within the central nervous system and requires preservation of non-neural structures such as the bones, joints, and ligaments. In disorders of the central nervous system, clinical evaluation reveals spasticity, ataxia, tremors or rigidity pointing toward stroke, myelopathy, cerebellar degeneration, or Parkinson's disease as the etiology of muscle weakness.

The presentation of elderly patients suffering from a primary muscle disorder is quite characteristic. Individuals report difficulty getting up from the floor, standing up from a chair, climbing stairs, and reaching up with the arms. Careful examination reveals weakness in the shoulder and hip girdle muscles while using the Medical Research Council (MRC) scale. When examining the strength of these patients, it is important to tailor the examiner's resistance with the patient's build. One way to ascertain the patient's weakness is through functional tests such as asking the patient to rise from a chair without arm support or to perform a squat. Pertinent negatives include lack of involvement of the mental status, cranial nerves (except for dysphagia), sensory system, and of the muscle stretch reflexes. Understandably, the latter may be reduced in severely weak muscles.

In this chapter, we review the differential diagnosis of proximal muscle weakness. We will then discuss the effects of aging on muscle, followed by a description of the idiopathic inflammatory myopathies (IIM). These are dermatomyositis (DM), polymyositis (PM), and inclusion body myositis (IBM). We will close by alluding to necrotizing myopathy (NM), hypothyroid myopathy, occulopharyngeal muscular dystrophy, and McArdles's disease.

Causes of Proximal Muscle Weakness

A primary disorder of muscle is highly likely in patients presenting with proximal muscle weakness. Table 1 lists conditions that mimic a myopathy. These are disorders of the anterior horn cell, nerve root, nerve plexus, peripheral nerve, and neuromuscular junction. Amyotrophic lateral sclerosis (ALS) may rarely present with only proximal weakness and is easily recognized due to the associated upper motor neuron signs. X-linked bulbospinal muscular atrophy presents in the fifth decade with proximal weakness, dysphagia, and muscle cramps. It is due to a triplet repeat expansion in the androgen-receptor gene. Distinguishing features are gynecomastia, hypogonadism, fasciculations, tremor, and a mild subclinical sensory neuropathy. Chronic inflammatory demyelinating polyneuropathy (CIDP) presents with proximal and distal muscle weakness. Though CIDP is a predominantly motor disorder, there are sensory symptoms and signs and hyporeflexia. Diabetic amyotrophy represents 1% of all diabetic neuropathies and might result infrequently in symmetric proximal leg weakness. Myasthenia gravis has a second peak in the sixth to seventh decade, presenting with fatigable weakness of the arms and legs. Though weakness may be proximal, patients often report diplopia, ptosis, and/or dysphagia. Proximal leg weakness with arreflexia and dysautonomia is the classic triad of the Lambert-Eaton mysathenic syndrome (LEMS). The latter is associated with an antibody to the voltage-gated P/Q type presynaptic calcium channel. The majority of LEMS patients have cancer, most frequently small cell lung cancer.

Table 2 lists various muscle disorders. While it is not uncommon for lipid lowering agents to cause muscle and joint pain, very few patients (0.5%) develop marked proximal weakness. Histopathology shows diffuse muscle fiber necrosis without a primary inflammatory component. Chronic high dose corticosteroid uptake may result in a myopathy associated with atrophy of type 2 muscle fibers. Intensive care unit patients are at risk for developing an acute quadriplegic myopathy with loss of thick filaments. Patients with glycolytic enzyme defects typically present with recurrent episodes of rhabdomyolysis but may at times present in later life with fixed proximal muscle weakness. Muscular dystrophies present usually in the younger age group, except for occulopharyngeal muscular dystrophy.

Sarcopenia

Sarcopenia refers to the age-related decline in skeletal muscle mass and strength. A more quantitative definition is the loss of fat free muscle mass of two or more standard deviations below the mean levels of sex- and age-matched normal subjects as measured by dual energy X-ray

Table 1 Myopathy Mimics

Anterior Horn Cell

Amyotrophic lateral sclerosis (ALS)

Kennedy disease (X-linked bulbospinal muscular atrophy)

Adult-onset spinal muscular atrophy

Poliomyelitis, West Nile virus

Nerve Root, Plexus, and Peripheral Nerve

Guillain-Barre syndrome

Chronic inflammatory demyelinating polyneuropathy

Multifocal motor neuropathy

Diabetic amyotrophy

Lymphomatous motor neuropathy

Neuromuscular Junction

Myasthenia Gravis

Lambert-Eaton myasthenic syndrome

Table 2 Muscle Disorders

Idiopathic Inflammatory Myopathies:	Sarcopenia :Age-related muscle loss
Dermatomyositis	
Polymyositis	
Inclusion body myositis	
Necrotizing myopathy	
Toxic Inflammatory Myopathies:	**Medical Conditions:**
D-Penicillamine	Hyperthyroid
Interferon alpha	Hypothyroid
L-tryptophan	Hyperparathyroid
Cimetidine	Hypoparathyroid
Phenytoin	Acromegaly
	Amyloidosis
Toxic Nectrotizing Myopathies:	**Mitochondrial:**
Statin	Progressive external ophtalmoparesis +
Fibrate	Mitochondrial neurogastointestinal Encephalopathy syndrome
Ezetimibe	
Alcohol	
Cyclosporine	
Other Toxic Myopathies:	**Metabolic:**
Corticosteroids	Acid maltase deficiency
Chloroquine	Myophosphorylase deficiency (McArdle's disease)
Amiodarone	
Cyclosporine	
Vincristine	
AZT	
Nutritional:	**Dystrophy:**
Acute quadriplegic myopathy	Myotonic dystrophy type 1 & 2
Vitamin D deficiency	Occulopharyngeal muscular dystrophy
	Limb girdle muscular dystrophy

absorptiometry (Melton 2000). The prevalence of sarcopenia increases with aging from 10% in the eighth decade to 20% in the ninth decade (Castillo 2003; Gillette-Guyonnet 2003).

Pathophysiology

Physical inactivity is the most readily reversible cause of sarcopenia. Additional contributing factors are complex and include age-dependent motor neuron loss, altered protein metabolism, inflammation, hormonal dysfunction, as well as oxidative and mitochondrial stress.

Aging is associated with reduced skeletal muscle mass and increased lipid and fibrous tissue content in muscle (Cree 2004; Forsberg 1991). This progressive process begins in the sixth decade of life (Melton 2000; Noppa 1980). With aging, lower muscle mass is linked to reduced isometric torque (Klitgaard 1990). In a 12-year longitudinal study of aged men, 90% of the strength loss of 1.4 %/year was attributable to the reduction in muscle cross-sectional area (Frontera 2000). Though both muscle fiber types are affected by aging, atrophy is most pronounced in type II fibers (Aniansson 1986). Furthermore, there is a decrease in the proportion of type II fibers (Jakobsson 1990). These changes may in part be explained by attrition in the number of motor neurons.

While data provides conflicting results about the effects of aging on protein breakdown, there is ample evidence to support the assertion that sarcopenia is associated with a reduction in protein synthetic rate (Yarasheski 1993). In older adults, knee extension strength and muscle mass correlated with myosin protein synthesis rates (Balagopal 1997). Furthermore, the mitochondrial protein synthesis rates and electron transport chain activity decline with aging (Rooyackers 1996).

Several causes for the reduction in mitochondrial enzyme activity are associated with aging. In addition to the down-regulation of genes involved in mitochondrial function (Melov 2007; Zahn 2006), there is an increase in the proportion of mitochondrial deoxyribonucleic acid (mtDNA) deletions in aged human skeletal muscle (Kovalenko 1997; Parise 2005). The latter is most pronounced in type I fibers (Pesce 2005).

It has been proposed that free radicals from electron transfer induce mtDNA mutations. The mtDNA mutations are associated with an increased proportion of cytochrome c oxidase (COX) deficient muscle fibers (Kovalenko 1997; Parise 2005), both of which are concentrated in foci of muscle atrophy (Aiken 2002; Lee 1998).

The role of apoptosis in sarcopenia is unclear. However, mitochondria can activate apoptosis through an increase in cytochrome-c (Stachowiak 1998). Release of the latter has been demonstrated together with a marked reduction in type II fibers mitochondrial content (Chabi 2008).

Genetic Contributions

Age-related changes in motor neurons and skeletal muscle fibers affect neuromuscular function and strongly influence the expression of neuromuscular disease. While attrition of motor units is primarily related to denervation (Lexell 1988; Lexell 1997), skeletal muscle alteration has been also described. Disuse (Castillo 2003), increased oxidation of myosin by free radicals (Lowe 2001; Lowe 2004), and increase in glycated myosin (Syrovy 1992) contribute to the decline in muscle mass and/or function. Both the synthetic rate of myosin (Proctor 1998) and the protein degradation (ubiquitin proteasome pathway) during muscle atrophy (Ferrington 2005) are decreased in aged rat muscle. Increased circulating levels of TNF-alpha, a pro-inflammatory cytokine, may increase the rate of free radical formation (Reid 2001). Furthermore, age is associated with reduced expression of a protective chaperone protein (Heat Shock Protein 70) in response to oxidative stress.

Older muscle fibers have impaired regenerative capacity due to the lower differentiation capacity of myoblasts. The latter is regulated by multiple myogenic regulatory factors. Of note, satellite cells from old animals can regenerate better when transplanted in young animals supporting the importance of circulating factors (Carlson 1989).

Myostatin inhibits proliferation, DNA synthesis, and protein synthesis in adult muscle cells. Gene transcription of the latter is decreased by resistance training and increased with aging (Yarasheski 2002) or prolonged bed rest. Insulin-like growth factor 1 (IGF-1) stimulates myoblast proliferation and differentiation and promotes skeletal muscle hypertrophy and glycolytic metabolism. IGF-1 and myostatin operate in a coordinated manner to regulate the proliferation, differentiation, and quiescence of satellite cells. The anabolic effects of IGF- and testosterone are attenuated by elevation in cytokine levels (TNF-alpha & IL-6). In rats, caloric restriction attenuates any fluctuations in TNF-alpha levels and lessens the degree of age-associated muscle atrophy (Phillips 2005).

Disuse results in muscle fiber atrophy, especially involving type 2 fibers (Degens 2006; Salmons 1981). Resistance training increases muscle mass and strength (Narici 2006; Roman 1993). Exercise training reduces the levels of TNF-alpha (Kovalenko 1997) and the frequency of apoptosis (Siu 2004). The exercise response is inversely related to the levels of TNF-alpha (Bruunsgaard 2004; Greiwe 2004). There is evidence, however, of an impaired response in old age which may be caused by an attenuated activation of the mTOR pathway after exercise (Parkington 2004) and impaired satellite cells differentiation (Charge 2004).

Clinical Presentation

After 60 years of age, the maximal mechanical force output of skeletal muscles gradually declines by as much as 30%–50% (Larsson 1979; Larsson 1997). As a result of sarcopenia, up to 25% of individuals older than 75 years suffer from functional impairments (Tarnopolsky 2007). Sarcopenia results in leg muscle weakness compromising the ability of older individuals to stand up from a chair or climb stairs. Sarcopenia often leads to impaired activities of daily living including independent ambulation and increased risk of falling. On neurologic examination, hip flexion weakness is mild. Functional testing demonstrates difficulty rising from a squatted or seated position without assistance. Laboratory investigation including creatine kinase, thyroid function tests and electromyography are normal. Muscle histopathology demonstrates clusters of atrophic angular muscle fibers and fiber type grouping as well as atrophy of mainly type 2 fibers (Jennekens 1971; Larsson 1979; Serratrice 1968; Tomonaga 1978). This may be due in large part to the progressive loss of active motor units and perhaps a switch to slower fiber type.

Treatment

Resistance Exercise Training

Resistance activity typically consists of a low repetition number of high intensity contractions of muscle fibers at 50% to 75% of one maximal repetition. Type II muscle fiber area increased in aged men and women after a 12-week regimen of resistance exercise training (Campbell 1999; Frontera 1988). Others identified an additional increase in type I muscle fiber area (Brose 2003). Long-term resistance exercise training in the elderly performed three times per week results in biceps and quadriceps muscle strength, histology, and chemistry that is similar to young subjects (Klitgaard 1990).

Data suggest a contribution of mitochondrial mechanisms to the beneficial effects of resistance training. A 14-week resistance exercise training program resulted in a significant increase in muscle COX enzyme activity (Parise 2005). Recently, skeletal muscle biopsies prior to exercise training showed an enrichment of genes associated with mitochondrial aging (Melov 2007). Exercise training reversed the transcriptional signature of aging back to that of younger levels for most genes. This effect of exercise may be due to the recruitment and fusion of dormant satellite cells which enjoy an intact complement of mitochondria.

A recent controlled trial extended the benefits of resistance training to frail nursing home residents (Fiatarone 2004). In this study, muscle strength, gait velocity and stair-climbing power improved in response to resistance training. Furthermore, the large strength gain in contrast with the modest change in muscle area suggested that improved neural recruitment may account for most of the functional improvement (Fiatarone 1994; Slivka 2008).

Resistance Exercise Training Combined with Supplements

In a prospective placebo-controlled study of a 14-week resistance training in individuals older than 65 years, the addition of creatine monohydrate (CrM) 5 grams daily provided added benefits. As expected, the resistance exercise training placebo recipients showed significant increases in all strength measures, muscle fiber area, and functional endpoints, including the number of chair stands in 30 seconds, timed 30 meter walk test, and timed 14-stair climb performance (Brose 2003). The CrM group additionally had significantly greater increases in fat-free mass and total body mass, and a greater increase in isometric knee extension strength, as compared to placebo recipients. In a similar randomized double-blind study, the effects of CrM (5 g/day) and conjugated linoleic acid (CLA 6g/d) were compared to placebo in 39 elderly community dwelling subjects following six months of resistance exercise training. Exercise training improved all measures of functional capacity and strength, with greater improvement for the CrM+CLA group in most measures of muscular endurance and in isokinetic knee extension strength. The combination of CrM and CLA may have a role in enhancing some of the beneficial effects of resistance training (Tarnopolsky 2007).

Endurance Exercise Training

Endurance training is an aerobic activity of sufficient intensity (50% to 85% of peak rate of oxygen consumption) and long duration (30 minutes). Some evidence suggests that endurance training may attenuate the progression towards sarcopenia in addition to the certain cardiovascular benefits. Endurance training is associated with an increase in muscle capillary density (Harris 2005). Endurance training for eight weeks improved insulin sensitivity as well as muscle fat oxidative capacity (Rimbert 2004). Being physically active correlates with higher mitochondrial enzyme levels including COX when compared to the sedentary state. Myosin heavy chain I mRNA and protein content increased in response to endurance exercise training (Short 2005). More recently, SIRT3 expression, a mitochondrial sirtuin linked to lifespan-enhancing effects of caloric restriction, was found to be increased by endurance exercise (Lanza 2008).

Idiopathic Inflammatory Myopathy
Epidemiology

Idiopathic inflammatory myopathy is divided into three major subtypes which include dermatomyositis (DM), polymyositis (PM), and inclusion body myositis (IBM) (Amato 1997; Dalakas 2003). These subtypes are clinically, histologically, and pathologically distinct (Table 3). The incidence of these disorders is approximately one in 100,000 per year. Other subtypes include necrotizing myopathy, overlap syndromes (inflammatory myopathy occurring in a patient with a connective tissue disorder such as mixed connective tissue disease), granulomatous myositis, and eosinophilic myositis.

Dermatomyositis
Clinical Presentation

Dermatomyositis affects children and adults. Adult DM generally manifests as subacute progressive painless proximal weakness, a skin rash, or both. Juvenile DM may present similarly or as an acute or subacute febrile illness followed by skin, muscle, or sometimes multisystem involvement. The pattern of proximal limb weakness in DM is not specific and does not distinguish DM from many other myopathies. Significant muscle asymmetry or prominent distal (forearm or lower leg) weakness should prompt consideration for inclusion body myositis (discussed later). Another consideration is sarcoidosis, for which clinical involvement similar to DM has been recognized (Kubis 1998).

DM can also affect the skin in various ways. A heliotrope rash (purplish discoloration) can occur on the eyelids. An erythematous rash can affect the face, neck, and anterior chest ("V-sign"), upper back

Table 3 Idiopathic Inflammatory Myopathies: Clinical and Laboratory

	Typical Age of Onset	Rash	Pattern of Weakness	Creatine Kinase	Muscle Biopsy	Cellular Infiltrate	Response to Immuno-suppressive Therapy	Common Associated Conditions
Dermatomyositis	Childhood and adult	Yes	Proximal > distal	Elevated (up to 50 × normal)	Perimysial and perivascular inflammation; perifascicular atrophy; MAC	CD4+T-cells; B cells; plasmacytoid dendritic cells	Yes	Malignancy, myocarditis, ILD, CTD, vasculitis (juvenile)
Polymyositis	Adult	No	Proximal > distal	Elevated (up to 50 × normal)	Endomysial inflammation	CD8+T-cells; macrophages; myeloid dendritic cells	Yes	Malignancy, Myocarditis, ILD, CTD
Inclusion Body Myositis	Elderly (>50)	No	Finger flexors, knee extensors	Normal or mildly elevated (<10 × normal)	Rimmed vacuoles; endomysial inflammation	CD8+T-cells; macrophages; myeloid dendritic cells	No	Autoimmune disorder
Necrotizing Myopathy	Adult and elderly	No	Proximal > distal	Elevated (> 10 × normal)	Necrotic muscle fibers; absent inflammatory infiltrate	None	Yes	Malignancy, CTD, drug-induced

Adapted and modified from AA Amato and RJ Barohn. Idiopathic inflammatory myopathies. *Neurol Clin* 1997;15:615–648.

("shawl sign"), elbows (see Figure 1a), or knees. Gottron's papules (see Figure 1b), a purple, scaly rash, can appear on the hands. "Mechanic's hands" occur when the skin on the dorsal and ventral surfaces of the hands become thickened and cracked. Subcutaneous calcinosis often occurs in juvenile DM but is uncommon in adult DM. Cutaneous symptoms in DM have a high impact on lowering quality of life in patients and include prominent pruritus (Shirani 2004; Hundley 2006).

Associated Conditions

In addition to skin abnormalities, DM is also associated with two other important clinical syndromes; interstitial lung disease (ILD) and cancer. ILD is present in at least 10% of adult DM patients and may occur in childhood DM. Malignancy has been estimated to be associated with 6% to 45% of adult patients with DM, with age-associated increased risk particularly in patients older than 40 years. The most common associated malignancy in older women is ovarian cancer

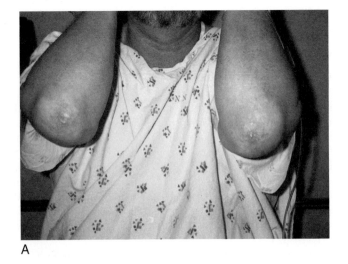

A

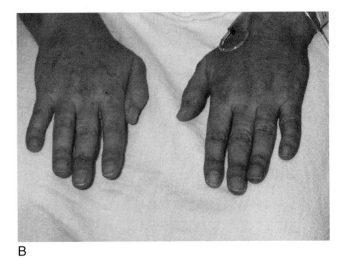

B

Figure 1a Violaceous erythematous scaly rash on elbows. See Figure 37.1a on the color insert.

Figure 1b Skin rash in DM—Gottron's papules. See Figure 37.1b on the color insert.

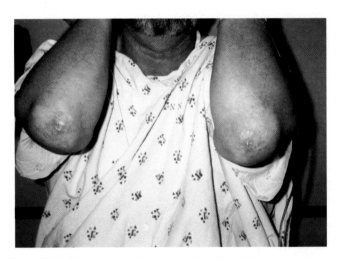

Figure 37.1a Violaceous erythematous scaly rash on elbows.

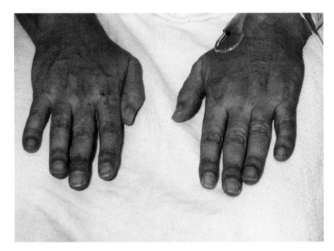

Figure 37.1b Skin rash in DM—Gottron's papules.

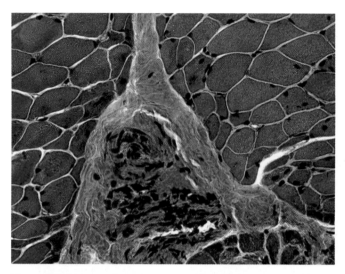

Figure 37.2 Hematoxylin and eosin stained muscle cross-section of quadriceps demonstrating parivascular inflammation and perifasicular atrophy. Photo courtesy of Sozos Papasozomenous.

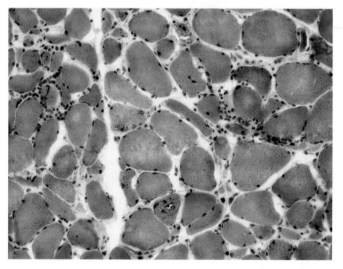

Figure 37.4 Hematoxylin and eosin-stained biceps muscle biopsy of a patient with inclusion body myositis. This demonstrates inflammatory cells invading non-necrotic muscle fiber, vacuolated muscle fibers, myofiber necrosis and regeneration.

(Scaling 1979), but the most common malignancy in men is small cell lung cancer.

Electrocardiographic abnormalities include conduction defects and arrhythmias which may occur in juvenile and adult DM. Pericarditis, myocarditis, and congestive heart failure can occasionally develop. Inflammation of the skeletal and smooth muscles of gastrointestinal tract can lead to dysphagia and delayed gastric emptying. Arthritis is typically symmetrical and involves both large and small joints.

Laboratory Testing

Serum CK level is elevated in more than 90% of patients with DM, and the level can be as high as 50 times the normal value. Normal serum CK may be present in patients with progressive disease and does not exclude the diagnosis. When elevated serum CK is present in DM, reductions generally occur with treatment and increase with relapse. For complete evaluation for any malignancy, several tests should be considered. A complete physical evaluation should be done, including skin examination. Women need breast and pelvic evaluations, and men need testicular and prostate examinations. The physician should also consider blood studies, such as complete blood count, liver function tests, lactate dehydrogenase, prostate-specific antigen, stool for occult blood, CT (chest, abdomen, and pelvis), and colonoscopy. We advocate a pelvic sonogram to better evaluate for ovarian malignancy.

Additional evaluation of adult patients with DM should be performed because of its association with interstitial lung disease. Pulmonary function tests, chest CT, and laboratory testing for the presence of antihistidyl tRNA synthetase antibodies (Jo-1 antibodies) should be considered in all patients with DM. An effective predictor of response to treatment and prognosis in DM may be myositis-specific antibodies (MSAs), which are associated with specific HLA haplotypes. Most patients have only one type of MSA. However, most patients with inflammatory myopathy do not have an MSA. Furthermore, the relevance of MSAs on treatment and prognosis have not been studied prospectively. The pathogenic relationship these antibodies have with inflammatory myopathies is unknown.

The MSAs include the cytoplasmic antibodies directed against Mi-2 and Mas antigens and against translational proteins such as various tRNA synthetases and the antisignal recognition particle. The Jo-1 antibody is the most common antisynthetase and is associated with ILD and arthritis. It is seen in up to 20% of patients with inflammatory myopathy. The other antisynthetases are much less common and are each seen in fewer than 2% to 3% of patients with inflammatory myopathy. The presence of Jo-1 antibodies has been associated with only a moderate response to treatment and a poor long-term prognosis. However, the associated ILD is responsible for the less favorable prognosis—not just the presence of Jo-1 antibodies. We lack prospective trials to demonstrate treatment outcomes of patients with myositis-ILD with anti-Jo-1 antibodies and similar patients without these antibodies.

Nonsynthetase Mi-2 antibodies are found in 15% to 20% DM. Mi-2 is a 240-kd nuclear protein of unknown function. The Mi-2 antibodies are associated with acute onset, erythematous rash, good response to therapy, and favorable prognosis. However, it is not known whether DM patients with Mi-2 antibodies respond differently than DM patients without the antibody.

Antibodies to the signal recognition particle (SRP) are known to be specific to PM and NM. IIM patients with SRP antibodies usually present with rapidly progressive proximal weakness and often respond poorly to steroid therapy (Kao 2004).

Electrophysiology

Electromyography (EMG) shows increased insertional and spontaneous activity with fibrillation potentials, positive sharp waves, and occasionally pseudo-myotonic and complex repetitive discharges. Polyphasic motor unit action potentials are of small duration and low amplitude. Motor unit action potentials (MUAPs) show early recruitment.

In addition, EMG may also be useful in previously responsive myositis patients, who become weakened due to type 2 muscle fiber atrophy from disuse or chronic steroid therapy. Isolated type 2 muscle fiber is not associated with any abnormal spontaneous activity on EMG.

MRI

Magnetic resonance imaging (MRI) occasionally provides information on the pattern of muscle involvement by looking at the cross-sectional area of axial and limb muscles. MRI may demonstrate signal abnormalities in affected muscles secondary to inflammation and edema or replacement by fibrotic tissue. Some have advocated MRI as a guide to determine which muscle to biopsy.

Muscle Pathology

Muscle biopsies from DM patients demonstrate perifascicular atrophy and perimysial inflammatory cells (see Figure 2). The inflammatory infiltrate is composed primarily of macrophages, B cells, and CD4+ cells. Endomysial inflammation is scant. When present, it surrounds non-necrotic and necrotic myofibers. An early histological abnormality in DM is deposition of the C5b-9 or membrane attack complex around small blood vessels (Kissel 1986; Emslie-Smith 1990). This deposition on small vessels precedes inflammation and other structural abnormalities in the muscle on light microscopy and is fairly specific for DM.

Polymyositis

It is difficult to classify patients with acquired myopathies whose weakness improves with immunosuppressive therapies and relapses with taper of such therapy but lack the rash and pathological features of DM. Polymyositis is an exclusionary diagnosis in patients who do not have an alternate muscle or nerve disease.

Clinical Presentation

PM usually affects patients over the age of 20 years and is more common in females (Amato 1997; Dalakas 2003; Bohan 1975).

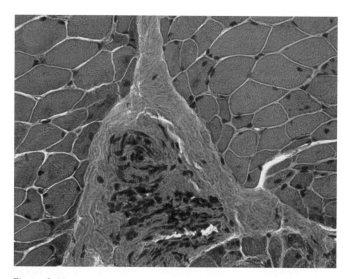

Figure 2 Hematoxylin and eosin stained muscle cross-section of quadriceps demonstrating parivascular inflammation and perifasicular atrophy. Photo courtesy of Sozos Papasozomenous. See Figure 37.2 on the color insert.

Diagnosis is often delayed compared with DM. Patients have neck flexor and symmetric proximal arm and leg weakness, which typically develops over the period of several weeks or months. Distal muscles may also become involved but are not as weak as the more proximal muscles. Myalgias and tenderness are common presentations. Dysphagia reportedly occurs in approximately one-third of patients secondary to oropharyngeal and esophageal involvement. Mild facial weakness occasionally may be demonstrated on examination. Sensation is normal, and muscle stretch reflexes are usually preserved.

Associated Conditions

The cardiac and pulmonary complications of PM are reported to be similar to those of DM. Myocarditis, which presents primarily as conduction abnormalities and less commonly as congestive heart failure, affects up to one-third of patients. Interstitial lung disease has been reported to occur in at least 10% of PM patients with at least half having the Jo-1 antibody. Polyarthritis has been reported in up to 45% of patients with PM at the time of diagnosis. The risk of malignancy with PM is lower than seen in DM, but it may be slightly higher than expected in the general population.

Laboratory Testing

Serum CK level is elevated 5-fold to 50-fold in the majority of PM patients.

Serum CK level may be useful in monitoring response to therapy, but only in conjunction with physical examination. CK does not correlate with the degree of weakness. Sedimentation rate is normal in at least half the patients and does not correlate with disease activity. A positive ANA is reported in 16% to 40% of patients with PM.

Electrophysiology

EMG findings are identical to those seen in DM and indicate an irritative myopathy.

Muscle Pathology

The histological features of PM are different from DM. The predominant histological features in PM are variability in fiber size, scattered necrotic and regenerating fibers, and endomysial inflammation that invades non-necrotic muscle fibers. The endomysial inflammatory cells consist primarily of activated CD8+ (cytotoxic) T cells, and macrophages.

All of the invaded and some of the noninvaded muscle fibers may express major histocompatibility complex class one, which is not normally present in the sarcolemma of muscle fibers.

Therapy for DM and PM

Patients with DM and PM with muscle weakness are usually treated with systemic immunosuppressive therapies. High doses of corticosteroids are typically used initially to control the disease and are then slowly tapered. When the disease cannot be controlled on lower doses of prednisone (20 mg or less), the dose is increased and second agents, typically either methotrexate or azathioprine, are introduced for long-term control. Then the corticosteroid taper is repeated, hoping to achieve disease control with low-dose corticosteroids. Adjuvant immune suppressive therapy is also recommended in patients with severe disease, those refractory to high dose steroids, and those who experience marked adverse events while on steroids.

Glucocorticoids can be used in a wide range of regimens, but one typical regimen for adults is prednisone 1 mg/kg/d until definite and satisfactory improvement in strength occurs, usually within one to three months of treatment. Slow tapering by 10 mg/month will then bring patients down typically to a dose of 20 mg/day after six months from the initiation of therapy. Patients without the comorbidities of diabetes or hypertension can be managed with alternate day therapy.

Methotrexate is typically used for patients whose disease cannot be controlled on sufficiently low doses of corticosteroids. Methotrexate is given once per week in divided doses, with one common approach starting at 7.5 mg/week. The dose may be increased by 2.5 mg/week, to as much as 20 mg/week orally. Folic acid 1 mg/day is given daily to reduce the mucocutaneous adverse event incidence. Laboratory monitoring is required, including monthly complete blood count, differential count, and liver function tests.

Azathioprine, like methotrexate, has a better long-term side effect profile than corticosteroids. Dosing can start at 50 mg/d and can be increased weekly by 50 mg to reach a total dose of 2 to 3 mg/kg/day. Dose reduction is required for patients on allopurinol or ACE inhibitors, due to increased risk of leukopenia. Monthly blood counts and liver function tests are required to monitor adverse effects due to azathioprine.

Intravenous immunoglobulin is useful for some patients with DM and PM. It can be used as initial treatment in severely affected patients with a goal of more rapid improvement, occasionally as maintenance therapy in otherwise refractory patients, or to reduce long-term corticosteroid use. Dosing is 2 g/kg total initially, given divided over two to five days, and then infusions are repeated every two to four weeks, with a total dosage of 1 to 2 g/kg/month.

Other treatment options include cyclophosphamide, cyclosporine, tacrolimus, chlorambucil, and mycophenolate. Plasma exchange has not shown to be of benefit in a controlled trial (Miller 1992). Rituximab has been used in refractive PM and DM with positive results (Noss 2006). A clinical trial is ongoing to clarify the role of rituximab in PM and DM.

Inclusion Body Myositis

After sarcopenia, inclusion body myositis is the next most common myopathy after age 60. Although onset over age 60 has been emphasized, symptom onset before age 60 is common (18% to 20% of patients) (Lotz 1989; Badrising 2005).

Frequently, diagnosis of IBM has been delayed by a mean of five to eight years from symptom onset (Lotz 1989; Badrising 2000; Lindberg 1994; Sayers 1992).

Clinical Presentation

The clinical presentation of IBM is quite distinct from that of other inflammatory myopathies. Atrophy and weakness of wrist and finger flexors (see Figure 3a) and quadriceps (see Figure 3b) are distinctive, and the physical examination should focus on careful testing of these muscle groups. Comparison of wrist and finger extensors with corresponding flexors may demonstrate greater involvement of the flexors and asymmetry. Relative preservation of the deltoid muscles, compared with the wrist flexors, can be impressive and in marked contrast to the pattern of weakness seen in DM and PM. Severe biceps muscle weakness, compared to preserved brachioradialis, and severe deep finger flexor weakness, but uncommonly involved adductor pollicis, have been reported (Lotz 1989). Involvement of the tibialis anterior muscle may occur in 10% of IBM. Dysphagia can be a significant problem with a prevalence estimated as high as 66% (Lotz 1989).

Associated Conditions

Autoimmune disorders such as systemic lupus erythematosus, Sjögren's syndrome, thrombocytopenia, and sarcoidosis have been reported in up to 15% with IBM. There is no increased risk of myocarditis, malignancy, or ILD associated with IBM.

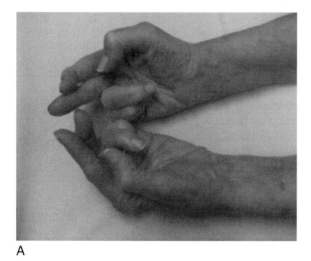

Figure 3a Finger flexor weakness in IBM.

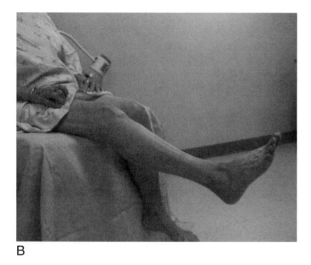

Figure 3b Thigh atrophy and quadriceps muscle weakness in IBM.

Laboratory Testing

Serum CK level may be normal or elevated, usually less than ten times above the normal limit. ANA is positive in 20% of IBM patients. IBM patients have a high prevalence of the HLA DR3 phenotype (*0301/0302).

Electrophysiology

Nerve conduction studies reveal electrophysiological evidence of a sensory neuropathy in 30% of the cases. Electrodiagnostic study findings are similar to those found in PM and DM. However, in one out of three IBM cases, the motor unit potentials are mixed myopathic and neuropathic. This is due to reinnervation of denervated muscle fiber in this chronic disease.

Muscle Pathology

The presence of multiple myofibers surrounded by inflammatory cells and many myofibers with rimmed vacuoles is highly supportive of a pathological diagnosis of IBM (see Figure 4). The presence of cytomembranous whorls and 15–18 nm diameter cytoplasmic tubulofilamentous inclusions on electron microscopy is also highly supportive of a diagnosis of IBM. Patients who have typical clinical

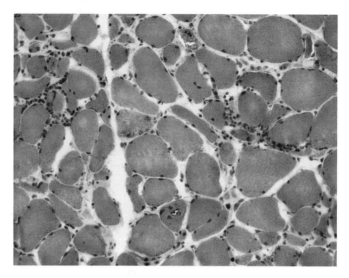

Figure 4 Hematoxylin and eosin-stained biceps muscle biopsy of a patient with inclusion body myositis. This demonstrates inflammatory cells invading non-necrotic muscle fiber, vacuolated muscle fibers, myofiber necrosis and regeneration. See Figure 37.4 on the color insert.

features but few inflammatory cells or few rimmed vacuoles can be more difficult to diagnose. Some patients who have steroid-responsive PM syndromes can have a few rimmed vacuoles (van der Meulen 2001).

Therapy

Treatment approaches for IBM have been ineffective. IBM does not respond to prednisone. No benefit has been seen in controlled trials with beta-interferon (Muscle Study Group 2004; Muscle Study Group 2001) after three months of intravenous immunoglobulin (IVIg) without (Dalakas 1997) and with prednisone (Dalakas 2001), and after 48 weeks of methotrexate (Badrising 2002).

A trial of six months of IVIg did not result in definitive improvement, although some effects may have been present (Walter 2000). Antithymocyte globulin (Lindberg 2003) in a pilot trial demonstrated some benefit. Oxandrolone, an androgen receptor agonist, had a borderline significant effect in improving whole-body strength and a significant effect in upper extremity strength (Rutkove 2002).

Necrotizing Myopathy

In addition to the above-mentioned subtypes of inflammatory myopathy, another emerging steroid-responsive inflammatory myopathy is "necrotizing myopathy."

Necrotizing myopathy (NM) is a unique immune-mediated myopathy with specific pathological features distinct from polymyositis and other inflammatory myopathies. It is an increasingly recognized immune-mediated myopathy.

Clinical Presentation

Necrotizing myopathy manifests in patients over the age of 30, with female gender preponderance. It usually presents with subacute, progressive onset of proximal muscle weakness. Weakness generally develops more rapidly as compared to polymyositis. Some patients complain of myalgias. Dysphagia has been reported in NM. Patients without an underlying connective tissue disorder, cancer, or toxic myopathy are considered to have idiopathic myopathy.

Associated Conditions

Malignancy and connective tissue disorders are frequently associated with NM. Gastrointestinal tract adenocarcinoma and small and non-small cell carcinoma of the lung are the common malignancies. Certain medications, especially statins, have been associated with necrotizing myopathy (Table 2).

Laboratory Testing

Serum CK level is often highly elevated, more than 10 times the normal limit. ANA is positive in those with underlying connective tissue disorder. NM patients should also be screened for an underlying malignancy.

Electrophysiology

EMG demonstrates increased insertional activity, positive sharp waves, and fibrillation potentials. MUAPs are usually of short duration and low amplitude with early recruitment similar to other inflammatory myopathies.

Muscle Pathology

Muscle histopathology plays a critical role in the diagnosis of NM. The most prominent feature of muscle biopsy is the absence of inflammatory infiltrates and the presence of scattered necrotic myofibers. Features of microangiopathy with thick "pipestem" vessels and microvascular deposits of complement membrane attack complex have been described (Allison 1991).

Therapy

Necrotizing myopathy is usually resistant to therapy, particularly if there is an underlying malignancy or toxic myopathy. However, immunosuppressants such as prednisone, methotrexate, and azathioprine are the mainstay of treatment. Most patients usually require corticosteroids and a second-line agent. Appropriate medication monitoring should be undertaken while using immunosuppressants.

Other Muscle Disorders

Oculopharyngeal Muscular Dystrophy (OPMD)

Clinical Presentation

OPMD is an autosomal dominant disorder. It is caused by expansion of a short GCG repeat on chromosome 14q11.1 in the PABN1 gene. It usually manifests in the fourth to sixth decade of life. Most patients present with progressive bilateral ptosis without diplopia. However, occasionally they may have unilateral ptosis or diplopia. The extraocular muscles are involved in nearly half of the patients.

Approximately one-fourth of patients develop dysphagia, which may lead to recurrent aspiration pneumonia. Mild facial weakness and mild proximal or distal limb weakness may occur with disease progression. A history of similar symptoms in relatives usually exists although a prior OPMD definitive diagnosis may not have been established. It is necessary to obtain a detailed family history specifically asking for complaints of weakness when suspecting a hereditary disorder like OPMD. Patients have a normal life span.

Associated Conditions

There is no specific disorder associated with OPMD.

Laboratory Testing

Serum CK level is normal or mildly elevated. OPMD is a clinical diagnosis. A genetic test is available and is essential in patients without a clear family history of OPMD.

Electrophysiology

EMG usually reveals short duration, low amplitude MUAPs usually without evidence of increased insertional activity or irritative features. These findings are not specific to OPMD.

Muscle Pathology

Muscle biopsy reveals fiber size variability, central nuclei, and increased adipose and endomysial connective tissue. Rimmed vacuoles may be found but are not a constant feature. On electron microscope, intranuclear tubofilamentous inclusions with a diameter of 8.5 nm and up to 0.25 μm length arranged in tangles or palisades can be identified.

Therapy

No medical treatment is available. Supportive treatment includes eyelid crutches, ptosis surgery, criocopharyngral myotomy, or percutaneous endogastric tube placement. Patients benefit from genetic counseling.

Hypothyroid Myopathy

Hypothyroidism increases in prevalence and incidence among the elderly. It is important for the clinician to appreciate myopathy associated with hypothyroidism in older individuals.

Clinical Presentation

Patients present with proximal arm and leg weakness with myalgias, cramps, and fatigue. In severe cases, the respiratory muscles may be involved (Martinez 1989). Clinical examination shows delayed relaxation of the muscle stretch reflexes. Myoedema is observed in approximately one-third of patients (Salick 1967).

Associated Conditions

As the name indicates, it is associated with hypothyroidism. There is no other associated disorder reported.

Laboratory Testing

Serum CK level ranges from 10 to 100 times the upper limit of normal. Thyroid function test are abnormal.

Electrophysiology

Nerve conduction study may be abnormal if there is an extremely rare polyneuropathy, though causal association is uncertain. EMG is usually normal due to involvement of mostly type 2 fibers but may show short duration and low amplitude MUAPs.

Muscle Pathology

Patients with myopathy must be routinely screened for thyroid dysfunction. Therefore, these patients usually do not require a muscle biopsy. Previous reports have described fiber size variability, central nuclei, and myofiber atrophy predominantly of type 2 fibers on muscle biopsy. Ring fibers, glycogen accumulation, vacuoles, and increased connective tissue may also be identified (Laycock 1991, Evans 1990).

Therapy

Correction of underlying hypothyroidism is the key treatment. However, some patients have residual weakness even a year after being euthyroid.

McArdle's Disease

Most metabolic myopathies are disorders of infancy, childhood, and early adulthood. Individuals typically present with exercise intolerance and episodes of myoglobinuria. However, onset of McArdle's disease (myophosphorylase deficiency) has been reported as late as the eighth decade of life, presenting as a proximal limb-girdle syndrome

(Engel 1963; Hewlett 1978; Kost 1980; Pourmand 1983; Felice 1992; Wolfe 2000). Most individuals present with exercise intolerance. Serum CK level is typically elevated between attacks and surges during attacks of weakness. The non-ischemic forearm exercise test demonstrates a lack of adequate rise of lactic acid despite normal increase in venous ammonia level. EMG shows myopathic MUAPs or may be normal. Muscle biopsy reveals the characteristic finding of glycogen accumulation in the subsarcolemmal and intermyofibrillar area. Staining for myophosphorylase is absent. Ingestion of sucrose prior to exercise improved exercise tolerance in a single-blind, randomized, placebo-controlled, crossover study (Vissing 2003).

In the past, the avoidance of exercise has been recommended in McArdle's disease, which we now know leads to further deconditioning. Endurance training carries the potential to increase capillary density, vascular conductance, and mitochondrial oxidative capacity (Saltin 1980). Eight patients tolerated well a 14-week program of cycle training at 60% to 70% of maximal heart rate (Haller 2006). The subjects had increased average work capacity, oxygen uptake, cardiac output, and citrate synthase enzyme level. The authors concluded moderate aerobic exercise is an effective means of improving exercise capacity in McArdle's disease due to the increase in the circulatory delivery and mitochondrial metabolism of bloodborne fuels.

Summary

The most common inflammatory myopathy in the elderly is IBM. It is unclear of IBM is primarily a degenerative disorder or an inflammatory muscle disease. IBM presents with proximal leg and distal arm weakness and has no known effective treatment. This is different from PM and DM which typically present with proximal arm and leg weakness. This clinical distinction is important given the availability of efficacious therapy for PM and DM, and to a large extent NM.

In developed countries, the population is aging, leading to a larger number of patients with sarcopenia. Resistance exercise training is the most effective intervention and can partially reverse the age-associated decline in muscle function. There is promising data to suggest that adding CrM and CLA may enhance the effect of resistance exercise in sarcopenia.

References

Aiken J, Bua E, Cao Z, et al. Mitochondrial DNA deletion mutations and sarcopenia. *Ann N Y Acad Sci* 2002;959:412–423.

Amato AA and Barohn RJ. Idiopathic inflammatory myopathies. *Neurol Clin* 1997;15:615–648.

Aniansson A, Hedberg M, Henning GB, et al. Muscle morphology, enzymatic activity, and muscle strength in elderly men: A follow-up study. *Muscle Nerve* 1986;9:585–591.

Badrising UA, Maat-Schieman M, van Duinen SG, et al. Epidemiology of inclusion body myositis in the Netherlands: A nationwide study. *Neurology* 2000;55:1385–1387.

Badrising UA, Maat-Schieman ML, Ferrari MD, et al. Comparison of weakness progression in inclusion body myositis during treatment with methotrexate or placebo. *Ann Neurol* 2002;51:369–372.

Badrising UA, Maat-Schieman ML, van Houwelingen JC, et al. Inclusion body myositis. Clinical features and clinical course of the disease in 64 patients. *J Neurol* 2005;252(12):1448–1454.

Balagopal P, Rooyackers OE, Adey DB, et al. Effects of aging on in vivo synthesis of skeletal muscle myosin heavy-chain and sarcoplasmic protein in humans. *Am J Physiol* 1997;273:E790–800.

Bohan A and Peter JB. Polymyositis and dermatomyositis (second of two parts). *N Eng J Med* 1975;292:403–407.

Brose A, Parise G, and Tarnopolsky MA. Creatine supplementation enhances isometric strength and body composition improvements following strength exercise training in older adults. *J Gerontol A Biol Sci Med Sci* 2003;58:11–19.

Bruunsgaard H, Bjerregaard E, Schroll M, and Pedersen BK. Muscle strength after resistance training is inversely correlated with baseline levels of soluble tumor necrosis factor receptors in the oldest old. *J Am Geriatr Soc* 2004; 52:237–241.

Campbell WW, Joseph LJ, Davey SL, et al. Effects of resistance training and chromium picolinate on body composition and skeletal muscle in older men. *J Appl Physiol* 1999;86:29–39.

Carlson BM and Faulkner JA. Muscle transplantation between young and old rats: Age of host determines recovery. *Am J Physiol* 1989; 256:C1262–1266.

Castillo EM, Goodman-Gruen D, Kritz-Silverstein D, et al. Sarcopenia in elderly men and women: the Rancho Bernardo study. *Am J Prev Med* 2003;25:226–231.

Chabi B, Ljubicic V, Menzies KJ, et al. Mitochondrial function and apoptotic susceptibility in aging skeletal muscle. *Aging Cell* 2008;7:2–12.

Charge SB and Rudnicki MA. Cellular and molecular regulation of muscle regeneration. *Physiol Rev* 2004;84:209–238.

Cree MG, Newcomer BR, Katsanos CS, et al. Intramuscular and liver triglycerides are increased in the elderly. *J Clin Endocrinol Metab* 2004;89:3864–3871.

Dalakas MC and Hohlfeld R. Polymyositis and dermatomyositis. *Lancet* 2003;362:971–982.

Dalakas MC, Koffman B, Fujii M, et al. A controlled study of intravenous immunoglobulin combined with prednisone in the treatment of IBM. *Neurology* 2001;56:323–327.

Dalakas MC, Sonies B, Dambrosia J, et al. Treatment of inclusion-body myositis with IVIg: a double-blind, placebo-controlled study. *Neurology* 1997;48:712–716.

Degens H and Alway SE. Control of muscle size during disuse, disease, and aging. *Int J Sports Med* 2006; 27:94–99.

Emslie-Smith AM, and Engel AG. Microvascular changes in early and advanced dermatomyositis: a quantitative study. *Ann Neurol* 1990;27:343–356.

Emslie-Smith AM, and Engel AG. Necrotizing myopathy with pipestem capillaries, microvascular deposition of complement membrane attack complex (MAC), and minimal cellular infiltration. *Neurology* 1991;41:936–939.

Engel WK, Everman EL, and Williams HE. Late-onset type of skeletal-muscle phosphorylase deficiency. *N Engl J Med* 1963; 268:135–137.

Evans RM, Watanabe I, and Singer PA. Central changes in hypothyroid myopathy: a case report. *Muscle Nerve* 1990;13:952–956.

Felice KJ, Schneebaum AB, and Royden Jones H. McArdle's disease with late-onset symptoms: case report and review of the literature. *J Neurol Neurosurg Psychiatry* 1992;55:407–408.

Ferrington DA, Husom AD, and Thompson LV. Altered proteasome structure, function, and oxidation in aged muscle. *FASEB J* 2005; 19:644–646.

Fiatarone MA, O'Neill EF, Ryan ND, et al. Exercise training and nutritional supplementation for physical frailty in very elderly people. *N Engl J Med* 1994;330:1769–1775.

Forsberg AM, Nilsson E, Werneman J, et al. Muscle composition in relation to age and sex. *Clin Sci (Lond)* 1991;81:249–256.

Frontera WR, Hughes VA, Fielding RA, et al. Aging of skeletal muscle: a 12-yr longitudinal study. *J Appl Physiol* 2000;88: 1321–1326.

Frontera WR, Meredith CN, O'Reilly KP, et al. Strength conditioning in older men: skeletal muscle hypertrophy and improved function. *J Appl Physiol* 1988;64:1038–1044.

Gillette-Guyonnet S, Nourhashemi F, Andrieu S, et al. Body composition in French women 75+ years of age: the EPIDOS study. *Mech Ageing Dev* 2003;124(3):311–316.

Greenberg SA, Pinkus GS, Amato AA, and Pinkus JL. Myeloid dendritic cells in inclusion-body myositis and polymyositis. Muscle Nerve 2007;35(1):17–23.

Greiwe JS, Cheng B, Rubin DC, et al. Resistance exercise decreases skeletal muscle tumor necrosis factor alpha in frail elderly humans. FASEB J 2001;15:475–482.

Haller RG, Wyrick P, Taivassalo T, and Vissing, J. Aerobic conditioning: an effective therapy in McArdle's disease. Ann Neurol 2006;59(6):922–928.

Harris BA. The influence of endurance and resistance exercise on muscle capillarization in the elderly: a review. Acta Physiol Scand 2005;185:89–97.

Hewlett RH and Gardner-Thorpe C. McArdle's disease—what limit to the age of onset? S Afr Med J 1978;55:60–63.

Hundley JL, Carroll CL, Lang W, et al. Cutaneous symptoms of dermatomyositis significantly impact patients' quality of life. J Am Acad Dermatol 2006;54:217–220.

Jakobsson F, Borg K, and Edström L. Fibre-type composition, structure and cytoskeletal protein location of fibres in anterior tibial muscle. Comparison between young adults and physically active aged humans. Acta Neuropathol 1990;80:459–468.

Jennekens FG, Tomlinson BE, and Walton N. Histochemical aspects of five limb muscles in old age. An autopsy study. J Neurol Sci 1971;14:259–276.

Kao AH, Lacomis D, Lucas M et al. Anti-signal recognition particle autoantibody in patients with and patients without idiopathic inflammatory myopathy. Arthritis Rheum 2004;50:209–15.

Kissel JT, Mendell JR, and Rammohan KW. Microvascular deposition of complement membrane attack complex in dermatomyositis. N Engl J Med 1986;314:329–334.

Klitgaard H, Mantoni M, Schiaffino S, et al. Function, morphology and protein expression of ageing skeletal muscle: a cross-sectional study of elderly men with different training backgrounds. Acta Physiol Scand 1990;140:41–54.

Kost GJ and Verity MA. A new variant of late-onset myophosphorylase deficiency. Muscle Nerv 1980;3:195–201.

Kovalenko SA, Kopsidas G, Kelso JM, and Linnane AW. Deltoid human muscle mtDNA is extensively rearranged in old age subjects. Biochem Biophys Res Commun 1997;232:147–152.

Kubis N, Woimant F, Polivka M, et al. A case of dermatomyositis and muscle sarcoidosis in a Caucasian patient. J Neurol 1998;245:50–52.

Lanza IR, Short DK, Short KR, et al. Endurance exercise as a countermeasure for aging. Diabetes 2008 Nov;57(11):2933–42.

Larsson L, Grimby G, and Karlsson J. Muscle strength and speed of movement in relation to age and muscle morphology. J Appl Physiol 1979;46:451–456.

Larsson L, Li X, Yu F, and Degens H. Age-related changes in contractile properties and expression of myosin isoforms in single skeletal muscle cells. Muscle Nerve 1997;5:S74–S78.

Laycock MA and Pascuzzi RM. The neuromuscular effects of hypothyroidism. Semin Neurol 1991;11:288–294.

Lee CM, Lopez ME, Weindruch R, and Aiken JM. Association of age-related mitochondrial abnormalities with skeletal muscle fiber atrophy. Free Radic Bioi Med 1998;25:964–972.

Lexell J. Evidence for nervous system degeneration with advancing age. J Nutr 1997; 127:1011S–1013S.

Lexell J, Taylor CC, and Sjöström M. What is the cause of the ageing atrophy? Total number, size and proportion of different fiber types studied in whole vastus lateralis muscle from 15- to 83-year-old men. J Neurol Sci 1988;84:275–294.

Lindberg C, Persson LI, Bjorkander J, and Oldfors A. Inclusion body myositis: clinical, morphological, physiological and laboratory findings in 18 cases. Acta Neurol Scand 1994;89:123–131.

Lindberg C, Trysberg E, Tarkowski A, and Oldfors A. Anti-T-lymphocyte globulin treatment in inclusion body myositis: a randomized pilot study. Neurology 2003;61:260–262.

Lotz BP, Engel AG, Nishino H, et al. Inclusion body myositis. Observations in 40 patients. Brain 1989;112(Pt 3): 727–747.

Lowe DA, Surek JT, Thomas DD, and Thompson LV. Electron paramagnetic resonance reveals age-related myosin structural changes in rat skeletal muscle fibers. Am J Physiol Cell Physiol 2001; 280:C540–C547.

Lowe DA, Warren GL, Snow LM, et al. Muscle activity and aging affect myosin structural distribution and force generation in rat fibers. J Appl Physiol 2004; 96:498–506.

Martinez FJ, Bermudez-Gomez M, and Celli BR. Hypothyroidism. A reversible cause of diaphragmatic dysfunction. Chest 1989;96: 1059–1063.

Melov S, Tarnopolsky MA, Beckman K, et al. Resistance exercise reverses aging in human skeletal muscle. PLoS ONE 2007;2:e465.

Melton LJ 3rd, Khosla S, Crowson CS, et al. Epidemiology of sarcopenia. J Am Geriatr Soc 2000;48:625–630.

Miller FW, Leitman SF, Cronin M, et al. Controlled trial of plasma exchange and leukapheresis in polymyositis and dermatomyositis. N Engl J Med 1992;326:1380–1384.

Muscle Study Group. Randomized pilot trial of high-dose betaINF-1a in patients with inclusion body myositis. Neurology 2004;63:718–720.

Muscle Study Group. Randomized pilot trial of betaINF1a (Avonex) in patients with inclusion body myositis. Neurology 2001;57:1566–1570.

Narici MV and Maganaris CN. Adaptability of elderly human muscles and tendons to increased loading. J Anat 2006; 208:433–443.

Noppa H, Andersson M, Bengtsson C, et al. Longitudinal studies of anthropometric data and body composition. The population study of women in Götenberg, Sweden. Am J Clin Nutr 1980;33:155–162.

Noss EH, Hausner-Sypek DL, and Weinblatt ME. Rituximab as therapy for refractory polymyositis and dermatomyositis. J Rheumatol 2006;33(5):1021–1026.

Parise G, Brose AN, and Tarnopolsky MA. Resistance exercise training decreases oxidative damage to DNA and increases cytochrome oxidase activity in older adults. Exp Gerontol 2005;40:173–180.

Parkington JD, LeBrasseur NK, Siebert AP, and Fielding RA. Contraction-mediated mTOR, 70S6k, and ERK1/2 phosphorylation in aged skeletal muscle. J Appl Physiol 2004; 97:243–248.

Pesce V, Cormio A, Fracasso F, et al. Age-related changes of mitochondrial DNA content and rnitochondrial genotypic and phenotypic alterations in rat hind-limb skeletal muscles. J Gerontol A Bioi Sci Med Sci 2005;60:715–723.

Phillips T and Leeuwenburgh C. Muscle fiber specific apoptosis and TNF-alpha signaling in sarcopenia are attenuated by life-long calorie restriction. FASEB J 2005;19:668–670.

Pourmand R, Sanders DB, and Corwin. Late-onset McArdle's disease with unusual electromyographic findings. Arch Neurol 1983;40:374–377.

Proctor DN, Balagopal P, and Nair KS. Age-related sarcopenia in humans is associated with reduced synthetic rates of specific muscle proteins. J Nutr 1998; 128:351S–355S.

Reid MB and Li YP. Tumor necrosis factor-alpha and muscle wasting: a cellular perspective. Respir Res 2001;2:269–272.

Rimbert V, Bouie Y, Bedu M, et al. Muscle fat oxidative capacity is not impaired by age but by physical inactivity: association with insulin sensitivity. FASEB J 2004;18:737–739.

Roman WJ, Fleckenstein J, Stray-Gundersen J, et al. Adaptations in the elbow flexors of elderly males after heavy- resistance training. J Appl Physiol 1993;74:750–754.

Rooyackers OE, Adey DB, Ades PA, Nair KS. Effect of age on in vivo rates of mitochondrial protein synthesis in human skeletal muscle. Proc Natl Acad Sci USA 1996;93:15364–15369.

Rutkove SB, Parker RA, Nardin RA, et al. A pilot randomized trial of oxandrolone in inclusion body myositis. *Neurology* 2002;58(7):1081–1087.

Salick Al, Pearson CM. Electrical silence of myoedema. *Neurology* 1967;17:899–901.

Salmons S, Henriksson J. The adaptive response of skeletal muscle to increased use. *Muscle Nerve* 1981;4:94–105.

Saltin B, Rowell L.B. Functional adaptations to physical activity and inactivity. *Fed Proc* 1980;39:1506–1513.

Sayers ME, Chou SM, Calabrese LH. Inclusion body myositis: analysis of 32 cases. *J Rheumatol* 1992;19:1385–1389.

Scaling ST, Kaufman RH, Patten BM. Dermatomyositis and female malignancy. *Obstet Gynecol* 1979;54(4):474–477.

Serratrice G, Roux H, Aquaron R. Proximal muscle weakness in elderly subjects. Reports of 12 cases. *J Neural Sci* 1968;7:275–299.

Shirani Z, Kucenic MJ, Carroll CL, et al. Pruritus in adult dermatomyositis. *Clin Exp Dermatol* 2004;29:273–276.

Short KR, Vittone JL, Bigelow ML, et al. Changes in myosin heavy chain mRNA and protein expression in human skeletal muscle with age and endurance exercise training. *J Appl Physiol* 2005;99:95–102.

Siu PM, Bryner RW, Martyn JK, Alway SE. Apoptotic adaptations from exercise training in skeletal and cardiac muscles. *FASEB J* 2004;18:1150–1152.

Slivka D, Raue U, Hollon C, et al. Single muscle fiber adaptations to resistance training in old (>80 yr) men: evidence for limited skeletal muscle plasticity. *Am J Physiol Regul Integr Comp Physiol* 2008;295:R273–280.

Stachowiak O, Dolder M, Wallimann T, Richter C. Mitochondrial creatine kinase is a prime target of peroxynitrite-induced modification and inactivation. *J Bioi Chem* 1998;273: 16694–16699.

Syrovy I, Hodny Z. Non-enzymatic glycosylation of myosin: effects of diabetes and ageing. *Gen Physiol Biophys* 1992; 11: 301–307.

Tarnopolsky M, Zimmer A, Paikin J, Safdar et al. Creatine monohydrate and conjugated linoleic acid improve strengtl and body composition following resistance exercise in older adults. *PLoS GNE* 2007;2:e991.

Tomonaga, M. Histochemical and ultrastructural changes in senile human skeletal muscle. *J Am Geriatr Soc* 1977;25:125–131.

·van der Meulen MF, Hoogendijk JE, Moons KG, et al. Rimmed vacuoles and the added value of SMI-31 staining in diagnosing sporadic inclusion body myositis. *Neuromuscul Disord* 2001;11: 447–451.

Vissing J, Haller RG. The effect of oral sucrose on exercise tolerance in patients with McArdle's disease. *N Engl J Med* 2003;349:2503–2509.

Walter MC, Lochmuller H, Toepfer M, et al. High-dose immunoglobulin therapy in sporadic inclusion body myositis: a double-blind, placebo-controlled study. *J Neurol* 2000;247:22–28.

Wolfe GI, Baker NS, Haller RG, et al. McArdle's disease presenting with asymmetric, late-onset arm weakness. *Muscle Nerve* 2000;23:641–645.

Yarasheski KE, Bhasin S, Sinha-Hikim I, et al. Serum myostatin-immunoreactive protein is increased in 60-92 year old women and men with muscle wasting. *J Nutr Health Aging* 2002;6(5):343–8.

Yarasheski KE, Zachwieja JJ, Bier DM. Acute effects of resistance exercise on muscle protein synthesis rate in young and elderly men and women. *Am J Physiol* 1993;265:E210–214.

Zahn JM, Sonu R, Vogel H, et al. Transcriptional profiling of aging in human muscle reveals a common aging signature. *PLoS Genet* 2006;2:e115.

38 Peripheral Motor and Sensory Neuropathies in Aging

Jennifer A. Tracy and P. James B. Dyck

Introduction

Peripheral neuropathies are a significant cause of disability in the general population; their manifestations can range from mild discomfort or numbness in the feet to severe weakness requiring assistance in activities of daily living. Peripheral neuropathy is more common with advancing age. In general, it affects 1–2% of the general population, and an Italian study found a prevalence of 6.98% in people 65 years of age or older (Baldereschi et al. 2007). Diabetes mellitus is one of the pre-eminent causes of peripheral neuropathy in western populations (whereas leprosy is for the world) but the differential is extensive and includes hereditary, nutritional, metabolic, inflammatory, and compressive etiologies. Despite the wide range of known causes, many cases of peripheral neuropathy remain idiopathic even with intensive investigation. Investigation of suspected neuropathy in the elderly can be complicated by the processes of normal aging; for instance, absence of Achilles tendon reflexes (Vrancken et al. 2006) or reduced sural nerve responses on nerve conduction studies (Esper et al. 2005) in an elderly patient are not necessarily abnormal. The elderly are more likely to experience several risk factors for the development of neuropathy, including the presence of diabetes mellitus, monoclonal gammopathy-associated disease, the regular use of pharmacologic agents (such as anti-neoplastic agents) that can precipitate neuropathy, vitamin deficiency and malnutrition. Once neuropathy is established, treatment regimens, whether immunomodulatory or symptomatic, can be complicated by the higher rate of comorbidities in elderly patients.

Pathophysiology

The pathophysiology of neuropathy is diverse, and we will discuss the putative mechanisms of common causes of neuropathy in the elderly. Before addressing these, however, it is important to discuss the changes that take place in nerve as part of the normal process of aging. A clear understanding of these changes is important so that pathology is not diagnosed where none exists, and to understand how the older population may be more vulnerable to other neuropathic stressors.

There is extensive data in the literature regarding changes on nerve conduction studies that occur with normal aging. There is evidence that nerve conduction velocities decrease with aging (Lafratta et al. 1964; Lafratta et al. 1966; Rivner et al. 2001). A study of healthy people separated by age group, 60–69, 70–79, and 80–89 years old, found a statistically significant decrease in distal tibial and sural amplitudes across decade groups even among the elderly (Falco et al. 1994). Vibratory sensation is decreased with advancing age (Martina et al. 1998). Pain, warmth and cold thresholds also increase at the foot with age (Lautenbacher et al. 1991). Low et al. (1997) performed systematic autonomic testing on normal subjects of different ages and found reduced heart rate response to deep breathing, Valsalva ratio, and sudomotor responses, with greater orthostatic blood pressure reduction with aging.

Much pathologic data of changes in nerve with age derives from animal models. Knox et al. (1989) found changes of myelin balloon formation, myelin splitting and infolding, reduplication, and remyelination in nerves of older rats. A study of posterior tibial nerve crush injury in rats of varying ages showed slower functional recovery in older animals (Belin et al. 1996). Verdu et al. (1995) crushed, sectioned, or sectioned and sutured the sciatic nerve of mice of varying ages, and measured motor and sudomotor reinnervation over time; both speed and efficacy of reinnervation was reduced in older animals. An autopsy study of human sural nerves showed a reduction in large myelinated fiber density with advanced age (Tohgi et al. 1977). Jacobs et al. (1985) showed a reduction of both myelinated and unmyelinated axon density in human sural nerve with increasing age. Reductions with age have also been found in the number of myelinated fibers in human spinal roots (Corbin et al. 1937). It is clear there is a decline in sensory perception and in electrophysiologic and pathologic markers of nerve function in healthy aging.

Inherited Neuropathies

There are many genetic syndromes of peripheral neuropathy—among the best known are HMSN (hereditary motor and sensory neuropathy) type I and II, and HSAN (hereditary sensory and autonomic neuropathy). HMSN type I is characterized primarily by demyelination, whereas HMSN type II has a primarily axonal pathology. Both subtypes show length-dependent weakness and sensory loss, usually without pain as a prominent feature. Hereditary sensory and autonomic neuropathy (HSAN), particularly HSAN type I, may present later in life, commonly with painful, burning feet (Dyck et al. 1983; Klein et al. 2005). Often, the family history in HSAN is hard to find even when it is autosomal dominant. This is due to incomplete penetrance and to the fact that it often presents later in life. Multiple gene mutations have been identified as causes for HMSN types I and II and HSAN I, and several subtypes of these classifications have been identified. Hereditary neuropathy with liability to pressure palsies can manifest as a mild peripheral neuropathy, with coexisting mononeuropathies at common sites of compression. In the elderly, history is generally revealing for this diagnosis, as it is likely the patient would have experienced episodes of compressive neuropathies over the years. However, these cases can be asymptomatic. Hereditary spastic paraparesis may also have an accompanying neuropathy, in addition to spasticity (Klein 2007). Spinocerebellar ataxias can present late in life with prominent neuropathic features, especially with large fiber sensory neuropathy (e.g. decreased vibration and proprioception) but on examination some elements of spasticity or ataxia are usually found (Manto 2005). Testing is available commercially and through research labs for the many gene abnormalities associated with neuropathy.

It is clear, however, that there is familial clustering of many neuropathy cases without a specific known genetic abnormality. It is extremely important to take a detailed family history in patients with neuropathy—not only asking whether there is a history of neuropathy or neuromuscular disease, but also directly addressing symptoms such as painful, burning feet in the family. Other clues include high arches, hammertoes, foot ulcers, or amputations (without other clearly defined etiologies). Some patients blame neuropathic pain on arthritis and "poor circulation," and have never had formal evaluation for neuropathy. Directly asking accompanying family members about symptoms or even examining them can be helpful in assessing the likelihood of hereditary neuropathy. Family history, however, should not dissuade one from a detailed neurologic evaluation, as hereditary and acquired neuropathies can coexist, and it is important to assess for treatable causes of neuropathy.

Diabetic Neuropathy

Diabetes mellitus is a common disease, and its complications increase with length of hyperglycemic exposure (Dyck et al. 2005). Diabetes mellitus is associated with a number of different types of neuropathy, with differing mechanisms that include inflammatory, ischemic, compressive, and metabolic. The most common type is diabetic sensorimotor polyneuropathy, with symmetric length-dependent distribution that is predominantly sensory, with loss of sensation, pain, and/or paresthesias. Problematic motor involvement is rare, and only about 1% of type 2 diabetic patients have severe enough neuropathy that they are unable to walk on their heels, so significant weakness on exam should prompt a search for etiologies other than diabetes mellitus. The development of diabetic sensorimotor polyneuropathy is associated with the development of other complications of diabetes, such as retinopathy and nephropathy (Dyck et al. 1993). Diabetic sensorimotor polyneuropathy is common and affects about half of patients with both type 1 and type 2 diabetes mellitus, but is only symptomatic in a small percentage of patients (Dyck et al. 1993). Nerve conduction abnormalities slowly worsen over time in diabetic patients until the diagnosis of diabetic polyneuropathy is made (Dyck et al. 2005). This type of diabetic neuropathy appears to be caused by microvascular damage, which may be the result of chronic glycemic exposure; evidence for this includes thickening of the endothelial basement membranes in nerve (Giannini et al. 1994).

Several studies have been performed to attempt to moderate the nerve damage caused by diabetes mellitus. The Diabetes Control and Complications Trial Research Group (1995) studied diabetic patients over a mean of 6.5 years, randomizing them to conventional treatment or intensive treatment with either insulin infusions or frequent insulin injections; the results were remarkable: a 64% risk reduction for confirmed clinical neuropathy and 44% risk reduction for abnormal nerve conduction studies in the intensively treated group. Other agents used to treat diabetic sensorimotor polyneuropathy include antioxidants such as alpha-lipoic acid (Ametov et al. 2003; Nagamatsu et al. 1995; Ziegler et al. 1999), with some studies suggesting efficacy and others not. Recombinant nerve growth factor, which may enhance the survival of small fiber neurons, was also tested in diabetic polyneuropathy patients, with some improvement in neuropathy impairment score in the lower limb (Apfel et al. 1998), but a larger trial (1019 patients) over 48 weeks showed no significant difference in the same parameter between treated and untreated patients (Apfel et al. 2000). The best

evidence at this time is for the benefit of tight glucose control for the prevention of diabetic sensorimotor polyneuropathy.

Mononeuropathies occur more commonly in patients with diabetes mellitus. This is especially true for carpal tunnel syndrome, which is present in a symptomatic form in 11%, and in an asymptomatic form in 22% of type 1 diabetic patients (Dyck et al. 1993). Symptomatic carpal tunnel syndrome is present in 6% and asymptomatic carpal tunnel syndrome in 29% of type 2 diabetic patients (Dyck et al. 1993). Mononeuropathies frequently occur in combination and so it is not uncommon to have a patient with both median neuropathy at the wrist (carpal tunnel syndrome) and ulnar neuropathy at the elbow (sometimes bilaterally). In fact, in patients with diabetic sensorimotor polyneuropathy who have problematic symptoms in the upper limbs, those symptoms are more likely to be secondary to mononeuropathies than to the polyneuropathy (Tracy et al. 2005).

There is growing concern about the potential role glucose impairment (defined as a two hour glucose level of 140 mg/dL to 199 mg/dL after a 75 gram oral glucose load) plays in the development of peripheral neuropathy. Singleton et al. (2001) studied 107 patients with an idiopathic symmetrical distal peripheral neuropathy; of the 72 patients who had an oral glucose tolerance test performed, 50% had impaired glucose tolerance (IGT). These patients had predominantly sensory symptoms, with pain occurring in almost all of the IGT subjects. Several other studies have found similar rates of small fiber predominant neuropathy in patients with glucose impairment (Hoffman-Snyder et al. 2006; Sumner et al. 2003). Hughes et al. (2004) studied patients with idiopathic axonal neuropathy and did not find an association between IGT and neuropathy. While there is a suggestion that IGT may be important in the development of neuropathy, further study needs to be done. In fact, with the markedly increased rates of obesity in the Western world, it is not clear that the rates of glucose impairment in the elderly patients with idiopathic small fiber neuropathy are very different from other elderly Western patients. A population-based study of patients with glucose impairment is in progress in Olmsted County, Minnesota to see if the rate of peripheral neuropathy is increased.

Diabetic lumbosacral radiculoplexus neuropathy (DLRPN), also known as diabetic amyotrophy, proximal diabetic neuropathy, and diabetic polyradiculopathy, is a potential complication of diabetes mellitus that occurs more commonly in elderly patients (average age is the mid-60s). Its mechanism is different from that of diabetic sensorimotor polyneuropathy and the population most at risk is also different. It affects approximately 1% of diabetic patients (Dyck et al. 1993). It is more common in patients with type 2 diabetes mellitus, and tends to occur in patients with better glucose control and a lower body mass index than typical community-based diabetic patients (Dyck et al. 2002). This disorder typically presents with acute to subacute onset of severe lower extremity pain, usually in the hip or thigh region, and is unilateral or asymmetric in severity (Dyck et al. 1999). It is often associated with weight loss. Pain usually starts to improve in conjunction with the development of weakness. Nerve conduction studies and electromyography are consistent with an axonal-predominant process, and CSF protein is usually elevated. Over time, this condition tends to spontaneously improve though some residual deficit is common. In Dyck et al.'s study (1999) of 33 patients with DLRPN, after prolonged follow-up three continued to require the use of a wheelchair, but 16 others required some other type of assistive device. Footdrop is usually the most refractory deficit, and most patients have marked improvement in proximal weakness and pain over time. The pathology of this disorder is inflammatory-immune, and shows ischemic injury (multifocal fiber loss, perineurial thickening, new vessel formation, and injury neuroma) that is caused by microvasculitis (small vessel destruction, inflammation, and hemosiderin-laden macrophages). Findings suggestive of microvasculitis were found in about one-half of Dyck's cases. The optimal management of this disorder is yet to be established, though immunomodulatory agents such as corticosteroids would be a logical strategy given the pathological findings. Dyck et al. (2006) carried out a prospective double-blinded placebo controlled trial of methylprednisolone, 1 gram intravenously, weekly for 12 weeks, in patients with DLRPN, and found that the treated patients had a significant improvement in pain and positive sensory symptoms; however, the primary endpoint of time to improvement in the neuropathy impairment score in the lower limbs (NIS-LL) was not statistically significant between the two groups. The lack of significant difference may be related to the protracted time between symptom onset and study entry—it is possible that had treatment been started earlier in the disease process, results may have been more favorable. Nonetheless, the reduction in pain and sensory symptoms with treatment was marked and significantly better than controls, and the practice of the authors is still to treat DLRPN with methylprednisolone unless there are contraindications.

Chronic Inflammatory Demyelinating Polyradiculoneuropathy (CIDP)

In 1958, James Austin described a patient with a relapsing polyneuropathy that was responsive to steroids, an entity that most likely represented CIDP (Austin 1958). The first large series of patients clinically described with this entity were considered to have chronic inflammatory polyradiculoneuropathy (CIP) in 1975 (Dyck et al. 1975); ultimately, after demyelination was recognized as a key feature, the name was changed to CIDP. This disorder is distinguished from acute inflammatory demyelinating polyradiculoneuropathy (AIDP, or Guillain-Barré syndrome) by its progression over a period of at least eight weeks. CIDP may present either in a relapsing form, in which there is significant resolution of symptoms/signs between episodes, or as a progressive disorder. AIDP should reach its maximal level of deficit by four weeks after onset; a group of patients with worsening greater than four weeks but less than eight weeks has been dubbed subacute inflammatory demyelinating polyradiculoneuropathy (SIDP) (Hughes et al. 1992; Oh et al. 2003). It is unclear to many investigators whether the latter entity is clinically unique, or if these patients really fall into the far ends of AIDP or CIDP.

The most easily recognized form of CIDP is a motor-predominant symmetrical syndrome with relative equality of proximal and distal weakness, and is slowly progressive or relapsing. Nerve conduction studies reveal prolonged distal latencies and F-wave latencies, reduced conduction velocities, and often show temporal dispersion and conduction block. Multiple different research criteria have been proposed for the diagnosis of CIDP (Cornblath et al. 1991; Barohn et al. 1989; AHS of AAN AIDS Task Force 1991; JTF of the EFNS and PNS 2005; Saperstein et al. 2001). Cerebrospinal fluid usually is acellular but reveals elevated protein. MRI can show hypertrophic nerve roots, though this is not an invariable finding, and may reflect duration of disease (Midroni et al. 1999). Nerve biopsies vary in their utility. Because CIDP is often a proximal and motor-predominant process, a distal sensory nerve such as the commonly biopsied sural nerve may not yield diagnostic information. This problem is compounded by the fact that most pathology laboratories do not do teased fiber preparations, and so demyelination may be missed. Thus the biopsy can be relatively normal, it may show evidence of increased inflammation (epineurial or endoneurial), or it may show frank

onion-bulbs (stacks of Schwann cell processes due to chronic demyelination and remyelination). The onion bulbs are usually in a mixed pattern which can help differentiate CIDP from a hereditary demyelinating neuropathy, which usually shows diffuse (generalized) onion-bulbs (Tracy et al. 2008). Teased fiber evaluation can be particularly useful and may show increased axonal degeneration (secondary) as well as increased rates of segmental demyelination and remyelination.

Treatment of CIDP is with immunomodulatory therapy, most commonly corticosteroids, intravenous immunoglobulin (IVIG), and/or plasma exchange (PLEX). The choice of appropriate agent should be made after careful consideration of comorbidities, side effect profile, and cost. Corticosteroids have adverse side effects which can include weight gain, hyperglycemia, osteopenia/osteoporosis, and cataract formation, and long-term immunosuppression can result in increased risk of infection, which make them less suitable for many elderly patients, particularly for long-term use. IVIG and PLEX are more expensive; among other side effects IVIG and PLEX, there is an increased risk of associated thrombotic events. However, considering the costs of side effect management, the use of IVIG and PLEX may be less expensive in the long-term for many patients. There remain questions as to relative efficacy. Dyck et al. (1982) performed a randomized controlled trial which showed efficacy of corticosteroids. A Cochrane review cited the previously mentioned trial in addition to other series as support, albeit with weak evidence-based medicine data, for the benefit of corticosteroids in CIDP (Mehndiratta et al. 2001). IVIG has proved beneficial in the management of CIDP in several studies (van Doorn et al. 1990; Hahn et al. 1996; Mendell et al. 2001; Hughes et al. 2008). A Cochrane review of IVIG in CIDP showed efficacy (van Schaik et al. 2002). Plasma exchange has been found to be beneficial in the treatment of CIDP (Dyck et al. 1986; Hahn et al. 1996); a Cochrane review of PLEX in CIDP has shown short-term benefit in approximately two-thirds of treated patients but it is noted that there is little long-term data available (Mehndiratta et al. 2008). A trial comparing the relative efficacy of IVIG and plasma exchange found no significant difference between the two treatments in neurological disability score, weakness score, or summated compound muscle action potentials (Dyck et al. 1994).

While "classic" CIDP is described above, there are many variants described in the literature which should be considered. The Lewis-Sumner syndrome, also known as multifocal CIDP, or multifocal acquired demyelinating sensory and motor neuropathy (MADSAM) can present with focal or multifocal involvement of a nerve, plexus, or even root (Lewis et al. 1982). While outwardly this syndrome may seem to resemble multifocal motor neuropathy, evidence is more convincing that it is a CIDP variant, such as the sensory involvement, frequency of elevated CSF protein, lack of GM1 antibody positivity, and the relative treatment responsiveness (Saperstein et al. 1999). Dyck et al. (2002) described six patients with lower limb mononeuropathies, which pathologically were consistent with CIDP; the authors have described these as chronic inflammatory demyelinating mononeuropathy (CIDM). Sinnreich and colleagues described an entity called chronic inflammatory sensory polyradiculopathy (CISP), in which only sensory nerve roots are affected. This syndrome presents as a sensory ataxia, with diminished or absent deep tendon reflexes. Nerve conduction studies are typically normal, but somatosensory evoked potentials often show slowing at the root level; MRI may show selective enlargement of nerve roots, and CSF protein is usually elevated. Sensory rootlet biopsies have shown loss of large myelinated fibers, scattered endoneurial inflammatory cells and onion bulb formation. The authors argue that CISP is a form of sensory CIDP. These patients have shown remarkable improvement with immunotherapy (Sinnreich et al. 2004).

Monoclonal Protein-associated Neuropathy

The finding of a monoclonal protein in a patient with peripheral neuropathy may be incidental but warrants further investigation. An abnormal monoclonal protein can be found in 3% of people over the age of 50, and in 5% of people over the age of 70 (Kyle et al. 1972), and in most cases this will represent monoclonal gammopathy of undetermined significance (MGUS). In patients with idiopathic peripheral neuropathy, approximately 10% will have a monoclonal protein in their blood (Kissel et al. 1996). There is a known entity of MGUS-associated neuropathy, but a monoclonal protein in the context of neuropathy may also represent amyloid, POEMS syndrome (polyneuropathy, organomegaly, endocrinopathy, M-spike, and skin changes), multiple myeloma, or lymphoma (including Waldenstrom's macroglobulinemia). There is a suggestion in the literature that there is a separate entity of MGUS-associated CIDP but this needs to be further defined.

MGUS-associated neuropathy has been given increased attention. In some cases, a specific antibody directed against myelin associated glycoprotein (MAG) has been identified (Braun et al. 1982). Gosselin et al. (1991) studied patients with IgM, IgG, and IgA MGUS with neuropathy, and found that IgM neuropathies had greater sensory loss, ataxia, nerve conduction abnormalities, and a greater likelihood of CMAP temporal dispersion. Furthermore, they found a higher frequency of the IgM subtype in the MGUS neuropathy patients than is found in MGUS patients without neuropathy, suggesting a particular pathogenicity of the IgM subtype. Of note, they did not find a difference in severity between patients with IgM anti-MAG versus those with an IgM that was not directed against MAG. Suarez et al. (1993) reported similar findings, with greater sensory loss, abnormal nerve conduction studies and overrepresentation of IgM monoclonal proteins in the neuropathy patients. There is also evidence that patients with the IgM subtype respond less well to immunotherapy than do patients with the IgG or IgA subtypes (Dyck et al. 1991).

There is evidence of pathogenicity of anti-MAG, and passive transfer of anti-MAG has induced demyelination in animal models (Hays et al. 1987; Tatum 1993). Gosselin et al. (1991) made the observation that motor distal latencies tended to be more prolonged in patients with IgM rather than IgG or IgA MGUS neuropathies. Katz et al. (2000) distinguished between what he considered a classic form of CIDP with primarily motor proximal and distal findings, and a distal acquired demyelinating symmetric (DADS) phenotype, with length-dependent sensory greater than motor involvement. They found that while 22% of patients with "classic" CIDP had an M-protein, almost two-thirds of those with a DADS phenotype had an IgM kappa monoclonal protein, and two-thirds of those had activity to MAG.

A pattern of demyelinating neuropathy with marked prolongation of distal latencies has been found in anti-MAG neuropathy, and this may help distinguish it from other types of demyelination polyneuropathies, both hereditary and acquired (Kaku et al. 1994), and calculation of the terminal latency index may be particularly useful in this distinction (Cocito et al. 2001; Lupu et al. 2007).

The anti-MAG phenotype is characterized by sensory predominance and sensory ataxia. Nobile-Orazio et al. (2000) analyzed long-term data on 25 patients with anti-MAG neuropathy with a mean followup of 8.5 years and found that at last followup or time of death, 44% were disabled by severe hand tremor and/or gait ataxia. It appears likely that patients with IgM related neuropathies, anti-MAG or otherwise, may

have a poorer response to immunotherapy than either CIDP or MGUS neuropathy patients (Dyck et al. 1991; Nobile-Orazio et al. 1988). One study showed a 47% response rate to immunotherapy, in most cases mild, and only 1 of 19 patients treated had a prolonged response to treatment (Nobile-Orazio et al. 2000). Management strategies are varied, and many immunomodulatory therapies have been attempted (Mariette et al. 1997; Blume et al. 1995), but results have not yielded definitive treatment algorithms (Lunn et al. 2008). Rituximab, a chimeric antibody against CD20 on B cells, has been employed with some success in these patients (Renaud et al., 2006). After treatment with rituximab, there is a rapid decrease in circulating peripheral B cells; they reappear after about six months, but are still below baseline levels at ten months (Dalakas et al. 2008). Rituximab has shown efficacy in reducing disability in anti-MAG neuropathy as well as in decreasing anti-MAG titers (Dalakas et al. 2007).

Amyloidosis is in the differential diagnosis for peripheral neuropathy with a monoclonal protein. While amyloidosis can be hereditary, associated with the deposition of abnormal proteins such as transthyretin and gelsolin, the more common cause in the elderly is primary (monoclonal protein-associated) amyloidosis. This condition is caused by overproduction of a monoclonal immunoglobulin light chain (lambda in two-thirds), and subsequent deposition in an insoluble form in tissue, causing local organ or tissue dysfunction. The kidney, heart, liver, and nerve are often significantly affected. The median age of onset is 65 years old. Symptoms usually reflect the tissue in which amyloid is deposited, and these can include congestive heart failure, nephrotic syndrome, and hepatomegaly. Systemic symptoms such as weight loss, fatigue, and malaise are common. Fifteen percent of patients with amyloidosis will develop an associated neuropathy, which is usually length-dependent with sensory (usually very painful) greater-than-motor involvement; autonomic involvement, with orthostatic hypotension and decreased sweat output, is common. Amyloid neuropathy often is found with concomitant carpal tunnel syndrome (Gertz et al. 1999).

Prognosis is guarded with amyloid neuropathy; cardiac involvement predicts a much poorer outcome, with a median survival of 4 6 months. Median survival is 30 months without cardiac involvement. Treatment strategies include autologous stem cell transplantation, which may increase survival (Dispenzieri et al. 2004), as well as melphalan and prednisone (Kyle et al. 1997).

POEMS syndrome includes dysfunction of multiple organ systems (polyneuropathy, organomegaly, endocrinopathy, monoclonal protein, and skin changes), associated with either osteosclerotic myeloma or Castleman's disease and the overproduction of a monoclonal protein. From one large study, the median age at clinical presentation is 51 years old, and the median survival is 165 months (Dispenzieri 2007). Peripheral neuropathy is the usual presenting complaint, though many of the other findings are present on initial evaluation if carefully sought. The neuropathy usually presents with length-dependent sensory symptoms, large-fiber predominant, followed by weakness, which is severe in half the cases (Dispenzieri 2007). Other findings associated with POEMS syndrome include thrombocytosis, polycythemia, papilledema, weight loss, and fatigue. In the vast majority of cases, the associated monoclonal protein is lambda subtype. In a large Mayo Clinic series, 97% of patients had bone lesion(s) detected on skeletal bone survey—nearly all sclerotic (Dispenzieri et al. 2003).

Studies of nerve conduction testing of patients with POEMS have shown more uniform conduction velocity slowing with decreased likelihood of conduction block and temporal dispersion compared with CIDP patients (Sung et al. 2002; Mauermann et al. 2008). Nerve biopsies have shown both axonal degeneration and primary demyelination (Vital et al. 2003; Koike et al., 2000), and ultrastructural studies have shown uncompacted myelin lamellae at a low percentage in many cases (Vital et al. 1994; Vital et al. 2003).

It has been observed that this syndrome is associated with elevated levels of vascular endothelial growth factor (VEGF), which may be produced by the bone lesions or enlarged lymph nodes of POEMS, and VEGF is likely causative for many of the organ-specific manifestations of the disorder (Watanabe et al. 1998; Dyck et al. 2006). High serum VEGF levels are associated with greater nerve endoneurial blood vessel numbers (Dyck et al. 2006) and abnormalities (Scarlato et al. 2005).

Treatment for POEMS syndrome depends upon the extent of disease. In a solitary plasmacytoma, irradiation is likely the best strategy. For more extensive disease, chemotherapy (Kuwabara et al. 1997) and peripheral blood stem cell transplantation should be considered. Peripheral blood stem cell transplantation has resulted in significant improvement or stabilization of disease in many patients, but the morbidity may be high (Dispenzieri et al. 2004), including an up to 50% rate of engraftment syndrome (Dispenzieri et al. 2008). There is increasing interest in the use of anti-VEGF antibodies for the treatment of POEMS syndrome, with case reports indicating efficacy (Badros et al. 2005; Dietrich et al. 2008), but concerns have been raised about the safety of rapidly decreasing VEGF levels because of ensuing blood vessel cell apoptosis and capillary leakage syndrome (Samaras et al. 2007; Straume et al. 2006), and further research needs to be performed.

Lymphoma (usually B cell) or other lymphoproliferative disorders (such as Waldenstrom's macroglobulinemia) can be associated with peripheral neuropathy. This can involve either focal invasion of a nerve(s) or can occur as a paraneoplastic (often predominantly demyelinating) diffuse symmetrical neuropathy. These entities should be considered in the context of an abnormal monoclonal protein, particularly if B symptoms exist. Data on direct lymphomatous invasion of nerve is limited. A review of 23 patients with neurolymphomatosis found that the most common presentation was brachial plexopathy (seven patients); the second most common presentation was an asymmetrical polyradiculoneuropathy (Taghavi et al. 2007). Neurolymphomatosis can occur as the initial manifestation of lymphoma or in the context of a previously known diagnosis of lymphoma. It is important to recognize the presence of neurolymphomatosis, as the treatment of the underlying lymphoma may be different in these cases. The nerve may act as a safe haven for lymphoma cells and high-dose chemotherapy with an agent such as methotrexate, which crosses the blood-nerve barrier, may be needed. If this diagnosis is strongly suspected, serious consideration should be given to a nerve biopsy—preferably a nerve affected clinically, by EMG, and by MRI abnormalities. AIDP and CIDP presentations in the context of lymphoma have also been reported (Kelly et al. 2005).

Waldenstrom's macroglobulinemia (WM) (lymphoplasmacytic lymphoma) has been associated with peripheral neuropathy; a study by Nobile-Orazio et al. (1987) of 26 patients with macroglobulinemia identified peripheral neuropathy in 46%. Other estimates are lower, in the range of 10% (Dimopoulos et al. 2000). A study of WM patients with neuropathy separated them into 2 groups—patients with a monoclonal protein reactive with myelin antigens (especially anti-MAG) and a second group with the monoclonal protein not reactive to myelin antigens. In the first group, a distal sensory predominant symmetric neuropathy was generally the first manifestation of their disease; proprioception was significantly affected, and motor dysfunction occurred later in the course. In the second group, a sensorimotor peripheral neuropathy was still the most common neuropathic presentation, but in 7 of 15 patients, these symptoms developed after the diagnosis of WM had been made (Dellagi et al. 1983). Moon et al.

(2008) reported on electrophysiological features distinguishing WM-associated neuropathy from IgM-MGUS associated neuropathy, with 72% of WM neuropathy patients showing evidence of an axonal neuropathy, and 70% of IgM-MGUS neuropathy patients showing evidence of a demyelinating neuropathy. These findings are useful in a large series but may not be able to differentiate the cause in individual cases.

Medication-related Neuropathy

Statins are commonly prescribed cholesterol-lowering drugs which act by inhibiting the enzyme HMG-CoA reductase. Initially prescribed mainly for coronary disease and hyperlipidemia, they have an additional benefit in decreasing the risk of ischemic stroke and transient ischemic attack (Collins et al. 2004). It is well-known that statins can cause a myopathy, which is generally reversible upon discontinuation of the medication (Armitage 2007). However, there is increasing recognition of a possible neuropathic effect as well. A large population-based study in the United Kingdom revealed a mildly increased incidence of idiopathic peripheral neuropathy in current statin users, but the confidence interval was wide, and the authors recommended interpretation with caution (Gaist et al. 2001). A large study in Denmark identified an odds ratio linking polyneuropathy to statin use of 3.7 (95% CI: 1.8-7.6). The authors conclude that statin use may increase the risk for developing polyneuropathy (Gaist et al. 2002). Concerns were raised about whether the underlying disease, hyperlipidemia, may itself have caused predisposition to neuropathy, and the association of neuropathy and statins remains controversial (Dyck et al. 2002).

Many other medications are associated with development of a peripheral neuropathy. Many types of chemotherapy for cancer can result in neuropathy, which is often length-dependent and painful (Windebank et al. 2008). Platinum compounds such as cisplatin can cause a sensory neuronopathy (Krarup-Hansen et al. 2007), with apoptosis of dorsal root ganglia (McDonald et al. 2005), and many patients who receive a course of cisplatin chemotherapy will develop a clinical neuropathy. A Cochrane review of agents to prevent the neurotoxic effect of platinum drugs concluded that there was insufficient data to suggest that amifostine, diethyldithiocarbamate, glutathione, Org 2766, or Vitamin E limits neurotoxicity of platinum drugs if given concurrently (Albers et al. 2007).

Taxanes (e.g. paclitaxel, docetaxel) act by inducing polymerization of microtubules, thereby causing abnormal structure and dysfunction. They are another frequently prescribed class of drugs for chemotherapy. Lipton et al. (1989) found that 16 of 61 patients in phase I trials of Taxol (paclitaxel) developed a sensory-predominant neuropathy (but only in patients receiving doses over 200 mg/m^2); electrophysiologic studies were consistent with a mixed axonal and demyelinating process. A study of 186 patients in phase I and II trials for docetaxel who received serial neurologic exams showed that 11% developed a sensorimotor peripheral neuropathy (New et al. 1996). Another study showed 20 of 41 patients receiving docetaxel developed peripheral neuropathy, usually mild and sensory, with worse outcomes with greater cumulative dose (Hilkens et al. 1996).

Other agents that cause peripheral neuropathy include the vinca alkaloids (vincristine, vinblastine). Vincristine has been shown to cause direct axonal injury in an in vitro model (Silva et al. 2006). A study of patients who developed vincristine-related neuropathy found the initial sign was reduced ankle-jerks followed by paresthesias and other sensory abnormalities, and lastly weakness; most of these findings improved markedly upon reduction or discontinuation of the medication (Casey et al. 1973).

Other drug therapies associated with peripheral neuropathy include amiodarone (Pellissier et al. 1984; Fraser et al. 1985), isoniazid (Chua et al. 1983), colchicine (Kuncl et al. 1987), and thalidomide (Chaudhry et al. 2003).

Alcohol-related Neuropathy

The diagnosis of alcohol-related neuropathy can be difficult, as many patients are unwilling to fully disclose issues of substance use and abuse. An Italian study assessing polyneuropathy and its risk factors showed a prevalence of 1.6% in screened patients with no known risk factors, but revealed a prevalence of 12.5% in patients who had a coexisting diagnosis of alcoholism (Beghi et al. 1998). A study of 296 alcoholic patients admitted for detoxification revealed that 16.2% reported symptoms of polyneuropathy; however, 48.6% of the patients had evidence of polyneuropathy based on nerve conduction studies, suggesting a more widespread problem than initially recognized in patients with severe alcoholism (Vittadini et al. 2001). Zambelis et al. (2005) performed nerve conduction studies, quantitative sensory testing, and neuropathy symptoms and neurologic disability scores on 98 alcohol-dependent patients, and diagnosed 58.2% with a peripheral neuropathy; most had large and small fiber dysfunction; neuropathy was significantly more common in men and was significantly correlated with patient age and years of alcohol abuse. The most common finding on nerve conduction studies was a reduced sural nerve conduction velocity, followed closely by a reduced amplitude sural sensory action potential. Clinically, patients with alcoholic polyneuropathy have a slowly progressive length-dependent neuropathy with more prominent small fiber than large fiber sensory symptoms; pain is common (Koike et al. 2003). An analysis of 18 male patients with alcoholic neuropathy revealed that eight had coexisting autonomic symptoms and eight had evidence of cerebellar ataxia (Koike et al. 2001). Worsened nerve conduction parameters are correlated with higher total lifetime exposure to alcohol (Monforte et al. 1995). Many authors have felt that alcoholic neuropathy is due to nutritional deficiency. Some have argued that it is due to a direct toxic effect. Koike et al. (2003) reported that sural nerve biopsies show loss of small fibers. The authors argued that in thiamine deficiency, there is more commonly large-fiber loss, and so felt that a direct toxic effect may be more likely. The ultimate cause of alcoholic neuropathy has yet to be determined.

Vitamin B12 Deficiency

Vitamin B12 deficiency is relatively common among older adults, with one study showing 13% of a community-based study of adults at least 75 years old with deficiency (Hin et al. 2006). Another study of 100 consecutive patients aged 65 years or older in a primary care office revealed that 16% of them had vitamin B12 levels 200 pg/mL or less (Yao et al. 1992). Vitamin B12 is taken in through the diet, mainly through meat, eggs, and milk. After ingestion, B12 is separated from bound proteins by the acidic gastric environment, then binds with intrinsic factor in the stomach; the vitamin B12-intrinsic factor complex which then binds to a receptor in the terminal ileum and is absorbed. Passive diffusion can lead to additional absorption of the vitamin with high dose ingestion. It serves as an important cofactor for DNA synthesis and for beta oxidation of fatty acids. Mechanisms for deficiency may include poor diet or decreased absorption due to reduced stomach pH from aging or the use of H2 blockers or proton pump inhibitors. Decreased absorption can occur in pernicious anemia, in which antibodies to parietal cells will result in decreased intrinsic factor production, and blocking antibodies further exacerbate the condition (Kumar 2007). There is a suggestion that atrophic gastritis related to *Helicobacter pylori* may result in B12 deficiency as well (Baik et al. 1999).

A small study by Geerling et al. (2000) showed significantly lower vitamin B12 levels in Crohn's disease patients within six months of their diagnosis versus matched controls. Other resective bowel surgeries, such as performed for inflammatory bowel disease, may increase the risk for vitamin B12 as well as other vitamin deficiencies.

A macrocytic anemia can be seen in vitamin B12 deficiency and can be a clue for this diagnosis. However, the absence of this finding should not dissuade one from this diagnosis. Lindenbaum et al. (1988) identified 141 patients with neuropsychiatric manifestations of vitamin B12 deficiency, and found that 34 of them had a normal hematocrit, 25 had a normal MCV, and 19 had both normal hematocrit and MCV.

The classical neurologic syndrome associated with vitamin B12 deficiency is subacute combined degeneration, with dorsal column and peripheral nerve dysfunction. Cognitive impairment is also common with vitamin B12 deficiency. Healton et al. (1991) reviewed a large cohort of patients with vitamin B12 deficiency with related neurologic disorders and found that just over 60% of these patients developed neurologic symptom onset after the age of 60; the most common initial complaint was paresthesia, usually in the feet or feet and hands. Patients frequently have sensory ataxia. In 31 of the 153 neurologic encounters documented, the neurologic examination was normal despite symptoms. The most common finding on examination was large-fiber sensory disturbance, with limb weakness only occurring in 16 of the 153 encounters. Overall, 40.5% of the neurologic syndromes were myelopathy and/or neuropathy. Eighteen of the encounters described involved "mental impairment."

Evidence of a sensorimotor axonal peripheral neuropathy is found with nerve conduction studies and electromyography, and somatosensory evoked potentials usually show abnormal central interpeak latencies (more commonly in the lower limbs) (Fine et al. 1990). Imaging studies may show abnormally increased T2 signal in the posterior columns of the spinal cord (Pittock et al. 2002; Timms et al. 1993; Ravina et al. 2000). Treatment should be initiated with vitamin B12 replacement—either oral or intramuscular depending on whether the cause of deficiency is related to intake or absorption. Many cases, replaced initially with B12 IM injection in the presence of clearly associated neurological symptoms, can then be transitioned to oral maintenance.

Thiamine Deficiency

Thiamine, or vitamin B1, is important for carbohydrate and protein metabolism. It is found in grains and meats, and many foods in the United States are fortified with thiamine. Deficiency states can occur either with decreased dietary intake or with intestinal malabsorption.

The most commonly known complications of thiamine deficiency are central, with Wernicke's encephalopathy (ataxia, confusion and ophthalmoplegia) and Korsakoff's syndrome (a syndrome of anterograde amnesia) (Sechi et al. 2007). However, peripheral manifestations can occur, which include a painful, length-dependent axonal peripheral neuropathy (with or without accompanying congestive heart failure) (Kumar 2007). Ohnishi et al. (1980) reviewed seven sural nerve biopsies of patients with thiamine deficiency in neuropathy, and found that the primary pathologic change was increased axonal degeneration on teased fibers, with a mean frequency of axonal degeneration of 37.5% of fibers evaluated.

Copper Deficiency

Copper serves as a prosthetic group in metalloenzymes, and is important for electron transfer in mitochondria; it also serves an important role in iron metabolism. Dietary sources include whole grains, cereals, nuts, and organ meats. It is absorbed in an active transport process in the stomach and small intestine; with high intake, passive transport also occurs. Causes for deficiency varyand can include deficient zinc intake as well as malabsorption after gastric bypass surgery (Kumar et al. 2004).

Kumar et al. (2004) described the clinical and electrophysiologic features of 13 patients with a copper-deficiency myelopathy; all had a sensory ataxia and lower extremity spasticity. All eight patients who had SSEPs performed demonstrated impaired central conduction. All 13 of their patients had a sensory-predominant polyneuropathy, which tended to be milder than the myelopathy. Wilson's disease was ruled out in all patients. Seven of these patients had evidence of anemia at the time of evaluation. Oral supplementation with copper prevented further progression of the neurologic syndrome with only mild improvement (Kumar et al. 2004).

MRI findings have been reported that are similar to that seen in vitamin B12-associated subacute combined degeneration, with increased T2 signal in the posterior columns of the spinal cord (Kumar et al. 2006; Goodman et al. 2006).

With the growing incidence of obesity in the population and resulting increase in bariatric surgery, it must be recognized that malabsorption of many vitamins and minerals can occur post-surgically, particularly when compliance with post-surgical vitamin and dietary supplementation is poor. Thaisetthawatkul et al. (2004) retrospectively reviewed records of 435 patients with bariatric surgery and identified 16% with evidence of peripheral neuropathy post-surgically. These authors identified three patterns of neuropathy occurring in patients after bariatric surgery: mononeuropathy, sensory predominant polyneuropathy, and radiculoplexus neuropathy. The mononeuropathies were associated with diabetes mellitus, whereas the sensory predominant polyneuropathies were associated with nutritional deficiencies (rapid weight loss, low albumin, not taking vitamin supplements, and dumping syndrome). Nerve biopsies showed an increased rate of axonal degeneration and perivascular inflammatory infiltrates. Overall, nutritional deficiencies, especially in the sensory predominant subtype, probably played a pathophysiological role.

Vasculitic Neuropathy

Vasculitic neuropathy should be differentiated into neuropathies associated with systemic vasculitic, autoimmune, or rheumatologic disorders or into isolated vasculitic neuropathies. Wegener's granulomatosis (WG), polyarteritis nodosa (PAN), Churg-Strauss syndrome (CSS), and microscopic polyangiitis (MPA) are examples of systemic vasculitic disorders which can cause neuropathies. Rheumatoid arthritis, Sjögren's syndrome, and other connective tissue disorders are rheumatologic disorders that can also have associated neuropathies. In addition, some infectious diseases (such as cytomegalovirus) can produce a vasculitic neuropathy. There are also isolated vasculitides which specifically affect nerve (further separated into necrotizing vasculitis and microvasculitis). These may or may not be associated with other disease, such as diabetes mellitus (as in the case of diabetic lumbosacral radiculoplexus neuropathy). The identification of a vasculitic neuropathy should prompt a careful search for evidence of other organ system involvement, as those complications may be life-threatening and treatable.

Classically, nerve vasculitis has been thought of as a mononeuritis multiplex with vasculitic lesions affecting individual nerves in a stepwise fashion. While that clinical presentation is very suggestive of vasculitis, it may also present as a length-dependent peripheral neuropathy.

WG is a form of systemic granulomatous vasculitis that affects small vessels (arterioles, venules, and capillaries); in addition to peripheral nerve, airways, lungs, and kidneys are commonly involved. A study of 128 patients with WG over 19 months with close evaluation found that 50% had evidence of either central or nervous system dysfunction. 24% of patients had a distal symmetrical polyneuropathy, and 19.5% developed multiple mononeuropathies (de Groot et al. 2001). A Mayo Clinic study of 324 patients with WG found that 16% had a peripheral neuropathy; in this group multiple mononeuropathies were by far the most common subtype, with distal symmetric polyneuropathy the second most common presentation (Nishino et al. 1993). There is some evidence that, in general, the peripheral neuropathy associated with WG is milder and occurs later in the disease course than in patients with either CSS or MPA (Cattaneo et al. 2007), though sometimes it can be the initial manifestation of the disease (de Groot et al. 2001).

PAN is a systemic vasculitis affecting mainly small and medium-sized arteries, with skin, kidneys, heart, and peripheral nerve as common sites of involvement. Approximately 60% of patients with PAN will develop multiple mononeuropathies (Stone 2002). CSS is a systemic vasculitis with involvement of small and medium-sized blood vessels, and asthma, eosinophilia, and peripheral neuropathy are common. Patients with CSS may present with a painful multiple mononeuropathy phenotype, which over time develops into an asymmetrical-appearing peripheral neuropathy, with significant axonal loss; nerve biopsy will often show epineurial necrotizing vasculitis (Hattori et al. 1999). MPA affects arterioles, venules, and capillaries; skin, kidney, and peripheral nerve are often affected. Patients with microscopic polyangiitis with peripheral neuropathy most commonly have multiple mononeuropathies (80%), or less often, a distal symmetric polyneuropathy pattern. The majority of cases present subacutely, with pain and/or paresthesias, typically lower-extremity predominant, with evidence of axonal loss (both by electrophysiology and pathology) and vasculitis on nerve biopsy (Sugiura et al. 2006). Hattori et al. (2002) showed that neuropathic symptoms, electrophysiologic parameters, and sural nerve biopsy findings were similar in CSS and MPA, but that there were more systemic complications and worse survival in MPA.

Peripheral neuropathy is common in rheumatologic disorders. One study of patients with rheumatoid arthritis showed that 23% of the 92 patients evaluated had a peripheral neuropathy, with the most common pattern a pure sensory neuropathy, followed by a sensorimotor peripheral neuropathy; they found that the most important independent risk factor for neuropathy in these patients was age (Albani et al. 2006). Rheumatoid arthritis-associated vasculitic neuropathy can present as multiple mononeuropathies also. In one such case that came to autopsy, Dyck et al. described the classical pathologic features of necrotizing vasculitis involving peripheral nerve. The authors reviewed 15,000 sections of L5 nerve root through lumbosacral plexus down to the peroneal and tibial nerves. They showed vasculitis occurred at all levels of the nerve but that infarcts of the nerve did not occur until the watershed zones of the nerve (mid-sciatic level) (Dyck et al. 1972).

A study of 62 patients with Sjögren's syndrome found that while 17 were felt to have a peripheral neuropathy after clinical exam, 34 (55%) had abnormalities consistent with neuropathy on nerve conduction studies, most commonly motor neuropathy, followed in frequency by sensory neuropathy, then sensorimotor neuropathy (Goransson et al. 2006). Mellgren et al. (1989) reviewed 33 cases and 11 nerve biopsies of patients with Sjögren's syndrome and found that symmetric sensorimotor peripheral neuropathy and symmetric sensory peripheral neuropathy were the most common presentations; of interest, they noted that one-fourth of patients had another type of neuropathy as well, including autonomic neuropathy, mononeuropathy, or cranial neuropathy. Biopsy findings showed primarily axonal degeneration and inflammation, with features consistent with microvasculitis in a majority of biopsies.

Even in the absence of meeting full criteria for Sjögren's syndrome, neuropathy in the context of sicca may prove to be a discrete entity from an inflammatory basis. Grant et al. (1997) identified 54 patients with both sicca complex and peripheral neuropathy; the most common patterns were sensory neuropathy and sensory polyganglionopathy. Twenty-seven of these patients had nerve biopsies, 19 of which showed abnormal degrees of inflammation; only one of these showed definite necrotizing vasculitis and another showed probable necrotizing vasculitis. It is not yet clear whether immunotherapy is beneficial in these patients.

Other important vasculitic neuropathies are those that are confined to peripheral nerve and do not have more widespread involvement of other tissues. Dyck et al. (1987) and Kissel et al. (1985) described vasculitis involving only the peripheral nerves. In Dyck's series of vasculitic neuropathy found on nerve biopsy, 20 of 65 had symptoms limited to peripheral nerve, a non-systemic vasculitic neuropathy (Dyck et al. 1987). In this group, the most common patterns of nerve involvement were multiple mononeuropathies, and asymmetric neuropathy; the authors suggest that prednisone may have been helpful in slowing the rate of progression in these patients.

Sarcoidosis

Sarcoidosis is a multi-system disorder characterized by the presence of non-caseating granulomatous inflammation. It only involves the nervous system in about 5% of cases. In cases with neurologic involvement, 50–75% will have a cranial neuropathy and 15% will have a peripheral neuropathy (Stern et al. 1985). Burns et al. (2006) studied 57 patients with peripheral nerve sarcoidosis (cases all had non-caseating granulomas found at the same time as neuropathy), and found that the most common patterns of nerve involvement were polyradiculoneuropathy (22) followed by polyneuropathy (19). Most patients presented with a sensory predominant syndrome, with positive neuropathic symptoms found in nearly all patients, some type of neuropathic pain complaint in 46, and weakness in 21. An important finding was that only a minority of patients had elevated angiotensin-converting enzyme (ACE) levels or calcium levels, so the absence of these markers should not dissuade one from the diagnosis of peripheral nerve sarcoidosis. If sarcoidosis of the nerve is considered, a thorough evaluation for more systemic evidence of sarcoidosis should be pursued, with particular attention to the presence of lung involvement. Nerve biopsy should be considered for diagnosis if a more easily biopsied lesion elsewhere is not identified. Corticosteroids are the usual treatment for sarcoidosis, and other steroid-sparing agents may also be employed (Baughman et al. 2008).

Autonomic Neuropathy

Autonomic neuropathy can occur in an isolated form, or in conjunction with other types of neuropathy. Autonomic functions include regulation of heart rate and blood pressure, maintenance of GI motility, and sweating. Symptoms of autonomic dysfunction may include lightheadedness, overheating (from decreased sweating), constipation, diarrhea, or sexual dysfunction. A concern with aging is that many commonly prescribed medications can have autonomic side effects, and careful evaluation of the patient's medication list is essential. The autonomic system can be damaged at the central or peripheral nervous system level. Neurodegenerative disorders such as multiple system atrophy and Parkinson's disease can have associated autonomic dysfunction. At a more isolated peripheral level, diabetes mellitus often causes a limited autonomic neuropathy. Some autonomic neuropathies are caused by autoimmune mechanisms (Suarez et al. 1994), and a subgroup of these is paraneoplastic. Vernino et al. (2000) studied sera from 46 patients with subacute idiopathic or paraneoplastic autonomic neuropathy and found that 41% of them had antibodies to the ganglionic acetylcholine receptor; levels were higher in more severely affected patients. Several reports indicate responsiveness of this entity to immunomodulatory therapy such as intravenous immunoglobulin (Modoni et al. 2007) and plasma exchange (Schroder et al. 2005).

Inherited neuropathies can be a frequent cause of autonomic dysfunction, and entities such as hereditary sensory and autonomic neuropathy (HSAN) should be considered, particularly if there are symptoms of painful or burning feet. The autonomic involvement of these can be as limited as reduced sweating in the feet or it can be more widespread.

Laboratory testing for autonomic dysfunction includes an autonomic reflex screen, which includes tilt-table, sudomotor evaluation, heart rate-deep breathing assessment, and Valsalva ratio. A thermoregulatory sweat test can also help diagnose an autonomic neuropathy, as well as whether it is a distal or patchy neuropathic process. Combining results from the quantitative sudomotor axonal reflex test (QSART) and the thermoregulatory sweat test can help distinguish between preganglionic (normal QSART) and postganglionic (reduced QSART) autonomic processes.

Management of an autonomic neuropathy can be symptomatic, with agents such as midodrine, fludrocortisone, and pyridostigmine for management of orthostatic hypotension, as well as behavioral strategies, such as use of compressive support hose, abdominal binders, judicious use of caffeine and avoidance of alcohol. It is important to determine if an autonomic neuropathy is part of a more widespread disorder which can be treated (such as diabetes mellitus or amyloid) or may have important prognostic significance (such as multiple system atrophy). This can usually be determined through careful history and physical examination.

Infectious Causes of Neuropathy

Herpes zoster infection, or "shingles," is caused by reactivation of varicella zoster virus in a sensory ganglion, and more commonly occurs in elderly and/or immunosuppressed individuals. It appears as a painful vesicular rash in a dermatomal distribution; pain can occur before the onset of rash. The incidence is estimated to be 214 per 100,000 person years, but increases markedly with age, with an estimated 1424 cases per 100,000 person-years in people 75 years of age or older (Donahue et al. 1995). Many patients are left with residual post-herpetic neuralgia (PHN), pain in the distribution of the skin lesions. One study showed a prevalence of 8% of PHN 30 days after the onset of zoster, and 4.5% at 60 days. However, the outcomes were worse with age; there was a 27.4-fold increased prevalence in PHN at 60 days in patients 50 years of age or older compared to those younger than 50 (Choo et al. 1997). Risk factors for development of PHN include advanced age, acute pain severity, severe rash, and time between development of rash and medical consultation (Opstelten et al. 2007).

Diagnosis is usually made on clinical grounds, with identification of the classical appearance of a zoster rash. Treatment can be initiated with antiviral medications, such as acyclovir, famciclovir, or valacyclovir. Oral steroids are often added in an attempt to reduce the risk of post-herpetic neuralgia. A trial of 40 patients over the age of 50 with herpes zoster randomized to either prednisolone or carbamazepine showed that the prednisone-treated patients developed post-herpetic neuralgia significantly less frequently (15%) than did the car-bamazepine treated patients (65%) (Keczkes et al. 1980). Other studies have failed to show an effect of steroids in the reduction of PHN (Esmann et al. 1987) (Clemmensen et al. 1984).

A varicella immunization has been made available for adults 60 years or older, and has been recommended by the Advisory Committee on Immunization Practices (ACIP) regardless of the patient's past history of varicella exposure (either chickenpox or shingles) as long as no contraindications exist (Harpaz et al. 2008).

Leprosy is the most common cause of peripheral neuropathy in the world. It is much less common in Western countries. It typically presents with multiple sensory mononeuropathies and involves cooler parts of the skin (Agarwal et al. 2005). Other infectious diseases that can cause peripheral neuropathy in the elderly include Lyme disease and HIV; the geographic location or origin of the patient as well as their social history should be considered. Hepatitis should also be considered, especially with co-existing cryoglobulinemia.

Diagnostic Evaluation

A thorough diagnostic workup is important in these patients to establish that peripheral neuropathy is indeed the correct diagnosis and to rule out other conditions that can mimic it (including local trauma, plantar fasciitis, peripheral vascular disease, degenerative disk disease, or cervical spondylosis). If the feet are most affected, and particularly when the process is asymmetric, a careful foot examination is warranted; some foot deformities may indicate an underlying arthritic process, and X-rays may help confirm this. Focal areas of pain can indicate plantar fasciitis or areas of fracture or sprain. Abnormal peripheral pulses, color change, history of exercise-induced pain, or known history of other vascular disease should prompt vascular studies. History of back trauma, back pain, shooting pain, or paresthesias down the thigh/leg should prompt careful consideration of primary back disease, and any evidence of spasticity or other upper motor neuron involvement should trigger evaluation of spinal cord disease. These are only a few of the common mimickers of peripheral nerve disease, and others should be considered in individual cases.

Routine serological studies in a patient with chronic neuropathy should include complete blood count, fasting glucose, glycosylated hemoglobin, renal, thyroid, and liver function tests, vitamin B12, methylmalonic acid, folate, and a monoclonal protein study (including immunofixation). Anti-nuclear antibodies, antibodies to extractible nuclear antigens, and rheumatoid factor should be performed in any patient with suspected underlying rheumatologic disease. Sedimentation rate can be useful but is nonspecific.

As previously noted, there remains controversy as to the role of glucose impairment in the development of peripheral neuropathy. In cases where the etiology of the neuropathy is indeterminate, a glucose tolerance test should be considered. In cases of suspected nutritional deficiency or excess, individual vitamin or mineral levels, such as copper, vitamin E, vitamin B6, and thiamine can be checked. In patients with known history of cancer or suspected cancer, serologic paraneoplastic testing can be performed. Urine heavy metal screen should be done in patients with suspected toxic neuropathy. In cases with a strong family history, genetic testing should be considered.

Nerve conduction studies and electromyography should be performed on all patients with suspected peripheral neuropathy. These studies are most helpful in patients with prominent weakness or large fiber sensory loss—these studies can be completely normal in cases of small fiber neuropathy. When available, specific testing for small fiber dysfunction can be a useful adjunct. Formal autonomic testing includes assessment of sudomotor, cardiovagal, and adrenergic function.

Using quantitative sudomotor axon reflex testing (QSART), heart rate-deep breathing, Valsalva maneuver, and tilt-table testing can help isolate involved areas of the nervous system, and can help predict which treatments can be useful. Quantitative sensory testing can discriminate between different populations of sensory fibers affected (large fiber-vibration, small fiber-cooling, and unmyelinated fiber-heat-pain). Thermoregulatory sweat testing can help isolate areas of anhidrosis and predict underlying disease (e.g. ganglionopathy versus distal small fiber neuropathy). Some neurologists have found assessment of epidermal nerve fibers using skin biopsy to be helpful in the diagnosis of peripheral neuropathy (Ebenezer et al. 2007).

Results of the preceding workup should help direct further study. In particular, presence of a monoclonal protein should result in referral to hematology, as well as consideration of bone marrow evaluation, urine monoclonal protein study, and fat aspirate for amyloid. Any abnormalities on paraneoplastic evaluation should lead to an aggressive search for malignancy.

Focal neuropathies may require a different workup. Clear compressive neuropathies, such as carpal tunnel syndrome and ulnar neuropathy at the elbow, may require only NCS/EMG, if there are no features that suggest a worrisome underlying etiology. Alternatively, focal neuropathic processes such as mononeuropathies which are not at common sites of compression, or plexopathies may warrant dedicated MRI imaging of the affected structure. High resolution (e.g. 3 Tesla) imaging across a suspected area of pathology can be useful in these cases.

Nerve biopsy can be a very helpful tool for determining the etiology of a peripheral neuropathy. However, it is an invasive test, and the risks and benefits of the procedure should be carefully weighed in each patient. It should be reserved for patients who have already had a thorough workup for neuropathy without an identified etiology. It should be limited to patients who are severely affected by their neuropathy (e.g. sensory ataxia, marked weakness) and/or to cases in which the suspected diagnosis has important treatment and prognostic implications. If the results are unlikely to affect management, it should not be performed. The choice of nerve should be carefully considered. The most common site for biopsy is the sural nerve, which provides sensation to the lateral foot. In most cases of peripheral neuropathy, this is an ideal nerve to biopsy as it is distal (and more likely to show pathology in length-dependent processes), purely sensory (will not cause motor deficit after biopsy), and easily harvested (performed under local anesthesia). This is not an ideal nerve to biopsy if the neuropathic process is proximal-predominant, upper-limb-predominant, or motor-predominant. Other commonly biopsied nerves include superficial peroneal nerve, superficial radial nerve, and greater auricular nerve, and these should be considered if the distributions they supply are more severely affected than the sural nerve distribution.

Fascicular nerve biopsies of large nerve, plexus, or root are performed under limited circumstances, such as evidence of focal mass, thickening, and/or enhancement of a limited area of nerve, in a patient with significant deficit and with high suspicion of a treatable underlying disease process, such as malignancy or vasculitis. Depending on the nerve chosen, fascicular nerve biopsies have the potential to leave residual motor deficit, and typically require general anesthesia to be performed, so careful consideration should be made of risk versus benefit for each patient (Dyck et al. 2006).

Treatments

There are two types of treatments available. First, there are treatments directed against the specific disease mechanism, and second, there are treatments directed against the patient's symptoms. We have discussed treatment strategies for each of the peripheral neuropathy subtypes described above, with targeted treatment, when possible, for the given etiology. For many patients with peripheral neuropathy, no specific treatable cause is identified and they struggle with troublesome weakness, numbness, and neuropathic pain. At present, if there is no underlying treatable mechanism of disease, there is no symptomatic pharmacologic treatment that is effective for either the weakness or numbness of an idiopathic polyneuropathy; rehabilitative services are crucial and often very effective in improving the mobility, function, and quality of life of these patients.

There are several treatments available for neuropathic pain, both behavioral and pharmacological. We emphasize with patients the importance of maintaining physical activity. Even in patients struggling with severe pain, some degree of physical exercise is often possible and desirable. Pool therapy can be helpful, as can walking and biking (often stationary biking). In patients with severe sensory loss in the feet, we tend to discourage activity with repetitive pounding of the feet, because of the risk of painless injury. Emphasis on physical exercise is critical for overall health maintenance, but weight reduction can often help improve mobility and regular stretching exercise can help prevent contractures in these patients.

When possible, over the counter pharmacologic and topical preparations should be used, in an attempt to reduce side effects and limit medication interactions in elderly patients. These medications include aspirin, acetaminophen, ibuprofen, and capsaicin cream. To avoid systemic absorption, a compounding pharmacy can be asked to prepare cream or gel preparations of a combination of agents such as amitriptyline, ketamine, and/or lidocaine, to be applied to the painful areas; lidocaine patches can also be useful if the affected area is small enough. Commonly prescribed neuropathic pain medications with a relatively mild side effect profile are gabapentin and pregabalin. Amitriptyline and nortriptyline may produce bothersome side effects in some patients, particularly because of their anticholinergic properties, but the side effect of sedation may actually be beneficial in a low bedtime dose in patients with severe nighttime pain. Duloxetine, a serotonin and norepinephrine reuptake inhibitor, is helpful for some types of neuropathic pain. Multiple other agents for neuropathic pain are available, with varying side effect profiles and interactions. Particular care should be taken to evaluate patients for evidence of renal or hepatic dysfunction before starting a medication, and some patients may benefit from a screening EKG before initiating certain medications, such as tricyclic antidepressants. Potential drug interactions should be assessed as well. Whatever medication is chosen for neuropathic pain, starting at a low dose with gradual titration is ideal in the elderly patient.

Regardless of the underlying etiology, care of the affected limb(s) is important. A serious complication of skin insensitivity due to neuropathy is local damage and ulcerations, which with poor healing, can lead to amputations. A particular risk is damage to feet from painless injuries, and patients should be cautioned to check their feet regularly, to have shoes carefully fitted, and to reduce risk of injury in their daily lives. As the symptoms progress, referral to physical medicine specialists should be considered for shoe and brace prosthetic/orthotic devices to support safe and efficient ambulation.

Future Direction

There is much information yet to be learned about etiology, manifestations, and treatment of peripheral neuropathies in the elderly. The best treatment, when possible, is prevention. Emphasis on healthful lifestyle, appropriate routine medical screening tests, and aggressive management of underlying medical conditions will be helpful in reducing the risk of developing neuropathy. Better treatments for pain control are needed to improve the quality of life of neuropathy patients.

Research continues to be done on growth factors to induce healing of nerve, but thus far, results have been mixed, and are not at a stage of clinical usefulness for our patients.

Summary

There is a greater incidence of peripheral neuropathy with advancing age, likely related to the frequency of general medical disease. Diabetes mellitus is a common cause, and the range of diabetic neuropathies is wide. Inherited neuropathy also will often present in old age, especially HSAN. Other important etiologies include medication-related, nutritional, monoclonal protein-associated, autoimmune, vasculitic, and infectious. Still others remain idiopathic. A thorough investigation—clinical, serological, and electrophysiologic—is required to assess for treatable conditions, and to determine prognosis. Management is individualized, with treatments available in some cases to address the underlying etiology, and others symptomatic. In the elderly population, risks and benefits of each intervention should be carefully weighed, and care must be taken to provide a rational management strategy given each patient's general medical health.

References

Ad hoc subcommittee of the American Academy of Neurology AIDS task force. Research criteria for the diagnosis of chronic inflammatory demyelinating polyradiculoneuropathy. *Neurology* 41: 617–618. 1991.

Agarwal A, Pandit L, Dalal M, and Shetty JP. Neurological manifestations of Hansen's disease and their management. *Clinical Neurology & Neurosurgery* 107(6): 445–454. 2005.

Albani G, Ravaglia S, Cavagna L, Caporali R, Montecucco C, and Mauro A, Clinical and electrophysiological evaluation of peripheral neuropathy in rheumatoid arthritis. *Journal of the Peripheral Nervous System* 11(2): 174–175. 2006.

Albers J, Chaudhry V, Cavaletti G, and Donehower R. Interventions for preventing neuropathy caused by cisplatin and related compounds. *Cochrane Database of Systematic Reviews.* (1): CD005228. 2007.

Ametov AS, Barinov A, Dyck PJ et al. The sensory symptoms of diabetic polyneuropathy are improved with alpha-lipoic acid. The Sydney trial. *Diabetes Care* 26(3): 770–776. 2003.

Anonymous. The effect of intensive diabetes therapy on the development and progression of neuropathy. The Diabetes Control and Complications Trial Research Group. *Annals of Internal Medicine* 122(8): 561–568. 1995.

Apfel SC, Kessler JA, Adornato BT et al. Recombinant human nerve growth factor in the treatment of diabetic polyneuropathy. *Neurology* 51(3): 695–702. 1998.

Apfel SC, Schwartz S, Adornato BT, et al. Efficacy and safety of recombinant human nerve growth factor in patients with diabetic polyneuropathy. A randomized controlled trial. *JAMA* 284: 2215–2221. 2000.

Armitage J. The safety of statins in clinical practice. *Lancet* 370: 1781–1790. 2007.

Austin JH. Recurrent polyneuropathies and their corticosteroid treatment: With five-year observations of a placebo-controlled case treated with corticotrophin, cortisone and prednisone. *Brain* 81: 157. 1958.

Badros A, Porter N, and Zimrin A. Bevacizumab therapy for POEMS syndrome. *Blood* 106(3): 1135. 2005.

Baik HW and Russell RM. Vitamin B12 deficiency in the elderly. *Annu Rev Nutr* 19: 357–377. 1999.

Baldereschi M, Inzitari M, Di Carlo A, Farchi G, Scafato E, and Inzitari D. ILSA Working Group. Epidemiology of distal symmetrical neuropathies in the Italian elderly. *Neurology* 68(18): 1460–1467. 2007.

Barohn RJ, Kissel JT, Warmolts JR, and Mendell JR. Chronic inflammatory demyelinating polyradiculoneuropathy: clinical characteristics, course, and recommendations for diagnostic criteria. *Archives of Neurology* 46(8): 878–884. 1989.

Braun PE, Frail DE, Latov N. Myelin-associated glycoprotein is the antigen for a monoclonal IgM in polyneuropathy. *Journal of Neurochemistry* 39: 1261–1265. 1982.

Baughman RP, Costabel U, and du Bois RM. Treatment of sarcoidosis. *Clinics in Chest Medicine* 29(3): 533–548. 2008.

Beghi E, Monticelli ML, and the Italian General Practitioner Study Group (IGPST). Chronic symmetric symptomatic polyneuropathy in the elderly: A field screening investigation of risk factors for polyneuropathy in two Italian communities. *Journal of Clinical Epidemiology* 51(8): 697–702. 1998.

Belin BM, Ball DJ, Langer JC, Bridge PM. Hagberg PK, and Mackinnon SE. The effect of age on peripheral motor nerve function after crush injury in the rat. *Journal of Trauma-Injury Infection & Critical Care* 40(5): 775–777. 1996.

Blume G, Pestronk A, and Goodnough LT. Anti-MAG antibody associated polyneuropathies: Improvement following immunotherapy with monthly plasma exchange and IV cyclophosphamide. *Neurology* 45: 1577–1580. 1995.

Burns TM, Dyck PJB, Aksamit AJ, and Dyck PJ. The natural history and long-term outcome of 57 limb sarcoidosis cases. *Journal of the Neurological Sciences* 244(1-2): 77–87. 2006.

Casey EB, Jelliffe AM, Le Quesne PM, and Millett YL. Vincristine neuropathy. Clinical and electrophysiological observations. *Brain* 96: 69–86. 1973.

Cattaneo L, Chierici E, Pavone L, et al. Peripheral neuropathy in Wegener's granulomatosis, Churg-Strauss syndrome and microscopic polyangiitis. *Journal of Neurology, Neurosurgery & Psychiatry* 78(10): 1119–1123. 2007.

Chaudhry V. Cornblath D, Corse A, Freimer A, Simmons-O'Brien E, and Vogelsang G. Thalidomide-induced neuropathy. *Neurology* 59: 1872–1875. 2002.

Choo PW, Galil K, Donahue JG, Walker AM, Spiegelman D, and Platt R. Risk factors for postherpetic neuralgia. *Archives of Internal Medicine* 157(11): 1217–1224. 1997.

Chua CL, Ohnishi A, Tateishi J, and Kuroiwa Y. Morphometric evaluation of degenerative and regenerative changes in isoniazid-induced neuropathy. *Acta Neuropathologica* 60(3-4): 183–193. 1983.

Clemmensen OJ and Andersen KE. ACTH versus prednisone and placebo in herpes zoster treatment. *Clinical and Experimental Dermatology* 9: 557–563. 1984.

Cocito D, Isoardo G, Ciaramitaro P, et al. Terminal latency index in polyneuropathy with IgM paraproteinemia and anti-mag antibody. *Muscle and Nerve* 24(10): 1278–1282. 2001.

http://www.cdc.gov/diabetes/pubs/pdf/ndfs_2007.pdf

Collins R, Armitage J, Parish S, Sleight P, and Peto R (Heart Protection Study Collaborative Group). Effects of cholesterol-lowering with simvastatin on stroke and other major vascular events in 20536 people with cerebrovascular disease or other high-risk conditions. *Lancet* 363(9411): 757–767. 2004.

Corbin KB and Gardner ED. Decrease in number of myelinated fibers in human spinal roots with age. *Anat Rec* 68: 63–74. 1937.

Cornblath DR, Feasby TE, Hahn AF, et al. Research criteria for diagnosis of chronic inflammatory demyelinating polyneuropathy (CIDP). *Neurology* 41: 617–618. 1991.

Dalakas MC. Inhibition of B cell functions: implications for neurology. *Neurology* 70(23): 2252–2260. 2008.

Dalakas MC, Rakocevic G, Salajegheh MK, et al. A double blind placebo controlled study of Rituximab in patients with anti-MAG antibody demyelinating polyneuropathy. *Neurology* 68(suppl):A214. 2007.

De Groot K, Schmidt DK, Arit AC, Gross WL, and Reinhold-Keller E. Standardized neurologic evaluations of 128 patients with Wegener granulomatosis. *Archives of Neurology* 58(8): 1215–1221. 2001.

Dellagi K, Dupouey P, Brouet JC, et al. Waldenstrom's macroglobulinemia and peripheral neuropathy: A clinical and immunologic study of 25 patients. *Blood* 62(2): 280–285. 1983.

Dietrich PY and Duchosal MA. Bevacizumab therapy before autologous stem-cell transplantation for POEMS syndrome. *Annals of Oncology* 19(3): 595. 2008.

Dimopoulos P, Panayiotidis LA, Moulopoulos P, Sfikakis P, and Dalakas M. Waldenstrom's macroglobulinemia: Clinical features, complications, and management. *Journal of Clinical Oncology* 18(1): 214–226. 2000.

Dispenzieri A. POEMS syndrome. *Blood Reviews* 21(6): 285–289. 2007.

Dispenzieri A and Gertz MA. Treatment options for POEMS syndrome. *Current Opinion on Pharmacotherapy* 6(6): 945–53. 2005.

Dispenzieri A, Kyle RA, Lacy MQ, et al. POEMS syndrome: Definitions and long-term outcome. *Blood* 101(7): 2496–2506. 2003.

Dispenzieri A, Lacy MQ, Hayman SR, et al. Peripheral blood stem cell transplant for POEMS syndrome is associated with high rates of engraftment syndrome. *European Journal of Haematology* 80(5): 397–406. 2008.

Dispenzieri A, Moreno-Aspitia A, Suarez GA, et al. Peripheral blood stem cell transplantation in 16 patients with POEMS syndrome, and a review of the literature. *Blood* 104: 3400–3407. 2004.

Dispenzieri A, Kyle RA, Lacy MQ, et al. Superior survival in primary systemic amyloidosis patients undergoing peripheral blood stem cell transplantation: A case-control study. *Blood* 103(10): 3960–3963. 2004.

Donahue JG, Choo PW, Manson JE, and Platt R. The incidence of herpes zoster. *Archives of Internal Medicine* 155(15): 1605–1609. 1995.

Dyck PJ, Benstead TJ, Conn DL, Stevens JC, Windebank AJ, and Low PA. Nonsystemic vasculitic neuropathy. *Brain* 110 (Pt 4): 843–853. 1987.

Dyck PJ, Conn DL, and Okazaki H. Necrotizing angiopathic neuropathy. Three-dimensional morphology of fiber degeneration related to sites of occluded vessels. *Mayo Clinic Proceedings* 47(7): 461–475. 1972.

Dyck PJ, Daube J, O'Brien P, et al. Plasma exchange in chronic inflammatory demyelinating polyradiculoneuropathy. *New England Journal of Medicine* 314(8): 461–465. 1986.

Dyck PJ, Engelstad J, and Dispenzieri A. Vascular endothelial growth factor and POEMS. *Neurology* 66(1): 10–12. 2006.

Dyck PJ, Kratz KM, Karnes JL, et al. The prevalence by staged severity of various types of diabetic neuropathy, retinopathy, and nephropathy in a population-based cohort: The Rochester Diabetic Neuropathy Study. *Neurology* 43(4): 817–824. 1993

Dyck PJ, Lais AC, Ohta M, et al. Chronic inflammatory polyradiculoneuropathy. *Mayo Clinic Proceedings* 50: 621. 1975.

Dyck PJ, Litchy WJ, Kratz KM, et al. A plasma exchange versus immune globulin infusion trial in chronic inflammatory demyelinating polyradiculoneuropathy. *Annals of Neurology* 36: 838–845. 1994.

Dyck PJ, Low PA, and Stevens JC. "Burning feet" as the only manifestation of dominantly inherited sensory neuropathy. *Mayo Clinic Proceedings* 58: 426–429. 1983.

Dyck PJ, Low PA, Windebank AJ, et al. Plasma exchange in polyneuropathy associated with monoclonal gammopathy of undetermined significance. *New England Journal of Medicine* 325: 1482–1486. 1991.

Dyck PJ, O'Brien PC, Litchy WJ et al. Monotonicity of nerve tests in diabetes. Subclinical nerve dysfunction precedes diagnosis of polyneuropathy. *Diabetes Care* 28(9): 2192–2200. 2005.

Dyck PJ, O'Brien PC, Oviatt KF, et al. Prednisone improves chronic inflammatory polyradiculoneuropathy more than no treatment. *Annals of Neurology* 11(2): 136–141. 1982.

Dyck PJB and Dyck PJ. Chronic inflammatory demyelinating mononeuropathy (CIDM): a focal form of CIDP? *Neurology* 58: A303. 2002.

Dyck PJB and Dyck PJ. Is statin use associated with polyneuropathy? *Journal Watch Neurology* Vol. 4, 10: 77–78. 2002.

Dyck PJB, Norell JE, and Dyck PJ. Microvasculitis and ischemia in diabetic lumbosacral radiculoplexus neuropathy. *Neurology* 53(9): 2113–2121. 1999.

Dyck PJB, O'Brien P, Bosch EP, et al. The multicenter, double-bind controlled trial of IV methylprednisolone in diabetic lumbosacral radiculoplexus neuropathy. *Neurology* 66(5 Suppl 2): A191.

Dyck PJB, Spinner RJ, Amrami KK, Klein CJ, Engelstd JK, and Dyck PJ. Targeted fascicular biopsy of proximal nerves with MRI abnormality usually diagnostically informative. *Annals of Neurology* 60 (Suppl 10): S14–15. 2006.

Dyck PJB and Windebank AJ. Diabetic and nondiabetic lumbosacral radiculoplexus neuropathies: new insights into pathophysiology and treatment. *Muscle & Nerve* 25(4): 477–491. 2002.

Ebenezer GJ, Hauer P, Gibbons C, McArthur JC, and Polydefkis M. Assessment of epidermal nerve fibers: a new diagnostic and predictive tool for peripheral neuropathies. *Journal of Neuropathology & Experimental Neurology* 66(12): 1059–1073. 2007.

Esmann V, Kroon S, Peterslund NA, et al. Prednisolone does not prevent post-herpetic neuralgia. *Lancet* ii:126-129. 1987.

Esper GJ, Nardin RA, Benatar M, Sax TW, Acosta JA, and Raynor EM. Sural and radial sensory responses in healthy adults: Diagnostic implications for polyneuropathy. *Muscle & Nerve* 31(5): 628–632. 2005.

Falco FJ, Hennessey WJ, Goldberg G, and Braddom RL. Standardized nerve conduction studies in the lower limb of the healthy elderly. *American Journal of Physical Medicine & Rehabilitation* 73(3): 168–174. 1994.

Fine EJ, Soria E, Paroski MW, Petryk D, and Thomasula L. The neurophysiological profile of vitamin B12 deficiency. *Muscle & Nerve* 13(2): 158–164. 1990.

Fraser AG, McQueen IN, Watt AH, and Stephens MR. Peripheral neuropathy during long-term high-dose amiodarone therapy. *Journal of Neurology, Neurosurgery & Psychiatry* 48(6): 576–578. 1985.

Gaist D, Garcia Rodriguez LA, Huerta C, Hallas J, and Sindrup SH. Are users of lipid-lowering drugs at increased risk of peripheral neuropathy? *European Journal of Clinical Pharmacology* 56(12): 831–933. 2001.

Gaist D, Jeppesen U, Andersen M, Garcia Rodriguez LA, Hallas J, and Sindrup SH. Statins and risk of polyneuropathy: A case-control study. *Neurology* 58(9): 1333–1337. 2002.

Geerling BJ, Badart-Smook A, Stockbrugger RW, and Brummer RJ. Comprehensive nutritional status in recently diagnosed patients with inflammatory bowel disease compared with population controls. *European Journal of Clinical Nutrition* 54(6): 514–521. 2000.

Gertz MA, et al. Amyloidosis. *Bailliere's Best Practice in Clinical Haematology* 18(4): 709–727. 2005.

Gertz MA, et al. Amyloidosis: Recognition, confirmation, prognosis, and therapy. *Mayo Clinic Proceedings* 74(5): 490–494. 1999.

Giannini C and Dyck PJ. Ultrastructural morphometric abnormalities of sural nerve endoneurial microvessels in diabetes mellitus. *Annals of Neurology* 36: 408–415. 1994.

Goodman BP, Chong BW, Patel AC, Fletcher GP, and Smith BE. Copper deficiency myeloneuropathy resembling B12 deficiency: Partial resolution of MR imaging findings with copper supplementation. *Ajnr: American Journal of Neuroradiology* 27(10): 2112–2114. 2006.

Goransson LG, Herigstad A, Tjensvoll A, Harboe E, Mellgren SI, and Omdal R. Peripheral neuropathy in primary Sjogren syndrome: A population-based study. *Archives of Neurology* 63(11): 1612–1615. 2006.

Gosselin S, Kyle RA, and Dyck PJ. Neuropathy associated with monoclonal gammopathies of undetermined significance. *Annals of Neurology* 30(1): 54–61. 1991.

Grant IA, Hunder GG, Homburger HA, and Dyck PJ. Peripheral neuropathy associated with sicca complex. *Neurology* 48(4): 855–862. 1997.

Hahn AF, Bolton CF, Pillay N, et al. Plasma-exchange therapy in chronic inflammatory demyelinating polyneuropathy. A double-blind, sham-controlled, cross-over study. *Brain* 119 (Pt 4): 1055–1066. 1996.

Hahn AF, Bolton CF, Zochodne D, and Feasby TE. Intravenous immunoglobulin treatment in chronic inflammatory demyelinating polyneuropathy. A double-blind, placebo-controlled, cross-over study. *Brain* 119(Pt 4): 1067–1077. 1996,

Harpaz R, Ortega-Sanchez IR, and Seward JF. Advisory Committee on Immunization Practices (ACIP) Centers for Disease Control and Prevention (CDC). Prevention of herpes zoster: Recommendations of the Advisory Committee on Immunization Practices (ACIP). *Morbidity & Mortality Weekly Report. Recommendations & Reports* 57(RR-5): 1–30. 2008.

Hattori N, Ichimura M, Nagamatsu M, et al. Clinicopathological features of Churg-Strauss syndrome-associated neuropathy. *Brain* 122 (Pt 3): 427–439. 1999.

Hattori N, Mori K, Misu K, Koike H, Ichimura M, and Sobue G. Mortality and morbidity in peripheral neuropathy associated Churg-Strauss syndrome and microscopic polyangiitis. *Journal of Rheumatology* 29(7): 1408–1414. 2002.

Hays AP, Latov N, Takatsu M, and Sherman WH. Experimental demyelination of nerve induced by serum of patients with neuropathy and an anti-MAG IgM M-protein. *Neurology* 37(2): 242–256. 1987.

Healton EB, Savage DG, Brust JCM, Garrett TJ, and Lindenbaum J. Neurologic aspects of cobalamin deficiency. *Medicine* 70(4): 229–245. 1991.

Hilkens PHE, Verweij J, Stoter G, Vecht CJ, van Putten WKJ, and can den Bent MJ. Peripheral neuropathy induced by docetaxel. *Neurology* 46(1): 104–108. 1996.

Hin H, Clarke R, Sherliker P, et al. Clinical relevance of low serum vitamin B12 concentrations in older people: The Banbury B12 study. *Age & Ageing* 35(4): 416–422. 2006.

Hoffman-Snyder C, Smith BE, Ross MA, Hernandez J, and Bosch EP. Value of the oral glucose tolerance test in the evaluation of chronic idiopathic axonal polyneuropathy. *Archives of Neurology* 63(8): 1075–1079. 2006.

Hughes RAC, Donofrio P, Bril V, et al., and on behalf of the ICE Study Group. Intravenous immune globulin (10% caprylate-chromatography purified) for the treatment of chronic inflammatory demyelinating polyradiculoneuropathy (ICE study): A randomized placebo-controlled trial. *Lancet Neurology* 7(2): 136–144. 2008.

Hughes RA, Sanders E, Hall S., et al. Subacute idiopathic demyelinating polyradiculoneuropathy. *Archives of Neurology* 49: 612. 1992.

Hughes RA, Umapathi T, Gray IA, et al. A controlled investigation of the cause of chronic idiopathic axonal polyneuropathy. *Brain* 127: 1723–1730. 2004.

Jacobs JM and Love S. Qualitative and quantitative morphology of human sural nerve at different ages. *Brain* 108 (Pt 4): 897–924. 1985.

Joint task force of the EFNS and PNS. European Federation of Neurological Societies/Peripheral Nerve Society guideline on management of chronic inflammatory demyelinating polyradiculoneuropathy. *Journal of the Peripheral Nervous System* 10: 220–228. 2005.

Kaku DA, England JD, and Sumner AJ. Distal accentuation of conduction slowing in polyneuropathy associated with antibodies to myelin-associated glycoprotein and sulphated glucuronyl paragloboside. *Brain* 117(5): 941–947. 1994.

Katz JS, Saperstein DS, Gronseth G, Amato AA, and Barohn RJ. Distal acquired demyelinating symmetric neuropathy. *Neurology* 54(3): 615–620. 2000.

Keczkes K and Basheer AM. Do corticosteroids prevent post-herpetic neuralgia? *British Journal of Dermatology* 102(5): 551–555. 1980.

Kelly JJ and Karcher DS. Lymphoma and peripheral neuropathy: A clinical review. *Muscle & Nerve* 31(3): 301–313. 2005.

Kissel JT and Mendell JR. Neuropathies associated with monoclonal gammopathies. *Neuromuscular Disorders* 6(1): 3–18. 1996.

Kissel JT, Slivka AP, Warmolts JR, and Mendell JR. The clinical spectrum of necrotizing angiopathy of the peripheral nervous system. *Annals of Neurology* 18: 251–257. 1985.

Klein CJ. The inherited neuropathies. *Neurologic Clinics* 25(1): 173–208. 2007.

Klein CJ and Dyck PJ. HSANs: Clinical features, pathologic classifications, and molecular genetics. In Dyck PJ, Thomas PK (eds.) *Peripheral neuropathy, 4th edition.* Philadelphia: Elsevier Saunders. 2005.

Knox CA, Kokmen E, and Dyck PJ. Morphometric alteration of rat myelinated fibers with aging. *Journal of Neuropathology and Experimental Neurology* 48(2): 119–139. 1989.

Koike H, Iijima M, Sugiura M, et al. Alcoholic neuropathy is clinicopathologically distinct from thiamine-deficiency neuropathy. *Annals of Neurology* 54: 19–29. 2003.

Koike H, Mori K, Misu K, Hattori N, Ito H, Hirayama M, and Sobue G. Painful alcoholic polyneuropathy with predominant small-fiber loss and normal thiamine status. *Neurology* 56(12): 1727–1732. 2001.

Koike H and Sobue G. Crow-Fukase syndrome. *Neuropathology* 20: S69–S72. 2000.

Krarup-Hansen A, Helweg-Larsen S, Schmalbruch H, Rorth M, and Krarup C. Neuronal involvement in cisplatin neuropathy: Prospective clinical and neurophysiological studies. *Brain* 130(Pt4): 1076–1088. 2007.

Kumar N. Nutritional neuropathies. *Neurologic Clinics* 25: 209–255. 2007.

Kumar N, Ahlskog JE, and Gross JB Jr. Acquired hypocupremia after gastric surgery. *Clinical Gastroenterology & Hepatology* 2(12): 1074–1079. 2004.

Kumar N, Ahlskog JE, Klein CJ, and Port JD. Imaging features of copper deficiency myelopathy: A study of 25 cases. *Neuroradiology* 48(2): 78–83. 2006.

Kumar N, Gross JB Jr, and Ahlskog JE. Copper deficiency myelopathy produces a clinical picture like subacute combined degeneration. *Neurology* 63(1): 33–39. 2004.

Kuncl RW, Duncan G, Watson D, Alderson K, Rogawski MA, and Peper M. Colchicine myopathy and neuropathy. *New England Journal of Medicine* 316(25): 1562–1568. 1987

Kyle RA, Finkelstein S, Elveback LR, and Kurland LT. Incidence of monoclonal proteins in a Minnesota community with a cluster of multiple myeloma. *Blood* 40:719–724. 1972.

Kuwabara S, Hattori T, Shimoe Y, and Kamitsukasa I. Long term melphalan-prednisolone chemotherapy for POEMS syndrome. *Journal of Neurology, Neurosurgery & Psychiatry* 63(3): 385–387. 1997.

Kyle RA, et al. A trial of three regimens for primary amyloidosis: Colchicine alone, melphalan and prednisone, and melphalan, prednisone, and colchicine. *New England Journal of Medicine* 336(17): 1202–1207. 1997.

LaFratta CW and Canestrari RE. A comparison of sensory and motor nerve conduction velocities as related to age. *Archives of Physical Medicine & Rehabilitation* 47: 286–290. 1966.

LaFratta CW and Smith OH. A study of the relationship of motor nerve conduction velocity in the adult to age, sex and handedness. *Archives of Physical Medicine & Rehabilitation.* 45: 407–412. 1964.

Lautenbacher S and Strian F. Similarities in age differences in heat pain perception and thermal sensitivity. *Functional Neurology* 6(2): 129–135. 1991.

Lewis RA, Sumner AJ, Brown MJ, and Asbury AK. Multifocal demyelinating neuropathy with persistent conduction block. *Neurology* 32: 958–964. 1982

Lindenbaum J, Healton EB, Savage DG, et al. Neuropsychiatric disorders caused by cobalamin deficiency in the absence of anemia or macrocytosis. *New England Journal of Medicine* 318(26): 1720–1728. 1988.

Lipton RB, Apfel SC, Dutcher JP, et al. Taxol produces a predominantly sensory neuropathy. *Neurology* 39(3): 368–373. 1989.

Low PA, Deng JC, Opfer-Gehrking TL, Dyck PJ, O'Brien PC, and Slezak JM. Effect of age and gender on sudomotor and cardiovagal function and blood pressure response to tilt in normal subjects. *Muscle & Nerve* 20(12): 1561–1568. 1997.

Lunn MPT and Nobile-Orazio E. Immunotherapy for IgM anti-myelin-associated glycoprotein paraprotein-associated peripheral neuropathies. *The Cochrane Library* 2. 2008.

Lupu VD, Mora CA, Dambrosia J, Meer J. Dalakas M, and Floeter MK. Terminal latency index in neuropathy with antibodies against myelin-associated glycoproteins. *Muscle and Nerve* 35(2): 196–202. 2007.

Manto MU. The wide spectrum of spinocerebellar ataxias. *The Cerebellum* 4: 2–6, 2005.

Mariette X, Chastang C, Clavelou P, Louboutin JP, Leger JM, and Brouet JC. A randomized clinical trial comparing interferon-alpha and intravenous immunoglobulin in polyneuropathy associated with monoclonal IgM. The IgM-associated Polyneuropathy Study Group. *Journal of Neurology, Neurosurgery & Psychiatry* 63(1): 28–34. 1997.

Martina IS, van Koningsveld R, Schmitz PI, van der Meche FG, and can Doorn PA. Measuring vibration threshold with a graduated tuning fork in normal aging and n patients with polyneuropathy. European Inflammatory Neuropathy Cause and Treatment (INCAT) group. *Journal of Neurology, Neurosurgery & Psychiatry* 65(5): 743–747. 1998.

Mauermann ML, Suarez G, Sorenson E, Dispenzieri A, and Dyck PJB. Uniform slowing with lack of conduction block and temporal dispersion may distinguish POEMS neuropathy from CIDP. *Neurology* 70 (Supp 1): A114. 2008.

McDonald ES, Randon KR, Knight A, and Windebank AJ. Cisplatin preferentially binds to DNA in dorsal root ganglion neurons in vitro and in vivo: A potential mechanism for neurotoxicity. *Neurobiology of Disease* 18(2): 305–313. 2005.

Mehndiratta MM and Hughes RA. Corticosteroids for chronic inflammatory demyelinating polyradiculoneuropathy. *Cochrane Database of Systematic Reviews* (3): CD002062. 2001.

Mehndiratta MM, Hughes RAC, and Agarwal P. Plasma exchange for chronic inflammatory demyelinating polyradiculoneuropathy. *Cochrane Database of Systematic Reviews* (2). 2008.

Mellgren SI, Conn DL, Stevens JC, and Dyck PJ. Peripheral neuropathy in primary Sjogren's syndrome. *Neurology* 39(3): 390–394. 1989.

Mendell JR, Barohn RJ, Freimer ML, et al. Working Group on Peripheral Neuropathy. Randomized controlled trial of IVIg in untreated chronic inflammatory demyelinating polyradiculoneuropathy. *Neurology* 56(4): 445–449. 2001.

Midroni G, de Tilly LN, Gray B, and Vajsar J. MRI of the cauda equine in CIDP: Clinical correlations. *Journal of the Neurological Science* 170(1): 36–44. 1999.

Modoni A, Mirabella M, Madia F, et al. Chronic autoimmune autonomic neuropathy responsive to immunosuppressive therapy. *Neurology* 68: 161–162. 2007.

Monforte R, Estruch R, Valls-Sole J, Nicolas J, Villalta J, and Urbano-Marquez A. Autonomic and peripheral neuropathies in patients with chronic alcoholism. A dose-related toxic effect of alcohol. *Archives of Neurology* 52(1): 45–51. 1995.

Moon JS, Mauermann ML, Zeldenrust SR, Dispenzieri A, Stevens SR, and Klein CJ. Nerve conductions help distinguish the neuropathies of Waldenstrom's macroglobulinemia (WM) from IgM monoclonal gammopathy of undetermined significance (IgM-MGUS). *Annals of Neurology* 64 (Suppl 12): M22. 2008.

Nagamatsu M, Nickander KK. Schmelzer JD, et al. Lipoic acid improves nerve blood flow, reduces oxidative stress, and improves distal nerve conduction in experimental diabetic neuropathy. *Diabetes Care* 18(8): 1160–1167. 1995.

New PZ, Jackson CE, Rinaldi D, Burris H, and Barohn RJ. Peripheral neuropathy secondary to docetaxel. *Neurology* 46(1): 108–111. 1996.

Nishino H, Rubino FA, DeRemee RA, Swanson JW, and Parisi JE. Neurological involvement in Wegener's granulomatosis: An analysis of 324 consecutive patients at the Mayo Clinic. *Annals of Neurology* 33(1): 4–9. 1993

Nobile-Orazio E., Baldini L, Barbieri S, et al. Treatment of patients with neuropathy and anti-MAG IgM M-proteins. *Annals of Neurology* 24(1): 93–97. 1988.

Nobile-Orazio E, Marmiroli P, Baldini L, et al. Peripheral neuropathy in macroglobulinemia: Incidence and antigen-specificity of M proteins. *Neurology* 37(9):1506–1514, 1987.

Nobile-Orazio E., Meucci N, Baldini L, Di Troia A, and Scarlato G. Long-term prognosis of neuropathy associated with anti-MAG IgM M-proteins and its relationship to immune therapies. *Brain* 123(4): 710–717. 2000.

Oh SJ, Kurokawa K, de Almeida DF, et al. Subacute inflammatory demyelinating polyneuropathy. *Neurology* 61: 1507. 2003.

Ohnishi A, Tsuji S, Igisu H, et al. Beriberi neuropathy. Morphometric study of sural nerve. *Journal of the Neurological Sciences* 45(2-3): 177–190. 1980.

Opstelten W, Zuithoff NP, van Essen GA, et al. Predicting postherpetic neuralgia in elderly primary care patients with herpes zoster: Prospective prognostic study. *Pain* 132 Suppl1: 552–559. 2007.

Pellissier JF, Pouget J, Cros D, De Victor B, Serratrice G, and Toga M. Peripheral neuropathy induced by amiodarone chlorhydrate. A clinicopathological study. *Journal of the Neurological Sciences* 63(2): 251–266. 1984.

Pittock SJ, Payne TA, and Harper CM. Reversible myelopathy in a 34-year-old man with vitamin B12 deficiency. *Mayo Clinic Proceedings* 77: 291–294. 2002.

Ravina B, Loevner LA, and Bank W. MRI findings in subacute combined degeneration of the spinal cord: A case of reversible cervical myelopathy. *AJR: American Journal of Roentgenology* 174(3): 863–865. 2000.

Renaud S, Fuhr P, Gregor M, et al. High-dose rituximab and anti-MAG-associated polyneuropathy. *Neurology* 66(5): 742–744. 2006.

Rivner MH, Swift TR, and Malik K. Influence of age and height on nerve conduction. *Muscle & Nerve* 24(9): 1134–1141. 2001.

Samaras P, Bauer S, Stenner-Liewen F, et al. Treatment of POEMS syndrome with bevacizumab. *Haematologica* 92(10): 1438–1439. 2007.

Saperstein DS, Katz JS, Amato AA, et al. Clinical spectrum of chronic acquired demyelinating polyneuropathy. *Muscle & Nerve* 24: 311–3324. 2001.

Saperstein DS, Amato AA, Wolfe GI, et al. Multifocal acquired demyelinating sensory and motor neuropathy: the Lewis-Sumner syndrome. *Muscle & Nerve* 22(5): 560–566. 1999.

Scarlato M, Previtali SC, Carpo M, et al. Polyneuropathy in POEMS syndrome: Role of angiogenic factors in the pathogenesis. *Brain* 128: 1911–1920. 2005.

Schroeder C, Vernino S, Birkenfeld AL, et al. Plasma exchange for primary autoimmune autonomic failure. *New England Journal of Medicine* 353: 1585–1590. 2005.

Sechi G and Serra A. Wernicke's encephalopathy: New clinical settings and recent advances in diagnosis and management. *Lancet Neurology* 6(5): 442–455. 2007.

Silva A, Wang Q, Wang M, Ravula SK, and Glass JD. Evidence for direct axonal toxicity in vincristine neuropathy. *Journal of the Peripheral Nervous System* 11(3): 211–216. 2006.

Singleton JR, Smith AG, and Bromberg MB. Increased prevalence of impaired glucose tolerance in patients with painful sensory neuropathy. *Diabetes Care* 24(8): 1448–1453. 2001.

Sinnreich M, Klein CJ, Daube JR, Engelstad J, Spinner RJ, and Dyck PJB. Chronic immune sensory polyradiculopathy: A possibly treatable sensory ataxia. *Neurology* 63(9): 1662–1669. 2004.

Stern BJ, Krumholz C, Johns PS, and Nassim J. Sarcoidosis and its neurological manifestations. *Archives of Neurology* 42: 909–917. 1985.

Stone JH. Polyarteritis nodosa. *Journal of the American Medical Association* 288(13): 1632–1639. 2002.

Straume O, Bergheim J, Ernst P, Badros A, and Jaccard A. Bevacizumab therapy for POEMS syndrome. *Blood* 107: 4972–4974. 2006.

Suarez GA, Fealey RD, Camilleri M, and Low PA. Idiopathic autonomic neuropathy: Clinical, neurophysiologic, and follow-up studies on 27 patients. *Neurology* 44: 1675–1682. 1994.

Suarez GA and Kelly JJ. Polyneuropathy associated with monoclonal gammopathy of undetermined significance: Further evidence that IgM-MGUS neuropathies are different than IgG-MGUS. *Neurology* 43(7): 1304–1308. 1993.

Sugiura M, Koike H, Ijima M, et al. Clinicopathologic features of nonsystemic vasculitic neuropathy and microscopic polyangiitis-associated neuropathy: A comparative study. *Journal of the Neurological Sciences* 241(1-2): 31–37. 2006.

Sumner CJ, Sheth S, Griffin JW, Cornblath DR, and Polydefkis M. The spectrum of neuropathy in diabetes and impaired glucose tolerance. *Neurology* 60(1): 108–111. 2003.

Sung JY, Kuwabara S, Ogawara K, Kanai K, and Hattori T. Patterns of nerve conduction abnormalities in POEMS syndrome. *Muscle & Nerve* 26: 189–193. 2002.

Taghavi V, Dyck PJ, Spinner RJ, et al. Clinical and neuropathological characteristics of peripheral nerve lymphoma. *Journal of the Peripheral Nervous System* 12(suppl 1): 85. 2007.

Tatum AH. Experimental paraprotein neuropathy, demyelination by passive transfer of human IgM anti-myelin-associated glycoprotein. *Annals of Neurology* 33(5): 502–506. 1993.

Thaisetthawatkul P, Collazo-Clavell ML, Sarr MG, Norell JE, and Dyck PJ. A controlled study of peripheral neuropathy after bariatric surgery. *Neurology* 63(8): 1462–1470. 2004.

Timms SR, Cure JK, and Kurent JE. Subacute combined degeneration of the spinal cord: MR findings. *AJNR: American Journal of Neuroradiology* 14(5): 1224–1227. 1993.

Tohgi H, Tsukagoshi H, and Toyokura Y. Quantitative changes with age in normal sural nerves. *Acta Neuropathologica (Berl.)* 38: 213–220. 1977.

Tracy JA, Dyck PJ, Engelstad JK, and Dyck PJB. Pattern of onion-bulb formation preductive of inflammatory or inherited hypertrophic neuropathy. *Neurology* 70 (11 Suppl 1): A313. 2008.

Tracy JA, Dyck PJB, Harper CM, and Dyck PJ. Hand symptomatology in diabetes usually due to mononeuropathy, not polyneuropathy. *Annals of Neurology* 58 (suppl 9): S36. 2005.

Van Doorn PA, Brand A, Strengers PF, Meulstee J, and Vermeulen M. High-dose intravenous immunoglobulin treatment in chronic inflammatory demyelinating polyneuropathy: A double-blind, placebo-controlled, crossover study. *Neurology* 40: 209–212. 1990.

van Schaik IN, Winer JB, de Haan R, and Vermeulen M. Intravenous immunoglobulin for chronic inflammatory demyelinating polyradiculoneuropathy. *Cochrane Database of Systematic Reviews* Issue 2. Art. No.: CD001797. DOI: 10.1002/14651858.CD001797. 2002.

Verdu E, Buti M, and Navarro X. The effect of aging on efferent nerve fibers regeneration in mice. *Brain Research* 696(1-2): 76–82. 1995.

Vernino S, Low PA, Fealey RD, Steward JD, Rarrugia G, and Lennon VA. Autoantibodies to ganglionic acetylcholine receptors in autoimmune autonomic neuropathies. *New England Journal of Medicine* 343: 847–855. 2000.

Vital C, Gherardi R, Vital A, et al. Uncompacted myelin lamellae in poluneuropathy, organomegaly, endocrinopathy, M-protein and skin changes syndrome. Ultrastructural study of peripheral nerve biopsy from 22 patients. *Acta Neuropathologica* 87(3): 302–307. 1994.

Vital C, Vital A, Ferrer X, et al. Crow-Fukase (POEMS) syndrome: A study of peripheral nerve biopsy in five new cases. *Journal of the Peripheral Nervous System* 8: 136–144. 2003.

Vittadini G, Buonocore M, Colli G, Terzi M, Fonte R, and Biscaldi G. Alcoholic polyneuropathy: A clinical and epidemiological study. *Alcohol & Alcoholism* 36(5): 393–400.2001.

Vrancken AFJE, Kalmijn S, Brugman F, Rinkel GJE, and Notermans NC. The meaning of distal sensory loss and absent ankle reflexes in relation to age: A meta-analysis. *Journal of Neurology* 253(5): 578–589. 2006.

Watanabe O, Maruyama I, Arimura K, et al. Overproduction of vascular endothelial growth factor/vascular permeability factor is causative in Crow-Fukase (POEMS) syndrome. *Muscle & Nerve* 21: 1390–1397. 1998.

Windebank AJ and Grisold W. Chemotherapy-induced neuropathy. *Journal of the Peripheral Nervous System* 13(1): 27–46. 2008.

Yao Y, Yao SL, Yao SS, Yao G, and Lou W. Prevalence of vitamin B12 deficiency among geriatric outpatients. *Journal of Family Practice* 35(5): 524–528. 1992.

Zambelis T, Karandreas N, Tzavellas E, Kokotis P, and Liappas J. Large and small fiber neuropathy in chronic alcohol-dependent subjects. *Journal of the Peripheral Nervous System* 10: 375–381. 2005.

Ziegler D, Hanefeld M, Ruhnau KJ, et al. Treatment of symptomatic diabetic polyneuropathy with the antioxidant alpha-lipoic acid (ALADIN III study group). *Diabetes Care* 22(8): 1296–1301. 1999.xia Research Alliance. *FA beginner's primer.* http://www.curefa.org/primer.html. Accessed July 17, 2009.

7
Disease States in the Elderly

39 Stroke

Sandeep Kumar and Louis Caplan

Stroke is a leading cause of death and severe disability. It is an even greater problem in the elderly population because the incidence of stroke increases steeply with age (Marini et al. 2001). The risk of stroke almost doubles in both men and women for each successive decade after 55. As the proportion of elderly individuals increase, the morbidity and mortality of stroke is expected to rise substantially (Marini et al. 2001; Murray and Lopez 1997; Bonita R, et al. 1993). This also implies that physicians and other health care providers will increasingly be entrusted with the task of caring for very elderly stroke victims, a group that remains under investigated with regards to cerebrovascular disease and stroke. Elderly stroke patients show some important differences as compared to their younger counterparts. They are more likely to be physically frail, have more coexisting medical problems, have different risk factor profiles, and may respond differently to stroke treatment and prevention strategies. The purpose of this chapter is to familiarize the reader with fundamental aspects of stroke epidemiology, pathophysiology and risk factors, clinical presentation, and treatment options with particular emphasis on the elderly and very elderly stroke patients.

Risk Factors and Preventive Implications

There are several established risk factors for stroke. The risks posed by some of them can be influenced by appropriate medical intervention and are thus termed modifiable risk factors such as hypertension and diabetes. Other risk factors such as age and genetic make-up are considered non-modifiable risks. This section discusses the important modifiable risk factors for both ischemic and hemorrhagic strokes. Available data in the elderly stroke sub-population is also discussed in this context as is the impact of modifying these risk factors in this group of patients.

Hypertension

Hypertension is a major risk factor for both ischemic strokes and intracerebral hemorrhages. The risk of stroke increases continuously above blood pressure levels of 115/75 mmHg (WHO report 2002). The relationship between elevated blood pressure and stroke is strong and almost two-thirds of the stroke burden globally is attributed to non-optimal blood pressure (i.e. greater than 115/75 mmHg). This relationship, however, decreases with age (Lawes et al. 2004) for reasons that remain unclear. It is possible that older individuals harbor other comorbid conditions putting them at risk for additional cardiovascular complications, thereby affecting the influence of blood pressure on stroke.

It is well recognized that blood-pressure reduction is effective in preventing stroke and other vascular events (Lawes et al. 2004). However, it not established whether achieving optimal blood pressure control in patients 80 years of age or older with antihypertensive treatment is beneficial. Hypertension affects blood vessels and body organs over time. Some individuals have delayed diagnosis and treatment of elevated blood pressure. Achieving normotension during the geriatric ages may not protect them from the effects of earlier vascular damage. Treating older patients with medications can also expose them to drug-related complications. A retrospective analysis of elderly patients (80 years or older) with hypertension who were treated with antihypertensives revealed that individuals with systolic blood pressure below 140 mmHg had shorter survival after adjustment for known predictors of death (Oates et al. 2007). A meta-analysis which analyzed treatment of hypertension specifically in this age group suggested that the benefits might be offset by possible adverse effects from treatment (Gueyffier et al. 1999). However, a recently concluded trial of blood pressure control in the very elderly, which aimed to achieve blood pressure levels of 150/80 mmHg or lower, demonstrated a clear benefit of treatment in patients over 80 years of age. The study did not answer the question whether the benefit of blood pressure control was offset at particular blood pressure levels. It remains unclear whether there exists an optimal blood pressure range for this age group. The trial results, nevertheless, have important clinical relevance since high blood pressure is common especially in the very elderly and its treatment can reduce the risks of stroke and other vascular events.

Atrial Fibrillation

Atrial fibrillation (AF) is a common cardiac arrhythmia, encountered more frequently in the elderly. The prevalence of AF increases from less than 1% in patients younger than 60 years to almost 10% in patients over the age of 80 years (As et al. 2001). Both chronic and paroxysmal AF are associated with high risk of ischemic strokes, at rates which are comparable to each other (Hart et al. 2000). In general it has been estimated that AF increases the risk of stroke by four to five folds (Wolf et al. 1991). Strokes resulting from AF are usually larger and much more likely to be lethal or cause severe impairments (Lin et al. 1996). The risk of stroke from non valvular AF increases with increasing age, presence of hypertension, congestive heart failure, diabetes, and prior ischemic strokes or TIAs (Albers et al. 2001). Atrial fibrillation therefore is a very potent risk factor for disabling strokes especially in the older population.

The role of antithrombotic agents in preventing stroke from AF has been studied in a number of clinical trials. Chronic treatment with adjusted dose warfarin was found to be superior to placebo or aspirin, though aspirin was more effective than placebo in some earlier studies (AF Investigators 1994). One of the dreaded complications of treatment with warfarin is bleeding, especially intracerebral hemorrhage. The risk of bleeding is higher in the elderly population, particularly in those individuals prone to falls. The systematic review as part of the UK National Institute for Health and Clinical Excellence (NICE) management guidelines for AF identified the following patient characteristics as risk factors for anticoagulation- related bleeding complications: advanced age, uncontrolled hypertension, history of myocardial infarction or ischemic heart disease, cerebrovascular disease, anemia or a history of bleeding, and the concomitant use of other drugs such as antiplatelet drugs. There is little consensus on the factors that constitute an absolute contraindication to anticoagulation, and treatment with antithrombotics often has to be tailored depending on an individual patient's profile. However, even in the very elderly age group, the bleeding risks are dwarfed by the thromboembolic complications from AF. The Birmingham Atrial Fibrillation Treatment of the Aged Study (BAFTA) specifically addressed this issue and demonstrated that the risk of bleeding from warfarin is over-estimated in the elderly population and is comparable to that of aspirin (Mant J et al. 2007). Furthermore, the overall risk of all strokes including hemorrhages was significantly lower in the warfarin group. These results suggest that warfarin is the preferred treatment for stroke prophylaxis in the elderly unless there is a compelling contraindication to anticoagulation. Warfarin treatment should be carried out in conjunction with scrupulous monitoring of patient's INR and regulation of blood pressure.

Carotid Stenosis

Carotid arteries in the neck are common sites for atherosclerosis, especially in the elderly and constitute a major risk factor for ischemic strokes. The risk of stroke increases with increasing degrees of stenosis. However, the strongest determinant of subsequent stroke risk is the presence of symptoms attributable to the carotid lesion. The risk of an ipsilateral ischemic stroke from a carotid stenosis greater than 50% is in the range of 20–30% during the first 30 days after a TIA or minor stroke (Fairhead et al. 2005). The risk of stroke during a 30-day period in a patient with a similar degree of asymptomatic stenosis has been estimated to be around 0.2%. Additional factors that have a bearing on stroke risk include age, gender, plaque morphology, presence of asymptomatic strokes in the carotid distribution on imaging studies, presence of contralateral stenosis or occlusion. Using data from ECST (European Carotid Surgery Trial), models for predicting risk of stroke from a symptomatic carotid stenosis have been published (Rothwell 1999).

The role of carotid endareterctomy (CEA) has been analyzed in multiple large scale clinical trials for treatment of carotid stenosis. Endarterectomy has been found to be superior to medical therapy for moderate to severe carotid stenosis-producing symptoms (NASCET Collaborators 1991; ECST Collaborative Group 1998). For asymptomatic stenosis, there is no clear advantage of surgery to medical management alone. The purported advantage of surgery is offset by procedural complications unless the surgical risk is extremely low. It is also unclear whether the benefits of carotid surgery reported in these trials can be extrapolated to the elderly since patients over 80 years of age were excluded from participating. Medicare data from the 1980s show a three- to fourfold increase in morbidity and mortality in patients over the age of 75 or 80 years who underwent carotid surgery (Winslow et al. 1988; Fisher et al. 1989). However, multiple single-center series have shown that CEA can be performed in the elderly without an increase in risk (Schneider et al. 2000; O'Hara et al. 1998; Ballotta et al. 1999). Benefit from CEA increased with age in the pooled analysis of trials in patients with recently symptomatic stenosis, particularly in patients over 75 years, mainly due to their high risk of stroke while on medical treatment (Rothwell et al. 2005). In addition, a recent systematic review of all published surgical case series reported no increase in the operative risk of stroke and death in patients aged over 75 years and only a small increase in operative mortality at age >85 years (Bond et al. 2005). These data suggest that using age alone as a criterion for withholding surgical treatment is not justified. Emerging less invasive intervention techniques such as carotid angioplasty and

stenting may potentially decrease the risk of revascularization further. The recently published results from the SAPPHIRE trial, which compared endarterectomy and stenting (with emboli protection device) for carotid artery disease in patients at high surgical risk, showed that the procedural risks between the two techniques were similar (SAPPHIRE Investigators 2008). In contrast, an increased risk of complications in elderly patients was seen during the Carotid Revascularization Endarterectomy vs. Stenting Trial (CREST) lead-in phase (Hobson et al. 2004). As these techniques evolve and mature with time, a decrease in complications from these novel procedures can be anticipated.

Diabetes

Patients with diabetes are at a two- to five-fold increased risk for stroke compared with those without diabetes (Manson et al. 1991; Stamlet et al. 1993). Presence of hypertension, smoking, and atrial fibrillation further increases the stroke risk in diabetic patients. Glucose intolerance increases with age and it is not uncommon for diabetes to develop in the later years of life (Selvin et al. 2006). Older individuals with diabetes are at a significantly higher risk of developing vascular complications including stroke compared to non-diabetics. They are also as a group less likely to be adequately treated for diabetes (Selvin et al. 2006).

Patients with diabetes are usually managed with oral hypoglycemics and less frequently insulin therapy. Lifestyle modifications including weight reduction, regular exercise, blood pressure control, and correction of dyslipidemia are also a major thrust of treatment. Treatment of diabetes in older populations is complicated by coexisting medical conditions, cognitive impairment, and overall physical fragility. Older patients are also more likely to develop complications from medical treatment including hypoglycemia and a less aggressive control of hyperglycemia has been recommended to offset treatment-related complications (Nathan et al. 2006).

Cholesterol

Elevated cholesterol levels are a risk factor for vascular events though high cholesterol levels have not been significantly associated with stroke risk in epidemiological studies (Prospective Studies Collaboration 1995). On the other hand, cholesterol-lowering medicines such as statins appear to have a protective effect in decreasing risk of stroke. In a metaanalysis involving more than 90,000 patients enrolled in trials exploring effect of statins, it was reported that LDL cholesterol and not total cholesterol levels was closely related with subsequent stroke risks in patients with cerebrovascular disease (Amerenco et al. 2004). It has been assumed that statins reduce the incidence of subsequent stroke by their effect on LDL cholesterol. Statins also have a pleotropic effect on the vascular endothelium and may also be neuroprotective, increasing the brain's resistance to ischemia. Statins can also be effective in reducing stroke risks in patients with arterial plaque disease and normal cholesterol levels. The benefit of pravastatin in reducing vascular events in the elderly population was investigated in the PROSPER trial (Shephard et al. 2002). Pravastatin use was associated with a significant decrease in risk of coronary disease but no effect on stroke was found. However, a recent pooled analysis of nine trials encompassing 19,569 patients with an age range of 65 to 82 years, found significant reductions in stroke risk in this age group. Elderly stroke patients may benefit from use of cholesterol-lowering medicines such as statins. These drugs appear to be underutilized in this age group.

Smoking

Smoking is a major risk factor for both ischemic and hemorrhagic stroke (Wolf et al. 1991; Broderick et al. 2003). The risk of stroke almost doubles with smoking after adjusting for other risk factors. Exposure to environmental tobacco smoke also increases the risk of stroke substantially (Bonita et al. 1999). Smoking contributes to increased risk via its acute effects on thrombus generation and more chronic effects which promote atherosclerosis. Smoking represents the strongest fully reversible stroke risk factor; cessation of smoking immediately and rapidly decreases the risk of stroke (Burns 2003) A significant number of elderly continue to smoke, and the majority of them are long term, heavy smokers (Orleans et al. 1991). Older smokers can have significant health benefits from quitting, including improvements in circulation and pulmonary functions and decrease in risk for cardiac disease and stroke. Patients should be strongly advised to stop smoking. Patient counseling, nicotine supplements and other pharmacological therapies can be helpful; one strategy is to counsel patients about smoking cessation and offering the above adjunctive treatment at every clinical encounter.

Stroke Subtypes and Pathophysiology

Stroke is a heterogeneous disorder but can be broadly subdivided into two major categories-ischemia and hemorrhage. Ischemia causes neuronal damage by depriving brain tissues of blood supply which is a major source of oxygen, glucose, and other nutrients. Ischemia can be generalized when there is a cardiac pump failure or circulatory collapse, but is more often focal when a supplying artery is obstructed by an atheroma, thrombosis, or an embolus. Hemorrhage, on the other hand, results from leakage of blood, either from rupture of an aneurysm at the surface of the brain into the subarachnoid space or from smaller arteries or arterioles directly into the brain parenchyma.

Cerebral Ischemia

Neurons in the brain and their supporting cells are very susceptible to damage in the setting of inadequate blood supply or hypoxia. Neurological dysfunction occurs if cerebral blood flow (CBF) falls below approximately 18 to 20 mL/100 g of tissue per minute. CBF of less than 10 mL/100 g of tissue per minute can cause infarction within a few minutes (Latchaw et al. 2003). This infarcted tissue represents an area of irreversible damage and is also known as the ischemic core. The ischemic core is surrounded by functionally impaired, but structurally intact tissue known as the penumbra. Within the ischemic penumbra, a cascade of biochemical events starts with energy depletion and is followed by disruption of ion homoeostasis, release of glutamate, calcium channel dysfunction, release of free radicals, membrane disruption, inflammatory changes, and necrotic and apoptotic cell death (Dirnagl et al. 1999). The infarct core contains tissue that is unsalvageable and represents the terminal events of the ischemic cascade. The penumbra, on the other hand, is brain tissue that can potentially be salvaged from ischemic injury.

The ischemic penumbra is thus the major target for acute therapeutic interventions since its recovery is associated with neurological improvement. Newer brain imaging techniques such as brain MRI with diffusion perfusion mapping are helpful in delineating infarcted from penumbral tissue. The mismatch between the volumes of brain with reduced perfusion is shown on perfusion-weighted imaging, and the volume of brain showing cellular swelling, the ischemic core, is shown on diffusion-weighted imaging. Mismatch between large perfusion deficit seen on perfusion-weighted image (PWI) and infarct core seen on diffusion-weighted image (DWI) represents penumbral tissue which is potentially salvageable. DWI/PWI mismatch can be used to identify patients who are most likely to benefit from new interventions in acute ischemic stroke.

There are three main underlying mechanisms of cerebral ischemia—thrombosis, embolism, and hypoperfusion. Thrombosis usually occurs in larger blood vessels which are typically narrowed by atherosclerosis and can result in complete vessel occlusion and interruption of blood flow. Progressive vascular stenosis can also decrease perfusion to an arterial bed especially in setting of global hypoperfusion caused by low blood pressure or pump failure. Thrombus formed in the proximal circulation such as the heart, aorta, or major extracranial blood vessels such as the carotid or vertebral arteries can dislodge and embolize, blocking a cerebral blood vessel. Occasionally, cholesterol plaques, tumor cells, and infected material can embolize similarly and lodge itself into a cerebral artery or its branches.

Large Artery Occlusive Disease

Atherosclerosis is a generalized process that leads to progressive arterial stenosis and occlusion due to gradual build up of arterial plaque. The plaque itself serves as a nidus for adhesion and aggregation of platelet clumps leading to thrombosis. Progressive narrowing of the vessel wall causes turbulence of blood flow, further promoting plaque growth and ulceration. Thrombosis of the small residual lumen often is the culminating event which produces symptoms, although occlusion may occur without producing any symptoms (Caplan and Pessin 1988) if collateral blood flow is adequate. Recently formed blood clots are less organized and loosely attached to the arterial wall and thus more susceptible to propagate or embolize distally, causing symptoms.

Atherosclerosis usually affects the large arteries of the neck especially at the origin of the internal carotid artery (ICA) at the carotid bifurcation and the vertebral artery origin from the subclavian artery. Other frequent but less common sites for stenosis includes the carotid siphon, proximal portions of the middle cerebral artery (MCA), intracranial portions of the vertebral artery, and the basilar artery. The distribution of atherostenosis shows significant gender and racial differences. Men, especially Caucasians, have lesions that predominantly affect the origins of the ICA and vertebral arteries extracranially, while women, blacks, and people of Asian descent have predominantly intracranial disease (Caplan et al. 1986).

Cerebral Embolism of Cardiac Origin

Cardiac embolism is estimated to account for at least 30% of ischemic strokes. This is not surprising since the brain receives a large proportion of the cardiac output, putting it at risk for materials dislodged proximally from the heart or aorta (Figure 1). Certain cardiac disorders like atrial fibrillation, atrial or left ventricular thrombus, prosthetic heart valves, cardiomyopathy, valvular vegetations such as infective endocarditis, or marantic endocarditis increase the risk for recurrent embolism. Other less likely sources of embolism includes patent foramen ovale, especially when associated with an interseptal aneurysm, atrial septal defect, mitral annulus calcification, and valvular strands.

Recurrent infarction in different vascular territories is very suggestive of cardiogenic embolism. Systemic embolism also occurs but is not well recognized. Most emboli in the anterior circulation lodge in the middle cerebral artery or its branches, causing surface infarcts (Caplan et al. 1983). About 20% of the emboli go to the posterior circulation, typically causing cerebellar or posterior cerebral territory artery infarction. Thrombus is the most common embolic material (Marder et al. 2006). Its predisposition to rapid dissolution probably increases the risk of subsequent hemorrhage. While cardiac thromboemboli frequently occlude cerebral artery stems or major branches, microemboli, such as air, fat, and cholesterol crystals, may travel to smaller terminal branches and cause smaller infarcts or watershed distribution strokes.

Embolism from Aorta

Cerebral embolism from the proximal portions of the aortic arch is an important cause of ischemic strokes. Prevalence of aortic atheromatous disease correlates with overall atherosclerotic burden. Plaque thickness as assessed by transesophageal echocardiogram shows that plaques greater than 4 mm in size pose a much higher risk of stroke (Amarenco et al. 1994). Furthermore, plaques that also show evidence of ulceration, are mobile, and are greater than 4 mm in size (complex plaques) indicate unstable lesions and are associated with a higher stroke risk (Stroke Prevention in Atrial Fibrillation Investigators Committee on Echocardiography 1998). The embolic material from a complex aortic plaque is usually a thrombus but the plaque can also give rise to cholesterol crystal embolism. The latter is more likely to occur during catheterization and during surgical clamping of the aorta, leading to both cerebral and systemic embolization.

Lacunar Infarction

Lacunes are small, deep infarcts caused by degenerative changes within the small penetrating arteries to the internal capsule, basal ganglia, cerebral white matter, and pons. Lipohyalinosis is the pathological term for the arterial lesions producing lacunes, which predominantly affects the media of small arteries. Unlike atherosclerosis, lipohyalinosis is not subintimal and arterial thrombosis is not prominent. Junctional microatheroma located at the origin of the small penetrating arteries can also lead to vessel occlusion. Approximately two-thirds of the patients with lacunes have hypertension and in 32%, an association with diabetes has been reported (Mohr et al. 1982).

The relative distribution of these stroke subtypes in an elderly population has not been studied systematically. Observation from a large hospital cohort shows that older stroke patients were more likely to present with large anterior circulation infarcts compared to their younger counterparts. Lacunar infarcts appeared to be slightly less common in this age group but a large number of very elderly stroke patients were placed in the "unclassifiable stroke subtype" category possibly because fewer imaging studies were undertaken in the very elderly patients (Di Carlo et al. 1999).

Hemorrhagic Stroke

The two major categories of hemorrhagic strokes are subarachnoid hemorrhage (SAH) and intracerebral hemorrhage (ICH). The usual cause of SAH is rupture of an aneurysm or a vascular malformation

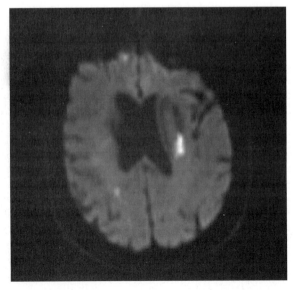

Figure 1 Diffusion weighted imaging sequences in patient with bi-hemispheric acute infarcts in different vascular territories suggestive of a proximal source of embolism.

leading to spillage of blood in the subarachnoid space. In aneurysmal SAH, the leakage of blood occurs under a higher pressure and frequently leads to increased intracranial pressure, hydrocephalus, and vasospasm. In contrast, ICH is usually caused by rupture of smaller arteries or arterioles directly into the brain parenchyma. Hypertension and amyloid angiopathy are the most common causes. Mechanical destruction and tissue displacement from an enlarging hematoma are probably the main mechanisms of cellular injury occur after an ICH. Inflammation and impairment of cerebral blood flow (CBF) around the blood clot likely contribute to delayed neuronal death.

Subarachnoid Hemorrhage

SAH accounts for 8–10% of strokes. Contrary to common perceptions, SAH is common in the elderly population (Sacco et al. 1984). The majority of patients with SAH harbor a saccular aneurysm which causes bleeding. These aneurysms form at the bifurcation of large arteries and are probably caused by a combination of congenital and degenerative changes. The most common sites for aneurysm formation are the ICA-posterior communicating artery junction, anterior cerebral artery-anterior communicating artery junction, and the bifurcation of the middle cerebral artery within the anterior circulation. Posterior circulation aneurysms are less common and involve the basilar bifurcation and the vertebral artery-posterior inferior cerebellar artery junction.

Rupture of arteriovenous malformation (AVM) can also cause bleeding in the subarchnoid space, though this more often bleeds into the brain parenchyma. Bleeding from AVMs is usually less brisk than that occurring from an aneurysm since it is under lower pressure. Presence of blood in the cerebrospinal fluid can produce vasoconstriction which can be localized or more diffuse leading to ischemia, brain edema, and infarction. The morbidity and mortality from SAH remains quite high.

Intracerebral Hemorrhage

The risk of intracerebral hemorrhage increases with age and is quite common in patients in their seventh and eight decades. The most common cause for ICH is hypertension. Hypertension causes degenerative changes in the vessels wall of the small penetrating arteries and arterioles, leading to microaneurysm formation and rupture. In a large number of patients however, acute increases in blood pressure causes rupture of these small penetrating arteries that had no prior vascular damage (Caplan 1988). Rupture of these small blood vessels exerts a sudden but local pressure effect on surrounding capillaries and arterioles, causing them in turn to break (Fisher 1971).

Amyloid angiopathy is another frequent cause of hemorrhage in the elderly. This disorder affects small arteries and arterioles in the meninges and cerebral white and gray matter. Vascular amyloid, like the amyloid plaques in Alzheimer disease (AD), is mainly composed of Aβ, a 39- to 43-amino acid proteolytic fragment of amyloid precursor protein. In milder forms, amyloid accumulates at the border of the media and adventitia of the vessel, whereas in more advanced cases there is total replacement of the smooth muscle media with amyloid accompanied by changes in vessel wall including microaneurysm formation, concentric splitting of the vessel wall, chronic inflammatory infiltrates, and fibrinoid necrosis (Vinters 1987). Most ICHs due to amyloid angiopathy are in the subcortical white matter. Hemorrhages can be multiple and are prone to recur.

Clinical Syndromes

Detailed studies of stroke syndromes in elderly and very elderly patients are currently lacking. Elderly stroke patients may present with a less than typical clinical picture and recognition of symptoms and signs of stroke can be challenging. They are more likely to be living alone or be institutionalized and there may be a delay in seeking medical attention. In addition they may have preexisting functional or cognitive impairment, which makes new signs and symptoms harder to detect. Falls, decreased mobility, lethargy, confusion, incontinence, and swallowing and speech difficulties are often the presenting symptoms that prompt hospital referral. A high index of suspicion is therefore necessary to accurately diagnose and manage these patients. Knowledge of clinical stroke syndromes can be very helpful in this regard. This section describes the major clinical syndromes seen with both ischemic and hemorrhagic strokes in the adult population.

Ischemic Strokes

Internal Carotid Artery

Almost half to three-fourths of carotid artery distribution strokes are preceded by TIAs (Mohr et al. 1981). Recognition of TIAs is therefore crucial since they serve as warning signs of an impending stroke and also provide an opportunity for timely therapeutic intervention. Internal carotid artery disease can manifest with either ocular or hemispheric symptoms.

The most common ocular symptoms include transient monocular blindness (TMB) or amaurosis fugax. Patients with TMB usually describe their visual symptoms as a shade or curtain falling from above or as a dimming, darkening, or blurring of vision. These attacks typically last between several seconds to minutes. Rarely, some patients describe a shade moving from side to side, which has been attributed to an anomalous central retinal artery branching whereby a single stem vessel supplies the superior and inferior nasal quadrants of the retina. Patients with severe bilateral carotid occlusive disease may develop visual loss after exposure to bright light. Retinal infarcts usually present with an altitudinal field cut.

Hemispheric ischemia most commonly affects the MCA distribution. The usual symptoms are numbness, weakness of the face, arm or leg, and aphasia or behavioral symptoms depending on the hemisphere affected. The arm is the most commonly affected part (Caplan and Pessin 1988). Hemispheric TIAs are often not stereotyped and vary between different episodes. The presence of both ipsilateral retinal symptoms and contralateral hemispheric symptoms is virtually diagnostic of ICA disease. Rarely, when the PCA (posterior cerebral artery) is supplied by the ICA, ICA occlusion can result in isolated PCA

territory infarctions, causing a hemianopia. Tight, unilateral ICA stenosis can also produce a perfusion insufficiency leading to watershed infarctions. Ischemia in a watershed territory causes weakness and numbness in the proximal segments of the arm and leg, sparing the face. Dominant hemispheric lesions can produce transcortical aphasias and non-dominant lesions may results in hemi-neglect. Low perfusion from a tight ICA stenosis or occlusion may also produce "limb shaking TIAs," which result in brief, involuntary, coarse, irregular wavering or trembling movements of the arm-hand alone or the hand and leg together.

Middle Cerebral Artery

MCA territory ischemia can result from embolism or local atherostenosis (Figure 2). The resulting ischemia can affect both the deep and cortical territories of the MCA, causing contralateral hemiplegia, hemianesthesia, and homonymous hemianopia. Associated behavioral disturbances include aphasia and apraxia or impaired awareness of clinical deficits. The deep lenticulostriate distribution infarcts usually produce varying degrees of hemiparesis with or without sensory abnormalities. Upper division infarcts produce contralateral hemiparesis, affecting the face and arm to a greater degree than the leg. Associated language disturbance or apraxia may occur if the dominant hemisphere is involved, or neglect with impaired awareness of deficits when the non-dominant hemisphere is involved. Isolated involvement of the inferior division produces a Wernicke's type of aphasia without any accompanying motor deficits when the non-dominant hemisphere is affected and behavioral disturbances with lesions of the non-dominant hemisphere.

Anterior Cerebral Artery

Anterior cerebral artery distribution strokes are less frequent and are usually produced by embolism. The clinical manifestations usually include contralateral hemiparesis and sensory loss predominantly affecting the leg and often sparing the hand and face. Occasionally, akinetic mutism, apraxia, amnestic syndromes and urinary incontinence may result as well.

Vertebral Artery

Vertebral artery origin is a common site for atherosclerosis. Plaque formation at the vertebral artery origin may result in development of a thrombus which can subsequently embolize to the ipsilateral vertebral or the basilar artery and its posterior cerebral artery branches (Caplan

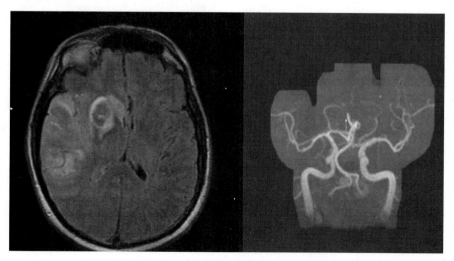

Figure 2 Large sub-acute right MCA territory infarction seen on FLAIR sequences in a patient with atrial fibrillation. Note the signal changes in the right caudate head indicative of early hemorrhagic transformation. The MRA on the right shows recanalization of the occluded R-MCA.

et al. 1992). Atherosclerosis often involves the intracranial portions of the vertebral artery. This segment of the vessel is also susceptible to trauma leading to dissection or inflammatory changes as it pierces the dura. The most common symptoms are those of lateral medullary dysfunction or cerebellar infarction. The corresponding clinical features include ipsilateral cerebellar ataxia, vertigo, nystagmus, dysphagia, dysphonia, hypoesthesia for pain and temperature sensation on the contralateral body, and Horner's syndrome. Cerebellar infarctions due to VA occlusion commonly involve the inferior and posterior regions, an area supplied by branches of the posterior inferior cerebellar arteries (PICA). Symptoms include sudden onset of vertigo, gait instability, nausea, and vomiting.

Basilar Artery

Atherostenosis most commonly affects the proximal portions of the artery but can also involve the middle and distal segments (Pessin and Caplan 1987). A wide spectrum of clinical symptoms and signs can result from basilar disease including hemiparesis, quadriparesis, limb ataxia, gaze palsies, bulbar weakness, disturbance of consciousness, as well as respiratory dysfunction. Although basilar occlusion can lead to devastating deficits, some patients show good recovery (Caplan 1979).

Lacunar Syndromes

The clinical presentation in lacunar infarction varies according to the perforating artery involved. The most common clinical presentations include pure motor hemiparesis, pure sensory stroke, and ataxic hemiparesis. Pure motor hemiparesis results from ischemia to the pons or internal capsule and results in unilateral weakness of the face, arm, and leg without sensory visual, cognitive, or behavioral abnormalities. Pure sensory stroke is usually due to infarction of the lateral thalamus or posterior limb of the internal capsule and results in numbness and parasthesias in the face, arm, trunk, and leg without any associated weakness, visual, cognitive, or behavioral abnormalities. The syndrome of ataxic hemiparesis is due to infarction in the rostral portions of the internal capsule or the pons and produces a cerebellar type incordination most marked in the upper extremity and homolateral weakness predominantly affecting the leg.

The diagnosis of lacunar infarction is based on the presence of risk factors, nature of clinical signs and symptoms, and results of neuroimaging tests. The absence of any history of hypertension or diabetes should weigh against the diagnosis of lacunar infarction. The presence of prominent headache, vomiting, or a decreased level of consciousness also makes lacunar disease unlikely. The clinical signs and symptoms should be compatible with a small, deep lesion with corresponding lesions on neuroimaging studies. A superficial infarct or a large deep infarct in the territory that would account for the symptoms excludes the diagnosis of lacunar infarction.

Hemorrhagic Stroke

Intracerebral Hemorrhage

Hypertension is the most common cause of intracerebral hemorrhage. Cerebral amyloid angiopathy (CAA), anticoagulant-related hemorrhages, and trauma are the other important causes of hemorrhage in the elderly (Kase and Caplan 1994). In most cases of ICH, the bleeding is under arteriolar or capillary pressure and not as brisk as in SAH, explaining why the symptoms evolve gradually. The first signs are focal, corresponding to the site of bleeding and as the hematoma expands substantially it leads to an increase in intracranial pressure producing headache, vomiting, and decrease in level of consciousness.

Hypertensive ICH predominantly occurs in the deep portions of the cerebral hemispheres, the putamen accounting for 35% to 50% of all cases (Kase et al. 1982; Kuntiz et al. 1984). The cerebellum, subcortical

white matter, thalamus, and pons are other common sites. Putaminal hemorrhage can cause a dense flaccid hemiplegia with hemisensory loss along with conjugate gaze palsy, aphasia, and neglect. Thalamic hemorrhages tend to produce a severe hemisensory loss with accompanying hemiparesis, gaze palsies (vertical, horizontal or pseudo-sixth), and small nonreactive pupils. Ventricular extension can cause obstructive hydrocephalus. Cerebellar hemorrhage is characterized by sudden onset of postural and gait instability, nausea, vomiting, and dizziness. Hematoma expansion can lead to brain stem compression producing facial weakness, impaired corneal reflex, or horizontal gaze palsy ipsilateral to the hemorrhage. It may also produce obstructive hydrocephalus. Pontine hemorrhages can involve the tectum or the tegmentum and can present with impaired consciousness and signs of cranial nerve and long tract involvement.

Almost 25% of intracerebral hemorrhages involve the subcortical white matter or the gray white matter junction. Lobar hemorrhages have been associated with hypertension, arteriovenous malformations, tumor, or coagulopathies. In the elderly, cerebral amyloid angiopathy is a leading cause of lobar hemorrhages. Although definite diagnosis of CAA requires pathological examination, amyloid angiopathy is likely in individuals older than 55 years of age who have multiple hemorrhages, restricted to lobar, cortical, or corticosubcortical regions, in the absence of other cause of hemorrhage.

Evidence of microhemorrhages in the cortical-subcortical junction on (Figure 3) T2*-weighted gradient-echo MR images (Tsushima et al. 2003) and extensive leukoariosis in the periventricular and subcortical white matter have been shown to be associated with recurrent lobar ICH. Clinical findings correspond to the site and location of the bleed. Smaller hemorrhages may cause focal impairments, whereas a larger bleed may result in impairment of consciousness including coma. Recurrent hemorrhages may lead to increasing disabilities and dementia.

Treatment of Acute Stroke

Early recognition of stroke symptoms is crucial for its successful management. A significant percentage of stroke patients deteriorate rapidly

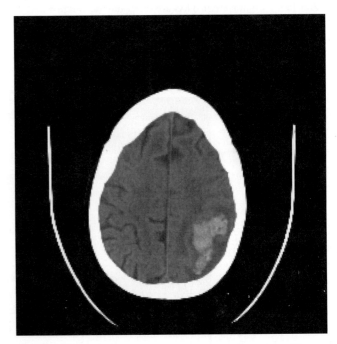

Figure 3 Acute lobar hemorrhage of the left frontal lobe in an 83-year-old man with right sided hemiparesis.

and benefits of acute ischemic therapies wane with passage of time. Concerted educational efforts directed at health care personnel in recognition of stroke symptoms have been helpful in increasing awareness about stroke and importance of prompt medical evaluation. In spite of educational efforts, the general public is still largely lacking in knowledge of stroke symptoms and medical attention is delayed in an overwhelmingly large proportion of stroke patients. It is hoped that greater emphasis on public education will be helpful in eliminating delays. Stroke recognition is a bigger problem in elderly patients because of their often solitary existence, cognitive impairment, and preexisting handicaps, making it harder to recognize emergence of new symptoms early.

Intracerebral Hemorrhage

The initial evaluation of ICH at the hospital involves assessment of the patient's presenting symptoms and associated activities at onset, time of stroke onset, age, and other risk factors. The physical examination focuses on level of consciousness and associated neurological deficits as well as evaluation of airway, breathing, circulation, and vital signs. Brain imaging is a crucial part of the emergent evaluation. Computed tomography (CT) and magnetic resonance scans are equally effective in detecting the presence of hemorrhage, estimating its size and location, and hematoma enlargement. CT may be superior at demonstrating associated ventricular extension, whereas magnetic resonance imaging (MRI) is superior at detecting underlying structural lesions and delineating the amount of perihematomal edema and herniation. Vascular imaging with CT angiography, MR angiograms, or conventional angiograms should be undertaken in hemorrhages in unusual locations such as primary intraventricular hemorrhage. Blood tests, especially prothrombin time or international normalized ratio (INR), and activated partial thromboplastin time are important to detect underlying coagulopathy.

Patients with elevated intracranial pressures (ICP) may respond to simple measures such as elevation of the head of the bed, analgesia, and sedation. More aggressive therapies to decrease elevated ICP, such as osmotic diuretics (mannitol and hypertonic saline solution), drainage of CSF via ventricular catheter, neuromuscular blockade, and hyperventilation, are sometimes warranted in select patients and often require concomitant monitoring of ICP and blood pressure with a goal to maintain CPP >70 mm Hg (Broderick et al. 2007). Patients with ICH also frequently have elevated blood pressure which requires judicious control. Trials are currently underway investigating blood pressure goals in patients with acute ICH. In the absence of any more concrete data, a mean arterial pressure range of 110 mm Hg or target blood pressure of 160/90 mm Hg has been suggested (Broderick et al. 2007). A significant number of elderly patients develop ICH on warfarin therapy. This requires rapid reversal of the coagulation defect to minimize further hematoma growth. Administration of vitamin K_1, fresh frozen plasma (FFP), prothrombin complex concentrate, or rFVIIa is usually used to correct this defect. Prothrombin complex concentrate, factor IX complex concentrate, and rFVIIa normalize the laboratory elevation of the INR very rapidly and with lower volumes of fluid than FFP but pose a greater risk of thromboembolism.

The role of hematoma evacuation by surgery was studied in the International Surgical Trial in Intracerebral Haemorrhage (STICH) trial. Eligible patients were randomized within 72 hours and operated on within 96 hours of symptom onset for a clot >2 cm in diameter. The results did not show any advantage of surgery over medical management (Mendelow et al. 2005). Routine surgical evacuation of intracerebral hematomas is therefore not indicated. Newer surgical techniques such as endoscopic aspiration, thrombolytic therapy, and aspiration of clots does show some promise but needs further testing. There is, however, general agreement that patients with cerebellar hemorrhage >3 cm who are deteriorating neurologically or who have brain stem compression and/or hydrocephalus from ventricular obstruction should have surgical removal of the hemorrhage as soon as possible.

Subarachnoid Hemorrhage

Subarachnoid hemorrhage can be a devastating event and carries a high mortality rate. Patients with depressed level of consciousness, older age and increased hematoma size have a more unfavorable prognosis. Non-contrast CT scans are very sensitive for detecting SAH especially within the first 12 hours after SAH (van der Wee et al. 1995) but thereafter its sensitivity declines with time. Lumbar puncture is necessary in those individuals who have a high clinical suspicion of SAH but have a normal scan. Most patients require additional vascular imaging with CTA or MRA, which can detect aneurysms 3–5 mm or larger. A conventional angiogram has higher resolution and detects smaller aneurysms and other vascular malformation. Patients with SAH are at a higher risk of rebleeding, increased ICP, and vasospasm causing cerebral infarcts. Systemic complications such as cardiac arrhythmias, myocardial infarction and impaired regulation of salt and blood volume are not uncommon. Patients require close monitoring of their neurological and cardiovascular status and are usually monitored in the intensive care units.

General management measures include bed rest and analgesia to diminish hemodynamic fluctuations and decrease risk of rebleeding. Blood pressure is carefully controlled, especially in patients with untreated aneurysms. Patients with SAH can develop high ICP which can compromise cerebral perfusion, and measurements of cerebral perfusion pressure (CPP) with a ventriculostomy may be required for judicious BP management. Nimodipine, a calcium channel antagonist, is used to prevent vasospasm. Following aneurysm obliteration, hyperdynamic therapy, including modest hemodilution, induced hypertension (with pressor agents such as phenylephrine or dopamine), and hypervolemia (so-called "triple-H" therapy), has been used to try to prevent vasospasm.

Treatment of cerebral aneurysm is usually done by craniotomy with clipping or by endovascular techniques using detachable platinum coils. Elderly SAH patients have been observed to have poorer outcomes (Kassell et al. 1990) and may not tolerate surgery well. However, data regarding surgical and endovascular treatment options in the elderly patients with aneurysmal SAH are scant. Some studies have shown a more favorable outcome after endovascular approaches in this patient population (Ryttlefors et al. 2008; Johansson et al. 2004).

Acute Ischemic Stroke

Accurate history, which often involves close questioning of patient's relatives and care-givers about time of stroke onset and associated activity along with a careful exam to discern clinical deficits, forms the initial part of stroke assessment. Blood tests, electrocardiogram, and radiological evaluations are performed promptly while the patient is in the emergency room. Patients usually undergo an urgent head CT scan to rule out ICH and to look for early signs of ischemia. Brain CTA or brain MRI can be very helpful in providing additional information about vascular occlusions and presence or absence of penumbral tissue which can further guide management. The initial management involves correction of any hemodynamic instability, blood glucose, and treatment of fever. High blood pressure is usually not treated in the initial 24 hours unless the SBP is greater than 220 and/or DBP is greater than 120 mmHg. High blood pressure probably augments blood flow to the penumbral tissue and rapid lowering of blood pressure has been shown to worsen outcomes. However, patients with cardiac ischemia, aortic dissection, or heart failure should have their blood pressure lowered. Similarly, candidates for thrombolytic therapy should be treated with antihypertensive and their blood pressures lowered to <185/110 mmHg (Adams et al. 2007).

Thrombolytic therapy with tPA has been found to be effective in improving functional outcomes after acute ischemic strokes (NINDS Study Group 1995; Wardlaw et al. 2003; Hacke et al. 2008). Newer methods such as catheter-based thrombolysis, mechanical thrombolysis, and clot retraction devices are currently being evaluated in the stroke population. The major complication arising from these treatments is intracerebral hemorrhage that can be fatal. The risk of hemorrhage after IV tPA in the original NINDS trial was reported to be around 6%. However, concern remains in extrapolating these figures to elderly populations since few patients over 80 years were enrolled in the thrombolytic trials. In-hospital mortality and risks for hemorrhage increase with age in tPA-treated patients (Hacke et al. 2004). However, it is also true that overall mortality and morbidity of stroke is higher in elderly stroke patients (Di Carlo et al. 1999) and these patients may derive benefit from thrombolytic and other novel stroke treatments. A recent systemic review has concluded that patients older than 80 years of age fared poorly after intravenous thrombolytic therapy as compared to individuals less than 80 (Engelter et al. 2006). However, a poorer outcome in this age group was not explained by increased rates of ICH since the incidence of bleeding was similar between the two age groups. More likely, older patients had comorbidities and preexisting functional impairments which had a greater influence on their outcomes. It is also unclear whether age-related physiological changes or changes in drug pharmacokinetics make thrombolytic therapy less effective in this age group. Further research is warranted to answer these questions. In the interim, excluding elderly patients from thrombolytic therapy on the basis of age alone is not justified. This is especially relevant since elderly stroke patients are more likely to be left with severe handicaps after a stroke.

In summary, stroke is a very common cause of disability and death in the elderly. There are many precursors to stroke which can be addressed in a preventative fashion. The early recognition of stroke symptoms and the diagnosis and tailored treatment of individual stroke syndromes is the best hope for a good outcome. The presence of many co-morbid medical conditions, and common preexisting cognitive and functional impairment cause overall mortality and morbidity of stroke to be higher in elderly stroke patients.

References

Adams HP Jr, del Zoppo G, Alberts MJ, et al. Guidelines for the early management of adults with ischemic stroke: A guideline from the American Heart Association/American Stroke Association Stroke Council, Clinical Cardiology Council, Cardiovascular Radiology and Intervention Council, and the Atherosclerotic Peripheral Vascular Disease and Quality of Care Outcomes in Research Interdisciplinary Working Groups: The American Academy of Neurology affirms the value of this guideline as an educational tool for neurologists. *Circulation* 2007; 115:e478e534.

Afilalo J, Duque G, Steele R, et al. Statins for secondary prevention in elderly patients: A hierarchical Bayesian meta-analysis. *JACC* 2008; 51: 37–45.

Albers GW, Dalen JE, Laupacis A, Manning WJ, Petersen P, and Singer DE. Antithrombotic therapy in atrial fibrillation. *Chest* 2001; 119(suppl):194S–206S.

Amarenco P, Cohen A, Tzourio C, et al. Atherosclerotic disease of the aortic arch and the risk of ischemic stroke. *N Engl J Med* 1994; 331: 1474–1479.

Amarenco P, Labreuche J, Lavalle´e P, and Touboul PJ. Statins in stroke prevention and carotid atherosclerosis systematic review and up-to-ate meta-analysis. *Stroke* 2004; 35:2902–2909.

AS Go, EM Hylek, KA Phillips, LE Henault, JV Selby and DE Singer. Prevalence of diagnosed atrial fibrillation in adults. National implications for rhythm management and stroke prevention: The AnTicoagulation and Risk Factors in Atrial Fibrillation (ATRIA) Study. *JAMA* 2001; 285: 2370–2375.

Atrial Fibrillation Investigators. Risk factors for stroke and efficacy of anti-thrombotic therapy in atrial fibrillation: Analysis of pooled data from five randomized controlled trials. *Arch Intern Med* 1994; 154: 1449–1457.

Ballotta E, Da Giau G, and Saladini M. Carotid endarterectomy in symptomatic and asymptomatic patients aged 75 years or more: Perioperative mortality and stroke risk rates. *Ann Vasc Surg* 1999; 123:158–163.

Bond R, Rerkasem K, Cuffe R, and Rowell PM. A systematic review of the associations between age and sex and the operative risks of carotid endarterectomy. *Cerebrovasc Dis* 2005; 20:69–77.

Bonita R, Duncan J, Truelsen T, Jackson RT, and Beaglehole R. Passive smoking as well as active smoking increases the risk of acute stroke. *Tob Control* 1999; 8: 156–160.

Broderick JP, Viscoli CM, Horwitz RI et al. Hemorrhagic Stroke Project Investigators. Major risk factors for aneurysmal subarachnoid hemorrhage in the young are modifiable. *Stroke* 2003; 34: 1375–1381.

Broderick J, Connolly S, Zuccarello M, et al. Guidelines for the management of spontaneous intracerebral hemorrhage in adults: 2007 update: A guideline from the American Heart Association/American Stroke Association Stroke Council, High Blood Pressure Research Council, and the Quality of Care and Outcomes in Research Interdisciplinary Working Group. *Circulation* 2007; 116:e391–e413.

Burns DM. Epidemiology of smoking-induced cardiovascular disease. *Prog Cardiovasc Dis* 2003; 46: 11–29.

Caplan LR, Hier DB, and D'Cruz I. Cerebral embolism in the Michael Reese Stroke Registry. *Stroke* 1983; 14: 530–536.

Caplan LR. Occlusion of the vertebral or basilar artery. *Stroke* 1979; 10: 277–282.

Caplan LR, Gorelick PB, and Hier DB. Race, sex, occlusive vascular disease: A review. *Stroke* 1986; 17: 648–55.

Caplan LR and Pessin MS. Symptomatic carotid artery disease and carotid endarterectomy. *Annu Rev Med* 1988; 39:273–299.

Caplan LR. Intracerebral hemorrhage revisited. *Neurology* 1988; 38: 624–627.

Caplan LR, Amerenco P, Rosengart A, et al. Embolism from vertebral artery origin occlusive disease. *Neurology* 1992; 42: 1505–1512.

Di Carlo A, Lamassa M, Pracucci G et al. Stroke in the very old: Clinical presentation and determinants of 3-month functional outcome: a European perspective. European BIOMED Study of Stroke Care Group. *Stroke* 1999; 30: 2313–9.

Dirnagl U, Iadecola C and Moskowitz MA. Pathobiology of ischaemic stroke: An integrated view. *Trends Neurosci* 1999; 22: 391–397.

Engelter ST, Bonati LH, and Lyrer PA. Intravenous thrombolysis in stroke patients of >80 versus <80 years of age—a systematic review across cohort studies. *Age and Ageing* 2006; 35: 572–580.

European Carotid Surgery Trialists Collaborative Group: Randomised trial of endarterectomy for recently symptomatic carotid stenosis: Final results of the MRC European Carotid Surgery Trial (ECST). *Lancet* 1998; 351:1379–87.

Fairhead JF, Mehta Z, and Rothwell PM: Population-based study of delays in carotid imaging and surgery and the risk of recurrent stroke. *Neurology* 2005; 65:371–5.

Fisher CM. Pathological observations in hypertensive cerebral hemorrhage. *J Neuropathol Exp Neurol* 1971; 30: 536–550.

Fisher ES, Malenka DJ, Solomon NA, et al. Risk of carotid endarterectomy in the elderly. *Am J Public Health* 1989; 79:1617–1620.

Gueyffier F, Bulpitt C, Boissel JP, et al. Antihypertensive drugs in very old people: A subgroup meta-analysis of randomized controlled trials. *Lancet* 1999; 353:793–6.

Guidelines for improving the care of the older person with diabetes mellitus. California Healthcare Foundation/American Geriatrics Society Panel on Improving #Care for Elders with Diabetes. 2003; 51(5 Suppl Guidelines):S265–80.

Gurm HS, Yadav JS, Cutlip DE; SAPPHIRE Investigators. Long-term results of carotid stenting versus endarterectomy in high-risk patients. *N Engl J Med* 2008 Apr 10; 358(15):1572–9.

Hacke W, Donnan G, Fieschi C et al. Association of outcome with early stroke treatment: pooled analysis of ATLANTIS, ECASS, and NINDS rt-PA stroke trials. *Lancet* 2004; 363: 768–74.

Hacke W, Kaste M, Toni D et al. Thrombolysis with alteplase 3 to 4.5 hours after acute ischemic stroke. *N Engl J Med* 2008 25; 359(13):1317–29.

Hart R, Pearce L, Rothbart M et al. Stroke with intermittent atrial fibrillation: Incidence and predictors during aspirin therapy. Stroke Prevention in Atrial Fibrillation Investigators. *J Am Coll Cardiol* 2000; 35: 183–187.

Hobson RW, Howard VJ, Roubin GS, et al. Carotid artery stenting is associated with increased complications in octogenarians: 30-day stroke and death rates in the CREST lead-in phase. *J Vasc Surg* 2004; 40:1006–1011.

Hughes M and Lip GY. Guideline Development Group, National Clinical Guideline for Management of Atrial Fibrillation in Primary and Secondary Care, National Institute for Health and Clinical Excellence. Stroke and thromboembolism in atrial fibrillation: A systematic review of stroke risk factors, risk stratification schema and cost effectiveness data. *Thromb Haemost* 2008; 99: 295–304.

Johansson M, Norback O, Enblad P, et al. Clinical outcome after endovascular coil embolization in elderly patients with subarachnoid hemorrhage. *Neuroradiology* 2004; 46:385–391.

Kase CS, Williams JP, and Mohr JP. Lobar intracerebral hematomas: Clinical and CT analysis in 22 cases. *Neurology* 1982; 32: 1146–1150.

Kase CS and Caplan LR. *Intracerebral hemorrhage.* Boston: Butterworth-Heinemann; 1994.

Kassell NF, Torner JC, Haley EC Jr, Jane JA, Adams HP, and Kongable GL. The International Cooperative Study on the Timing of Aneurysm Surgery. Part 1: Overall management results. *J Neurosurg* 1990; 73:18–36.

Kuntiz SC, Gross CR, Wolf PA et al. The pilot stroke data bank: Definitions, design and data. *Stroke* 1984. 15; 740–746.

Latchaw RE, Yonas H, Hademenos G et al. Guidelines and recommendations for perfusion imaging in cerebral ischemia: A scientific statement for healthcare professionals by the writing group on perfusion imaging, from the Council on Cardiovascular Radiology of the American Heart Association. *Stroke* 2003; 34: 1084–1104.

Lawes CM, Bennett DA, Feigin VL, and Rodgers A. Blood pressure and stroke: An overview of published reviews. *Stroke* 2004; 35:1024.

Lin H, Wolf PA, D'Agostino RB et al. Stroke severity in atrial fibrillation. The Framingham Study. *Stroke* 1996; 27:1760–1764.

Manson JAE, Colditz GA, Hennekens CHA, et al. A prospective study of maturity-onset diabetes mellitus and risk of coronary heart disease and stroke in women. *Arch Intern Med* 1991; 151: 1141–1147.

Mant J, Hobbs FDR, Fletcher K, et al. on behalf of the BAFTA Investigators. Warfarin versus aspirin for stroke prevention in an elderly community population with atrial fibrillation (the Birmingham Atrial Fibrillation Treatment of the Aged Study, BAFTA: A randomized controlled trial. *Lancet* 2007; 370: 493–503.

Marder V, Chute D, Starkman S et al. Analysis of thrombi retrieved from cerebral arteries of patients with acute ischemic stroke. *Stroke* 2006; 37: 2086–2093.

Marini C, Triggiani L, Cimini N, et al. Proportion of older people in the community as a predictor of increasing stroke incidence. *Neuroepidemiology* 2001; 20:91–95.

Mendelow AD, Gregson BA, Fernandes HM, et al. Early surgery versus initial conservative treatment in patients with spontaneous supratentorial intracerebral haematomas in the International Surgical Trial in Intracerebral Haemorrhage (STICH): A randomised trial. *Lancet* 2005; 365: 387–397.

Mohr JP, Caplan LR, Melski JW et al. The Harvard co operative stroke registry-a prospective registry. *Neurology* 1978; 28: 274.

Mohr JR, Kase CS, Wolf PA, Kunitz S et al. Lacunes in the NINCDS Pilot Stroke Data Bank. *Ann Neurol* 1982; 12: 84.

Nathan DM, Buse JB, Davidson MB, et al. Management of hyperglycemia in type 2 diabetes: A consensus algorithm for the initiation and adjustment of therapy: A consensus statement from the American Diabetes Association and the European Association for the Study of Diabetes. *Diabetes Care* 2006; 29:1963–1972.

NINDS—The National Institute of Neurological Disorders and Stroke rt-PA Stroke Study Group. Tissue plasminogen activator for acute ischemic stroke. *N Engl J Med* 1995; 333:1581–7.

North American Symptomatic Carotid Endarterectomy Trial Collaborators. Beneficial effect of carotid endarterectomy in symptomatic patients with high-grade carotid stenosis. *N Eng J Med* 1991; 325: 445–53.

Oates DJ, Berlowitz DR, Glickman ME, Silliman RA, and Borzecki AM. Blood pressure and survival in the oldest old. *J Am Geriatr Soc* 2007; 55:383–8.

O'Hara PJ, Hertzer NR, Mascha EJ, et al. Carotid endarterectomy in octogenarians: Early results and late outcome. *J Vasc Surg* 1998; 27:860–871.

Orleans CT, Rimer BK, Cristinzio S, Keintz MK, and Fleisher L. A national survey of older smokers: Treatment needs of a growing population. *Health Psychol* 1991; 10(5):343–51

Pessin MS and Caplan LR. Basilar artery stenosis-middle and distal segments. *Neurology* 1987; 37:1742–1746.

Prospective Studies Collaboration. Cholesterol, diastolic blood pressure, and stroke: 13 000 strokes in 450 000 people in 45 prospective cohorts. *Lancet* 1995; 346:1647–1653.

Rothwell PM, Warlow CP, on behalf of the ECST Collaborators. Prediction of benefit from carotid endarterectomy in individual patients: a risk-modelling study. *Lancet* 1999; 353:2105–10.

Rothwell PM, Eliasziw M, Gutnikov SA, Warlow CP, and Barnett HJ. Carotid Endarterectomy Trialists Collaboration Endarterectomy for symptomatic carotid stenosis in relation to clinical subgroups and timing of surgery. *Lancet* 2004; 363:915–24.

Russo LS. Carotid system transient ischemic attacks-clinical, racial and angiographic correlations. *Stroke* 1981; 12:470.

Ryttlefors M, Enblad P, Molyneux, M, et al. International Subarachnoid Aneurysm Trial of Neurosurgical Clipping Versus Endovascular Coiling Subgroup Analysis of 278 Elderly Patients. *Stroke* 2008; 39:2720–2726.

Sacco RL, Wolf PA, Bharucha N, et al. Subarachnoid hemorrhage: Natural history, prognosis and precursive factors in the Framingham study. *Neurology* 1984; 34: 847–854.

Schneider JR, Droste JS, Schindler N, et al. Carotid endarterectomy in octogenarians: comparison with patients' characteristics and outcomes in younger patients. *J Vasc Surg* 2000; 31:927–935.

Selvin E, Coresh J, and Brancati F. The burden and treatment of diabetes in elderly individuals in the U.S. *Diabetes Care* 29:2415–2419, 2006.

Stamler J, Vaccaro O, Neaton JD, and Wentworth D. Diabetes, other risk factors, and 12 year cardiovascular mortality for men screened in the Multiple Risk Factor Intervention Trial. *Diabetes Care* 1993; 16: 434–444.

Shepherd J, Blauw GJ, Westendorp RG et al. PROspective Study of Pravastatin in the Elderly at Risk. Pravastatin in elderly individuals at risk of vascular disease (PROSPER): A randomised controlled trial. *Lancet* 2002; 360:1623–1630.

Stroke Prevention in Atrial Fibrillation Investigators Committee on
  Echocardiography. Transesophageal echocardiography correlates of
  thromboembolism in high-risk patients with nonvalvular atrial
  fibrillation. *Ann Intern Med* 1998; 128: 639–647.

Tsushima Y, Aoki J, and Endo K. Brain microhemorrhages detected on
  T2*-weighted gradient-echo MR images. *AJNR Am J Neuroradiol*
  2003; 24: 88–96.

Van der Wee N, Rinkel GJ, Hasan D, and van Gijn J. Detection of
  subarachnoid haemorrhage on early CT: Is lumbar puncture still
  needed after a negative scan? *J Neurol Neurosurg Psychiatry* 1995 Mar;
  58:357–9.

Vinters HV. Cerebral amyloid angiopathy. A critical review. *Stroke* 1987;
  18: 311–324.

Wardlaw JM, Zoppo G, Yamaguchi T, and Berge E. Thrombolysis for acute
  ischaemic stroke. *Cochrane Database Syst Rev* 2003: 3: CD000213.

Winslow CM, Solomon DH, Chassin MR, et al. The appropriateness of
  carotid endarterectomy. *N Engl J Med* 1988; 318:721–727.

Wolf PA, Abbott RD, and Kannel WB. Atrial fibrillation as an
  independent risk factor for stroke: The Framingham Study. *Stroke*
  1991; 22:983–988.

Wolf PA, D'Agostino RB, Belanger AJ, and Kannel WB. Probability of
  stroke: A risk profile from the Framingham Study. *Stroke* 1991; 22:
  312–318.

World Health Organization. *The World Health Report 2002: Reducing
  Risks, Promoting Healthy Life*. Geneva, Switzerland: World Health
  Organization; 2002.

40 Epilepsy and the Elderly

Anne C. Van Cott and Mary Jo Pugh

Introduction

Although many consider epilepsy a condition of childhood, the highest incidence of new onset epilepsy occurs in individuals over the age of 60. The annual of incidence of epilepsy rises with each decade over 60 years (see Figure 1).

Seizures can be either provoked or unprovoked. Metabolic disturbances and alcohol withdrawal are common causes of acute provoked seizures and treatment is directed towards the underlying provoking medical condition. In contrast, the diagnosis of *epilepsy* is made when a patient experiences recurrent *unprovoked* seizures; in this chapter, we will review the topic of epilepsy in the elderly; please see chapter 20 for information on metabolic disturbances and alcohol withdrawal. We will discuss: a) the type of epilepsy older individuals experience, b) the causes of new onset epilepsy in the elderly, c) the diagnostic evaluation of the older patient with spells of alteration in level of consciousness, and d) the treatment of epilepsy in the elderly (Van Cott and Pugh 2008).

Types of Seizures

One of the major developments in the field of epilepsy has been the adoption of the International Classification of Epileptic Seizures (ICES) which recognizes two major categories of seizures: those that begin locally in a specific region of the brain and then spread (partial seizures) and those that are widespread with no identifiable focal origin at onset (generalized seizures) (Commission on Classification and Terminology of the International League Against Epilepsy 1989). In contrast to children who commonly present with generalized seizures, the majority of older individuals who develop new onset epilepsy experience *partial* seizures. Partial seizures are subdivided based on the impact of the seizure on consciousness. *Simple* partial seizures are typically brief (less than a minute) and consciousness is preserved, although communication skills may be impaired. During a simple partial seizure, a patient may experience abnormalities of movement (e.g. twitching), emotions (e.g. fear), or sensations (e.g. visual disturbances) that correspond to the affected region of the brain. In the past, the term *aura* was used to describe the warning feeling sensed by some patients during a simple partial seizure before the onset of alteration of consciousness due to spread of the abnormal epileptic discharge in the brain signaling the evolution to a complex partial seizure.

During a complex partial seizure, consciousness is altered. Typical complex partial seizures last one to three minutes, and involve a larger area of the brain on EEG. Often starting with a blank stare, patients can develop non-purposeful movements (automatisms), such as chewing or fumbling with objects. It has been proposed that elderly patients have atypical symptoms because, in contrast to younger patients, complex partial seizures are more likely to be extratemporal in origin (Ramsay and Pryor 2000). Confused and frequently still ambulatory, these patients are at risk for falls and injuries. Partial seizures can spread and evolve into generalized tonic clonic (previously called grand mal seizures).

Status epilepticus (SE), defined as a) more than 30 minutes of continuous seizure activity or b) two or more sequential seizures without full recovery of consciousness between seizures (Epilepsy Foundation of America 1993), is common in older individuals. The incidence of SE in individuals over the age of 60 (86/100,000) is almost twice that of the general population (Waterhouse and DeLorenzo 2001). Mortality associated with SE in the geriatric population is high: 38% in those over the age of 60 and over 50% in those over the age of 80 (Sung and Chu 1989). Cerebrovascular disease is the most commonly identified cause of convulsive SE in the elderly (Sung and Chu 1989).

Clinicians need to maintain a heightened awareness of nonconvulsive status epilepticus (NCSE) which describes a spectrum of status epilepticus not associated with overt motor convulsions. It is common in elderly patients and is particularly challenging to diagnose. NCSE is a term most often applied to patients who are severely obtunded or comatose with minimal or no motor activity, often with serious illness. The term has also been used to describe individuals who are awake, ambulatory, but confused and found to have electrographic seizures on EEG. NCSE requires EEG testing to diagnose appropriately (Brenner 2004).

Etiology of Seizures

It is not surprising that partial seizures are the most common type of seizures in the elderly, since stroke is the most commonly identified cause of new onset epilepsy in the geriatric population. Risk factors for the development of post-stroke epilepsy include: hemorrhage, cerebral cortical involvement, and a history of acute symptomatic seizures

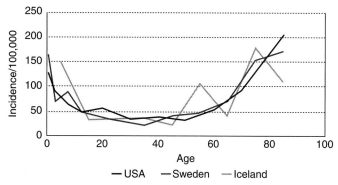

Figure 1 Incidence of unprovoked seizures in developed countries.

(Lancman, Golimstok, Norscini, et al. 1993). Unfortunately, there is no way of determining which stroke patients will develop seizures, and there is no role for prophylactic antiepileptic drug (AED) therapy since the far majority of stroke patients do not go on to develop epilepsy. Degenerative brain disorders, head trauma, and brain tumor (both primary and metastatic) are the other most frequently identified etiologies of new onset seizures in the elderly. Alzheimer's disease is a risk factor for epilepsy; between 9% to 16% of Alzheimer's patients will develop a seizure disorder, typically in the later stages of the illness (Hauser, Morris, Heston, et al. 1986; McAreavey, Ballinger, and Fenton 1992; Hesdorffer, Hauser, Annegers, et al. 1996). Despite recent advances in neuroimaging, one-third to one-half of older patients experience "cryptogenic" seizures, where the exact cause is unknown (Ramsay, Rowan, and Pryor 2004; Hauser, Annegers, and Kurland 1993; Loiseau, Loiseau, Duche et al. 1990; Stephen and Brodie 2000; Bergey 2004). Some researchers propose that CNS vascular disease is the cause of most of the cryptogenic cases since stroke risk factors (hypertension, hypercholesterolemia, coronary artery disease, and peripheral vascular disease) are associated with seizures, in the absence of stroke on neuroimaging studies (Li, Breteler, de Bruyne, et al. 1997; Ng, Hauser, Brust et al. 1993). A recent study using national VA databases to identify risk factors for geriatric epilepsy compared clinical characteristics in older individuals with new onset epilepsy to a matchedseizure-free group. Cerebrovascular disease and dementia had the strongest relationship with new onset epilepsy. Interestingly, individuals with both cerebrovascular disease and dementia diagnoses were more likely by a factor of *four* to have new onset epilepsy suggesting an additive effect of these two conditions. After controlling for underlying variables, hypertension, diabetes, hypercholesterolemia, coronary artery disease, and peripheral vascular disease were not found to be independent risk factors for the development of new onset epilepsy in this geriatric veteran cohort (Pugh, Knoefel, Mortensen, et al. 2009). If possible, identification of the cause of new onset epilepsy in the elderly is important since it might implicate a treatable, previously unidentified neurological and/or systemic illness. In addition, determining the etiology and type of seizures in an elderly individual with new onset epilepsy will help determine future medical and neurological interventions for that patient.

Clinical Diagnosis

Frequently, it is difficult to establish the diagnosis of epilepsy in the older individual. As already discussed, most seizures in elderly patients are focal in onset with less obvious and more nonspecific symptoms than in younger individuals (Hauser, Annegers, and Kurland 1993; Hiyoshi and Yagi 2000; Rowan, Kelly, Bergey, et al. 2005; Tinuper, Provini, Marini, et al. 1996). The possibility of seizures should be considered in any older individual who presents with intermittent confusional states. It has been suggested that symptoms during a seizure may be atypical in elderly patients because the seizure focus is often extra-temporal (Ramsay and Pryor 2000), making the clinical diagnosis even more challenging. The health care provider needs to interview not only the patient about his symptoms, but any available witnesses who have seen the individual's spells of alteration in level of consciousness. The older patient may not experience a classic aura (e.g. déjà vu, olfactory hallucination) associated with temporal lobe seizures (Tinuper, Provini, Marini, et al. 1996; Kellinghaus, Loddenkemper, Dinner, et al. 2004). Instead, older patients tend to report nonspecific changes before loss of consciousness such as lightheadedness, dizziness, and muscle cramps. Witnesses will often describe episodic confusion accompanied by a blank stare, clumsiness, or non-purposeful movements. Postictal confusion is frequently longer (hours) in

Table 1 "Spells" in the Elderly

- ◆ Transient ischemic attacks
- ◆ Syncope
- ◆ Cardiovascular events
- ◆ Dementia
- ◆ Non-epileptic events
- ◆ Metabolic disorders
- ◆ Medications

duration than is witnessed in younger patients. Often the diagnosis of epilepsy is not established until the patient has a secondarily generalized tonic-clonic seizure.

The first clinical consideration that needs to be addressed is whether the patient has had an epileptic seizure. The differential diagnosis for spells of alteration in level of consciousness in the elderly is broad (Table 1) and includes transient ischemic attacks (TIAs) and syncope.

TIAs usually present with negative symptoms that are not often seen with seizures, such as numbness and weakness. In addition, although a TIA can cause focal neurological symptoms, it is not typically associated with generalized confusion. During a TIA, motor symptoms consist of weakness. During a seizure, motor symptoms are more often than not repetitive movements. The duration of the spell may prove helpful distinguishing tool, since seizures typically last no more than three minutes, whereas TIA symptoms may last longer (minutes to hours) (Sirven 2001).

Syncope, especially cardiogenic syncope, should be considered in the differential for epilepsy. Questions regarding pallor, palpitations, diaphoresis, chest discomfort, and dyspnea frequently provide additional clues indicative of a cardiovascular event. The development of lightheadedness, dizziness, nausea, and fatigue upon standing or sitting upright suggest orthostatic intolerance and serve as clinical clues to the diagnosis of syncope. It is important for the clinician to remember that syncope can be accompanied by brief clonic activity due to brain hypoperfusion. In contrast to seizure activity, muscle twitching with syncope is mostly clonic or myoclonic (not tonic) and involves the distal extremeties (not axial). While rare with syncope, injury (e.g. tongue/cheek biting, falling) is common with seizures. People with convulsions often fall forward or backward during the phase of tonic rigidity sustaining injury to the forehead, chin, or occipital area. Headache, confusion, and urinary incontinence are common with seizures, but rare with syncope. Focal neurological findings on examination are sometimes present with seizures, but not with syncope (Sirven 2001; Leppik 2006).

Diagnostic Evaluation

If the spells are epileptic in nature, the examination should search for provoking factors. Seizures caused by metabolic disturbance (e.g. hypoglycemia), medications (e.g. bupropion), medication withdrawal (e.g. benzodiazepines), or substance abuse (e.g. alcohol) are treated by addressing the underlying medical issue; AED treatment is typically not prescribed. Since both drug (medication or illicit) toxicity and metabolic abnormalities can provoke seizures and lower seizure threshold in epileptic patients, patients with acute seizures should have a toxicology screen and serum analyzed for electrolytes, BUN, creatinine, glucose, calcium, magnesium, and liver function tests. If AED therapy is an option, a simultaneous complete blood count, differential, and platelets can rule out infection and provide baseline data if AED therapy is considered. Since stroke is the most common etiology for new onset epilepsy in the elderly, laboratory evaluation for stroke risk factors (e.g. hemoglobin A1C, lipid panel) should be considered.

Because a structural lesion is the most common cause of epilepsy in the elderly, neuroimaging studies should be obtained. A CT scan may be of value in an emergency setting to assess for a focal mass that requires emergent intervention (e.g. intracranial hemorrhage, tumor). In a recent study investigating the treatment of epilepsy in the elderly, only 18% of patients had normal CT scans of the brain (Rowan, Ramsay, Collins, et al. 2005). MRI with contrast should be pursued in most cases, especially if the older individual has complaints suggesting a focal abnormality, has a focal neurological exam, or an abnormal EEG suggestive of a partial seizure disorder caused by a CNS structural lesion.

The Quality Standards Subcommittee of the American Academy of Neurology considers EEG part of the routine neurodiagnostic evaluation of adults presenting with an apparent unprovoked first seizure. The guidelines site evidence that a routine EEG can predict the risk of seizure recurrence. Interictal epileptiform abnormalities (e.g. sharp waves, spikes, polyspikes) are suggestive of a seizure tendency. An EEG performed while a patient is asleep, as well as during wakefulness, increases the diagnostic yield of the EEG. It is important to remember that a normal EEG does not eliminate epilepsy as a diagnosis. For adults presenting with a first seizure, epileptiform abnormalities (Figure 2) are present in 23% of patients and were predictive of seizure recurrence. However, a routine EEG in elderly patients with epilepsy has limited values, since it has been reported to be a less sensitive in detecting interictal epileptiform discharges than in children and adults with seizure disorders (Drury and Beydoun 1998a). Non-specific EEG abnormalities, such as intermittent focal slowing, are common, being reporting in up to 38% of older individuals without seizures (Drury and Beydoun 1998b; McBride, Shih, and Hirsch 2002).

An electro-clinical seizure on EEG confirms the diagnosis of epilepsy in an individual with stereotypical spells, but these are rarely recorded during the course of a routine EEG. Closed-circuit television (CCTV)-EEG monitoring, also called Video-EEG monitoring, which has proven invaluable in the diagnosis and classification of epileptic syndromes in younger patients, tends to be underused in the elderly population. Recently, it has been reported that video-EEG monitoring leads to a definitive diagnosis in the majority of elderly patients referred for epilepsy monitoring within days of admission (McBride, Shih, and Hirsch 2002; Lancman, O'Donovan, Dinner, et al. 1996; Duncan, Sander, Sisodiya, et al. 2006; Behrouz, Heriaud, and Benbadis 2006). Events attributable to treatable medical conditions and non-epileptic "psychogenic" seizures have been described in the older population and are readily diagnosed with video EEG monitoring (Drury, Selwa, Schuh, et al. 1999; McBride, Shih, and Hirsch 2002; Lancman, O'Donovan, Dinner, et al. 1996; Duncan, Sander, Sisodiya, et al. 2006; Behrouz, Heriaud, and Benbadis 2006).

Treatment

Although neurosurgical intervention and vagal nerve stimulation are therapeutic options for older adults with refractory seizures (Grivas, Schramm, Kral, et al. 2006; Sirven, Malamut, O'Connor, et al. 2000), medications remain the mainstay of therapy for epilepsy in the geriatric population. AEDs are classically separated into the older/established AEDs and the newer AEDs that have primarily been approved by the FDA as add-on therapy (Table 2). Despite lack of FDA approval, many clinicians use the newer agents as monotherapy for treatment of new onset epilepsy because of their theoretical advantages (Table 3). The older antiepileptic drugs (AEDs), especially phenobarbital and phenytoin, have fallen out of favor for treatment of the elderly primarily because of their side effect profile. Many neurologists advocate the use of the newer AEDs (e.g. lamotrigine, gabapentin, levetiracetam) since they are effective and better tolerated in the older individual with a seizure disorder.

The normal aging process has a considerable influence on the pharmaokinetics of drugs in the elderly. Physiological alterations associated with aging that impact the metabolism of AEDs include decreased plasma protein binding, increased volume of distribution, decreased hepatic drug metabolism and renal clearance, and altered GI absorption (Perucca, Berlowitz, Birnbaum, et al. 2006; Gidal 2006).

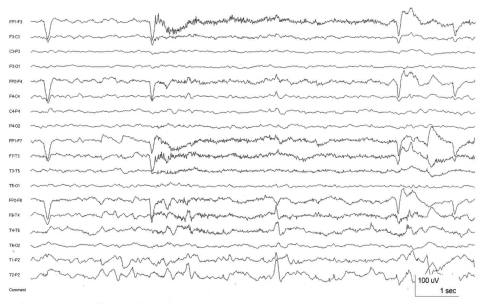

Figure 2 Right temporal sharp waves in a 65-year-old man with a history of a right middle cerebral infarct. Interictal epileptiform abnormalities that suggest a seizure tendency are less common with advancing age.

Table 2 Antiepileptic Drugs

Older AEDs	Newer AEDs
Phenobarbital	Felbamate
Primidone	Lamotrigine+
Phenytoin	Topiramate*+
Carbamazepine	Tiagabine
Valproic acid	Gabapentin+
	Levetiracetam
	Oxcarbazepine*+
	Zonisamide
	Pregabalin
	Lacosamide

*Approved by FDA as initial monotherapy for adults

+AAN/AES guidelines initial monotherapy

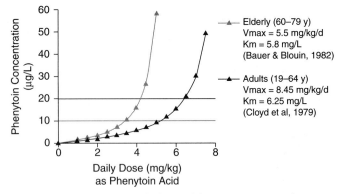

Figure 3 Phenytoin levels are higher in older patients compared to adults. Cloyd 1997.

Pharmacokinteic problems are more likely to occur with the older, established agents that are more highly protein bound, more commonly hepatically metabolized, and renally excreted (Faught 1999; Perucca, Berlowitz, Birnbaum, et al. 2006). AED treatment is further complicated in the geriatric epilepsy population since these patients are usually taking other medications for concurrent diseases (Lackner, Cloyd, Thomas, et al. 1998). Many AEDs impact metabolizing enzymes; and induction and inhibition of these systems can lead to clinically significant drug interactions. The theoretical advantages of the newer AEDs, in conjunction with recently published clinical trials (Brodie, Overstall, and Giorgi 1999; Rowan, Ramsay, Collins, et al. 2005), have led many experts to consider several of the newer AEDs as optimal treatment for older individuals with epilepsy (http://www.sign.ac.uk/guidelines/fulltext/70/index.html; Semah, Picot, Derambure, et al. 2004; Karceski, Morrell, and Carpenter 2005). In addition, phenobarbital and phenytoin are now believed by many epilepsy experts to be "suboptimal" AEDs for older patients due to their side effect profiles and potential for drug interactions. While it is possible that some patients may have good seizure control with low-dose phenobarbital, the associated adverse effects (e.g. cognitive decline, forgetfulness, gait disturbance) led the U.S. National Committee on Quality Assurance to identify phenobarbital as a drug to be avoided in the elderly (http://www.ncqa.org/Programs/HEDIS/NDC_2006/Drugs%20to%20be%20Avoided.xls).

Phenytoin's non linear kinetics can result in a narrowed therapeutic window (Rowan. and Ramsay 1997) leading to a greatly increased risk of overt toxicity. In addition, in older individuals, a very small increase in dose or altered absorption can result in a broad variability in phenytoin serum levels leading to potential toxicity or breakthrough seizure activity (see Figure 3).

Table 3 Theoretical Advantages of Newer AEDs

- Effective
- Fewer adverse reactions
- Fewer dose-related side effects
- Less drug interactions
- Fewer problems with metabolism and excretion
- Ease of use

In one recent study of elderly nursing home residents, phenytoin levels were highly variable, even when doses were unchanged and medication administration was regulated (Birnbaum, Hardie, Leppik, et al. 2003). Clinicians must also remember that phenytoin is a highly protein bound AED. A routine serum phenytoin level is a total level that represents the sum of the protein bound phenytoin and the protein unbound (or free) phenytoin in the blood. It is the "free" phenytoin, which enters the brain, controls seizures, and can produce neurotoxic side effects. In older individuals with low albumin levels, the free drug level may be increased relative to the total level and lead to dose-related toxicity. Measuring free phenytoin levels may provide a more effective guide to dose adjustment than routine total serum phenytoin levels if phenytoin must be used. Despite recommendations, phenytoin remains the most widely prescribed AED in the US and is commonly used in the geriatric population, including those in nursing homes (Ruggles, Haessly, and Berg 2001; Pugh, Cramer, Knoefel, et al. 2004). In a recent study that examined the changes in US prescribing patterns for the treatment of new onset epilepsy in older individuals between 2000 and2004, there was a consistently steady decline in the use of phenobarbital. However, phenytoin remained the most commonly used AED and the decrease of its use was only modest (70.6% to 66.1%) over the four year study (Pugh, Van Cott, Cramer, et al. 2008).

Several international neurological organizations have established recommendations or guidelines for the treatment of epilepsy in children and adults, but few specifically address the treatment of the geriatric population with epilepsy (http://www.sign.ac.uk/guidelines/fulltext/70/index.html; French, Kanner, Bautista, et al. 2004; National Collaborating Center for Primary Care 2004). This is because only a few clinical trials specifically studied antiepileptic drug (AED) treatment in the elderly (Leppik 2006). A recent review by the International League Against Epilepsy (Glauser, Ben-Menachem, Bourgeois, et al. 2006), identified only two randomized studies that examined the efficacy and tolerability of AED therapy in the elderly (Rowan, Ramsay, Collins, et al. 2005; Brodie, Overstall, and Giorgi 1999). In those two studies, elderly patients were randomized to different AED treatments. As with most AED clinical trials, the primary study outcome measure was retention of subjects over a period of time (1–2 years). In the first study, lamotrigine was compared to carbamazepine in a 24-week study in 150 older patients. Patients on lamotrigine had a higher completion rate (71% versus 42%), seizure free rate (39%versus 21%), and fewer number of side effects (n=102 versus 48) (Brodie, Overstall, and Giorgi 1999). In the second study, three treatment groups were used to compare lamotrigine, gabapentin, and carbamazepine in 593 elderly patients with epilepsy. Early teminators (44.2%, 51%, and 64.5% respectively) and terminations due to adverse drug reactions (12.1%,

21.6%, and 31% respectively) were less common in those taking lamotrigine or gabapentin compared with carbamazepine. There was no significant difference in the seizure-free rates at 12 months (Rowan, Ramsay, Collins, et al. 2005). A more recent study comparing lamotrigine and extended release carbamazepine in 185 epilepsy patients over 65 years old found no differences between groups in study completion, time to drug withdrawal, seizure remission, or treatment-emergent adverse events after 40 weeks (Saetre, Perucca, Isojarvi, et al. 2007). Retention rates, or the number of patients who completed the study, reflect both withdrawal due to either intolerable side effects or inadequate seizure control. All studies found that older patients were more likely to withdraw because of side effects and advocated the use of the newer AEDs (lamotrigine and gabapentin monotherapy) over carbamazepine in older patients with new onset epilepsy. However, some warn against drawing firm conclusions from short duration drug trials in epilepsy. Short term studies emphasizing dropout as an endpoint tend to favor drugs with lower side effects, even if they may be less effective (French and Chadwick 2005).

Starting at a low dose and titrating the AED slowly is strongly advocated by experts (Leppik 2006). In the largest randomized clinical trial to date (Rowan, Ramsay, Collins, et al. 2005) using the newer AEDs, gabapentin was started at 300mg/day and increased by 300mg/day every three days to a target dose of 1,500mg/day (tid dosing); lamotrigine was titrated at 25mg/day for two weeks, 50 mg/day for two weeks and 100mg/day for one week, followed by 150mg/day (bid dosing). These doses were not fixed throughout the study and incremental increases above the target were allowed at any time if seizure control was inadequate. Conversely, incremental decreases were permitted if the patient experienced toxicity. Interestingly, actual total daily doses of the study drugs approached target doses. At 52 weeks, mean dosages were 1,422 +/- 288 mg/day and 152 +/- 33mg/day for gabapentin and lamotrigine, respectively.

At the end of January 2008, the FDA issued an alert indicating that antiepileptic drug (AED) treatment is associated with increased risk for suicidal ideation, attempt, and completion. This decision was based on an analysis of suicidal ideation and behavior in placebo-controlled clinical studies of 11 antiepileptic drugs used in the treatment of epilepsy, psychiatric disorders, and other conditions (including migraine and neuropathic pain) (http://www.fda.gov/cder/drug/InfoSheets/HCP/antiepilepticsHCP.htm). The FDA recommended that health care professionals should closely monitor all patients who are currently taking or starting any AED for behavioral changes. Health care providers were instructed to inform patients, their families, and caregivers of the potential for an increase in the risk of suicidality. The FDA also advised providers to balance the clinical need for these medications with the elevated risk for suicidality. Recently, Avorn (2008) suggested the AED-suicidality controversy reveals the limitations of ascertaining adverse events in randomized controlled trials designed specifically to meet the requirements for FDA approval. A recent study utilized data from VA and Medicare databases and focused specifically on veterans 66 years and older and demonstrated that the stongest predictor of suicide-related behaviors for older patients newly treated with AED Monotherapy was a prior diagnosis of affective disorder (VanCott, Cramer, and Copeland, 2010).

Conclusion

Epilepsy is a common neurological disorder in elderly patients. Partial seizures (both simple and complex) are the most frequent seizure type and can be difficult to diagnose. Obtaining a precise history, including events observed by witnesses, is invaluable. Video-EEG monitoring may prove diagnostically useful. Phenobarbital and phenytoin are

suboptimal AEDs for new onset epilepsy in the elderly. Newer agents (lamotrigine and gabapentin) and extended release carbamazepine should be considered as treatment options.

References

Avorn, J.: Drug warnings that can cause fits—communicating risks in a data-poor environment. *N Engl J Med* 359:991–4, 2008.

Behrouz, R., Heriaud, L., amd Benbadis, S.R.: Late-onset psychogenic nonepileptic seizures. *Epilepsy Behav* 8:649–50, 2006.

Bergey, G.K.: Initial treatment of epilepsy: Special issues in treating the elderly. *Neurology* 63:S40–8, 2004.

Birnbaum, A., Hardie, N.A., Leppik, I.E., et al.: Variability of total phenytoin serum concentrations within elderly nursing home residents. *Neurology* 60:555–9, 2003.

Brenner, R.P.: EEG in convulsive and nonconvulsive status epilepticus. *J Clin Neurophysiol* 21:319–31, 2004.

Brodie, M.J., Overstall, P.W., and Giorgi, L.: Multicentre, double-blind, randomised comparison between lamotrigine and carbamazepine in elderly patients with newly diagnosed epilepsy. The UK Lamotrigine Elderly Study Group. *Epilepsy Res* 37:81–7, 1999.

Cloyd, J.C.: Commonly used antiepileptic drugs: age-related pharmacokinetics. In *Seizures and epilepsy in the elderly*, (Rowan, A.J., Ramsay, R.E., editors). Butterworth-Heinemann, Newton, MA, pp 219–28, 1997.

Drury, I. and Beydoun, A.: Interictal epileptiform activity in elderly patients with epilepsy. *Electroencephalogr Clin Neurophysiol* 106: 369–73, 1998a.

Drury, I. and Beydoun, A.: Seizures and epilepsy in the elderly revisited. *Arch Intern Med* 158: 99–100, 1998b.

Drury, I., Selwa, L.M., Schuh, L.A., et al.: Value of inpatient diagnostic CCTV-EEG monitoring in the elderly. *Epilepsia* 40:1100–2, 1999.

Duncan, J.S., Sander, J.W., Sisodiya, S.M., et al.: Adult epilepsy. *Lancet* 367:1087–100, 2006.

Faught, E.: Epidemiology and drug treatment of epilepsy in elderly people. *Drugs Aging* 15:255–69, 1999.

French, J.A. and Chadwick, D.W.: Antiepileptic drugs for the elderly: using the old to focus on the new. *Neurology* 64:1834–5, 2005.

French, J.A., Kanner, A.M., Bautista, J., et al.: Efficacy and tolerability of the new antiepileptic drugs I: Treatment of new onset epilepsy: Report of the Therapeutics and Technology Assessment Subcommittee and Quality Standards Subcommittee of the American Academy of Neurology and the American Epilepsy Society. *Neurology* 62:1252–60, 2004.

Gidal, B.E.: Drug absorption in the elderly: Biopharmaceutical considerations for the antiepileptic drugs. *Epilepsy Res* 68:65–9, 2006.

Glauser, T., Ben-Menachem, E., Bourgeois, B., et al.: ILAE treatment guidelines: evidence-based analysis of antiepileptic drug efficacy and effectiveness as initial monotherapy for epileptic seizures and syndromes. *Epilepsia* 47:1094–120, 2006.

Grivas, A., Schramm, J., Kral, T., et al.: Surgical treatment for refractory temporal lobe epilepsy in the elderly: Seizure outcome and neuropsychological sequels compared with a younger cohort. *Epilepsia* 47:1364–72, 2006.

Hauser, W.A., Annegers, J.F., Kurland, L.T.: Incidence of epilepsy and unprovoked seizures in Rochester, Minnesota: 1935–1984. *Epilepsia* 34:453–68, 1993.

Hauser, W.A., Morris, M.L., Heston, L.L., et al.: Seizures and myoclonus in patients with Alzheimer's disease. *Neurology* 36:1226–30, 1986.

Hesdorffer, D.C., Hauser, W.A., Annegers, J.F., et al.: Dementia and adult onset unprovoked seizures. *Neurology* 46:727–30, 1996.

Hiyoshi, T. and Yagi, K.: Epilepsy in the elderly. *Epilepsia* 41:31–5, 2000.

Karceski, S., Morrell, M.J., Carpenter, D.: Treatment of epilepsy in adults: Expert opinion, 2005. *Epilepsy Behav* 7:S1–64, 2005.

Kellinghaus, C., Loddenkemper, T., Dinner, D.S., et al.: Seizure semiology in the elderly: A video analysis. *Epilepsia* 45:263–7, 2004.

Lackner, T.E., Cloyd, J.C., Thomas, L.W., et al.: Antiepileptic drug use in nursing home residents: Effect of age, gender, and comedication on patterns of use. *Epilepsia* 39:1083–7, 1998.

Lancman, M.E., Golimstok, A., Norscini, J., et al.: Risk factors for developing seizures after a stroke. *Epilepsia* 34:141–3, 1993.

Lancman, M.E., O'Donovan, C., Dinner, D., et al.: Usefulness of prolonged video-EEG monitoring in the elderly. *J Neurol Sci* 142:54–8, 1996.

Leppik, I.: Antiepileptic drug trials in the elderly. *Epilepsy Res* 68: 45–8, 2006.

Leppik, I.E.: *Contemporary diagnosis and management of the patient with epilepsy*, Ed 6th. Handbooks in Health Care, Newton, PA, 2006, pp 1–251.

Li, X., Breteler, M.M., de Bruyne, M.C., et al.: Vascular determinants of epilepsy: The Rotterdam Study. *Epilepsia* 38:1216–20, 1997.

Loiseau, J., Loiseau, P., Duche, B., et al.: A survey of epileptic disorders in southwest France: Seizures in elderly patients. *Ann Neurol* 27:232–7, 1990.

McAreavey, M.J., Ballinger, B.R., Fenton, G.W.: Epileptic seizures in elderly patients with dementia. *Epilepsia* 33:657–60, 1992.

McBride, A.E., Shih, T.T., Hirsch, L.J.: Video-EEG monitoring in the elderly: A review of 94 patients. *Epilepsia* 43:165–9, 2002.

National Collaborating Center for Primary Care: The epilepsies: The diagnosis and management of the epilepsies in adults and children in primary and secondary care. London: National Institute for Clinical Excellence; 2004.

NCQA. HEDIS 2006 draft NDC lists public comment–September 2–30. 2005. http://www.ncqa.org/Programs/HEDIS/NDC_2006/ Drugs%20to%20be%20Avoided.xls.

Ng, S.K., Hauser, W.A., Brust, J.C., et al.: Hypertension and the risk of new-onset unprovoked seizures. *Neurology* 43:425–8, 1993.

Commission on Classification and Terminology of the International League Against Epilepsy. Proposal for revised classification of epilepsies and epileptic syndromes. *Epilepsia* 30:389–99, 1989.

Epilepsy Foundation of America: Treatment of convulsive status epilepticus. Recommendations of the Epilepsy Foundation of America's Working Group on Status Epilepticus. *JAMA* 270:854–9, 1993.

Perucca, E., Berlowitz, D., Birnbaum, A., et al.: Pharmacological and clinical aspects of antiepileptic drug use in the elderly. *Epilepsy Res* 68:49–63, 2006.

Pugh, M.J., Cramer, J., Knoefel, J., et al.: Potentially inappropriate antiepileptic drugs for elderly patients with epilepsy. *J Am Geriatr Soc* 52:417–22, 2004.

Pugh, M.J., Knoefel, J.E., Mortensen, E.M., et al.: New-onset epilepsy risk factors in older veterans. *J Am Geriatr Soc* 57(2): 237–42, 2009.

Pugh, M.J., Van Cott, A.C., Cramer, J.A., et al.: Trends in antiepileptic drug prescribing for older patients with new-onset epilepsy: 2000-2004. *Neurology* 70:2171–8, 2008.

Ramsay, R.E. and Pryor, F.: Epilepsy in the elderly. *Neurology* 55:S9–14; discussion S54–8, 2000.

Ramsay, R.E., Rowan, A.J., Pryor, F.M.: Special considerations in treating the elderly patient with epilepsy. *Neurology* 62:S24–S29, 2004.

Rowan, A.J., Kelly, K.M., Bergey, G.K., et al.: Epilepsy later in life: managing the unique problems of seizures in the elderly. *Geriatrics* Special Supplement:3–21, 2005.

Rowan, A.J., Ramsay, R.E., Collins, J.F., et al.: New onset geriatric epilepsy: A randomized study of gabapentin, lamotrigine, and carbamazepine. *Neurology* 64:1868–73, 2005.

Ruggles, K.H., Haessly, S.M., and Berg, R.L.: Prospective study of seizures in the elderly in the Marshfield Epidemiologic Study Area (MESA). *Epilepsia* 42:1594–9, 2001.

Saetre, E., Perucca, E., Isojarvi, J., et al.: An international multicenter randomized double-blind controlled trial of lamotrigine and sustained-release carbamazepine in the treatment of newly diagnosed epilepsy in the elderly. *Epilepsia* 48:1292–302, 2007.

Scottish Intercollegiate Guidelines Network. Diagnosis and management of epilepsy in adults. 1997. http://www.sign.ac.uk/guidelines/ fulltext/70/index.html.

Semah, F., Picot, M.C., Derambure, P., et al.: The choice of antiepileptic drugs in newly diagnosed epilepsy: A national French survey. *Epileptic Disord* 6:255–65, 2004.

Sirven, J.I.: Acute and chronic seizures in patients older than 60 years. *Mayo Clin Proc* 76:175–83, 2001.

Sirven, J.I., Malamut, B.L., O'Connor, M.J., et al.: Temporal lobectomy outcome in older versus younger adults. *Neurology* 54:2166–70, 2000.

Stephen, L.J. and Brodie, M.J.: Epilepsy in elderly people. *Lancet* 355:1441–6, 2000.

Sung, C.Y. and Chu, N.S.: Status epilepticus in the elderly: Etiology, seizure type and outcome. *Acta Neurol Scand* 80:51–6, 1989.

Tinuper, P., Provini, F., Marini, C., et al.: Partial epilepsy of long duration: Changing semiology with age. *Epilepsia* 37:162–4, 1996.

U.S. Food and Drug Administration: Center for Drug Evaluation and Research. Information for healthcare professionals: Suicidality and antiepileptic drugs. 2008. http://www.fda.gov/cder/drug/InfoSheets/ HCP/antiepilepticsHCP.htm.

Van Cott, A.C. and Pugh, M.J.: Epilepsy and the elderly. *Annals of Long Term Care: Clinical Care and Aging* 16:28–32, 2008.

VanCott, A.C., Cramer, J.C., Copeland, L.A., et al.: Suicide-related behaviors in older patients with new anti-epileptic drug use: data from the VA hospital system. *BMC Medicine* 8:4, 2010.

Waterhouse, E.J. and DeLorenzo, R.J.: Status epilepticus in older patients: Epidemiology and treatment options. *Drugs Aging* 18:133–42, 2001.

41 Head Injury in the Elderly

David A. Olson

Introduction

Head injury is any alteration in consciousness caused by an impact to the head. Given such a broad definition, head injury outcomes can range from the inconsequential to the devastating. For example, in the United States, 1.4 million people are head injured each year, but only about 235,000 require hospital admission. Those over 65 years of age are disproportionately affected. In 2003, head injuries resulted in hospitalization for 234 elderly per 100,000 persons compared to 99.9 per 100,000 persons of all ages, and deaths from head injuries in the elderly were twice that of the general population (Rutland-Brown et al. 2006). Similarly, rates of hospitalization for those 85 and over were quadruple those between 65 and 74 years of age (Coronado et al. 2005).

The majority of traumatic brain injuries in the elderly, roughly two-thirds in a 1999 study, are from falls, with motor vehicle accidents a distant second (Coronado et al. 2005). Furthermore, medical comorbidities, such as diabetes, hypertension, and cardiac disease, are more likely to occur in those elderly injured in falls compared to those injured in motor vehicle accidents (Coronado et al. 2005). Finally, as the United States' population ages, fall-related head injuries are increasing, creating a major public health threat (Thomas et al. 2008) (Figure 1). In Oklahoma, for example, head injury rates in the elderly increased 79% from 1992 to 2003, primarily secondary to falls (Fletcher et al. 2007).

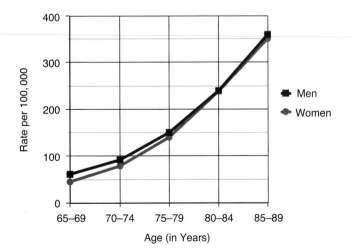

Figure 1 Fall-related traumatic brain injury non-fatal hospitalizations among older adults by age and sex in the United States in 2005. (Adapted from Thomas et al., 2008)

Pathophysiology

Head injury is a complex process involving gross, structural brain perturbations as well as biochemical abnormalities (Table 1). In addition, immediate pathologies such an intracranial bleeding and contusions are often complicated by secondary injuries like loss of oxygen and blood flow. Increased intracranial pressure, herniations, and accompanying cerebral infarctions are also secondary injuries.

Mechanical forces can cause direct injury to the brain or result in contracoup injuries in which the brain pushes into the calvarium on the side opposite the point of impact. Acceleration, deceleration, and rotational forces damage white matter tracts through shear injury or axonal breakage. Such damage is termed diffuse axonal injury and primarily affects the subcortical white matter, corpus callosum, and brain stem (Leclercq et al. 2001). Indeed, a recent Australia/New Zealand study of 635 patients with head injuries of all severities reported 28% had a CT-identified mass lesion (bleed or contusion), while 73% had associated axonal injury (Myburgh et al. 2008). In the last decade or so, antibodies against amyloid precursor protein have been used to identify such axonal damage, even in cases of mild head injury (Blumbergs et al. 1995). Elderly patients, however, more often have low impact injuries and are possibly less affected by axonal injury.

Post-traumatic cerebral infarctions are also common. A recent review of 353 patients with moderate to severe head injury showed that 12% developed infarctions identified on follow-up CT scans, usually within two weeks of the inciting trauma. Decreased sensorium, craniotomies, hypotension, and herniation syndromes all produced increased infarction risk, but increased age did not. Patients with infarctions, not surprisingly, did worse, with increased in-hospital mortality and lower functional outcomes after three months (Tian et al. 2008).

Vasospasm was not examined in the above study, but is common and could readily yield to frank infarction. The previously mentioned 635 patient study found 32% of admission head CT scans revealed subarachnoid hemorrhages, hemorrhages which, when occurring from an aneurysmal source, are commonly associated with vasospasm (Myburgh et al. 2008). Post-traumatic vasospasm, though, is a well-recognized entity and has been associated with, although not exclusively, traumatic subarachnoid bleeds. Serial transcranial Doppler examinations in 299 patients with mild to severe head trauma recently found 45% with Doppler evidence of spasm (Oertel et al. 2005). While no outcome measures were gathered for this study, at least one older study of 70 patients with mild, moderate, and severe head injuries reported that transcranial Doppler vasospasm resulted in 2.21 greater likelihood of a worse six month outcome compared to patients without vasospasm, even after controlling for age and injury severity (Lee et al. 1997).

Following head injury, a cascade of neurochemical changes ensues. Glutamate is released extracellularly, likely potentiated by the shutting down of astrocytic transporters. The extracellular glutamate can lead

Table 1 Immediate and Delayed Sequelae of Traumatic Brain Injury

Immediate	Delayed (Secondary)
Direct Impact	Increased Intracranial Pressure
Bleeding	Herniation
Axotomy/Axonal Shearing	Hypoxia
	Vasospasm
	Infarction
	Brain Hypermetabolic State
	Excitotoxicity
	Inflammation
	Apoptosis

to massive depolarization of neurons with subsequent elevations of intracellular calcium as well as other ionic fluxes, which ultimately lead to brain edema, raised intracranial pressure, and herniation. Cell death and ATP depletion also occur (Yi and Hazell 2006).

Immune dysregulation and cytokine release in head injury has also come under increased scrutiny in the last decade. Although serum and cerebrospinal fluid measurements of immune modulators have been performed, more recent work has used microdialysis catheters with diameters of around 330 μm, which are inserted into the cortex away from the site of injury and measure molecules of interest. Using this technique, interleukin-6 levels correlated with improved six month outcomes in 14 patients with severe head injuries, indicating that possibly interleukin-6 is somehow neuroprotective (Winter et al. 2004). Similarly, measurements of microdialysated cytokines in 15 severely head-injured patients found that elevations in an endogenous interleukin-1 receptor antagonist correlated with a favorable six month outcome (Hutchinson et al. 2007).

Apoptosis or programmed cell death is also initiated after head trauma. Proteinases called caspaces activate endonucleases which break down nuclear DNA. Utilizing immunological methods to identify caspaces and an enzymatic method of locating DNA break sites, pathologists have been able to identify apoptosis in post-mortem human brains following head injuries. Apoptosis was present in subjects of all ages and did not increase with age (Dressler et al. 2007). Other researchers have correlated head injury severity to cerebrospinal fluid elevations of caspace-3 in patients up to 65 years of age (Uzan et al. 2006).

This structural and biochemical damage from head injury, when occurring in the elderly, manifests in the context of a virtual procrustean bed of pre-existing pathologies and disabilities. The Centers for Disease Control (CDC) reports that the average 75 year old in the United States takes five different prescription medications and has at least three chronic health conditions (CDC 2004). In the setting of head injury, this obviously creates a highly complex clinical scenario, particularly when comparing it to one of the prototypical young adult, head-injured male. Indeed, clinical practice guidelines have recently come under harsh criticism because they often are applied noncontextually and neglect to speak to elderly patients with multiple medical comorbidities (Boyd et al. 2005).

Genetic Contributions

Studies of genetic influences on head injury in humans are limited and generally have examined non-elderly populations. Although the APO e4 allele was originally described as a marker of decreased survivorship

and functionally worse outcomes after head injuries in humans in the 1990s (Friedman et al. 1999), recent research has, at least in part, failed to replicate these early dismal associations. While earlier research had focused on six month outcomes, a more recent study following 108 moderately to severely head-injured patients with a mean age of 34 years found after a three year period, contrary to most prior studies, significantly improved outcomes for those patients possessing at least one APO e4 allele (Willemse-van Son et al. 2008). Nonetheless, a recent meta-analysis of 14 cohort studies examining all grades of head injury severity found patients with the APO e4 allele experienced a poorer six month outcome after traumatic brain injury than those possessing other ApoE isoforms (Zhou et al. 2008).

An allelic variant of catechol-O-methyltransferase (COMT), which theoretically results in less cortical dopamine, has been correlated with frontal dysfunction, as evidence by increased perseverative responses on the Wisconsin Card Sorting Test, in younger head-injured patients possessing this variant compared to those lacking it (Lipsky et al. 2005). A polymorphism in the pro-apototic gene p53, which may be triggered by trauma and promotes programmed cell death, has been associated with worsening six month functional outcomes for 90 nonelderly severely head-injured patients, although mortality remained unaffected (Martinez-Lucas et al. 2005). Post-traumatic brain hemorrhages have been correlated with interleukin polymorphisms in nonelderly patients with head injury, presumably because these genetic variants code for a propensity for inflammation which damages and weakens blood vessel walls (Hadjigeorgiou et al. 2005).

CACNA1A mutations in the calcium channel gene (such mutations have also been associated with spinocerebellar ataxia 6 and familial hemiplegic migraine) have been correlated with trauma-induced malignant cerebral edema in three patients, possibly because such a mutation predisposes to mechanically-induced depolarizations, which cause massive, abrupt ionic cellular influxes and consequent cytotoxic edema (Kors et al. 2001).

The genetic underpinnings of head injury are only beginning to be understood. Advances in technology should enable researches to examine polymorphisms more rapidly and in a more cost-effective manner than at present. In addition, different genetic variants may influence head injury recovery at different times; for example, early inflammatory responses would be expected to influence recovery in a different manner and temporal course than long-term neuronal repair in the rehabilitation phase. Furthermore, focal contusions and bleeds are a different process than diffuse axonal injuries, and genetic contributions are accordingly expected to be dissimilar (Diaz-Arrastia and Baxter 2006). Finally, although an understanding is beginning to emerge of how these factors influence head injury outcomes in younger adults, there is a dearth of research into how these factors play a role in the head-injured elderly.

Presentation

For the most part, elderly patients presenting with head injuries are straightforward. There is a history of a fall or injury, and there are physical exam findings such as ecchymoses or lacerations suggesting or corroborating trauma.

Sometimes, however, there are limited clues. The patient may have a pre-existing dementia and may not recall the trauma. The patient may present with new onset or worsening confusion, but the mental status changes are attributed to another medical problem; for example, an elderly patient immobilized after a fall may become volume depleted or dehydrated and develop not only electrolytic changes, but also an infection, and both of these entities may be assumed to be etiologic of the mental status changes, thereby masking the head injury. Indeed, in a recent study of abnormal CT scans in the elderly with head injuries, 20% of patients exhibited no external signs of trauma (Mack et al. 2003). Furthermore, the history may be fabricated and the head injury component downplayed by caregivers who, having engaged in elder abuse, are trying to avoid detection (Lachs and Pillemer 2004).

Alternatively, a patient may present with a history and physical exam concordant with head trauma, even exhibiting focal findings, but these findings could ultimately be secondary not to head trauma but to ischemia in the setting of a missed arterial dissection. Indeed, such a presentation lead to the disqualification of one patient recently enrolled in a study of progesterone treatment in acute head injury (Wright et al. 2007).

Finally, there are patients who talk and die. Traditionally, these patients have been children and younger people presenting awake and alert following head injury but who quickly decline and lose consciousness due to the sudden development of malignant cerebral edema; conversely older patients may present similarly affected by a rapidly expanding, arterial-fed epidural hematomas. More recently, acute subdurals and focal contusions were etiologic in 15 such patients, over half between the ages of 70 and 94 years, who presented with lucidity and the ability to speak but subsequently deteriorated within 30 minutes to 12 hours with death eventually ensuing. Lack of proper levels of medical observation as well as inattention to coagulopathies were believed to be contributory (Goldschlager, Rosenfeld, and Winter 2007).

Diagnosis

History

The history is, of course, of utmost importance. Usually, this is obtained by the patient or a close family member or witness. The mechanism of injury is significant. For example, pedestrians struck by a moving vehicle have a greater chance of death or impaired cognitive and motor functioning at hospital discharge compared to motor vehicle occupants (Haider et al. 2008). Head injuries sustained in an assault also portend a poor prognosis (Wagner et al. 2000).

If the patient is seen in the emergency room, the data sheet from the emergency responders contains historical as well as initial exam data, including the first Glasgow Coma Scale (GCS). This is a 15 point, near-universally employed scale that scores the level of alertness (1 to 4), best verbal response (1 to 5), and best motor response (1 to 6) (Table 2). A score of 13 to 15 implies a mild head injury, 9 to 12 a moderate one, and 8 or less a severe one. Although this scoring has a generic usefulness in predicting patient outcomes, several researchers believe that the GCS underestimates head injury severity in the elderly because of unique factors which delay symptom onset such as frequent low impact falls, pronounced brain atrophy, and a propensity for venous bleeding (Yap et al. 2008).

If the patient is seen in the office several weeks after the initial injury, information on the initial GCS is unlikely to be immediately available. In this case, the estimated duration of post-traumatic amnesia, defined as the time from the injury to the laying down of continuous memory, is another way of grading head injury severity. This measure is not only reliable several weeks after the event, but may also be more accurate in predicting functional outcomes in the elderly. Less than 24 hours of post-traumatic amnesia is graded mild, while one to four weeks is severe (Yap et al. 2008).

Physical Exam

The general physical exam should include looking for bruising about the orbits (raccoon eyes) or behind the ears (Battle's sign), which may

Table 2 Glasgow Coma Scale Abbreviated Scoring

Eye Opening (Points)	Verbal Response (Points)	Motor Response (Points)
Spontaneous opening (4)	Oriented (5)	Obeys commands (6)
Opens to verbal command (3)	Confused conversation (4)	Purposeful to pain (5)
Opens to pain (2)	Inappropriate responses, discernable words (3)	Withdrawals from pain (4)
None (1)	Incomprehensible speech (2)	Flexion of arms (3)
	None (1)	Extension of arms (2)
		None (1)

indicate a skull fracture. Ten to thirty percent of patients with skull base fractures develop cerebrospinal fluids leaks with an attendant 10% to 50% risk of meningitis (Yilmazlar et al. 2006). Such leaks clinically manifest as clear fluid discharging from the nose or ears. Glucose testing is no longer recommended because of poor specificity and sensitivity, but confirmatory testing with a transferrin unique to the CNS, beta-2 transferrin, is available (Abuabara 2008).

Cranial nerve findings are not uncommon in more severe injuries. Olfaction is frequently affected with an incidence between 5% and 65% depending on injury severity, but this is seldom tested at the bedside. Anosmia is associated with occipital fractures with contracoup frontal injuries; the impact theoretically causes a shearing of the olfactory nerve (Swann et al. 2006).

Optic nerve damage is more unusual and occurs in 0.5% to 5% of patients with head trauma. Painless loss of vision ensues, but spontaneous recovery may occur in up to 30% of patients (Wu et al. 2008). Fixed, dilated pupils, on the other hand, when combined with a GCS of 3, equated with no chance of survival among 173 head-injured patients (Tien et al. 2006).

Oculomotor palsies may imply increased intracranial pressure if there is lateral gaze paresis from a sixth nerve palsy, but uncal herniation is also common, wherein the temporal lobe presses on the ipsilateral third nerve resulting in eye deviation laterally due to the unopposed action of the abducens. Internuclear ophthalmoplegia is more unusual and may represent extra-axial compression on the brainstem or even ischemia, and in isolation this is usually a benign prognostic indicator (Doe and Jay 2006).

Facial nerve palsy occurred in about 5% of head injured patients with over half of those afflicted older than 60 years. Spontaneous and complete recovery eventuated in 30% (Odebode and Ologe 2006). Rare delayed facial paralysis has been also reported in head injury (Napoli and Panagos 2005). When combined with ipsilateral hearing loss, a facial paralysis almost always implicates a temporal bone fracture.

Hearing loss could also occur in isolation and may represent not only eighth nerve damage, but even structural damage to the ossicles (Basson and van Lierop 2008). Tinnitus may manifest as a sequelae of such injury, but when pulsatile and combined with conjunctival hyperemia, a post-traumatic carotid cavernous fistula is likely operative (Lerut et al. 2007).

Swallowing is commonly affected with up to 65% of patients with severe head injury demonstrating an impaired gag reflex and 90% demonstrating oral and pharyngeal pathology on videofluoroscopy.

Fortunately, dysphagia typically improves at discharge from neurore-habilitation with 72% of patients able to sustain on oral feedings alone (Terre and Mearin 2007).

Motorically, in the acute setting, focal findings could represent extra-axial bleeds, contusions, infarctions, or even a herniation syndrome. Flexor or extensor posturing implies increased intracranial pressure or diffuse intracranial injuries. In the recovery phase, less than antigravity strength in the upper or lower extremities as well as impaired balance predicts lack of independence in self-care activities one year after discharge (Duong et al. 2004).

Cognitively, bedside testing may initially focus on levels of alertness and command following, but later more subtle assessments are important. The major cognitive domains are readily testable at the bedside and include attention, language, verbal memory, visual spatial skills, and executive functioning, although the latter, while commonly impaired, is more difficult to assess. The Luria hand sequencing fist, chop, slap test is anecdotally useful, but overall the quality of the patient's responses, whether impulsive, disinhibited, or perseverative, offer an approximate assessment of the patient's executive abilities (Figure 2). Indeed, neuropsychological testing has documented impaired attention, memory, and executive functioning even 10 years after the initial brain injury (Draper and Ponsford 2008).

Affective changes occur as well after closed head injuries, and rates of depression have been documented as high as 77% (Flanagan et al. 2006). Older patients may be more prone to depression after head injuries than younger patients (Blicher and Nielsen 2008).

Imaging

Criteria for neuroimaging in the elderly after head injury should be liberal. Certainly, in the setting of obvious severe trauma, persistently impaired cognition, or focal motor findings, an urgent head CT is needed to exclude neurosurgically treatable pathologies: subdurals, epidurals, contusions, and edema may be visualized.

In milder head injuries, the decision may appear more complicated, and decision rules have been generated, but even in these cases, those aged 60 years or greater mandate immediate CT imaging (Smits et al. 2007). Indeed, in a study of 133 patients older than 59 years who experienced mild head injuries, absolutely no useful clinical or exam predictors of CT-identified intracranial pathology could be identified (Mack et al. 2003). In a more recent study of 106 consecutive patients over the age of 70 years presenting with confusion, the only patient with a non-focal neurologic exam and an abnormal head CT was injured in a fall (Hardy and Brennan 2008).

Follow-up imaging is, of course, needed in those patients with unexplained clinical deterioration, but routine CT follow-up imaging is controversial. Because over one half of patients with traumatic intracerebral hemorrhages demonstrate expansion of their lesions on follow-up CT scans within the first 24 hours, early repeat scanning is prudent (Narayan et al. 2008). Some authors have estimated that such serial CT scanning is cost-effective as well, especially in the elderly who have a higher risk of delayed bleeding (Stein et al. 2008). MRI scanning employing FLAIR, diffusion, and gradient echo sequences is also important in the face of persistent, unexplained motoric or cognitive deficits because such imaging is more sensitive to microbleeds as well as diffuse axonal injury and because unexpected pathologies may be indentified, such as ischemia strokes (Topal et al. 2008).

Diffuse tensor imaging, which examines water diffusion along white matter tracts, may soon migrate out of the research environment and into clinical practice. This methodology can delineate axonal damage in patients with head injuries even when conventional MRI imaging is unremarkable. For example, a study of 21 younger patients with mild head injuries disclosed multiple diffusion abnormalities in cortical projection fibers along with actual discontinuity of fiber tracts in 19% despite normal conventional brain MRI scans (Rutgers et al. 2008).

Functional imaging utilizing fluoro-2-deoxyglucose positron emission tomography is still more of a research tool, but recent studies have shown hypometabolism in the cingulate gyrus of 12 patients aged 18 to 50 years with moderate head injuries who demonstrated inattention, poor working memory, and executive dysfunction on neuropsychological testing (Nakashima et al. 2007). These same researchers found hypometabolism in the right cingulate and bilateral medial frontal regions, which correlated with full scale IQ scores, in 36 head-injured patients aged 20 to 50 years who had sustained diffuse axonal damage (Kato et al. 2007).

Labs

Electrolytic disturbances are of major importance with altered sodium levels occurring in up to 50% of comatose, head-injured patients (Tisdall et al. 2006). Hyponatremia may imply volume depletion, the syndrome of inappropriate antidiuretic hormone (SIADH), or cerebral salt wasting, the latter occurring in volume depleted patients by the release of a natriuretic hormone. Increased serum sodium levels, on the other hand, implicate pure dehydration or diabetes insipidus.

Hypomagnesemia has been documented in up to 85% of head injured patients during the course of their acute treatment. Magnesium blocks excitotoxins and its depletion could theoretically worsen brain injury. Although a recent trial of magnesium treatment in moderate or severe head injuries demonstrated no clinical benefit, this trial was potentially confounded by the aggression repletion of low serum magnesium levels in the controls, and the authors note that careful magnesium repletion may itself confer benefit (Temkin et al. 2007).

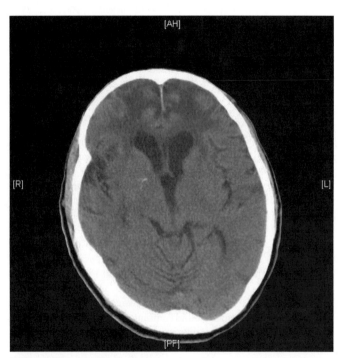

Figure 2 Marked frontal encephalomalacia from a remote head injury in a 65-year-old man with seizures and disinhibited, sexually inappropriate behavior.

Because brain trauma releases thromboplastin, which dysregulates the coagulation process, and damages the cerebral endothelium, which activates platelets and the clotting cascade, a coagulopathy may occur. Of 224 patients aged 27 to 54 years with isolated head trauma, 17% developed prolonged prothrombin or partial thromboplastin times during their initial hospitalization (Zehtabchi et al. 2008). Such hemostatic defects may contribute to the delayed intracranial bleeding seen in patients with head injuries.

In contrast to conventional laboratories, an ideal serum marker for head injury has been sought because such a marker would offer several advantages to current clinical and radiographic assessments: It could potentially identify head injury where the history is unobtainable, quantify severity, and possibly even correlate with long term outcomes. Unfortunately, such markers when found have usually lacked specificity.

S100 is a protein found mainly in the astroglia and Schwann cells. A recent study of 59 patients aged 8 to 80 years with severe head injuries correlated elevated serum S100 levels with one year outcomes: the higher the level, the less favorable the outcome (Nylen et al. 2008). However, S100 is non-specific and elevations have been documented in hypoperfused, critically ill patients (Routsi et al. 2006) as well as non-head injured soccer players (Straume-Naesheim et al. 2008).

Neuron-specific enolase is a protein found primarily in neurons and is leaked into the extracellular space with injury, making this a potentially more specific marker of brain injury. In a study of 169 patients aged 1 to 75 years with all degrees of head injury severity, serum elevations of neuron-specific enolase correlated with worsening head injury and higher levels were seen in those patients who died within 30 days of their injury (Guzel et al. 2008). Still, this marker is non-specific, and elevations have been documented in hypoperfusion and extra-cranial trauma (Pelinka et al. 2005).

Finally, glial fibrillary acidic protein is a cytoskeletal component of the astroglia and has been found to be elevated in the serum of 39 head-injured patients compared to 12 non-head injured, general trauma controls. Glial fibrillary acidic protein elevations on the second day of the hospitalization correlated with increased mortality (odd ratio 1.45) (Lumpkins et al. 2008). Further work will be needed to clarify the specificity of this marker.

Treatments Available

Acute

Both medical and surgical treatments may improve outcomes. In the 1980s, secondary brain injury factors such as hypoxia, hypoglycemia, and hypotension were identified, and subsequent practice has focused on ameliorating these clinical parameters through the dissemination of evidence-based guidelines (Brain Trauma Foundation 1996), although when these secondary injury factors are present, they still portend a poor outcome. A 2003 review of 81 severely head-injured patients correlated hyperglycemia, hypothermia, and hypotension with increased in-house mortality, while hypoxia correlated with longer hospital and ICU stays (Jeremitsky et al. 2003). Indeed, the 2008 Australia/New Zealand study documented a 22% incidence of hypotensive events along with a 32% incidence of hypoxia. The authors of this study sheepishly note that their overall mortality and unfavorable outcome data are comparable to the pre-guideline era, and they attribute this to not only the aging population, but to this high incidence of secondary brain injury (Myburgh et al. 2008). Paradoxically, hypoxia reduction through in-field intubation has been controversial and at least one major study failed to show improved outcomes with this intervention (Wang et al. 2004). Initial attention is, nevertheless, directed at airway control and prevention of secondary injury due to hypotension or other cardiovascular problems.

Prevention of hypoxia and hypotension are of course paramount, but blood transfusions, curiously, may worsen outcomes. For example, a 2008 review of 1150 head injured patients admitted over a 7 1/2 year period identified mortality (odds ratio 2.19) and medical complications (odds ratio 3.67) increases in those patients undergoing blood transfusions, even after controlling for anemia. Infection risk, vasospasm, and microvascular obstruction from the increased rigidity of stored red blood cells were some hypothesized mechanisms for the unexpectedly worse outcomes (Salim et al. 2008).

Nutritional support is not only common sense, but of extreme importance because head injury produces a hypermetabolic state in the brain. A recent retrospective study of 797 patients with severe head injuries, including a large proportion of the elderly, demonstrated that those patients who were not fed in the first 5 to 7 days had a 2 to 4 times greater mortality rate compared to those patients with early feedings, even after controlling for age, hypotension, CT abnormalities, and non-reactive pupils (Hartl et al. 2008).

Phenytoin has been shown to prevent early post-traumatic seizures within the first two weeks of head injuries, but no effect on long-term outcome has been documented (Temkin et al. 1990). Because phenytoin has numerous side effects (2.5% develop allergic reactions early on), levetiracetam has been seen as an appealing alternative. In a prospective study of 32 patients with severe head injuries compared to historic phenytoin-treated controls, no differences in clinical seizures were documented; however, levetiracetam-treated patients had more frequent epileptiform discharges on EEG, and further study is warranted before abandoning phenytoin as a first line agent (Jones et al. 2008). Phenytoin is usually discontinued after 1 to 2 weeks unless further seizure activity supervenes.

Raised intracranial pressure often complicates head injuries. The brain is an enclosed space with blood, tissue, and cerebrospinal fluid. Brain swelling, increased blood flow, hematomas, or cerebrospinal fluid outflow blockages all can raise the intracranial pressure. Too much pressure exacerbates ischemia and can eventually result in herniation syndromes and death. Higher intracranial pressures are commonly associated with worse outcomes.

Direct treatment of raised intracranial pressures have included head of bed elevation, mild hyperventilation, osmotic diuretics (mannitol or hypertonic saline), direct cerebrospinal fluid drainage, sedatives, or even barbituate coma. Decompressive craniectomy is advocated in patients refractory to conventional management; although no randomized, controlled trials have yet been published (two such trials are ongoing). Published studies to date have traditionally excluded older patients (Schirmer et al. 2008), and a recent Cochrane Database review found no empirical support for decompressive craniectomies (Sahuquillo and Arikan 2006).

One retrospective study, however, of 55 patients undergoing decompressive craniectomy for refractory intracranial pressure (ICP) increases included patients of all ages (eleven patients were greater than 65 years) and found that although no patients over 65 years with a GCS of 3 to 5 attained a good outcome, four older patients with GCS scores greater than 6 did, leading the authors to conclude that age alone should not be a factor to exclude patients from this procedure (Pompucci et al. 2007).

Focusing solely on increased intracranial pressure has generated controversy. Although a 2008 analysis found that the intensity and duration of increased intracranial pressure significantly correlated with poor six month outcomes, the magnitude of this effect was small (odds ratio 1.02) and of dubious clinical import (Vik et al. 2008).

Furthermore, a large study of severe head injury in a younger population reported intracranial pressure monitoring was associated with an actual 45% reduction in survival, even after controlling for pupillary abnormalities, injury severity, and hypotension (Shafi et al. 2008).

Alternative approaches have focused on maintaining an adequate cerebral perfusion pressure. Cerebral perfusion pressure is obtained by subtracting the intracranial pressure from the mean arterial pressure. This should prevent secondary brain ischemic injuries. Approaches to maintain the cerebral perfusion pressure usually employ the use of vasopressors to keep the systemic blood pressure elevated. Retrospective studies have found improved outcomes in patients whose cerebral perfusion pressures measured greater than 60 mm Hg (Huang et al. 2007), and clinical guidelines now advocate such perfusion pressure therapy (White and Venkatesh 2008).

Fluid resuscitation aims to augment perfusion pressure and albumin, by increasing oncotic pressure, was hoped to not only increase cerebral perfusion, but also to prevent extravasation of fluids into brain parenchyma, which could aggravate edema. Unfortunately, a post hoc analysis of a double blind, randomized study of 460 patients with head injuries of all severities, including 91 patients over 55 years of age, found a higher 24 month mortality for 4% albumin infusions compared to saline infusions given during the patients' initial intensive care hospitalization (SAFE investigators 2007).

The brain maintains its blood flow by vasoconstricting or vasodilating in response to changes in systemic pressure. This ability to autoregulate may be compromised in the elderly. A study of 358 patients between 16 and 87 years old who presented with head injuries of all severities found not only worse outcomes in the aged, but also decreased intracranial pressures and increased perfusion pressures. The latter two factors should actually portend better outcomes for the elderly, but intracranial ultrasound vasculature measures of cerebral blood flow documented deteriorating autoregulation in these patients, and this was hypothesized to account for the observed age-associated outcome decline (Czosnyka et al. 2005).

Surgery is generally performed for the extra-axial bleeds, namely subdural and epidural hematomas, especially if the bleed produces mass effect or is otherwise symptomatic. Subdurals occur in about 30% of severe head injuries and arise from tearing of bridging veins, which in the elderly is exacerbated by brain atrophy, which expands this potential space and creates a tensile force on the bridging veins (Figure 3). Forty-six percent of patients aged 65 or older developed post-traumatic subdurals in a recent study compared to only 28% of their younger counterparts (Mosenthal et al. 2002). Occasional arterial causes of subdurals have also been documented (Matsuyama et al. 1997). Epidurals occur in less than 1% of cases and are caused by breakage of the middle meningeal artery with consequent rapid arterial bleeding and progression. Even with prompt neurosurgical evacuation, these lesions can be deadly with a recent retrospectively assigned mortality rate of 26% for all comers, and as usual those patients who were older did worse even with surgery (Tallon et al. 2008). The decision of if and when to operate ultimately lies in the domain of neurosurgical judgment, and hard and fast clinical decision rules do not presently apply.

Non-surgical treatment of acute intracranial hematomas with volumes of at least 2 milliliters demonstrated a dose-dependent trend toward regression when recombinant Factor VIIa was administered acutely to 61 patients with head trauma compared to 36 non-treated controls. More deep venous thromboses were identified in the treated group, however, and further study is needed (Narayan et al. 2008). Others have advocated using recombinant Factor VIIa to reverse coagulopathies prior to neurosurgical intervention in patients with severe head injuries (Stein et al. 2008).

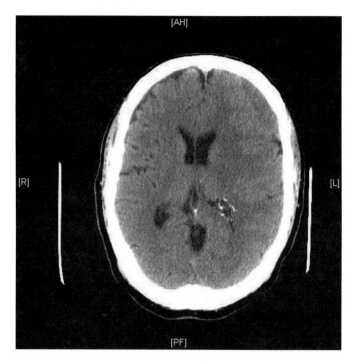

Figure 3 Left frontal isodense subdural in a septuagenarian with effortful speech and anemia after a fall.

The elderly are also afflicted with chronic subdural hematomas, which are usually of low density on CT scans, but may cause symptoms based on their localization or mass effect. The hematoma may sustain itself with the autoproduction of anti-clotting factors. Although occurring in less than 1% of the elderly, chronic subdurals are frequently encountered both in the outpatient setting as well as in the hospital. A twist drill craniostomy technique with drainage has been updated in recent years and is now performed under local anesthesia with minimal complications. For example, of 42 retrospectively studied patients between the ages of 65 to 97 years of age with chronic subdurals and mass effect, 88% achieved a good recovery at one week (Ramnarayan et al. 2008). Still, long term recurrences with this technique are problematic and more definitive studies are needed (Weigel, Schmiedek, and Krauss 2003).

Neuroprotective treatments for the human head-injured have been disappointing, despite the attainment of positive outcomes with such treatments in laboratory animal models. In the last decade, acute interventions such as hypothermia, intravenous magnesium, steroids, cannabinoids, and calcium channel blockers have all failed to demonstrate benefit in clinical trials. Intravenous progesterone has shown efficacy in an aged rodent model of head injury (Cutler et al. 2007) as well as in a recent younger aged human phase II trial, where progesterone not only did not cause harm but also reduced mortality by 57% compared to placebo, although worse clinical outcomes were measured at 30 days in the severely head injured subgroup (Wright et al. 2007).

The immunomodulator cyclosporine, when infused in a small group of younger patients with severe head injuries, demonstrated a trend toward improved six month functional outcomes (Hatton et al. 2008). Rosuvastatin may also be an immunomodulator, and when administered subacutely in the course of mild head injuries in younger patients with intracranial lesions on CT scans, resulted in improved memory and orientation in treated patients examined four months after their injury (Tapia-Perez et al. 2008).

Recently, a 15 day infusion of branch-chain amino acids within 90 days of head injury lessened clinical disability in predominately middle-aged adults compared to controls who received a general protein mixture infusion. The branch-chain amino acids were hypothesized to provide substrates for neurotransmitters as well as for ATP generation (Aquilani et al. 2008). Confirmatory studies of such novel interventions are obviously needed and will hopefully be performed, but even if phase III trials demonstrate benefit, the particular safety and efficacy of these agents in elderly head-injured patients will likely remain unexplored.

Natural Progression of Disease

Many factors, of course, determine the outcome of head-injured patients, including their medical comorbidities, pre-injury medications, mechanism and severity of head injuries, and medical and surgical treatments. Outcomes, not surprisingly, also depend on the particular outcome measures examined and when in the course of the head injury and rehabilitation these measurements took place.

Medications taken prior to head injuries have increasingly come under focus. Warfarin, as well as antithrombotics, has been inconsistently implicated. For example, in a study of 309 moderately head-injured patients with ages ranging from 30 to 75 years, patients with coagulopathy, defined as an INR greater than 1.3, had a 4.48 greater likelihood of a poor six month outcome than patients with normal INR values (Fabbri et al. 2008). Another study retrospectively reviewed 109 elderly, head-injured patients who were taking aspirin, clopidogrel, or both prior to the injury and compared them with 42 head injured controls. Those on the antithrombotics were more likely to have larger hemorrhages and more likely to die from smaller ones than the controls (Ivascu et al. 2008). A larger retrospective study examining 416 head injured patients with ages greater than 50 years who reported taking aspirin, plavix, or warfarin prior to admission actually found higher aggregate mortality rates in older patients who were not taking Coumadin or antithrombotics, despite the fact that the subgroup on warfarin actually had the highest mortality rate at 34% (Fortuna et al. 2008). Some of the discrepancies between these studies could reflect that medication usage was assessed with self-report, and elderly non-compliance with outpatient medications may be as high as 66% (Vik et al. 2004). Measures of platelet function and INR values may be more accurate.

More recently, pre-injury beta blockers have been associated with a trend toward lesser mortality in 568 head-injured patients over the age of 64 years compared to non-head injured general trauma controls (Neideem et al. 2008). Another retrospective analysis of 303 general trauma patients identified beta blocker treatment prior to or during hospitalization as a significant marker of lessened mortality (odds ratio 0.2) for those patients with head injuries (Saman et al. 2007). Despite their potential for hypotension, beta blockers may halt the catecholamine surge which occurs after head injury and contributes to the brain hypermetabolic state.

Recreational pharmaceuticals are also influential. Alcohol and amphetamine use as identified with admission toxicology screens was recently associated with significantly decreased mortality in 483 patients with severe head injuries. Neuroprotective effects may be at work, although clouding of the initial GCS by substance abuse temper these results (O'phelan et al. 2008).

More general outcome examinations were employed by the recent New Zealand/Australia prospective study of 635 patients with all degrees of head injury, which utilized a 12 month dichotomized Glasgow Outcome Scale whereby outcomes are either graded poor (dead, vegetative, or severely disabled) or good (moderately disabled but independent in daily activities or normal): overall mortality was 29% and favorable outcomes were achieved in 59% of

patients of all ages (Myburgh et al. 2008). By contrast, another study of 191 patients over the age of 65 with all degrees of head injury retrospectively found that those elderly presenting with a GCS less than 11 (approximating those with severe and moderate injuries) had invariably poor outcomes at the time of discharge from the hospital, while the overall mortality was comparable at 34% (Ritchie et al. 2000). Longer term outcomes in this study, unfortunately, were not measured.

Even mild head injuries may have lasting detrimental effects in the elderly. For example, a recent prospective study of the mildly head-injured compared 44 patients over 65 years of age with 187 younger patients and observed that at acute hospital discharge 23% of the elderly exhibited severe disability compared to only 9% of their younger counterparts, and good functional six month outcomes occurred in only 63% of the elderly compared to 80% of the younger group (Mosenthal et al. 2004). Similarly, only 21% of 52 patients aged greater than 54 years with mostly mild head injuries achieved good functional outcomes after six months (Yap et al. 2008). Finally, long-term outcomes are also likely compromised. One hundred forty-three patients between the ages of 40 to 85 with head injuries of all severities were compared to 285 younger head injured patients, and despite the older cohort having less severe initial head injuries, the older patients suffered more disability on both cognitive and functional independence measures five years after the initial injury (Marquez de la Plata et al. 2008).

In summary, the elderly experience an overall increase in mortality after closed head injuries (Table 3). However, those who survive do show gradual improvements in functioning, and even if current measurements, such as the dichotomized Glasgow Outcome Scale, fail to show that most elderly achieve functional independence after head injuries, substantive gains, nevertheless, have been achieved on selected functional measures. Such gains may help lessen their caregivers' burdens.

Rehabilitative/Psychological

Primary Pharmacological Interventions

No major studies have focused exclusively on the elderly head injured. The acetylcholinesterase inhibitor donepezil has been frequently studied as a cognitive enhancer in patients with head injuries, but most studies are non-randomized and employ small numbers of patients (Ballesteros et al. 2008). One exceptional double blind, placebo-controlled study of 18 closed head-injured patients between 19 and 57 years of age treated within 2 to 24 months of their injury showed a significant improvement in attention and memory during a ten week treatment phase (Zhang et al. 2004). Similar limitations pervade the medication trials of methylphenidate in head injury, but this medication, too, has demonstrated improved attention and disability rating scores after a 30 day treatment period in a double-blind, placebo-controlled study of 23 patients between the ages of 16 to 64 years (Plenger et al. 1996).

Because of their limited side effects, the serotonin re-uptake inhibitors are preferred for the treatment of depression in the setting of closed head injury (Flanagan et al. 2006). Sertraline, for instance, has shown efficacy in a non-randomized eight week trial in patients with mild closed head injuries between 24 to 54 years of age (Fann et al. 2000). Pharmacologic control of agitation is more difficult with little empiric guidance available, although a recent review has suggested that, in general, beta-blockers have shown more efficacy here than other classes of medications (Fleminger et al. 2006). However, beta-blockers are poorly tolerated in the elderly, and the author prefers quetiapine for its sedative qualities and lack of clinically important

Table 3 Selected Contemporary Studies of Functional Outcomes of Head Injury in the Elderly

Researchers	Number of Patients/ Number of Elderly Patients	Initial Severity(GSC)	Outcome Measures	Time of Outcome Assessment after Injury	Outcome
MyBurgh et al. (2008)	635/NA	Median GCS: 7	Death; Extended Glasgow Outcome Score (eGOS)	12 month	Death: 29%; Favorable: 59%
Ritchie et al. (2000)	191/191	Median: 13–15	Death; Glasgow Outcome Scale (GOS)	Hospital discharge	Death: 33.5%; Good: 47.6 %
Frankel et al. (2006)	534/267 aged 55 and over	Mean: 12	Disability rating scale (DRS); Function independence measure (FIM)	Rehabilitation discharge	81% of elderly discharged home
Mosenthal et al. (2004)	231/44 aged 65 and over	Mean: 13	GOS; FIM	6 months	Good: 63% of elderly; 80% of young
Marquez de la Plata (2008)	428/143 aged 40 to 85	Mean: 8 younger; 10 older	DRS: eGOS; FIM	5 years	Older patients with greater disability ratings
Yap et al. (2008)	52 aged 55 and over	43% 13-15	Barthel Index; GOS	6 months	Good: 21%

parkinsonian side effects, but blood pressure monitoring is imperative given quetiapine's hypotensive effects.

The treatment of spasticity in the elderly is also problematic because of the potentially sedating effects of medications, but baclofen or tizanidine would be customary choices. Botulinum toxin could also be employed (Richardson et al. 2000). Spasticity treatment should emphasize control of pain and improved flexibility for hygiene because overzealous pharmacologic treatment of spasticity may destabilize ambulation.

Other Interventions

Constraint-induced therapy has been used in small numbers of primarily younger patients with traumatic brain injuries with promising results. The unaffected limb is restrained, typically in a mitten, while use of the affected limb is encouraged. Such therapy for two weeks resulted in both objective and subjective improvements in the affected upper limb in 22 patients with a mean age of 39 years, although after two years a 21% decline in function was noted (Shaw et al. 2005). Neuronal plasticity, whereby uninjured brain takes over the functioning of damaged brain regions, is the hypothesized mechanism, and this has been supported with functional MRI and transcranial magnetic stimulation studies.

Increased therapy intensity, defined as the total number of rehabilitative therapy hours divided by the length of stay, has been also correlated with improved motor outcomes in a large study of 491 predominately younger patients with all severities of head injuries (Cifu et al. 2003). Curiously, both speech and physical therapy were significant predictors of improved motor outcomes at discharge from rehabilitation, while no therapeutic modalities demonstrably contributed to cognitive gains. Another prospective study of 135 patients with severe head injuries and a mean age of 40 years who entered an early, multimodal rehabilitation program, involving expeditious transfer from an intensive care setting to a 1.5 to 3 hour per day therapy program, resulted in 62% of these patients achieving good to excellent outcomes after three months, improving more than expected based on historic controls (Choi et al. 2008).

More research is clearly needed to address the head-injured elderly with multiple co-morbidities and determine not only when to begin therapy and what therapies to employ, but why certain treatment modalities are more effective than others.

Future Directions

Head injury in the elderly is incompletely understood. The entire process takes place in an already compromised system secondary to both aging and multiple medical comorbidities. Compromised central nervous system reserve was hypothesized to account for the worse performance on cognitive testing in head-injured patients with premorbid neurologic injuries compared to their premorbidly pristine counterparts, despite comparable severities of the head injuries in both groups at the time of the testing (Ropacki and Elias 2003). Similarly, in another study, longer posttraumatic amnestic durations were correlated with less education and lower pre-injury IQ scores (Dawson et al. 2007). Unfortunately, while central nervous system reserve remains a practical framework at the bedside and can perhaps help explain the substantial declines which occur from historically modest head injuries in the elderly, it lacks quantitative rigor and the capacity to offer outcome predictions for individual patients. Perhaps newer biomarkers and improved neuroimaging methods will enable more precise use of the central nervous system reserve construct.

Some researchers have physiologically located such central nervous system reserve, at least in part, in the generation of new neurons in the hippocampus (Kemperman 2008). Adult neurogenesis as well as anatomic plasticity is only beginning to be understood, but offers a new realm of treatment options as pharmacologic enhancers of restoring neurologic functioning are developed. Axonal growth promoters and agents to counter growth-inhibiting factors are also in the works (Priestley 2007). Neurogenesis and plasticity could also be achieved with stem cell implantations, which could potentially not only differentiate into the phenotype of the trauma-damaged cells, but also provide growth factors and other elements which enhance neuroprotection and regeneration (Maegele and Schaefer 2008).

Finally, neuroprosthetics is gaining ground. Monkeys have been successful at feeding themselves with a robotic limb activated by their own motor cortical firing patterns (Velliste et al. 2008). Such prostheses would benefit not only countless elderly with paralysis from head injuries, but paralysis from other neurologic and non-neurologic etiologies. Unfortunately, brain injury is usually diffuse, and cognitive impairments are unlikely to be amenable to such prostheses. Nevertheless, deep brain stimulation of the hypothalamus and fornix has produced enhancement of mnemonic functioning in a solitary patient treated for morbid obesity (McKhann 2008); this modality offers obvious future therapeutic potential for cognitively impaired elderly brain-injured patients as well.

Summary

Head injuries in the elderly are problematic and inexorably increasing. They are physiologically complex injuries which cause both immediate mechanical damage as well as delayed cellular destruction. The manifestations of head injuries are influenced by not only the pre-existing genotype of the patient, but also their medical comorbidities. Although acute mortality may be worse in the elderly compared to younger patients, ultimately a large proportion of the elderly can return to some measure of independence. Careful medical attention as well as pharmacologic and physiatric rehabilitation allows maximal recovery. Advances in neuroscience along with neuroimaging, biomarkers, and rehabilitative techniques will hopefully translate into improved outcomes at the bedside.

References

Abuabara A.: Cerebrospinal fluid rhinorrhoea: Diagnosis and management. *Med Oral Patol Oral Cir Bucal* 12(5): E397–400, 2007.

Aquilani R., Boselli M., Boschi F., et al.: Branched-chain amino acids may improve recovery from a vegetative or minimally conscious state in patients with traumatic brain injury: A pilot study. *Arch Phys Med Rehabil* 89(9): 1642–7, 2008.

Ballesteros J., Guemes I., Ibarra N., et al.: The effectiveness of donepezil for cognitive rehabilitation after traumatic brain injury: A systematic review. *J Head Trauma Rehabil* 23(3): 171–80, 2008.

Basson O.J. and van Lierop A.C.: Conductive hearing loss after head trauma: Review of ossicular pathology, management and outcomes. *J Laryngol Otol* 19: 1–5, 2008.

Blicher J.U. and Nielsen J.F.: Does long-term outcome after intensive inpatient rehabilitation of acquired brain injury depend on etiology? *Neurorehab* 23(2): 175–83, 2008.

Blumbergs P.C., Scott G., Manavis J., et al.: Topography of axonal injury as defined by amyloid precursor protein and the sector scoring method in mild and severe closed head injury. *J Neurotrauma* 12(4): 565–72, 1995.

Boyd C.M., Darer J., Boult C., et al.: Clinical practice guidelines and quality of care for older patients with multiple comorbid diseases: Implications for pay for performance. *JAMA* 294(6): 716–24, 2005.

Brain Trauma Foundation. Guidelines for the management of severe head injury. *J Neurotrauma* 13: 639–734, 1996.

Centers for Disease Control: The State of Aging and Health in America 2004. www.cdc.gov (accessed on November 30, 2008).

Choi J.H., Jakob M., Stapf C., et al.: Multimodal early rehabilitation and predictors of outcome in survivors of severe traumatic brain injury. *J Trauma* 65(5): 1028–35, 2008.

Cifu D.X., Kreutzer J.S., Kolakowsky-Hayner S.A., et al.: The relationship between therapy intensity and rehabilitative outcomes after traumatic brain injury: A multicenter analysis. *Arch Phys Med Rehabil* 84: 1441–48, 2003.

Coronado V.G., Thomas K.E., Sattin R.W., et al.: The CDC traumatic brain injury surveillance system: Characteristics of persons aged 65 years and older hospitalized with a TBI. *J Head Trauma Rehabil* 20(3): 215–228, 2005.

Cutler S.M., Cekic M., Miller D.M., et al.: Progesterone improves acute recovery after traumatic brain injury in the aged rat. *J Neurotrauma* 24(9): 1475–86, 2007.

Czosnyka M, Balestreri M. Steiner L., et al.: Age, intracranial pressure, autoregulation, and outcome after brain trauma. *J Neurosurg* 102: 450–454, 2005.

Dawson K.S., Batchelor J., Meares S., et al.: Applicability of neural reserve theory in mild traumatic brain injury. *Brain Inj* 21(9): 943–9, 2007.

Diaz-Arrastia R. and Baxter V.K.: Genetic Factors in outcome after traumatic brain injury: What the human genome project can teach us about brain trauma. *J Head Trauma Rehabil* 21(4): 361–74, 2006.

Doe J.W. and Jay W.M.: Traumatic unilateral internuclear ophthalmoplegia. *Semin Ophthalmol* 21(4): 245–53, 2006.

Draper K. and Ponsford J.: Cognitive functioning ten years following traumatic brain injury and rehabilitation. *Neuropsychology* 22(5): 618–24, 2008.

Dressler J., Hanisch U., Kuhlisch E., et al.: Neuronal and glial apoptosis in human traumatic brain injury. *Int J Legal Med* 121: 365–375, 2007.

Duong T.T., Englander J., Wright J., et al.: Relationship between strength, balance, and swallowing deficits and outcome after traumatic brain injury: A multicenter analysis. *Arch Phys Med Rehabil* 85(8): 1291–7, 2004.

Fabbri A., Servadei F., Marchesini G., et al.: Early predictors of unfavorable outcome in subjects with moderate head injury in the emergency department. *J Neurol Neurosurg Psychiatry* 79(5): 567–73, 2008.

Fann J.R., Uomoto J.M., and Katon W.J.: Sertraline in the treatment of major depression following mild traumatic brain injury. *J Neuropsychiatry Clin Neurosci* 12(2): 226–32, 2000.

Flanagan S. R., Hibbard M.R., Riojordan B., et al.: Traumatic brain injury in the elderly: Diagnostic and treatment challenges. *Clin Geriatr Med* 22(2): 449–68, 2006.

Fleminger S., Greenwood R.J., and Oliver D.L.: Pharmacological management for agitation and aggression in people with acquired brain injury. *Cochrane Database Syst Rev* Oct 18 (4): CD003299, 2006.

Fletcher A.E., Khalid S., and Mallonee S.: The epidemiology of severe traumatic brain injury among persons 65 years of age and older in Oklahoma, 1992–2003. *Brain Injury* 21(7): 691–699, 2007.

Fortuna G. R., Mueller E.W., James L.E., et al.: The impact of preinjury antiplatelet and anticoagulant pharmacotherapy on outcomes in elderly patients with hemorrhagic brain injury. *Surgery* 144: 598–605, 2008.

Frankel J.E., Marwitz J.H., Cifu D.X., et al.: A follow-up of older adults with traumatic brain injury: taking into account decreasing length of stay. *Arch Phys Med Rehabil* 87(1): 57–62, 2006.

Friedman G., Froom P., Sazbon L., et al.: Apolipoprotein E-epsilon4 genotype predicts a poor outcome in survivors of traumatic brain injury. *Neurology* 52(2): 244–8, 1999.

Goldschlanger T., Rosenfeld J.V., and Winter C.D.: 'Talk and die' patients presenting to a major trauma centre over a 10 year period: A critical review. *J Clin Neurosci* 14(7): 618–23, 2007.

Guzel A., Uygur E. Tatli M., et al.: Serum neuron-specific enolase as a predictor of short-term outcome and its correlation with Glasgow Coma Scale in traumatic brain injury. *Neurosurg Rev* 31: 439–445, 2008.

Hadjigeorgiou G.M., Paterakis K., Dardiotis E., et al.: IL-1RN and IL-1B gene polymorphisms and cerebral hemorrhagic events after traumatic brain injury. *Neurology* 65: 1077–1082, 2005.

Haider A.H., Chang D.C., Haut E.R., et al.: Mechanism of injury predicts patient mortality and impairment after blunt trauma. *J Surg Res* (in press), 2008.

Hardy J.E. and Brennan N.: Computerized tomography of the brain for elderly patients presenting to the emergency department with acute confusion. *Emergency Medicine Australasia* 20: 420–24, 2008.

Hartl R., Gerber L.M., Ni Q., et al.: Effect of early nutrition on deaths due to severe traumatic brain injury. *J Neurosurg* 109(1): 50–6, 2008.

Hatton J., Rosbolt B., Empey P., et al.: Dosing and safety of cyclosporine in patients with severe brain injury. *J Neurosurg* 109(4): 699–707, 2008.

Huang S.J., Hong W.C., Han Y.Y., et al.: Clinical outcome of severe head injury in different protocol-driven therapies. *J Clin Neurosci* 14(5): 449–54, 2007.

Hutchinson P.J., O'Connell M.T., Rothwell N.J., et al.: Inflammation in human brain injury: Intracerebral concentrations of IL-1alpha, IL-1beta, and their endogenous inhibitor IL-1ra. *Journal of Neurotrauma* 24: 1545–1557, 2007.

Ivascu F.A., Howells G.A., Junn F.S., et al.: Predictors of mortality in trauma patients with intracranial hemorrhage on preinjury aspirin or clopidogrel. *J Trauma* 65: 785–8, 2008.

Jeremitsky E., Omert L., Dunhan C., et al.: Harbingers of poor outcome the day after severe brain injury: Hypothermia, hypoxia, and hypoperfusion. *J Trauma* 54(2): 312–319, 2003.

Jones K.E., Puccio A.M., Harshman K.J., et al.: Levetiracetam versus phenytoin for seizure prophylaxis in severe traumatic brain injury. *Neurosurg Focus* 25(4): 1–5, 2008.

Kato T., Nakayama N., Yasokawa Y., et al.: Statistical image analysis of cerebral glucose metabolism in patients with cognitive impairment following diffuse traumatic brain injury. *J Neurotrauma* 24(6): 919–26, 2007.

Kempermann G.: The neurogenic reserve hypothesis: What is adult hippocampal neurogenesis good for? *Trends Neurosci* 31(4): 163–9, 2008.

Kors E.E., Terwindt G.M., Vermeulen F.L.M.G., et al.: Delayed cerebral edema and fatal coma after minor head trauma: Role of the CACNA1A calcium channel subunit gene and relationship with familial hemiplegic migraine. *Ann Neurol* 49: 753–760, 2001.

Lachs M.S. and Pillemer K.: Elder abuse. *The Lancet* 364: 1263–72, 2004.

Leclercq P.D., McKenzie J.E., Graham D.I., et al.: Axonal injury is accentuated in the caudal corpus callosum of head-injured patients. *Journal of Neurotrauma* 18(1): 1–9, 2001.

Lee J.H., Martin N.A., Alsina G., et al.: Hemodynamically significant cerebral vasospasm and outcome after head injury: A prospective study. *J Neurosurg* 87: 221–223, 1997.

Lerut B., De Vuyst C., Ghekiere J., et al.: Post-traumatic pulsatile tinnitus: The hallmark of a direct carotico-cavernous fistula. *J Laryngol Otol* 121(11): 1103–7, 2007.

Lipsky R.H., Sparling M.B., Ryan L.M., et al.: Association of COMT Val158Met genotype with executive functioning following traumatic brain injury. *J Neuropsychiatry Clin Neurosci* 17: 465–71, 2005.

Lumpkins K.M., Bochichio G.V., Keledjian K., et al.: Glial fibrillary acidic protein is highly correlated with brain injury. *J Trauma* 65: 778–82, 2008.

Mack L.R., Chan S.B., Silva J.C., et al.: The use of head computed tomography in elderly patients sustaining minor head trauma. *The Journal of Emergency Medicine* 24(2): 157–162, 2003.

Maegele M. and Schaefer U.: Stem cell-based cellular replacement strategies following traumatic brain injury. *Minimally Invasive Therapy* 17(2): 119–31, 2008.

Marquez de la Plata C.D., Hart T., Hammond F.M., et al.: Impact of age on long-term recovery from traumatic brain injury. *Arch Phys Med Rehabil* 89: 896–903, 2008.

Martinez-Lucas P., Moreno-Cuesta J., Garcia-Olmo D.C., et al.: Relationship between the Arg72Pro polymorphism of p53 and outcome for patients with traumatic brain injury. *Intensive Care Med* 31(9): 1168–73, 2005.

Matsuyama T., Shimomura T., Okumura Y., et al.: Acute subdural hematomas due to rupture of cortical arteries: A study of the points of rupture in 19 cases. *Surgical Neurology* 47(5): 423–7, 1997.

McKhann G.M.: Memory enhancement by hypothalamic/fornix deep brain stimulation. *Neurosurgery* 62(4): N8, 2008.

Mosenthal A.C., Lavery R.F., Addis, M., et al.: Isolated traumatic brain injury: Age is an independent predictor of mortality and early outcome. *The Journal of Trauma* 52(5): 907–11, 2002.

Mosenthal A.C., Livingston D.H., Lavery R.F., et al.: The effect of age on functional outcome in mild traumatic brain injury: 6-month report of a prospective multicenter trial. *J Trauma* 56: 1042–1048, 2004.

Myburgh J.A., Cooper D.J., Finfer S.R., et al.: Epidemiology and 12-month outcomes from traumatic brain injury in Australia and New Zealand. *J Trauma* 64(4): 854–62, 2008.

Nakashima T., Nakayama N., Miwa K., et al.: Focal brain glucose hypometabolism in patients with neuropsychologic deficits after diffuse axonal injury. *AJNR* 28(2): 236–42, 2007.

Napoli A.M. and Panagos P.: Delayed presentation of traumatic facial nerve (CN VII) paralysis. *J Emerg Med* 29(4): 421–4, 2005.

Narayan R.K., Maas A.L.R., Servadel F., et al.: Progression of traumatic intracerebral hemorrhage: a prospective observational study. *Journal of Neurotrauma* 25: 629–639, 2007.

Narayan R.K., Maas A. I., Marshall L.F., et al.: Recombinant factor VIIa in traumatic intracerebral hemorrhage: Results of a dose-escalation clinical trial. *Neurosurgery* 62(4): 776–86, 2008.

Neideen T., Lam M. and Brasel K.J.: Preinjury beta blockers are associated with increased mortality in geriatric trauma patients. *J Trauma* 65(5): 1016–20, 2008.

Nylen K., Ost M., Csajbok L.Z., et al.: Serum levels of S100B, S100A1B, and S100BB are all related to outcome after severe traumatic brain injury. *Acta Neurochir (Wien)* 150(3): 221–7, 2008.

Odebode T.O and Ologe F.E., Facial nerve palsy after head injury: Case incidence, causes, clinical profile and outcome. *J Trauma* 61(2): 388–91, 2006.

Oertal M., Boscardin W.J., Obrist W.D., et al.: Posttraumatic vasospasm: The epidemiology, severity, and time course of an underestimated phenomenon: A prospective study performed in 299 patients. *J Neurosurg* 103(5): 812–24, 2005.

O'phelan K., McArthur D.L., Chang C.W., et al.: The impact of substance abuse on mortality in patients with severe traumatic brain injury. *J Trauma* 65(3): 674–677, 2008.

Pelinka L.E., Hertz H., Mauritz W., et al.: Nonspecific increase of systemic neuron-specific enolase after trauma: Clinical and experimental findings. *Shock* 24(2): 119–123, 2005.

Plenger P.M., Dixon C.E., Castillo R.M., et al.: Subacute methylphenidate treatment for moderate to moderately severe traumatic brain injury: A preliminary double-blind placebo-controlled study. *Arch Phys Med Rehabil* 77(6): 536–40, 1996.

Pompucci A., De Bonis P., Pettorini B., et al.: Decompressive craniectomy for traumatic brain injury: Patient age and outcome. *Journal of Neurotrauma* 24(7): 1182–1188, 2007.

Priestley J.V.: Promoting anatomical plasticity and recovery of function after traumatic injury to the central or peripheral nervous system. *Brain* 130: 895–897, 2007.

Ramnarayan R., Arulmurugan B., Wilson P.M., et al.: Twist drill craniostomy with closed drainage for chronic subdural haematoma in the elderly: An effective method. *Clin Neurol Neurosurg* 110(8): 774–778, 2008.

Richardson D., Sheean G., Werring D., et al.: Evaluating the role of botulinum toxin in the management of focal hypertonia in adults. *J Neurol Neurosurg Psychiatry* 69(4): 499–506, 2000.

Ritchie P.D., Cameron P.A., Ugoni A.M., et al.: A study of the functional outcome and mortality in elderly patients with head injuries. *J Clin Neurosci* 7(4): 301–304, 2000.

Ropacki M.T. and Elias J.W.: Preliminary examination of cognitive reserve theory in closed head injury. *Archives of Clinical Neuropsychology* 18: 643–654, 2003.

Routsi C., Stamataki E., Nanas S., et al.: Increased levels of serum S100B protein in critically ill patients without brain injury. *Shock* 26: 20–24, 2006.

Rutgers D. R., Toulgoat F., Cazejust J., et al.: White matter abnormalities in mild traumatic brain injury: A diffusion tensor imaging study. *AJNR* 29: 514–519, 2008.

Rutland-Brown W., Langlois J.A., and Thomas K.E.: Incidence of traumatic brain injury in the United States, 2003. *J Head Trauma Rehabil* 21(6): 544–548, 2006.

SAFE Study Investigators: Saline or albumin for fluid resuscitation in patients with traumatic brain injury. *NEJM* 357: 874–84, 2007.

Sahuaquillo J. and Arikan F.: Decompressive craniectomy for the treatment of refractory high intracranial pressure in traumatic brain injury. *Cochrane Database Syst Rev* Jan 25(1): CD003983, 2006.

Salim A., Hadjizacharia P., DuBose J., et al.: Role of anemia in traumatic brain injury. *J Am Coll Surg* 207(3): 398–405, 2008.

Saman A. Campion E.M., Hemmila M.R., et al.: Beta-blocker use is associated with improved outcomes in adult trauma patients. *J Trauma* 62(1): 56–62, 2007.

Schirmer C.M., Ackil A.A., and Malek A.M.: Decompressive craniectomy. *Neurocrit Care* 8(3): 456–470, 2008.

Shafi S., Diaz-Arrastia R., Madden C., et al.: Intracranial pressure monitoring in brain-injured patients is associated with worsening of survival. *J Trauma* 64(2): 335–340, 2008.

Shaw S.E., Morris D.M., Uswatte G., et al.: Constraint-induced movement therapy for recovery of upper-limb function following traumatic brain injury. *J Rehabil Res Dev* 42(6): 769–78, 2005.

Smits M., Dippel D.W.J., Steyerberg E.W., et al.: Predicting intracranial traumatic findings on computed tomography in patients with minor head injury: The CHIP prediction rule. *Ann Intern Med* 146: 397–405, 2007.

Stein D.M., Dutton R.P., Kramer M.E., et al.: Recombinant factor VIIa: Decreasing time to intervention in coagulopathic patients with severe traumatic brain injury. *J Trauma* 64(3): 620–627, 2008.

Stein S.C., Fabbri A., and Servadei F.: Routine serial computed tomographic scans in mild traumatic brain injury: When are they cost-effective? *J Trauma* 65(1): 66–72, 2008.

Straume-Naesheim T.M., Andersen T.E., Jochum M., et al.: Minor head trauma in soccer and serum levels of S100B. *Neurosurgery* 62(6): 1297–1305, 2008.

Swann I.J., Bauza-Rodriguez B., Currans R., et al.: The significance of post-traumatic amnesia as a risk factor in the development of olfactory dysfunction following head injury. *Emerg Med J* 23: 618–621, 2006.

Tallon J.M., Ackroyd-Stolarz S., Karim S.A., et al.: The epidemiology of surgically treated acute subdural and epidural hematomas in patients with head injuries: A population-based study. *Can J Surg* 51(5): 339–345, 2008.

Tapia-Perez J.H., Sanchez-Aguillar M., Torres-Corzo J.G., et al.: Effect of rosuvastatin on amnesia and disorientation after traumatic brain injury. *J Neurotrauma* 25(8): 1011–1017, 2008.

Temkin N.R., Dikmen S.S., Wilensky A.J., et al.: A randomized, double-blind study of phenytoin for the prevention of post-traumatic seizures. *NEJM* 323(8): 497–502, 1990.

Temkin N.R., Anderson G.D., Winn H.R., et al.: Magnesium sulfate for neuroprotection after traumatic brain injury: A randomized controlled trial. *Lancet Neurology* 6: 29–38, 2007.

Terre R. and Mearin F.: Prospective evaluation of oro-pharyngeal dysphagia after severe traumatic brain injury. *Brain Injury* 21: 1411–1417, 2007.

Thomas KE, Stevens JA, Sarmiento K, et al.: Fall-related brain injury deaths and hospitalizations among older adults - United States, 2005. *Journal of Safety Research* 39: 269–272, 2008.

Tian H.L., Geng Z., Cui Y.H., et al.: Risk factors for posttraumatic cerebral infarction in patients with moderate or severe head trauma. *Neurosurg Rev* 31(4): 431–437, 2008.

Tien H.C., Cunha J.R., Wu S.N., et al.: Do trauma patients with a Glasgow Coma Scale score of 3 and bilateral fixed and dilated pupils have any chance of survival? *J Trauma* 60 (2):274–280, 2006.

Tisdall M., Crocker M., Watkiss J., et al.: Disturbances of sodium in critically ill adult neurologic patients: A clinical review. *J Neurosurg Anesthesiol* 18(1): 57–63, 2006.

Topal N.B., Hakyemez B., Erdogan C., et al.: MR imaging in the detection of diffuse axonal injury with mild traumatic brain injury. *Neurol Res* 30(9): 974–978, 2008.

Uzan M., Eraman H., Tanriverdi T., et al.: Evaluation of apoptosis in the cerebrospinal fluid of patients after severe head injuries. *Acta Neurochir (Wien)* 148(11): 1157–1164, 2006.

Velliste M., Perel S., Spalding M.C., et al.: Cortical control of a prosthetic arm for self-feeding. *Nature* 453(7198): 1098–1101, 2008.

Vik A., Nag T., Fredriksli O.A., et al.: Relationship of "dose" of intracranial hypertension to outcome in severe traumatic brain injury. *J Neurosurg* 109(4): 678–684, 2008.

Vik S.A., Maxwell C.J., and Hogan D.B.: Measurement, correlates, and health outcomes of medication adherence among seniors. *Ann Pharmacother* 38: 303–312, 2004.

Wagner A.K., Sasser H.C., Hammond F.M., et al.: Intentional traumatic brain injury: Epidemiology, risk factors, and associations with injury severity and mortality. *J Trauma* 49(3): 404–410, 2000.

Wang H.E., Peitzman A.B., Cassidy L.D., et al.: Out-of-hospital endotracheal intubation and outcome after traumatic brain injury. *Ann Emerg Med* 44(5): 439–450, 2000.

Weigel R., Schmiedek P., and Krauss J.K.: Outcome of contemporary surgery for chronic subdural haematoma: Evidence based review. *J Neurol Neurosurg Psychiatry* 74(7): 937–943, 2003.

White H. and Venkatesh B.: Cerebral perfusion pressure in neurotrauma: A review. *Anesth Analg* 107(3): 979–988, 2008.

Willemse-van Son A.H.P., Ribbers G.M., Hop W.C.J., et al.: Association between apolipoprotein-E4 and long-term outcome after traumatic brain injury. *J Neurol Neurosurg Psychiatry* 79: 426–430, 2008.

Winter C.D., Pringle A.K., Clough G.F., et al.: Raised parenchymal interleukin-6 levels correlate with improved outcomes after traumatic brain injury. *Brain* 127:315–320, 2004.

Wright D.W., Kellermann A.L., Hertzberg V.S., et al.: ProTECT: A randomized clinical trial of progesterone for acute traumatic brain injury. *Annals of Emergency Medicine* 49 (4): 391–402, 2007.

Wu N., Yin Z.Q., and Wang Y.: Traumatic optic neuropathy therapy: An update of clinical and experimental studies. *J Int Med Res* 36(5): 883–889, 2008.

Yap S.G.M. and Chua K.S.: Rehabilitation outcomes in elderly patients with traumatic brain injury in Singapore. *The Journal of Head Trauma Rehabilitation* 23(3): 158–163, 2008.

Yi J. and Hazell A.S., Excitotoxic mechanisms and the role of astrocytic glutamate transporters in traumatic brain injury. *Neurochemistry International* 48: 394–403, 2006.

Yilmazlar S., Arsian E., Kocaeli H., et al.: Cerebrospinal fluid leakage complicating skull base fractures: Analysis of 81 cases. *Neurosurg Rev* 29(1): 64–71, 2006.

Zehtabchi S., Soghoian S., Liu Y., et al.: The association of coagulopathy and traumatic brain injury in patients with isolated head injury. *Resuscitation* 76: 52–56, 2008.

Zhang L., Plotkin R.C., Wang G., et al.: Cholinergic augmentation with Donepezil enhances recovery in short-term memory and sustained attention after traumatic brain injury. *Arch Phys Med Rehabil* 85: 1050–1055, 2004.

Zhou W., Xu D., Peng X., et al.: Meta-analysis of APOE4 allele and outcome after traumatic brain injury. *J Neurotrauma* 25(4): 279–290, 2008.

42 Language Changes Associated with Aging

Loraine K. Obler, Martin L. Albert, Avron Spiro, III, Mira Goral, Elena Rykhlevskaia, JungMoon Hyun, Christopher B. Brady, and David Schnyer

Many language abilities do not change with advancing age; however, certain ones do (Burke 2006; Burke and MacKay 1997; Burke et al. 2000; Cortese et al. 2003; Kemper et al. 1992; Kemper and Sumner 2001; Wingfield and Stine-Morrow 2000). Research over the past 30 years in the Language in the Aging Brain (LAB) project at the VA Boston Healthcare System (Boston University School of Medicine, Martin Albert and Loraine Obler, co-PIs) has documented numerous language processes that do not change with age (e.g., at the levels of phonology, morphology, discourse when memory demands are not great), and has focused on the two aspects of language skills whose vulnerability to normal aging poses the greatest problems for elders and those who communicate with them: lexical retrieval in language production and sentence processing (e.g., Au et al. 1995; Connor et al. 2004; Goral et al. 2007; Goral et al. in press; Obler et al. 1985; Obler and Albert 1999).

Crucially, however, not all elders have difficulty with lexical retrieval or sentence processing (e.g., Wingfield and Grossman 2006). Moreover, the degree to which concomitant age-related cognitive and sensory changes contribute to language difficulties is not well understood. To explain these observations, we have proposed the hypothesis that age-related declines in certain language functions are mediated by brain-based changes in executive system functions associated with declining vascular health. In this chapter we review literature on age-related changes in lexical retrieval and sentence processing, considering, in particular, clinically relevant cognitive-related, health-related, and brain-related aspects of these changes.

Lexical Processes in Aging

Although there is general consensus that lexical-retrieval skills (i.e., locating intended lexical items in order to speak them) decline with age (Au et al. 1995; Barresi et al. 2000; Burke et al. 1991; Feyereisen 1997; Kaplan et al. 1983; Nicholas et al. 1985), cognitive aging researchers continue to debate whether this decline is a normal part of aging. Most studies of lexical retrieval have used picture-naming tasks (e.g., the Boston Naming Test: Kaplan, Goodglass and Weintraub 1983) as well as verbal fluency tasks, and recently an idiom production task (Conner et al. submitted). However, not all lexical-retrieval tasks and items appear to be equally sensitive to age-related change (Goral et al. 2007). On verbal fluency tests (where participants are asked to list as many words of a certain type in one minute), which require a different type of lexical search than picture-naming tasks, large age differences have been found on semantic fluency tasks (e.g., animal list generation), with relatively smaller or no differences found on phonemic fluency tasks (e.g., Boone et al. 1990; Parkin and Walter 1991; Whelihan and Lesher 1985). Troyer et al. (1997) showed that age differences in fluency performance are related to older adults being less able to switch among semantic subcategories (e.g., switching from birds to mammals during tests of animal fluency).

Using longitudinal data on the Boston Naming Test collected over 20 years from participants aged 30 to 94, we examined change in lexical retrieval with age, adjusting for gender, education, and their interactions, comparing the results of random-effects longitudinal and traditional cross-sectional models (Connor et al. 2004). Random-effects modeling revealed significant linear and quadratic change in lexical retrieval with age; it also showed an interaction between gender and education, indicating poorest performance for women with less education. Cross-sectional analyses revealed a similar pattern but produced greater estimates of change with age than did longitudinal analyses. Based on the longitudinal analysis, we found that decline in naming ability starts earlier than reported previously. Longitudinal studies show that naming abilities peak in the 30s, and problems with naming thereafter increase progressively with advancing age, with more rapid decline starting in the mid-60s, somewhat less obviously for individuals with higher education (Goral et al. 2007).

To further study the change in lexical-retrieval skills in adulthood (Goral et al. 2007), we used a mixed models approach to refine our understanding of the acceleration of decline in object naming with increasing age. In this study, we dissociated lexical-retrieval performance on picture naming (ANT and BNT) and verbal fluency (category and letter fluency) tasks. While ANT and BNT show a non-linear, accelerated decline with increasing age, verbal fluency tasks do not. Within verbal fluency tasks, we see a dissociation, with semantic fluency showing a linear, non-accelerating decline with increasing age. By contrast, letter fluency skills first increase and then decline in adulthood, but without acceleration. Vocabulary increases with age, as others have found. This series of analyses adds to our understanding of age-related lexical retrieval deficits, as we now see that different retrieval processes (picture naming, category-based list generation, and phoneme-based list generation) show different trajectories of decline and may therefore have different underlying causes. Future research should focus on possible differences in underlying neural mechanisms to account for these differences in age-related decline in lexical retrieval.

It now appears that older adults show increased variability of responses in discourse-level lexical retrieval (Obler et al. 2007): To broaden our understanding of the contexts in which older adults experience lexical retrieval difficulties, we created a discourse-level lexical retrieval task, using the picture book *'Frog, Where Are You?'* Participants were asked to narrate the story, and include in their narration the salient items (33 objects and 24 actions) we had circled in the book. Responses were coded as correct, incorrect, or acceptable alternates (which were not the expected target response yet were not incorrect). Acceptable alternates were further divided into nonspecific (e.g. animal for deer) or specific (e.g., lake for pond). In a study of 143 participants ages 45–95, we found that the older adults were significantly less likely to produce the expected target response for both actions and objects. In addition, we found that older adults were more likely than younger adults to produce off-target nouns, whether specific or non-specific, but there was no significant difference for verbs. This study provides evidence that older adults have difficulty retrieving specific words even in the context-rich environment of discourse.

Although there is now consensus that older adults experience lexical retrieval deficits, it is unclear how these deficits are related to specific components of lexical search mechanisms (e.g., Belke and Meyer 2007; Shafto et al. 2007). We have proposed that components of executive and other cognitive functions that decline with age, especially those linked to vascular risk factors, underlie difficulties with lexical search mechanisms. To assess this hypothesis, we have employed tasks that vary in search requirements: the Action Naming Test (ANT) and Boston Naming Test (BNT), which require the retrieval of specific lexical items in response to picture stimulus, letter fluency tasks requiring retrieval of words beginning with a single letter, and semantic fluency tasks requiring the retrieval of items from a semantic category. In addition, we use a Rapid Automatized Naming (RAN) task that requires the inhibition of semantically-related items and may be likely to elicit perseverative responses. Such tasks should permit us to determine the extent to which the executive functions are linked to naming abilities.

The literature on possible age-related changes in lexical access during sentence processing suggests little or no age-related change (e.g., Griffin and Spieler 2006; Kemper and Liu 2007; Spieler and Griffin 2006; Stern et al. 1991), although some studies (e.g., Wingfield et al. 1991; Howard et al. 1986; Sommers 1996) show problems with lexical and/or semantic activation. Age-related delays in lexical access (e.g., Laver and Burke 1993) likely contribute to age-related problems with sentence processing; frontal lobe recruitment for elders' speech recognition has been postulated to play a role (Eckert et al. 2008).

Indeed, we have found that frontal brain regions are associated with individual differences in naming in older adults (Obler et al. 2010). To explore structural brain correlates of lexical retrieval we collected structural magnetic resonance imaging(MRI) as well as diffusion tensor images of the brain from 23 adults (aged 56–79 years). The Boston Naming Test (BNT) and Action Naming Test (ANT) were administered to these participants, yielding reaction time and accuracy scores for each subject. Voxel-base morphometry analysis (VBM; Ashburner and Friston 2000) was conducted on structural MR images to measure individual differences in local concentration of brain tissue in a voxel-wise fashion. As found by others (e.g. Smith et al. 2007), age was negatively correlated with local density of gray matter in temporal, cingulate, occipital, and orbitofrontal regions. The local density of white matter was negatively correlated with age in symmetric areas of periventricular white matter.

Performance on the naming tests correlated with gray matter volume as follows: ANT accuracy correlated with left mid-frontal, right angular, and right middle temporal gyri volumes; BNT response time for trials on which participants got the correct response correlated with left planum temporale and left mid-frontal gyrus volumes. As well, VBM identified white matter areas that differentiate between better and worse performers on the ANT test. Reaction time on ANT was negatively correlated with local density of white matter in periventricular matter and arcuate fasciculus in left hemisphere, as well as with portions of corona radiata ascending to right postcentral gyrus. The effects of age on both white and gray matter were symmetrical, whereas areas showing correlation with performance on lexical retrieval tasks were largely lateralized. Significant effects were found only in white matter, supporting a connectivity-based view of age-related language impairment (Obler et al. 2010).

To further investigate white matter correlates of lexical retrieval in elderly adults, region-of-interest diffusion tensor tractography was performed using BioImage Suite (2008). Streamline tractography (Jackowski 2005) was seeded from six regions of interests, including the three regions that showed peak correlations of white matter density with ANT reaction time, as well as their three homologous counterparts. The fibers originated from the seed regions of interest clustered well into distinct groups of fibers identified as arcuate fasciculus, portions of internal capsule, and posterior corona radiata ascending to postcentral gyrus. Coefficient of lateralization was computed as a difference in the number of fibers that originate from homologous seed regions. Reaction time on ANT was significantly lower in participants with greater left-sided lateralization in both arcuate fasciculus and periventricular white matter areas.

The use of diffusion tensor tractography allowed for the detailed analysis of anatomical connectivity related to lexical retrieval deficits showed by elderly adults. The specific mechanism by which impaired structural connectivity affects language performance is likely explained by subsequent impairments in functional communication among language areas of the brain. We conclude that changes in both structural and functional connectivity in the aging brain determine their concurrent contribution to decline in language function.

Moreover, it appears that presence or absence of hypertension predicts naming performance in older adults (Albert et al. 2009): To explore the effect of health-related factors on lexical retrieval in older adults, we administered the Action Naming Test (ANT) and Boston Naming Test (BNT) to 284 adults ages 55–85. Using regression analyses, we showed that, after accounting for the effects of age, race, gender, and education, hypertension was associated with accuracy on the BNT such that hypertensive participants were less accurate than normotensives. No differences were found on the ANT; diabetes was not associated with either task. These studies provide evidence that 1) hypertension is related to naming performance in different stimulus contexts (both picture naming and descriptive naming) and 2) there is a dissociation between two key cardiovascular risk factors (hypertension and diabetes) with regard to their effect on naming.

One further health parameter appears associated with naming at this time: Metabolic syndrome is associated with impairment in aspects of naming and sentence processing. Using data collected from 289 of our study pool participants aged 55 to 84, we computed both ATP/NCEP (Expert Panel 2001) and AHA/NHLBI (Grundy et al. 2005) definitions of metabolic syndrome. We found neither race nor age differences in incidence of metabolic syndrome, but women had a lower prevalence (17%, 31%) than did men (35%, 49%) by ATP/NCEP and AHA/NHLBI criteria, respectively. Preliminary analyses, after adjustment for demographics, suggest that those with metabolic syndrome have worse performance on action naming, but not object naming, and also on processing sentences with both embedded clauses and with multiple negations.

In sum, data indicate that lexical retrieval difficulties begin as early as the 30s, progress slowly until the mid-60s, and then make a more rapid dip. These changes are greater for people with poor education (probably due to reduced cognitive reserve), and (for reasons as yet undetermined) for women. Lexical retrieval deficits in aging are linked to cerebrovascular risk factors (especially hypertension and metabolic syndrome), and our neuroimaging findings suggest that these deficits are related to frontal system functions.

Sentence-level Processes in Aging

The second language domain in which age-related decline has been demonstrated is that of processing auditorily presented complex verbal material. The lexical retrieval difficulty of normal aging is well-known, of course, but the difficulty with auditory comprehension has been less widely appreciated clinically, despite considerable research literature on this topic. Although changes in comprehension with advancing age have been reported for extended and paragraph-length prose (e.g., Byrd 1985; Stine and Wingfield 1990; Wingfield et al. 1989; Hasher and Zacks 1988), sentences (e.g., Davis and Ball 1989; Obler et al. 1991; Stine 1990; Waters and Caplan 2001), words (e.g., Gordon-Salant and Fitzgibbons 1995; Marshall et al. 1996; Stern et al. 1991; Wingfield et al. 1991) and phonemes (Humes et al. 1993; Wingfield et al. 1991), most salient in daily life is age-related difficulty in comprehending auditorily presented sentences in discourse in less than ideal conditions. Older adults are able to make good use of linguistic context, normal prosody, and semantic probability, but demonstrate difficulty when the redundancy that characterizes normal auditory sentence comprehension situations decreases and the processing load increases (Davis and Ball 1989; DeDe et al. 2004; Obler et al. 1985, 1991; Pichora-Fuller and Souza 2003; Tun 1998; Waters and Caplan 2001; Wingfield et al. 1991). Our review of this literature highlights three types of tasks with which age differences have been found: syntactically-complex sentences, illogical or implausible sentences, and noise overlay.

With respect to syntactically-complex sentences, Obler et al. (1991) found that older adults had more difficulty than young adults processing a variety of auditorily presented, syntactically complex sentences. Most problematic were the two types of structures we chose as exemplars of syntactic complexity: those containing two negatives and those with embedded clauses. Similar results for older adults have been reported in studies of reading comprehension (Stine-Morrow et al. 2000), auditory sentence comprehension (Waters and Caplan 2001), and sentence processing (e.g., Zurif et al. 1995) when structures such as subject-relative (SR; e.g., The dog that chased the cat ran down the street.) and object-relative (OR; e.g., The cat that the dog chased ran down the street.) embedded sentences were used. More recent data confirm that some older adults produce more errors and are slower in processing Multiple Negatives tests (MN) and Embedded Sentences (ES) (Goral et al. in press).

Obler et al. (1991) further found that older adults made disproportionately more errors relative to younger adults on implausible sentences (e.g., The small boy attacked the huge mugger in the park.) than on plausible ones (e.g., The fierce wolf attacked the lost sheep in the woods.). Preliminary analyses of accuracy data confirm an interaction between age and plausibility in OR and SR sentences but suggest that the relationship between age and plausibility is task-dependent. Preliminary accuracy data from the Multiple Negations task show no interaction between age and plausibility while in the SPIN task, which is administered in both high- and low-noise conditions, age interacts with plausibility only in the low-noise condition (Goral et al. 2006).

Noisy Conditions

Many hearing science studies have shown that presbycusis is related to auditory comprehension difficulties in older adults (Bergman 1980; Corso 1977; Humes and Roberts 1990); however, even older adults with no significant hearing impairment experience difficulties with comprehending speech in various conditions (Gordon-Salant and Fitzgibbons 1995; Tun 1998). In addition, tasks in which stimuli are acoustically distorted, unnaturally fast, or where one must attend to speech when there are others talking in the environment cause older adults disproportionate difficulty (Peelle and Wingfield 2005; Wingfield et al. 2003; Wingfield et al. 2005; 2006). Therefore, the sensory declines experienced by older adults, particularly deficits in frequency and temporal resolution, and a loss of acuity for high frequency sounds, complicate the comprehension process (Wingfield, Tun, and McCoy 2005).

An obvious and useful consequence of these observations for the benefit of older patients (but not always practiced in a busy doctor's office) is to reduce background noise, and speak slowly and clearly.

Executive Systems Functions

Wingfield and Grossman (2006) suggested that older adults may have differing brain-based capacities for compensating for impaired language skills, and that those who perform as well as younger individuals on language comprehension tasks can better compensate. Executive functions, such as inhibition and set-shifting skills, have been shown to decline with age (e.g., Hasher, Lustig, and Zacks 2007; Moscovitch and Winocur 1992; Wecker et al. 2000) but new understanding of how these changes interact with sentence processing is underway (see Hasher and Zacks 1988; Darowski et al. 2008; Burke and Shafto 2008). We examined age and executive function abilities as predictors of accuracy on exemplar syntactic sentence-processing tasks and found that, whereas all participants (older and younger) demonstrated increased difficulty on the more complex sentence structures, after correction for hearing, age predicted accuracy on our Embedded Sentences but not Multiple Negatives tests. Executive function as measured by perseverative errors on the WCST predicted performance on both sentence processing tests. Working memory span also predicted performance: Those with better WM span were more accurate than those with lower span; Stroop interference did not predict accuracy on either task. Furthermore, we found that individuals with low scores on both EF and WM demonstrated lower accuracy scores than those with only low EF or only low WM performance. Thus, among older adults, not only age, but also executive system function (in addition to working memory) predicts performance on sentence-processing tasks (Goral et al. in press).

In the cognitive aging literature, researchers have tended to focus on working memory explanations for age-related problems with sentence processing; however, the degree to which the relevant working memory system is specialized for verbal processing is not settled. Waters and Caplan (2001; Waters et al. 1995), for example, have argued that general working memory capacity and overall verbal memory load are not associated with performance on syntactic processing and that only "post-interpretive" processes are affected by working memory load. Their separate-sentence-interpretation resource theory stands in contrast to single-resource theories (e.g., Grossman 1999; Just and Carpenter 1992; Salthouse 1988a, 1988b, 1991) and theories of deficits of resource allocation (e.g., Stine-Morrow et al. 2000) or decreased attention and inhibition (e.g., Hasher and Zacks 1988; Stoltzfus et al. 1996). Wingfield and Grossman (2006) proposed a two-component model of sentence comprehension: a core sentence processing component and an associated network of brain regions that support the working memory and other resources needed for comprehension of long or syntactically complex sentences.

Complementary to these studies is our study of auditory sentence processing in aging in which we assessed ability to process English sentences spoken with non-native accents. Following a study with college-age adults (Goral et al. 2000), we tested young and older adults (Shah et al. 2005), and older adults with and without Alzheimer's dementia (AD) (Shah et al. 1997, 1998), and showed that older adults diagnosed with differing degrees of AD had progressively more difficulty repeating sentences spoken in accented English than did the control group. In contrast, neurologically intact older adults performed worse, overall, than young adults but did not show proportionately more difficulty with the accented as compared to the unaccented material.

In sum, auditory comprehension of spoken language declines in aging but not for everyone, and not under all listening conditions.

One challenge for future research will be to specify with greater precision the conditions that cause increased comprehension difficulties for elderly persons, be they environmental, health related, or brain related.

Age-related Decline in Language Skills: Cognition, Health, and the Brain

Although the age-related changes in lexical and sentence-level performance noted above are well-documented, relatively little work has examined these language changes within the larger context of the cognitive neuroscience of aging, including our current understandings of age-related changes in health and disease, as related to brain function. Cabeza (2004) pointed out all would agree that the cognitive changes associated with aging must result from changes in brain. Yet over the past 30 years, the study of language in aging has focused on discrete aspects of the problem, with relatively little emphasis on integration across the domains of cognitive aging, age-related changes in the brain, and age-related changes in language, and with even less focus on the crucial role of health and disease in aging.

Language, Aging, and Cognition

Despite some notable earlier work (e.g., Kemper et al. 1989; Stine et al. 1986), only during the past decade or so have studies begun to evaluate the explanatory power of theories of cognitive aging to account for age-related language changes. Because most studies of language in aging have focused on a single model to explain specific findings, there is a dearth of studies examining multiple indicators of change in language, although the review by Wingfield and Stine-Morrow (2000) indicates that such studies are warranted.

Cognitive aging theories have sought to explain various aspects of age-related cognitive decline, suggesting that decline is due to reductions in processing speed (Salthouse et al. 1996), sensory and cognitive function due to a "common cause" (Baltes and Lindenberger 1997; Lindenberger, Scherer, and Baltes 2001), executive functions (Dempster 1992; Moscovitch and Winocur 1992; West 1996), and working memory (Wingfield et al. 1988). Models that posit declines in executive functions as mediators of cognitive aging (Dempster 1992; Moscovitch and Winocur 1992; West 1996) have received a considerable amount of attention (e.g., Band et al. 2002; Greenwood 2000; Jurado and Rosselli 2007; Kennedy and Raz 2009; West 2000). Executive functions "consist of those capacities that enable a person to engage successfully in independent, purposive, self-serving behavior" (Lezak 1995, p. 42); examples pertinent to the study of language in aging include inhibition of pre-potent responses, concept formation, shifting of cognitive set, initiation, and output monitoring (Jurado and Rosselli 2007; Lezak 1995; Miyake et al. 2000). Our recent findings agree with previous findings that working memory also plays a role in sentence processing (Goral et al. in press), perhaps because of age-related changes in medial temporal regions that may result from declining vascular health (Obler et al. 2010).

Language, Aging, and Health

A major lacuna in research on language in aging has been the relation of age-related changes in health to changes in language. Wingfield et al. (2005) have clearly pointed out the important role of sensory decline, while Spiro (2001, 2007) and his colleagues (Aldwin, Spiro, and Park 2006) have emphasized health as a developmental phenomenon of particular interest in the study of aging, especially cognitive aging (Spiro and Brady 2008).

Regarding potential etiological factors for age-related neuropathology of frontal cortex and other cortical and subcortical regions, vascular disease risk factors (e.g., age, hypertension, diabetes, metabolic syndrome, inflammation) have been suggested to produce the pattern of neuropathology seen in nondemented older adults (Brady et al. 2001, 2005; Llewellyn et al. 2008). Vascular (cardiovascular and cerebrovascular) disease risk factors predispose even relatively healthy older adults to ischemic changes in the brain, primarily in the periventricular white matter, basal ganglia, and pons, prior to the development of frank vascular disease (e.g., Alves de Morales et al. 2002; McPherson and Cummings 1997; Pantoni and Garcia 1997; Raz et al. 2000; 2003). A large proportion of this white matter pathology is apparent on MRI scans and occurs in the ascending and descending pathways between the frontal cortex and the basal ganglia and brain stem, as well as in connections between frontal and other cortical regions (e.g., Chui and Willis 1999; Goldberg and Bilder 1987; Pugh and Lipsitz 2002). Furthermore, this white matter pathology may interrupt the integrity of frontal-subcortical circuits thought to be important to frontally mediated cognitive functions (Cummings 1993; Gunning-Dixon and Raz 2000; Marshall et al. 2006; Oosterman et al. 2004; McPherson and Cummings 1997). Other similar evidence suggests a link between white matter changes and specific stroke risk factors such as hypertension (e.g., Raz et al. 2003; Soderlund et al. 2003; Swan et al. 1998), diabetes (e.g., Jongen et al. 2005; Ylikoski et al. 1995), and cardiac disease (e.g., Breteler et al. 1994). Indeed, there is growing behavioral evidence linking executive and working-memory dysfunction to vascular risk factors such as hypertension (e.g., Elias et al. 1997; Raz et al. 2007; Waldstein et al. 1996), diabetes (e.g., Knopman et al. 2001; Kuo et al. 2005) and heart disease (Dywan et al. 1992; Jefferson, Poppas, Paul, and Cohen 2006; Thayer, et al. 2009).

Language, Aging, and the Brain

Age-related structural (anatomical) changes in the brain have been shown by both structural MRI and diffusion tensor imaging (DTI). Overall tissue loss, cortical thinning, and the reduction of white matter integrity are observed along the anterior-posterior gradient, with frontal areas being most vulnerable to aging (Raz 2000; Resnick et al. 2003; Sullivan and Pfefferbaum 2006). These structural frontal changes have two important clinical implications: On the one hand, overall brain decline (especially in specialized areas) leads to additional resource recruitment from contralateral (compensatory plasticity) or frontal (executive control) regions. On the other hand, frontal regions degrade the fastest, compromising overall compensatory mechanisms. Gray matter reduction, being prevalent in frontal lobes, seems to affect executive functions the most, with verbal function being relatively spared (Park et al. 2001; Raz 2000). White matter changes are linked to deficits in speed (possibly due to demyelinization) and executive functions (Gunning-Dixon and Raz 2000; Rabbitt et al. 2007).

Perhaps because of frontal degradation, the compensatory recruitment of frontal/prefrontal cortex does not always aid performance. While some studies show effective compensation, others show quite the opposite: The poorer performers on an attention task had more evidence of bilateral over-recruiting. Those same poor performers who showed no effective compensatory over-recruitment also had frontal white matter deficits, revealed by structural MR images (Colcombe et al. 2005). In another study, elders with bilateral activation performed worse on a working memory task than those with lateralized activity, and these same participants reportedly had smaller corpus callosum (Leaver et al. submitted). These two studies reveal an important link between the efficiency of compensatory functional reorganization in elderly brains and the preservation of white matter, a substrate for neural communication. It is possible that the compensatory involvement of frontal lobes is not always effective due to the impaired anatomical connectivity which adversely affects communication between (and within) the executive frontal/prefrontal network and the specialized task-related networks. The "cerebral disconnection" hypothesis of age-related cognitive decline is now being actively explored with advanced imaging methodologies such as DTI (Charlton, et al. 2006).

The specific brain mechanisms underlying age-related language decline have not been thoroughly investigated using in-vivo brain imaging. Wingfield and Grossman (2006) reported an fMRI study that showed significant up-regulation of dorsolateral prefrontal cortex (DLPFC) in poor elderly performers on a complex sentence comprehension task. This increased DLPFC over-activation accompanied under-recruitment of perisylvian and temporo-parietal "core language" regions, compared to good elderly comprehenders. By contrast, good comprehenders performed just as well as young subjects, accounted for by additional recruitment of temporo-parietal regions. These findings suggest that the compensatory mechanisms for age-related decline of language functions might be similar to those in other cognitive functions, such as working memory or attention. In a recent study using neuroimaging techniques, Takahashi et al. (2007) demonstrated that memory-related areas in the left dorsolateral prefrontal cortex (DLPFC) and the left ventrolateral prefrontal cortex (VLPFC) each connect with memory-related areas in the left temporal cortex. The fact that compensatory mechanisms are not always effective may be explained by the impaired communication between frontal and "core language" regions. Stamatakis and Tyler (2006), for example, found reduced fronto-temporal connectivity in functional networks of elderly participants, inferred from fMRI recorded during morphological processing.

It is certainly plausible that this impaired functional connectivity was caused by an underlying lack of anatomical connectivity, possibly due to white matter damage. Our preliminary findings show that there is structural decline in dorsolateral and fronto-temporal connectivity linked to poor performance on a lexical retrieval task.

It remains to be determined whether a lexical retrieval task shows the phenomenon of bilateral over-recruitment in poorly performing elderly. If so, one might ask whether this inefficiency can be explained by the lack of communication among the core language areas and frontal resource network regions. We suspect that structural and, subsequently, functional connectivity impairments (especially in the prefrontal cortex) are important factors contributing to inefficient top-down regulation of language function, as people get older.

Language in Older Adults: Cognition, Health, and the Brain

Given that executive functions and the executive or processing component of working memory are thought to be largely mediated by the frontal cortex (e.g., Baddeley and Hitch 1994; Stuss and Benson 1986; but see Collette and Van der Linden 2002, who argue that posterior regions are engaged as well), researchers who posit executive dysfunction as a mediator of cognitive aging have argued that executive dysfunction is an indicator of relatively greater age-related frontal system dysfunction. Whereas neuroanatomic evidence of relatively greater age-related neuropathology in the frontal cortex has been questioned (e.g., Morrison and Hof 1997), age-related diffuse changes in the cerebral white matter that provide connections between the frontal cortex and other cortical and subcortical regions are firmly established (e.g., Chui 1999; Goldberg 1987; Pantoni and Garcia 1997). Neuroimaging evidence (e.g., Alexander and Stuss 2000; Kennedy and Raz 2009; Raz 2000; Raz et al. 1998, 2003) suggests that age-related volumetric changes in frontal and white matter structures, as seen in structural

magnetic resonance imaging (MRI), are linked to age-related changes in several cognitive domains, most notably executive functions and working memory. In future research, relations among age-linked changes in lexical processing, sentence-level processing, executive system dysfunction, vascular health, and prefrontal connectivity merit further integrated study. Note: in this chapter we have been stressing the importance of integration of data from several fields that touch on issues of age-related language decline.

In sum, the findings of 1) selective lexical decline with aging (i.e., preserved vocabulary knowledge, letter fluency, and use of clustering in verbal fluency tasks, in contrast to declining semantic fluency, switching in verbal fluency, and the ability to call up specific items in confrontation naming); 2) selective decline in sentence processing (i.e., increased difficulty with auditorily presented complex material in the absence of redundancy in contrast to preserved performance on material presented with maximized redundancy); and 3) the emerging evidence for the role of executive functions (in addition to working memory) in the tasks that do show decline, lead us to posit that health-related changes in executive function abilities are at least partially responsible for age-related decline in language skills.

Lexical retrieval and complex sentence processing are the two linguistic skills most prone to change with aging. Many attempts to explain these changes have focused on cognitive contributions, drawing explanatory theories from models of cognitive aging. However, such models alone do not fully explain language changes in aging. Findings from our lab suggest, rather, that health-related factors and brain-related factors, integrated with cognitive factors, are required for a more comprehensive explanation of language changes in normal aging.

Such studies provide diagnostic and intervention strategies that can optimize functional communication of older adults by clarifying the borders of normal and pathologic language function in the elderly. With regard to clinical intervention on behalf of elderly patients, research observations such as those reviewed here can be used to reassure patients that their language function is normal (if it is), and can be used by conversation partners and speech language pathologists to gauge the limits of a person's language ability, and to compensate appropriately. We conclude that aging does not automatically result in decline in all aspects of communicative capability. Indeed, research reviewed here offers the means by which communication partners and caretakers of elderly individuals can enable them to improve and enrich their communication in everyday life.

Acknowledgments

This research was supported in part by Grant AG14345 (PI: Martin L. Albert) from the National Institute on Aging, and by Merit Review grants to Avron Spiro and Christopher Brady by the Clinical Science Research and Development Service, US Department of Veterans Affairs. We thank all our participants and Manuella (Rossie) Clark-Cotton, Keely Sayers, Joshua Berger, Dalia Cahana-Amitay, and Mallory Finley for their invaluable help.

References

Albert, M. L., Spiro, A. R., Sayers, K., et al. Effects of health status on word finding in aging. *Journal of the American Geriatrics Society, 57,* 2300–2305, 2009.

Aldwin, C. M., Spiro, A. III, and Park, C.L. (2006). Health, behavior, and optimal aging: A life span developmental perspective. In J. E. Birren and K. W. Schaie (Ed.), *Handbook of the psychology of aging* (pp. 85–104). Burlington, MA: Elsevier.

Alexander, M.P., and Stuss, D.T. (2000). Disorders of frontal lobe functioning. *Seminars in Neurology, 20*, 427–437.

Alves de Morales, S., Szklo, M., Knopman, D., and Sato, R. (2002). The relationship between temporal changes in blood pressure and changes in cognitive function. Atherosclerosis Risk in Communities (ARIC) study. *Preventive Medicine*, San Diego, CA-EUA, 35, 258–263.

Ashburner, J., and Friston, K. J. (2000). Voxel-based morphometry: The methods. *NeuroImage, 11*, 805–821.

Au, R., Joung, P., Nicholas, M., Obler, L.K., Kass, R. and Albert, M.L. (1995). Naming ability across the adult life span. *Aging and Cognition, 2*, 300–311.

Baddeley, A. D. and Hitch, G. J. (1994). Developments in the concept of working memory, *Neuropsychology, 8*, 485–493.

Baltes, P.B., and Lindenberger, U. (1997). Emergence of a powerful connection between sensory and cognitive functions across the adult life span: A new window to the study of cognitive aging? *Psychology and Aging, 12*, 12–21.

Band, G.P.H., Riddernikhof, K.R., and Segalowitz, S. (2002). Explaining neurocognitive aging: Is one factor enough? *Brain and Cognition, 49*, 259–267.

Barresi, B., Nicholas, M., Connor, L.T., Obler, L.K., and Albert, M.L. (2000). Semantic degradation and lexical access in age-related naming failures. *Aging, Neuropsychology, and Cognition, 7*, 169–178.

Belke, E., & Meyer, A.S. (2007). Single and multiple object naming in healthy aging. *Language and Cognitive Processes, 22*, 1178-1211.

Bergman, M. (1980). *Aging and the perception of speech*, (45–47). Baltimore: University Park Press.

Boone, K.B., Miller, B.L., Lesser, I.M., Hill, E., and D'Elia, L.F. (1990). Performance on frontal lobe tests in healthy, older individuals. *Developmental Neuropsychology, 6*, 215–224.

Brady, C. B., Spiro, A. III, and Gaziano, J.M. (2005). Effects of age and hypertension status on cognition: The Veterans Affairs Normative Aging Study. *Neuropsychology, 19*, 770–777.

Brady, C. B., Spiro, A. III, McGlinchey-Berroth, R., Milberg, W. and Gaziano, J.M. (2001). Stroke risk predicts verbal fluency decline in healthy older men: Evidence from the Normative Aging Study. *Journals of Gerontology: Psychological Sciences and Social Sciences, Series B, 56*, 340–346.

Breteler, M.M.B., Van Swieten, J.C., Bots, M.L., et al. (1994). Cerebral white matter lesions, vascular risk factors, and cognitive function in a population-based study: The Rotterdam Study. *Neurology, 44*, 1246–1252.

Burke, D. (2006). Representation and aging. In E. Bialystok and F.I.M. Craik (Eds.), *Lifespan cognition: Mechanisms of change* (pp. 397). New York, NY: Oxford University Press.

Burke, D.M., and Shafto, M. A. (2008). Language and aging. In: T. A. Salthouse (Ed.). The handbook of aging and cognition (pp. 373–443). New York: Psychology Press.

Burke, D. M., and MacKay, D. (1997). Memory, language and ageing. *Philosophical Transactions of the Royal Society of London, Biological Sciences, 352*, 1845–1856.

Burke, D. M., MacKay, D.G., and James, L.E. (2000). Theoretical approaches to language and aging. In T. P. E. Maylor (Ed.), *Models of cognitive aging* (pp. 204–237). New York, NY: Oxford University Press.

Burke, D.M., MacKay, D.G., Worthley, J.S., and Wade, E. (1991). On the tip of the tongue: What causes word finding failures in young and older adults? *Journal of Memory and Language, 30*, 542–579.

Byrd, M. (1985). Age differences in the ability to recall and summarize textual information. *Experimental Aging Research, 11*, 87–91.

Cabeza, R. (2004). Neuroscience frontiers of cognitive aging: Approaches to cognitive neuroscience of aging. In R. A. Dixon, L. Backman & L.-G. Nilsson (Eds.), *New frontiers in cognitive aging*. Oxford: Oxford University Press.

Charlton, R., Barrick, T., McIntyre, D., et al. (2006). White matter damage on diffusion tensor imaging correlates with age-related cognitive decline. *Neurology, 66*, 217–222.

Chui, H., and Willis, L. (1999). Vascular diseases and the frontal lobes. In B.L. Miller and J.L. Cummings (Eds.), *The human frontal lobes*. New York: The Guilford Press.

Colcombe, S.J., Kramer, A. F., Erickson, K. I. and Scalf, P. (2005). The implications of cortical recruitment and brain morphology for individual differences in inhibitory function in aging humans. *Psychology & Aging, 20*, 363–375.

Collette, F., and Van der Linden, M. (2002). Brain imaging of the central executive component of working memory. *Neuroscience & Biobehavioral Reviews, 26*, 105–125.

Conner, P.S., Hyun, J., O'connor, B., Anema, I., et al. (submitted). Age-related differences in idiom production in adulthood.

Connor, L.T., Spiro, A., Obler, L.K. and Albert, M.L. (2004). Change in object naming ability during adulthood. *Journal of Gerontology: Psychological Sciences, 5*, 203–209.

Corso, J. (1977). Auditory perception and communication. In J.E. Birren and K.W. Schaie (Eds.), *Handbook of psychology and aging*. New York: Van Nostrand Reinhold.

Cortese, M., Balota, D., Sergent-Marshall, S., and Buckner, R. (2003). Spelling via semantics and phonology: Exploring the effects of age, Alzheimer's disease, and primary semantic impairment. *Neuropsychologia, 41*, 952–967.

Cummings, J.L. (1993). Frontal subcortical circuits and human behavior. *Archives of Neurology, 50*, 873–880.

Darowski, E. S., Helder, E., Zacks, R. T., Hasher, L. and Hambrick, D. Z. (2008). Age-related differences in cognition: The role of distraction control. *Neuropsychology, 22*(5), 638–644.

Davis, G.A., and Ball, H.E. (1989). Effects of age on comprehension of complex utterances in adulthood. *Journal of Speech and Hearing Research, 32*, 143–150.

DeDe, G., Caplan, D., Kemtes, K., and Waters, G. (2004). The relationship between age, verbal working memory, and language comprehension. *Psychology and Aging, 19*, 601–616.

Dempster, F. N. (1992). The rise and fall of the inhibitory mechanism: Toward a unified theory of cognitive development and aging. *Developmental Review, 12*, 47–75.

Dywan, J., Segalowitz, S., and Unsal, A. (1992). Speed of information processing, health, and cognitive performance in older adults. *Developmental Neuropsychology, 8*, 473–490.

Eckert, M. A, Walczak, A., Ahlstrom, J., Denslow, S., Horwitz, A., and Dubno, J. R. (2008). Age-related effects on word recognition: Reliance on cognitive control systems with structural declines in speech-responsive cortex. *Journal of the Association for Research in Otolaryngology, 9*, 252–259.

Elias, P.K., Elias, M.F., D'Agostino, R.B., and Cupples, L.A. (1997). NIDDM and blood pressure as risk factors for poor cognitive performance. *Diabetes Care, 20*, 1388–1395.

Expert Panel on Detection, Evaluation, and Treatment of High Blood Cholesterol in Adults. (2001). Executive summary of the Third report of the National Cholesterol Education Program (NCEP) Expert Panel on Detection, Evaluation, and Treatment of High Blood Cholesterol in Adults (Adult Treatment Panel III). *JAMA. 285*, 2486–2497.

Feyereisen, P. (1997). A meta-analytic procedure shows and age-related decline in picture naming: Comments on Goulet, Ska, and Kahn. *Journal of Speech, Language, and Hearing Research, 40*, 1328–1333.

Goldberg, E., and Bilder, R.M. (1987). The frontal lobes and hierarchical organization of cognitive control. In E. Perecman (Ed.), *The frontal lobes revisited* (pp. 159–187). Hillsdale, NJ: Lawrence Erlbaum Associates.

Goral, M., Clark-Cotton, M., Spiro, A. III, Obler, L. K., Verkuilen, J., and Albert, M. L. (in press). The contribution of set shifting and working memory to sentence processing in older adults. Experimental Aging Research.

Goral, M., Levy, E., Obler, L., and Cohen, E. (2006). Cross-language lexical connections in the mental lexicon: Evidence from a case of trilingual aphasia. Brain and Language, 98, 235–247.

Goral, M., Obler, L.K. and Galletta, E. (2000). Factors underlying comprehension of accented English. In L.T. Connor & L.K. Obler (Eds.), Neurobehavior of language and cognition: Studies of normal aging and brain damage. (pp. 23–42). Norwell, MA: Kluwer Academic Publishers.

Goral, M., Spiro, A. III, Albert, M.L., Obler, L.K., and Connor, L.T. (2007). Change in lexical retrieval skills in adulthood. The Mental Lexicon, 2, 215–238.

Gordon-Salant, S., and Fitzgibbons, P.J. (1995). Recognition of multiply degraded speech by young and elderly listeners. Journal of Speech and Hearing Research, 38, 1150–1156.

Greenwood, P.M. (2000). The frontal aging hypothesis evaluated. Journal of the International Neuropsychological Society, 6, 705–726.

Griffin, Z.M., and Spieler, D.H. (2006). Observing the what and when of language production for different age groups by monitoring speakers' eye movements. Brain & Language, 99(3), 272–288.

Grossman, M. (1999). Sentence processing in Parkinson's disease. Brain and Cognition, 40, 387–413.

Grundy, S. M., Cleeman, J. I., Diniels, S. R., et al. (2005). AHA/NHLBI Diagnosis and management of the metabolic syndrome: An AHA/NHLBI scientific statement. Circulation, 112, 2735–2752.

Gunning-Dixon, F.M., and Raz, N. (2000). The cognitive correlates of white matter abnormalities in normal aging: A quantitative review. Neuropsychology, 14, 224–232.

Hasher, L., Lustig, C., and Zacks, R. T. (2007). Inhibitory mechanisms and the control of attention. In A. R. A. Conway, C. Jarrold, M. and, A. Miyake, J. N. Towse (Eds.), Variation in working memory (pp.227–249). New York: Oxford University Press.

Hasher, L. and Zacks, R.T. (1988). Working memory, comprehension, and aging: A review and a new view. In G.H. Bower (Ed.), The psychology of learning and motivation (pp. 193–225). San Diego, CA: Academic Press.

Howard, D. V., Shaw, R. S., and Heisey. J. G. 1986. Aging and the time course of semantic activation. Journal of Gerontology, 41, 195–203.

Humes, L.E. and Roberts, L. (1990). Speech-recognition difficulties of the hearing-impaired elderly: The contribution of audibility. Journal of Speech and Hearing Research, 33, 726–735.

Humes, L.E., Nelson, K.J., Pisoni, D.B. and Lively, S.E. (1993). Effects of age on serial recall of natural and syntactic speech. Journal of Speech and Hearing Research, 36, 634–639.

Jackowski, M., Kao, C. Y., Qiu, M., Constable, R. T., and Staib, L. H. (2005). White matter tactography by anisotropic wavefront evolution and diffusion tensor imaging. Medical Image Analysis, 9, 427–440.

Jefferson, A. L., Poppas, A., Paul, R. H., and Cohen, R. A. (2006). Systemic hypoperfusion is associated with executive dysfunction in geriatric cardiac patients. Neurobiology of Aging, 28, 477–483.

Jongen, C., van der Grond, J., Kappelle, L. J., Biessels, G. J. Viergever, M. A., and Pluim, J. P. W. on behalf of the Utrecht Diabetic Encephalopathy Study Group, (2007). Automated measurement of brain and white matter lesion volume in type 2 diabetes mellitus, Diabetologia, 50, 1509–1516.

Jurado, M.B., and Rosselli, M. (2007). The elusive nature of executive functions: A review of our current understanding. Neuropsychology Reviews 17, 213–33.

Just, M.A., and Carpenter, P.A. (1992). A capacity theory of comprehension: Individual differences in working memory. Psychological Review, 99, 122–149.

Kaplan, E., Goodglass, H., and Weintraub, S. (1983). The Boston Naming Test (pp.395–400). Philadelphia: Lea & Febiger.

Kemper, S., and Craik, F.I.M. (1992). Language and aging. In F.I.M. Craik and T.A. Salthouse (Eds.), Handbook of aging and cognition (pp. 213–270). Hillsdale, NY: Erlbaum.

Kemper, S., and Liu, C. (2007). Eye movements of young and older adults during reading. Psychology & Aging, 22, 84–93.

Kemper, S., and Sumner, A. (2001). The structure of verbal abilities in young and older adults. Psychology and Aging, 16, 312–322.

Kemper, S., Kynette, D., Rash, S., Sprott, R., and O'Brien, K. (1989). Life-span changes to adults' language: Effects of memory and genre. Applied Psycholinguistics, 10, 49–66.

Kennedy, K.M. and Raz N. (2009). Aging white matter and cognition: Differential effects of regional variations in diffusion properties on memory, executive functions, and speed. Neuropsychologia, 47, 916–927.

Knopman, D.S., Boland, L.L., Mosley, T., et al. (2001). Cardiovascular risk factors and cognitive decline in middle-aged adults. Neurology, 56, 42–48.

Kuo, H. K., Jones, R. N., Milberg, W. P., et al. (2005). Effect of blood pressure and diabetes mellitus on cognitive and physical functions in older adults: A longitudinal analysis of the advanced cognitive training for independent and vital elderly cohort. Journal of the American Geriatrics Society. 53, 1154–1161.

Laver, G. D., and Burke, D. M. (1993). Why do semantic priming effects increase in old age? A meta-analysis. Psychology and aging, 8, 34–43.

Leaver, E., Rykhlevskaia, E., Wee, E., Gratton, G., Fabiani, M. (submitted). Corpus callosum size and age-related decline in working memory.

Lezak, M.D. (1995). Neuropsychological assessment. New York, Oxford University Press.

Lindenberger, U., Scherer, H., and Baltes, P.B. (2001). The strong connection between sensory and cognitive performance in old age: Not due to sensory acuity reductions operating during cognitive assessment. Psychology and Aging, 16, 196–205.

Llewellyn, D.J., Lang, I.A., Xie, J. Huppert, F.A., Melzer, D., and Langa, K. (2008). Framingham stroke risk profile and poor cognitive function: A population-based study. BMC Neurology, 8, 8–12.

Marshall, G. A., Hendrickson, R., Kaufer, D. I., Ivanco, L. S., and Bohnen, N. I. (2006). Cognitive correlates of brain MRI subcortical signal hyperintensities in non-demented elderly. International Journal of Geriatric Psychiatry, 21, 32–35.

Marshall, N. B., Duke, L. W., and Walley, A. C. (1996). Effects of age and Alzheimer's disease on recognition of gated spoken words. Journal of Speech and Hearing Research, 39, 724–733.

McPherson, S.E. and Cummings, J.L. (1997). Vascular dementia: Clinical assessment, neuropsychological features and treatment. In P.D. Nussbaum (Ed.), Handbook of neuropsychology and aging (pp. 177–188). New York: Plenum Press.

Miyake, A., (2001). Individual differences in working memory. Introduction to the special section. Journal of Experimental Psychology, 130, 163–168.

Morrison, J.H. and Hof, P.R. (1997). Life and death of neurons in the aging brain. Science, 278, 412–419.

Moscovitch, M., and Winocur, G. (1992). The neuropsychology of memory and aging. In F. I.M. Craik and T.A. Salthouse (Eds.). The handbook of aging and cognition (pp. 315–372). Hillsdale, NJ: Lawrence Erlbaum Associates.

Nicholas, M., Obler, L.K., Albert, M., and Goodglass, H. (1985). Lexical retrieval in healthy aging. Cortex, 21, 595–606.

Obler, L. and Albert, M.L. (1999). Verb naming in normal aging. Applied Neuropsychology, 6, 57–67.

Obler, L. K., Clark-Cotton, M. R., Spiro, R., et al. (2007, October). Compensation for age-related lexical-retrieval problems in discourse. Poster presented at the Aging and Communication conference, Bloomington, ID.

Obler, L.K., Fein, D., Nicholas, M. and Albert, M.L. (1991). Auditory comprehension and aging: Decline in syntactic processing. *Applied Psycholinguistics, 12*, 433–452.

Obler, L.K., Nicholas, M., Albert, M.L. and Woodward, S. (1985). On comprehension across the adult lifespan. *Cortex, 21*, 273–280.

Obler, L.K., Rykhlevskaia, E., Schnyer, D., et al. (2010). Bilateral brain regions associated with naming in older adults. *Brain Language*, 113, 113–123.

Oosterman, J. M., Sergeant, J. A., Weinstein, H. C., and Scherder, E. J. (2004). Timed executive functions and white matter in aging with and without cardiovascular risk factors. *Reviews in the Neurosciences, 15*, 439–462.

Pantoni, L., and Garcia, J.H. (1997). Pathogenesis of leukoaraiosis: A review. *Stroke, 28*, 652–659.

Park, D. C., Polk, T. A., Mikels, J. A., Taylor, S. F., and Marshuetz, C. (2001). Cerebral aging: Integration of brain and behavioral models of cognitive function. *Dialogues in Clinical Neuroscience: Cerebral Aging, 3*, 151–165.

Parkin, A.J., and Walter, B.M. (1991). Aging, short-term memory, and frontal dysfunction. *Psychobiology, 19*, 175–179.

Peelle, J.E., and Wingfield, A. (2005). Dissociations in perceptual learning revealed by adult age differences in adaptation to time-compressed speech. *Journal of Experimental Psychology: Human Perception and Performance, 31*, 1315–1330.

Pichora-Fuller, M. K., and Souza, P.E. (2003). Effects of aging on auditory processing of speech. *International Journal of Audiology, 42*, 11–16.

Pugh, K. G., and Lipsitz, L. A. (2002). The microvascular frontal-sub cortical syndrome of aging. *Neurobiology of Aging, 23*, 421–431.

Rabbitt, P., Scott, M., Lunn, M., et al. (2007). White matter lesions account for all age-related declines in speed but not in intelligence. *Neuropsychology, 21*, 363–370.

Raz, N. (2000). Aging of the brain and its impact on cognitive performance: Integration of structural and functional findings. In F. I. M. Craik and T. A. Salthouse (Eds.), *The handbook of aging and cognition* (pp.1–90). Mahwah, NJ: Lawrence Erlbaum Associates.

Raz, N., Gunning-Dixon, F.M., Head, D., Dupuis, J.H., and Acker, J.D. (1998). Neuroanatomical correlates of cognitive aging: Evidence from structural magnetic imaging. *Neuropsychology, 12*, 95–114.

Raz, N., Rodrigue, K. M., and Acker, J. D. (2003). Hypertension and the brain: Vulnerability of the prefrontal regions and executive functions. *Behavioral Neuroscience, 117*, 1169-1180.

Raz, N., Rodrigue, K. M., Kennedy, K. M., & Acker, J. D. (2007). Vascular health and longitudinal changes in brain and cognition in middle-aged and older adults. *Neuropsychology, 21*, 149–157.

Resnick, S. M., Pham, D. L., Kraut, M. A., Zonderman, A. B., and Davatzikos, C. (2003). Longitudinal magnetic resonance imaging studies of older adults: A shrinking brain. *Journal of Neuroscience, 23*, 3295–3301.

Salthouse, T. A., Fristoe, N., and Rhee, S. H. (1996). How localized are age-related effects on neuropsychological measures? *Neuropsychology, 10*, 272–285.

Salthouse, T.A. (1988a). Resource-reduction interpretation of cognitive aging. *Developmental Review, 8*, 238–272.

Salthouse, T.A. (1988b). The role of processing resources in cognitive aging. In M.L. Howe and C.J. Brainerd (Eds.), *Cognitive development in adulthood* (pp. 185–239). New York: Springer-Verlag.

Salthouse, T.A. (1991). *Theoretical perspectives on cognitive aging*. Hillsdale, NJ: Erlbaum.

Shafto, M. A., Burke, D. M., Stamatakis, E. A., Tam, P. P., and Tyler, L. K. (2007). On the tip-of-the-tongue: Neural correlates of increased word-finding failures in normal aging. *Journal of Cognitive Neuroscience, 19*, 2060–2070.

Shah, A., Schmidt, B.T., Goral, M., and Obler, L.K. (2005). Age effects in processing bilinguals' accented speech. In J. Cohen, K. McAlister, K.

Rolsta and J. MacSwan (Eds.), *ISB4: Proceedings of the 4th International symposium on bilingualism* (pp.2115–2121). Somerville: Cascadilla Press.

Smith, C. D., Chebrolu, H., Wekstein, D. R., Schmitt, F. A., and Markesbery, W. R. (2007). Age and gender effects on human brain anatomy: A voxel-based morphometric study in healthy elderly. *Neurobiology of Aging, 28(7)*, 1075–1087.

Soderlund, H., Nyberg, L., Adolfsson, R., Nilsson, L. G., and Launer, L. J. (2003). High prevalence of white matter hyperintensities in normal aging: Relation to blood pressure and cognition. *Cortex, 39*, 1093–1105.

Sommers, M. S. (1996). The structural organization of the mental lexicon and its contribution to age-related declines in spoken-word recognition. *Psychology and Aging, 11*, 333–341.

Spieler, D.H., and Griffin, Z.M. (2006). The influence of age on the time course of word preparation in multiword utterances. *Language & Cognitive Processes, 21*, 291–321.

Spiro, A. III, and Brady, C.B. (2008). Integrating health into cognitive aging research and theory. In S.M. Hofer and D.F. Alwin (Eds.), *The handbook of cognitive aging: Interdisciplinary perspectives*. Newbury CA: Sage Publications.

Stamatakis, E. A., and Tyler, L. K. (2006). Language lateralization as a function of age. *Journal of Cognitive Neuroscience, 18*, Suppl. A128.

Stern, C., Prather, P., Swinney, D., and Zurif, E. (1991). The time course of automatic lexical access and aging. *Brain and Language, 40*, 359–372.

Stine, E.A.L. (1990). On-line processing of written text by younger and older adults. *Psychology and Aging, 5*, 68–78.

Stine, E.A.L., and Wingfield, A. (1990). How much do working memory deficits contribute to age differences in discourse memory? *European Journal of Cognitive Psychology, 2*, 289–304.

Stine, E.A.L., Wingfield, A., and Poon, L. (1986). How much and how fast: Rapid processing of spoken language in later adulthood. *Psychology and Aging, 1*, 303–311.

Stine-Morrow, E. A. L., Ryan, S., and Leonard, S. (2000). Age differences in on-line syntactic processing. *Experimental Aging Research, 26*, 315–322.

Stoltzfus, E.R., Hasher, L., and Zacks, R.T. (1996). Working memory and aging: Current status of the inhibitory view. In R. Richardson (Ed.), *Working memory and cognition*. New York: Oxford University Press.

Stuss, D.T., and Benson, D.F. (1986). *The frontal lobes*. New York: Raven Press.

Sullivan, E.V., and Pfefferbaum, A. (2006). Diffusion tensor imaging and aging. *Neuroscience & Biobehavioral Reviews, 30*,749–761.

Swan, G.E., Decarli, C., Miller, B.L., et al. (1998). Association of midlife blood pressure to late-life cognitive decline and brain morphology. *Neurology, 51*, 986–992.

Takahashi, E., Ohki, K., and Kim, D.-S. (2007). The anatomical network underlying the human memory system. *NeuroImage, 34*, 827–838.

Thayer, J. F., Hansen, A. L., Saus-Rose, E., and Johnsen, B. H. (2009). Heart rate variability, prefrontal neural function, and cognitive performance: The neurovisceral integration perspective on self-regulation, adaptation, and health. *Annals of Behavioral Medicine, 37*, 141–153.

Troyer, A.K., Moscovitch, M., and Winocur, G. (1997). Clustering and switching as two components of verbal fluency: Evidence from younger and older healthy adults. *Neuropsychology, 11*, 138-146.

Tun, P. (1998). Fast noisy speech: Age differences in processing rapid speech with background noise. *Psychology and Aging, 13*, 424–434.

Waldstein, S.R., Jennings, J.R., Ryan, C.M., et al. (1996). Hypertension and neuropsychological performance in men: Interactive effects of age. *Health Psychology, 15*, 102–109.

Waters, G.S. and Caplan, D. (2001). Age, working memory, and on-line syntactic processing in sentence comprehension. *Psychology and Aging, 16*, 128–144.

Waters, G.S., Caplan, D., and Rochon, E. (1995). Processing capacity and sentence comprehension in patients with Alzheimer's disease. *Cognitive Neuropsychology, 12*, 1–30.

Wecker, N., Kramer, J., Wisniewski, A., Delis, D., and Kaplan, E. (2000). Age effects on executive ability. Neuropsychology, 14, 409–414.

West, R. (2000). In defense of the frontal lobe hypothesis of cognitive aging. *Journal of the International Neuropsychological Society, 6,* 727–729.

West, R.L. (1996). An application of prefrontal cortex function theory to cognitive aging. *Psychological Bulletin, 120,* 272–292.

Whelihan, W.M., and Lesher, E.L. (1985). Neuropsychological changes in frontal function with aging. *Developmental Neuropsychology, 1,* 371–380.

Wingfield, A., and Grossman, M. (2006). Language and the aging brain: Patterns of neural compensation revealed by functional brain imaging. *Journal of Neurophysiology, 96,* 2830–2839.

Wingfield, A., & Stine-Morrow, E.A.L. (2000). Language and speech. In F.I.M. Craik, & T.A. Salthouse (Eds.) *The handbook of aging and cognition.* Mahwah, NJ: Lawrence Erlbaum Associates.

Wingfield, A., Aberdeen, J.S., & Stine, E. (1991). Word onset gating and linguistic context in spoken word recognition by young and elderly adults. *Journal of Gerontology: Psychological Sciences, 3,* 127-129.

Wingfield, A., Lahar, C.J., and Stine, E.A.L. (1989). Age and decision strategies in running memory for speech: Effects of prosody and linguistic structure. *Journal of Gerontology: Psychological Sciences, 44,* 106–113.

Wingfield, A., Lindfield, K. C., and Kahana, M. J. (1998). Adult age differences in the temporal characteristics of category free recall. *Psychology and Aging, 13,* 256–266.

Wingfield, A., Peelle, J. E., and Grossman, M. (2003). Speech rate and syntactic complexity as multiplicative factors in speech comprehension by young and older adults. *Aging, Neuropsychology, and Cognition, 10,* 310–322.

Wingfield, A., Stine, E.A.L., Lahar, C.J., and Aberdeen, J.S. (1988). Does the capacity of working memory change with age? *Experimental Aging Research, 14,*103–107.

Wingfield, A., Tun, P.A., and McCoy, S.L. (2005). Hearing loss in older adulthood: What it is and how it interacts with cognitive performance. *Current Directions in Psychological Science, 14,* 144–148.

Ylikoski, A., Erkinjunti, T., Raininko, R., Sarna, S., Sulkava, R., and Tilvis, R. (1995). White matter hyperintensities on MRI in the neurologically nondiseased elderly: Analysis of cohorts of consecutive subjects aged 55 to 85 years living at home. *Stroke, 26,* 1171–1177.

Zurif, E., Swinney, D., Prather, P., Wingfield, A., and Brownell, H. (1995). The allocation of memory resources during sentence comprehension: Evidence from the elderly. *Journal of Psycholinguistic Research, 24,* 165–182.

43 Normal Pressure Hydrocephalus

Winnie C.W. Pao and Neill R. Graff-Radford

This study was funded in part by grant P50 AG16574 and by the Robert and Clarice Smith and Abigail Van Buren Alzheimer's Disease Research Program. With permission this chapter is based in part on one in the Neurologic Clinic 2007.

Introduction

Doctors find the management of normal pressure hydrocephalus (NPH) difficult; the diagnosis is often uncertain and treatment with shunt surgery carries a significant risk. With the aim of highlighting the useful but largely anecdotal, information available on NPH, this chapter will discuss: epidemiology, reasons why the diagnosis is difficult, differential diagnosis, features of the history, examination, neuropsychological assessment, radiological evaluation and special tests that may help clinicians with management. Further, we shall discuss the relationship of systemic hypertension and head size to the pathogenesis of NPH.

Epidemiology

There are a few studies in the literature that address the incidence and prevalence of NPH. One involved the evaluation of all elderly persons in the Republic of San Marino (smallest independent country, in Italy), and found 2 of 396 persons with idiopathic normal pressure hydrocephalus (INPH), a 0.5% prevalence of persons over 65 (Casmiro, Benassi et al. 1989). In a door-to-door survey of parkinsonism, Trenkwalder et al.(Trenkwalder, Schwarz et al. 1995) found 4/982 with NPH, with a prevalence of 0.5%. In a stable population of 220,000 in the Norwegian county of Vestfold, all patients with signs and symptoms of INPH were recruited. Sixty-three patients fulfilled diagnosis criteria for possible INPH, and 48 for probable INPH. They estimated a minimal prevalence of probable INPH of 117.9/100,000 (0.12%) for individuals 65 years or above (Brean and Eide 2008). In a study from Japan, they mailed a questionnaire to 2,516 persons over 65 years, and 2352 responded. Of these, they randomly selected 240 (10%) to undergo evaluation and 200 had MRI imaging. Forty could not have MRI because of physical limitations. Of the 200, 170 had neurological and neuropsychological testing. They found 5 (2.9%) with INPH (Hiraoka, Meguro et al. 2008). In the 2006 US census there were 37 million persons 65 and older. If the estimated prevalence is between 0.12% and 2.9%, there is an estimated prevalence of 44,400 to 1,073,000 persons with INPH. Another way to estimate the US prevalence is from the study by Clarfield and colleagues (Clarfield 2003), who report in a meta analysis of 37 dementia studies, a 1% NPH prevalence in more than 5,000 dementia patients. Based on this study and the estimated 4–6 million persons in the US with dementia (Hebert, Scherr et al. 2003) there would be about 40,000 to 60,000 with NPH.

Regarding incidence of NPH, the best study is from Brean and colleagues who estimated the incidence in Norway to be 5.5/100,000/yr for probable and 7.3/100,000/yr for possible INPH (Brean and Eide 2008).

Why the Diagnosis Is Difficult

Doctors find the diagnosis and treatment of patients with NPH particularly difficult. The reasons for this are: no combinations of the cardinal findings (gait difficulty, cognitive decline, incontinence of urine, and enlarged ventricles) are pathognomonic for the diagnosis; each of the cardinal symptoms and combinations of these cardinal symptoms are exceedingly common in the elderly and have many causes (see below); all of the diagnostic tests so far described give both false positive and false negative results; the surgical treatment carries significant short and long-term risks, and we do not know the cause or pathogenesis of many NPH cases.

Let's look at each of the cardinal findings:

1. Gait difficulty: One study found that 20% of persons 75 and older had gait abnormality and this was related to future development of dementia (Verghese, Lipton et al. 2002).

2. Cognitive decline: One study estimated that 4.5 million persons over 65 had Alzheimer's disease (AD) in the US in 2000 (Hebert, Scherr et al. 2003).

3. Incontinence: In 2006, Anger and colleagues (Anger, Saigal et al. 2006) reported the overall prevalence of incontinence in older women is 38% and Stothers and colleagues (Stothers, Thom et al. 2005) reported a prevalence of 17% in men over age 60.

4. Enlarged ventricles: Barron and colleagues (Barron, Jacobs et al. 1976) showed that ventricle size increases with age and Jack and colleagues have shown ventricle size increases faster in AD compared to controls (Jack, Shiung et al. 2004).

Thus it is clear that all the cardinal features are common in the elderly and have many causes.

Differential Diagnosis

When evaluating the patient, keep in mind practical differential diagnoses, as listed in Table 1, which helps focus the history and examination.

Clinical Evaluation

General Factors

The clinician should evaluate the patient's general medical health because this may be important when considering surgery. Factors that theoretically could aggravate hydrocephalus include systemic hypertension (see belowfor a discussion of the association of hydrocephalus and hypertension) and a recent head injury (which is particularly pertinent

Table 1 Differential Diagnosis of NPH

- Combinations of ventriculomegaly, dementia and factors affecting gait (e.g. cervical spondylosis, large joint arthritis, peripheral neuropathy, impaired vision, vestibular dysfunction, antipsychotics)
- Vascular dementia including subcortical ischemic encephalopathy or Binswanger's disease
- Parkinson's disease dementia and enlarged ventricles
- Parkinsonian syndromes (Lewy body disease, corticobasal degeneration, progressive supranuclear palsy and multiple system atrophy) and enlarged ventricles
- Frontotemporal dementia with caudate atrophy

in individuals with gait difficulty). Evaluate for sleep apnea, congestive heart failure, lung disease, and obesity, all of which could increase jugular venous pressure and decrease CSF flow into the cerebral venous sinuses. If the patient is on long-term anticoagulants, such as Coumadin for atrial fibrillation, take this into account for the theoretical increased risk of brain hemorrhage during and after surgery. Look for evidence of arthritis of the hips and knees, cervical myelopathy, lumbar stenosis and radiculopathy, visual impairment, vestibular dysfunction, and peripheral neuropathy, all of which could impair gait.

History Related to Hydrocephalus

There are several specific questions that should be asked when taking a history from these patients and their families.

Ask how long the patient has demonstrated symptoms of dementia. If this is more than two years, it is less likely that the patient will respond to surgery (Petersen, Mokri et al. 1985; Graff-Radford, Godersky et al. 1989). Note that the question is not how long the patient has had gait abnormality but how long the patient has been demented. In our series this question predicted 5/7 unimproved and 21/23 improved patients (Graff-Radford, Godersky et al. 1989).

Ask which started first, gait abnormality or dementia. If the gait abnormality began before or at the same time as dementia, then there is a better chance for successful response to surgery; whereas, if dementia started before gait abnormality, shunting is less likely to help. In our series this question predicted 3/7 unimproved and 23/23 improved patients (Graff-Radford, Godersky et al. 1989). Note, this observation had been previously reported by Fisher (Fisher 1977).

Ask if the patient abused alcohol because alcohol abuse is a poor prognostic indicator (De Mol 1985).

Ask if there are secondary causes for hydrocephalus such as subarachnoid hemorrhage, meningitis, prior brain surgery, and head injury. If any of these are present, the chances of improvement with surgery are better (Black, Ojemann et al. 1985; De Mol 1985; Petersen, Mokri et al. 1985).

Ask if the patient has a large head size as evidenced by needing a large hat. This may indicate that the patient suffers from congenital hydrocephalus that has become symptomatic in later life (Graff-Radford and Godersky 1989; Krefft, Graff-Radford et al. 2004). We have found that 10–20% of persons diagnosed with so called idiopathic normal pressure hydrocephalus (INPH) have large heads, indicating that they may have congenital hydrocephalus that becomes symptomatic in later life (Graff-Radford and Godersky 1989; Krefft, Graff-Radford et al. 2004).

Examination

On examination, the following issues should be addressed.

Measure the head circumference. If greater than 59 cm in males or 57.5 cm in females, suspect that the patient could have an element of congenital hydrocephalus that has become symptomatic in later life (Graff-Radford and Godersky 1989; Krefft, Graff-Radford et al. 2004).

Look for signs of diseases that may mimic NPH (see Table 1). These include Alzheimer's disease with extrapyramidal features, Parkinson's disease dementia, Parkinsonian syndromes (PSP, CBD, and MSA), diffuse Lewy body disease, frontotemporal dementia, cerebrovascular disease, and phenothiazine use. Also look for cervical spondylosis with spinal cord compression, lumbar stenosis or radiculopathy, arthritis of the hips and knees, and multiple factors that impair gait abnormality (as might occur in diabetics with peripheral neuropathy and visual impairment; or alcoholics with peripheral neuropathy and cerebellar atrophy; or the elderly with vestibular and visual dysfunction and arthritis.)

Neuropsychology

Look for evidence of aphasia. If there is evidence of aphasia (e.g. anomia) this is a poor prognostic indicator for surgical success (De Mol 1985; Graff-Radford, Godersky et al. 1989).

Ogino and colleagues (Ogino, Kazui et al. 2006) compared 42 AD with 21 NPH patients matched for age, gender and Mini-Mental State Examination score (Folstein, Folstein et al. 1975). The NPH patients scored better on orientation and on the delayed recall of the Wechsler Memory Scale-Revised (WMS-R) (Wechsler 1987), but significantly lower on the attention and concentration subtests of the WMS-R and on the digit span, arithmetic, block design, and digit symbol substitution subtest of the Wechsler Adult Intelligence Scale-Revised (Wechsler 1997). Hellstrom and colleagues compared 58 INPH patients (33 without and 25 with vascular risk factors) with 108 healthy individuals. The NPH patients performed worse on tests of reaction time, tests using motor skills, verbal memory, attention, and timed tests. Interestingly, those with vascular risk factors were worse than those without, indicating that the white matter damage associated with vascular risk factors may make the neuropsychological profile worse (Hellstrom, Edsbagge et al. 2007).

Chaudhry and colleagues looked at the prognostic value of neuropsychometric testing. They carried out a prospective study of 60 patients (70.6 +/– 12.1 years, mean duration of symptoms 3.5 years) with NPH on neuropsychometric testing. In the results, 74% showed significant cognitive improvement 3–6 months post-shunt. Factors predicting good outcome were: 1. improvement on cognitive tests after a trial of controlled CSF drainage, 2. younger age, 3. being female, 4. baseline Wechsler Memory Scale immediate recall score < 1 SD below normal, 5. improvement in Ray Auditory Verbal Learning Test (RAVLT) by at least five points. However, some patients expected not to improve on the basis of these factors, improved significantly on cognitive tests and reported substantial gains in everyday functioning (Chaudhry, Kharkar et al. 2007). As is typical in prognostic NPH studies, there are both false positives and negatives.

In summary, patients with aphasia have a poorer prognosis for shunt surgery while patients with milder memory impairment do better. Those with vascular risk factors have greater impairment.

Radiological Evaluation

Diagnosis of probable INPH under the published guidelines for NPH (Bergsneider, Black et al. 2005) is based on clinical history, brain imaging, physical findings, and physiological criteria (see Table 2).

Table 2 Probable INPH (This is based upon the published guidelines for NPH (69))

The diagnosis of probable INPH is based on clinical history, brain imaging, physical findings, and physiological criteria

I. History

History should be corroborated by an informant

a. Insidious onset (versus acute)

b. Start after 40 years

c. Minimum duration of 3–6 months

d. No secondary causes (head trauma, intracerebral hemorrhage, meningitis, or other known cause of secondary hydrocephalus)

e. Progression over time

f. No other neurological, psychiatric, or medical condition that are sufficient to explain the presenting symptoms

II. Brain Imaging

Brain imaging study (CT or MRI) after onset must show evidence of

a. Ventricular enlargement not entirely attributable to cerebral atrophy or congenital enlargement (Evan's index >0.3 or comparable measure, equivalent to ventriculomegaly > 95 percentile)

b. No macroscopic obstruction of CSF flow

c. At least one of the following supportive features

   1. Enlargement of the temporal horns of the lateral ventricles not attributable to hippocampal atrophy

   2. Callosal angle of 40 degrees or more

   3. Evidence of altered brain water content, including periventricular signal changes on CT and MRI not attributable to microvascular ischemic changes or demyelination

   4. An aqueductal or fourth ventricular flow void on MRI

Other brain imaging findings

   1. Brain imaging study performed before onset of symptoms showing smaller ventricular size or without evidence of hydrocephalus

   2. Radionucleotide cisternogram showing delayed clearance of radiotracer over the cerebral convexities after 48–72h.

   3. Cine MRI study or other technique showing increased ventricular flow rate

   4. A SPECT-acetazolamide challenge showing decreased periventricular perfusion that is not altered by acetazolamide

III. Clinical

By classic definition, findings of gait/balance disturbance must be present plus at least one other area of impairment in cognition and urinary symptoms or both

With respect to gait and balance, at least two of the following should be present and not entirely attributable to other conditions.

a. Decreased step height

b. Decreases step length

c. Decreased cadence

d. Increased trunk sway

e. Widened standing base

f. Toes turned outward on walking

g. Retropulsion (spontaneous or provoked)

Table 2 Continued

h. En bloc turning (turning requires three or more steps for 180 degrees)

With respect to cognition there must be documented impairment (adjusted for age and education) and/or decrease in performance on a cognitive screening instrument (such as the Mini Mental Status Examination) or evidence of at least two of the following on examination that is not fully attributable to other conditions.

a. Psychomotor slowing

b. Decreased fine motor speed

c. Difficulty dividing or maintaining attention

d. Impaired recall, especially for recent events

e. Executive dysfunction, such as impairment in multistep procedures, working memory, formulation of abstract/similarities, insight

f. Behavioral or personality change

To document symptoms in the domains of urinary continence, one of the following should be present

a. Episodic or persistent urinary incontinence and not attributable to urological disorders

b. Persistence of urinary incontinence

c. Persistence of fecal incontinence

Or any two of the following be present

a. Urinary urgency as defined by perception of a pressing need to void

b. Urinary frequency as defined by more than six episodes in an average 12-hour period despite normal fluid intake

c. Nocturia as defined by need to urinate more that two times in an average night

IV. Physiological

CSF pressure opening in the range of 5–18mm Hg (or 70–245 mmH2O) as determined by a lumbar puncture or a comparable procedure. Appropriately measure pressures that are significantly higher or lower are not consistent with a probable NPH diagnosis.

Possible INPH

I. History

Reported symptoms may

   a. Have a subacute or indeterminate mode of onset

   b. Begin at any age after childhood

   c. May have less than three months of indeterminate duration

   d. May follow events such as mild head trauma, remote history or intracerebral hemorrhage, or childhood and adolescent meningitis, or other conditions that in the judgment of the clinician are not likely to be casually related

   e. Coexist with other neurological, psychiatric, or general medical disorders but in the judgment of the clinician not be entirely attributed to these conditions

   f. Be nonprogressive or not clearly progressive

II. Brain Imaging

Ventricular enlargement consistent with hydrocephalus but associated with any of the following

   a. Evidence of cerebral atrophy of sufficient severity to potentially explain ventricular size

   b. Structural lesions that may influence ventricular size

Table 2 Continued

III. Clinical

Symptoms of either

   a. Incontinence and/or cognitive impairment in the absence of an observable gait or balance disturbance

   b. Gait disturbance or dementia alone

IV. Physiological

Opening pressure not available or pressure outside the range of required for probable INPH.

Unlikely INPH

1. No evidence of ventriculomegaly

2. Signs of increased intracranial pressure such as papilledema

3. No component of the clinical triad of INPH

4. Symptoms explained by other causes (e.g. spinal stenosis)

Computerized Tomography (CT)

Since the advent of CT, the documentation of ventriculomegaly has become easier. A patient has ventriculomegaly (above the 95th percentile) when the modified Evan's ratio (maximum width of the frontal horns / measurement of the inner table of the cranium at the same place) is greater than 0.31 (Gyldenstad 1977). The ventricles normally enlarge with age (Barron, Jacobs et al. 1976), a point to be taken into account when diagnosing hydrocephalus. There is slow ventricular enlargement to age 60 years and then the rate of enlargement increases. In Barron's study (Barron, Jacobs et al. 1976), the mean ventricular size was 5.2% (percent of intracranial area) in the decade 50 to 59 years, 6.4% 60 to 69 years, 11.5% 70 to 79 years and 14.1% 80 to 89 years.

In one study, the greater the sulcal enlargement the less the chance of improvement with surgery (Borgesen and Gjerris 1982). However, patients might still improve with surgery, even if there is sulcal enlargement and hydrocephalus. Borgesen and Gjerris (1982) measured the largest sulcus in the high frontal or parietal region and found that if the cortical sulci were less than 1.9 mm, 17 of 17 patients shunted improved; if the sulci were 1.9 to 5 mm, 17 of 20 shunted improved; and if the sulci were 5mm or more, 15 of 27 shunted improved.

Magnetic Resonance Imaging (MRI)

MRI is an excellent method for evaluating patients with possible symptomatic hydrocephalus and is the neuroimaging study of choice in NPH patients. It has the advantage of being able to visualize relevant structures in the posterior fossa including cerebral aqueduct stenosis, cerebellar tonsil herniation, and infarctions in the brain stem. Further, MRI can be used to obtain volumetric measures of medial temporal lobe structures, a technique that has been shown to be useful in separating Alzheimer disease patients from normal elderly controls (Jack, Petersen et al. 1992). Voxel-based MRI may also be useful in differentiating between INPH, AD, and normal controls (Ishii, Kawaguchi et al. 2008).

About 10–20% of patients with symptomatic hydrocephalus in the elderly may have congenital hydrocephalus that becomes symptomatic in later years (Graff-Radford and Godersky 1989; Krefft, Graff-Radford et al. 2004; Wilson and Williams 2007). A clinical clue to this is that the patient has a large head size. On MRI the ventricular enlargement shows no or little associated periventricular increased signal on T2-weighted imaging, indicating a chronic process. This raises the possibility that one of the causes of so called INPH is that patients born with hydrocephalus may become symptomatic later in life. In addition, rarely a cause for the congenital hydrocephalus may be found, such as an Arnold-Chiari malformation or aqueductal stenosis.

MRI Differentiation of NPH and Alzheimer's Disease

Traditionally, the presence of ventriculomegaly without sulcal enlargement has been a radiological finding felt to indicate NPH when accompanied by the typical clinical triad. However, studies by Holodny and colleagues (Holodny, George et al. 1998) and Kitagaki and colleagues (Kitagaki, Mori et al. 1998) both have pointed out the occasional occurrence of focally dilated sulci over the convexity or medial surface of a hemisphere in NPH patients, unlike the diffuse sulcal enlargement seen in Alzheimer's disease (Figure 1). The Kitagaki report (Kitagaki, Mori et al. 1998) also indicated significantly greater sylvian CSF volume in idiopathic NPH compared to AD patients. He felt this was a sign supportive of NPH, indicating a "suprasylvian block."

An area where MRI has the potential to be helpful for surgical prognosis is in volumetric measurements of certain structures in the temporal lobe. There is enlargement of the temporal horns of the lateral ventricles in both NPH and AD patients. Jack and colleagues (Jack, Petersen et al. 1992) developed a technique for measuring the volumes of structures in the anterior temporal lobe and hippocampal formation. Holodny and colleagues (Holodny, Waxman et al. 1998) measured the CSF volumes of the perihippocampal fissures (PHF) and the ventricular volumes. They showed that the PHFs were significantly enlarged in AD patients compared to NPH patients whereas the ventricles were larger in NPH. This was detectable both by visible inspection and computer volumetrics.

MR-based volumetric measurements of the hippocampal formation have been shown to be useful in discriminating between Alzheimer's disease and normal elderly controls (Jack, Petersen et al. 1992). Though Golomb and colleagues (Golomb, de Leon et al. 1994) found smaller hippocampal volumes in NPH patients compared to controls, Savolainen and colleagues (Savolainen, Laakso et al. 2000) only found a minor left side decrease. However, Savolainen importantly detected significantly larger hippocampi in NPH patients compared to AD patients. Ishii and colleagues used Voxel-based MRI found no difference in hippocampal size compared to AD cases. They analyzed 34 subjects each in probable INPH (based on 2005 guidelines), AD, and

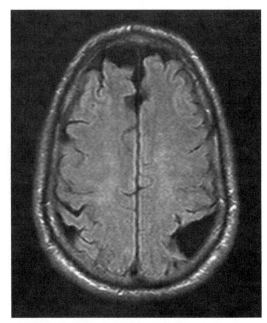

Figure 1 MRI demonstrating enlarged sulci with entrapped CSF. This is not atrophy but part of the so called "supra Sylvian block" sometimes seen in hydrocephalus.

normal control (Ishii, Kawaguchi et al. 2008). The most characteristic finding of NPH in their study was that the precuneus sulci were tighter than other regions (Figure 2). Adachi et al. reported "a cingulated sulcal sign" which may distinguish INPH from AD. They showed that on the paramedian sagittal MR plane of INPH scans, the anterior part of the cingulated sulcus is wider than the posterior part (Figure 2) (Adachi, Kawanami et al. 2006).

In summary, when looking at the CT or MRI, hydrocephalus must be present. The modified Evan's ratio should be greater than 0.31 (Gyldenstad 1977). Note if cortical atrophy is prominent. If there is extensive cortical atrophy, this reduces but does not eliminate the chance of improvement with surgery (Borgesen and Gjerris 1982; Petersen, Mokri et al. 1985). Avoid calling entrapped sulci or suprasylvian block brain atrophy (Holodny, George et al. 1998; Kitagaki, Mori et al. 1998).

Look for evidence of congenital hydrocephalus. For example, is there aqueductal stenosis or an Arnold-Chiari malformation and are the ventricles enlarged with little white matter abnormality indicating a chronic process (Graff-Radford and Godersky 1989; Krefft, Graff-Radford et al. 2004)?

The pattern of atrophy may be useful diagnostically (e.g., does it involve the medial temporal lobes as seen in Alzheimer's disease?). Look at the perihippocampal fissure which is larger in AD and also evaluate the anterior cingulated sulcus (enlarged in INPH) and the precuneus sulci (narrowed in INPH) (Figure 2).

Newer MRI techniques, such as Cine-MRI involving the analysis of a CSF flow void in the aqueduct of Sylvius were first thought to be helpful (Bradley, Whittemore et al. 1991; Bradley, Scalzo et al. 1996), but unfortunately have not been found to be so in subsequent studies (Krauss, Regel et al. 1997; Hakim and Black 1998; Dixon, Friedman et al. 2002).

Prognostic Studies for Shunt Outcome

A combination of tests and clinical symptoms has been used as selection criteria to better aid in predicting who will benefit from surgical shunting.

CSF Drainage Procedures

Lumbar Puncture

If the patient's gait improves after removing a large quantity of CSF by lumbar puncture (30 to 50 cc and this can be repeated daily), this person would be a good candidate for shunt surgery (Wikkelso, Andersson et al. 1986). Malm and colleagues found no predictive values of a spinal tap test (Malm, Kristensen et al. 1995) but Walchenbach and colleagues (Walchenbach, Geiger et al. 2002) found a poor sensitivity (9/35 cases with a positive test had improvement with shunt surgery) but a very good positive predictive value (9/9 with a positive test improved). One of the issues is that in both of these studies the gait was evaluated 4–6 hours after the LP. In patients that don't leak CSF after the LP the CSF is replaced at 0.3cc per minute so could be back to normal in two hours. Kilic and colleagues reported one of the largest studies regarding repeated LPs (one per day removing 30–40cc of fluid daily for three days) in suspected NPH patients. They did LPs in 155 persons and 129 improved who were then shunted. Following surgery, 111 of the 129 patients improved. In those who did not improve, they offered shunt revision and 10 of 18 accepted revision and three of these improved. Thus, 114 of 129 (88%) with a positive repeated LP test improved (Kilic, Czorny et al. 2007).

At this time it is reasonable to presume that a positive repeated LP test has a good positive predictive value but a completely accurate sensitivity cannot be calculated (in the Kilic study they did not shunt all with a negative LP but see later under lumbar external drainage (LED) because they came close by offering LED to all with negative LPs).

Lumbar External Drainage

A modification of this technique has also been reported and is continuous CSF drainage via a catheter placed in the lumbar CSF space (Haan and Thomeer 1988). In the guidelines for the diagnosis and management of INPH (Marmarou, Bergsneider et al. 2005) they based the guidelines on three studies (Haan and Thomeer 1988; Malm, Kristensen et al. 1995; Walchenbach, Geiger et al. 2002). These studies showed a range of sensitivity from 50% to 100%, specificity 60% to 100% and positive predictive value from 80% to 100%, negative predictive value from 36% to 100% and accuracy from 58% to 100%. In the Kilic study, 73 had external CSF drainage as the first choice and they also offered this to the 26 with a negative repeated LP test. Seventeen of the latter accepted. Fifty of the 73 and 7 of the 17 had a positive LED test. All these patients underwent shunt surgery and 51/57 improved. For the six who did not improve, revision of shunt surgery was proposed and five accepted. Of these, one improved. As a result, a total of 52/57 (91%) with a positive LED test improved. We can conclude that the LED test has a high positive predictive value but we can't accurately calculate the sensitivity because not all who had the test underwent shunt surgery.

In the one LED study (Walchenbach, Geiger et al. 2002), two of 38 developed meningitis, five pulled out their drains. In another study (Haan and Thomeer 1988), two of 22 had infections, four removed their drains, and three had root irritation. In the Kilic study, 11 of 90 undergoing LED developed meningitis and in 18 of 90 the drain had to

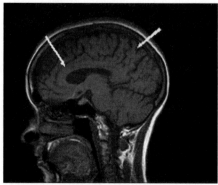

AD   INPH

Figure 2 Cingulate sulcal sign. Paramedian sagittal plane of MRI showing the anterior part of cingulate sulcus wider than the posterior (see arrows). This helps to distinguish INPH patients from AD.

be replaced. While this test is more sensitive than a large volume spinal tap, we would caution that it should be undertaken by an experienced team that can limit the complication rate.

CSF Infusion Tests

Resistance to CSF (Rcsf) absorption or its reciprocal, the conductance, can be determined by several methods (Katzman and Hussey 1970; Borgesen and Gjerris 1982). The idea is that the greater the pressure needed to obtain an amount of CSF absorption, the better the chance of patient improving with shunt surgery. Borgersen and Gjerris reported that a conductance of < 0.08 (Rcsf of 12.5 mmHg/ml/min) predicted a favorable outcome (Borgesen and Gjerris 1982). Boon and colleagues (Boon, Tans et al. 1997) reported the first multiple center, randomized study evaluating the predictive value for shunt surgery of measuring resistance to outflow of the cerebrospinal fluid. They enrolled 101 patients (both idiopathic and secondary, although they note most were idiopathic) and measured the resistance to outflow of CSF. They randomized the patients to receive either low- or medium-pressure valves. Outcome measures were an NPH scale (sum of gait and dementia measures) and the modified Rankin scale. Follow-up was at 1, 3, 6, 9, and 12 months. Intention to treat analysis was performed on all 101 patients and 57% showed improvement in the NPH scale and 59% in the modified Rankin scale at one year. When all known serious events unrelated to NPH that clearly interfered with neurological function were excluded, 95 patients were left. In these patients, 76% had a meaningful improvement on the NPH scale and 69% improved one grade on the modified Rankin scale. Using a cutoff of the resistance to CSF outflow of < 18 mmHg/ml/min, 20/59 had no improvement on the NPH scale. Above this cutoff, 3/36 had no improvement on the NPH scale.

The authors conclude that the Rcsf obtained by lumbar CSF infusion is a reliable method for selecting patients for shunt surgery if the Rcsf cutoff is 18 mmHg/ml/min or greater. Patients with an Rcbf less than 18 mmHg/ml/min should only undergo shunt placement when characteristic clinical features of NPH are present. Unfortunately, the majority of patients (>60%) under consideration for shunt surgery have an Rcsf of less than 18 mmHg/ml/min and this diagnostic test is not helpful in this group. In the guidelines Aygok, Marmarou et al. (2005) noted the data is limited and "the results, methods and thresholds are center specific and subject to wide variation."

CSF Pressure Monitoring

There have been reports of a significant relationship between measures of intracranial CSF pressure monitoring and surgical outcome for symptomatic hydrocephalus, e.g. in the Borgersen and Gjerris study and in our study (Borgesen and Gjerris 1982; Graff-Radford, Godersky et al. 1989) the greater the percentage of time B waves were present, the greater the chance of a good outcome. Pfisterer and colleagues looked at 92 patients with suspected NPH (74 INPH, 18 SNPH) who received continuous intraventricular pressure monitoring (CIPM) for 48 hrs including intraventricular steady-state infusion test to determine resistance to outflow. Shunting criteria required a basal ICP above 10mmHg and/or occurrence of A-waves and/or occurrence of B waves of more than 10% of recorded periods. When there were 5-10% B-waves present, they only shunted the patients if there was also a positive steady-state infusion test. Thirty-seven patients did not meet these criteria and were not shunted. Fifty-five patients met the criteria and were shunted with follow up for 1–10yrs (median 6.5). Gait improved in 96.1%, cognition in 77.1%, and urine control in 75.7%. They concluded that CIMP was helpful in choosing patients for shunt surgery (Pfisterer, Aboul-Enein et al. 2007). Williams and colleagues found that using a threshold of 25% of time B waves present, the

sensitivity in predicting surgical outcome was 78% but the specificity was 40% (Williams, Razumovsky et al. 1998).

From all the studies using only the percentage of time B waves present would be inadequate in predicting surgical outcome. The consensus guidelines (Marmarou, Bergsneider et al. 2005) notes that there is insufficient evidence to use pressure monitoring for prognostic purposes.

One point to be evaluated in the future is the prognostic value of continually measuring the CSF pressure and determining how long the pressure is high. In our series, the longer the pressure was more than 15 mm Hg, the better the chance of successful surgery (Graff-Radford, Godersky et al. 1989). This may be important because it implies that increased pressure may be pathogenic in symptomatic hydrocephalus. These data raise the issue about what is meant by normal pressure hydrocephalus. Does it mean normal pressure at one spinal tap or does it imply the pressure remains normal all the time? We do not know what 24-hour CSF pressure recordings in normal people show. It follows that we do not know if the pressure is normal or abnormal in those who respond to surgery but have CSF pressures greater than 15mmHg for a percentage of time.

CSF Biomarkers

N-acetylaspartate (NAA) is considered a marker of neuronal integrity exclusively confined to neuronal cells. Using proton magnetic resonance spectroscopy, Lenfeldt and colleagues evaluated NAA/Cr (creatine) in 16 NPH patients compared to 10 controls. The NPH patients also underwent lumbar external drainage (LED) (Dickson, Fujishiro et al. 2008). On average, those NPH patients who improved on LED had an NAA/Cr ratio closer to controls than those that did not improve. If we equate improvement on LED to a positive improvement with shunt, this study implies that persons with more viable neurons have a better chance of improving with shunt surgery. However, there was considerable overlap of NAA/Cr between the patients that responded to LED compared to those that did not. Also, the study sample is small, making it hard to generalize (Lenfeldt, Hauksson et al. 2008).

Two studies have evaluated CSF Aβ42 and tau levels in NPH (Agren-Wilsson, Lekman et al. 2007; Kapaki, Paraskevas et al. 2007). In both studiesCSF Aβ42 levels are lower in NPH cases than controls. In Kapaki and colleagues' study, Aβ42 was the same as AD cases while tau was lower in INPH than AD cases and the same as controls. The study by Agren-Wilsson and colleagues differs by showing that tau CSF levels were lower than controls. In summary, Aβ42 is lower in INPH than controls but the same as in AD, whereas total tau and phosphor-tau are either the same or lower in INPH than controls and are lower than in AD cases. Another interesting observation by Agren-Wilson and colleagues is that after shunting, follow-up CSF analysis shows a significant increase in several proteins including tau but no increase in Aβ42 in the lumbar CSF. Clearly further studies are needed to evaluate CSF biomarkers.

Flow Void on MRI as a Predictive Test of Surgical Outcome

In 1991, Bradley and coworkers (Bradley, Whittemore et al. 1991) retrospectively reviewed the MRI scans of 20 patients who had undergone ventriculoperitoneal shunt surgery for normal pressure hydrocephalus. They rated initial surgical outcome as excellent, good, or poor and correlated this with the extent of flow void in the cerebral aqueduct. They found a significant correlation (P<0.003) between extent of increased aqueduct flow void and initial surgical outcome. More specifically, eight out of ten with an increased CSF flow void score had an excellent or good response to surgery, whereas only one out of nine with a normal flow void score improved with surgery.

In a subsequent study of 18 NPH patients, Bradley and colleagues (Bradley, Scalzo et al. 1996) studied the CSF stroke volume (see his article for methods) and the CSF flow void score. The 12 with a CSF stroke volume of 42mL all improved, but of those with a CSF stroke volume of less than 42mL, three improved and three did not. Using the flow void score, four of fifteen improved patients had false negative tests and one of three unimproved patients had a false positive test.

Krauss and colleagues report that that the flow void in the cerebral aqueduct of 37 idiopathic NPH patients was not significantly different to that in 37 age-matched controls (Krauss, Regel et al. 1997). Further, the extent of the flow void extension into the 3rd, 4th, and lateral ventricles did not correlate with amount of improvement in these patients, but rather correlated with the width of the ventricles.

Hakim and Black (Hakim and Black 1998), in a small study of 12 patients of whom ten improved, found that the MRI-CSF flow studies were correct in six, but five had false negatives and one with false positive.

Dixon and colleagues also found in 49 patients that CSF flow through the cerebral aqueduct did not reliably predict those who improved with shunt surgery (Dixon, Friedman et al. 2002). These last three studies cast doubt on CSF flow as a diagnostic test in NPH.

Regional Cerebral Blood Flow (rCBF)

It has been reported that rCBF is decreased in the frontal areas in hydrocephalus (Jagust, Friedland et al. 1985), and in the parietotemporal areas in Alzheimer's disease (Mosconi 2005). On the presumption that many of the non-improved group have Alzheimer's disease (Bech and colleagues have shown more recently (Bech, Juhler et al. 1997) that 25% at time of shunt surgery brain biopsy shows AD pathology), we tried to differentiate those who will respond to shunt surgery from those who will not, based on the pattern of preoperative regional CBF (Graff-Radford, Rezai et al. 1987). To do this, we calculated the ratio of frontal over posterior regional blood flow, expecting a lower frontal-posterior ratio in true symptomatic hydrocephalus and a higher ratio in pseudo-symptomatic hydrocephalus patients who have Alzheimer's disease. In fact, this has been a good method in predicting surgical outcome: the ratio predicted 5/7 unimproved and 22/23 improved patients in our series (Graff-Radford, Godersky et al. 1989). Granado and colleagues (Granado, Diaz et al. 1991) also found that those suspected of NPH with an Alzheimer pattern did not improve but those with frontal hypoperfusion did. Unfortunately, a review of the literature on cerebral blood flow in NPH shows no clear cut use at this time (Owler and Pickard 2001).

Cisternography

The literature suggests there are numerous cases with a positive test (radioisotope seen within the ventricles 48–72 hours after being injected in the lumbar area) who do not improve with surgery and patients with equivocal or negative tests who do improve. Further, the test itself may be difficult to interpret (Black 1982). Black and colleagues (Black 1982), in a review of their experience with this test, found the following: Of eleven patients who had a positive test, nine improved and two did not; of the six patients who had mixed results, three improved and three did not; of the six who had negative results, four improved and two did not. They suggest a positive test is helpful but an equivocal or negative test is not. A more recent study by Vanneste and colleagues (Vanneste, Augustijn et al. 1992) reported that "cisternography did not improve the accuracy of combined clinical and computerized tomography in patients with presumed normal-pressure hydrocephalus."

White Matter Lesions and NPH

While some early reports using CT indicated the presence of 'transependymal flow' may be related to a good surgical prognosis (Borgesen and Gjerris 1982) (Borgesen and Gjerris's study reported 16 of 16 with periventricular hypodensity on CT improved with surgery), later studies did not confirm this or found the opposite. Bradley and colleagues (Bradley 2001) reported on MR images the presence or extent of deep white matter changes did not correlate with outcome. More recent studies by Kilic and colleagues (Kilic, Czorny et al. 2007), and Pfisterer and colleagues (Pfisterer, Aboul-Enein et al. 2007) also showed that PVH is not predictive of shunt outcome. However, Krauss and colleagues (Krauss, Regel et al. 1996) reported that the degree of improvement after shunt surgery depends on the extent and severity of white matter lesions, i.e., the more extensive the white matter lesions the less the improvement. In a subsequent report (Krauss, Regel et al. 1997), they compared the MRI findings in NPH to an age-matched control group and found that in both groups the periventricular white matter lesions correlated with the deep white matter lesions. In the control group the white matter lesions correlated significantly with age and the anterior horn index (frontal horn width divided by the horizontal intracranial width). In contrast, in the NPH group, there was no correlation of white matter lesions with age and there was a significant negative correlation between the white matter lesions and the frontal horn index, i.e., the wider the frontal horns the fewer white matter lesions present. They argue that the white matter lesions do not cause the hydrocephalus but that the common link between the frequent coexistence of idiopathic NPH and vascular encephalopathy (as evidenced by white matter lesions) is arterial hypertension. See below for further discussion on the association of systemic hypertension and NPH.

In a post mortem MRI study of autopsied brains and the histological analysis of the same brains, Munoz et al. (Munoz, Hastak et al. 1993) found the white matter changes seen on MRI correlate with decreased density of axons and myelinated fibers, diffuse vacuolation of white matter (so called spongiosis) and decreased density of glia. Infarctions were not common in these areas. While this study does not necessarily apply to the white matter changes seen in hydrocephalic patients, it does indicate that white matter MRI findings don't necessarily indicate irreversible periventricular infarctions, which would make shunt surgery unlikely to be effective.

A summary of prognostic factors related to shunt surgery are given in Table 3.

Probable and Possible NPH Criteria

Relkin and colleagues (Relkin, Marmarou et al. 2005) published the following criteria for probable and possible INPH. While these have not been tested prospectively they are based on an extensive review of the literature (Table 4). Extensive guidelines have also recently been published by Ishikawa and colleagues (Ishikawa, Hashimoto et al. 2008).

How to Assess Patient Improvement

Older studies measure patient improvement on a five-point rating scale (Black 1982; Borgesen and Gjerris 1982). This may be problematic because levels on the scale overlap and it is a subjective judgment into which level the patient falls. More recently, measures of outcome have included more objective measures of gait change (Graff-Radford, Godersky et al. 1989; Boon, Tans et al. 1997), scales measuring change

Table 3

Factors Favoring Clinical Improvement in NPH after Shunting

Secondary NPH
Gait disturbance preceding cognitive impairment
Mild impairment in cognition
Short duration of cognitive impairment
Clinical improvement (usually in gait) following lumbar puncture or continuous lumbar CSF drainage
Resistance to CSF outflow of 18 mm Hg/ml/min or greater during continuous lumbar CSF infusion test
Presence of B-waves for 50% of the time or greater during continuous lumbar CSF monitoring

Factors Weighing Against Clinical Improvement after Shunting

Moderate or severe cognitive impairment
Dementia present for two or more years
Cognitive impairment preceding gait disturbance
Presence of aphasia
History of ethanol abuse
MRI with diffuse cerebral atrophy

Factors of Uncertain Significance

MRI with significant white matter involvement
Long duration of gait abnormality
Absence of aqueductal flow void despite patent aqueduct (on MRI)
No clinical improvement after lumbar puncture
Cisternography
CBF measurements
CSF biomarkers

in Activities of Daily Living, such as the Katz Index (Graff-Radford, Godersky et al. 1989) or the Rankin Scale (Boon, Tans et al. 1997), both of which are sensitive to deficits in NPH.

A number of objective measurements of gait changes are available. One of them is the Computer Dyno Graphy (CDG) system that measures distribution of forces of reaction on the ground during walking. It measures particular phases of gait, regularity, and symmetry, and parameters such as ground reaction force as a function of time, time of single support, time of double support, and time of stance (Szczepek, Dabrowski et al. 2008). Another objective assessment program is GAITRite Portable Walkway and Gait Analysis System. It measures

Table 4   Complications of Shunt Surgery

Complications related to surgery and anesthesia such as myocardial infarction and deep vein thrombosis.

Acute intracerebral hemorrhage

Infection of the shunt

Subdural hematoma

Subdural hygroma (sometimes these may have a small hemorrhagic component)

Seizures

Shunt malfunction

Headache

Hearing loss

Tinnitis

Oculomotor palsies

Damage to intra abdominal organs

objective spatial and temporal gait parameters, which include velocity, mean normalized velocity, stride length, coefficient of variance of stride length, step length, cadence, double support time, base width, and functional ambulation profile (FAP: 0 to 100) (Williams, Thomas et al. 2008). Gait change can also be measured using the Tinetti scale on videotaped gait of the patient before and after intervention such as spinal tap or shunting.

Shunts

There is no good guidance in the literature to advise patients on the complication rate and the type of shunt that should be used. Some of the older studies report a complication rate from 30% to 40% (Black, Ojemann et al. 1985; Petersen, Mokri et al. 1985), but the complication rate has improved in recent studies (Bech, Waldemar et al. 1999; Kilic, Czorny et al. 2007; Pfisterer, Aboul-Enein et al. 2007; Greenberg and Williams 2008). The best way for doctors to be able to advise patients about the complication rate of shunt surgery is for them to become familiar with the complication rate at the center where they practice.

All complications are important but some affect patients more. A list of the more commonly encountered complications is given in Table 2 and is based on the surgical management chapter in the INPH guidelines (Bergsneider, Black et al. 2005). Prior to adjustable valves becoming available, one prospective study compared low and medium pressure valves. In this study, 35/49 patients receiving low pressure and 16/47 patients receiving medium pressure valves developed subdural collections. More patients in the LPV group improved compared to the MPV group (p<0.06). In recent years, the use of adjustable shunts has made the management of subdural hygromas and hematomas easier and allowed adjustment down of the opening pressure if the patient does not improve. Accurate information on shunt complications and which shunt to use is sorely needed.

Endoscopic Third Ventriculostomy

There are now several studies evaluating endoscopic third ventriculostomy (EVT) in NPH (Gangemi, Maiuri et al. 2004; Longatti, Fiorindi et al. 2004; Farin, Aryan et al. 2006; Dusick, McArthur et al. 2008). At this time we would not recommend this approach because the data is not convincing that it is as effective as the standard shunt procedures.

Long-term Outcome of INPH after Shunt Surgery

One of the crucial unknowns in NPH is if the person improves, how long they will stay improved. One study addressing this issue was published by Malm and colleagues (Malm, Kristensen et al. 2000). They found when they prospectively followed 84 surgically treated INPH patients, 64% were improved at three months but only 26% remained improved at three years. In Aygok and colleagues' (Aygok, Marmarou et al. 2005) study they followed 50 INPH patients and noted a decline in gait improvement from 90% at three months to 75% at three years but cognitive improvement remained steady at 80% at three months and three years and incontinence improved from 70% at three months to 82.5% at three years.

Histopathology of the Brains of Patients with INPH

In a unique study, Bech and colleagues (Bech, Juhler et al. 1997) reported their experience with 38 consecutive patients with INPH.

They monitored and performed absorption tests on all, but most importantly they performed brain biopsies on all. Twenty-nine of 38 patients fulfilled hydrodynamic criteria for shunt surgery (resistance to outflow of 10 Hg/ml/min with or without B activity for more than 50% of the monitoring period). Of the 29 individuals shunted, 27 had follow up and of these 9 (33.3%) improved, 10 (37%) remained stable, and 8 (29.6%) deteriorated. These results are not necessarily representative of all series in which INPH patients undergo shunt surgery, e.g. in our series more than 70% improved (Graff-Radford, Godersky et al. 1989) and in Boon and colleagues' series (Boon, Tans et al. 1997) 53% of the medium pressure valve group and 74% of the low pressure valve group improved. Nonetheless, the biopsy findings are of great interest. Only 12 of 25 had arachnoid fibrosis (not all biopsies had arachnoid tissue), 17 had normal parenchyma, 10 had Alzheimer disease and 8 had vascular disease.

There was no significant association of the presence or absence of arachnoid fibrosis with the hydrodynamic measures.

The Bech study has some important implications. Ten of 38 patients who were thought clinically possibly to have NPH, had biopsy verified AD. The criteria used to diagnose AD were conservative, that is, 10 neuritic plaques per high power field in the frontal lobe. It is possible that at autopsy several additional patients may have had AD. In a follow-up paper (Bech, Waldemar et al. 1999) Bech found no correlation between clinical outcome after shunting NPH patients and the presence or absence of AD pathology. Further, he also found that vascular disease and arachnoid fibrosis did not correlate with outcome. Golomb (Golomb, Wisoff et al. 2000) found AD pathology in 23 of 56 (41%) biopsied NPH patients. The NPH patients with concomitant AD had more impairment of gait and cognition than the "pure" NPH patients. Only 18% of the patients with Global Deterioration Scores (GDS) of three and below had AD positive biopsies, whereas 75% of those with GDS 6 or above were AD positive. There was comparable improvement in gait velocity in NPH patients regardless of the presence of AD pathology or not. No consistent cognitive improvement occurred in either group after shunting. Savolainen (Savolainen, Paljarvi et al. 1999) found concomitant AD pathology by biopsy in 31% of 51 consecutive NPH patients.

These three studies (Bech, Juhler et al. 1997; Savolainen, Paljarvi et al. 1999; Golomb, Wisoff et al. 2000) show that AD pathology is frequent in patients diagnosed with idiopathic NPH. Further, some of these patients have gait improvement after shunting. The implication is that NPH and AD may occur simultaneously in the same patient and families should be made aware of this. In Braak's classic study (Braak and Braak 1997) of autopsies of more than 2,000 persons from the medical examiner, the prevalence of AD pathology in the age group 71–75 was 30% and 76–80 was 40%, so the AD biopsy rate of NPH patients is similar to those patients not selected for being demented, i.e., from the medical examiner.

The Relationship of Idiopathic NPH and Systemic Hypertension

Several lines of evidence in the literature now point to a relationship between hydrocephalus and systemic hypertension.

Clinical and Autopsy Studies of NPH Patients

A number of postmortem examinations of NPH patients and case control studies have reported the association of systemic hypertension and NPH (Earnest, Fahn et al. 1974; Haidri and Modi 1977; Koto, Rosenberg et al. 1977; Shukla, Singh et al. 1980; Casmiro, D'Alessandro et al. 1989; Bech, Juhler et al. 1997). In our own series (Graff-Radford

and Godersky 1987) a significantly higher prevalence of systemic hypertension was found in INPH patients compared with matched, demented controls, and to the published prevalence of hypertension in the US population, matched for age. A more recent, much larger case control study (Krauss, Regel et al. 1996) of 65 INPH patients versus 70 matched control patients found a prevalence of 83% of systemic hypertension in the NPH patients compared to 36% in the control group. This was highly significant ($p<0.001$).

Boon (Boon, Tans et al. 1999) showed that cerebrovascular risk factors (hypertension, diabetes mellitus, cardiac disease, peripheral vascular disease, male gender, and advancing age) did not influence outcome after shunt placement. However, the presence of cerebrovascular disease (history of stroke, cerebral infarction noted on computerized tomography, or moderate-to-severe white matter hypodense lesions on CT) was an important predictor of poor outcome. Nonetheless, even though 74% of those without concomitant cerebrovascular disease improved with shunting, 49% with it also improved. In fact, four of the seven patients with the most severe white matter hypodense lesions responded favorably to shunting.

At this time regarding hypertension, subcortical arteriosclerotic encephalopathy (SAE), and NPH we have more questions than answers. Are hypertension, white matter changes, and cerebrovascular disease merely frequent concomitants of NPH? Do NPH and SAE represent a spectrum as suggested by Gallassi (Gallassi, Morreale et al. 1991)? Is one causative of the other?

Hydrocephalus Following Subarachnoid Hemorrhage

Another line of evidence showing that systemic hypertension and hydrocephalus may be related comes from the Cooperative Aneurysm Study (Graff-Radford, Torner et al. 1989). In over 3,000 patients with subarachnoid hemorrhage, it was found that a preoperative history of hypertension, the admission blood pressure measurement, and sustained hypertension during hospitalization after surgery, were all highly significantly related to patients developing hydrocephalus.

Hypertension in Patients with Aqueductal Stenosis

Greitz et al (Greitz, Levander et al. 1971) found a high prevalence of systemic hypertension in patients with hydrocephalus from aqueductal stenosis.

Hydrocephalus in the Spontaneously Hypertensive Rat

The association of hypertension and hydrocephalus are corroborated by reports in the animal literature. Ritter and Dinh (Greitz, Levander et al. 1971) showed that the spontaneously hypertensive rat develops hydrocephalus.

Experimental Models of Hydrocephalus, Ventricular Pulse Pressure, and Systemic Hypertension

Portnoy et al (Portnoy, Chopp et al. 1983) showed, in dogs, that infusing dopamine and norepinephrine led to increased systemic blood pressure, which, in turn, resulted in an increased CSF pressure and pulse pressure. Experimentally creating an increased CSF pulse pressure with an inflatable balloon in the lateral ventricle of sheep leads to hydrocephalus within hours (Pettorossi, Di Rocci et al. 1978). Bering and Salibi (Bering and Salibi 1959) performed seminal work on hydrocephalus in dogs. They tied off the jugular veins in the dogs and also measured the intraventricular pulse pressure. They concluded that the mechanism involved in the ventricular enlargement seemed to be a combination of at least two factors:

> "One was the possible failure of CSF absorption in the face of increased superior sagittal sinus venous pressure, and the other the increased intraventricular pulse pressure from the choroid plexus."

Thus, a body of information is accumulating that systemic hypertension and hydrocephalus are associated. It remains to be shown whether hypertension causes hydrocephalus or hydrocephalus causes hypertension, or both.

Retrograde Jugular Venous Flow

A recent paper reported the valves in the jugular veins are incompetent in INPH patients allowing retrograde flow (found in 19/20 INPH patients vs. 3/13 controls). While this is unlikely to be a good diagnostic test it may show a mechanism of pathogenesis (Kuriyama, Tokuda et al. 2008).

Conclusion

When confronted with a patient with possible normal pressure hydrocephalus, use the following systematic approach. Keeping in mind the differential diagnosis, look for pertinent factors in the history and examination and neuropsychological evaluation that have a bearing on diagnosis and surgical prognosis. On the MRI, look at the amount and pattern of atrophy and white matter changes. Perform between one and three spinal taps and evaluate the effect of this on the gait. At this time you may wish to advise about surgery. If your center performs external CSF drainage or intracranial pressure monitoring, this may be helpful. The patient and family must be aware of both the possible benefits and the risks of the surgery. If they choose surgery, follow the patient carefully to see if there is improvement and to detect possible surgical complications. If you are uncertain whether the patient should undergo surgery or the family and patient choose not to undergo surgery, make sure you have established a baseline from which you can follow the patient. Ideally, this includes a video of their gait, a brain MRI, and neuropsychological testing. Follow the patient at three-month intervals with serial videotaping of gait. Stability or deterioration of the gait often helps both the family and doctor decide on further action.

References

Adachi, M., T. Kawanami, et al. (2006). Upper midbrain profile sign and cingulate sulcus sign: MRI findings on sagittal images in idiopathic normal-pressure hydrocephalus, Alzheimer's disease, and progressive supranuclear palsy. *Radiat Med* 24(8): 568–572.

Agren-Wilsson, A., A. Lekman, et al. (2007). CSF biomarkers in the evaluation of idiopathic normal pressure hydrocephalus. *Acta Neurol Scand* 116(5): 333–339.

Anger, J. T., C. S. Saigal, et al. (2006). The prevalence of urinary incontinence among community dwelling adult women: Results from the National Health and Nutrition Examination Survey. *J Urol* 175(2): 601–4.

Aygok, G., A., Marmarou, et al. (2005). Three-year outcome of shunted idiopathic NPH patients. *Acta Neurochir Suppl* 95: 241–5.

Barron, S. A., L. Jacobs, et al. (1976). Changes in size of normal lateral ventricles during aging determined by computerized tomography. *Neurology* 26(11): 1011–3.

Bech, R. A., M. Juhler, et al. (1997). Frontal brain and leptomeningeal biopsy specimens correlated with cerebrospinal fluid outflow resistance and B-wave activity in patients suspected of normal-pressure hydrocephalus. *Neurosurgery* 40(3): 497–502.

Bech, R. A., G. Waldemar, et al. (1999). Shunting effects in patients with idiopathic normal pressure hydrocephalus; correlation with cerebral and leptomeningeal biopsy findings. *Acta Neurochir (Wien)* 141(6): 633–639.

Bergsneider, M., P. M. Black, et al. (2005). Surgical management of idiopathic normal-pressure hydrocephalus. *Neurosurgery* 57(3 Suppl): S29–39; discussion ii–v.

Bering, R. J. and B. Salibi (1959). Production of hydrocephalus by increased cephalic-venous pressure. *Archives of Neurology and Psychiatry* 81: 693–698.

Black, P. M. (1982). Normal-pressure hydrocephalus: Current understanding of diagnostic tests and shunting. *Postgrad Med* 71(2): 57–61, 65–67.

Black, P. M., R. G. Ojemann, et al. (1985). CSF shunts for dementia, incontinence, and gait disturbance. *Clin Neurosurg* 32: 632–651.

Boon, A. J., J. T. Tans, et al. (1997). Dutch Normal-Pressure Hydrocephalus Study: Prediction of outcome after shunting by resistance to outflow of cerebrospinal fluid. *J Neurosurg* 87(5): 687–693.

Boon, A. J., J. T. Tans, et al. (1999). Dutch Normal-Pressure Hydrocephalus Study: The role of cerebrovascular disease. *J Neurosurg* 90(2): 221–226.

Borgesen, S. E. and F. Gjerris (1982). The predictive value of conductance to outflow of CSF in normal pressure hydrocephalus. *Brain* 105(Pt 1): 65–86.

Braak, H. and E. Braak (1997). Frequency of stages of Alzheimer-related lesions in different age categories. *Neurobiol Aging* 18(4): 351–357.

Bradley, W. G. (2001). Normal pressure hydrocephalus and deep white matter ischemia: Which is the chicken, and which is the egg? *AJNR Am J Neuroradiol* 22(9): 1638–1640.

Bradley, W. G., Jr., D. Scalzo, et al. (1996). Normal-pressure hydrocephalus: Evaluation with cerebrospinal fluid flow measurements at MR imaging. *Radiology* 198(2): 523–529.

Bradley, W. G., Jr., A. R. Whittemore, et al. (1991). Marked cerebrospinal fluid void: Indicator of successful shunt in patients with suspected normal-pressure hydrocephalus. *Radiology* 178(2): 459–466.

Brean, A. and P. K. Eide (2008). Prevalence of probable idiopathic normal pressure hydrocephalus in a Norwegian population. *Acta Neurol Scand* 118(1): 48–53.

Casmiro, M., G. Benassi, et al. (1989). Frequency of idiopathic normal pressure hydrocephalus. *Arch Neurol* 46(6): 608.

Casmiro, M., R. D'Alessandro, et al. (1989). Risk factors for the syndrome of ventricular enlargement with gait apraxia (idiopathic normal pressure hydrocephalus): A case-control study. *J Neurol Neurosurg Psychiatry* 52(7): 847–852.

Chaudhry, P., S. Kharkar, et al. (2007). Characteristics and reversibility of dementia in normal pressure hydrocephalus. *Behav Neurol* 18(3): 149–158.

Clarfield, A. M. (2003). The decreasing prevalence of reversible dementias: An updated meta-analysis. *Arch Intern Med* 163(18): 2219–2229.

De Mol, J. (1985). [Prognostic factors for therapeutic outcome in normal-pressure hydrocephalus. Review of the literature and personal study]. *Acta Neurol Belg* 85(1): 13–29.

Dermaut, B., S. Kumar-Singh, et al. (2004). A novel presenilin 1 mutation associated with Pick's disease but not beta-amyloid plaques. *Ann Neurol* 55(5): 617–626.

Dickson, D. W., H. Fujishiro, et al. (2008). Evidence that incidental Lewy body disease is pre-symptomatic Parkinson's disease. *Acta Neuropathol* 115(4): 437–444.

Dixon, G. R., J. A. Friedman, et al. (2002). Use of cerebrospinal fluid flow rates measured by phase-contrast MR to predict outcome of ventriculoperitoneal shunting for idiopathic normal-pressure hydrocephalus. *Mayo Clin Proc* 77(6): 509–514.

Dusick, J. R., D. L. McArthur, et al. (2008). Success and complication rates of endoscopic third ventriculostomy for adult hydrocephalus: A series of 108 patients. *Surg Neurol* 69(1): 5–15.

Earnest, M. P., S. Fahn, et al. (1974). Normal pressure hydrocephalus and hypertensive cerebrovascular disease. *Arch Neurol* 31(4): 262–266.

Farin, A., H. E. Aryan, et al. (2006). Endoscopic third ventriculostomy. *J Clin Neurosci* 13(7): 763–770.

Fisher, C. M. (1977). The clinical picture in occult hydrocephalus. *Clin Neurosurg* 24: 270–284.

Folstein, M. F., S. E. Folstein, et al. (1975). Mini-mental state. A practical method for grading the cognitive state of patients for the clinician. *J Psychiatr Res* 12(3): 189–198.

Gallassi, R., A. Morreale, et al. (1991). Binswanger's disease and normal-pressure hydrocephalus. Clinical and neuropsychological comparison. *Arch Neurol* 48(11): 1156–1159.

Gangemi, M., F. Maiuri, et al. (2004). Endoscopic third ventriculostomy in idiopathic normal pressure hydrocephalus. *Neurosurgery* 55(1): 129–134; discussion 134.

Golomb, J., M. J. de Leon, et al. (1994). Hippocampal atrophy correlates with severe cognitive impairment in elderly patients with suspected normal pressure hydrocephalus. *J Neurol Neurosurg Psychiatry* 57(5): 590–593.

Golomb, J., J. Wisoff, et al. (2000). Alzheimer's disease comorbidity in normal pressure hydrocephalus: Prevalence and shunt response. *J Neurol Neurosurg Psychiatry* 68(6): 778–781.

Graff-Radford, N. R. and J. C. Godersky (1987). Idiopathic normal pressure hydrocephalus and systemic hypertension. *Neurology* 37(5): 868–871.

Graff-Radford, N. R. and J. C. Godersky (1989). Symptomatic congenital hydrocephalus in the elderly simulating normal pressure hydrocephalus. *Neurology* 39(12): 1596–1600.

Graff-Radford, N. R., J. C. Godersky, et al. (1989). Variables predicting surgical outcome in symptomatic hydrocephalus in the elderly. *Neurology* 39: 1601–1604.

Graff-Radford, N. R., K. Rezai, et al. (1987). Regional cerebral blood flow in normal pressure hydrocephalus. *J Neurol Neurosurg Psychiatry* 50(12): 1589–1596.

Graff-Radford, N. R., J. Torner, et al. (1989). Factors associated with hydrocephalus after subarachnoid hemorrhage. A report of the Cooperative Aneurysm Study. *Arch Neurol* 46(7): 744–752.

Granado, J. M., F. Diaz, et al. (1991). Evaluation of brain SPECT in the diagnosis and prognosis of the normal pressure hydrocephalus syndrome. *Acta Neurochir (Wien)* 112(3–4): 88–91.

Greenberg, B. M. and M. A. Williams (2008). Infectious complications of temporary spinal catheter insertion for diagnosis of adult hydrocephalus and idiopathic intracranial hypertension. *Neurosurgery* 62(2): 431–435; discussion 435–436.

Greitz, T., B. E. Levander, et al. (1971). High blood pressure and epilepsy in hydrocephalus due to stenosis of the aqueduct of Sylvius. *Acta Neurochir (Wien)* 24(3): 201–206.

Gyldenstad, C. (1977). Measurements of the normal ventricular system and hemispheric sulci of 100 adults with computerizes tomography. *Neuroradiology* 14: 183–192.

Haan, J. and R. T. Thomeer (1988). Predictive value of temporary external lumbar drainage in normal pressure hydrocephalus. *Neurosurgery* 22(2): 388–391.

Haidri, N. H. and S. M. Modi (1977). Normal pressure hydrocephalus and hypertensive cerebrovascular disease. *Dis Nerv Syst* 38(11): 918–921.

Hakim, R. and P. M. Black (1998). Correlation between lumbo-ventricular perfusion and MRI-CSF flow studies in idiopathic normal pressure hydrocephalus. *Surg Neurol* 49(1): 14–9; discussion 19–20.

Hebert, L. E., P. A. Scherr, et al. (2003). Alzheimer Disease in the US population: Prevalence estimates using the 2000 census." *Archives of Neurology August* 60(8): 1119–1122.

Hellstrom, P., M. Edsbagge, et al. (2007). The neuropsychology of patients with clinically diagnosed idiopathic normal pressure hydrocephalus. *Neurosurgery* 61(6): 1219–1226; discussion 1227–1228.

Hiraoka, K., K. Meguro, et al. (2008). Prevalence of idiopathic normal-pressure hydrocephalus in the elderly population of a Japanese rural community. *Neurol Med Chir (Tokyo)* 48(5): 197–199; discussion 199–200.

Holodny, A. I., A. E. George, et al. (1998). Focal dilation and paradoxical collapse of cortical fissures and sulci in patients with normal-pressure hydrocephalus. *J Neurosurg* 89(5): 742–747.

Holodny, A. I., R. Waxman, et al. (1998). MR differential diagnosis of normal-pressure hydrocephalus and Alzheimer disease: Significance of perihippocampal fissures. *AJNR Am J Neuroradiol* 19(5): 813–819.

Ishii, K., T. Kawaguchi, et al. (2008). Voxel-based analysis of gray matter and CSF space in idiopathic normal pressure hydrocephalus. *Dement Geriatr Cogn Disord* 25(4): 329–335.

Ishikawa, M., M. Hashimoto, et al. (2008). Guidelines for management of idiopathic normal pressure hydrocephalus. *Neurol Med Chir (Tokyo)* 48 Suppl: S1–23.

Jack, C. R., Jr., R. C. Petersen, et al. (1992). MR-based hippocampal volumetry in the diagnosis of Alzheimer's disease. *Neurology* 42(1): 183–188.

Jack, C. R., Jr., M. M. Shiung, et al. (2004). Comparison of different MRI brain atrophy rate measures with clinical disease progression in AD. *Neurology* 62(4): 591–600.

Jagust, W. J., R. P. Friedland, et al. (1985). Positron emission tomography with [18F]fluorodeoxyglucose differentiates normal pressure hydrocephalus from Alzheimer-type dementia. *J Neurol Neurosurg Psychiatry* 48(11): 1091–1096.

Kapaki, E. N., G. P. Paraskevas, et al. (2007). Cerebrospinal fluid tau, phospho-tau181 and beta-amyloid1-42 in idiopathic normal pressure hydrocephalus: A discrimination from Alzheimer's disease. *Eur J Neurol* 14(2): 168–173.

Katzman, R. and F. Hussey (1970). A simple constant-infusion manometric test for measurement of CSF absorption. I. Rationale and method. *Neurology* 20(6): 534–544.

Kilic, K., A. Czorny, et al. (2007). Predicting the outcome of shunt surgery in normal pressure hydrocephalus. *J Clin Neurosci* 14(8): 729–736.

Kitagaki, H., E. Mori, et al. (1998). CSF spaces in idiopathic normal pressure hydrocephalus: Morphology and volumetry. *AJNR Am J Neuroradiol* 19(7): 1277–1284.

Koto, A., G. Rosenberg, et al. (1977). Syndrome of normal pressure hydrocephalus: Possible relation to hypertensive and arteriosclerotic vasculopathy. *J Neurol Neurosurg Psychiatry* 40(1): 73–79.

Krauss, J. K., J. P. Regel, et al. (1996). Vascular risk factors and arteriosclerotic disease in idiopathic normal-pressure hydrocephalus of the elderly. *Stroke* 27(1): 24–29.

Krauss, J. K., J. P. Regel, et al. (1997). Flow void of cerebrospinal fluid in idiopathic normal pressure hydrocephalus of the elderly: Can it predict outcome after shunting? *Neurosurgery* 40(1): 67–73; discussion 73–74.

Krauss, J. K., J. P. Regel, et al. (1997). White matter lesions in patients with idiopathic normal pressure hydrocephalus and in an age-matched control group: A comparative study. *Neurosurgery* 40(3): 491–495; discussion 495–496.

Krefft, T. A., N. R. Graff-Radford, et al. (2004). Normal pressure hydrocephalus and large head size. *Alzheimer Dis Assoc Disord* 18(1): 35–37.

Kuriyama, N., T. Tokuda, et al. (2008). Retrograde jugular flow associated with idiopathic normal pressure hydrocephalus. *Ann Neurol* 64(2): 217–221.

Lenfeldt, N., J. Hauksson, et al. (2008). Improvement after cerebrospinal fluid drainage is related to levels of N-acetyl-aspartate in idiopathic normal pressure hydrocephalus. *Neurosurgery* 62(1): 135–141, discussion 141–142.

Longatti, P. L., A. Fiorindi, et al. (2004). Failure of endoscopic third ventriculostomy in the treatment of idiopathic normal pressure hydrocephalus. *Minim Invasive Neurosurg* 47(6): 342–345.

Malm, J., B. Kristensen, et al. (1995). The predictive value of cerebrospinal fluid dynamic tests in patients with idiopathic adult hydrocephalus syndrome. *Arch Neurol* 52(8): 783–789.

Malm, J., B. Kristensen, et al. (2000). Three-year survival and functional outcome of patients with idiopathic adult hydrocephalus syndrome. *Neurology* 55(4): 576–578.

Marmarou, A., M. Bergsneider, et al. (2005). The value of supplemental prognostic tests for the preoperative assessment of idiopathic normal-pressure hydrocephalus. *Neurosurgery* 57(3 Suppl): S17–28; discussion ii–v.

Mosconi, L. (2005). Brain glucose metabolism in the early and specific diagnosis of Alzheimer's disease. FDG-PET studies in MCI and AD. *Eur J Nucl Med Mol Imaging* 32(4): 486–510.

Munoz, D. G., S. M. Hastak, et al. (1993). Pathologic correlates of increased signals of the centrum ovale on magnetic resonance imaging. *Arch Neurol* 50(5): 492–497.

Ogino, A., H. Kazui, et al. (2006). Cognitive impairment in patients with idiopathic normal pressure hydrocephalus. *Dement Geriatr Cogn Disord* 21(2): 113–119.

Owler, B. K. and J. D. Pickard (2001). Normal pressure hydrocephalus and cerebral blood flow: A review. *Acta Neurol Scand* 104(6): 325–342.

Petersen, R. C., B. Mokri, et al. (1985). Surgical treatment of idiopathic hydrocephalus in elderly patients. *Neurology* 35(3): 307–311.

Pettorossi, V., C. Di Rocci, et al. (1978). Communicating hydrocephalus induced by mechanically increased amplitude of the intraventricular cerebrospinal fluid pulse pressure: Rationale and method. *Experimental Neurology* 59: 30–39.

Pfisterer, W. K., F. Aboul-Enein, et al. (2007). Continuous intraventricular pressure monitoring for diagnosis of normal-pressure hydrocephalus. *Acta Neurochir (Wien)* 149(10): 983–990; discussion 990.

Portnoy, H. D., M. Chopp, et al. (1983). Hydraulic model of myogenic autoregulation and the cerebrovascular bed: The effects of altering systemic arterial pressure. *Neurosurgery* 13(5): 482–498.

Relkin, N., A. Marmarou, et al. (2005). Diagnosing idiopathic normal-pressure hydrocephalus. *Neurosurgery* 57(3 Suppl): S4–16; discussion ii–v.

Savolainen, S., M. P. Laakso, et al. (2000). MR imaging of the hippocampus in normal pressure hydrocephalus: Correlations with cortical Alzheimer's disease confirmed by pathologic analysis. *AJNR Am J Neuroradiol* 21(2): 409–414.

Savolainen, S., L. Paljarvi, et al. (1999). Prevalence of Alzheimer's disease in patients investigated for presumed normal pressure hydrocephalus: A clinical and neuropathological study. *Acta Neurochir (Wien)* 141(8): 849–853.

Shukla, D., B. M. Singh, et al. (1980). Hypertensive cerebrovascular disease and normal pressure hydrocephalus. *Neurology* 30(9): 998–1000.

Stothers, L., D. Thom, et al. (2005). Urologic diseases in America project: Urinary incontinence in males–demographics and economic burden. *J Urol* 173(4): 1302–1308.

Szczepek, E., P. Dabrowski, et al. (2008). Gait disturbances in Computer Dyno Graphy examination in patients with normal pressure hydrocephalus before and after surgery. *Neurol Neurochir Pol* 42(1): 22–27.

Trenkwalder, C., J. Schwarz, et al. (1995). Starnberg trial on epidemiology of Parkinsonism and hypertension in the elderly. Prevalence of Parkinson's disease and related disorders assessed by a door-to-door survey of inhabitants older than 65 years. *Arch Neurol* 52(10): 1017–1022.

Vanneste, J., P. Augustijn, et al. (1992). Shunting normal-pressure hydrocephalus: Do the benefits outweigh the risks? A multicenter study and literature review. *Neurology* 42(1): 54–59.

Verghese, J., R. B. Lipton, et al. (2002). Abnormality of gait as a predictor of non-Alzheimer's dementia. *N Engl J Med* 347(22): 1761–1768.

Walchenbach, R., E. Geiger, et al. (2002). The value of temporary external lumbar CSF drainage in predicting the outcome of shunting on normal pressure hydrocephalus. *J Neurol Neurosurg Psychiatry* 72(4): 503–506.

Wechsler, D. (1987). *Wechsler Memory Scale-Revised*. New York: The Psychological Corporation.

Wechsler, D. (1997). *Wechsler Adult Intelligence Scale, 3rd Edition administration and scoring manual*. Orlando: The Psychological Corporation.

Wikkelso, C., H. Andersson, et al. (1986). Normal pressure hydrocephalus. Predictive value of the cerebrospinal fluid tap-test. *Acta Neurol Scand* 73(6): 566–573.

Williams, M. A., A. Y. Razumovsky, et al. (1998). Comparison of Pcsf monitoring and controlled CSF drainage diagnose normal pressure hydrocephalus. *Acta Neurochir Suppl* 71: 328–330.

Williams, M. A., G. Thomas, et al. (2008). Objective assessment of gait in normal-pressure hydrocephalus. *Am J Phys Med Rehabil* 87(1): 39–45.

Wilson, R. K. and M. A. Williams (2007). Evidence that congenital hydrocephalus is a precursor to idiopathic normal pressure hydrocephalus in only a subset of patients. *J Neurol Neurosurg Psychiatry* 78(5): 508–511.

44 Spinal Cord Injury and Dysfunction in the Elderly

K.J. Fiedler

Popular lore suggests that if you have the "right stuff," you can prevail and overcome any difficulty. Yet physical disability in combination with the environment present a handicap that penalizes the disabled person in comparison to the "nondisabled" person. Moreover, this penalty increases with age...

Roberta Trieschmann

Introduction

Regardless of its duration or interruption by ill health, *living* is effectively synonymous with *aging*. This is not only evident experientially (Trieschmann 1987), but also apparently occurs at the neuronal molecular level (de Magahaes and Sandberg 2005). So most people only gradually perceive aging as curtailing activities of daily life; in many cases its initial subtle impacts are first noted—and often cushioned—by family and associates. But there are others whose lives have already been irreducibly altered in youth or middle age when they were suddenly or sub-acutely "disabled," whether by paroxysmal injury or illness. When those individuals eventually grow old, the incremental insults of aging are not only added to that somatic burden, but also often reawaken the mental trauma of their first bout of functional loss. And there are still others, without prior calamitous ill health, whose gradual acceptance (or at least tolerance) of aging is interrupted by the sudden intrusion of a severe acquired disability.

Survivors of spinal cord injury or dysfunction (SCI/D), acquired at whatever age, are often perceived as embodying the extreme form of such intrusive physical disability. This is reflected in the common lay perception that they must endure a "life sentence," in contrast to the presumed "death sentence" implied by a diagnosis of, say, lung cancer. A perhaps shortsighted, but neither infrequent nor surprising, lay conclusion is that death is in fact preferable to such an existence.[1]

A medical text written at least four thousand years ago defined SCI as "an ailment not to be treated" (Smith 1862), presumably due to the ineluctable painfully protracted demise of the afflicted. This pessimistic perspective remained unchallenged for millennia: Just before World War II, one of the most authoritative neurologists of that era made it

quite clear that although a few [SCI] patients exceptionally might survive 2, 4, or 6 years, a fatal outcome from bedsores and urinary infections was inevitable, and he describes stages of recovery, stabilization and final decay as invariable (Foerster 1936).

But in the early 1940s, in response to the unconcealed influx of mostly young, and otherwise healthy, veterans returning to their homelands in the Allied countries with combat-acquired paraplegia or what was called quadriplegia in the US and tetraplegia in the UK and Australia, physicians not perceived as fit for active military duty (whether because of age, debility, or refugee status) successfully began to address those previously fatal complications (Munro 1940; Munro 1943). It is neither inconsequential nor trivial to note that the most influential of those physicians were called "Poppa" or "Pappy" by the SCI patients they continued to attend for the rest of their lives. And those predominantly male WWII veterans, all patients initially and most intermittently thereafter, became the first groups of individuals surviving with SCI that were statistically large enough to call "cohorts," enabling scientific progress from anecdotal to evidence-based practices. Only a few of them survive as of this writing—yet collectively their medical histories suggested and then largely defined the risks and prognoses, as well as framing the treatment attempts whether curative, preventative, or palliative, that comprise current medical practice in this field.

Today, even if SCI/D occurs in a person's seventh decade or later, the efficiency of emergency services and the efficacy of trauma and rehabilitation specialists make survival commonplace. Accordingly, those with late-life SCI/D are now a growing segment of the growing proportion of the elderly population living with disability and/or chronic disease. In contrast, those whose SCI/D occurred earlier in life, and whose innate and acquired qualities, along with fortunate access to care, had enabled them to achieve some degree of equilibrium with both somatic and environmental constraints, increasingly find themselves newly compromised by the often insidious effects of aging with a disability (McGlinchey-Berroth et al. 1995).

This chapter addresses both of these groups of potential—or actual—SCI/D patients. The risks for non-spinal cord disabled elderly to acquire SCI/D, and the subsequent risks, consequences, and care efforts for those individuals whose SCI/D may be either recent or remote, are outlined below.

Epidemiology

As in almost every discussion of epidemiology, that pertaining to SCI/D is initially confounded by inadequate clinical definitions, and ultimately constrained by inadequate data. The catchall phrase "SCI/D" is meant to encompass both traumatic and non-traumatic etiologies resulting in lesions of the spinal cord, but is itself ambiguous. The term *injury* may be intended as identical to direct *trauma* (i.e., acute, mechanical and exogenous) or it may be taken (with varying degrees of inclusion) to subsume other quasi-compressive etiologies, such as myelopathy due to degenerative disk or vertebral lesions—sometimes including even the neurological sequelae of so-called "pathological fractures" due to cancer metastatic to the spine.

The 'D' in the rubric SCI/D, which in this text stands for *dysfunction*, in other current usage represents *disorders* or *diseases*. Each of those not-quite-synonymous terms encompasses different clusters of etiologies; their superimposed Venn diagram would certainly show intersection (i.e., mutual inclusion) for infection, infarct, and CNS demyelinating processes, principally multiple sclerosis. However, further intersection with other diagnostic entities varies idiosyncratically from one categorizer to the next. Problematic entities whose inclusion or exclusion from the SCI/D group actually has little more than semantic import, due to their relative rarity, are exemplified by the hereditary spastic paraplegias, vasculitides (such as lupus erythematosus), infections (such as epidural abscess, Pott's disease, or the HTLVs), paraneoplastic "molecular mimicry" autoimmune entities, residual effects on the spinal cord of post-infectious pseudomyelomeningocele, the progressive degenerative effects of ankylosing spondylitis or rheumatoid arthritis, vitamin deficiencies (e.g., "sub-acute combined degeneration"), or the previously puzzling central nervous system (CNS) effects found in the victims of Guillain-Barre syndrome (GBS), particularly the proximal variants originally supposed to involve only "peripheral" cranial and cervico-brachial nerves, such as the syndrome initially described by Miller Fisher. These variants, along with classical GBS and Bickerstaff's brainstem encephalitis, are more recently perceived as comprising overlapping entities along a spectrum of autoimmune attacks on sub-populations of gangliosides found in both the peripheral and central nervous systems (Lo 2007).

More significant is the inclusion or exclusion of two other much more common causes of non-traumatic spinal cord disability: the motor neuron diseases [MNDs], principally amyotrophic lateral sclerosis [ALS] with its apparent recent increasing incidence among Gulf War veterans (Haley 2003), and the undeniably significant prevalence of spinal cord involvement in neoplastic disease, whether metastatic to the bony spinal column potentially causing compression of the cord or directly to the cord itself.

Other than to a scholarly systematist of biological classification (Senyk, Patil, and Sonnenberg 1989), why should such inclusion or exclusion matter? Accessibility to treatment (the true "bottom line" from a patient's perspective) is the issue here. Insurance coverage, both from the private sector and from the various governmentally funded workmen's compensation programs, varies relative to such categorization. Also notably, treatment in the Spinal Cord Injury Centers of the U.S. Veterans Affairs [VA] health care system, the largest dedicated SCI/D care program in the world, which is open to both service connected and non-service connected veterans, is so determined: Patients with multiple sclerosis and ALS are currently accepted, while those with metastatic disease to the spinal cord are specifically excluded (VHA Handbook 2005).

Overall, incidence and prevalence data on traumatic SCI *per se* are imprecise. A recent survey of pertinent worldwide publications found "insufficient" data to reliably estimate prevalence, and generously noted that incidence "lies between 10.4 and 83/million inhabitants per year" (Wyndaele and Wyndaele 2006). Statistical modeling in 1995 projected an increase in the number of acute SCI cases admitted to U.S. hospitals from ~11,500 in 1994 to ~13,400 in 2010; prevalence was expected to increase 20% over ten years, from ~201,000 in 1994 to ~247,000 in 2004. Age-adjusted post-hospitalization incidence was then ~38/million. These authors also noted, "… the veteran segment, which currently comprises 22% of the SCI population, is projected to decline" (Lasfargues et al. 1995). Online data give estimates of 30–60 new civilian U.S. cases of SCI per year as of 2007, and a prevalence of 183,000 to 230,000 cases, the equivalent of 700-900 per million population. Very roughly, this approximates to one person in every one hundred and fifty in the U.S. As overall risk-taking equilibrates between the sexes, incidence seems to be moving towards two males for each female; overall however, prevalence remains about 4:1 (Dawodu 2007).

Other than fatalities, quantitative data on U.S. troops' casualties sorted by functional system (e.g., SCI/D) in the current Afghanistan and Iraq wars do not appear to be generally accessible. Available anatomical wound location summaries show that "polytrauma"

(i.e., more than one location involved) is common, and extremity wounds predominate (70%), which is actually consistent for battlefield injuries since WW II (Zouris et al. 2006). In contrast, head and neck wounds are more common than previous conflicts, and thoracic wounds are less common, both at highly statistically significant levels (Owens et al. 2008). These data support the impression given through the news media that head and extremity wounds (i.e., body parts apparently not as well protected by current body armor) predominate; isolated SCI is apparently not common.

In the civilian arena, most traumatic SCIs continue to occur from motor vehicle accidents and falls, which predominate respectively in those under and over 50 years of age. The number of fall-induced cervical spine injuries in the elderly has shown an "alarming" rise in recent years (Kannus et al. 2007). Trauma from non-accidental interpersonal violence is also increasingly involved in civilian SCIs overall; this cause has gone from less than 15% in the 1970's to 25% or more in recent years (DeVivo, Krause, and Lammertse 1999). It is noteworthy that the specific etiology of SCI has no predictive effect on consequent morbidity and mortality, except for non-accidental violence. In the U.S., both perpetrators and victims of non-accidental violence are statistically more likely to be male, non-white, unemployed, and relatively less educated. These socio-economic factors undoubtedly contribute to the increased likelihood of early development of serious pressure sores and other complications requiring rehospitalization, and to the significantly higher risk of dying within two years of the injury, which continues as a modestly increased mortality risk thereafter (Zafonte and Dijkers 1999).

Iatrogenic SCI/D has been noted following spinal injections for pain, placement of epidural catheters, and more recently through an increasing number of reports of spinal cord compression by "fibrotic/inflammatory masses" provoked by intrathecal catheters and pumps (Peng and Massicotte 2004). Therapeutic spinal manipulation is sometimes suspected (by practitioners who do not include it in their therapeutic *armamentaria*, and often prejudiciously consider it quackery and/or assault) to be a significant cause of SCI/D, in addition to its more evident contribution to the incidence of arterial damage. (It is worth noting that to health care consumers, manipulative therapy is cheap, its consequences predictable, and is literally sensible; by and large, allopathic encounters have none of these virtues.) No prospective studies, large or small, appear to have been attempted to investigate this allegation. Meta-analysis of reported adverse reactions does reveal predominantly vascular problems (e.g., arterial dissection occurred in 18 of 42 reports from throughout Australia over six years; the denominator—the total number of such willingly manipulated Australians—is of course unknown [Ernst 2002]). There appears to be a single retrospective study of non-vascular adverse sequelae reporting on the 18 patients who presented to a neurosurgical practice over a six-year period complaining of "a quantitative worsening of symptoms immediately after spinal manipulative treatment." Myelopathy, paraparesis, cauda equina syndrome, and radiculopathy were identified; "eighty-nine percent required surgery." An unspecified number were found to have had previously undiagnosed "substantial" disk herniation, and three subsequently died from previously occult spinal malignancies. The authors suggest pre-manipulation screening by imaging techniques is more sensitive than plain X-rays (Oppenheim, Spitzer, and Segal 2006).

With regard to the epidemiology of non-traumatic SCI/D, the most common etiology—which, despite being more frequent than traumatic SCI and demyelinating disease taken together and which is relatively unfamiliar to most neurologists—is the complex and heterogeneous set of neoplastic diseases. Primary spinal cord tumors comprise very few of all CNS primaries (less than 12–15%), with an estimated incidence of 0.5–2.5 cases per 100,000. They also comprise very few of the total cases of neoplastic disease causing spinal cord compression; most (estimates vary from 85% to 97%) are metastatic and initially extradural. Estimates of metastases to the spine and/or cord vary from 5% to 30% of all cancer patients, with a 40-fold variation among different types of cancer. The most prevalent are lung, prostate, renal, and breast cancers; lymphoma, sarcoma, and multiple myeloma also frequently tend towards spinal cord metastasis; the least is pancreatic cancer (Huff 2007). Symptomatic spinal cord compression, appropriately termed "malignant," i.e., manifested by new back pain presaging paraplegia, occurs in 3–5% of cancer patients in the five years preceding death from cancer (Loblaw, Laperierre, and Mackillop 2003). In the U.S., this translates into an incidence of approximately 13,000 people per year.

The multiple riddles of the epidemiology of multiple sclerosis (MS) will not be summarized here, except to note that in "susceptible populations" the prevalence is approximately 100–150 per 100,000 population and rising (Hirst et al. 2008). There is no apparent collated data on the percentage of those with MS whose signs and symptoms are predominantly due to spinal cord lesions. Both the persistent distinction of "transverse myelitis" (once other inflammatory etiologies are ruled out) as a disease entity characterized by a single episode (Jacob and Weinshenker 2008), and the more recent distinction of neuromyelitis optica (NMO; previously called Devic's disease) largely because of the presence of a nominally specific antibody marker (Wingerchuk 2007), from the congeries of demyelinating syndromes lumped together under the rubric of MS, will only be clinically useful if they lead to etiologically-based specific treatments. Transverse myelitis remains without even a suggested course of treatment, and the protracted immunomodulation currently suggested for NMO does not meet such specific criteria.

Pathophysiology

Medical professionals as well as other speakers of colloquial English commonly use phrases such as "she broke her back," or "he's paralyzed because of a broken neck" in describing people with traumatic SCI/D. And in discussing the consequences of both traumatic and non-traumatic SCI/D, this is often followed by a phrase indicating that the person concerned "can't feel anything or move anything below [such-and-such a] level." As metaphors, these statements are unfortunately both compelling and communicative. In terms of pathophysiology, they are, of course, almost always totally erroneous.

It is only in the rare instance of a stabbing that successfully gets between vertebrae or a bullet that makes a direct hit, that the cord is literally "broken." Otherwise, even in combat situations, actual avulsion, laceration, or transection of the spinal cord is unusual. Cervical or thoracic gunshot wounds usually produce SCI by pressure transduced from the missile's cone of force passing through the thorax, affecting vessels and neurons within the cord. This, like the paroxysmal torque and extreme flexion and/or extension of the spine that occurs in accidents (whether in vehicles, sports or those resulting from falls), results in the actual common, and commonplace, cause of spinal cord "injury"—an hypoxic-ischemic insult in an enclosed space. The pathophysiological cascade of sequelae, over milliseconds to months, is no different than in any other tissue so afflicted. Pain and spasticity, discussed further below, are the obvious counterexamples to the implied total absence of feeling or movement below the level of the SCI.

Cervical spondylosis is the most common progressive disorder in the aging spine, and is perhaps the most common neurological disease in civilized populations. Associated disk protrusion, retrolisthesis, and osteophyte formation frequently lead to radiculopathy and often myelopathy (Shedid and Benzel 2007). Surgeons often find themselves in the unenviable position of trying to arrest this degenerative process; at best they can only expect to stop further progression, at worst, the patient may deteriorate during or following surgery, even without apparent operator error. Age-and SCI related calcium disorders (deposition in arteries and ligaments, loss from bones) compound these issues; they are discussed below.

A discussion of non-traumatic SCDpathophysiology is beyond the scope of this discussion, except to note that dissemination of metastatic neoplastic cells occurs hematogenously to the vertebral bodies, with subsequent expansion to the epidural space either through gross tumor invasion through the intervertebral foramina or via Batson's venous plexus. Consequently, most metastatic seeding to the spinal cord is thoracic (~70%), followed by lumbar (~20%), and cervical (~10%) (Spinazze, Caraceni, and Schrijvers 2005). It should be recalled that the thoracic spine and cord are relatively remote from both proximal and distal sources feeding the so-called anterior spinal artery (actually an arteriolar network): the vertebral arteries cephalad and the artery of Adamkiewicz caudad. This results in that region being effectively subject to "watershed" ischemia. Thus, thoracic trauma is more likely to produce complete than incomplete SCI, and blood-borne immunomodulation to that region is correspondingly reduced.

Genetic Contributions to SCI/D

The hereditary spastic paraplegias are a heterogeneous group of single-gene disorders; more than thirty different chromosomal loci have so far been identified. The conditions are of considerable theoretical interest due to the aspects of intracellular transport and trafficking of molecules and organelles their study has enabled (Soderblom and Blackstone 2006). They are so rare, however, that most clinicians will never encounter a patient with the disorder.

There are occasional cases of trauma, acute or repetitive, superimposed on occult spina bifida or other congenital defects, which result in a spinal cord injury that could therefore be said to have a genetic basis. Otherwise, there is no known genetic predisposition for traumatic SCI, unless there are as yet undetermined genes associated with being "accident-prone." This is not entirely a specious or ironic supposition: For many years prior to the increased incidence of SCI in the elderly, both medical and psychologically-oriented clinicians wondered if, aside from sharing what might be termed coincident states of youth, high testosterone, and frequent intoxication, the majority of SCI victims might not also share a genetically-based trait of "sensation seeking" (Ditunno, McCauley and Marquette 1985; Mawson et al. 1988). If true, this still unresolved speculation could help explain the frequent intemperate behavior that characteristically leads directly to the traumatic injury, as well as the apparent relatively high prevalence of pre-existing or coincident head injury (with its likely subsequent cognitive deficits) among this group. Intriguingly, recent work by anthropological geneticists suggests that the presence of certain alleles of human dopamine receptor polymorphisms may in fact confer "greater food and drug cravings, novelty-seeking, and ADHD symptoms" which, in the context of their study, are construed to be selectively advantageous for nomadic as opposed to sedentary populations (Eisenberg et al. 2008).

The genetic contributions favoring acquisition of non-traumatic SCI/D are generally accepted as simply unknown (e.g., "sero-negative" ankylosing spondylitis), unknown but controversially argued (e.g., the predisposing immune characteristics of people with one of the various entities now diagnostically lumped together as multiple sclerosis), or as yet incompletely understood although arguably on the way to elucidation (e.g., the genetic reasons for susceptibility to the various neoplastic and infectious diseases that afflict the spinal cord among other target organs). Current views may readily be found online.

Clinical Presentations

In a conscious, complaining patient, SCI/D typically presents as motor loss (ranging from subtle weakness to frank paralysis) and loss of sensation (ranging from "pins and needles" to anesthesia) in a paraplegic or quadriplegic distribution, i.e., deficits that are "transversely" (i.e., horizontally, so to speak)—and usually bilaterally—delimited, rather than the unilateral, vertical distribution of a hemiplegic stroke, or the focal and usually acral deficits characteristic of root or peripheral nerve lesions. The medical history will immediately or eventually suggest the etiology, particularly in the context of non-traumatic SCI/D.

Persistent pain is rarely the presenting sign except in the context of a known cancer patient with new back pain. Even in the absence of any neurological findings (which, if present, are likely to be unilateral), that person should have diagnostic magnetic resonance imaging performed as soon as possible since treatment (corticosteroids, radiation, possibly surgery) must be promptly initiated. The treatment goal here, even when the patient's estimated survival is numbered only in months, is to preserve ambulation, which is usually seen by patient and family as a major contributor to quality of life, second only to adequate pain relief (Abraham, Banffy, and Harris 2008).

In non-cancer patients, there may also be unrecognized quasi-subacute presentations, due to signs and symptoms that fluctuate or even alternate laterality, as is seen occasionally following incomplete cervical SCI. The otherwise healthy patient, presenting a day or two after what sounds like minor neck trauma, may complain only of occasional "stingers" or some other self-invented phrase describing L'Hermitte's sign, i.e., transient electric shock-like pains down (or very rarely up) the back or into one or the other (usually upper) extremity. They may be accompanied by equally fleeting upper extremity weakness, misinterpreted by the examining physician as unwillingness to use the painful limb (Bicknell and Fiedler 1992). Hyperreflexia and increased tone (so-called upper motor neuron signs, which would be better termed upper motor neuron lesion signs) may not yet have emerged; appropriate imaging, if considered and obtained, may reveal the injury—or, depending on the duration and extent of the injury, follow-up examination and sequential re-imaging may be needed before cord involvement can conclusively be ruled in or out (Levi et al. 2006).

With regard to most traumatic SCI however, the mechanism of injury speaks for itself: if not whiplashed in a motor vehicle accident (the adoption of chest-crossing seat belts skewed the prevalence of cord damage in an MVA from paraplegia to quadriplegia), then being "found down" as a consequence of falling. In most instances the mechanism of the fall, if not bluntly and/or shamefully recalled by the faller, is evident by the position and context where found: unless diving, the neck usually hyperextended, indoors catching the chin on the leading edge of the sink or the tub from slipping on a throw rug or the wet kitchen or bathroom floor; outdoors from mismanaging the stoop, the gravel, or muddy driveway on the way to the mailbox, or just a random pair of barely uneven patches—affording different proprioceptive and exteroceptive information (Gibson 1964/1982)—underfeet. In virtually every case the victim, perhaps already minimally impaired by mild ataxia whether from diabetes, parkinsonism, dysthyroid status, hypocyanocobalminemic, habitual ethanol or other substance use, or just idiosyncratically neuropathic, has previously fallen repeatedly and been repeatedly warned by family, if not also by the primary care physician. Not infrequently, this then sets the patient and family up for

persistent mutual recrimination and guilt, whose effects in turn may complicate rehabilitation.

If the event does not appear to have been unequivocally and truly accidental, then the question of intentional intoxication (alcohol or other substance abuse) needs to be pursued. Further inquiry of family as well as the patient is needed to elucidate prior history of the "sensation seeking" mentioned above—whether genetically based or not—often manifested in the elderly at the time of their "accident" by age-inappropriate activity: shingling or house-painting, hanging curtains, tending the swamp-cooler on a steeply pitched roof without proper precautions, pruning limbs high in a tree, overturning an all-terrain vehicle, wrestling with an ostensibly unloaded gun.

Diagnosis

The pitfalls in SCI/D diagnosis overall are an over-simplified differential and inadequate imaging, the dynamic and progressive nature of the pathophysiology with staggered presentation of its signs and symptoms, and the tendency of patient and physician(s) alike to confuse the pertinent orthopedic and neurological diagnoses.

Each SCI patient, or her/his family, can recall someone pointing at an X-ray or other medical image, saying, "See that? It's a C5 [or whatever level] fracture… you'll never walk again." Yet only after *spinal shock*[2] has passed will functional assessment actually define which spinal cord level is producing no less than 3/5 strength[3] in the majority of its supplied myotome. This functional level is generally accepted as naming the injury, whatever the sensory deficits may be. The terms *complete* or *incomplete* are added, reflecting absence or presence of retained sacral segment movements (e.g., voluntary anal contraction) or sensation. (Physiologists refer to preserved function on somatosensory evoked potentials in the absence of conscious sensation as *dyscomplete*, but this term has no clinical usage.)

But because there are eight named cervical cord levels (C1 through C8) but only seven numbered cervical vertebrae, and because, in adults, the cord ends (tails off, so to speak) distally in the upper lumbar area, there are several opportunities for an orthopedist and a neurologist to examine the same patient with an SCI, identify two different levels of injury, and both be correct. The orthopedist is focused on the bony lesion(s); the neurologist regards the fracture as no more than a possibly misleading marker. Hypoxic-ischemic injury to the cord has been observed to extend multiple levels below or above the vertebral damage, and of course may not be symmetrical transversely either.

Timing of imaging, as well as pre-existing morbidity, can lead to further confusion. The high incidence of missed fractures in the ankylosed spine, for example, which may be accompanied by a spinal epidural hematoma unnoticed on plain X-rays, suggests the range of imaging pitfalls (Jacobs and Fehlings 2008). CT, plain radiography, MRI and its variants (diffusion tensor weighted and fMRI), PET, and intraoperative spinal sonography (Lammartse et al. 2007), as well as EMG and transcranial magnetic stimulation (Takahashi et al. 2008), all have distinct contributions in SCI/D diagnostic and prognostic assessment.

During their training, most clinicians memorized a litany of eponyms for partial SCI (Brown-Sequard, anterior cord, posterior cord, conus medullaris and cauda equina syndromes), which generally have little prognostic value. The one of note among the elderly is the **central cord syndrome**, usually caused by cervical hyper-extension resulting from a fall (Weingarden and Graham 1989). As previously mentioned, age has enabled development of vascular and ligamentous calcification, which compromises the arterial branches entering the cord. If shock (decreased tissue perfusion) occurs in the fallen individual, circulation in the central portion of the cord diminishes, resulting in preferential necrosis of the medial corticospinal tracts. The clinical consequence is called "upside-down paraplegia" by patients, due to the greater functional loss in upper extremities than in the lower, although an overall picture of incomplete quadriplegia emerges.

The American Spinal Injury Association (ASIA) has devised a scale categorizing SCI.[4] Overall it does not have evident prognostic value, and in terms of its rubrics from "A" (complete injury) to "E" (normal), it does not consistently identify decreasing disability. It is not applicable to most SCDs. It does provide a uniform terminology, and accordingly has been widely accepted, particularly its "ASIA motor score" component that is used in many studies to quantify severity of injury.

Treatment

There is no cure for traumatic SCI, or for any of the non-traumatic spinal cord disorders other than infection. Treatment is therefore aimed at community reintegration, prevention of complications, reducing co-morbidity, and eventually provision of palliative care; these issues are addressed elsewhere in this chapter.

Natural Progression and Optimal Treatment Outcomes

The natural progression of SCDs (as opposed to SCI) predictably varies with their pathophysiology. MS in many cases maintains its remitting/relapsing pattern; some victims descend into the less punctuated, protracted decline of "secondary progression." It is mostly that group, currently understood to have progressed to predominantly axonal degeneration rather than recurrent episodic demyelination, because of non-remitting bowel and bladder dysfunction and weakness that requires power mobility, which becomes functionally paraplegic or quadriplegic. Those with MNDs usually endure a relatively short decline, typically culminating in respiratory failure; rarely an atypical patient will survive for years, ventilator dependent and requiring "max assist" with all activities of daily life. The other non-traumatic entities follow their discrete patterns, and of course the various cancers, their own predominantly inexorable and terminal courses.

In contrast, since the large-scale study of traumatic SCI started following World War II, it was deliberately perceived (by the patients at least) as having no natural progression. They had each sustained an individual—and to that extent different—injury, but the injuries were collectively static. Unlike patients with an illness, they weren't going to be involved in an ongoing disease process. After surviving long enough (it seemed to be a year or two) to become "stabilized," it was only their inherited or other (non-SCI) acquired risk factors that could possibly affect their future health.

This attitude was reflected ideologically—and politically—in the exclusive admission policy of the newly established SCI Centers within the national health care system of the U.S. VA (the Veterans' Administration, as it was then known).[5] Only veterans with combat-related traumatic SCI were admitted, treated, and subsequently followed, including federally mandated lifelong annual evaluations. Within a few years, veterans with non-service connected SCI (i.e., not acquired during military service) were included. However, it wasn't until the 1980s, when the inevitable demographic decrease in the numbers of surviving WWII vets became significant, that the concerned veterans' service organizations permitted admission of patients with spinal cord *disorders* (i.e., diseases such as multiple sclerosis). Roughly coincident with that concession, overt recognition also began regarding the progressive risks that specifically accompany aging with the sequelae of traumatic SCI.

In the US "civilian" (i.e., non-VA) health sector, whether or not avowedly for-profit, a number of rehabilitation hospitals emerged and found a niche in the 1960s and 1970s. A few of them became strongly academically affiliated and developed expertise in SCI/D health care delivery. With federal grant support, they also joined together collegially into what has become known as the Model Systems, creating a large database that has enabled many sophisticated medical, epidemiological, and psycho-social studies to be performed (Stover, DeVivo, and Go 1999). They were and still are principally focused on "acute" care, which in the domain of SCI/D extends not much longer than the first year post onset. Some have modest regular follow-up programs beyond that timeframe; others have further contact with discharged patients only if readmitted for complications like pressure sores.

The reason for expounding this bit of medical history is to point out the crucial difference between medical research studies on VA patients, predominantly consistently followed medically and psycho-socially by an integrated system of SCI/D care, and those on Model Systems patients, essentially getting only sporadic care from the SCI/D centers concerned. Intuitively, the measured outcomes would in some circumstances be similar, and in others would vary significantly; and in fact their resultant "evidence-based" recommendations are sometimes at odds. Apparently, no objective formal study of these foundational differences has ever been attempted; none has been published.

Based on mixed conclusions from studies conducted in both of these U.S. venues, as well as elsewhere in the world, the following paragraphs address alphabetically some of the health-related risks associated with surviving (or succumbing) with SCI/D. Several, like autonomic dysreflexia, are virtually unique to that condition and relatively unfamiliar to many clinicians, and are accordingly discussed in some detail. Others, such as urinary tract infections or the metabolic syndrome, are widespread particularly among the elderly. Because they are thoroughly addressed elsewhere in the medical literature, in this chapter their elucidation is focused on aspects specifically pertinent to people with SCI/D, to the limited extent currently known and thought to be clinically useful.

Autonomic Dysreflexia

All intact vertebrates mount an adrenergic reflexive response to noxious stimuli; those with proximal spinal cord injury show an exaggerated autonomic hyperreflexia that is protracted and may itself be life threatening (Sherrington 1906). The pathognomonic triad of headache, paroxysmal sweating and flushing above the level of the spinal cord injury, and raised blood pressure was first medically documented in 1917 (Head and Riddoch 1917); however, its causal relationship with visceral stimulation was not definitively established until the 1940s, when aggressive treatment of bladder infections in SCI patients was initiated, at that time including frequent bladder washing ("tidal drainage") along with the then newly discovered antibiotics (Guttmann and Whitteridge 1947).

This condition is properly termed **autonomic dysreflexia**, often familiarly abbreviated to "AD." Frankly, many SCI/D patients have encountered medical practitioners, often in emergency departments, who are essentially ignorant about this condition; accordingly, during their initial rehabilitation traumatic SCI patients are now routinely educated about AD, and provided with informative wallet cards to politely show such providers if necessary. It should be noted that blood pressures in the range of 90/60 are normal for an active, asymptomatic person with quadriplegia (provided their own individual aging has not endowed them with essential hypertension), so recording a pressure of 120/80 or thereabouts in the emergency room setting may further confuse a practitioner unfamiliar with AD, who may consider such a reading as "WNL" (within normal limits).

However, it is notable that even though recently rehabilitated people with traumatic SCI are more knowledgeable about AD than some health care professionals (and those with non-traumatic spinal cord disorders, who may also be at risk), 41% of a recently surveyed Canadian community-dwelling cohort with long-term chronic SCI

> "had not heard of AD. More concerning was that 22% of individuals with SCI reported symptoms consistent with unrecognized AD (McGillivray et al. 2009)."

Examples of known noxious triggers for AD, often but not exclusively occurring in insensate parts of the body below the level of injury, include the following listed in Table 1—some of which are intuitively obvious, others less so.

Recalling that lack of pain awareness ("… but they can't feel anything below the level of the injury") does not equate with failure of centripetal neuronal transmission, such stimuli trigger spinal cord and extra-spinal receptors, which in turn activate a sympathetic response "within 1–2 heartbeats" (Frankel and Mathias 1976). Animal models demonstrate that following SCI aberrant sprouting of afferent neuronal C-fibers occurs into the cord below the level of injury. Distension of pelvic viscera in particular increases the excitation of these afferent receptors, which in turn amplifies the activation of sympathetic preganglionic neurons (Rabchevsky 2006).

This produces the adrenergic signs mentioned above, along with stuffy nose (Guttmann's sign), piloerection, and tachycardia. Aortic baro- and chrono-receptors alert the medulla via vagal afferents; in response, a negative chronotropic message is usually—but not invariably—sent through a vagal efferent (which is notably external to the spinal cord) to the sympathetic chain, that promptly restores relative bradycardia.

Note that this autonomic reflex occurs in *everyone*—with or without SCI/D—who sustains any such painful stimulus. In persons without a spinal cord injury, or whose SCI is below T6, a negative barotropic efferent response from the medulla is routinely sent to the sympathetic chain intra-spinally through the intermediolateral column of Clarke, which counteracts the initial hypertensive response. But in persons with SCI/D at or above that level, this normal reflexive descending inhibitory message is blocked, and the systemic hypertension persists.

[It is failure of this otherwise ubiquitous protective reflex, due to blockade by the spinal cord lesion, which accounts for the term "*dys*reflexia."] If unresolved, this protracted hypertension has been known to cause retinal detachment, new-onset seizures, stroke and, very rarely, sudden death due to intracranial hemorrhage.

Treatment is initially empirical: sit the patient upright and loosen all clothing. Then search for—and alleviate—the cause. If urethral re-catheterization, digital rectal stimulation, or actual manual evacuation of feces is indicated, the patient should be pre-medicated topically with lidocaine jelly inserted into the urethra or rectum using small diameter tubing on a large bore syringe. Waiting 5–15 minutes for the local anesthetic to take effect before further manipulation will reduce further noxious stimulation of the viscera, and correspondingly decrease the potential for consequent exacerbation of the hypertension.

If no trigger for the AD episode can be readily identified or resolved, the currently approved pharmacological treatment in the United States, if judged necessary due to intolerable headache or malignant hypertension, is a "ribbon" of nitroglycerine paste an inch or two long, spread onto the patient's chest. Should the patient subsequently become overly hypotensive or bradycardic, the paste can readily be removed. Other acceptable medications, which should be used with appropriate caution for their individual relative contraindications, include nifedipine, captopril, hydralazine, and magnesium sulfate for acute episodes. Initially positive, but not yet sufficiently evidence-based, studies suggest trials of prazosin and prostaglandin E_2 drugs as regular preventative medications in individuals prone to frequent AD, and the *ad hoc* intra-vesicular usage of botulinum toxin and capsaicin before or during planned urological procedures (Krassioukov 2009).

Overall, the best treatment for autonomic dysreflexia is avoidance of the precipitating triggers such as bladder distention or fecal impaction.

Bladder and Renal Disease

Briefly summarized, if disease is permitted to ascend from the bladder to the kidneys in individuals with SCI/D, it moves from the domain of urology to that of internal medicine, which is to say, from bad to worse. This applies to urinary output (and its antecedent production), storage, infection, stones, and issues related to muscle tone, whether due to hypertonic reflux or hypotonic flaccidity.

The inappropriate term **"neurogenic" bladder** adds no clarity to neuropathic effects on the urinary system. Clinicians would do better to keep the knee-jerk in mind: an upper motor neuron (UMN) lesion (exemplified by stroke or proximal SCI) leads to a hyperactive reflexive jerk, provoked even by a minimal tap on the patellar tendon; a lower motor neuron (LMN) lesion (classically exemplified by polio infection of the anterior horn cells) leaves the limb flaccid and the reflex itself impossible to elicit. Similarly, the detrusor muscle (which comprises almost all of the quasi-spherical bladder wall), if deprived of descending inhibition by an UMN lesion, becomes over-reactive, irritable, and "non-compliant," prompted to contract and evacuate urine in response to only minimal increments in intra-vesicular volume. And since **detrusor-sphincter dyssynergia** (DSD), i.e., failure of the urethral gate to open synergistically when the wall contracts, is also a frequent neuropathic consequence of a spinal cord lesion, then the evacuated urine refluxes upstream, leading to distended, incompetent hydroureters and markedly increased risks for renal infection and stone formation.

In contrast, the bladder affected by a LMN lesion (e.g., cauda equina injury), will be flaccid and non-reactive to accumulated volumes of up to several liters, and will, even then, pass only "overflow" urine. The bladder will eventually become literally saggy and baggy - an enlarged, trabeculated trap for stagnant urine: a nidus for lower tract infection and stone formation. These neuropathic conditions can be objectively

Table 1 A Few of the Known Triggers for Autonomic Dysreflexia

Urinary retention	Tight garment,e.g., underwear
Fecal impaction	Tight shoelace
Occult fracture	Tight urinary leg-bag holder
Deep venous thrombosis	Pulmonary embolism
Rectal (or other) abscess	Sinusitis
Osteomyelitis	Arthritis (acute) or Charcot's joint
Cholelithiasis, -cystitis	Ingrown toenail
Sunburn/dehydration	Insect sting or bite
Uterine contraction	Retained tampon
Spinal instability	Diskitis
Urological procedures	Colonoscopy
General surgery	Functional electrical stimulation
Orthopedic and podiatric surgery	"Too much Thanksgiving dinner"
Etcetera	

documented by examining the intra-vesicular volume vs. pressure curves charted by urodynamics studies (UDS); however the marked variability of these cystometric measurements (with deviations of greater than 100% of the mean even within ranges defined as tightly as the 25th to the 75th percentiles) reduces their prognostic value in sequential studies of an individual patient (Chou, Ho, and Linsenmeyer 2006).

Diagnosis of **urinary tract infection (UTI)**, upper or lower, is notoriously problematic in persons with SCI/D. The major underlying confounding factor is that whether from continual use of an indwelling catheter or from regular intermittent ("clean" but not sterile) self-catheterization, many are chronically colonized. This concept may still be theoretically tenuous (Pordeus et al. 2008), but on a practical level it means they are carriers of urinary microbes that are not actually causing illness but are present in sufficient quantities to appear as though significant in laboratory culture and sensitivity (C&S) reports. A second common confounding factor is mistaking prostatitis for a bladder infection; suspecting this pitfall may be the only clinically defensible indication for ordering a serum prostate specific antigen (PSA) anymore.

So, if the patient presents febrile, complaining of the individual signs and symptoms that she or he has learned to be indicative of a UTI, and has "TNTC" white cells in the urinalysis (U/A), there is no quandary: empirical antibiotic treatment, guided if available by the most recent urine microbiogram, can be appropriately started pending a current C&S report. But if, as is more often the case, the patient has only mild to moderate malaise and a U/A showing 30 or fewer WBC/HPF, it is unlikely to be a UTI, and treatment (other than changing the catheter) should be withheld until further clues to the patient's discomfort emerge. Most challenging is the patient who presents febrile and with a serum leukocytosis, no egregious focal findings on exam, and a U/A with 30 or so WBC/HPF. Clinicians with relatively little SCI/D experience may be tempted to diagnose this as "urosepsis." Whether empirical antibiotics are started or not, after obtaining urine, blood, and sputum cultures it would be prudent to look carefully for other etiologies. It may take super-imposed CT and PET imaging to discover an occult osteomyelitis or other deep infection, once the common "silent" inflammations (facial sinusitis, peri-rectal abscess, cholecystitis, and smoldering scabbed-over or sub-cutaneous pressure sores) have been ruled out.

Calcium-related Bone Disorders

Heterotopic ossification (HO) is the formation of mature lamellar bone in soft tissue sites, i.e., outside and separate from the skeleton. It requires inductive signaling pathways, inducible osteoprogenitor cells, and an environment conducive to osteogenesis (Kaplan et al. 2004). Little is known about any of these processes, other than the empirical observation that HO frequently complicates treatment of burns, arthroplasties, fractures, and spinal and brain injuries while the patient is immobilized. A meta-analysis of pharmacological treatment yielded insufficient evidence to recommend the use of disodium etidronate or comparable agents, which apparently only delay—rather than prevent—the mineralization of HO (Haran, Bhuta, and Lee 2004). After mineralization is complete, as indicated by serial serum alkaline phosphatase determinations, surgical intervention may be indicated to relieve impaired joint function.

Bone demineralization (usually, but not thoughtfully, called osteopenia or osteoporosis) occurs in virtually every SCI patient, and is manifested in a markedly increased incidence of lower extremity fractures. The loss does not occur in supralesional bones, and in weight-bearing areas below the lesion (e.g., lumbar vertebrae) bone density is often increased compared to accepted norms (Jiang, Dai, and Jaing

2006). However, decreased levels of osteoprotegerin (a circulating marker of bone turnover) were found to be associated with severity of SCI (indicated by lower ASIA motor scores) but not with differences in mobility (walking vs. using a wheelchair) (Morse et al. 2008). Of recent note, bone loss in the aged is associated with depression, caused by stimulation of the sympathetic nervous system (Yirmiya et al. 2006). It is unknown if the relative loss of sympathetic tone in SCI/D at different levels of injury offsets this mechanism. Pharmacologic interventions for bone demineralization have included calcium, phosphate, vitamin D, calcitonin and, somewhat controversially because of potential side effects, biphosphonates. A recent systematic review of biphosphonate use found insufficient data to recommend its routine use in either acute or chronic SCI for fracture prevention (Bryson and Gorlay 2009).

Cardiovascular Disease

As more people with SCI/D age, the incidence of cardiovascular disease increases; this has been commonly ascribed to a relatively sedentary lifestyle and higher prevalence of traditional risk factors including obesity, lipid disorders, metabolic syndrome, and diabetes (Collins, Rodenbaugh, and DiCarlo 2006; Myers, Lee, and Kiratli 2007). This concept is in flux. Recently, although measurement of coronary artery calcification by imaging confirmed greater atherosclerosis than in matched non-SCI controls, the finding was significantly beyond that explained by the clustering of traditional risk factors (Orakzai et al. 2007). Another study, using recognized definitions of the metabolic syndrome and assessing coronary heart disease (CHD) risk by Framingham risk scoring (FRS) found both of these markedly *decreased* in SCI subjects compared with the general population; however, high-sensitivity C-reactive protein (CRP) values indicated 36.7% of the participants at high CHD risk (Finnie et al. 2008). The unresolved complexity of this observation is evident from the fact that CRP elevations in this population are known to correlate with obesity, use of motorized wheelchair mobility, and having had a pressure sore or urinary tract infection within the past year, but not with age, smoking, or SCI level or severity (Morse et al. 2008). As mortality from cardiovascular disease appears likely to overtake pulmonary disease as the major cause of death in those with SCI, considerable effort will continue to identify, and in turn palliate, risk factors specific to this population.

Depression

General psychological issues in the context of the subsequent rehabilitative process are discussed below; **depression**, whether manifested as a reactive state or a chronic trait, occurs so frequently in people with SCI/D it is addressed here specifically. Attitudes about emotional dependence on bodily input have been dichotomized for more than a century since William James proposed a "peripheral theory of emotion," arguing that lack of central representation of bodily responses would cause decreased "emotional colour" in people with somatic deficits such as those seen with SCI/D. Walter Cannon responded by stipulating that cognition (i.e., responses already learned and stored in the CNS) would make up for this reduced somatic afferent information, leaving emotional reactions essentially unchanged (Cobos et al. 2002). Current neuroscientific opinion, not surprisingly, postulates ongoing interaction between both visceral and cognitive inputs as framing emotional aspects of consciousness: different contexts evoking differing predominance (Damasio 1999).

Again in the seminal post-WWII era, a paraplegic American psychologist interviewed a cohort of fellow soldiers with SCI. Asked to compare their recalled pre-injury feelings with their post-injury emotional reactions, those with paraplegia noted little difference. Those with quadriplegia however made comments like, "The anger just doesn't have the heat to it that it used to. It's a mental kind of anger." Additionally, "sentimental" emotions expressed in body areas above the neck were perceived as more intense than pre-injury; all the men reported "increases in weeping, lumps in the throat, and getting choked up when saying good-bye, worshipping, or watching a touching movie" (Hohmann 1966).[6]

A recent functional MRI (fMRI) study comparing aversive fear conditioning in persons with SCI with non-SCI controls showed differences in emotion-related brain activity. Those with SCI showed enhanced anterior cingulate and peri-aquaductal grey matter responses, interpreted as reflecting central sensitization of the pain matrix. In addition,

"decreased subgenual cingulate activity may represent a substrate underlying affective vulnerability in SCI patients consequent on perturbation of autonomic control and afferent visceral representation" (Nicotra et al. 2006).

Such motivational and affective sequelae of SCI may be interpreted (by non-SCI persons) as behaviors implying clinical depression. It may be that our understanding of "depression," and perhaps other reified psychosomatic disorders, will undergo a paradigm shift by being redefined in terms of such up- or down-regulation of neural circuitry. This would at least have the merit of leaving behind the "statistical" approach to diagnosis that has made the DSM (I through IV) somewhat less than convincing to most non-behaviorally trained clinicians.

As in any group of elderly patients, treatment with bed-time tricyclic medications, taking advantage of their sedative effects, may cause troublesome anti-cholinergic side effects. Serotonergic drugs, trazodone, or MAOIs may interact with other medications commonly used by those with SCI/D, particularly opioids or the popular herbals ginseng or St. John's wort, to produce the so-called serotonin toxidrome ("storm") with its hypervigilant, hyperadrenergic, and hyperthermic signs and sequelae. Puzzling out the appropriate treatment brings to mind a colleague, locally regarded as one of the best-informed medication-oriented psychiatrists, who was queried, "How do **you** handle depression?" Sardonically he replied, "Not very well" (Li sansky 2005).

Fatigue and Deconditioning

Beyond the fatigue that follows an effort with the depletion of metabolic substrates that all of us experience, at times, there is a deeper, inchoate weariness that afflicts many of those with neuromuscular disorders: MS, MNDs, and SCI/D among them. It is apparently exacerbated relatively early in the aging process. As reported in one study of quality of life noted by people with SCI, it also has a puzzling inverse quality to it—in the sense that "those who experienced fewer disability-related problems were more likely to report a qualitative disadvantage in aging, and the younger members of the sample were more likely to report fatigue....Fatigue is a concern because of its relationship with perceived temporal disadvantage in aging, health problems, and disability problems. This finding highlights the need for clinical vigilance among those just beginning to experience the effects of aging" (McColl and Charlifue, 2003).

The filmmaker, writer, and sometime editor of *New Mobility*, Barry Corbet, who among other achievements had climbed Mt. Everest before a helicopter accident left him paraplegic at age thirty-one, noted as he turned fifty:

But now comes fatigue and it's fatigue that seems way out of proportion to what I see in my non-disabled peers. When that new fatigue combines with my old pain, my pain threshold drops, so it seems like more pain. That means more fatigue. The combination limits my sitting time, which limits what I do. It's a vicious cycle.

What it means for me is that my disability is taking more of my time. It means time, for me, has become the same thing as energy… That has meant elimination of almost all social life and recreation. It has meant less time with my friends and children, less travel and less work. It has meant less money earned (Corbet 1987).

Fatigue, superimposed on the physical limitations due to paraplegia or incomplete quadriplegia in a person with SC I/D, obviously contributes to deconditioning no matter how well motivated or previously fit.

Arm exercise is performed at a greater physiologic cost than is leg exercise; it is less efficient and effective in terms of both central and peripheral aspects of cardiovascular fitness. (Use of an arm bicycle is correspondingly unsuitable for a cardiac exercise-based stress test.) Lower extremity blood-pooling, as a result of loss of sympathetic tone and the absence of a "muscle pump" in the legs, results in relatively poor venous return. This can be ameliorated with various functional electrical stimulation (FES) devices, to achieve better aerobic performance (Philips et al. 1998). Unless so motivated, patients' acceptance of FES devices is not infrequently limited by feeling "that I'm being moved around like a puppet on strings."

Gastrointestinal (GI) Disorders

The **"silent acute abdomen"** is one of the few potential complications of SCI/D included in virtually all medical education. (Note parenthetically that apparently only a minority of U.S. medical schools has even a single lecture dedicated to SCI/D.) If only such educated awareness that **being insensate often leads to a delayed presentation for care** was readily generalized by clinicians regarding this population… GERD engenders pain complaints, but gastric and hepato-biliary and intestinal diseases often don't. Other pertinent signs and symptoms are unaffected by SCI/D, and, as implied above, any noxious GI lesion may evoke AD. People with SCI appear to be at increased risk to develop **gallstones**, but the incidence of biliary complications does not warrant prophylactic cholecystectomy (Moonka et al. 1999).

The major GI dysfunction due to SCI/D is neurogenic dysmotility, manifested primarily as **constipation**, with associated risks for fecal incontinence including "squirt around" apparent diarrhea or actual impaction causing intestinal obstruction, nausea and emesis, and AD. "Bowel care" and "bowel program" are accepted euphemisms for the individualized procedures necessary to initiate defecation and accomplish rectal evacuation. Appropriate diet, scheduled use of oral or rectal medications, and rectal stimulation ("dig stim") to evoke peristalsis are all usually necessary (Stiens, Bergman, and Goetz 1997). Eventual development of hemorrhoids and varying degrees of rectal prolapse are not uncommon. The mundane repeated need for prolonged assistance to achieve defecation (two or more hours every one to three days) is neither trivial if demanded from a family member, nor inexpensive if an attendant must be hired for this task. Recently, a three-week functional magnetic stimulation protocol has been shown to significantly improve SCI bowel dysfunction for at least three months; its longer term duration is as yet unknown (Tsai et al. 2009).

Gender and Sex-related Issues

In the context of neurologic and functional recovery following acute SCI, women appear to have more natural recovery in the first year after injury, as judged by serial improvement in ASIA motor scores. Men, however, achieve higher functional independence measure (FIM) scores by the time of discharge from initial rehabilitation (Sipski et al. 2004). In a separate retrospective study, men with incomplete SCI given testosterone replacement therapy showed higher motor scores on discharge than those not so treated (Clark et al. 2008). Subsequent rehabilitation and aging issues do not diverge significantly from traditional expression of gender roles in persons without SCI. Women with

SCI characterize their aging experience as "accelerated," while men with SCI characterize it as "complicated." Women report more effects of pain, fatigue, skin problems, and transportation issues. Men report more health problems (particularly diabetes) and need for more adaptive equipment changes (McColl et al. 2004). Routine gynecological assessment (e.g., mammography, Pap smears) and treatment (e.g., hormone replacement therapy) are not altered by SCI/D.

Sexual function is compromised, whatever the age, biological sex, or gender orientation of the person with SCI/D, by the probable obstacles of sensory loss and frequent, if not habitual, use of an indwelling catheter (whether urethral or supra-pubic), and of course in males, by often total erectile dysfunction (ED). Depending on the level of the lesion, there may be additional difficulties with embracing or other movement due to weakness and spasticity. As noted above, absence (or diminution) of peripheral somatic input to the brain appears to attenuate emotional framing of interpersonal responses.

Both men (Alexander, Sipski, and Findley 1993) and women (Sipski and Alexander 1993) have reported decreased sexual desire following SCI, but these surveys are admittedly confounded by coincident depression and somatic embarrassment in those questioned. Men with SCI who report strong sexual desire evince higher rates of depression when they conform to cultural norms emphasizing male sexual prowess. In contrast, men who report little sexual desire show lower rates of depression even if they endorse masculine norms for prowess (Burns et al. 2009). Women with SCI identified as having sexual dysfunction by structured self-report did not show any consistent pertinent hormonal abnormalities (Lombardi et al. 2007), suggesting an equivalent predominance of psychosocial factors contributing to sexual difficulties. In any case, it does not seem likely that individuals with SCI/D would be further affected in this regard more than any others by the additional influence of aging.

Counsel regarding exploring alternative methods of sexual excitation or "giving (and receiving) pleasure" is available from professionals, peers, and online (Lombardi et al. 2008). Use of injectable/intraurethral PGE1 analogs (e.g., alprostadil) or the oral PDE-5 inhibitors (e.g., sildenafil) for ED requires only the same precautions as with non-SCI/D patients; exacerbation of the infrequent spontaneous priapism (presumed due to parasympathetic predominance) noted in this population, usually in response to non-sexual stimuli such as a change in ambient temperature, has not been observed. Autonomic dysreflexia in those susceptible to it is also not routinely provoked by sexual intercourse, although in younger male patients seeking semen for artificial insemination electro-ejaculation may evoke it.

Hematological Disorders

Increased susceptibility to clotting and the sub-acute development of anemia are the two major blood-related risks for those with SCI/D. Work-up of the "anemia of chronic disease" is routine in this group; the only caveat is that replacement of iron (even if its deficiency is specifically indicated by appropriate testing) is unlikely to fully resolve the anemia if coincident pressure sores, osteomyelitis, or recurrent UTIs persist (Perkash and Brown 1986). Exclusion of occult bleeding is confounded by absent sensation and the common use of digital stimulation to produce bowel movements with consequent retained rectal bleeding, which may be "bright red" as expected, but may also be melanotic, causing "tarry stools" and positive FOBT cards. Colonoscopy may be indicated at an earlier age and higher frequency than in non-SCI/D groups, and its preparation is arduous in this population, often requiring pre-procedural hospitalization for 3–5 days for adequate bowel cleansing from "above and below."

Even after the usual period of total or relative immobilization following the onset of SCI/D, once they are active in rehabilitation or even reintegrated into community life, their lack of spontaneous movement of some parts of their bodies leaves this population forever at risk for deep venous thrombosis (DVT) and subsequent pulmonary embolism (PE). Wisely choosing and contextually changing among the common anticoagulants (warfarin, heparin, and enoxaparin) is a slowly acquired skill for the clinician, bringing to mind the neglected second half of Hippocrates' cliché (after the *vita brevis* tag): "...experience fleeting, judgment fallacious." If for no other than medico-legal reasons, in the applicable clinical settings, published guidelines should be followed (McKinney 2008).[7] But on the other hand, considering the risks of long-term anticoagulation in a population as susceptible to falls as those with SCI/D, as well as the logistical difficulties of requiring monitoring by venipuncture, there are no conclusive data-based guidelines to help answer the patients' recurrent question: "When can I quit taking this stuff?"

Immunity and Immunization

There is no consensus on alterations (if any) in immune status following traumatic SCI, nor the precise extent of those which undoubtedly accompany MS or neoplastic SCI/D. In general, CNS tissue has been characterized as "immunologically privileged," noting for example its tolerance of certain intracellular neurotrophic viruses rather than uniformly eliminating all infected neurons. This may result from evolutionary pressure to down-modulate immune responses in crucial tissues. Another insight into CNS immune privilege may be exemplified by the central canal of the spinal cord, which is generally regarded as a vestigial structure obliterated after birth. However, this obliteration is a pathological (necrotic) process rather than an involutional (apoptotic) event (Milhorat, Kotzen, and Anzil 1994), suggesting that selection has opposed even minimal programmed cord degeneration. Persons with quadriplegia or paraplegia with lesions above T_{10} invariably have sympathetic dysregulation; this has been significantly correlated with impaired phagocytic ability and decreased natural killer cell cytotoxicity (Compagnolo, Bartlett, and Keller 2000). Overall, it is as yet unclear if exogenous SCI/D *per se* brings about "tolerated" damage; it is clear that "the challenge remains to support beneficial immune cascades without causing additional damage, and vice versa" (Bechmann 2005).

Tetanus inoculation (with or without "big or little" diphtheria or pertussis antigens, depending on endemic regional indications) is indicated for people with SCI/D every ten years. It is also the only preventative "shot" many of this population will accept. One or more annual influenza vaccinations (depending on the number of currently prevalent strains), and exposure to pneumococcal vaccine (principally aimed at pneumonia prevention) are recommended. As of this writing, whether one or two inoculations are needed for the latter, and the age at which it should be initiated for people with SCI/D, remain debated topics. Similarly there are no current SCI/D patient data supporting or contraindicating "shingles vaccine" at this time.

Regardless of scientific disagreement over such issues, as well as over the degree and duration of immune compromise in this population, many people with SCI/D simply refuse these vaccinations. A few patients have credible histories of prior adverse reactions, but most appear to be influenced by the generally accepted relationship between recent inoculation and the onset of GBS—which they unscientifically transfer to their own status. Still others simply declare themselves unwilling to "put more germs into my body."

Infectious Disease

The propensity to over-diagnose UTIs in this population is discussed above; the need for clinical hypervigilance with regard to pneumonia is briefly mentioned below. Osteomyelitis is the third notable diagnostic infectious disease conundrum occurring in people with SCI/D—like an iceberg, it often lurks out of sight. It may emerge abruptly as a newly gaping, previously unsuspected pressure sore, linger in a bony prominence beneath a relatively insignificant but persistently recurrent ulcer, or stay hidden subcutaneously but provoke intermittent systemic signs of fever, malaise, and diffusely increased spasticity. Despite having a prevalence of only about 2 in 10,000 in the general population, it is often cited as one of the most threatening causes of non-focal, nagging back pain in the elderly (Broder and Snarski 2007), requiring timely diligence to distinguishing dangerous from benign causes.

In people with SCI/D, absent sensation often removes even this vague clue. Incidence and prevalence in this population are as obscure as its diagnosis, but it is a frequent cause of re-hospitalization. MRI and PET/CT imaging are as yet irresolute regarding osteomyelitis; radiologists not infrequently retreat behind the mantra of "clinical correlation is advised." Cultures obtained from contiguous pressure sores or other soft tissue infections are noncontributory; bone cultures themselves are inconclusive, yielding a similar number of bacterial isolates in patients with or without proven osteomyelitis, which can be definitively diagnosed only by direct pathological examination of the affected bone (Darouiche et al. 1994). Of course, sampling error adds further ambiguity; the cited study retrospectively showed the sensitivity and specificity of clinical evaluation to be only 33% and 60%, respectively. Equally sobering, the authors conclude that "it is possible that treatment of osteomyelitis may improve the outcome of associated pressure sores."

Any 21st century discussion of infection must mention methicillin-resistant *S. aureus* (MRSA). It is sufficient to say everyone with SCI/D, whether hospitalized or in the community, should be considered as colonized with it, until proven otherwise. Accordingly, it is a probable agent in any infected site or organ, and antibiotic treatment started empirically should adequately address it.

The Metabolic Syndrome

The co-morbid occurrence of obesity, hyper- and dyslipidemias, and diabetes mellitus, with the associated specters of hypertension and atherosclerosis, is variably defined as comprising "the" metabolic syndrome. As noted above in the paragraph on cardiovascular disease, there is controversy over its prevalence as a grouped entity in persons with SCI/D. Setting aside the visual illusion of "quad belly" (as it is known by some with SCI), which is apparent obesity due to lack of abdominal wall muscle tone, persons with SCI are indeed fatter using any accepted body mass index, and demonstrate less lean tissue, than controls; advancing age in this group is strongly associated with greater adiposity, while it is only mildly related in controls (Spungen et al. 2003). In contrast, no significant differences were observed in mass or body composition between ambulatory MS patients and controls (Lambert, Lee-Archer, and Evans 2002). SCI individuals are predisposed to excessive abdominal obesity, with correspondingly higher leptin levels and insulin resistance (Maruyama et al. 2008; Karlsson 1999). People with paraplegia who are clinically depressed have higher total and LDL cholesterol, as well as triglycerides, and greater adiposity than non-depressed SCI controls. This is not the case for depressed people with quadriplegia (Kemp et al. 2000), perhaps due to their loss of sympathetic tone. One can also speculate that this observation is related to the notion of "comfort food," coupled with the relative ease of paraplegic persons to raid the refrigerator.

A survey of U.S. veterans with SCI/D reported an overall prevalence of diabetes mellitus of 20%. This is roughly three times higher than in the general non-veteran population, but is similar to veterans overall (LaVela et al. 2006). It is not clear if this represents over- or under-diagnosis in the venues in which veterans and non-veterans receive health care, or if it implies that diabetes ought to be classified as a service-connected condition. Perhaps conclusively, a detailed meta-analysis of studies conducted worldwide from 1996–2007 concluded that the available evidence does not indicate that adults with spinal cord injuries are at a markedly greater risk for carbohydrate or lipid disorders than able-bodied adults, and that diagnostic/treatment thresholds should not be altered for this population (Wilt et al. 2008).

Pain

When it is appreciated as a sign (not a symptom) of inflammation, tissue compression, or some other active pathological process, pain is understandable and the patient is usually approached sympathetically by caregivers and empathetically by clinicians. But when it is repeatedly expressed without any discernible acute trigger, it becomes more likely to be perceived merely as a complaint, symptomatic of a desire for secondary gain and perhaps prescribed intoxication. "Take a couple of pain pills, and call another doctor in the morning." This ostensibly humorous fantasy of the SCI/D primary care physician—to shunt complaints about pain to another provider—reflects both the patient's undeniable anguish and the provider's frustration at failing to adequately relieve it. Transference and counter-transference may then take over, and mutually anger-provoking suspicions—and sometimes overt accusations—of drug-seeking and malicious withholding of narcotics further erode the doctor-patient relationship, and only exacerbate each party's pain.

People with SCI/D are prone to the short-term pains everyone encounters through minor trauma, exercise, and repetitive activities such as "pushing" a manual wheelchair. They may not be as focally localizable as before SCI/D, but they are usually clearly peripheral and describable in familiar language: "a burning feeling, or a cramp, an ache, a sharp or dull pressure..." They respond gratifyingly to rest, massage, topical heat or cold, perhaps even further gentle stretching or use, and minor medications.

But there are other feelings that are literally "hard to put into words," because there has been no prior experience to provide an accepted vocabulary for the exact sensations evoked: "No, it's not really burning or cramping or squeezing or stabbing or..." These central pains, which begin—and then persist—in the setting of SCI/D and occasionally stroke or other paroxysmal CNS damage, are literally neurogenic. The term is etiologically appropriate in this context, since it is aberrant neural circuitry that perpetuates (one might say perseverates) an acute pain long after its precipitating insult has healed or scarred over. One postulated mechanism is "senseless" long-term potentiation (LTP), predominantly in thalamic afferents and efferents. This LTP embodies learning, i.e., stores memories in neural circuits selected by Hebbian coincidence in firing, which when subsequently evoked by non-painful stimuli, are perceived anew as painful (Rygh et al. 2005). It has also been recently proposed that activated CNS glial cells participate in maintaining the pain sensation by altering neuronal excitability (Hansson 2006). Additionally, these activated glia appear to compromise the efficacy of morphine and other opioids (both endogenous and exogenous) for pain control. Accordingly, targeting glia and their pro-inflammatory products is expected to provide novel effective therapy for controlling clinical pain syndromes (Watkins et al. 2007), including the intractable chronic central pain characteristic of SCI/D.

The difficulties of pharmacological treatment of chronic pain are familiar to all clinicians; and of central pain to all neurologists. In the setting of SCI/D, appeal to surgical intervention such as pump placement (with its significant risks and problematic maintenance issues) for intrathecal delivery of medications seems to have proven as ineffective overall as the once vaunted dorsal column stimulators or dorsal root entry zone ablations of the past (Siddall 2002). While awaiting new treatments such as the anti-glials, perhaps it will be forgiven if this paragraph is closed with another bitter-sweet joke: "The only pain that's tolerable is somebody else's."

Pressure Sores

This term is preferentially used, rather than the common erroneous term "decubiti," ignorantly considered the plural of decubitus ulcer.[8] These pressure sores occur in skin and subcutaneous tissues subject to prolonged pressure between a bony prominence and a relatively hard surface, such as a seat cushion or mattress, no matter how resilient their design or manufacture. Classic studies defined the limiting pressure as 1.5 lb/in² (which approximately equals 10.3 kPa), and is about 80 mm Hg, i.e., just above arteriolar pressure (Trumble 1930). Most sensate people automatically shift position about every twenty minutes; without such adjustments, after ~2 hours irreversible necrosis occurs. Pressure sores were formerly not infrequently found in many "bed-bound" neurological patients, whether from unmedicated parkinsonian rigidity or chronic opisthotonos, or merely from being "warehoused" in institutions for those with developmental disabilities (Spillane 1968).

Nowadays they occur in individuals with SCI/D, principallydue to their reduced or absent capacity to either feel the premonitory numbness of pending ischemia, or to respond with regular automatic shifting of position. Yet education on diet and regular physical activity, including learning to perform specific pressure relief maneuvers every twenty minutes particularly when sitting and providing for regular turning when in bed, as well as maintaining a "healthy lifestyle," disappointingly don't really seem to affect the incidence or prevalence of these ulcers: they occur with almost equal frequency (about 17% of all medical complications) in the second year following traumatic SCI and more than thirty years later (Ditunno and Formal 1994). This suggests a more complex, poly-factorial etiology involving interactions between pressure-related compromise of tissue perfusion, shearing between adjacent tissue layers (e.g., fascia against muscle "pinching" blood vessels), friction translated differentially from epidermis to dermis, post-SCI disturbances of cutaneous axonal vascular reflexes exemplified by the loss of the normal triple response of Lewis (Appenzeller 1986), obesity, superficial moisture, opportunistic biofilms of pathogens, and the putative loss of a still undetermined trophic factor in denervated tissue. The concatenation of some or all of these factors into producing an actual pressure sore remains speculative (Stekelenburg 2008).

Consensus on staging of pressure sores, useful for communication regarding consultation or referral to specialized centers, comparison of treatment outcomes, and ultimately prognosis, has developed since 1975 into the following system (National Pressure Ulcer Advisory Panel), now internationally accepted.

Stage I: Intact skin with non-blanchable redness of a localized area usually over a bony prominence. Darkly pigmented skin may not have visible blanching; its color may differ from the surrounding area.

Stage II: Partial thickness loss of dermis presenting as a shallow open ulcer with a red-pink wound bed, without slough. May also present as an intact or open/ruptured serum-filled blister.

Stage III: Full thickness tissue loss. Subcutaneous fat may be visible but neither bone, tendon, or muscle are exposed. Slough may be present but does not obscure the depth of tissue loss. May include undermining and tunneling.

Stage IV: Full thickness tissue loss with exposed bone, tendon, or muscle. Slough or eschar may be present on some parts of the wound bed. Often include undermining and tunneling.

Unstageable: Full thickness tissue loss in which the base of the ulcer is covered by slough (yellow, tan, gray, green or brown) and/or eschar (tan, brown or black) in the wound bed.

Appropriate treatment of a pressure sore at any stage, aside from "getting off of it," is still far from being evidence-based; fads and anecdotal success stories fluctuate and occasionally recur. Fifty years ago, dressings soaked with saline or dilute Dakin's solution were popular. Bed-side lamps shining into open wounds, and decoctions of honey and poultices of herbal "stems and seeds" followed. Multiple dressings with and without poly-enzymatic activity have come and gone over the years; silver-containing preparations have similarly passed in and out (and back in again) of favor. Hyperbarometric O_2 insulations, and pulsatile wound irrigation have had their proponents, and most recently, constant suction of the ulcer bed at sub-atmospheric pressures using a "wound vac" under a variety of foams and occlusive dressings has prevailed. Special wound clinics, staffed by both medical and "alternative" specialists, have entered the fray in the medical marketplace; these are less competitively paralleled by the apparent recent increase in invited participation of nurse representatives of proprietary vendors on regular wound rounds in ostensibly not-for-profit hospital settings.

In anecdotal summary, on the SCI ward in which the writer works, we often still retreat to dressings soaked with saline or dilute Dakin's solution…. Perhaps it is no more than the net immuno-irritant effect of periodically changing treatments in a patient otherwise slow to heal, that eventually stimulates endogenous healing by what used to be called, admittedly somewhat teleologically, secondary intention (Morykwas et al. 1997).

If the patient is sufficiently well nourished, and the affected area hasn't been rendered bereft of vascular support by prior failed skin flaps, the plastic surgeon may agree to attempt surgical intervention. Post-op care requires a month or more supine in a Clinitron-type blown sand suspension bed (known plaintively to the patients as "the cat box" or, more ominously, "my casket"), with the concomitant somatic risks of infection, often speculative antibiotic treatment, and problematic maintenance of intravenous access. The consequent development of *C. difficile* toxin-associated diarrhea, with its augmented risk for recurrent wound breakdown in this population, is notoriously more frequent in institutionalized patients, and its unwelcome persistence or recurrence, due to resistance to antibiotic eradication, appears to disproportionately affect older patients (Calfee 2008). Providers should also anticipate the inevitable psychosocial risks of further prolongation of institutional care: pain and boredom, exacerbated by depression, likely to lead to drug-seeking; staff-splitting; and diverse complaints broadcast as widely as imagination, roommates, personal caregivers and family, spokespersons, and disgruntled staff can suggest.

Like most potential complications, the best (and least intrusive) treatment for a pressure sore is "simply" to avoid ever getting one.

Pulmonary Disease

As one person with SCI put it, "tobacco smoking is one of the few remaining vices I can indulge in." Accordingly, chronic obstructive pulmonary disease is frequent and persistent in these patients. SCI/D, of whatever etiology, by its nature as a neuromuscular impairment itself causes significant restrictive pulmonary disease. Their coexistence contributes to the epidemiological fact that for more than two decades pneumonia has been the most common cause of death in this population (Burns 2007). Upper respiratory infections and acute bronchitis are more likely to be precipitating factors for pneumonia than in the general population. Avoid watchful waiting—pulmonary reserve in this group is at best diminished, and often essentially non-existent. Consider your clinical suspicion as a virtual diagnosis, hospitalize promptly, re-discuss potential intubation issues, and treat early with broad antibiotic coverage.

Spasticity

The undesired movements and chronic muscular tension caused by spasticity (like the noxious sensations of myelopathic pain) contradict the oversimplified notion that a person with complete SCI/D can't move (or feel) below the level of the injury. All animal movements start and end with muscle-controlled posture, and when useful, make sense of afferent information (Partridge and Partridge 1993). In adult-onset spasticity (without the subsequent abnormal growth and development characteristic of, say, cerebral palsy) the loss of normal descending neuro-modulation results in apparently useless movement based on "senseless" afferent stimuli.

A century or more of physiological controversy over definitions (spasms vs. spasticity) (Maynard, Karunas, and Waring 1990), source (cerebral vs. spinal cord) (Young 1994), extent (basic vs. excess) (Michaelis 1976), contributing factors (CNS intrinsic vs. CNS extrinsic) (Ragnarsson 1992), muscle composition (mechanical vs. contractile alterations) (Dietz, Quintern, and Berger 1981), muscle groups affected (gravity-opposing vs. gravity-augmenting) (Edstrom, Grimby, and Jannerz 1973), and clinical assessment (scales vs. grading) (Hsieh et al. 2008) has led to neither a compelling explanation nor an effective treatment. People with SCI/D and their caregivers alike lump together the increased tone and associated pain, the spasms, the variable stiffness/resistance of limbs in response to speed and direction of attempted movement, eventual contractures, and the consequent further reduction of the patients' independence and ease of care, into a single clinical problem—"spasticity," from which prompt and lasting relief is demanded.

Exercise, "ranging," and other physical therapy modalities including functional electrical stimulation, best effected on a muscle-by-muscle basis (Gracies 2005), offer short-term reduction in symptoms. Currently favored medications have been in use for decades, or longer: baclofen and tizanidine are still popular; benzodiazepines and dantrolene are less commonly used today than previously. None are uniformly effective, all have troublesome side effects. Botulinum toxin injections, although conceptually appealing, have not proven widely effective. As of this writing, there are various new drugs being marketed, but none (so far) appear to be promising, perhaps sadly reaffirming one clinician's encapsulation of this problem more than thirty-five years ago:

> "…too often the patient's motivation, confidence, time, and money are dissipated by the ill-considered treatment of a vague neologism with a nostrum. That there is no substitute for the neurologist's own supportive observation of the individual patient in his effort to cope with real life performance handicaps seems to be a lesson that we never learn but never quite forget" (Landau 1974)

Sweating Disorders

The most frequent instance of "abnormal" sweating in a patient with SCI/D is the excessive adrenergic sweating above the level of the lesion coincident with autonomic dysreflexia, discussed above. In contrast, the inability to sweat normally below the level of the lesion as a cooling mechanism makes "spinal man" (or woman) effectively a poikilotherm; risk for sunstroke or other heat exposures is dangerously augmented. Elite wheelchair racing athletes have been known to take advantage of this property: by inducing AD through heat intolerance, they can "boost" (actually reduce) their performance times by as much as 10%, as a result of increased oxygen utilization (Bhambhani 2002).[9]

Hyperhydrosis is occasionally the presenting sign of syrinx, as discussed below. Night sweats, which may paradoxically occur below the level of the lesion, sometimes herald occult infection such as osteomyelitis or spinal abscess (Forlenza, Axelrod, and Grieco 1979). Soaking perspiration, beyond provoking embarrassment, is a risk factor for skin breakdown and/or intertriginous yeast infection. After excluding Graves' disease and pheochromocytoma, treatment options include glycopyrrolate cream, oral oxybutinin, propantheline, and clonidine, scopolamine patches, botulinum toxin injections (particularly if focal, e.g., axillary) and sympathectomy; all have drawbacks and relative contraindications.

Syrinx

With regard to pathology of the spinal cord, the most useful translation of this Greek word is "cyst."[10] Incidence and prevalence of its variants remain ill-described, since all are rare, and consequently studies of statistically significant series are few and far between. The most likely estimate seems to be that the post-traumatic variety eventually presents clinically in 3–5% of persons with SCI; MRIs done for other indications on asymptomatic persons (with or without SCI) show occult prevalence about twice that. Unproven and intriguing etiological theories abound, e.g., intramedullary cord pulsation of cerebrospinal fluid [CSF] induced by routinely alternating normal systolic and diastolic pressures (Anson, Benzel, and Awad 1997).

Syrinx may occur idiosyncratically, usually as a remnant of the embryologically overt central canal of the spinal cord. If it occurs within the conus medullaris (where it is known as a *ventriculus terminalis*) it may cause bladder or bowel sphincter incompetence. More commonly, being centrally located in the cord, the cyst primarily affects the crossing of the bilateral ascending spino-thalamic tracts, giving rise to the characteristic dissociated sensory deficit: loss of the so-called protopathic sensations (pain and temperature) with preservation of touch, pressure and the other epicritical sensations, which are relayed in the uninterrupted posterior column pathways. A syrinx may also rarely occur elsewhere in the cord in association with intramedullary neoplastic disease, frequently an ependymoma.

When a syrinx is identified in persons with established SCI presenting with "new" complaints of extremity or truncal pain, spasticity, sensorimotor loss, or very rarely, segmental hyperhidrosis, it is interpreted as post-traumatic. Since it may not present until months or years after the actual SCI, it is not clear if it is a tardive sequela of a separate but coincident trauma at the time of the original SCI, or if it somehow progressively develops *de novo* thereafter.

Except for possible additional invasive effects from the neoplastic variety, the signs and symptoms resulting from any syrinx are caused by its cystic contents (essentially normal, locally elaborated CSF) swelling it sufficiently to become a space-occupying lesion. Compression of adjacent neurons, neuropil, and vessels apparently produces the actual positive or negative signs; consequently in most cases if surgical treatment is undertaken, placement of a shunt to the adjacent sub-arachnoid space or a more distant poly-absorbent site (e.g., the retroperitoneal space or the pericardial sac) is effected. Conventional neurosurgical wisdom relates that a third of such procedures offer improvement, a third have no effect, and a third result in worsening (Vernon, Silver, and Symon 1983). No pre- or intra-operative parameters or other clinical criteria, including depiction by modern neuroimaging techniques, have as yet been identified that accurately predict an ameliorative, neutral, or pejorative outcome.

(Further) Trauma and Overuse Syndromes

Overall, subsequent injuries following initial rehabilitation for SCI and apparent community reintegration impact about 20% of people with SCI annually. Being younger, having an ASIA grade D (relatively incomplete) injury, higher sensation-seeking scores, and "heavy" use of ethanol or prescription medications for pain, spasticity, or sleep were associated with a greater likelihood of subsequent injury (Krause 2004). The risk for accidental fractures in infralesional demineralized bones in persons with SCI is discussed above; this is disproportionately increased in middle-aged patients but continues with further aging. For example, one study found femoral fractures to have greater incidence in people with SCI by factors of 104 and 24 at ages 50 and 70, respectively (Frisbie 1997). Another study comparing fracture incidence in veterans with SCI versus MS, noted that in both groups fracture risk was maximal in those with moderate (as opposed to either little or severe) motor impairment, but that having traumatic SCI further increased the risk ratio by 80% (Logan et al. 2008).

An occasional patient, perceiving himself to be without home or community social support, will self-inflict such "painless" fractures in order to obtain or prolong institutional care. In other cases, self-perception as having "useless" body parts below the level of SCI can lead to seemingly careless trauma with subsequent infection, eventually requiring amputation. One documented extreme case, in which the patient presented himself over several years to be "whittled on" by a series of apparently unsuspecting podiatric and orthopedic surgeons, led ultimately to having achieved a hip disarticulation on one lower extremity, and a hemi-pelvectomy on the other.

Less sensationally but more painfully, SCI/D persons with actual or effective paraplegia, after "pushing" themselves for years in manual wheelchairs, develop shoulder pain and rotator cuff injuries that require orthopedic intervention and, not infrequently, a change to power mobility. Not surprisingly, risks for this damage are increased age, duration of injury, daily wheelchair activity, and female gender (Lal 1998). Perhaps less intuitively obvious, persons with SCI who report lower subjective quality of life experience significantly higher levels of shoulder pain, but shoulder pain intensity in this group does not relate to involvement in general community activities (Gutierrez et al. 2007).

Rehabilitative/psychological Aspects

The potential for mutually enabled despondency between patients with newly diagnosed SCI/D and their families and friends is memorably implied by the ironic statement of a combat injured paraplegic WWII Army Chaplain (technically—and even more ironically—a non-combatant), who advised: "The first duty of the paraplegic patient is to cheer up his visitors" (Bull 1979).

In a recent study of people with SCI and chronic pain (N=190), cluster analysis revealed three groups, independent of sex, pain duration, and functional status: (1) "Dysfunctional" (34.6%) characterized by higher reported pain severity, life interference, affective distress, and lower levels of life control and activities; (2) "Interpersonally supported" (33.0%) characterized by moderately high reported pain severity, and higher life control and support from significant others and activities; and (3) "Adaptive copers" (32.4%) characterized by lower reported pain severity, life interference, affective distress, support from significant others, and higher life control (Widerstrom-Noga 2007). Beyond the issue of pain, this categorization of persons with SCI/D seems applicable to their general psychosocial reactive styles.

Long experience with people initially coping with SCI/D and their subsequent lifelong rehabilitative process suggests that all of them are continually dealing with depression, coupled with fear. In many patients of all three types described above, these moods are often obscured by denial and preoccupation with somatic adaptations in the first year or two after injury. In some "go-getters" of Group 3, these

linked potentially oppressive symptoms remain covert for years, until aging intrudes. This is exemplified by another quotation from Barry Corbet:

What are our expectations from aging with a disability? We do not know. Most of us do not think anyone else knows either, that is a constant refrain. Being part of a newly surviving population makes us nervous.

Do we have any complaints about our health care? Yes. What I heard over and over was that it is hard to find a dedicated cord injury doctor, it is hard to find a good family physician, it is hard to find someone who can make sense out of the information the specialists generate.

What do we fear as we age?... We fear loss of independence... For most of us, our independence was the principal accomplishment of our lives. It was the toughest and best thing we ever did. We coped with a catastrophic injury and an apathetic society and now we are afraid that we are going to lose what we fought for. (Corbet 1987)

Current studies in animal models on molecular level interventions for inhibition of fear, termed "learned safety," show involvement of hippocampal neurogenesis and down-regulation of dopaminergic and neuropeptidergic, but not the serotonergic, systems in the basolateral amygdala. These data suggest that learned safety is an animal model of a behavioral antidepressant that shares some neuronal hallmarks of pharmacological antidepressants (Pollak, Monie, and Kandel 2008). Noting that rehabilitation medicine has long been perceived as lacking a unifying basic science of its own (Frontera et al. 2006), perhaps we can begin to redress that embarrassing molecular deficit by re-framing the goals of "rehabilitation" and "community reintegration" as behaviors achievable through the acquisition of learned safety?

A seemingly minor indicator of the pervasive character of this fear is the common reluctance of the person with SCI/D to accept a new model when the need to replace familiar, but worn-out, equipment arises. The offered new power-wheelchair doesn't seem to fit, no matter how carefully measured; the new hand-controls to drive the adapted vehicle are not merely hard to get used to, but are judged insurmountably unsafe. Accepting such change appears to reawaken the dismay that accompanied the initial slow acceptance of the disability that led to the need for powered mobility or hand controls. In this context, note that a sip-and-puff (i.e., breath controlled) power wheelchair needed for independent mobility by a person with high quadriplegia costs at least $35,000 in 2010 U.S. dollars; with standing and stair-climbing options, about $85,000. (Activities most readers of this chapter do daily, at no extra cost....) And even with careful attention to maintenance, the device will need to be replaced about every six or seven years.

The additional, and deeper, dismay that loss of an older partner or longtime family caregiver evokes is often devastating, whether caused by age-related physical inability to perform the necessary tasks, or—far worse—by long-term burnout, illness, or death. It may present obliquely, for example, as a pressure sore that can no longer be cared for in the home; only as the need for hospitalization draws to a close, does the lack of a caregiver to return to become evident. The burdens of expense to hire a replacement, or acceptance of institutional care, are each clearly unwelcome and sometimes intolerable. Preventative efforts in support of aging caregivers need to be initiated well before such a crisis emerges, and should realistically encourage them to participate in their own health-promoting behaviors and increase their awareness and utilization of existing sources of support (Su, Amsters, and Carlson 2002).

The patient's expressed concern quoted above regarding finding a knowledgeable and dedicated primary care practitioner (PCP) is matched by consternation among medical educators and planners, who note spreading fiscal and attitudinal obstacles putting "primary care, the backbone of the nation's health care system,…at grave risk of collapse" (Bodenheimer 2006). People with SCI/D essentially are engaged in "rehab" all the rest of their lives, and this process is not infrequently interrupted by acute overt medical needs. Risks for subsequent illness include age, time since injury, and disability and handicap severity. A person with chronic SCI is more than twice as likely to be rehospitalized than a member of the general population, and stays in hospital three times as long. Urinary and pressure sore complications are the principal indications (Savic et al. 2000). And whether during the initial hospitalization or subsequent admissions for whatever indication, acquisition of hospital-acquired infections is significantly higher than in other groups (Evans et al. 2008).

The provision of such subsequent care can occur in diverse settings, usually dictated by a person's health insurance or eligibility for VA care. Comparison of care from disparate providers with that provided by specialized SCI/D programs (either regarding initial rehabilitation or subsequent care) is reflected subjectively in terms of patient satisfaction and objectively in terms of efficacy and efficiency. No satisfactory tool has yet been devised to genuinely assess satisfaction in the context of health care (Williams, Coyle, and Healy 1998). Measurable way-points for efficacy, exemplified by serial scoring on the Functional Independence Measure (FIM) are generally perceived as too simplistic and context-bound (Ota et al. 2001), and in settings where they are used to determine length of stay and/or reimbursement, are too susceptible to "gaming"; more suitable tools have not yet emerged.

"Bottom line" measures of health care efficiency with regard to SCI/D ultimately are framed in terms of life expectancy. Aside from the highly speculative issue of individual prognosis, reliable statistical calculations regarding life expectancy are clearly needed by the insurance industry. They are also of interest to litigators (and the experts they hire) seeking settlements for alleged legal responsibility for contributing to a plaintiff's SCI (Berkowitz et al. 1998).[11] This has resulted in a literature with many biases. But as a general rule, life expectancy for an otherwise healthy person with paraplegia is 80% of normal at age 20, but by age 80 the estimates fall to 50% of normal or lower (Anderson and Marion 2003). For those with quadriplegia, it appears to be 4–6 years shorter; and "those with incomplete lesions at any level can expect 8 more years than those with complete injuries" (McColl et al. 1997). In comparison, note that life expectancy with multiple sclerosis is typically reduced by only a few years, if at all (DeVivo 2004).

As recently as 2004, it occurred to an experienced group of SCI demographers (and was deemed publishable) that in addition to health parameters, consideration of economic and psycho-social factors would make computations of life expectancy more accurate (Krause, Devivo, and Jackson 2004). However, subsequent reappraisal showed the positive effect of favorable economics was much less than previously reported, and that interpretation of the effects of social integration is "complicated by questions of cause and effect" (Strauss et al. 2008). For many years, an anecdotal impression among concerned professionals has postulated that there has been a notable decrease in mortality from SCI in the first two years post-injury, and also a significant decline in mortality over the longer term following that initial period. The same group of analysts studied records of 30,822 patients followed from 1973 to 2004 in SCI Model Systems facilities; they contributed data on 323,618 person-years, and 4980 deaths occurred. There was a 40% decline in mortality during the first two years after SCI. However, the decline in mortality after the initial two-year post-injury period was small and not statistically significant (Strauss et al. 2006). The authors conclude,

"Improvements in critical care medicine after spinal cord injury may explain the marked decline in short-term mortality. In contrast, although

there have no doubt been improvements in long-term rehabilitative care, their effect in enhancing the life span of persons with SCI appears to have been overstated."

The only pertinent Cochrane Database systematic review to date finds "the current evidence does not enable conclusions to be drawn about the benefits or disadvantages of immediate referral versus late referral to spinal injury centers," and by inference, of their overall utility (Jones and Bagnall 2004). The issue mentioned above regarding the effect of lifelong care from a single unified system versus sporadic care from diverse providers has only been obliquely addressed, in an "independent report commissioned by the VA." It compared four VA SCI/D facilities, four Model Systems SCI/D facilities, four other facilities not associated with VA or Model Systems, and a "single payer" national health care system outside the U.S. Quality of care and clinical outcomes were not addressed. Analysis of program data showed that the VA and single payer models offer care at a lower cost to the individual, and that the VA provides more comprehensive coverage—"no other provider is as involved in the full continuum of care." The conclusion was perhaps predictably tautological:

"External comparisons should focus on Acute Rehabilitation, since that is the segment of the continuum of care most non-VA facilities provide" (Booz-Allen & Hamilton, Inc. 2000).

The ambiguities encountered in teasing apart social, political, and health care system contributions to clinical outcomes are evident from the findings of a careful study of international differences in aging with spinal cord injury. After controlling for age, level of lesion, and duration of disability, the following differences were noted: (1) Americans aging with SCI had a better psychological profile and fewer health and disability-related problems; (2) British aging with SCI had less joint pain and less likelihood of perceiving they were aging more quickly; and (3) Canadians aging with SCI had more health and disability-related complications (particularly bowel, pain, and fatigue problems) (McColl et al. 2002).

Whatever the results of sporadic political attempts at health care reform in the U.S., managed care (a fading euphemism for managed expenditures) will survive in spirit if not in name. "Do more with less!" will continue to be demanded of health care providers in every system of health care delivery. Rationalized as population-based, people with SCI/D, along with everyone else who can't personally afford a "boutique physician," are likely to endure further reduction in access to PCPs and specialists alike, and increasingly limited provision of medications, supplies, and durable medical equipment. Particularly with the advent of such constraints, allopathic clinicians must swallow possible resentment at "qigongization" or other appeals to alternative holistic medicine by patients seeking to utilize "mind control to prevent illness, heal existing physical and emotional problems, and promote health and happiness" (Trieschmann 1999).

Future Directions

"Cure not care!" has been the rallying cry of the activists among those with SCI/D since the concept of disability rights emerged in the 'sixties. Social networking sites on the Web specifically for those with SCI and various SCDs have emerged in the 2000s, allowing colloquial (and unrefereed) peer support on a previously unobtainable level.[12]

The scope of current basic and applied scientific efforts to achieve cure is summarized in this recent categorization of research utilizing animal models: A. Reduce the effects of damage (e.g., maintain circulation and oxygenation, reduce neurotoxins, inflammation and apoptosis); B. Encourage correct neuron connections (e.g., with cells, with matrix modifiers and "bridges," and nerve grafts); C. Enhance regeneration/axon growth (e.g., with antibodies and growth factors); D. Replace lost nerve cells (e.g., with fetal, stem, or olfactory cells, or by exogenous gene delivery); E. Inhibit scar/gliosis formation (e.g., with chondroitinases or decorin) and F. Reduce neurocircuit deficits (e.g., with channel or receptor blockers) (Donovan 2007). It is noteworthy that scientists doing this work are now motivated to include publications on appropriate long-term care of their paraplegic experimental animal subjects in their CVs (Santos-Benito, Munoz-Quiles, and Ramon-Cueto 2006).

Nanorobotics avoids any of the perceived ethical issues constraining some of the approaches listed above. One such emerging research field pertinent to SCI/D is operative neuromodulation (altering electrically or chemically the signal transmission in the nervous system by implanted devices), with its necessary engineering sub-discipline functional neuroprosthetics (the design and construction of devices to replace damaged neural circuitry) (Sakas et al. 2007). Perhaps most intriguing, because they attempt to bring together rehabilitation theory and CNS substance, are the efforts aimed at understanding and directing innate plasticity, whether in the context of activity-dependent "re-education of the spinal cord" (Wolpaw 2007), or in an appropriately "enriched environment" that promotes neural and astrocytic regeneration (Nilsson and Pekny 2007).

If and when one or more of the "cast of thousands" (Ramer, Ramer, and Steeves 2005) of proposed interventions proves successful in actually curing spinal cord injury or one or more of its disorders, general awareness won't even have to wait for online medical publication. It will be instantly texted and tweeted about until, a few hours later, it is the lead story on the evening news throughout the world!

Summary

SCI/D patients and their medical care providers must jointly address the additional problems the acquired disability superimposes on the fluctuating but inevitably degenerative course of normal living and aging. Even lacking development of true cures, opportunities for health maintenance through preventative and ultimately palliative care will repeatedly present themselves. The satisfaction providers can derive from their attentive and compassionate practice will be valid only if matched by the symptomatic relief and genuine comfort given the patient and his or her family, as they all collectively deal with the compelling embodiments of Euripides' classical adage: "Fear old age—for it does not come alone."

I would like to add a postscript from Dr. George Hohmann, who after 42 years of living with a disability [SCI] said this: "The good news is that we are. That we are….The good news is that we are still going about our lives and we're living."

I asked him how he was going to spend his dotage. He said, "I'm going to live."

- *Barry Corbet* (Corbet 1987)

Endnotes

[1] This pessimistic attitude is exemplified by two popular films: *Whose Life Is It Anyway?* (1981) in which the character played by Richard Dreyfuss commits suicide rather than endure life as a person with quadriplegia, and *Million Dollar Baby* (2004) in which the character played by Clint Eastwood "mercifully" kills the character played by Hilary Swank in order to spare her such a life.

[2] The clinical extent of "spinal shock" escapes precise delineation, and its pathophysiology still has no cogent explanation. Transient absence of motoric reflex responses and tone immediately following SCI progressing over time to hyperreflexia and spasticity is the hallmark, but basic cause and understanding of its increased duration correlated with phylogenetic complexity (hours to days in rats, days to weeks in cats, weeks to months in humans) remain obscure. See Smith PM, Jeffery ND. 2005. Spinal shock – comparative aspects and clinical relevance. *J Vet Intern Med* 19(6):788–793.

[3] The manual muscular testing (MMT) grades are: 0/5 - no evident response to a demand for contraction of a particular muscle; 1/5 - a "twitch" is visibly observed or palpated, but no effective contraction occurs; 2/5 - use of the muscle in a posture not affected by gravity is effective; 3/5 - use of the muscle in a posture where it just works against gravity is effective; 4/5 - use of the muscle in a posture affected by gravity is effective, but is constrained to some degree by additional external resistance; 5/5 - use of the muscle in a posture affected by gravity is effective, and is unaffected by further external resistance. Note that "5/5" is relative to demographic expectations, such that a healthy elderly person or a healthy infant can (and ideally should) demonstrate 5/5 responses.

[4] The ASIA scale is as follows: **A** - Complete: No sensory or motor function is preserved in sacral segments S4-S5; **B** - Incomplete: Sensory, but not motor, function is preserved below the neurologic level and extends through sacral segments S4-S5; **C** - Incomplete: Motor function is preserved below the neurologic level, and most key muscles below the neurologic level have muscle grade less than 3; **D** - Incomplete: Motor function is preserved below the neurologic level, and most key muscles below the neurologic level have muscle grade greater than or equal to 3; **E** - Normal: Sensory and motor functions are normal. URL:asia-spinalinjury.org/

[5] The lifelong care provided to eligible SCI/D veterans (whose entitlements vary with dates of service, service-relatedness of the complaint, and the fiscal responsiveness of any one Presidency/dominant Congress to the next) follows a theme from Abraham Lincoln's second presidential inaugural address in March, 1865 (a month before his assassination): "Let us strive … to bind up the nation's wounds, to care for him who shall have borne the battle…." After WWII, Gen. Omar Bradley, the last U.S. five-star general and first Chairman of the Joint Chiefs of Staff, was given command of the VA. He immediately focused on strengthening and expanding its medical system, famously pointing out to whining administrators: "We are dealing with Veterans, not procedures… with their problems, not ours."

[6] Hohmann G. 1966. Some effects of spinal cord lesions on experienced emotional feelings. *Psychophysiology* 3(2):143–156. This late published version does not include in full some interview data (e.g., the "above the neck" reports); these were however included in early versions of this paper still being circulated in mimeographed format at various VA SCI Centers in the early 1980's. The quoted passages are cited in Meyers DG. 2003. *Psychology*. New York: Worth Publishers.

[7] Also currently still e-published as authoritative "based on an interval survey of the literature" is *Prevention of thromboembolism in spinal cord injury*. 1998. Consortium for Spinal Cord Medicine/Paralyzed Veterans of America.

[8] Readers interested in etymological precision should note that *decubitus* is a fourth, rather than second, declension Latin noun; its plural is – not informatively – the same as its singular form, i.e., *decubitus*. That term was derived from the Roman practice of reclining at meals, leaning on one's elbow (*cubitum*); by extension it came to have the medical implication of being in a lying-down position, whether prone, supine, or "lateral," i.e., on one side or the other.

[9] The International Paralympics Committee has banned athletes from voluntarily inducing Autonomic Dysreflexia during competition.

[10] These lesions are also often referred to by the term *syringomyelia*, meaning "a cyst of the spinal cord." But everyone familiar with medical terminology will recognize that the root *myel-*, in addition to referring

to the spinal cord in such rubrics as "cervical myelopathy," when used in terms like "myelodysplastic syndrome" or "myelopoesis," implies something related to bone marrow. This double usage stems from the time of early medieval post-mortem anatomical studies, when both long bones and the spinal canal were first scientifically explored. The macroscopically similar yellowish stuff they both contained was named from the Greek word *myelos* – meaning yellow; the same color word was later applied to CNS *myelin*, denoting the visual contrast to the adjacent grey matter. To further add to this etymological morass, the actual Greek plural of *syrinx* is *syringes*. This plural has been adapted - and then colloquially singularized - into the familiar English word meaning a hollow container used to inject or suck up fluids. This term may be compared with the similar plural form *meninges*, which is the collective name for the connective tissues covering the central nervous system: the dura mater, arachnoid, and pia mater. These three layers are scarcely ever categorically referred to individually; to do so properly, each of them would correctly be called a *meninx*.

[11] Although the listed costs in dollars are out of date, this monograph remains useful for its thorough scope and inclusion of a validated individual patient survey instrument.

[12] See for example, archived or recent exchanges on suicide, or parenting from a wheelchair, or travel tips and accessibility on www.apparelyzed.com/forums/index.

References

Abraham JL, Banffy MB, and Harris MB. 2008. Spinal cord compression in patients with advanced metastatic cancer. *JAMA* 299(8):937–46.

Alexander CJ, Sipski ML, and Findley TW. 1993. Sexual activities, desire, and satisfaction in males pre- and post-spinal cord injury. *Arch Sex Behav* 22(3):217–28.

Anderson TW and Marion SA. 2003. Underestimation of life expectancy in elderly patients: the example of paraplegia. *British Columbia Med J* 45(4):178–82.

Anson JA, Benzel EC, and Awad IA. 1997. *Syringomyelia and the Chiari malformations.* Park Ridge, Ill.: American Association of Neurological Surgeons.

Appenzeller O. 1986. The influence of the nervous system on the triple response of Lewis. P. 222 in *Clinical autonomic failure: Practical concepts.* Amsterdam: Elsevier.

Bechmann I. 2005. Failed central nervous system regeneration: A downside of immune privilege? *Neuromolecular Med* 7(3):217–28.

Berkowitz M, O'Leary PK, Kruse DL, and Harvey C. 1998. *Spinal cord injury: An analysis of medical and social costs.* New York: Demos.

Bhambhani Y. 2002. Physiology of wheelchair racing in athletes with spinal cord injury. *Sports Med* 32(1):23–51.

Bicknell JM, Fiedler KJ. 1992. Unrecognized incomplete cervical spinal cord injury: Review of nine new and 28 previously reported cases. *Am J Emergency Med* 10:336–43.

Bodenheimer T. 2006. Primary care—will it survive? *NEJM* 355(9):861–64.

Booz-Allen & Hamilton, Inc. 2000. *Spinal cord injury & disorders: A comparison of program data collected across four modes of care.* Washington DC: VHA.

Broder J, and Snarski JT. 2007. Back pain in the elderly. *Clin Geriatr Med* 23(2):271–89.

Bryson JE, and Gorlay ML. 2009. Biphosphonate use in acute and chronic spinal cord injury: A systematic review. *J Spinal Cord Med* 32(3):215–25.

Bull A. 1979. Sir Ludwig Guttmann: From a grateful patient. *Paraplegia* 20:1–17.

Burns SP. 2007. Acute respiratory infections in persons with spinal cord injury. *Phys Med Rehabil Clin N Am* 18(2):203–216, v–vi.

Burns SM, Hough S, Boyd BL, and Hill J. 2009. Sexual desire and depression following spinal cord injury: Masculine sexual prowess as a moderator. *Sex Roles* 61: 120–29.

Calfee DP. 2008. Clostridium difficile: a reemerging pathogen. *Geriatrics* 63:(9):10–21.

Chou FH, Ho CH, and Linsenmeyer TA. 2006. Normal ranges of variability for urodynamic studies of neurogenic bladders in spinal cord injury. *J Spinal Cord Med* 29(1): 26–31.

Clark MJ, Petroski GF, Mazurek MO, et al. 2008. Testosterone replacement therapy and motor function in men with spinal cord injury: A retrospective analysis. *Am J Phys Med Rehabil* 87(4): 281–84.

Cobos P, Sanchez M, Garcia C, et al. 2002. Revisiting the James versus Cannon debate on emotion: Startle and autonomic modulation in patients with spinal cord injuries. *Biol Psychol* 61: 251–69.

Collins HL, Rodenbaugh DW, and DiCarlo SE. 2006. Spinal cord injury alters cardiac electrophysiology and increases the susceptibility to ventricular arrhythmias. *Prog Brain Res* 152:275–88.

Compagnolo DI, Bartlett JA, and Keller SE. 2000. Influence of neurological level on immune function following spinal cord injury: A review. *J Spinal Cord Med* 23(2):121–28.

Corbet B. 1987. *The Options Group: Perspectives on aging with spinal cord injury.* Golden Colorado: In cooperation with the American Spinal Injury Association.

Damasio A. 1999. *The feeling of what happens.* San Diego: Harcourt, Inc.

Darouiche RO, Landon GC, Klima M, Musher DM, and Markowski J. 1994. Osteomyelitis associated with pressure sores. *Arch Intern Med* 154(7):753–58.

Dawodu ST. 2007. Spinal cord injury: Definition, epidemiology, pathophysiology. URL:http://WebMD/*eMedicineSpecialties/ PhysicalMedicineandRehabilitation/SPINALCORDINJURY*.

de Malgahaes JP and Sandberg A. 2005. Cognitive aging as an extension of brain development: A model linking learning, brain plasticity, and neurodegeneration. *Mech Ageing Dev.* 126(10):1026–33.

Ditunno JF and Formal CS. 1994. Chronic spinal cord injury. *NEJM* 330(8):550–56.

DeVivo MJ. 2004. Aging with a neurodisability: Morbidity and life expectancy issues.

DeVivoMJ, Krause JS, and Lammertse DP. 1999. Recent trends in mortality and causes of death among persons with spinal cord injury. *Arch Phys Med Rehabil* 80(11):1411–1419.

Dietz V, Quintern J, and Berger W. 1981. Electrophysiological studies of gait in spasticity and rigidity: Evidence that altered mechanical properties of muscle contribute to hypertonia. *Brain* 104:431–49.

Ditunno PL, McCauley C, and Marquette C. 1985. Sensation-seeking behavior and the incidence of spinal cord injury. *Arch Phys Med Rehabil* 66(3):152–5.

Donovan WH. 2007. Spinal cord injury—past, present, and future. *J Spinal Cord Med* 30:85–100.

Edström L, Grimby L, and Jannerz J. 1973. Correlation between recruitment order of motor units and muscle atrophy pattern in upper motoneurone lesion: Significance of spasticity. *Cell Molec Life Sci* 29(5):560.

Eisenberg DTA, Campbell B, Gray PB, and Sorensen MD. 2008. Dopamine receptor genetic polymorphisms and body composition in undernourished pastoralists: An exploration of nutrition indices among nomadic and recently settled Ariaal men of northern Kenya. *BMC Evolutionary Biology* 8:173–85.

Ernst E. 2002. Manipulation of the cervical spine: A systematic review of case reports of serious adverse events, 1995–2001. *Med J Australia* 176(8):376–80.

Evans CT, LaVela S, Weaver FM, et al. 2008. Epidemiology of hospital-acquired infections in veterans with spinal cord injury and disorder *(sic)*. *Infect Control Hosp Epidemiol* 29:234–42.

Finnie AK, Buchholz AC, Martin Ginis KA, et al. 2008. Current coronary heart disease risk assessment tools may underestimate risk in community-dwelling persons with chronic spinal cord injury. *Spinal Cord* 46(9):608–615.

Frankel HL and Mathias CJ. 1976. The cardiovascular system in tetraplegia and paraplegia. In Vinken PJ, Bruyn GW, eds. *Injuries of the spine and spinal cord, Part II. (Handbook of Clinical Neurology, Volume 26.)* Amsterdam: North Holland Publishing Company.

Foerster O. 1936. *Symptomatologie der Erkrankungen des Rückenmarks und seiner Wurzeln.* In Bumke O, Foerster O, eds. *Handbuch der Neurologie,* vol. 5. Cited in Whitteridge D. 1983. Ludwig Guttmann 3 July 1899–18 March 1980. *Biograph. Mem. FRS.* 29:227–44. URL: http://www.jstor.org/stable/769803.

Forlenza SW, Axelrod JL, and Grieco MH. 1979. Pott's disease in heroin addicts. *JAMA* 241:379–80.

Frisbie JH. 1997. Fractures after myelopathy: The risk quantified. *J Spinal Cord Med* 20(1):66–69.

Frontera WR, Fuhrer MJ, Jette AM, et al. 2006. Rehabilitation medicine summit: Building research capacity Executive Summary. *J NeuroEngineering Rehabil* 3:1 *(sic).* URL: www.jneuroengrehab.com/content/3/1/1.

Gibson JJ. 1964/1982. The uses of proprioception and the detection of proprioceptive information. Pp. 164–70 in Reed E, Jones R, eds. 1982 *Reasons for realism: selected essays of James J. Gibson.* Hillsdale NJ: Lawrence Erlbaum Assoc.

Gracies JM. 2005. Pathophysiology of spastic paresis. II: Emergence of muscle overactivity. *Muscle Nerve* 31(5):552–71.

Gutierrez DD, Thompson L, Kemp B, et al. 2007. The relationship of shoulder pain intensity to quality of life, physical activity, and community participation in persons with paraplegia. *J Spinal Cord Med* 30(3):251–55.

Guttmann L and Whitteridge D. 1947. Effects of bladder distension on autonomic mechanisms after spinal cord injuries. *Brain* 70:361–404.

Haley RW. 2003. Excess incidence of ALS in young Gulf War veterans. *Neurology* 61:750–56.

Hansson E. 2006. Could chronic pain and spread of pain sensation be induced and maintained by glial activation? *Acta Physiol (Oxf)* 187(1-2):321–27.

Haran M, Bhuta T, and Lee B. 2004. Pharmacological interventions for treating acute heterotopic ossification. *Cochrane Database Syst Rev* (4):CD003321.

Head H and Riddoch G. 1917. The autonomic bladder, excessive sweating and some other reflex conditions, in gross injuries of the spinal cord. *Brain* 40:188–263.

Hirst CL, Ingram G, Pickersgill TP, et al. 2008. Increasing prevalence and incidence of multiple sclerosis in South East Wales. *J Neurol Neurosurg Psychiatry* October 17, 2008. [Epub ahead of print.]

Hohmann G. 1966. Some effects of spinal cord lesions on experienced emotional feelings. *Psychophysiology* 3(2):143–56.

Hsieh JT, Wolfe DL, Miller WC, and Curt A. 2008. Spasticity outcome measures in spinal cord injury: Psychometric properties and clinical utility. *Spinal Cord* 46(2): 86–95.

Huff JS. 2007. Neoplasms, spinal cord. *eMedicine.* URL: http://www.emedicine.com/emerg/topic337.htm.

Jacob A and Weinshenker BG. 2008. An approach to the diagnosis of acute transverse myelitis. *Semin Neurol* 28(1):105–20.

Jacobs WB and Fehlings MG. 2008. Ankylosing spondylitis and spinal cord injury: Origin, incidence, management, and avoidance. *Neurosurg Focus* 24(1):E12.

Jiang SD, Dai LY, and Jiang LS. 2006. Osteoporosis after spinal cord injury. *Osteoporos Int* 17(2):180–92.

Jones L and Bagnall A. 2004. Spinal injury centres (SICs) for acute traumatic spinal cord injury. *Cochrane Database Syst Rev* 18(4):CD004442.

Kannus P, Palvanen M, Niemi S, and Parkkari J. 2007. Alarming rise in the number and incidence of fall-induced cervical spine injuries among older adults. *J Gerontol A Biol Sci Med Sci.* 62(2):180–83.

Kaplan FS, Glaser DL, Hebela N, and Shore EM. 2004. Heterotopic ossification. *J Am Acad Orthop Surg* 12(2):116–25.

Karlsson AK. 1999. Insulin resistance and sympathetic function in high spinal cord injury. *Spinal Cord* 37(7):494–500.

Kemp BJ, Spungen AM, Adkins RH, et al. 2000. The relationship among serum lipid levels, adiposity, and depressive symptomatology in persons aging with spinal cord injury. *J Spinal Cord Med* 23(4):216–20.

Krause JS. 2004. Factors associated with risk for subsequent injuries after traumatic spinal cord injury. *Arch Phys Med Rehabil* 85(9): 1503–1508.

Krause JS, Devivo MJ, and Jackson AB. 2004. Health status, community integration, and economic risk factors for mortality after spinal cord injury. *Arch Phys Med Rehabil* 85(11):1764–73.

Krassioukov A, Warburton DE, Teasell R, and Eng JJ. 2009. A systematic review of the management of autonomic dysreflexia after spinal cord injury. *Arch Phys Med Rehabil* 90: 682–95.

Lal S. 1998. Premature degenerative shoulder changes in spinal cord injury patients. *Spinal Cord* 36(3):186–89.

Lambert CP, Lee Archer R, and Evans WJ. 2002. Body composition in ambulatory women with multiple sclerosis. *Arch Phys Med Rehabil* 83(11):1559–69.

Lammartse D, Dungan D, Dreisbach J, et al. 2007. Neuroimaging in traumatic spinal cord injury: An evidence-based review for clinical practice and research. *J Spinal Cord Med* 30(3):205–214.

Landau WM. 1974. Spasticity: the fable of a neurological demon and the emperor's new therapy. *Arch Neurol* 31: 217–219.

Lasfargues JE, Custis D, Morrone F, et al. 1995. A model for estimating spinal cord prevalence in the United States. *Paraplegia* 33(2): 62–68.

LaVela SL, Weaver FM, Goldstein B, et al. 2006. Diabetes mellitus in individuals with spinal cord injury or disorder. *J Spinal Cord Med* 29(4):387–95.

Levi AD, Hurlbert RJ, Anderson P, et al. 2006. Neurologic deterioration secondary to unrecognized spinal instability following trauma—a multicenter study. *Spine* 31(4):451–8.

Lisansky J. 2005. Personal communication.

Lo YL. 2007. Clinical and immunological spectrum of the Miller Fisher syndrome. *Muscle Nerve* 36 (5):615–27.

Loblaw DA, Laperierre NJ, and Mackillop WJ. 2003. A population-based study of malignant spinal cord compression in Ontario. *Clin Oncol (R Coll Oncol)* 15(4):211–7.

Logan WC Jr, Sloane R, Lyles KW, et al. 2008. Incidence of fractures in a cohort of veterans with chronic multiple sclerosis or traumatic spinal cord injury. *Arch Phys Med Rehabil* 89(2):237–43.

Lombardi G, Mondaini N, Macchiarella A, et al. 2007. Female sexual dysfunction and hormonal status in spinal cord injured patients. *J. Androl* 28(5):722–26.

Lombardi G, Macchiarella A, Cecconi F, et al. 2008. Sexual life of males over 50 years of age with spinal-cord lesions of at least 20 years. *Spinal Cord* 46(10):679–83.

Maruyama Y, Mizuguchi M, Yaginuma T, et al. 2008. Serum leptin, abdominal obesity and the metabolic syndrome in individuals with chronic spinal cord injury. *Spinal Cord* 46(7):494–99.

Mawson AR, Jacobs KW, Winchester Y, and Biundo JJ Jr. 1988. Sensation-seeking and traumatic spinal cord injury: Case-control study. *Arch Phys Med Rehabil* 69 (12): 1039–43.

Maynard FM, Karunas RS, and Waring WP. 1990. Epidemiology of spasticity following traumatic spinal cord injury. *Arch Phys Med Rehabil* 71:566–69.

McColl MA, Arnold R, Charlifue S, et al. 2003. Aging, spinal cord injury, and quality of life: Structural relationships. *Arch Phys Med Rehabil* 84(8):1137–44.

McColl MA, Charlifue S, Glass C, et al. 2002. International differences in ageing and spinal cord injury. *Spinal Cord* 40:128–36.

McColl MA, Charlifue S, Glass C, et al. 2004. Aging, gender, and spinal cord injury. *Arch Phys Med Rehabil* 85(3):363–67.

McColl MA, Walker J, Stirling P, et al. 1997. Expectations of life and health among spinal cord injured adults. *Spinal Cord* 35:818–28.

McGillivray CF, Hitzig SL, Craven C, et al. 2009. Evaluating knowledge of autonomic dysreflexia among individuals with spinal cord injury and their families. *J Spinal Cord Med* 32(1):54–62.

McGlinchey-Berroth R, Morrow L, Ahlquist M, Sarkarati M, and Minaker KL. 1995. Late-life spinal cord injury and aging with a long term injury: Characteristics of two emerging populations. *J Spinal Cord Med* 18(3):183–93.

McKinney D. 2008. Prevention of thromboembolism in SCI: Treatment and medication. URL: http://emedicine.medscape.com/article/322897. treatment. Also currently still e-published as authoritative "based on an interval survey of the literature" is *Prevention of thromboembolism in spinal cord injury*. 1998. Consortium for Spinal Cord Medicine/ Paralyzed Veterans of America.

Michaelis LS. 1976. Spasticity in spinal cord injuries. Pp. 477–87 in VinkenPJ, Bruyn GW, Braakman R, eds. *Injuries of the spine and spinal cord, Part II. (Handbook of clinical neurology, v. 26.)* New York: American Elsevier.

Milhorat TH, Kotzen RM, and Anzil AP. 1994. Stenosis of the central canal of spinal cord in man: Incidence and pathological findings in 232 autopsy cases. *J Neurosurg* 80(4):716–22.

Moonka R, Steins SA, Resnick WJ, et al. 1999. The prevalence and natural history of gallstones in spinal cord injured patients. *J Am Coll Surg* 189(3):274–81.

Morse LR, Nguyen HP, Jain N, et al. 2008. Age and motor score predict osteoprotegerin level in chronic spinal cord injury. *J Musculoskelet Neuronal Interact* 8(1):50–57.

Morse LR, Stolzmann K, Nguyen HP, et al. 2008. Association between mobility mode and C-reactive protein levels in men with chronic spinal cord injury. *Arch Phys Med Rehabil* 89(4):726–31.

Morykwas MJ, Argenta LC, Shelton-Brown EI, and McGuirt W. 1997. Vacuum-assisted closure: A new method for wound control: animal studies and basic foundation. *Ann Plastic Surgery* 38:553–62.

Munro D. 1940. Care of the back following spinal cord injuries: Consideration of bed sores. *NEJM* 223:391–98.

Munro D. 1943. Tidal drainage and cystometry in the treatment of sepsis associated with spinal cord injuries. *NEJM* 229:6–14.

Myers J, Lee M, and Kiratli J. 2007. Cardiovascular disease in spinal cord injury: An overview of prevalence, risk, evaluation, and management. *Am J Phys Med Rehabil* 86(2):142–52.

National Pressure Ulcer Advisory Panel. 2007. URL: http://www.npuap. org/pr2.htm.

Nicotra A, Critchley HD, Mathias CJ, and Dolan RJ. 2006. Emotional and autonomic consequences of spinal cord injury explored using functional brain imaging. *Brain* 129(3): 718–28.

Nilsson M and Pekny M. 2007. Enriched environment and astrocytes in central nervous system regeneration. *J Rehabil Med* 39(5):345–52.

Oppenheim JS, Spitzer DE, and Segal DH. 2006. Nonvascular complications following spinal manipulation. *Spine J.* 5(6):660–6.

Orakzai SH, Orakzai RH, Ahmadi N, et al. 2007. Measurement of coronary artery calcification by electron beam computerized tomography in persons with chronic spinal cord injury: Evidence for increased atherosclerotic burden. *Spinal Cord* 45(12):775–79.

Ota T, Akaboshi K, Nagata M, et al. 2001. Functional assessment of patients with spinal cord injury: Measured by the motor score and the Functional Independence Measure. *Spinal Cord* 34(9):531–35.

Owens BD, Kragh JF Jr, Wenke JC, et al. 2008. Combat wounds in operation Iraqi Freedom and operation Enduring Freedom. *J Trauma* 64(2):295–9.

Partridge LD and Partridge DL. 1993. *The nervous system: Its function and its interaction with the world.* Cambridge: MIT Press.

Peng P and Massicotte ZM. 2004. Spinal cord compression from intrathecal catheter-tip inflammatory mass: Case report and a review of etiology. *Res Anesth Pain Med* 29(3):237–42.

Perkash A and Brown M. 1986. Anemia in patients with traumatic spinal cord injury. *J Am Paraplegia Soc* 9(1-2):10–15.

Phillips WT, Kiratli BJ, Sarkarati M, et al. 1998. Effect of spinal cord injury on the heart and cardiovascular fitness. *Curr Probl Cardiol* 23(11):641–716.

Pollak DD, Monie FJ, and Kandel ER. 2008. An animal model of a behavioral intervention for depression. *Neuron* 60910;149–61.

Pordeus V, Szyper-Kravitz M, Levy RA, et al. 2008. Infections and autoimmunity: A panorama. *Clin Rev Allergy Immunol* 34:(3): 283–99.

Rabchevsky AG. 2006. Segmental organization of spinal reflexes mediating autonomic dysreflexia after spinal cord injury. *Prog Brain Res* 152:265–74.

Ragnarsson KT. 1992. Functional electrical stimulation and suppression of spasticity following spinal cord injury. *Bull NY Acad Med* 68:351–64.

Ramer LM, Ramer MS, and Steeves JD. 2005. Setting the stage for functional repair of spinal cord injures: A cast of thousands. *Spinal Cord* 43:134–61.

Rygh LJ, Svendsen F, Fiskå A, et al. 2005. Long-term potentiation in spinal nociceptive systems—how acute pain may become chronic. *Psychoneuroendocrinology* 30(10): 959–64.

Sakas DE, Panourias IG, Simpson BA, et al. 2007. An introduction to operative neuromodulation and functional neuroprosthetics, the new frontiers of clinical neuroscience and biotechnology. *Acta Neurochir Suppl* 97(1):3–10.

Santos-Benito FF, Munoz-Quiles C, and Ramon-Cueto A. 2006. Long-term care of paraplegic laboratory mammals. *J Neurotrauma* 3(3-4):521–36.

Savic G, Short DJ, Weitzenkamp D, et al. 2000. Hospital readmissions in people with chronic spinal cord injury. *Spinal Cord* 38:371–77.

Senyk O, Patil R, and Sonnenberg F. 1989. Systematic knowledge base design for medical diagnosis. *Applied Artificial Intelligence* 3(2/3):249–74.

Shedid D and Benzel EC. 2007. Cervical spondylosis anatomy: Pathophysiology and biomechanics. *Neurosurgery* 60(1 Suppl 1) :S7–13.

Sherrington CS. 1906. *The Integrative action of the nervous system.* New York: Charles Scribner's Sons.

Siddall PJ. 2002. Spinal drug administration in the treatment of spinal cord injury pain. Pp. 353–64 in Yezierski RP, Burcheil KJ, eds. *Spinal cord injury pain: Assessment, mechanisms, management.* Seattle: IASP Press.

Sipski ML and Alexander CJ. 1993. Sexual activities, response and satisfaction in women pre- and post-spinal cord injury. *Arch Phys Med Rehabil* 74(10):1025–9.

Sipski ML, Jackson AB, Gomez-Marin O, et al. 2004. Effects of gender on neurologic and functional recovery after spinal cord injury. *Arch Phys Med Rehabil* 85(11):1826–36.

Smith E. *Edwin Smith Surgical Papyrus.* ~ 2500-3000 B.C.E. Hieratic manuscript purchased by E. Smith in Luxor, Egypt, 1862. Translated into English by James Breasted, 1930. Text facsimile and translation at http://www.touregypt.net/edwinsmithsurgical.htm.

Soderblom C and Blackstone C. 2006. Traffic accidents: Molecular genetic insights into the pathogenesis of the hereditary spastic paraplegias. *Pharmacol Ther* 109(1–2):42–56.

Spillane JD. 1968. *An Atlas of clinical neurology.* London: Oxford University Press.

Spinazzé S, Caraceni A, and Schrijvers D. 2005. Epidural spinal cord compression. *Crit Rev Oncol Hematol.* 56(3):397–406.

Spungen AM, Adkins RH, Stewart CA, et al. 2003. Factors influencing body composition in persons with spinal cord injury: A cross-sectional study. *J Appl Physiol* 95(6):2398–2407.

Stekelenburg A, Gawlitta D, Bader DL, and Oomens CW. 2008. Deep tissue injury: How deep is our understanding? *Arch Phys Med Rehabil* 89:(7):1410–1413.

Stiens SA, Bergman SB, and Goetz LL. 1997. Neurogenic bowel dysfunction after spinal cord injury: clinical evaluation and rehabilitative management. *Arch Phys Med Rehabil* 78(3 Suppl):S86–102.

Stover SL, DeVivo MJ, and Go BK. 1999. History, implementation and current status of the National Spinal Cord Injury Database. *Arch Phys Med Rehabil* 80:1365–71.

Strauss DJ, Devivo MJ, Paculdo DR, and Shavelle RM. 2006. Trends in life expectancy after spinal cord injury. *Arch Phys Med Rehabil* 87(8):1079–85.

Strauss D, DeVivo M, Shavelle R, et al. 2008. Economic factors and longevity in spinal cord injury: A reappraisal. *Arch Phys Med Rehabil* 89(3): 572–74.

Su D, Amsters D, and Carlson G. 2002. The experiences and perceptions of older family caregivers of people with spinal cord injury living in the community: Service implications. *SCI Psychosocial Process* 15(3):125, 130–38.

Takahashi J, Hirabayashi H, Hashidate H, et al. 2008. Assessment of cervical myelopathy using transcranial magnetic stimulation and prediction of prognosis after laminoplasty. *Spine* 33(1):E15–20.

Trieschmann RB. 1987. *Aging with a disability*. New York: Demos Publications.

Trieschmann RB. 1999. Energy medicine for long-term disabilities. *Disabil Rehabil*. 21(5-6):269–76.

Trumble AC. 1930. The skin tolerance for pressure and pressure sores. *Med J Australia* 2:724–25.

Tsai PY, Wang CP, Chiu FY, et al. 2009. Efficacy of functional magnetic stimulation in neurogenic bowel dysfunction after spinal cord injury. *J Rehabil Med* 41(1):41–47.

Vernon JD, Silver JR, and Symon L. 1983. Post-traumatic syringomyelia: The results of surgery. *Paraplegia* 21(1): 37–46.

VHA Handbook 1176.1: Spinal cord injury and disorders system of care procedures. 2005. Washington, DC: Department of Veterans Affairs, Veterans Health Administration.

Watkins LR, Hutchinson MR, Ledeboer A, et al. 2007. Glia as the "bad guys": Implications for improving pain control and the clinical utility of opioids. *Brain Behav Immun* 21:131–46.

Weingarden SI and Graham PM. 1989. Falls resulting in spinal cord injury: Patterns and outcomes in an older population. *Paraplegia* 27(6):423–27.

Widerstrom-Noga EG, Felix ER, Cruz-Almeida Y, and Turk DC. 2007. Psychosocial subgroups in persons with spinal cord injuries and chronic pain. *Arch Phys Med Rehabil* 88(12):1628–35.

Williams B, Coyle J, and Healy D. 1998. The meaning of patient satisfaction: An explanation of high reported levels. *Soc Sci Med* 47(9):1351–59.

Wilt TJ, Carlson KF, Goldish GD, et al. 2008. Carbohydrate and lipid disorders and relevant considerations in persons with spinal cord injury. *Evid Rep Technol Assess (Full Rep)* (163):1–95.

Wingerchuk DM. 2007. Diagnosis and treatment of neuromyelitis optica. *Neurologist* 13(1):2–11.

Wolpaw JR. 2007. Spinal cord plasticity in acquisition and maintenance of motor skills. *Acta Physiol (Oxf)* 189(2):155–69.

Wyndaele M and Wyndaele JJ. 2006. Incidence, prevalence and epidemiology of spinal cord injury: What learns (*sic*) a worldwide literature survey? *Spinal Cord* 44(9):523–29.

Yirmiya R, Goshen I, Bajyo A, et al. 2006. Depression induces bone loss through stimulation of the sympathetic nervous system. *Proc Nat Acad Sci USA* 103(45): 16876–81.

Young RR. 1994. Spasticity: A review. *Neurol* 44(suppl 9):s12–20.

Zafonte RD and Dijkers M. 1999. Medical and functional sequelae of spinal cord injury caused by violence: Findings from the Model Systems. *Top SCI Rehab* 4:36–50.

Zouris JM, Walker GJ, Dye J, and Galarneau M. 2006. Wounding patterns for U.S. Marines and sailors during Operation Iraqi Freedom, major combat phase. *Mil Med* 171(3):246–52.

45 Brain Tumor in the Elderly

Robert Cavaliere and David Schiff

Introduction

The optimal treatment of elderly patients with glioblastoma (GBM) remains undefined. This is becoming an increasingly relevant issue as the demographics of this disease are changing. The incidence of GBM in the elderly is increasing. In addition, patient age greater than 60 forms the most rapidly growing segment of the general population. The exclusion of elderly patients from clinical trials as well as age bias and therapeutic nihilism limit the interpretation of the available data. Few prospective trials focusing on this population have been performed and the available data are derived from retrospective series flawed by significant selection bias. Furthermore, extrapolation of the results of clinical trials consisting of younger patients to an older population is not appropriate given the physiologic changes that accompany aging. The increased incidences of comorbidities among the elderly further distinguish this population from younger patients. These differences alter the risk-benefit ratio of treatment as the elderly may be more predisposed to toxicity. Despite phenotypic similarities, molecular and genetic abnormalities of GBM in younger and older populations are distinct. Such differences may alter the behavior and responsiveness of these tumors. The available treatments have only modest impact on survival, and prognosis remains poor even with aggressive therapy. The potential morbidity and cost to the patient may outweigh the survival advantage. Few trials have focused on the impact of treatment on patient symptoms and quality of life (QOL) as assessed by the patient. This, however, is perhaps the most important outcome in patients with cancer and limited survival.

Epidemiology

GBM is a high-grade, primary brain tumor that commonly affects the elderly. Age-specific incidence for GBM peaks at 13.74/100,000 person-years among those 65 to 74 years of age in the United States (CBTRUS)(1). The incidence of GBM is increasing among the elderly despite remaining relatively stable among the younger population (Fleury et al. 1997; Greig, Ries, and Yancik 1990; Werner, Phuphanich, and Lyman 1995). Werner et al. noted 16%, 30%, 36%, and 254% increases in age-specific incidence rates of malignant primary brain tumors among patients 70–74, 75–79, 80–84, and greater than 85 respectively between early and late 1980s (Figure 1). In comparison, incidence rates were stable for the population less than age 65 (Werner, Phuphanich, and Lyman 1995). Furthermore, the elderly are the most rapidly expanding segment of the population (Table 1). Thus, one can expect the number of cases of GBM to increase significantly in the years to come.

Limitations of Available Data

The treatment of GBM remains a challenge for neuro-oncologists. Despite advances in surgical techniques and radio- and chemotherapeutics, median survival has changed little since the 1970s; approximately one to two months with best supportive care and one year with aggressive treatment. Among the most important prognostic factors for survival is age, with almost all studies reporting survival among the elderly to be usually four to six months, well below that of younger

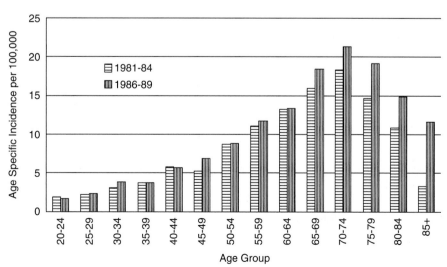

Figure 1 Age-specific incidence of primary brain tumors reported to Florida Cancer Data System.

Table 1 Projected Change in United States Population by Age Group Between 2000 and 2050

Age Group	Percent Change
20 – 44	25.8%
45 – 64	52.1%
65 – 84	131.4%
85+	388.9%

patients. Treatment of GBM consists of surgery, radiation therapy, and chemotherapy. Efficacy of these interventions has been demonstrated in both retrospective and prospective clinical trials. Data on the elderly, however, are limited as older patients are frequently excluded from clinical trials (Kornblith et al. 2002; Chang et al. 2002). For example, a recent positive, prospective randomized trial of radiation with or without concomitant temozolomide in the treatment of newly diagnosed GBM excluded patients older than 70 (Stupp et al. 2009; Stupp et al. 2005). The median age of patients enrolled on GBM clinical trials is 55 compared to 64, the median age of patients with GBM within the general population (Chang et al. 2002; Central Brain Tumor Registry of the United States 2005). In addition, prospective trials focusing specifically on this age group are rarely performed. Information gathered from retrospective reviews is compromised by selection bias as performance status, a powerful predictor of outcome, influences therapeutic decisions (Iwamoto et al. 2009; Iwamoto et al. 2005; Whittle

et al. 2002). For example, radiation therapy is withheld in 25% to 50% of patients on the basis of poor performance status (Mohan et al. 1998; Villa et al. 1998). Patients with better prognostic factors are more likely to undergo extensive surgery and treatment with chemotherapy (Whittle et al. 2002; Kurimoto et al. 2002; Iwamoto et al. 2008). Thus, it is difficult to separate treatment efficacy from underlying patient factors. Ageism and therapeutic nihilism (McKenna 1994) remain a significant barrier in the study of elderly with cancer. Older patients with cancer are offered less aggressive management than younger patients afflicted with similar diseases. Yet little data are available to support such differential treatment. Fear of increased toxicity from what otherwise are effective therapies have yet to be definitively substantiated.

The results of trials focusing on younger patients cannot be extrapolated to older patients. Older people differ from younger people in several important respects. Physiologic changes that accompany aging may predispose older people to the side effects of treatment. Aging is associated with decreased total body water, increased total body fat, and a decline in the concentration of plasma proteins, potentially altering drug distribution (Balducci L, and Extermann 1997; Vestal 1997). A consequence of aging is a decline in renal function and glomerular filtration rate that may lead to prolonged half-life of renally excreted medications (Balducci L, and Extermann 1997; Vestal 1997). A decrease in liver mass that accompanies aging may influence the metabolism of drugs cleared by the liver (Vestal 1997). Marrow cells are fewer and proliferative potential is lower among older patients (Denduluri and Ershler 2004). Diminished bone marrow reserve may predispose to myelotoxicity (Balducci, Hardy, and Lyman 2000).

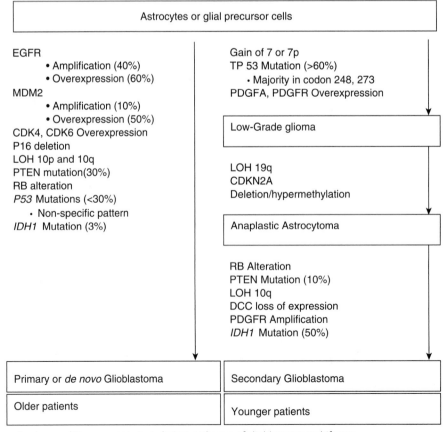

Figure 2 Molecular and genetic abnormalities present in two distinct pathways of glioblastoma multiforme.

Age-related decline in the immune system in conjunction with chemotherapy might predispose to reactivation of infections such as herpes
zoster (Denduluri and Ershler 2004). This is particularly true of
patients with brain tumors who are usually maintained on corticosteroids, which may further suppress T-cell function. Age-associated cognitive decline is a well-recognized, non-pathological consequence of
aging. "Normal" changes within the brain of the elderly may account
for this phenomenon. Idiopathic, pathological degeneration results in
several geriatric conditions including Alzheimer's disease and
Parkinson's disease. Comorbid conditions such as hypertension, diabetes, stroke, and heart disease, which increase in incidence with aging,
have direct consequences on the brain and its vasculature. As such, the
central nervous system (CNS) of the elderly may be more sensitive to
the direct effect of the tumor and its treatments. Thus, caution must
definitely be taken when extending the results of clinical trials in
younger patients to older patients.

GBM are a heterogenous group of tumors that arise from different
molecular pathways (Lang et al. 1994). Despite phenotypic similarity,
high-grade gliomas in the elderly are distinct from identical tumors in
younger patients. For example, GBM in younger patients are often
derived from pre-existing lower-grade tumors that have undergone
malignant progression. Such tumors are often referred to as secondary
GBM. In contrast, GBM in the elderly arise de novo as grade IV tumors
rather than from progression from lower grade tumors. Furthermore,
these tumors have distinct genetic and molecular abnormalities
(Ichimura et al. 2009; Ohgaki et al. 2004; Ohgaki and Kleihues 2007;
Reifenberger and Collins 2004) (Figure 2).

Treatment

A limited number of studies of elderly patients with high-grade gliomas have demonstrated a survival advantage when treated with surgery, radiation, and chemotherapy. Untreated, the median survival of
unselected elderly patients, typically defined as age greater than 70,
with GBM is 1.2 months (Mohan et al. 1998). By comparison, the
median survival reported in retrospective series of unselected older
patients undergoing a variety of treatments is only four to six months
(Iwamoto et al. 2008; Meckling et al. 1996; Mohan et al. 1998;
Patwardhan et al. 2004; Villa et al. 1998). In the palliative situation of
poor prognosis patients with high-grade gliomas, survival has to be
balanced against treatment morbidity and the effect on quality of life
(Kelly and Hunt 1994; Muacevic and Kreth 2003; Villa et al. 1965;
Vuorinen et al. 2003). Carefully selected older patients undoubtedly
benefit from aggressive treatment. Performance status, a measure of a
patient's global well being and function, has consistently been identified as the most important clinical factor to predict outcome in
patients. Specifically, a highly functioning, independent individual
with less impairment may benefit from aggressive therapy more than
someone more disabled.

Surgery

Surgery remains a critical part of the diagnosis and treatment of gliomas. Although widely accepted and routinely performed in the younger
population, surgery is less often undertaken in the elderly. Although
the appearance of a lesion on imaging may be suggestive of a particular
diagnosis, pathological confirmation is always necessary if treatment is
considered an option. Six of thirty elderly patients presumed to have a
high-grade glioma on pre-operative imaging were found to have alternative pathological diagnosis, including three patients with non-
neoplastic conditions (Vuorinen et al. 2003). What is less clear is whether
to pursue aggressive cytoreductive surgery or biopsy alone. In addition

to establishing a pathological diagnosis, tumor debulking allows for
rapid decompression in patients with tumors associated with significant mass effect. This allows for a more rapid and complete tapering of
corticosteroids. In certain instances, surgery may provide rapid symptom relief and improvement in performance status (Schiff and Shaffrey
2003). Extensive surgical resection may prolong survival relative to
stereotactic biopsy alone (Schiff and Shaffrey 2003), even among the
elderly (Fujimura et al. 2004; Kelly and Hunt 1994; Mohan et al. 1998;
Stummer et al. 2008; Vuorinen et al. 2003). In their retrospective
review of a prospectively maintained surgical database, Stummer et al.
found that the impact on survival conferred by complete resection was
similar between older (>60 years) and younger (≤60) patients, a hazard
ratio of .55 versus .61 respectively (Stummer et al. 2008). Yet despite
these benefits, older patients are less likely to undergo surgery
(Barnholtz-Sloan et al. 2006; Iwamoto et al. 2008). This may be attributed to a physician's perception of a lack of benefit or concerns of the
adverse effects and prolonged recovery among the elderly. In addition,
the survival advantage conferred by surgery is modest. Median survival of patients undergoing resection versus biopsy was 30 and 16.9
weeks respectively. Although this represents a 78% increased in survival, the absolute difference was only 13.1 weeks (Kelly and Hunt
1994). In the only prospective, randomized trial of surgery versus
biopsy in 30 older patients, median survival was 171 and 85 days in
favor of resection. Time to deterioration was not statistically different
between the two groups although a trend in favor of resection was
present (105 versus 72 days) (Vuorinen et al. 2003). Other studies,
however, have failed to demonstrate a survival advantage with more
extensive surgery (Meckling et al. 1996; Villa et al. 1998; Whittle et al.
2002). In addition, surgical morbidity among older patients undergoing craniotomy for brain tumors is approximately 30% to 35%
(Fujimura et al. 2004; Tomita and Raimondi 1981; Villa et al. 1998).
This is higher than reported morbidity in younger patients with similar conditions, about 20% (Cabantog and Bernstein 1994). Fadul et al.
found increasing age to be the single most important indicator of surgical mortality risk (Fadul et al. 1988). With advances in imaging and
surgical techniques, risk is lower but still significant (Fujimura et al.
2004). Furthermore, craniotomy requires longer hospitalization and
greater costs. Among 44 patients older than 80, mean duration of
intensive care and hospitalization was 10 and 34 days respectively.
Twenty-two percent of patients died or condition worsened relative to
pre-operative state (Pietila et al. 1999). Fujimara et al. compared post-
and pre- operative performance status in a cohort of older patients
undergoing craniotomy for high-grade gliomas. Overall, the number
of patients with a given performance status was unchanged following
surgery (Fujimura et al. 2004). Collectively, the data suggest that
aggressive resective surgery confers a palliative and survival advantage.
Patients, however, must be carefully selected and high-risk patients
managed with biopsy or supportive care.

Radiation Therapy

Cranial radiotherapy is the mainstay of treatment for gliomas. The
effectiveness of radiation therapy was first demonstrated in the late
1970s and has since been considered the standard of care (Walker et al.
1980). It is perhaps the most efficacious of the known treatments for
this tumor, extending survival to approximately 10 to 12 months.
There is some evidence to suggest, however, that gliomas in older
patients are more resistant to this intervention (Kita et al. 2009). In a
retrospective analysis of a cohort enrolled in two prospective clinical
trials, the odds ratio of a radiographic response was 0.80 per decade of
age in patients treated with radiation therapy (Barker et al. 2001).
Nonetheless, several studies have found radiation to prolong survival

Table 2 Typical Neurological Symptoms and Their Causes Associated with Cerebral Radiation Therapy

Syndrome	Symptoms	Onset After RT
Acute fatigue, encephalopathy	Worsening symptoms, headache	During treatment
Early delayed	Somnolence, poor concentration, impaired memory	Weeks to months
Late delayed	Focal deficits, seizures, elevated ICP	6 to 24 months
	Dementia, gait disturbance, incontinence	> 6 months

in older patients, from approximately two months in untreated patients to four to 10 months in those who received treatment (Meckling et al. 1996; Mohan et al. 1998; Villa et al. 1998; Whittle et al. 2002). More recently, in one of the few prospective, randomized studies in the elderly GBM population, the addition of radiation therapy to supportive care versus supportive care alone resulted in a 53% relative reduction in the risk of death. The median survival of patients treated with radiation therapy was 29.1 weeks versus 16.9 weeks receiving supportive care alone. Although performance status, quality of life scores, and measures of cognitive status declined over time, the difference between groups was not significant. Taken together, this study suggests that the addition of radiation therapy to supportive care prolonged survival and did not reduce health-related quality of life or cognitive function in elderly patients with GBM (Keime-Guibert et al. 2007). The benefit, however, was comparatively less compared to the results of studies in younger patients (Walker et al. 1980).

Despite the frequent use of radiotherapy in the treatment of gliomas in elderly patients, little is known about the impact on quality of life, side effects, and outcome of radiation in this population. Radiation treatment necessitates daily trips to a treatment facility. A "standard" schedule requires therapy five days per week for six weeks. This may be difficult for an elderly individual, especially those with diminished performance status and neurological impairment. Between 10% and 20% of elderly patients who initiate radiation therapy are unable to complete it because of their clinical status (Keime-Guibert et al. 2007; Mohan et al. 1998; Pierga et al. 1999; Villa et al. 1998). In addition, it requires the participation of a caregiver. Abbreviated regimens of radiation therapy that reduce the treatment period to two to four weeks are frequently employed to minimize this inconvenience. Two prospective, randomized studies of poor prognosis patients, including elderly patients, failed to demonstrate a difference in survival between those treated with a standard or shortened course of treatment (Phillips et al. 2003; Roa et al. 2004). Similarly, prospective, single arm studies of abbreviated regimens yielded survival similar to historical controls (Bauman et al. 1994; Chang et al. 2003; Ford et al. 1997; McAleese et al. 2003; Thomas et al. 1994). Yet, reduction in treatment times comes at the expense of a reduced radiation dose. Given the known dose-response of these tumors (Walker, Strike, and Sheline 1979), there is at least a theoretical loss of efficacy in pursuing this option.

Trends towards more favorable survival with conventional treatment have been noted in some series (McAleese et al. 2003; Mohan et al. 1998; Pietila et al. 1999). In addition, the use of larger fractions in several hypofractionated regimens potentially increases the risk of radiation toxicity (Clarke et al. 2008; Lutterbach and Ostertag 2005). Thus, although radiation may improve survival outcomes, the optimal regimen remains uncertain (Clarke et al. 2008).

The impact of radiation on patient symptomatology and performance status is limited. In one retrospective series, only 20% of symptomatic patients improved (Meckling et al. 1996). On the contrary, radiation therapy has damaging effects on normal brain that may adversely impact quality of life in elderly patients (Table 2). Although acute and early delayed toxicity are reversible, given the limited survival of these patients, any loss of quality survival is significant. In addition, treatment of these conditions necessitates the use of corticosteroids that carry significant side effects. Delayed toxicity typically develops beyond the median survival of older patients with this tumor. One may see this irreversible complication, however, soon after or even during treatment. Furthermore, as more effective treatment strategies improve survivors, the risk of delayed toxicity increases. The elderly may be at higher risk of brain damage (Constine et al. 1988; Corn et al. 1994; Crossen et al. 1994; Swennen et al. 2004). The coexistence of comorbidities such as cerebrovascular disease, stroke, hypertension, and diabetes as well as primary degenerative disorders (i.e., Alzheimer's and Parkinson's disease) are more common in older patients. These may further predispose the elderly to cerebral injury. Thus, studies focusing on quality of life and cognitive outcomes are needed to better define the relative impact of disease and treatment on patient outcomes.

Chemotherapy

Chemotherapy is the least well studied of the available treatment modalities. Clinical trials of chemotherapy for GBM demonstrated only minimal impact on survival (Fine et al. 1993). This has partly been attributed to the blood brain barrier that restricts entry into the CNS of many of the available chemotherapeutics. Drug regimens were often poorly tolerated, further limiting their benefit. With respect to the elderly population, physiologic changes that occur with aging raise the concern of increased toxicity. In addition, a decline in chemoresponsivness with age has been demonstrated in cell cultures (Rosenblum et al. 1982) and case series (Grant et al. 1995)(Table 3).

With the advent of less toxic therapies and improved supportive care, chemotherapy has become more feasible among older patients. Temozolomide, an oral alkylating agent with excellent bioavailability and safety profile, remains the standard for glioblastoma in younger patients. Its efficacy, when administered concomitant with and following radiation therapy, was demonstrated in a large phase III randomized study compared to radiation alone (Stupp et al. 2009; Stupp et al. 2005). Unfortunately, patients ≥ 70 were excluded from this study. Recursive portioning analysis, however, demonstrated that patients in

Table 3 Age Influences the Response to Chemotherapy and the Rate of Complication

Age	PR (%)	SD (%)	PD (%)	Complication (%)
< 40	38	38	25	13
40–59	15	46	39	19
> 60	6	28	66	35

PR partial response; SD stable disease; PD progressive disease

RPA class 5 and 6 (which historically includes a large proportion of elderly patients) derived little benefit from combined modality treatment (Mirimanoff et al. 2006). Concerns regarding toxicity and limited efficacy have limited the usage of this regimen among the elderly population. More recent studies, however, demonstrated more encouraging results (Brandes et al. 2009; Brandes et al. 2003; Combs et al. 2008; Minniti et al. 2008). Median overall survival, approximately 11 to 16 months, compared favorably to historical results. Furthermore, among patients with good prognostic factors (more extensive resection, favorable RPA class and performance status), median survival closely approximated that reported in younger populations. Hematological toxicity was also similar to what was reported in younger patients. Brandes et al. compared three different regimens: radiation alone versus radiation with procarbazine, CCNU, and vincristine or temozolomide. Median survival was 14.9 months in those treated with temozolomide versus 12.7 months and 11.2 months in the PCV and radiation alone arms respectively (Brandes et al. 2003). These results, however, should be taken with caution. The included population consisted mostly of the "young" elderly. In only one of the four studies was median age greater than 70 (Minniti et al. 2008). The median age in remaining studies (approximately 68 years) reflects a more broad definition of elderly (≥ 65). In addition, the patients included in these studies consisted of a prognistically more favorable population. For example, two studies included only patients that underwent tumor resection with a good performance status (Brandes et al. 2009; Brandes et al. 2003). Thus, to what extent these studies can be extrapolated to the general elderly population remains in question. Furthermore, treatment was associated with neurological toxicity. Minniti et al. reported neurological decline during or immediately after radiation in 12 of the 32 patients reported in their study (Minniti et al. 2008). Brandes et al. noted grade 2 or 3 mental status deterioration leading to significant disability in 56% of patients at a median of six months from the end of radiation (Brandes et al. 2009). In both studies, the decline was attributed to treatment in most cases.

Concerns regarding the neurotoxicity of radiation therapy have prompted studies of chemotherapy in lieu of radiation. Glantz et al. retrospectively reviewed 86 consecutive patients aged ≥ 70, of whom 32 received temozolomide in lieu of radiation. Survival was similar among the two groups, 4.1 and 6 months for radiation and temozolomide groups respectively, suggesting comparable efficacy (Glantz et al. 2003). A subsequent phase II study in a similar population demonstrated similar results (median overall survival 6.4 months) (Chinot et al. 2004) as did a more recent small pilot study (median survival 6.0 months) (Chamberlain and Chalmers 2007). Comparatively, at face value, this approach appears inferior to combined chemoradiation. However, patients enrolled in these studies were older (median age 75 to 79), with a worse performance status (median Karnofsky Performance Status 70). In addition, the majority of patients underwent biopsy only. These differences may account at least partially for the inferior results. Quality of life and cognitive status were not assessed. Additional study of chemotherapy with deferred radiotherapy is warranted.

Based on the available data, a definitive recommendation regarding the treatment of elderly patients with GBM is not feasible. Outcome is inferior to younger patients with similar disease and the risk of toxicity may be greater. Nonetheless, multimodality treatment does have a positive impact in some patients. Clearly, age alone should not dictate treatment. Stratifying patients based on performance status is critical in defining patients that may benefit from treatment. With respect to surgery, the feasibility of resection may be defined by the location of the tumor. The anatomic constraints of the central nervous system may limit the ability of neurosurgeons to resect a tumor and high-risk tumors should not be resected at the expense of clinical status. The medical status of a potentially surgical patient must be considered. All good performance status patients should be considered for radiation therapy, especially those who have undergone resection of their tumor. Ideally, the standard treatment schedule should be considered especially in those in a more prognostically favorable category. Whether to administer temozolomide concomitantly is uncertain, but should be considered. Temozolomide with deferred radiotherapy is the least explored of the available options. Although this may represent a compromise in terms of efficacy, it is a more convenient option with potentially less toxicity.

The Future

Overall survival has been the traditional endpoint of most clinical trials in oncology. The impact of treatment on quality of life (QOL), however, may offset any survival advantage. Yet QOL has only recently emerged as an outcome in clinical trials. Several disease specific (including brain tumor), validated instruments are available that allow patients to report subjective interpretations of their experience in a standardized fashion. Obstacles to QOL assessment remain, however. Few of the available scales have been validated in the elderly population. Yet the goals of treatment and concept of QOL may differ in this population relative to younger patients. In addition, the deficits of patients with brain tumors may prohibit them from filling out the forms. Completion of QOL questionnaires declines with age (Ballatori et al. 2001; Hjermstad et al. 1998). Although compliance with initial, baseline evaluation is high, participation declines over time (Ballatori et al. 2001). Often this is associated with disease progression and associated decline in performance status and consequently, QOL (Ballatori et al. 2001). QOL is given low priority by research teams and data are often not collected correctly or completely.

Economic outcomes are becoming increasingly relevant. The available therapies, supportive care, and surveillance come at great cost not only to society but to the patient as well. The elderly population generally have fixed incomes and reduced financial resources. The financial burden carried by the patient and family may result in significant stress and ultimately deplete surviving family members of life savings. As the elderly population grows and social security resources are depleted, health dollars may be distributed in a more restricted manner. Economic outcomes deserve more attention in the future from both societal and individual standpoints.

The role of comorbidities on the outcome of treatment of brain tumors has yet to be thoroughly examined. From a theoretical standpoint, those with underlying disease may be more susceptible to toxicity than otherwise healthy patients. This is particularly relevant in the elderly population in whom there is a greater incidence of comorbidities and polypharmacy. As such, comorbidities may influence outcomes and define prognostic groups. This knowledge may assist clinicians in developing treatment plans.

Alternative therapies are being developed that specifically target molecular and genetic abnormalities present within cancer cells. Unlike conventional cytotoxic therapies that affect all proliferating cells, these agents theoretically attack the machinery driving the malignant cells. Antiangiogenic therapy antagonizing the tumor-derived vasculature has recently shown some promise. In fact, treatment with bevacizumab, an anti-vascular endothelial growth factor monoclonal antibody, may be more efficacious in the elderly relative to younger patients (Kreisl et al. 2009). Although there may be some overlap with normal tissue, such therapies may be less toxic. To take full advantage of targeted therapies, we must continue to develop our understanding of the molecular biology of GBM. Ultimately, personalized therapy to an individual's tumor may maximize efficacy while minimizing toxicity. This is particularly important in the elderly population.

Until recently, little attention has been focused on this very challenging part of a very challenging disease. As efforts are increased and studies dedicated to better understand how disease and treatments interact with older patients with GBM, we will be better able to serve this ever-growing population.

References

Statistical report: Primary brain tumors in the United States, 1998–2002. *Central Brain Tumor Registry of the United States* 2005.

Balducci L and Extermann M. Cancer chemotherapy in the older patient: What the medical oncologist needs to know. *Cancer* 80: 1317–1322, 1997.

Balducci L, Hardy CL, and Lyman GH. Hemopoietic reserve in the older cancer patient: Clinical and economic considerations. *Cancer Control* 7: 539–547, 2000.

Ballatori E. Unsolved problems in evaluating the quality of life of cancer patients. *Ann Oncol* 12 Suppl 3: S11–13, 2001.

Barker FG, 2nd, Chang SM, Larson DA, Sneed PK, Wara WM, Wilson CB, and Prados MD. Age and radiation response in glioblastoma multiforme. *Neurosurgery* 49: 1288–1297; discussion 1297–1288, 2001.

Barnholtz-Sloan JS, Williams VL, Maldonado JL, Shahani D, Stockwell HG, Chamberlain M, and Sloan AE. Patterns of care and outcomes among elderly individuals with primary malignant astrocytoma. *J Neurosurg* 108: 642–648, 2008.

Bauman GS, Gaspar LE, Fisher BJ, Halperin EC, Macdonald DR, and Cairncross JG. A prospective study of short-course radiotherapy in poor prognosis glioblastoma multiforme. *Int J Radiat Oncol Biol Phys* 29: 835–839, 1994.

Brandes AA, Franceschi E, Tosoni A, et al. Temozolomide concomitant and adjuvant to radiotherapy in elderly patients with glioblastoma: Correlation with MGMT promoter methylation status. *Cancer* 115: 3512–3518, 2009.

Brandes AA, Vastola F, Basso U, et al. A prospective study on glioblastoma in the elderly. *Cancer* 97: 657–662, 2003.

Cabantog AM and Bernstein M. Complications of first craniotomy for intra-axial brain tumour. *Can J Neurol Sci* 21: 213–218, 1994.

Chamberlain MC and Chalmers L. A pilot study of primary temozolomide chemotherapy and deferred radiotherapy in elderly patients with glioblastoma. *J Neurooncol* 82: 207–209, 2007.

Chang EL, Yi W, Allen PK, Levin VA, Sawaya RE, and Maor MH. Hypofractionated radiotherapy for elderly or younger low-performance status glioblastoma patients: Outcome and prognostic factors. *Int J Radiat Oncol Biol Phys* 56: 519–528, 2003.

Chang SM, Barker FG, 2nd, Schmidt MH, et al. Clinical trial participation among patients enrolled in the Glioma Outcomes Project. *Cancer* 94: 2681–2687, 2002.

Chinot OL, Barrie M, Frauger E, et al. Phase II study of temozolomide without radiotherapy in newly diagnosed glioblastoma multiforme in an elderly population. *Cancer* 100: 2208–2214, 2004.

Clarke JW, Chang EL, Levin VA, Mayr NA, Hong E, Cavaliere R, and Lo SS. Optimizing radiotherapy schedules for elderly glioblastoma multiforme patients. *Expert Rev Anticancer Ther* 8: 733–741, 2008.

Combs SE, Wagner J, Bischof M, et al. Postoperative treatment of primary glioblastoma multiforme with radiation and concomitant temozolomide in elderly patients. *Int J Radiat Oncol Biol Phys* 70: 987–992, 2008.

Constine LS, Konski A, Ekholm S, McDonald S, and Rubin P. Adverse effects of brain irradiation correlated with MR and CT imaging. *Int J Radiat Oncol Biol Phys* 15: 319–330, 1988.

Corn BW, Yousem DM, Scott CB, et al. White matter changes are correlated significantly with radiation dose. Observations from a randomized dose-escalation trial for malignant glioma (Radiation Therapy Oncology Group 83-02). *Cancer* 74: 2828–2835, 1994.

Crossen JR, Garwood D, Glatstein E, and Neuwelt EA. Neurobehavioral sequelae of cranial irradiation in adults: A review of radiation-induced encephalopathy. *J Clin Oncol* 12: 627–642, 1994.

Denduluri N, and Ershler WB. Aging biology and cancer. *Semin Oncol* 31: 137–148, 2004.

Fadul C, Wood J, Thaler H, Galicich J, Patterson RH, Jr., and Posner JB. Morbidity and mortality of craniotomy for excision of supratentorial gliomas. *Neurology* 38: 1374–1379, 1988.

Fine HA, Dear KB, Loeffler JS, Black PM, and Canellos GP. Meta-analysis of radiation therapy with and without adjuvant chemotherapy for malignant gliomas in adults. *Cancer* 71: 2585–2597, 1993.

Fleury A, Menegoz F, Grosclaude P, et al. Descriptive epidemiology of cerebral gliomas in France. *Cancer* 79: 1195–1202, 1997.

Ford JM, Stenning SP, Boote DJ, et al. A short fractionation radiotherapy treatment for poor prognosis patients with high grade glioma. *Clin Oncol (R Coll Radiol)* 9: 20–24, 1997.

Fujimura M, Kumabe T, Tominaga T, Jokura H, Shirane R, and Yoshimoto T. Routine clinical adoption of magnetic resonance imaging was associated with better outcome after surgery in elderly patients with a malignant astrocytic tumour: A retrospective review. *Acta Neurochir (Wien)* 146: 251–255, 2004.

Glantz M, Chamberlain M, Liu Q, Litofsky NS, and Recht LD. Temozolomide as an alternative to irradiation for elderly patients with newly diagnosed malignant gliomas. *Cancer* 97: 2262–2266, 2003.

Grant R, Liang BC, Page MA, Crane DL, Greenberg HS, and Junck L. Age influences chemotherapy response in astrocytomas. *Neurology* 45: 929–933, 1995.

Greig NH, Ries LG, Yancik R, and Rapoport SI. Increasing annual incidence of primary malignant brain tumors in the elderly. *J Natl Cancer Inst* 82: 1621–1624, 1990.

Hjermstad MJ, Fayers PM, Bjordal K, and Kaasa S. Using reference data on quality of life—the importance of adjusting for age and gender, exemplified by the EORTC QLQ-C30 (+3). *Eur J Cancer* 34: 1381–1389, 1998.

Ichimura K, Pearson DM, Kocialkowski S, et al. IDH1 mutations are present in the majority of common adult gliomas but rare in primary glioblastomas. *Neuro Oncol* 11: 341–347, 2009.

Iwamoto FM, Cooper AR, Reiner AS, Nayak L, and Abrey LE. Glioblastoma in the elderly: the Memorial Sloan-Kettering Cancer Center Experience (1997–2007). *Cancer* 115: 3758–3766, 2009.

Iwamoto FM, Reiner AS, Panageas KS, Elkin EB, and Abrey LE. Patterns of care in elderly glioblastoma patients. *Ann Neurol* 64: 628–634, 2008.

Keime-Guibert F, Chinot O, Taillandier L, et al. Radiotherapy for glioblastoma in the elderly. *N Engl J Med* 356: 1527–1535, 2007.

Kelly PJ, and Hunt C. The limited value of cytoreductive surgery in elderly patients with malignant gliomas. *Neurosurgery* 34: 62–66; discussion 66–67, 1994.

Kita D, Ciernik IF, Vaccarella S, Franceschi S, Kleihues P, Lutolf UM, and Ohgaki H. Age as a predictive factor in glioblastomas: Population-based study. *Neuroepidemiology* 33: 17–22, 2009.

Kornblith AB, Kemeny M, Peterson BL, et al. Survey of oncologists' perceptions of barriers to accrual of older patients with breast carcinoma to clinical trials. *Cancer* 95: 989–996, 2002.

Kreisl TN, Kim L, Moore K, et al. Phase II trial of single-agent bevacizumab followed by bevacizumab plus irinotecan at tumor progression in recurrent glioblastoma. *J Clin Oncol* 27: 740–745, 2009.

Kurimoto M, Nagai S, Kamiyama H, et al. Prognostic factors in elderly patients with supratentorial malignant gliomas. *Neurol Med Chir (Tokyo)* 47: 543–549; discussion 549, 2007.

Lang FF, Miller DC, Koslow M, and Newcomb EW. Pathways leading to glioblastoma multiforme: A molecular analysis of genetic alterations in 65 astrocytic tumors. *J Neurosurg* 81: 427–436, 1994.

Lutterbach J and Ostertag C. What is the appropriate radiotherapy protocol for older patients with newly diagnosed glioblastoma? *J Clin Oncol* 23: 2869–2870, 2005.

McAleese JJ, Stenning SP, Ashley S, et al. Hypofractionated radiotherapy for poor prognosis malignant glioma: Matched pair survival analysis with MRC controls. *Radiother Oncol* 67: 177–182, 2003.

McKenna RJ, Sr. Clinical aspects of cancer in the elderly. Treatment decisions, treatment choices, and follow-up. *Cancer* 74: 2107–2117, 1994.

Meckling S, Dold O, Forsyth PA, Brasher P, and Hagen NA. Malignant supratentorial glioma in the elderly: Is radiotherapy useful? *Neurology* 47: 901–905, 1996.

Minniti G, De Sanctis V, Muni R, et al. Radiotherapy plus concomitant and adjuvant temozolomide for glioblastoma in elderly patients. *J Neurooncol* 88: 97–103, 2008.

Mirimanoff RO, Gorlia T, Mason W, et al. . Radiotherapy and temozolomide for newly diagnosed glioblastoma: Recursive partitioning analysis of the EORTC 26981/22981-NCIC CE3 phase III randomized trial. *J Clin Oncol* 24: 2563–2569, 2006.

Mohan DS, Suh JH, Phan JL, Kupelian PA, Cohen BH, and Barnett GH. Outcome in elderly patients undergoing definitive surgery and radiation therapy for supratentorial glioblastoma multiforme at a tertiary care institution. *Int J Radiat Oncol Biol Phys* 42: 981–987, 1998.

Muacevic A, and Kreth FW. Quality-adjusted survival after tumor resection and/or radiation therapy for elderly patients with glioblastoma multiforme. *J Neurol* 250: 561–568, 2003.

Ohgaki H, Dessen P, Jourde B, et al. Genetic pathways to glioblastoma: A population-based study. *Cancer Res* 64: 6892–6899, 2004.

Ohgaki H and Kleihues P. Genetic pathways to primary and secondary glioblastoma. *Am J Pathol* 170: 1445–1453, 2007.

Patwardhan RV, Shorter C, Willis BK, et al. Survival trends in elderly patients with glioblastoma multiforme: Resective surgery, radiation, and chemotherapy. *Surg Neurol* 62: 207–213; discussion 214–205, 2004.

Phillips C, Guiney M, Smith J, Hughes P, Narayan K, and Quong G. A randomized trial comparing 35Gy in ten fractions with 60Gy in 30 fractions of cerebral irradiation for glioblastoma multiforme and older patients with anaplastic astrocytoma. *Radiother Oncol* 68: 23–26, 2003.

Pierga JY, Hoang-Xuan K, Feuvret L, et al. Treatment of malignant gliomas in the elderly. *J Neurooncol* 43: 187–193, 1999.

Pietila TA, Stendel R, Hassler WE, Heimberger C, Ramsbacher J, and Brock M. Brain tumor surgery in geriatric patients: A critical analysis in 44 patients over 80 years. *Surg Neurol* 52: 259–263; discussion 263–254, 1999.

Reifenberger G, and Collins VP. Pathology and molecular genetics of astrocytic gliomas. *J Mol Med* 82: 656–670, 2004.

Roa W, Brasher PM, Bauman G, et al. Abbreviated course of radiation therapy in older patients with glioblastoma multiforme: A prospective randomized clinical trial. *J Clin Oncol* 22: 1583–1588, 2004.

Rosenblum ML, Gerosa M, Dougherty DV, et al. Age-related chemosensitivity of stem cells from human malignant brain tumours. *Lancet* 1: 885–887, 1982.

Schiff D and Shaffrey ME. Role of resection for newly diagnosed malignant gliomas. *Expert Rev Anticancer Ther* 3: 621–630, 2003.

Stummer W, Reulen HJ, Meinel T, et al. Extent of resection and survival in glioblastoma multiforme: Identification of and adjustment for bias. *Neurosurgery* 62: 564–576; discussion 564–576, 2008.

Stupp R, Hegi ME, Mason WP, et al. Effects of radiotherapy with concomitant and adjuvant temozolomide versus radiotherapy alone on survival in glioblastoma in a randomised phase III study: 5-year analysis of the EORTC-NCIC trial. *Lancet Oncol* 10: 459–466, 2009.

Stupp R, Mason WP, van den Bent MJ, et al. Radiotherapy plus concomitant and adjuvant temozolomide for glioblastoma. *N Engl J Med* 352: 987–996, 2005.

Swennen MH, Bromberg JE, Witkamp TD, Terhaard CH, Postma TJ, and Taphoorn MJ. Delayed radiation toxicity after focal or whole brain radiotherapy for low-grade glioma. *J Neurooncol* 66: 333–339, 2004.

Thomas R, James N, Guerrero D, Ashley S, Gregor A, and Brada M. Hypofractionated radiotherapy as palliative treatment in poor prognosis patients with high grade glioma. *Radiother Oncol* 33: 113–116, 1994.

Tomita T and Raimondi AJ. Brain tumors in the elderly. *Jama* 246: 53–55, 1981.

Vestal RE. Aging and pharmacology. *Cancer* 80: 1302–1310, 1997.

Villa S, Vinolas N, Verger E, et al. Efficacy of radiotherapy for malignant gliomas in elderly patients. *Int J Radiat Oncol Biol Phys* 42: 977–980, 1998.

Vuorinen V, Hinkka S, Farkkila M, and Jaaskelainen J. Debulking or biopsy of malignant glioma in elderly people—a randomised study. *Acta Neurochir (Wien)* 145: 5–10, 2003.

Walker MD, Green SB, Byar DP, et al. Randomized comparisons of radiotherapy and nitrosoureas for the treatment of malignant glioma after surgery. *N Engl J Med* 303: 1323–1329, 1980.

Walker MD, Strike TA, and Sheline GE. An analysis of dose-effect relationship in the radiotherapy of malignant gliomas. *Int J Radiat Oncol Biol Phys* 5: 1725–1731, 1979.

Werner MH, Phuphanich S, and Lyman GH. The increasing incidence of malignant gliomas and primary central nervous system lymphoma in the elderly. *Cancer* 76: 1634–1642, 1995.

Whittle IR, Basu N, Grant R, Walker M, and Gregor A. Management of patients aged >60 years with malignant glioma: Good clinical status and radiotherapy determine outcome. *Br J Neurosurg* 16: 343–347, 2002.

46 Multiple Sclerosis in the Elderly
Tanuja Chitnis and Howard L. Weiner

Introduction

Multiple sclerosis (MS) is an immune-mediated, demyelinating, and degenerative disease of the central nervous system. MS generally starts in early adulthood with the majority of cases presenting between 25–35 years of age. Onset between 18 and 49 is termed adult-onset MS (AOMS). Rarely, MS presents in the extremes of the age spectrum, from the very young to the very old. It is recognized that MS can present in the elderly, and onset after age 50 is termed late-onset MS (LOMS). The clinical and radiological features of late onset MS will be discussed here. Another topic relevant to the aging population are the issues that patients with established adult-onset MS face when they enter their 50s and 60s. Important changes in the immune system, nervous system, and endocrine system that occur during senescence may modify the underlying mechanisms of MS, resulting in changes in the clinical features. In this chapter, we will review the available literature on the MS disease course in the elderly, its underlying mechanisms and management approaches.

Biological Changes During Senescence and Effect on MS

Biological differences in the elderly compared to young adult may explain why MS-onset is rare after 50 years of age. Moreover, given that the lifespan of the typical MS patient is close to the normal lifespan, the majority of patients with established adult-onset MS will survive well into their 60s and 70s, making biological changes that occur during senescence relevant to disease course during this period. During the period around age 50, the immune, nervous, and endocrine systems undergo critical changes, which can affect the disease course of MS patients as well as response to treatment. Although there are few studies specifically exploring the effect of biological changes in the elderly MS patient, we will review current knowledge of immune, CNS, and endocrine alterations in senescence and their potential effects on disease course and treatment.

Immune System During Senescence

T cells are thought to play a key role in the initiation of MS (Chitnis 2007). Antigen-presenting cells present antigen and provide costimulation to T cells (Chitnis and Khoury 2003). B cells may play a role in antigen presentation and B cell antibody production may increase tissue damage within the CNS (Antel and Bar-Or 2006). Macrophages invade the CNS and release damaging factors including cytokines and nitric oxide, which may also be produced by resident CNS microglia (Jack, Ruffini et al. 2005). During senescence there are significant changes that occur in both the innate and adaptive branches of the immune system that may limit the initiation and progression of some autoimmune or immune-mediated processes relevant to MS.

Here, we will summarize the literature describing changes in the immune system during senescence.

Thymic involution results in a decrease in circulating T cells in the elderly (Taub and Longo 2005). The ratio of naïve:memory T cells decreases with age (Cossarizza, Ortolani et al. 1996). A significant reduction in repertoire diversity of B and T cells is present in the elderly (Gorczynski, Kennedy et al. 1984; Weksler 2000; Vallejo 2006; Goronzy, Lee et al. 2007). The general decline in immunoglobulin repertoire is associated with decreased B cell class switching induced by CD40 and BAFF (Frasca, Riley et al. 2005; Frasca, Riley et al. 2007). However, the frequency of certain immunoglobulin subtypes may be altered with age (Paganelli, Quinti et al. 1992). An increase in the expression of natural killer cell (NK) receptors and killer cell immunoglobulin-like receptors (KIR) is found on T cells, and has been postulated to compensate for the loss of TCR diversity (Vallejo 2006).

T cell hyporesponsiveness is well described in aging models and in humans (Castle, Uyemura et al. 1999), and has been ascribed to both a change in effector populations as well as regulatory T cell function. Changes in costimulatory molecule expression including an increase in CTLA4 expression and a decrease in CD28 expression during aging may contribute to hyporesponsive T cells (Leng, Bentwich et al. 2002). In addition, hyporesponsivness is associated with alterations in T cell signaling (Chakravarti, Chakravarti et al. 1998). There is considerable controversy regarding the changes occurring in regulatory T cell populations in aging models, and it has been suggested that these differences may be dependent on the specific animal model studied (Thomas, Mellanby et al. 2007). A reduction in frequency and function of CD4+CD25+Foxp3+ regulatory T cells and TGF-beta-producing Tr3 cells has been demonstrated in aged mice (Gorczynski, Alexander et al. 2007), while another study demonstrated reduced suppressive function, and an increase in frequency of CD4+CD25+ regulatory T cells compared to younger animals (Zhao, Sun et al. 2007). In contrast, other investigators found no change in numbers and function of CD4+CD25+Foxp3+ regulatory T cells, and suggest instead that decreased T cell function during aging is due to hyporesponsiveness in the CD4+CD25- responder population (Nishioka, Shimizu et al. 2006). Additional studies suggest that the CD4+CD25-CD103+ T cells from aged animals can themselves induce suppression (Shimizu and Moriizumi 2003; Shimizu and Moriizumi 2003). Studies in humans are limited, and one report describes an increase in the frequency and suppressive function of CD4+CD25+ T cells in elderly healthy individuals (Rosenkranz, Weyer et al. 2007).

Studies are in general agreement that in animal models, peripheral innate immunity is suppressed during senescence (Solana, Pawelec et al. 2006). Macrophages from aged mice show impairment in the expression of most toll-like receptors and production of pro-inflammatory cytokines (Renshaw, Rockwell et al. 2002; Gomez, Nomellini et al. 2008). However, some studies in humans found significantly increased production of pro-inflammatory cytokines IL-6, TNF-α and IL-1β (Fagiolo, Cossarizza et al. 1993), and increased antigen-presenting function (Castle, Uyemura et al. 1999), suggesting a state of activation. It has been suggested that this dichotomy between mouse and human studies may be due to selection bias in the human population for those suffering from chronic diseases. Other studies using well-screened cohorts of healthy individuals found no difference in IL-6 production (Beharka, Meydani et al. 2001), and decreased production of IL-12 in dendritic cells from the elderly (Uyemura, Castle et al. 2002). It is thus unclear whether innate immune changes occurring with age differ between humans and mice, and further studies, which control for the presence of chronic diseases in the elderly, are required.

Animal models of MS in aged animals are generally less susceptible to induction of experimental autoimmune encephalomyelitis (EAE), a model for multiple sclerosis disease. Older Balb/c mice were more resistant to active EAE disease induction by myelin basic protein or proteolipid protein compared to younger animals (Endoh, Rapoport et al. 1990). This was associated with decreased T cell proliferation and cytokine production. Adoptive transfer experiments demonstrated that APC function was intact in older animals, but that T cell function was defective. There are no studies in human MS patients evaluating immune function in elderly MS patients and those with LOMS.

Senescence and the Central Nervous System

In contrast to the general finding that peripheral immune responses are suppressed during senescence, immune responses are generally enhanced in the aging brain and central nervous system. This may be particularly relevant to the mechanisms of disease progression in MS, which are believed to be mediated to a large extent, by endogenous CNS inflammation (Kutzelnigg, Lucchinetti et al. 2005; Weiner 2008).

The most widely observed change in the aged brain is an activated phenotype and enhanced reactivity of microglial cells. In addition, more hypertrophied and reactive astrocytes are observed in the brains of aged animals (Landfield, Rose et al. 1977). Toll-like receptor 1, 2, 4, 5, and 7 transcripts localized to monocytes were found to be up-regulated in the aged mouse brain while expression of TLR3, TLR6, and TLR8 was unchanged and TLR9 was down-regulated (Letiembre, Hao et al. 2007). Glial cells from aged animals have been shown to produce increased levels of pro-inflammatory cytokines. In contrast to neonatal microglia and astrocytes, mixed glial cells from 18–20 month old rats were unable to rescue neurons from A-beta-induced toxicity and expressed increased levels of nitric oxide and IL-1β (Yu, Go et al. 2002). One study has demonstrated more frequent dendritic cells and CD3+ T cells in the perivascular spaces and meninges of aged mice as well as in white matter tracts including the corpus callosum (Stichel and Luebbert 2007). This may be attributable to enhanced blood brain barrier vascular permeability associated with senescence (Saija, Princi et al. 1990; Plateel, Teissier et al. 1997). Changes in blood brain barrier structure include a decrease in tight junction transmembrane protein occludin in 24-month-old rats compared to 12-month-old rats (Mooradian, Haas et al. 2003). A reduction in lymphocyte expression of the homing molecule integrin alpha4beta7 and its specific receptor MAdCAM-1 on vascular endothelial cells in the intestine is described in aged animals (Schmucker, Owen et al. 2002).

Neurodegenerative and regenerative mechanisms may be important in disease progression and recovery in MS (Chitnis, Imitola et al. 2005). Studies using the cuprizone model in mice have found that axonal loss is increased in older mice (Irvine and Blakemore 2006). In addition, remyelination in this model is impaired in older animals compared to younger animals. This is due to less downregulation of

oligodendrocyte differentiation inhibitors in older animals, regulated in part by recruitment of histone deacetylases to promoter regions (Shen, Sandoval et al. 2008).

Endocrine System and Senescence

Probably the most important biological changes that occur during senescence are in the endocrine system. Age-associated alterations in the endocrine system likely affect the immune and nervous system and contribute to the changes described above. In women, menopause, defined as permanent cessation of menstruation for at least one year, reflects the inability of ovaries to produce the hormones progesterone and estradiol as a result of complete oocyte astresia, resulting in changes to the endometrium, as well as skeletal and dermatological changes. This process occurs over the period of several years, and may therefore have different consequences than surgical- or chemotherapy-induced ovariectomy.

There is some literature documenting immune changes in relation to menopause and hormone replacement therapy (HRT). One study found a significant decrease in naive T cells and an increase in memory/activated T cells in subjects sampled at late post-menopause compared to those at early post-menopause (Kamada, Irahara et al. 2000). The percentage of lymphocytes in women on HRT was significantly higher than that in untreated women at late post-menopausal stage, however there was no difference in the proportion of activated or memory T cells. Studies of lipopolysaccharide-activated T cells found higher production of IFN-γ in postmenopausal women compared with that of younger women, whereas the production of IL-10 increased gradually with age, in parallel with the postmenopausal period (Deguchi, Kamada et al. 2001). Levels of IFN-γ, IL-2, IL-4, and IL-10 were significantly lower in HRT-treated post-menopausal women than untreated subjects (Kamada, Irahara et al. 2001). Menopause was associated with a decrease in B cells, but HRT was associated with an increase in B cell subsets, but no immunoglobulin production (Kamada, Irahara et al. 2001). Reproductive senescent-derived microglia cultures had higher basal expression of NO and MMP-9 activity as compared to those from young adult microglial cultures (Johnson, Bake et al. 2006). Dye extravasation was almost two to three times greater in the olfactory bulb and hippocampus of senescent animals as compared to their young counterparts. Interestingly, estrogen treatment significantly increased dye extravasation in the hippocampus of senescent animals, but decreased dye extravasation in younger animals (Johnson and Sohrabji 2005). The mechanisms of this change are undefined, but may be related to differential expression of tight junction-related proteins in older age animals, as described above. There are currently no published studies examining the effects of menopause or HRT on immune responses in MS.

Genetics

The gene mostly frequently linked with MS is HLA DRB1 (Stewart, McLeod et al. 1981), with DRB1*1501 (Haines, Ter-Minassian et al. 1996) being the most frequently involved allele. Recently, a large genome-wide study identified IL-2R and IL-7R alleles as risk alleles for multiple sclerosis (Hafler, Compston et al. 2007). DRB1*1501 homozygosity is associated with earlier onset of MS (Barcellos, Oksenberg et al. 2002). Many efforts have focused on identifying genotypes associated with increased disease severity. The APOE gene locus has been widely studied, and some studies found an association of APOE4 with a more severe relapse phenotype (Evangelou, Jackson et al. 1999; Fazekas, Strasser-Fuchs et al. 2001), and others found an association with cognitive deficits (Parmenter, Denney et al. 2007), while other studies found no association with disease severity measures (Burwick, Ramsay et al. 2006; Sedano, Calmarza et al. 2006). Larger studies to evaluate the effect of MS risk alleles on age at onset and modification of disease course are underway.

Late Onset MS

Late onset multiple sclerosis (MS) is generally defined as first symptom-onset after the age of 50 years. The prevalence of late-onset MS has been reported as 3.4% (Delalande, De Seze et al. 2002), 4.6% (Polliack, Barak et al. 2001), 4.7% (Tremlett and Devonshire 2006), 9.4% (Noseworthy, Paty et al. 1983), 9.6% (Martinelli, Rodegher et al. 2004), and 12% (Phadke 1990). Very late onset MS (VLOMS), with onset at or after age 60 (Azzimondi, Stracciari et al. 1994), is even more rare, with a reported prevalence of 0.45% (Delalande, De Seze et al. 2002) and 0.6% (Hooge and Redekop 1992). The oldest age at MS onset reported in the medical literature is 87 years (Takeuchi, Ogura et al. 2008), and this particular patient presented with a tumefactive lesion. Another case of a with onset at 82 years of age presented with a large spinal cord lesion (Abe, Tsuchiya et al. 2000). Although MS may come to clinical attention after age 50, it remains to be determined whether this is the first pathologic manifestation of the disease. Significant evidence from migration studies suggests that events prior to puberty may play an important role in disease pathogenesis. In addition, autopsy studies have demonstrated lesions consistent with MS in patients with no prior history of clinical symptoms, suggesting that clinical symptoms only occur in a proportion of all cases.

There is limited information available regarding the demographic features of LOMS. Gender ratios are reported in the literature as 1.72:1 (Polliack, Barak et al. 2001) and 1.8:1 (Phadke 1990), and reflect a slight decrease in female:male ratios compared to typical adult-onset MS. There is little data describing race and ethnicity in LOMS patients. Most patients with LOMS do not have a family history of MS (Lyon-Caen, Izquierdo et al. 1985).

Clinical Presentation and Disease Course

LOMS and VLOMS (Hooge and Redekop 1992) frequently present with a primary progressive course, and in one major series, are reported at an incidence of 83% in comparison to patients with onset before age 29, who presented with a relapsing-remitting course almost exclusively (Kis, Rumberg et al. 2008). LOMS patients who present with a relapsing course generally develop a secondary progressive course shortly after diagnosis. Motor symptoms are the most common clinical presentation of LOMS (Cazzullo, Ghezzi et al. 1978; Lyon-Caen, Izquierdo et al. 1985; Polliack, Barak et al. 2001; Martinelli, Rodegher et al. 2004), with an incidence of 54% reported in one series (Delalande, De Seze et al. 2002). Optic neuritis presentations are uncommon (Lyon-Caen, Izquierdo et al. 1985). Up to 20% of patients in one series presented with a major depressive episode (Polliack, Barak et al. 2001). Compared to typical adult-onset MS, LOMS patients progress more rapidly to a disability score (EDSS) of 6, which indicates the need for unilateral assistance with gait, with reported disease durations of 27.7 years in AOMS compared to 16.9 years in LOMS (Tremlett and Devonshire 2006). However, despite this more rapid progression, LOMS patients typically have fewer deficits at any given age than patients with AOMS. Rate of progression does not seem to differ between those who present with a relapsing versus progressive subtype.

Common symptoms of MS, which may occur independently of relapses, include fatigue, depression, bladder dysynergia and incontinence, bowel constipation and incontinence and pain syndromes. Symptomatic therapies are available and are outlined below; however, frequent use raise issues regarding polypharmacy in the elderly.

Diagnosis

The diagnosis of multiple sclerosis generally rests on the demonstration of demyelinating lesions with dissemination in space and time. The McDonald guidelines (McDonald, Compston et al. 2001; Polman, Reingold et al. 2005) are used for diagnosis for multiple sclerosis and include the Barkhof MRI diagnostic criteria. Oligoclonal bands may aid in the diagnosis, particularly in cases with two or fewer MRI lesions, or in cases of suspected primary progressive MS; however, oligoclonal bands are not necessary for diagnosis in most cases. Oligoclonal bands are reported as present at similar frequencies in LOMS and adult-onset MS (Kis, Rumberg et al. 2008), and may help in distinguishing from other diagnostic possibilities.

Brain MRI T2 lesion distribution in LOMS is generally similar to adult-onset MS (Kis, Rumberg et al. 2008); however, one study has found that spinal cord lesions are more frequent (81% vs. 48%), and cerebellar lesions more rare in LOMS (11% vs. 44%) (Kis, Rumberg et al. 2008). Gadolinium-enhancing lesions are significantly more rare in LOMS. A study of 20 established LOMS patients found that the Barkhof MRI diagnostic criteria were 85% sensitive and 65% specific in detecting cases of suspected LOMS (de Seze, Delalande et al. 2005). It was suggested that spinal cord MRI may be an important distinguishing factor from other diseases, and should be performed in all suspected cases.

The differential diagnosis of LOMS may be challenging and includes stroke and vascular syndromes, hypertension-related disorders, primary or secondary vasculitis, cancer, compressive myelopathies, metabolic diseases, and degenerative and nutritional disorders (See Table 1). A clinical history consistent with a relapsing disorder with subacute onset of lesions may suggest MS rather than stroke. Cases of primary progressive MS may be more challenging to diagnose, and ancillary testing including MRI and CSF is very helpful. Brain MRI including diffusion-weighted sequences is essential and may be effective in differentiating MS from stroke. The demonstration of ovoid T2 lesions in areas characteristic for MS such as the periventricular white matter and corpus callosum, and fulfillment of the Barkhof criteria may indicate MS as opposed to lacunar strokes. Spine MRI is essential in ruling out compressive myelopathies, which are common in the elderly. A standard bloodwork panel which includes B12, folate, ANA, ESR, and Lyme titer should be obtained in all patients. CSF analysis for oligoclonal bands and elevated IgG index may be helpful in distinguishing LOMS from other disorders, particularly stroke. CSF cytology should be performed in cases in which CNS lymphoma is suspected. In cases of tumor-like lesions, advanced imaging techniques such as MR spectroscopy and PET imaging may be useful in differentiating tumefactive MS from CNS tumor (Butteriss, Ismail et al. 2003; Enzinger, Strasser-Fuchs et al. 2005). A systemic scan for primary malignancies should also be considered in such cases. Brain biopsy may also be considered (Lucchinetti, Gavrilova et al. 2008) in diagnostically challenging cases, in which definitive diagnosis will change management.

Treatment

Disease-modifying treatment protocols specific for late-onset MS have not been defined. Phase II and III trials of standard first-line therapies beta-interferons (1993; Paty and Li 1993; Jacobs, Cookfair et al. 1996; 1998; Li and Paty 1999) and glatiramer acetate (Johnson, Brooks et al. 1995; Wolinsky, Narayana et al. 2001) have included patients up to the age of 65; however, subgroup analyses for LOMS have not been published. Beta-interferons and glatiramer acetate initiated during the relapsing-remitting phase of disease are effective in reducing relapses and new MRI lesion formation; however, generally have little effect in

Table 1 Differential Diagnosis of Late-onset Multiple Sclerosis

Cerebrovascular:

Ischemic stroke

Small vessel lacunar infarcts

Primary vasculitis

Secondary vasculitis

Anterior spinal artery syndrome

Neoplastic:

Astrocytoma

Glioma

Primary CNS lymphoma

Metastases

Nutritional/Metabolic:

Vitamin B12 deficiency

Vitamin E deficiency

Non-insulin dependent diabetes mellitus (NIDDM)

Hypothyroidism

Degenerative:

Late-onset spinocerebellar syndromes

Adrenomyeloneuropathy

Adult-onset leukodystrophy

Structural abnormalities:

Compressive myelopathy

Arnold-Chiari syndrome

Syringomyelia

Inflammatory:

Acute disseminated encephalomyelitis (ADEM)

Transverse myelitis

Temporal arteritis

Sarcoidosis

Systemic lupus erythematosus

Rheumatoid arthritis

Behcet's disease

Lymphomatoid granulomatosis

Infectious:

HIV

HTLV-1

Lyme disease

Herpes encephalitis

Progressive multifocal leukoencephalopathy

Syphilis

preventing disease progression, unless initiated very early in the disease course (Kappos, Polman et al. 2006). Beta-interferons initiated during the secondary progressive phase of disease had little to no effect on disease progression (1998; 2001; Kappos, Weinshenker et al. 2004; Panitch, Miller et al. 2004). Given the natural history of LOMS, which has an

early proclivity to secondary progression, the primary goal of therapy should be prevention of disease progression. Unfortunately, few therapies accomplish this goal, with the exception of drugs with strong effects on relapse reduction, which likely leads to an overall reduction in the risk of disability. Phase III data from clinical trials of Tysabri demonstrated a strong effect on relapse reduction and slowing of disease progression (Polman, O'Connor et al. 2006; Rudick, Stuart et al. 2006). As well, Phase II studies of Campath-1H show a significant reduction in disease progression compared to a beta-interferon (Coles, Compston et al. 2008). However, both drugs have significant side effects, which in the case of Tysabri, includes progressive multifocal leukoencephalopathy (Mullen, Vartanian et al. 2008; Panzara, Bozic et al. 2008) and a possible association with melanoma (Mullen, Vartanian et al. 2008; Panzara, Bozic et al. 2008). Side effects of Campath-1H include immune thrombocytopenic purpura and thyroid disease (Coles, Compston et al. 2008). A recent trial of pulse high dose intravenous steroids administered for five days every four months demonstrated a reduction in the proportion of patients with sustained disease progression and brain atrophy (Zivadinov, Rudick et al. 2001). However, elderly patients are particularly susceptible to side effects of long-term high dose steroids including osteoporosis, hypertension and peptic ulcer disease. Novantrone is an FDA-approved medication for worsening or progressive MS; however, its side effects include cardiomyopathy and lymphoma, raising concerns for its use in the elderly (van de Wyngaert, Beguin et al. 2001; Hartung, Gonsette et al. 2002). Cyclophosphamide is an alkylating agent that has been used extensively, including by our group for worsening MS (Weiner, Mackin et al. 1993; Hohol, Olek et al. 1999; Perini, Calabrese et al. 2006). Subgroup analyses suggest that initiation during the relapsing remitting or early secondary progressive phase yields better results than late initiation (Weiner, Mackin et al. 1993; Hohol, Olek et al. 1999; Perini, Calabrese et al. 2006). However, it has also been suggested that younger age may predispose to better outcomes (Gonsette, Demonty et al. 1977; Hommers, Lamers et al. 1980; Weiner, Mackin et al. 1993). Cyclophosphamide can lead to bladder cancer, but is not associated with cardiomyopathy, making it a potentially more tolerable treatment in the elderly population.

Although incomplete recovery from relapses may lead to accumulation of step-wise disability, the mechanisms of non-relapse related disease progression are likely different and may involve mechanisms of neurodegeneration and activation of an endogenous CNS inflammatory cascade which are not specifically targeted by the available MS therapies (Imitola, Chitnis et al. 2006; Weiner 2008). Newer therapies which target these mechanisms (Chitnis, Imitola et al. 2005) are required to halt disease progression and to slow or reverse secondary progressive MS.

There are no FDA-approved therapies for primary progressive MS. Clinical trials in PPMS have largely been unsuccessful in slowing disease progression. These include trials using beta-interferon, Novantrone. The PROMISE trial of Copaxone in PPMS patients demonstrated slowing of progression only in a subgroup of male patients (Wolinsky, Narayana et al. 2007). Rituximab only showed benefit in patients under the age of 51 years, and those with enhancing lesions on MRI, suggesting that inflammatory mechanisms are being targeted (WCTRIMS 2008). Since the pathogenic mechanisms of PPMS may be similar to those in SPMS, therapies targeting neurodegeneration and endogenous CNS inflammation may be beneficial.

A constellation of chronic symptoms commonly appear during the course of MS. These include fatigue, depression, bladder dysynergia and incontinence, bowel constipation and incontinence and pain syndromes. Symptomatic treatments targeting these symptoms are listed in Table 2.

Table 2 Symptomatic Treatments for Multiple Sclerosis in the Elderly

Bowel and Bladder

Oxybutynin (immediate/extended release and patch) 5mg bid–5mg qid
  Side Effects: Dry mouth, drowsiness, urinary retention

Tolterodine 2mg bid
  Side Effects: Mild dry mouth, drowsiness

Amitriptyline 25–100mg in divided doses
  Side Effects: Dry mouth, fatigue, confusion, orthostatic hypotension, urinary retention, arrhythmia

Darifenacin 7.5mg–15mg daily
  Side Effects: Dry mouth, fatigue, confusion, orthostatic hypotension, urinary retention, arrhythmia

Trospium 20mg twice a day
  Side Effects: Dry mouth, fatigue, confusion, orthostatic hypotension, urinary retention, arrhythmia

Fatigue

Amantidine 100mg bid–100mg tid
  Side Effects: Nausea, dizziness, insomnia

Methylphenidate (10–60mg in divided doses); (18–36mg daily)
  Side Effects: Hepatic dysfunction, insomnia, seizures, anorexia

Fluoxetine 20mg qAM–20mg bid or other selective serotonin reuptake inhibitors
  Side Effects: Anxiety, anorexia, dizziness

Modafinil 200–400mg qAM
  Side Effects: Headache, nausea, rhinitis, nervousness, decreased efficacy of oral contraceptives

Pain Treatment

Phenytoin 100mg bid–100mg qid
  Side Effects: Nystagmus, ataxia, dysarthria, confusion, nausea, rash, hepatic injury

Carbamezepine 200mg bid–200mg qid
  Side Effects: Dizziness, drowsiness, ataxia, nausea, leukopenia, rash, hepatic injury, hyponatremia

Amitriptyline or Nortriptyline 10mg qhs–150mg qhs
  Side Effects: Dry mouth, fatigue, confusion, orthostatic hypotension, urinary retention, arrhythmia

Gabapentin 100mg–600mg qid
  Side Effects: Dizziness, headache, drowsiness

Pregabalin 50mg–100mg tid
  Side Effects: Drowsiness, dizziness, edema, dry mouth, rare rhabdomyolysis

Duloxetine 30–60mg qd
  Side effects: GI side effects, blurred vision, dry mouth, muscle pain, fatigue

Spasticity

Baclofen 5mg tid–20mg qid or higher
  Side Effects: Drowsiness, dizziness, fatigue, weakness

Diazepam 2.5mg tid–10mg qid
  Side Effects: Drowsiness, dizziness, ataxia

Dantrolene 25mg qid–100mg qid
  Side Effects: Drowsiness, dizziness, weakness, diarrhea, hepatic injury

Tizanidine 2mg tid–12mg tid
  Side Effects: Drowsiness, dry mouth, orthostatic hypotension

Intrathecal Baclofen up to 800mcg/day
  Side Effects: Drowsiness, dizziness, nausea, hypotension, weakness

Table 2 Continued

Depression

Prozac 10mg–40mg daily
  Side Effects: Weight gain, sexual side effects, agitation, insomnia

Sertraline 50mg–200mg daily
  Side Effects: Sexual side effects, loss of appetite, GI side effects, agitation, insomnia

Escitalopram citrate 10mg–20mg daily
  Side Effects: Sexual side effcts, nausea, diarrhea, agitation, insomnia

Citalopram 20mg–60mg daily
  Side Effects: syncope, lightheadedness, tremor, hallucinations, sexual side effects

Venlafaxine 37.5mg–225mg long-acting forms given once daily
  Side Effects: tachycardia, hypotension, sexual side effects, nausea, weight loss

Bupropion 100mg–300mg in divided doses
  Side Effects: lowers seizure threshold, nausea, constipation, headache, insomnia, rare Stevens-Johnson syndrome

Rehabilitation/psychosocial Support

Physical therapy is an important component of MS treatment, particularly in situations of progressive disability. Targeted assessment of gait and need for walking aids are particularly important. The physician should be alert for any changes in condition that may require retraining. Occupational therapy to help with adaptation to changing physical abilities and to evaluate home safety should be considered.

Cognitive impairment occurs in 35–65% of MS patients, and its incidence increases with age and disease duration. Indeed, it may be difficult to distinguish the effects of MS on cognitive decline from Alzheimer's disease (AD). There may be areas of overlap in terms of cognitive impairment in the MS and AD population, however in one study, AD patients demonstrated more severe impairment overall, and more difficulty with learning, memory, and verbal skills, while MS patients had greater relative impairment in attention, and incidental and psychomotor functions (Filley, Heaton et al. 1989). However, despite these differences in more established patients, early AD may be missed in the MS patient. Interestingly, a pathological study found no difference in the incidence of AD in MS patients and healthy controls, and no difference in the density of amyloid-beta plaques between the two groups (Dal Bianco, Bradl et al. 2008). If acute cognitive impairment ensues, testing for reversible causes of dementia should be considered. Acetylcholinesterase inhibitors, which slow cognitive decline in AD, have been shown to be effective in reducing MS-associated cognitive impairment, and in particular memory in small studies (Krupp, Christodoulou et al. 2004; Tsao and Heilman 2005; Christodoulou, Melville et al. 2006).

Depression is a common symptom in MS, and may be a result of the disease itself or medications, particularly beta-interferons. Counseling or antidepressants should be considered in persistent cases.

Adult-onset MS During Senescence

Multiple Sclerosis in the Elderly

Clinical Presentation

MS is a progressive disorder, and natural history data indicate that the majority of patients who present with an initial relapsing-remitting course will go on to develop secondary progressive MS (SPMS), thus making it likely that the majority of elderly MS patients will fall into this category. Primary progressive MS affects between 10–15% of MS patients, while 5% experience a progressive-relapsing course (Lublin and Reingold 1996). There are very few publications describing the clinical course and management of established MS in the elderly population. Since MS affects women in a 2:1 ratio, and women tend to live longer than men, a higher proportion of elderly MS patients will be women. Relapses become less frequent during the secondary progressive stage of MS; however, increasing difficulty with gait, balance, and bladder and bowel function pose significant challenges for the advanced MS patient. Disability levels correlate most strongly with current age, with later age at onset contributing to increased rate of disability progression (Trojano, Liguori et al. 2002). Cognitive impairment due to MS increases with age (Amato, Portaccio et al. 2006), and overlap with Alzheimer's disease may be present in some patients. Depression and anxiety are common in the MS population, and may be caused by the disease or reaction to increasing disability, as well as MS medications.

Diagnosis

The MRI picture of the elderly adult-onset MS patient typically demonstrates numerous and sometimes confluent lesions in the brain. Spinal cord lesions are frequently present. One study has demonstrated that gadolinium-enhancing lesions were less frequent in patients over the age of 50 years, compared to those under 40 years of age (Tortorella, Bellacosa et al. 2005), likely reflecting the differences between the RRMS and SPMS stages.

Treatment

The management of established MS in the aging population is as described in the preceding section on LOMS. Since disease-modifying treatments are generally ineffective in advanced secondary and primary progressive MS, maximizing symptomatic treatments and optimizing mobility and safety is generally the mainstay of therapy. A listing of common MS-associated symptoms and treatments are listed in Table 2. However, the side effects of symptomatic treatments and polypharmacy issues should be evaluated carefully.

Injurious falls are common in the elderly MS population and in one study were reported with an incidence of 50% (Peterson, Cho et al. 2008). For this and other reasons, maximizing gait stability and home safety through physical therapy and occupational therapy are essential. Driving may also be more challenging with increasing disability. Driving evaluations and rehabilitation should be considered in such cases.

Co-morbidities may play a role in the course and management of elderly MS patients. Cardiac disease, advanced pulmonary disease, and osteoporosis may increase disability and risk of falls. Poly-pharmacy and side effects of MS medications should be taken into account.

A common question that arises is the effect of menopause on MS. Unfortunately, only limited studies in this area exist. A questionnaire-based study of perimenopausal women found that 40% of women reported worsening of their MS symptoms related to menopause, whereas 56% reported no change and 5% a decrease in symptoms (Holmqvist, Wallberg et al. 2006). A similar study in 19 post-menopausal women found that 54% reported a worsening of symptoms with menopause, and 75% of those who tried hormone replacement therapy (HRT) reported some benefit (Smith and Studd 1992). To our knowledge, no studies have formally assessed the effects of menopause on disease course or MRI measures of disease severity in MS patients. Moreover, there are no studies evaluating effects of HRT or disease-modifying treatments in the post-menopausal population.

Summary and Future Directions

Late-onset MS is an increasingly recognized disorder; however, a broad differential diagnosis must be considered. Giving the increasing size of the aging population and longevity of MS patients due to improved medical care and treatments, there is an increasing population of elderly MS patients. These groups are more likely to have progressive forms of MS, likely due to the effects of the senescent immune system and CNS. Treatment of MS in the elderly populations must carefully consider efficacy and side effects of medications. Supportive management strategies are essential, and comorbidities should be considered. Further studies are required to elucidate the effects of hormones and menopause on the disease course of MS in the elderly, as well as understanding the effects and safety of MS treatments in this age group.

References

1993 (1993). "Interferon beta-1b is effective in relapsing-remitting multiple sclerosis. I. Clinical results of a multicenter, randomized, double-blind, placebo-controlled trial. The IFNB Multiple Sclerosis Study Group." *Neurology* **43**(4): 655–61.

1998 (1998). "Placebo-controlled multicentre randomised trial of interferon beta-1b in treatment of secondary progressive multiple sclerosis. European Study Group on interferon beta-1b in secondary progressive MS." *Lancet* **352**(9139): 1491–7.

1998 (1998). "Randomised double-blind placebo-controlled study of interferon beta-1a in relapsing/remitting multiple sclerosis. PRISMS (Prevention of Relapses and Disability by Interferon beta-1a Subcutaneously in Multiple Sclerosis) Study Group." *Lancet* **352**(9139): 1498-504.

2001 (2001). "Randomized controlled trial of interferon- beta-1a in secondary progressive MS: Clinical results." *Neurology* **56**(11): 1496-504.

Abe, M., K. Tsuchiya, et al. (2000). "Multiple sclerosis with very late onset: a report of a case with onset at age 82 years and review of the literature." *J Spinal Disord* **13**(6): 545-9.

Amato, M. P., E. Portaccio, et al. (2006). "The Rao's Brief Repeatable Battery and Stroop Test: normative values with age, education and gender corrections in an Italian population." *Mult Scler* **12**(6): 787-93.

Antel, J. and A. Bar-Or (2006). "Roles of immunoglobulins and B cells in multiple sclerosis: from pathogenesis to treatment." *J Neuroimmunol* **180**(1-2): 3-8.

Azzimondi, G., A. Stracciari, et al. (1994). "Multiple sclerosis with very late onset: report of six cases and review of the literature." *Eur Neurol* **34**(6): 332-6.

Barcellos, L. F., J. R. Oksenberg, et al. (2002). "Genetic basis for clinical expression in multiple sclerosis." *Brain* **125**(Pt 1): 150-8.

Beharka, A. A., M. Meydani, et al. (2001). "Interleukin-6 production does not increase with age." *J Gerontol A Biol Sci Med Sci* **56**(2): B81-8.

Burwick, R. M., P. P. Ramsay, et al. (2006). "APOE epsilon variation in multiple sclerosis susceptibility and disease severity: some answers." *Neurology* **66**(9): 1373-83.

Butteriss, D. J., A. Ismail, et al. (2003). "Use of serial proton magnetic resonance spectroscopy to differentiate low grade glioma from tumefactive plaque in a patient with multiple sclerosis." *Br J Radiol* **76**(909): 662-5.

Castle, S. C., K. Uyemura, et al. (1999). "Age-related impaired proliferation of peripheral blood mononuclear cells is associated with an increase in both IL-10 and IL-12." *Exp Gerontol* **34**(2): 243-52.

Castle, S. C., K. Uyemura, et al. (1999). "Antigen presenting cell function is enhanced in healthy elderly." *Mech Ageing Dev* **107**(2): 137-45.

Cazzullo, C. L., A. Ghezzi, et al. (1978). "Clinical picture of multiple sclerosis with late onset." *Acta Neurol Scand* **58**(3): 190-6.

Chakravarti, B., D. N. Chakravarti, et al. (1998). "Effect of age on mitogen induced protein tyrosine phosphorylation in human T cell and its subsets: down-regulation of tyrosine phosphorylation of ZAP-70." *Mech Ageing Dev* **104**(1): 41-58.

Chitnis, T. (2007). "The role of CD4 T cells in the pathogenesis of multiple sclerosis." *Int Rev Neurobiol* **79**: 43-72.

Chitnis, T., J. Imitola, et al. (2005). "Therapeutic strategies to prevent neurodegeneration and promote regeneration in multiple sclerosis." *Curr Drug Targets Immune Endocr Metabol Disord* **5**(1): 11-26.

Chitnis, T. and S. J. Khoury (2003). "Role of costimulatory pathways in the pathogenesis of multiple sclerosis and experimental autoimmune encephalomyelitis." *J Allergy Clin Immunol* **112**(5): 837-49; quiz 850.

Christodoulou, C., P. Melville, et al. (2006). "Effects of donepezil on memory and cognition in multiple sclerosis." *J Neurol Sci* **245**(1-2): 127-36.

Coles, A. J., D. A. Compston, et al. (2008). "Alemtuzumab vs. interferon beta-1a in early multiple sclerosis." *N Engl J Med* **359**(17): 1786-801.

Cossarizza, A., C. Ortolani, et al. (1996). "CD45 isoforms expression on CD4+ and CD8+ T cells throughout life, from newborns to centenarians: implications for T cell memory." *Mech Ageing Dev* **86**(3): 173-95.

Dal Bianco, A., M. Bradl, et al. (2008). "Multiple sclerosis and Alzheimer's disease." *Ann Neurol* **63**(2): 174-83.

de Seze, J., S. Delalande, et al. (2005). "Brain MRI in late-onset multiple sclerosis." *Eur J Neurol* **12**(4): 241-4.

Deguchi, K., M. Kamada, et al. (2001). "Postmenopausal changes in production of type 1 and type 2 cytokines and the effects of hormone replacement therapy." *Menopause* **8**(4): 266-73.

Delalande, S., J. De Seze, et al. (2002). "[Late onset multiple sclerosis]." *Rev Neurol (Paris)* **158**(11): 1082-7.

Endoh, M., S. I. Rapoport, et al. (1990). "Studies of experimental allergic encephalomyelitis in old mice." *J Neuroimmunol* **29**(1-3): 21-31.

Enzinger, C., S. Strasser-Fuchs, et al. (2005). "Tumefactive demyelinating lesions: conventional and advanced magnetic resonance imaging." *Mult Scler* **11**(2): 135-9.

Evangelou, N., M. Jackson, et al. (1999). "Association of the APOE epsilon4 allele with disease activity in multiple sclerosis." *J Neurol Neurosurg Psychiatry* **67**(2): 203-5.

Fagiolo, U., A. Cossarizza, et al. (1993). "Increased cytokine production in mononuclear cells of healthy elderly people." *Eur J Immunol* **23**(9): 2375-8.

Fazekas, F., S. Strasser-Fuchs, et al. (2001). "Apolipoprotein E epsilon 4 is associated with rapid progression of multiple sclerosis." *Neurology* **57**(5): 853-7.

Filley, C. M., R. K. Heaton, et al. (1989). "A comparison of dementia in Alzheimer's disease and multiple sclerosis." *Arch Neurol* **46**(2): 157-61.

Frasca, D., R. L. Riley, et al. (2005). "Humoral immune response and B-cell functions including immunoglobulin class switch are downregulated in aged mice and humans." *Semin Immunol* **17**(5): 378-84.

Frasca, D., R. L. Riley, et al. (2007). "Aging murine B cells have decreased class switch induced by anti-CD40 or BAFF." *Exp Gerontol* **42**(3): 192-203.

Gomez, C. R., V. Nomellini, et al. (2008). "Innate immunity and aging." *Exp Gerontol* **43**(8): 718-28.

Gonsette, R. E., L. Demonty, et al. (1977). "Intensive immunosuppression with cyclophosphamide in multiple sclerosis. Follow up of 110 patients for 2-6 years." *J Neurol* **214**(3): 173-81.

Gorczynski, R. M., C. Alexander, et al. (2007). "An alteration in the levels of populations of CD4+ Treg is in part responsible for altered cytokine production by cells of aged mice which follows injection with a fetal liver extract." *Immunol Lett* **109**(2): 101-12.

Gorczynski, R. M., M. Kennedy, et al. (1984). "Altered lymphocyte recognition repertoire during ageing. III. Changes in MHC restriction patterns in parental T lymphocytes and diminution in T suppressor function." *Immunology* **52**(4): 611-20.

Goronzy, J. J., W. W. Lee, et al. (2007). "Aging and T-cell diversity." *Exp Gerontol* **42**(5): 400-6.

Hafler, D. A., A. Compston, et al. (2007). "Risk alleles for multiple sclerosis identified by a genomewide study." *N Engl J Med* **357**(9): 851-62.

Haines, J. L., M. Ter-Minassian, et al. (1996). "A complete genomic screen for multiple sclerosis underscores a role for the major histocompatability complex. The Multiple Sclerosis Genetics Group." *Nat Genet* **13**(4): 469-71.

Hartung, H. P., R. Gonsette, et al. (2002). "Mitoxantrone in progressive multiple sclerosis: a placebo-controlled, double-blind, randomised, multicentre trial." *Lancet* **360**(9350): 2018-25.

Hohol, M. J., M. J. Olek, et al. (1999). "Treatment of progressive multiple sclerosis with pulse cyclophosphamide/methylprednisolone: response to therapy is linked to the duration of progressive disease." *Mult Scler* **5**(6): 403-9.

Holmqvist, P., M. Wallberg, et al. (2006). "Symptoms of multiple sclerosis in women in relation to sex steroid exposure." *Maturitas* **54**(2): 149-53.

Hommers, O. R., K. J. Lamers, et al. (1980). "Effect of intensive immunosuppression on the course of chronic progressive multiple sclerosis." *J Neurol* **223**(3): 177-90.

Hooge, J. P. and W. K. Redekop (1992). "Multiple sclerosis with very late onset." *Neurology* **42**(10): 1907-10.

Imitola, J., T. Chitnis, et al. (2006). "Insights into the molecular pathogenesis of progression in multiple sclerosis: potential implications for future therapies." *Arch Neurol* **63**(1): 25-33.

Irvine, K. A. and W. F. Blakemore (2006). "Age increases axon loss associated with primary demyelination in cuprizone-induced demyelination in C57BL/6 mice." *J Neuroimmunol* **175**(1-2): 69-76.

Jack, C., F. Ruffini, et al. (2005). "Microglia and multiple sclerosis." *J Neurosci Res* **81**(3): 363-73.

Jacobs, L. D., D. L. Cookfair, et al. (1996). "Intramuscular interferon beta-1a for disease progression in relapsing multiple sclerosis. The Multiple Sclerosis Collaborative Research Group (MSCRG)." *Ann Neurol* **39**(3): 285-94.

Johnson, A. B., S. Bake, et al. (2006). "Temporal expression of IL-1beta protein and mRNA in the brain after systemic LPS injection is affected by age and estrogen." *J Neuroimmunol* **174**(1-2): 82-91.

Johnson, A. B. and F. Sohrabji (2005). "Estrogen's effects on central and circulating immune cells vary with reproductive age." *Neurobiol Aging* **26**(10): 1365-74.

Johnson, K. P., B. R. Brooks, et al. (1995). "Copolymer 1 reduces relapse rate and improves disability in relapsing-remitting multiple sclerosis: results of a phase III multicenter, double-blind placebo-controlled trial. The Copolymer 1 Multiple Sclerosis Study Group." *Neurology* **45**(7): 1268-76.

Kamada, M., M. Irahara, et al. (2001). "Transient increase in the levels of T-helper 1 cytokines in postmenopausal women and the effects of hormone replacement therapy." *Gynecol Obstet Invest* **52**(2): 82-8.

Kamada, M., M. Irahara, et al. (2000). "Effect of hormone replacement therapy on post-menopausal changes of lymphocytes and T cell subsets." *J Endocrinol Invest* **23**(6): 376-82.

Kamada, M., M. Irahara, et al. (2001). "B cell subsets in postmenopausal women and the effect of hormone replacement therapy." *Maturitas* **37**(3): 173-9.

Kappos, L., C. H. Polman, et al. (2006). "Treatment with interferon beta-1b delays conversion to clinically definite and McDonald MS in patients with clinically isolated syndromes." *Neurology* **67**(7): 1242-9.

Kappos, L., B. Weinshenker, et al. (2004). "Interferon beta-1b in secondary progressive MS: a combined analysis of the two trials." *Neurology* **63**(10): 1779-87.

Kis, B., B. Rumberg, et al. (2008). "Clinical characteristics of patients with late-onset multiple sclerosis." *J Neurol* **255**(5): 697-702.

Krupp, L. B., C. Christodoulou, et al. (2004). "Donepezil improved memory in multiple sclerosis in a randomized clinical trial." *Neurology* **63**(9): 1579-85.

Kutzelnigg, A., C. F. Lucchinetti, et al. (2005). "Cortical demyelination and diffuse white matter injury in multiple sclerosis." *Brain* **128**(Pt 11): 2705-12.

Landfield, P. W., G. Rose, et al. (1977). "Patterns of astroglial hypertrophy and neuronal degeneration in the hippocampus of ages, memory-deficient rats." *J Gerontol* **32**(1): 3-12.

Leng, Q., Z. Bentwich, et al. (2002). "CTLA-4 upregulation during aging." *Mech Ageing Dev* **123**(10): 1419-21.

Letiembre, M., W. Hao, et al. (2007). "Innate immune receptor expression in normal brain aging." *Neuroscience* **146**(1): 248-54.

Li, D. K. and D. W. Paty (1999). "Magnetic resonance imaging results of the PRISMS trial: a randomized, double-blind, placebo-controlled study of interferon-beta1a in relapsing-remitting multiple sclerosis. Prevention of Relapses and Disability by Interferon-beta1a Subcutaneously in Multiple Sclerosis." *Ann Neurol* **46**(2): 197-206.

Lublin, F. D. and S. C. Reingold (1996). "Defining the clinical course of multiple sclerosis: results of an international survey. National Multiple Sclerosis Society (USA) Advisory Committee on Clinical Trials of New Agents in Multiple Sclerosis." *Neurology* **46**(4): 907-11.

Lucchinetti, C. F., R. H. Gavrilova, et al. (2008). "Clinical and radiographic spectrum of pathologically confirmed tumefactive multiple sclerosis." *Brain* **131**(Pt 7): 1759-75.

Lyon-Caen, O., G. Izquierdo, et al. (1985). "Late onset multiple sclerosis. A clinical study of 16 pathologically proven cases." *Acta Neurol Scand* **72**(1): 56-60.

Martinelli, V., M. Rodegher, et al. (2004). "Late onset multiple sclerosis: clinical characteristics, prognostic factors and differential diagnosis." *Neurol Sci* **25 Suppl 4**: S350-5.

McDonald, W. I., A. Compston, et al. (2001). "Recommended diagnostic criteria for multiple sclerosis: guidelines from the International Panel on the diagnosis of multiple sclerosis." *Ann Neurol* **50**(1): 121-7.

Mooradian, A. D., M. J. Haas, et al. (2003). "Age-related changes in rat cerebral occludin and zonula occludens-1 (ZO-1)." *Mech Ageing Dev* **124**(2): 143-6.

Mullen, J. T., T. K. Vartanian, et al. (2008). "Melanoma complicating treatment with natalizumab for multiple sclerosis." *N Engl J Med* **358**(6): 647-8.

Nishioka, T., J. Shimizu, et al. (2006). "CD4+CD25+Foxp3+ T cells and CD4+CD25-Foxp3+ T cells in aged mice." *J Immunol* **176**(11): 6586-93.

Noseworthy, J., D. Paty, et al. (1983). "Multiple sclerosis after age 50." *Neurology* **33**(12): 1537-44.

Paganelli, R., I. Quinti, et al. (1992). "Changes in circulating B cells and immunoglobulin classes and subclasses in a healthy aged population." *Clin Exp Immunol* **90**(2): 351-4.

Panitch, H., A. Miller, et al. (2004). "Interferon beta-1b in secondary progressive MS: results from a 3-year controlled study." *Neurology* **63**(10): 1788-95.

Panzara, M. A., C. Bozic, et al. (2008). "More on melanoma with transdifferentiation." *N Engl J Med* **359**(1): 99; author reply 99-100.

Parmenter, B. A., D. R. Denney, et al. (2007). "Cognitive impairment in patients with multiple sclerosis: association with the APOE gene and promoter polymorphisms." *Mult Scler* **13**(1): 25-32.

Paty, D. W. and D. K. Li (1993). "Interferon beta-1b is effective in relapsing-remitting multiple sclerosis. II. MRI analysis results of a multicenter, randomized, double-blind, placebo-controlled trial. UBC MS/MRI Study Group and the IFNB Multiple Sclerosis Study Group." *Neurology* **43**(4): 662-7.

Perini, P., M. Calabrese, et al. (2006). "Mitoxantrone versus cyclophosphamide in secondary-progressive multiple sclerosis: a comparative study." *J Neurol* **253**(8): 1034-40.

Peterson, E. W., C. C. Cho, et al. (2008). "Injurious falls among middle aged and older adults with multiple sclerosis." *Arch Phys Med Rehabil* **89**(6): 1031-7.

Phadke, J. G. (1990). "Clinical aspects of multiple sclerosis in north-east Scotland with particular reference to its course and prognosis." *Brain* **113 (Pt 6)**: 1597-628.

Plateel, M., E. Teissier, et al. (1997). "Hypoxia dramatically increases the nonspecific transport of blood-borne proteins to the brain." *J Neurochem* **68**(2): 874-7.

Polliack, M. L., Y. Barak, et al. (2001). "Late-onset multiple sclerosis." *J Am Geriatr Soc* **49**(2): 168-71.

Polman, C. H., P. W. O'Connor, et al. (2006). "A randomized, placebo-controlled trial of natalizumab for relapsing multiple sclerosis." *N Engl J Med* **354**(9): 899-910.

Polman, C. H., S. C. Reingold, et al. (2005). "Diagnostic criteria for multiple sclerosis: (2005) revisions to the "McDonald Criteria"." *Ann Neurol* **58**(6): 840-6.

Renshaw, M., J. Rockwell, et al. (2002). "Cutting edge: impaired Toll-like receptor expression and function in aging." *J Immunol* **169**(9): 4697-701.

Rosenkranz, D., S. Weyer, et al. (2007). "Higher frequency of regulatory T cells in the elderly and increased suppressive activity in neurodegeneration." *J Neuroimmunol* **188**(1-2): 117-27.

Rudick, R. A., W. H. Stuart, et al. (2006). "Natalizumab plus interferon beta-1a for relapsing multiple sclerosis." *N Engl J Med* **354**(9): 911-23.

Saija, A., P. Princi, et al. (1990). "Aging and sex influence the permeability of the blood-brain barrier in the rat." *Life Sci* **47**(24): 2261-7.

Schmucker, D. L., T. M. Owen, et al. (2002). "Expression of lymphocyte homing receptors alpha4beta7 and MAdCAM-l in young and old rats." *Exp Gerontol* **37**(8-9): 1089-95.

Sedano, M. I., P. Calmarza, et al. (2006). "No association of apolipoprotein E epsilon4 genotype with faster progression or less recovery of relapses in a Spanish cohort of multiple sclerosis." *Mult Scler* **12**(1): 13-8.

Shen, S., J. Sandoval, et al. (2008). "Age-dependent epigenetic control of differentiation inhibitors is critical for remyelination efficiency." *Nat Neurosci*.

Shimizu, J. and E. Moriizumi (2003). "Aging-dependent generation of suppressive CD4+CD25-R123loCD103+ T cells in mice." *Eur J Immunol* **33**(9): 2449-58.

Shimizu, J. and E. Moriizumi (2003). "CD4+CD25- T cells in aged mice are hyporesponsive and exhibit suppressive activity." *J Immunol* **170**(4): 1675-82.

Smith, R. and J. W. Studd (1992). "A pilot study of the effect upon multiple sclerosis of the menopause, hormone replacement therapy and the menstrual cycle." *J R Soc Med* **85**(10): 612-3.

Solana, R., G. Pawelec, et al. (2006). "Aging and innate immunity." *Immunity* **24**(5): 491-4.

Stewart, G. J., J. G. McLeod, et al. (1981). "HLA family studies and multiple sclerosis: A common gene, dominantly expressed." *Hum Immunol* **3**(1): 13-29.

Stichel, C. C. and H. Luebbert (2007). "Inflammatory processes in the aging mouse brain: participation of dendritic cells and T-cells." *Neurobiol Aging* **28**(10): 1507-21.

Takeuchi, T., M. Ogura, et al. (2008). "Late-onset tumefactive multiple sclerosis." *Radiat Med* **26**(9): 549-52.

Taub, D. D. and D. L. Longo (2005). "Insights into thymic aging and regeneration." *Immunol Rev* **205**: 72-93.

Thomas, D. C., R. J. Mellanby, et al. (2007). "An early age-related increase in the frequency of CD4+ Foxp3+ cells in BDC2.5NOD mice." *Immunology* **121**(4): 565-76.

Tortorella, C., A. Bellacosa, et al. (2005). "Age-related gadolinium-enhancement of MRI brain lesions in multiple sclerosis." *J Neurol Sci* **239**(1): 95-9.

Tremlett, H. and V. Devonshire (2006). "Is late-onset multiple sclerosis associated with a worse outcome?" *Neurology* 67(6): 954-9.

Trojano, M., M. Liguori, et al. (2002). "Age-related disability in multiple sclerosis." *Ann Neurol* 51(4): 475-80.

Tsao, J. W. and K. M. Heilman (2005). "Donepezil improved memory in multiple sclerosis in a randomized clinical trial." *Neurology* 64(10): 1823; author reply 1823.

Uyemura, K., S. C. Castle, et al. (2002). "The frail elderly: role of dendritic cells in the susceptibility of infection." *Mech Ageing Dev* 123(8): 955-62.

Vallejo, A. N. (2006). "Age-dependent alterations of the T cell repertoire and functional diversity of T cells of the aged." *Immunol Res* 36(1-3): 221-8.

van de Wyngaert, F. A., C. Beguin, et al. (2001). "A double-blind clinical trial of mitoxantrone versus methylprednisolone in relapsing, secondary progressive multiple sclerosis." *Acta Neurol Belg* 101(4): 210-6.

Weiner, H. L. (2008). "A shift from adaptive to innate immunity: a potential mechanism of disease progression in multiple sclerosis." *J Neurol* 255 **Suppl** 1: 3-11.

Weiner, H. L., G. A. Mackin, et al. (1993). "Intermittent cyclophosphamide pulse therapy in progressive multiple sclerosis: final report of the Northeast Cooperative Multiple Sclerosis Treatment Group." *Neurology* 43(5): 910-8.

Weksler, M. E. (2000). "Changes in the B-cell repertoire with age." *Vaccine* 18(16): 1624-8.

Wolinsky, J. S., P. A. Narayana, et al. (2001). "United States open-label glatiramer acetate extension trial for relapsing multiple sclerosis: MRI and clinical correlates. Multiple Sclerosis Study Group and the MRI Analysis Center." *Mult Scler* 7(1): 33-41.

Wolinsky, J. S., P. A. Narayana, et al. (2007). "Glatiramer acetate in primary progressive multiple sclerosis: results of a multinational, multicenter, double-blind, placebo-controlled trial." *Ann Neurol* 61(1): 14-24.

Yu, W. H., L. Go, et al. (2002). "Phenotypic and functional changes in glial cells as a function of age." *Neurobiol Aging* 23(1): 105-15.

Zhao, L., L. Sun, et al. (2007). "Changes of CD4+CD25+Foxp3+ regulatory T cells in aged Balb/c mice." *J Leukoc Biol* 81(6): 1386-94.

Zivadinov, R., R. A. Rudick, et al. (2001). "Effects of IV methylprednisolone on brain atrophy in relapsing-remitting MS." *Neurology* 57(7): 1239-47.

47 Sleep Disorders in Aging

Amanda A. Beck and Frank M. Ralls

Introduction

Sleep may be favorably viewed as a period of welcome disconnect from the active world, to restore alertness and energy and perhaps to dream. Sleep is vital to health and well-being. It is driven by strong homeostatic and circadian rhythms, and these will overcome higher cortical functions attempting to avoid sleep for prolonged periods. This simple process of sleep is, however, heavily influenced by both expectations and influences which are psychological, social, and cultural in nature. The normal process of aging interacts with illness, medication, and substance use to produce multiple sleep disorders which elders complain about; notably, difficulty falling asleep, staying asleep, early morning awakening, and excessive daytime sleepiness. These interactions also result in life threatening conditions such as obstructive sleep apnea, central sleep apnea and hypoventilation, which may cause fewer subjective complaints early on but contribute significantly to overall morbidity and mortality.

This chapter reviews the physiological changes in sleep with advancing age, circadian rhythm disorders, and insomnia; sleep disorders found in psychiatric disorders such as depression and anxiety; and in medical disorders such as gastroesophageal disease, asthma, chronic obstructive pulmonary disease, and cardiac disease. The last section covers sleep-related breathing disorders. Movement disorders in sleep are discussed in Chapter 29.

Effects of Aging on Adult Sleep and Sleep Architecture

The total amount of sleep that people get does not change dramatically in advanced age. Older adults report sleeping about 7–8 hours per night similar to the amount reported by younger adults (Stepnowsky and Ancoli-Israel 2008; Foundation NS 2010).

While it is clear to all that sleep is distinct from being awake, it is only with advent of advanced monitoring, notably polysomnography (PSG), that we describe sleep not as a homogenous state but as two distinct states: REM (rapid eye movement sleep) and NREM (non-rapid eye movement sleep) and components therein. Until recently, the scoring system of Rechschaffen and Kales (Stepnowsky and Ancoli-Israel 1968) was used to divide NREM sleep into Stage 1, 2 (commonly known as light sleep), 3, and 4 (commonly known as deep sleep). The difference in scoring stage 3 and 4 was based only on the percentage of slow wave sleep in a 30 second scored epoch of sleep. In 2007, the American Academy of Sleep Medicine published the Scoring Manual, which changed the criteria so that Stage 1 is labeled NREM1 (N1), Stage 2 is labeled NREM 2 (N2), and Stages 3 and 4 are combined and labeled NREM 3 (N3), while REM remains unchanged (Iber 2007).

Normal healthy well-slept young adults exhibit four or five alternating cycles of NREM and REM sleep across a prototypic night of sleep.

A cycle of NREM followed by REM is called a "sleep cycle." This is characterized by a sequential descent from lighter sleep (N1 and N2) into deep sleep (N3) and then an ascent to N2, and sometimes N1 ending in a period of REM.

NREM 1 is characterized by a decreased alpha rhythm (8–12 Hz), increasing theta (4–7 Hz), and slow rolling eye movements, and represents a transitional state usually lasting only a few minutes at the onset of sleep. NREM 2 is characterized by the presence of K complexes, and, in young adults, spindle activity (12–16 Hz), with a background of theta activity typically lasting 10–25 minutes. This is followed by a gradual build up of NREM 3, also known as slow wave sleep, and is characterized by high amplitude slow wave activity (> 75mV, 0.5–2.0 Hz) termed delta waves. A cluster of body movements often signal the more rapid return to N2, lasting 5–10 minutes. Then sleep transitions abruptly into REM sleep characterized by rapid eye movement and relative muscle atonia. The first REM of the night is often brief, lasting only 1–5 minutes, and often lacks the required eye movements, complicating the identification and scoring of this initial cycle.

Sleep cycles typically last from 90 to 110 minutes, the first is shorter (70 to 100 minutes) and later cycles range from 90 to 120 minutes. Spending 30 minutes or less from lights out to sleep onset (sleep latency) is considered normal. The time from sleep onset to REM sleep (REM latency) is usually within 70 to 90 minutes after sleep onset. NREM 3 dominates the cycles in the first third of the night and REM in the last third of the night. A healthy young adult spends about 75–80% of total sleep time (TST) in NREM sleep. Normally in young adults wake-after-sleep-onset (WASO) occupies less than 5% of the TST, N1 2% to 5%, N2 45% to 55%, N3 13% to 20%, with REM then 20% to 25% (Carskadon 2005).

While sleep architecture changes with advancing age from young adulthood though old age, the changes are not consistently progressive. The percentage of N3 decreases dramatically from teenage years to middle age. Thereafter, there is a much slower decline until about age 60 when it stabilizes at about 5–10% of total sleep time. N1 shows a minor increase and REM shows only a minor decrease to approximately 18%. Thus, NREM 2 occupies the vast majority of sleep. Latency to sleep onset increases. The number of arousals continues to increase with advancing age, resulting in more fragmented sleep as well as lighter sleep and more episodes of WASO Sleep efficiency (time asleep/time in bed) is typically 90% or above in healthy younger adults in the laboratory setting while that of healthy elders is more commonly 80% to 85%. While reasons for a daytime rest period are myriad, including cultural mores, seeking relief of pain, etc., it is likely that much of napping in elders is to compensate for the sleep loss during the nocturnal period.

Klerman and Dijk (2008) compared sleep propensity in 18 older and 35 younger subjects for 3–5 days and found in the absence of social and circadian restraints, sleep was 1.5 hours shorter in older (7.4 + 0.4 hours) than in younger subject (8.9 + 0.4 hours). The total sleep time for a 24-hour period in older adults may not decline, but elders may spend more time in bed at night attempting to obtain a greater total amount of sleep; sleep may become polyphasic with more frequent daytime naps to accomplish the same purpose.

The electroencephalogram (EEG) in sleep and wakefulness changes with aging. A study of the effect of aging on waking EEG of very healthy elders found the dominant posterior alpha rhythm of wake was higher than 8 HZ in those younger than 84 years, but between 7 and 8 HZ in 1/4 of the 22 older subjects. Intermittent focal slowing in the temporal regions was seen in 50%, which correlated with white matter hyperintensities on magnetic resonance imaging (MRI) (Oken and Kaye 1992). Fast beta activity in the EEG increases with age, especially in women (Brenner et al. 1995). Intermittent rhythmic delta is maximal over the frontal regions and can be seen in normal elders at sleep onset, differentiated from pathological slowing by its disappearance in deeper stages of sleep (Katz and Horowitz 1982). Slowing of alpha rhythm below 8 HZ intermixed with theta and delta activity is seen in the waking EEG of elders with dementia. Some have attributed slowing of the alpha rhythm in elders to age-related changes in cerebral blood flow (Obrist et al. 1963).

EEG patterns of sleep are also affected by aging even among healthy elders (Bliwise 1993; Dijk at al. 2001; Landolt et al. 1996). The amplitude, amount, and frequency of sleep spindles decrease. Frequency is reduced from 13–14 Hz to 12 Hz. The amplitude of slow wave activity in NREM 3 decreases with age and is attributed to reduction of neuronal synchronization in the neocortex, increasing skull thickness, and/or changes in the subarachnoid space. REM density (number of eye movements per minute of REM sleep) decreases with advancing age even among healthy elders (Darchia et al. 2003; Ficca et al. 2004; Ficca et al. 1999), and was shown by Spiegel et al. (1999) to correlate with reduced cognitive impairment in elders at 14 year follow-up.

Circadian Rhythm

The term circadian is taken from the Greek circa (about) and dien (day). Circadian rhythms are generated by a circadian pacemaker located in the suprachiasmatic nucleus (SCN) of the hypothalamus (Edgar et al. 1993). These rhythms are found in every physiologic and behavioral process including sleep, wakefulness, daily temperature fluctuations and endocrine cycles. The SCN consists of approximately 20,000 neurons located in the anterior hypothalamus. The basic mechanism by which the SCN generates and maintains a rhythm is via an autoregulatory feedback loop in which gene products regulate their own expression through phosphorylation and dephosphorylation. The feedback loop consists of four main proteins: period (PER), cryptochrome (CRY), and the transcriptional factors CLOCK and BMAL1. CLOCK and BMAL1 combine and form a complex that activates the transcription of CRY and PER genes to increase the production of the proteins CRY (CRY1 and CRY2) and PER (PER1, PER2, and PER3). These in turn inhibit the activity of the transcriptional factors CLOCK and BMAL1 and shut off their own transcription. Once CRY and PER levels drop off through degradation, the cycle is restarted by activation of the CLOCK and BMAL1 complex (Takimoto et al. 2005). Polymorphisms in the PER3 gene have been associated with increased predisposition to Delayed Sleep Phase Syndrome (DSPS), a condition whereby the individual falls asleep at progressively later times at night (Wyatt 2004). Advanced sleep phase syndrome (ASPS) is associated with a hypophosphorylation in the PER2 gene and affected individuals suffer from an abnormal advancement of the major sleep period.

Patients with ASPS usually report sleep onset of 6–9 PM and early morning awakening of 1–5AM (Reid 2001).

A consistent finding in aging is phase advance, related to going to bed earlier. This coincides with the nadir of endogenous body temperature occurring earlier, and often with earlier initiation of hormone cycles. Van Coevorden (1991) and coworkers found that the cycles of cortisol and thyroid stimulating hormone occurred 1–1.5 hours earlier in elders as compared to younger subjects. Growth hormone release is tightly coupled with the first third of the night and was found to be phase advanced along with sleep onset in elders. Dampened circadian amplitude of circulating growth hormone, thyroid stimulating hormone, and melatonin have also been reported (van Cauter et al. 1996). Some authors have suggested that the phase advance found in elders is secondary to a shortened period of the circadian oscillator (Tau), but research on this in published studies reveal inconsistent results.

Melanopsin-containing retinal ganglion cells are especially sensitive to blue wave light (450–495 nm) and constitute the major photoreceptors for the circadian clock and thus promote wakefulness (Rollag et al. 2003). It has been suggested that aging may decrease the circadian response to light because of cataracts or yellowing of the lens, which markedly reduces transmission of blue light (Dillon et al. 2004). Some studies have shown a decline in melatonin level with age while another study has shown the impact of light to suppress melatonin release at night is reduced with age (Dillon et al. 2004). Photic information from the retina reaches the SCN via the retinohypothalamic tract. The SCN send regulatory signals to other sleep and wake promoting centers in the ventrolateral preoptic nuclei (VLP) and the locus coerulus (LC) via neural pathways such as the dorsomedial and subparaventricular zones of the hypothalamus (Saper et al. 2005).

Circadian amplitude refers to the difference between peak and nadir of a particular sleep/wake related variable and determines the robustness of its influence. Human studies have shown decreased amplitude in body temperature rhythms in older men but less so in older women (Touitou 2001; Richardson et al. 1982; Vitiello et al. 1986). One study reported reduced circadian amplitude thought to be caused by a reduction in the nocturnal nadir of cortisol rather than, as expected, by a decrease in daytime peak cortisol level (van Coevorden et al. 1991). Not all studies have shown consistent results in the changes in melatonin and core body temperature amplitude changes, suggesting that factors other than chronological age serve as stronger influences (Naylor and Zee 2006).

The inherent circadian oscillator has an endogenous period or Tau. It is close to the standard 24-hour day but most studies have found it to be a little longer at about 24.2 hours. Multiple external factors called "zeitgebers" derived from the German term for "time givers" contribute to synchronizing these rhythms into a steady "entrained state." Light exposure is the most important zeitgeber but physical activity is also important in humans. Without daily adjustments by zeitgebers, the human daily cycle would gradually prolong, causing a drift backward around the clock.

Circadian phase refers to timing of the circadian-related event with respect to the external clock. Phase advance occurs when these events come earlier than would be normal and phase delay when these come later than would be normal based on healthy young adults. A consistent finding in aging is phase advance of the typical time in bed and out of bed (Monk, Buysse, and Reynolds 1995; Monk, Buysse, and Reynolds 1992). This coincides with advances in the nadir of endogenous body temperature and often with advances in hormone rhythms. Van Coevorden (Van Coevorden 1991) and coworkers found that the rhythms of cortisol and thyroid stimulating hormone all occurred 1 to 1.5 hours earlier in elderly as compared to younger subjects. Growth hormone release is tightly coupled with the first third of the night and was found to be advanced along with sleep onset in elders most likely due to sleep onset timing (Monk, Buysse, and Reynolds 1992; Benloucif, Masana, and Dubocovich 1997). Some authors have suggested that the phase advance found in elders is secondary to a shortened Tau or endogenous day. However, this literature is primarily in animal studies and has shown inconsistent results (Valentinuzzi et al. 1997; Possidente, McEldowney, and Pabon 1995; Van Reeth et al. 1992).

The physiologic propensity for sleep is determined by two opposing processes: circadian factors and homeostatic factors. Circadian factors determine the timing, duration, and characteristic of sleep. Homeostasis refers to the need to compensate for prior sleep deprivation and is dependent directly on the prior amount of time awake as well as any sleep debt left from prior nights. The melatonin and body temperature rhythms exert significant influences on sleepiness. Melatonin is a lipid-soluble hormone released from the pineal gland that has sleep-promoting effect. Melatonin is secreted throughout the night, but levels begin to rise approximately two hours before habitual sleep time. Plasma levels usually peak in the early morning hours and then progressively fall. Light exposure shuts down melatonin release. Body temperature falls during the night with its nadir during the second half of the usual nocturnal period. Maximum sleep propensity occurs at the time of temperature minimum. The nadir is generally between 3 and 5 AM with a small decline generally seen in early to mid-afternoon. Subjective sleepiness is interpreted by an individual's perception and is dependent on motivational, situational, and behavioral factors such as caffeine ingestion, in addition to circadian and homeostatic factors.

In simple terms, a circadian rhythm disorder is the inability to fall asleep at the "right time." The ability to shift circadian rhythms to new demands with new zeitgebers is impaired with aging. This is most noticeable with shift work and jet lag. In a study by Harma (Harma et al. 1994) on shift work, younger workers reported decreased sleepiness and crew members on long haul flight operations aged 50–60 averaged 3.5 times as much sleep loss. Laboratory experiments showed slower ability to change core body temperatures. Some but not all have reported a decreased effect of bright light exposure in phase shifting in elders. However, there is evidence that exercise is still effective in human elders in shifting dim light melatonin onset (DLMO) (Monk et al. 2000; Klerman et al. 2001; Baehr et al. 2003). Elders often decreased exposure to bright light, physical activity, and occupational and social obligations, which are effectively used by young adults as synchronizers for their circadian rhythm. Institutional living and cognitive dysfunction furthereduce the ability of elders to compensate for intrinsic deficits in their circadian rhythm (Ancoli-Israel et al. 1997).

Some studies have shown efficacy in using bright light therapy in elders with sleep maintenance insomnia and early morning awakening (Campbell, Dawson, and Anderson 1993; Lack et al. 2005). Ancoli-Israel has devoted extensive effort to environment interventions, particularly bright light exposure, that improve the robustness of circadian rhythms and result in more effective sleep and daytime alertness (Ancoli-Israel et al. 2002; Ancoli-Israel et al. 2003). Others found that structured physical activity resulted in improved nighttime sleep (Naylor et al. 2000; Benloucif et al. 2004; King et al. 1997). King found that following a bedtime routine and increasing exposure to only 30 minutes of sunlight a day, resulted in improved night sleep and decreased daytime sleeping. Melatonin has proven effective in reducing sleep onset latency in melatonin deficient elders but the role for its use and that of the melatonin agonist agomelatine to produce significant phase shifts in broader populations is still unclear (Brzezinski et al. 2005; Pandi-Perumal et al. 2005).

Insomnia

Insomnia is described as the inability to fall asleep, or to stay asleep, or early morning awakening resulting in daytime impairment. Complaints are more common in women and increase with advancing age (Foundation NS 2003). Prevalence overall is 40% greater in women than men. Complaints are stable through adulthood (16%) for both combined, and there is a marked increase after age 70 (23%) for men and after age 80 for women (41%) (Lichstein et al. 2006). This sharp rise is less likely in African Americans (Durrence and Lichstein 2006). It is generally thought that older adults are more likely to have sleep maintenance insomnia because of laboratory findings of lighter and more fragmented sleep. However, all types of insomnia including delayed sleep onset and early morning awakenings are observed in older adults (Foundation NS 2003). While patients with primary or psychophysiological insomnia complain of fatigue, difficulty with attention, concentration, memory, and incompletion of tasks (Buysse et al. 2007), objective measures of neurocognitive testing, MSLT (the propensity to fall asleep) or MWT (ability to stay awake) are not increased in this group. Objective sleepiness per se is more likely in patients with comorbid insomnia. The data associating insomnia and poor sleep in general with poor health, decreased physical functioning, increased falls, cognitive impairment, and increased mortality has recently been reviewed (Ancoli-Israel et al. 2009).

Insomnia may be an acute reaction to danger or stress. As such it serves a survival advantage. When it becomes chronic and a self-fulfilling prophecy, it becomes dysfunctional. Chronic insomnia may be primary in nature or co-morbid with other disorders such as depression, anxiety, pain, medical illness, neurological illness, substance or medication use, sleep apnea, and movement disorders.

Hyperarousal is the basis of primary insomnia. This may be a conditioned response to negative stimuli in the sleep environment or a fundamental trait that is continuous (Morin 2009). The hallmarks of psychophysiological insomnia are learned beliefs and conditioned behaviors which result in increased tension, which in turn is incompatible with the relaxation needed for sleep onset. Several conceptual models have been used to explain the development of chronic primary insomnia (Perlis and Pigeon 2005). Spielman (Speilman and Glovinski 1987) describes predisposing, precipitating, and perpetuating factors which help to explain the risk of some individuals for chronic primary insomnia. One common predisposing factor is a "worry-prone personality." The occurrence of a precipitating factor marks a change from healthy sleep to insomnia. These major stressful events such as illness, hospitalization, or loss of spouse occur more frequently in advanced age and likely contribute to rapid increase in complaints of insomnia in advanced age and likely contribute to the significant increase in insomnia in advanced age. Perpetuating factors maintain the pattern of insomnia. These include beliefs that a certain amount of sleep is needed, excessive emphasis on the negative consequences of changing sleep patterns, the expectation that sleep must remain as it was many years ago, and attempts to stay in bed longer to obtain more sleep. Insomnia may be chronic and unrelenting but more likely is intermittent and varies according to the degree of life stress.

Insomnia in elders is multifactoral. It is important to delineate causes which are age associated, those which began earlier and have persisted into advancing age, and those which are the result of social, psychological, and physical disability occuring with advanced age. Assessment involves differentiating those normal age-related changes in sleep from potentially treatable causes of insomnia (Morgan 2000). Treatment should focus on the factors most amenable to change and those perceived by the patient as important.

Treatment is based on a working partnership between the patient and the clinician. The goal is to improve sleep so that overall well-being and function are improved. However, insomnia is a chronic disorder. The patient will become a better sleeper but may not achieve the sleep quality of an individual not predisposed to insomnia and is at risk for recurrent symptoms.

Treatment for insomnia includes psychological and behavioral treatments such as cognitive behavioral therapy (CBT) as well as the judicious use of hypnotics. Some studies indicate that CBT is as effective as medication in treating insomnia with the benefit of fewer side effects (Moran 1993). Treatment for comorbid insomnia adds the treatment of the associated condition and its features contributing to poor sleep.

The ideal hypnotic induces sleep rapidly, sustains sleep, preserves normal sleep architecture, and leaves the individual feeling well rested in the morning. It does not contribute to cognitive, psychomotor, or motivational deficits during the day. It maintains potency for months or years, has low toxicity, (Buysse 2000) and is affordable.

Sleep-promoting medications are the most common prescribed treatments for insomnia in all ages but use is much more common in community-dwelling elders (3% to 21% for men and 7% to 29% for women) (Ohayon et al. 1998) compared to only 2% to 4% for younger adults (Maggi et al. 1998). The U.S. Federal Drug Administration officially recognizes nine drugs in two classes for the treatment of insomnia. All but one are in the class of benzodiazepine receptor agonists (BZRAs), the "classic benzodiazepines" estazolam, flurazepam, quazepam, temazepam and triazolam; and the more selective and rapid onset "Z" drugs, shorter acting zaleplon (T1/2=1 hr), zolpidem (T1/2 = 2.5 hours), and longer acting escopiclone (T1/2 =6 hours). A relative zopiclone has been approved outside of the U.S. for many years. These drugs target the gama-aminobutyric acid (GABA) type A receptor, the predominant inhibitory receptors in the brain. However, GABA A has two receptor subtypes referred to an omega 1 and omega 2. The "Z" drugs interact preferentially with omega 1 receptors which have a hypnosedative action. Benzodiazepines interact with both omega 1 and omega 2, which leads to the adverse effects on cognitive performance and memory (Terzano et al. 2003). Classic benzodiazepines have been associated with reduced slow wave sleep and REM and with residual sedation. Discontinuation of these drugs may result in rebound insomnia (hypnotic dependent insomnia). Both classes of BZRAs have demonstrated efficacy in treating late-life insomnia (Stepnowsky and Ancoli-Israel 2008; Chasens et al. 2007; Dolder, Nelson, and McKinsey 2007; Ancoli-Israel et al. 2005; Gottlieb 1990; Kupfer and Reynolds 1997). Most BZRAs are indicated for short-term use (several weeks). Zaleplon has a very short half life and may be useful in initiating sleep or returning a patient to sleep after awakening. A one-year open label clinical trial with zaleplon showed persistentffectiveness with a favorable safety profile (Chasens et al. 2007). Long acting escopiclone and the modified release form of zolpidem are indicated for sleep onset and maintenance insomnia and have been approved for continued use for six months. Ramelteon is the only drug in its class, and though structurally unrelated to melatonin, is a melatonin type 1 (MT1) and type 2 (MT2) agonist. Its main value has been to reduce sleep onset latency, but its effects overall have been modest (Haimov et al. 1995; Roth, Stubbs, and Walsh 2005). However, there is no evidence of tolerance, withdrawal, rebound insomnia, cognitive or psychomotor impairment, or daytime sedation. Because of this favorable safety and tolerability profile, it may be attractive for use in elders; it has the additive benefit that it is not a scheduled substance by the FDA. Some bizarre sleep-related behaviors (sleepwalking, sleep eating, sleep driving, sleep sex, hallucinations, and amnesic events) have been

reported primarily with the BZRAs, resulting in an FDA warning in 2007 for all primary benzodiazepine receptor agonists, as well as ramelteon. This risk is increased when the drugs are combined with other sedatives, alcohol, or used in higher-than-recommended doses. No reports thus far have implicated increased age as a risk for these adverse events. However, it is prudent to reduce the dose with advanced age and vital to warn patients of these potential side effects. Melatonin is available over the counter, rapidly absorbed, and has a short half life. It has shown some value in treating sleep onset disorders in elders, particularly in those who are melatonin deficient. Melatonin is also helpful in producing phase shifts for night workers. It is useful as a means to entrain circadian rhythms in totally blind individual who cannot use environmental cues. The only side effect observed has been sedation (Buscemi et al. 2005).

Sedating antidepressants such as tricyclic antidepressant (TCAs), trazadone, and mirtazipine are some of the most commonly prescribed agents for chronic insomnia. This is in spite of minimal data regarding efficacy and lack of FDA indication. They have been used for neuropathic pain control with the desired side effect of sedation. Their sedating properties are probably mediated by their agonistic effects on histamine type 1 (H1), serotonin type 2 (5HT2), and alpha adrenergic type 1 receptors. While TCAs in low doses have been reported helpful in primary insomnia, they can impact sleep architecture, most notably reduction of REM sleep. REM atonia may be lost, and sleep disorders already a problem in older adults such as restless legs syndrome and periodic limb movement disorder may be increased (Wilson and Argyropoulos 2005). Orthostatic hypotension and prolonged QT syndrome are side effects which can be highly lethal in accidental or intentional overdose. Dry mouth, constipation, and other anticholinergic effects are common limiting complaints. Trazadone has historically been one of the most frequently prescribed hypnotics, usually in low doses of 50–100 mg at bedtime. There is a wide safety profile, given that antidepressant doses are 300–500 mg/day. A morning hangover and excessive daytime sleepiness can be limiting factors. However, its cost is low, access is not restricted as a scheduled substance, and there is no labeling preventing long-term uses. One study in younger adults comparing trazadone to zolpidem showed efficacy of both in the first week of use (Walsh and Erwin 1998). The most consistent architectural finding has been an increase in SWS which could be useful in elders. Mirtazipine has emerged as a popular hypnotic for use in elders. The sedative effect of mirtazipine is strong at low dose (5–15 mg) as well as in the antidepressant therapeutic range of 15–45 mg. There are relatively few data on its use in insomnia, especially in elders. Atypical antipsychotics such as quetiapine and olzanapine have also been used increasingly for insomnia and are effective in treating insomnia comorbid with psychiatric illness. There is an increased risk for weight gain, abnormal glucose metabolism including insulin resistance and diabetes, as well as daytime sedation and sudden onset diabetic ketoacidosis. In addition, all atypical antipsychotics carry a "black box" warning for sudden death in elderly patients with dementia.

Several anticonvulsants acting on the GABA system have been used for insomnia. As a group, they have low toxicity and are not controlled substances. They can also be used for their sedative side effects while treating a primary disorder. Gabapentin has been shown to improve insomnia in an open label study of alcoholics with insomnia (Karam-Hage and Brower 2003)and increases slow wave sleep in normal adults (Foldvary-Schaefer 20002). There is little direct data on insomniacs and elders. Side effects include daytime sedation, cognitive slowing, dizziness, and leucopenia.

Pregabalin approved for the treatment of fibromyalgia was also designed as a GABA analog. When compared to alprazolam, both reduced sleep latency and decreased REM amount. Pregabalin lead to significant increase in slow wave sleep. Side effects are similar to gabapentin (Hindmarch, Dawson, and Stanley 2005). Tiagabine inhibits GABA reuptake through inhibition of the GABA transporter. In one of the few placebo-controlled studies in elder insomniacs, doses of 4–8 mg increased slow wave sleep and 6–8 mg decreased awakenings. However daytime sleepiness and adverse events were worse (Roth, Wright, and Walsh 2005; Walsh et al. 2005).

Self-medication with alcohol and over-the-counter drugs (OTC) is frequent in individuals of any age with insomnia. Antihistamines such as diphenhydramine and doxyalamine are in almost all OTC sleep aides. Mild sedation has been found in the limited studies on these agents. However, the significant anti-cholinergic side effect profile of dry mouth, dizziness, constipation and urinary retention, cognitive impairment, confusion, tinnitus, increased intraocular pressure, and daytime hangover make these unwise choices for elders in particular.

Cognitive behavioral therapy (CBT) is a set of methods involving the patient directly in the process of improving in insomnia. It requires the active participation of the patient, including inter-session homework, so that cognitive impairment may limit its success. Many clinical trials have demonstrated the ability of older adults to successfully participate in CBT. A meta-analysis by Irwin (Irwin, Cole, and Nicassio 2006 73B) compared the efficacy of CBT in middle age to older patients. While stronger treatment effects were seen in sleep efficiency and total sleep time for younger patients, there was no difference between age groups in improvement in sleep quality, sleep onset latency, and waking after sleep onset. While both medication and CBT can be beneficial, changes made through CBT are more likely to persist once active treatment with either is discontinued.

The most widely used techniques in older adults are progressive relaxation, passive relation, stimulus control which limits bedroom use to sleep and sex, sleep restriction which limits time in bed to little more than that actually spent sleeping (Speilman and Glovinski 2007; Bootzin 2000), sleep compression which prescribes a gradual reduction of time in bed (Lichstein et al. 2001), cognitive therapy which changes self-defeating thoughts, and sleep education and sleep hygiene which produce functional sleep behaviors and discourage dysfunctional ones (Reidel 2000). Irwin et al.'s (2006) meta-analysis compared the efficacy of CBT in middle age and older patients. While stronger treatment effects were seen in sleep efficiency and total sleep time for the younger patients, there was no difference between age groups' improvement in sleep quality, sleep onset latency, and wake after onset (Irwin, Cole, and Nicassio 2006). Overall, CBT has proven to be as effective as medication with fewer side effects (Engle-Friedman et al. 2001).

Sleep in Psychiatric and Medical Disorders

Insomnia and hypersomnia are prominent findings in many psychiatric and medical disorders. Comorbid insomnia was previously thought best treated by targeting the underlying conditions. There is mounting evidence that comorbid insomnia has a bidirectional relationship with its associated illnesses. This means that treatments which also directly target the insomnia are vital in enhancing the treatment of the underlying psychiatric illness. Both CBT and medication can be effective components of therapy, although the use of CBT may be impaired by the cognitive impairments of the psychopathology (Rybarczyk et al. 2005). Exploiting the side effects of psychiatric pharmacotherapy can be an effective means of comprehensive treatment, e.g., using sedating antidepressants, antipsychotics, and mood stabilizers when insomnia

is a prominent co-morbidity (NIH State of the Science Conference Statement 2005; Stepanski and Rybarczyk 2006).

Treatment of co-morbid fatigue and hypersomnia is a source of larger debate. Until recently, stimulants (norepinephrine/dopamine reuptake inhibitors and agonists) were the only professional treatments available for hypersomnia and fatigue. The risk of abuse and potent adverse side effects limited their use. With the release of modafinil and armodafinil, the pressure for use in multiple fatigue-related illnesses has increased. The science has not yet confirmed the safe use of these substances in the sleepiness and fatigue of comorbid disorders especially in elders. Hopefully, further investigation will clarify these issues.

Depression and anxiety are significant causes of morbidity and functional impairment in both the medically healthy and medically impaired population over 65. Insomnia has a stronger association with depression in the primary care setting than any other medical condition (Katz and McHorney 2002). Insomnia as a new complaint in elders also predicts depression in the near future even in those not currently depressed (Almeida and Pfaff 2005; Livingston, Blizard, and Mann 1993). About 8% of people in the general population complain of hypersomnia and that in itself is also predictive of depression, particularly bipolar affective disorder and seasonal affective disorder (Breslau et al. 1996). Elders who report daytime sleepiness are also more likely to report symptoms of depression. Objective findings in the sleep laboratory show disturbances in older people in general consistent with those of younger depressed people (Benca et al.1992). Risk of new onset depression is increased in the older population with the increased burden of ill health bereavement and caregiving. Most anxiety disorders in elders are a continuation of those seen earlier in life with the exception of some increase in agoraphobia (Barczi 2006). Generalized anxiety disorder and age-emergent anxiety have the same basis of hyperarousal commonly found in people who have not been diagnosed with an anxiety disorder (Barczi 2006).

While the prevalence of alcohol, nicotine, and caffeine abuse declines with age, these continue to be a source of illness and contributors to poor sleep. Community rates of alcohol dependence in the geriatric population are estimated at 2% of men and 1% women. This is much higher at 4% in the clinic population and 23% in the hospital population. Overlap of excessive alcohol and nicotine use is common (Grant 1997; Atkinson 2000). Acute alcohol ingestion initially decreases sleep latency and increases sleep continuity but as it metabolizes during the night it leads to fragmented sleep. Alcohol also lowers the tone of upper airway muscles and raises arousal threshold, potentially worsening sleep apnea.

Pain or discomfort in the broad sense is probably the most common mechanism for disturbed sleep. In the general population aged 55–84, 19% reported that pain disrupted their sleep a few times a week and 12% reported almost nightly disruption (Foley et al. 2004). For those with chronic pain seeking professional care, more than half complain of insomnia (Latham and Davis 1994). Osteoarthritis is one of the most common chronic diseases in older adults, affecting 50–80%. Nearly 60% of those with arthritis experience pain during the night with the vast majority of those reporting difficulty staying asleep and, to a lesser extent, difficulty getting to sleep or awakening too early (MacLean 2001; Wilcox et al. 2000). Cognitive behavioral therapy has been demonstrated effective in this group of patients.

Gastroesophageal reflux (GERD) increases in frequency with age and obesity. Nocturnal reflux can cause sleep disruption and patients may not even be aware of the cause. Since nocturnal cough and hoarseness can also be unrecognized symptoms of GERD, the prevalence is likely significantly underestimated. Obstructive sleep apnea increases the likelihood of GERD and the inflammation from pharyngeal acid exposure increases the likelihood of obstructive sleep apnea.

Chronic obstructive pulmonary disease (COPD) leads to disrupted sleep from increased work of breathing and hypoxia. Such patients complain both of insomnia and daytime hypersomnia. Overlap syndrome refers to the coexistence of chronic obstructive pulmonary disease and obstructive sleep apnea. The prevalence of overlap syndrome in Veterans Administration studies can be as high as 40% (Mapel, Dedrick, and Davis 2005). Oxygen therapy in COPD can correct hypoxia but underlying mechanical factors persist resulting in persistent sleep disturbance (O'Brien and Whitman 2005). Some obese elders also overlap obstructive sleep apnea with obesity hypoventilation and some are unfortunate enough to have both of these overlap with COPD as well. Treatment with positive airway pressure (PAP) therapy improves sleep quality and daytime sleepiness. However, even optimal treatment is not curative and significant impairment may persist.

As the prevalence of chronic illness increases with advancing age, the number of medications taken also increases. Studies of elders in outpatient setting demonstrate that after age 65, 57% of women and 44% of men use at least five medications and that 12% of both women and men use more than ten medications. The most common classes of medications are anti-hypertensives and diuretics, anti-inflammatory agents (NSAIDs), and hypnotics (Kaufman et al. 2002).

Although aimed to alleviate distress, the following medications can impact sleep negatively and produce distress that neither patient nor clinician anticipated. Medications with histamine 1 (H1) antagonism have a greater likelihood for sedation and cognitive impairment in elders. These include antihistamines, antispasmodics, antipsychotics, antiemetics and anti-parkinsonian drugs. Commonly used drugs in this class are OTC allergy medications, OTC hypnotics, and prescription antidepressants (tricyclic antidepressants, mirtazipine) and oxybutynin. Dopamine agonists can produce excessive sleepiness and sleep attacks. Anticonvulsant agents often used to ameliorate pain produce more sleepiness in older adults. Opiate analgesics being used more commonly for non-malignant pain have sedation and respiratory suppression as a major side effect in elders. The synergistic effects when used in combination with other sedating agents are particularly problematic. Other medications disrupt sleep, resulting in insomnia, notably corticosteroids and beta agonists used in exacerbations of asthma and COPD. While depression can cause insomnia, some stimulating antidepressants can contribute as well, notably SSRIs (fluoxetine, sertraline, etc), SNRIs (venlafaxine, duloxetine, etc), and buproprion. Although stimulants are contraindicated in elders, some are still used as adjunctive therapy for depression and for residual daytime sleepiness in treated sleep apnea. Great caution is recommended in the use of these in elders to avoid precipitating or exacerbating symptoms not only of sleep disruption, but delirium and cardiovascular illness as well.

Sleep Disordered Breathing

The respiratory system consists of central controllers in the medulla aided by supra medullary components and chemoreceptors, pulmonary and upper airway receptors, the thoracic bellows consisting of respiratory and other thoracic muscles, nerves and bones, and the upper and lower airways themselves. These components are closely integrated. Breathing is controlled during wakefulness by two separate and independent systems, the metabolic or autonomic and the voluntary or behavioral. Both metabolic and voluntary systems operate during wakefulness. Breathing during sleep is entirely dependent on the inherent rhythmicity of the autonomic respiratory control system in the medulla. The reticular activating system exerts a tonic influence on brainstem respiratory neurons while variable influences come from variable activities such as swallowing and speech (Chokroverty 2009).

The function of ventilation is to maintain blood gas homeostasis with normal partial pressures of oxygen (PO_2) and carbon dioxide (PCO_2). The hypoxic ventilatory response is mediated through the carotid body. The hypercapnic drive is mediated through the medullary chemoreceptors and to a lesser extent through the carotid body chemoreceptors. Both hypoxia and hypercapnea stimulate breathing but the sensitivity with which they do this is quite different. The hypoxic response displays a hyperbolic curve that shows a sudden increase in ventilation when PO_2 falls below 60 mm HG. However, the hypercapnic ventilator drive is linear. When the PCO_2 falls below an individual's unique level, the apnea threshold, breathing stops. When the PCO_2 level rises above this, ventilation resumes. The absolute PCO_2 value which is the apnea threshold varies widely among individuals (Douglas 2005). This results from individual chemoreceptor sensitivity (a mutation in Phox2B, has been shown to cause reduced chemosensitivity from medications such as propofol and diseases such as CHF (Eckert et al. 2007).

Ideally, there is appropriate balance and compensation, but overshoot can occur with oscillation between hypo and hyperventilation and appears as a waxing and waning of the tidal volume in a pattern similar to Cheyne-Stokes breathing. This "transitional breathing" is normal for a very short period at the onset of sleep and may occur after arousal from sleep. The change in stimulation between wakefulness and sleep, and reduction in chemosensitivity at onset of sleep, contribute to this phenomenon.

During NREM sleep, ventilation falls secondary to a reduction in tidal volume that is due in a large part to increased upper airway resistance to airflow, resulting from hypotonia of the pharyngeal dilator muscles. After sleep onset, PCO_2 rises 2–8 mm HG, PO_2 decreases by 3–10 mm HG and arterial saturation (SAO_2) decreases by less than 2% (Douglas et al. 1992). As sleep deepens, respiration becomes stable and rhythmic and depends entirely on the metabolic control system. Hypoxic ventilatory response is decreased in men but not women in NREM sleep but is significantly decreased in both men and women during REM sleep (Schafer 2006). Hypercapnic ventilatory response also decreases by 20–50% during NREM sleep and even further in REM (Gothe et al. 1981; Douglas et al. 1982). As a result, increasing amounts of CO_2 are needed to stimulate ventilation and functional alveolar hypoventilation occurs. Intercostal muscles become hypotonic during sleep and atonic during REM. Phasic activity of the diaphragm is maintained but tonic activity is reduced during REM (McNicholas 1997; Hudgel and Hamilton 1994). Normal individuals also have a nocturnal increase in bronchoconstriction (Hetzel and Clark 1980). These cumulative changes render sleep, and REM sleep in particular, hazardous for those with predispositions to destabilization of breathing, upper airway closure, neuromuscular weakness, reactive airway disease, or the need for accessory muscle use.

Sleep-disordered breathing (SDB) is most commonly applied to apnea syndromes. However, it more broadly overlaps with other causes of nocturnal hypoventilation. This can occur from exogenous restrictive lung disease of obesity, neuromuscular disease, or rib cage deformity such as kyphosis commonly seen in elders. It can also occur from endogenous causes such as restrictive pulmonary diseases, nocturnal asthma, and chronic obstructive pulmonary disease.

Obstructive sleep apnea (OSA) occurs when there is sufficient increase in upper airway resistance during sleep to significantly impede airflow, producing turbulence during inspiration and closure or near closure at the end of exhalation. Meanwhile attempts to breathe continue.

Obstruction is due to reduced muscle tone of the airway dilator muscles: genioglossus, geniohyoid, tensor veli palatini, and posterior cricoarytenoid muscles, as well as the diaphragm and intercostal muscles. Obstruction, therefore, may occur at the level of the soft palate, base of tongue, or hypopharyngeal area and often occurs on multiple levels (Launois et al. 1993). Classic symptoms of obstructive sleep apnea are cessation of breathing followed by increasing loud snoring and then arousal. This arousal may range from only EEG defined arousal to wild flailing and vocalizations. In uncomplicated cases, witnessed periods of apnea coupled with "heroic snoring" (snoring audible to sleepers two bedrooms away is pathognomonic of OSA).

Central sleep apnea (CSA) occurs when no airflow occurs while the throat is open and there is no attempt to breathe. Symptoms of central apnea commonly seen are a cessation of breathing following by quiet return to deeper breathing with mild snoring during the hyperneic phase. The hyperventilatory phase is observed as the classic symptom of congestive heart failure, paroxysmal nocturnal dyspnea. Mixed apnea is a combination of these, most commonly a central component followed by an obstructive component (White 2005).

The 2007 American Academy of Sleep Medicine (AASM) Manual specifies that an apnea must last ten seconds or more and airflow must drop to 90% of its previous flow volume, i.e., there is 10% or less air flow remaining. A hypopnea is defined as an event lasting ten seconds or more with a reduction in airflow of 30% from previous flow, with a 4% drop in SaO_2, resulting in arousal. This is consistent with the Centers for Medicare and Medicaid (CMS) definition. An alternative definition for hypopnea (AASM) is a reduction of flow to 50% of previous flow with a 3% drop in SaO_2 resulting in an arousal. Upper airway resistance syndrome (UARS) is a milder form of obstructive sleep apnea in which there is mild resistance to flow in the upper airway, resulting in increased work of breathing and recurrent arousals from sleep. People with UARS commonly complain of insomnia as well as excessive daytime sleepiness (Guilleminault et al. 1993).

The gold standard for measurement of sleep disordered breathing is the in-laboratory standard polysomnography (PSG), which includes sensors for EEG activity, EMG activity of chin and legs, EOG activity for eye movements, EKG, oxygen saturation monitoring, pressure transducer to measure resistance to flow, thermister to measure airflow based on temperature changes between inhalation and exhalation, and respiratory bands to measure movement of the ribs and abdomen. Additional sensors may be added to address more specific questions. Ambulatory PSG with a more limited number of channels is being developed for diagnostic use in typical obstructive apnea patients without other complications. Severity of apnea is reported primarily with the apnea/hypopnea Index (AHI) defined as the frequency of apneas plus hypopneas per hour of sleep. The obstructive or central nature can be easily determined from standard PSG measures. However, hypopneas are more common events and cannot be truly classified as obstructive or central in nature without esophageal manometry to measure increasingly negative intrathoracic pressure consistent with upper airway obstruction. Apnea is described as obstructive if the majority of events are obstructive apneas and resistance to flow can be determined in the hypopneas. Apnea is described as central apnea if the majority of apneas are central in nature or there is predominant pattern of oscillatory breathing. More recently complex sleep-disordered breathing to describe a pattern across the night which is sometimes predominantly central in nature, sometimes obstructive, and often mixed has gained acceptance (Gilmartin, Daly, and Thomas 2005). The correct recognition of these patterns has become increasingly important with respect to understanding etiology and prescribing successful treatment.

In clinical practice, the AASM standards of practice are used. An AHI less than 5 is considered normal, 5–15 mild, 15–30 moderate, and above 30 severe (Gilmartin, Daly, and Thomas 2005). This includes obstructive, central, and mixed apneas in one index. Oxygen minimum is considered an interpretation of results but is not an essential component of the index. In epidemiological studies, various AHIs cutoffs have been used to define the presence of sleep apnea and the criteria often include an associated clinical consequence such as excessive daytime sleepiness. The prevalence of SDB increases with age and is more frequent in men than women. In middle age, from 30–60, the prevalence is estimated at between 2% for women and 4% for men (Young, Peppard, and Gottlieb 2002). The estimates of sleep-disordered breathing are much higher in older adults with a very broad range reported from 5% to 90% depending on the techniques employed, the population studied, and the definition of severity. Ancoli-Israel and coworkers reported a 44% prevalence of an AHI = 20 and 24% for an AHI >40 in a large community based sample of people 65–95 years old (Ancoli-Israel et al. 1991; Enright et al. 1996). In comparison, the Sleep Heart Health Study was designed specifically to find the consequences of sleep-disordered breathing. It evaluated a group of community-dwelling people from 40–98 years old. The prevalence of AHI ³15 increased each decade but flattened after age 60 to about 34%. Ancoli-Israel found the presence of AHI >20 to be 50% in demented elders and several other authors have reported higher prevalence in demented elders as well (Ancoli-Israel et al. 1991).

Risk factors for obstructive sleep apnea include male gender and obesity. Additionally family history, craniofacial structure (which predisposes to a small airway), smoking, ethnic background associated with mid-face hypoplasia and the use of alcohol and sedating medication all increase the risk. In middle age adults, 40% of those with a body mass index over 40 and 50% of those with a BMI over 50 had significant apnea (Kripke et al. 1997). The highest rates of progression in apnea with aging were among obese men. Menopause is also a risk factor with post-menopausal women having an SDB rate more like men of a similar age compared to premenopausal women or post menopausal women on estrogen replacement (Young et al. 2003; Shahar et al. 2003; Bixler et al. 2001). Risk factors for central and complex sleep disordered breathing include congestive heart failure, neuromuscular disease, and the use of narcotic respiratory suppressant medication. Methadone is particularly problematic, with Wang reporting a 30% prevalence of central sleep apnea in chronic users of methadone (Wang et al. 2005).

While sleep-disordered breathing has been associated with increased mortality in elders, it is probable that its role in mediating cardiovascular disease is the culprit in this association. While sleep-disordered breathing with recurrent arousals and sympathetic surges is an established risk factor for hypertension in younger adults, a weaker correlation has been found in elders. The Sleep Heart Health Study showed SDB increases the risk of CVD, defined as coronary artery disease, congestive heart failure, or stroke, by a third in middle age adults but not in elders (Haas et al. 2005). A number of studies have found a higher prevalence SDB, particularly an increase in central sleep apnea, in patients with congestive heart failure and more severe AHIs are significant predictors of poor outcome in this group. Improvement in the degree of heart failure improves the severity of the SDB (Verrier 2002). While it is likely that treatment of the sleep-disordered breathing has a positive effect on CHF, no studies thus far have reported on this effect. Hopefully, research in this treatment will demonstrate this efficacy in the near future.

A number of studies have documented the increased prevalence of SDB in patients who have suffered a stroke compared with age and gender-matched controls. The presence of SDB in the setting of acute stroke is an independent risk factor for mortality (Yaggi et al. 2007; Bassetti, Milanova, and Gugger 2006). SDB frequently persists after resolution of clinical stroke symptoms (Martinez-Garcia, Soler-Cataluna, and Ejarque-Martinez 2009). The Sleep Heart Health Study has also demonstrated the strong relationship between SDB and cardiac arrhythmia including atrial fibrillation, nonsustained ventricular tachycardia, and complex ventricular ectopy. With advanced age, however, the strength of these relationships weakens (Mehra et al. 2006).

There is a great interest in the association between SDB and impaired glucose homeostasis, insulin sensitivity, and diabetes. The Wisconsin Sleep Study cohort showed an elevation in type II diabetes for an AHI >15 when adjusted for age, gender, and BMI (Dopp, Reichmuth, and Morgan 2007). The Sleep Heart Health Study found SDB more common in diabetics but this association was explained by higher body mass index (BMI) (Resnick et al. 2003). Treatment trials with CPAP for a mean of 85 days in younger adults reduced HbA1c levels and increased insulin sensitivity. This effect was predominant in non-obese patients (Babu et al. 2005). The impact on glucose metabolism in older adults has not yet been determined.

Impairment in attention and concentration is the most consistent finding in cognitive impairment associated with SDB (Aloia et al. 2004). Sleepiness as a result of sleep fragmentation and sleep deprivation appears to be more closely associated with cognitive deficits than either severity of AHI or oxygen nadir (Dopp, Reichmuth, and Morgan 2007). In dementia of Alzheimer's type, SDB is increased with increasing severity of disease. Patients with Parkinson's disease have increased prevalence of SDB as neuronal degeneration progresses (Ancoli-Israel et al. 1991).

One of the challenges of diagnosis and treatment of SDB in the elderly is that symptoms of the disease are often misinterpreted as normal changes of aging. This includes snoring, an intermittent breathing pattern, excessive daytime sleepiness, and napping. Embarrassment about snoring may preclude elders, especially women, from mentioning this problem. Elders may have a bed partner whose hearing is impaired and therefore will not complain about snoring or apnea, or they live alone and are not even aware of the problem.

Symptoms of sleep-disordered breathing deserve routine evaluation in the clinical setting. However, elders with excessive sleepiness and high risk comorbid conditions such as multi-drug hypertension, diabetes, morbid obesity, and congestive heart failure deserve special attention. Evaluation of severity is similar to that of younger patients, with polysomnography producing the most credible results. However, more education and family involvement may be necessary. Overnight home oximetry may demonstrate the extent of oxygen deprivation to patients and their families and thereby facilitate collaboration in diagnosis and treatment. A short daytime "nap" to introduce the laboratory and CPAP may be helpful to desensitize patients to the procedures for diagnosis and treatment. A full night diagnostic study followed by an in-person discussion with the elder and family about treatment options may be needed more so than with younger patients. Medicare has approved the use of ambulatory polysomnography done in the patient's home for diagnosis of obstructive sleep apnea. This may seem more convenient for elders. However, many systems are cumbersome and confusing for the patient and family to use correctly at home. Additionally, ambulatory PSG is only indicated for patients with high probability of uncomplicated obstructive sleep apnea. Many elders are at risk for complex sleep apnea due to comorbid medical illness, making ambulatory PSG both practically and clinically limited in its usefulness.

Standard therapy for obstructive sleep apnea remains continuous positive airway pressure (CPAP) therapy, which delivers a constant pressure though a mask providing an air stint to the upper airway especially at the end of expiration when it is most vulnerable to collapse. If ventilation is also required, bi-level positive (BPAP) airway pressure is used. This produces a higher pressure with inhalation to deliver air deeper into closed small airways and then a significantly lower pressure on exhalation to allow passive recoil of the lungs to expel more carbon dioxide while maintaining adequate pressure for end exhalation stinting. Over recent years, many improvements have been made to continuous and bi-level positive airflow generators to include smaller units with integrated heated humidification, pressure relief with exhalation, auto-titrating units designed to increase or decrease pressure based on resistance to flow, and battery packs for travel. For patients with central apnea and complex sleep-disordered breathing, adaptive servo-ventilation has become available (Allam et al. 2007). These units have a set exhalation stint pressure determined in the sleep laboratory and then a computer algorithm in the unit adjusts flow to maintain minute ventilation with a back-up rate for prolonged central apnea. The mask interface between the machine and the patient has grown to more than 100 types ranging from those sitting at the tip of the nose to those covering most of the face. Improvements in these various devices continue to be made frequently. Therefore, patients who might not have been successful in using PAP therapy in the past may find success with the newer modalities. There are those who feel that the diagnosis and treatment of apnea is intolerable to elders in general and particularly those with dementia or neurological disease. However, clinical evidence indicates a high proportion of symptomatic elders can be successful particularly when treatment gives them relief of symptoms such as excessive daytime sleepiness and nocturnal dyspnea.

Standard alternatives to PAP therapy are oral appliance and upper airway surgery. An oral appliance is constructed by a mold of the patient's upper and lower jaw, generally with a mechanism to advance the mandible a few millimeters and produce more space in the upper airway. This is more effective in thin patients with milder apnea. Difficulty with temporomandibular joint disease and edentulousness make this treatment less useful for elders but no studies have addressed elders specifically. Surgery of the upper airway is frequently uvulopalatopharyngoplasty coupled with advancement of the jaw by hyoid suspension and genioglossus advancement or base of tongue reduction. Upper airway surgery is restricted to obstructive sleep apnea, has not been as successful as CPAP therapy, and is considered salvage therapy for those unable to use either PAP or dental appliance therapy. No definitive studies have been done on surgical treatment in elders and elders are often reticent to consider a surgery of this type.

Oxygen supplementation alone is often requested by elders who are unwilling or unable to tolerate PAP therapy. Given data that suggests that severity of the AHI in elders may not have the same clinical consequences that it has in younger adults, this is not an unreasonable thought. In cases where hypoxia is the predominant problem versus apnea with arousals, and in- laboratory studies demonstrate improvement in oxygenation without significant worsening in apnea length or hypoventilation, then oxygen therapy alone is a reasonable therapeutic choice.

Summary

In summary, there are many and reliable changes in sleep with aging; these changes are compounded by multiple medical diagnoses, the very common presence of multiple prescription medications and the nearly universal use of OTC sedatives and hypnotics by the elderly. The diagnosis of insomnia is complicated and requires quite a detailed, focused history. Improvement of sleep can be made with counseling on sleep hygiene, elimination of potentially offending medications, use of cognitive behavioral therapy and judicious prescription of hypnotic medication. A polysomnogram may or may not be needed for the diagnosis and treatment of insomnia. On the other hand, sleep disordered breathing usually requires a polysomnogram for an accurate diagnosis of obstructive or central sleep apnea leading to a precise recommendation for continuous or bi-level positive (BPAP) airway pressure assistance during sleep. Alternative treatments are available since many elderly do not tolerate well the recommended breathing devices.

References

Allam JS, Olson EJ, Gay PC, Morgenthaler TI. Efficacy of adaptive servoventilation in treatment of complex and central sleep apnea syndromes. *Chest.* Dec 2007;132(6):1839-1846.

Almeida OP and Pfaff JJ. Sleep complaints among older general practice patients: association with depression. *Br J Gen Pract.* Nov 2005;55(520):864-866.

Aloia MS, Arnedt JT, Davis JD, Riggs RL, and Byrd D. Neuropsychological sequelae of obstructive sleep apnea-hypopnea syndrome: A critical review. *J Int Neuropsychol Soc.* Sep 2004;10(5):772-785.

Ancoli-Israel S. Sleep and its disorders in aging populations. *Sleep Med.* Sep 2009;10 Suppl 1:S7-11.

Ancoli-Israel S, Gehrman P, Martin JL, et al. Increased light exposure consolidates sleep and strengthens circadian rhythms in severe Alzheimer's disease patients. *Behav Sleep Med.* 2003;1(1):22-36.

Ancoli-Israel S, Klauber MR, Butters N, Parker L, and Kripke DF. Dementia in institutionalized elderly: Relation to sleep apnea. *J Am Geriatr Soc.* Mar 1991;39(3):258-263.

Ancoli-Israel S, Klauber MR, Jones DW, et al. Variations in circadian rhythms of activity, sleep, and light exposure related to dementia in nursing-home patients. *Sleep.* Jan 1997;20(1):18-23.

Ancoli-Israel S, Kripke DF, Klauber MR, Mason WJ, Fell R, and Kaplan O. Sleep-disordered breathing in community-dwelling elderly. *Sleep.* Dec 1991;14(6):486-495.

Ancoli-Israel S, Martin JL, Kripke DF, Marler M, and Klauber MR. Effect of light treatment on sleep and circadian rhythms in demented nursing home patients. *J Am Geriatr Soc.* Feb 2002;50(2):282-289.

Ancoli-Israel S, Richardson GS, Mangano RM, Jenkins L, Hall P, and Jones WS. Long-term use of sedative hypnotics in older patients with insomnia. *Sleep Med.* Mar 2005;6(2):107-113.

Atkinson R. Substance abuse. In: Coffe C, Cummings, J., ed. *Textbook of geriatric neuropsychiatry*: American Psychiatry Press; 2000:367-400.

Babu AR, Herdegen J, Fogelfeld L, Shott S, and Mazzone T. Type 2 diabetes, glycemic control, and continuous positive airway pressure in obstructive sleep apnea. *Arch Intern Med.* Feb 28 2005;165(4):447-452.

Baehr EK, Eastman CI, Revelle W, Olson SH, Wolfe LF, and Zee PC. Circadian phase-shifting effects of nocturnal exercise in older compared with young adults. *Am J Physiol Regul Integr Comp Physiol.* Jun 2003;284(6):R1542-1550.

Barczi SR, TMJ. *Co-morbidities, psychiatric, medications and substances.* Vol 1: Elsevier; 2006.

Bassetti CL, Milanova M, and Gugger M. Sleep-disordered breathing and acute ischemic stroke: Diagnosis, risk factors, treatment, evolution, and long-term clinical outcome. *Stroke.* Apr 2006;37(4):967-972.

Benca RM, Obermeyer WH, Thisted RA, and Gillin JC. Sleep and psychiatric disorders. A meta-analysis. *Arch Gen Psychiatry.* Aug 1992;49(8):651-668; discussion 669-670.

Benloucif S, Masana MI, and Dubocovich ML. Light-induced phase shifts of circadian activity rhythms and immediate early gene expression in the suprachiasmatic nucleus are attenuated in old C3H/HeN mice. *Brain Res.* Jan 30 1997;747(1):34-42.

Benloucif S, Orbeta L, Ortiz R, et al. Morning or evening activity improves neuropsychological performance and subjective sleep quality in older adults. *Sleep.* Dec 15 2004;27(8):1542-1551.

Bixler EO, Vgontzas AN, Lin HM, et al. Prevalence of sleep-disordered breathing in women: Effects of gender. *Am J Respir Crit Care Med.* Mar 2001;163(3 Pt 1):608-613.

Bliwise DL. Sleep in normal aging and dementia. *Sleep.* Jan 1993;16(1):40-81.

Bootzin RR. *Stimulus control*: Sage; 2000.

Brenner RP, Ulrich RF, and Reynolds CF, 3rd. EEG spectral findings in healthy, elderly men and women—sex differences. *Electroencephalogr Clin Neurophysiol.* Jan 1995;94(1):1-5.

Breslau N, Roth T, Rosenthal L, and Andreski P. Sleep disturbance and psychiatric disorders: A longitudinal epidemiological study of young adults. *Biol Psychiatry.* Mar 15 1996;39(6):411-418.

Brzezinski A, Vangel MG, Wurtman RJ, et al. Effects of exogenous melatonin on sleep: A meta-analysis. *Sleep Med Rev.* Feb 2005;9(1):41-50.

Buscemi N, Vandermeer B, Hooton N, et al. The efficacy and safety of exogenous melatonin for primary sleep disorders. A meta-analysis. *J Gen Intern Med.* Dec 2005;20(12):1151-1158.

Buysse DJ, CFRI. *Pharmacologic treatment* First Edition: Sage; 2000.

Buysse DJ, Thompson W, Scott J, et al. Daytime symptoms in primary insomnia: A prospective analysis using ecological momentary assessment. *Sleep Med.* Apr 2007;8(3):198-208.

Campbell SS, Dawson D, and Anderson MW. Alleviation of sleep maintenance insomnia with timed exposure to bright light. *J Am Geriatr Soc.* Aug 1993;41(8):829-836.

Carskadon MA, Ed. *Normal human sleep: An overview.* Fourth ed. Philadelphia: Saunders; 2005. Kryger M.H. RT, Dement W.C., ed. Principles and practices of sleep medicine.

Chasens ER, Sereika SM, Weaver TE, and Umlauf MG. Daytime sleepiness, exercise, and physical function in older adults. *J Sleep Res.* Mar 2007;16(1):60-65.

Chokroverty S. *Physiologic changes in sleep.* 3rd ed: Elsevier; 2009.

Cohen-Zion M, Stepnowsky C, Marler, Shochat T, Kripke DF, and Ancoli-Israel S. Changes in cognitive function associated with sleep disordered breathing in older people. *J Am Geriatr Soc.* Dec 2001;49(12):1622-1627.

Darchia N, Campbell IG, and Feinberg I. Rapid eye movement density is reduced in the normal elderly. *Sleep.* Dec 15 2003;26(8):973-977.

Dijk DJ, Duffy JF, and Czeisler CA. Age-related increase in awakenings: Impaired consolidation of non-REM sleep at all circadian phases. *Sleep.* Aug 1 2001;24(5):565-577.

Dillon J, Zheng L, Merriam JC, and Gaillard ER. Transmission of light to the aging human retina: Possible implications for age related macular degeneration. *Exp Eye Res.* Dec 2004;79(6):753-759.

Dolder C, Nelson M, and McKinsey J. Use of non-benzodiazepine hypnotics in the elderly: Are all agents the same? *CNS Drugs.* 2007;21(5):389-405.

Dopp JM, Reichmuth KJ, and Morgan BJ. Obstructive sleep apnea and hypertension: Mechanisms, evaluation, and management. *Curr Hypertens Rep.* Dec 2007;9(6):529-534.

Douglas NJ. *Respiratory physiology, control of ventilation.* 4th ed: Elsevier; 2005.

Douglas NJ, White DP, Pickett CK, Weil JV, and Zwillich CW. Respiration during sleep in normal man. *Thorax.* Nov 1982;37(11):840-844.

Douglas NJ, White DP, Weil JV, et al. Hypoxic ventilatory response decreases during sleep in normal men. *Am Rev Respir Dis.* Mar 1982;125(3):286–289.

Durrence HH and Lichstein KL. The sleep of African Americans: A comparative review. *Behav Sleep Med.* 2006;4(1):29–44.

Eckert DJ, Jordan AS, Merchia P, and Malhotra A. Central sleep apnea: Pathophysiology and treatment. *Chest.* Feb 2007;131(2):595–607.

Edgar DM, Dement WC, and Fuller CA. Effect of SCN lesions on sleep in squirrel monkeys: Evidence for opponent processes in sleep-wake regulation. *J Neurosci.* Mar 1993;13(3):1065–1079.

Engle-Friedman M, Bootzin RR, Hazlewood L, and Tsao C. An evaluation of behavioral treatments for insomnia in the older adult. *J Clin Psychol.* Jan 1992;48(1):77–90.

Enright PL, Newman AB, Wahl PW, Manolio TA, Haponik EF, and Boyle PJ. Prevalence and correlates of snoring and observed apneas in 5,201 older adults. *Sleep.* Sep 1996;19(7):531–538.

Ficca G, Gori S, Ktonas P, Quattrini C, Trammell J, and Salzarulo P. The organization of rapid eye movement activity during rapid eye movement sleep is impaired in the elderly. *Neurosci Lett.* Nov 19 1999;275(3):219–221.

Ficca G, Scavelli S, Fagioli I, Gori S, Murri L, and Salzarulo P. Rapid eye movement activity before spontaneous awakening in elderly subjects. *J Sleep Res.* Mar 2004;13(1):49–53.

Foldvary-Schaefer N, De Leon Sanchez I, Karafa M, Mascha E, Dinner D, and Morris HH. Gabapentin increases slow-wave sleep in normal adults. *Epilepsia.* Dec 2002;43(12):1493–1497.

Foley D, Ancoli-Israel S, Britz P, and Walsh J. Sleep disturbances and chronic disease in older adults: Results of the 2003 National Sleep Foundation Sleep in America Survey. *J Psychosom Res.* May 2004 ;56(5):497–502.

Foundation NS. Sleep in America Poll 2003: *Sleep in Aging.* 2003. Accessed January 21, 2010.

Gilmartin GS, Daly RW, and Thomas RJ. Recognition and management of complex sleep-disordered breathing. *Curr Opin Pulm Med.* Nov 2005;11(6):485–493.

Gothe B, Altose MD, Goldman MD, and Cherniack NS. Effect of quiet sleep on resting and CO_2-stimulated breathing in humans. *J Appl Physiol.* Apr 1981;50(4):724–730.

Gottlieb GL. Sleep disorders and their management. Special considerations in the elderly. *Am J Med.* Mar 2 1990;88(3A):29S–33S.

Grant BF. Prevalence and correlates of alcohol use and DSM-IV alcohol dependence in the United States: Results of the National Longitudinal Alcohol Epidemiologic Survey. *J Stud Alcohol.* Sep 1997;58(5):464–473.

Guilleminault C, Stoohs R, Clerk A, Cetel M, and Maistros P. A cause of excessive daytime sleepiness. The upper airway resistance syndrome. *Chest.* Sep 1993;104(3):781–787.

Haas DC, Foster GL, Nieto FJ, et al. Age-dependent associations between sleep-disordered breathing and hypertension: Importance of discriminating between systolic/diastolic hypertension and isolated systolic hypertension in the Sleep Heart Health Study. *Circulation.* Feb 8 2005;111(5):614–621.

Haimov I, Lavie P, Laudon M, Herer P, Vigder C, and Zisapel N. Melatonin replacement therapy of elderly insomniacs. *Sleep.* Sep 1995;18(7):598–603.

Harma MI, Hakola T, Akerstedt T, and Laitinen JT. Age and adjustment to night work. *Occup Environ Med.* Aug 1994;51(8):568–573.

Hetzel MR and Clark TJ. Comparison of normal and asthmatic circadian rhythms in peak expiratory flow rate. *Thorax.* Oct 1980;35(10):732–738.

Hindmarch I, Dawson J, and Stanley N. A double-blind study in healthy volunteers to assess the effects on sleep of pregabalin compared with alprazolam and placebo. *Sleep.* Feb 1 2005;28(2):187–193.

Hudgel DW and Hamilton HB. Respiratory muscle activity during sleep-induced periodic breathing in the elderly. *J Appl Physiol.* Nov 1994;77(5):2285–2290.

Iber C, Ancoli-Israel S, Chesson A, and Quan SF, for the American Academy of Sleep Medicine. *The AASM manual for the scoring of sleep and associated events: Rules, terminology and technical specifications,* 1st *ed.* Westchester, IL: American Academy of Sleep Medicine; 2007.

Irwin MR, Cole JC, and Nicassio PM. Comparative meta-analysis of behavioral interventions for insomnia and their efficacy in middle-aged adults and in older adults 55+ years of age. *Health Psychol.* Jan 2006;25(1):3–14.

Karam-Hage M and Brower KJ. Open pilot study of gabapentin versus trazodone to treat insomnia in alcoholic outpatients. *Psychiatry Clin Neurosci.* Oct 2003;57(5):542–544.

Katz RI and Horowitz, GR. Electroencephalogram in the septuagenarian: Studies in a normal geriatric population. *J Am Geriatr Soc.* 1982;3:273.

Katz DA and McHorney CA. The relationship between insomnia and health-related quality of life in patients with chronic illness. *J Fam Pract.* Mar 2002;51(3):229–235.

Kaufman DW, Kelly JP, Rosenberg L, Anderson TE, and Mitchell AA. Recent patterns of medication use in the ambulatory adult population of the United States: The Slone survey. *JAMA.* Jan 16 2002;287(3):337–344.

King AC, Oman RF, Brassington GS, Bliwise DL, and Haskell WL. Moderate-intensity exercise and self-rated quality of sleep in older adults. *A randomized controlled trial. JAMA.* Jan 1 1997;277(1):32–37.

Klerman EB and Dijk DJ. Age-related reduction in the maximal capacity for sleep—implications for insomnia. *Curr Biol.* Aug 5 2008;18(15):1118–1123.

Klerman EB, Duffy JF, Dijk DJ, and Czeisler CA. Circadian phase resetting in older people by ocular bright light exposure. *J Investig Med.* Jan 2001;49(1):30–40.

Kripke DF, Ancoli-Israel S, Klauber MR, Wingard DL, Mason WJ, and Mullaney DJ. Prevalence of sleep-disordered breathing in ages 40-64 years: A population-based survey. *Sleep.* Jan 1997;20(1):65–76.

Kupfer DJ and Reynolds CF, 3rd. Management of insomnia. *N Engl J Med.* Jan 30 1997;336(5):341–346.

Lack L, Wright H, Kemp K, and Gibbon S. The treatment of early-morning awakening insomnia with 2 evenings of bright light. *Sleep.* May 1 2005;28(5):616–623.

Landolt HP, Dijk DJ, Achermann P, and Borbely AA. Effect of age on the sleep EEG: Slow-wave activity and spindle frequency activity in young and middle-aged men. *Brain Res.* Nov 4 1996;738(2):205–212.

Latham J and Davis BD. The socioeconomic impact of chronic pain. *Disabil Rehabil.* Jan-Mar 1994;16(1):39–44.

Launois SH, Feroah TR, Campbell WN, et al. Site of pharyngeal narrowing predicts outcome of surgery for obstructive sleep apnea. *Am Rev Respir Dis.* Jan 1993;147(1):182–189.

Lichstein KL, SKC, Nau, SD. et al. Insomnia in the elderly. In: Ancoli-Israel, ed. *Sleep medicine clinics.* Vol 12006:221–229.

Lichstein KL, Riedel BW, Wilson NM, Lester KW, and Aguillard RN. Relaxation and sleep compression for late-life insomnia: A placebo-controlled trial. *J Consult Clin Psychol.* Apr 2001;69(2):227–239.

Livingston G, Blizard B, and Mann. Does sleep disturbance predict depression in elderly people? A study in inner London. *Br J Gen Pract.* Nov 1993;43(376):445–448.

MacLean CH. Quality indicators for the management of osteoarthritis in vulnerable elders. *Ann Intern Med.* Oct 16 2001;135(8 Pt 2):711–721.

Maggi S, Langlois JA, Minicuci N, et al. Sleep complaints in community-dwelling older persons: Prevalence, associated factors, and reported causes. *J Am Geriatr Soc.* Feb 1998;46(2):161–168.

Mapel DW, Dedrick D, and Davis K. Trends and cardiovascular co-morbidities of COPD patients in the Veterans Administration Medical System, 1991–1999. *COPD.* Mar 2005;2(1):35–41.

Martinez-Garcia MA, Soler-Cataluna JJ, Ejarque-Martinez L, et al. Continuous positive airway pressure treatment reduces mortality in patients with ischemic stroke and obstructive sleep apnea: A 5-year follow-up study. *Am J Respir Crit Care Med.* Jul 1 2009;180(1):36–41.

McNicholas WT. Impact of sleep in respiratory failure. *Eur Respir J.* Apr 1997;10(4):920–933.

Mehra R, Benjamin EJ, Shahar E, et al. Association of nocturnal arrhythmias with sleep-disordered breathing: The Sleep Heart Health Study. *Am J Respir Crit Care Med.* Apr 15 2006;173(8):910–916.

Monk TH, Buysse DJ, Carrier J, and Kupfer DJ. Inducing jet-lag in older people: directional asymmetry. *J Sleep Res.* Jun 2000;9(2):101–116.

Monk TH, Buysse DJ, Reynolds CF, 3rd, Jarrett DB, and Kupfer DJ. Rhythmic vs homeostatic influences on mood, activation, and performance in young and old men. *J Gerontol.* Jul 1992;47(4): P221–227.

Monk TH, Buysse DJ, Reynolds CF, 3rd, Kupfer DJ, and Houck PR. Circadian temperature rhythms of older people. *Exp Gerontol.* Sep-Oct 1995;30(5):455–474.

Morgan M. *Sleep and aging*: Sage; 2000.

Morin CM. *Insomnia, psychological assessment and management*: Guilford; 1993.

Morin CM. *Nature and treatment of insomnia*. 3rd ed: Elsevier; 2009.

Naylor E, Penev PD, Orbeta L, et al. Daily social and physical activity increases slow-wave sleep and daytime neuropsychological performance in the elderly. *Sleep.* Feb 1 2000;23(1):87–95.

Naylor Z and Zee, PC. Circadian rhythm alterations with aging. In: Ancoli-Israel, ed. *Sleep medicine clinics.* Vol 12006:187–196.

NIH State of the Science Conference statement on Manifestations and Management of Chronic Insomnia in Adults statement. *J Clin Sleep Med.* Oct 15 2005;1(4):412–421.

O'Brien A and Whitman K. Lack of benefit of continuous positive airway pressure on lung function in patients with overlap syndrome. *Lung.* Nov–Dec 2005;183(6):389–404.

Obrist WD, Sokoloff L, Lassen NA, Lane MH, Butler RN, and Feinberg I. Relation of EEG to cerebral blood flow and metabolism in old age. *Electroencephalogr Clin Neurophysiol.* Aug 1963;15:610–619.

Ohayon MM, Caulet M, Priest RG, and Guilleminault C. Psychotropic medication consumption patterns in the UK general population. *J Clin Epidemiol.* Mar 1998;51(3):273–283.

Oken BS and Kaye JA. Electrophysiologic function in the healthy, extremely old. *Neurology.* Mar 1992;42(3 Pt 1):519–526.

Pandi-Perumal SR, Zisapel N, Srinivasan V, and Cardinali DP. Melatonin and sleep in aging population. *Exp Gerontol.* Dec 2005;40(12): 911–925.

Perlis M and Pigeon WR. Etiology and pathophysiology of insomnia: Elsevier; 2005.

Possidente B, McEldowney S, and Pabon A. Aging lengthens circadian period for wheel-running activity in C57BL mice. *Physiol Behav.* Mar 1995;57(3):575–579.

Rechtschaffen A and Kales A. *A manual of standardized terminology, techniques, and scoring system for sleep stages of human subjects.* Bethesda, MD: National #Institute of Neurological Disease and Blindness; 1968.

Reid KJ, Chang AM, Dubocovich ML, Turek FW, Takahashi JS, and Zee PC. Familial advanced sleep phase syndrome. *Arch Neurol.* Jul 2001;58(7):1089–1094.

Reidel BW. *Sleep hygiene*: Sage; 2000.

Resnick HE, Redline S, Shahar E, et al. Diabetes and sleep disturbances: Findings from the Sleep Heart Health Study. *Diabetes Care.* Mar 2003;26(3):702–709.

Richardson GS, Carskadon MA, Orav EJ, and Dement WC. Circadian variation of sleep tendency in elderly and young adult subjects. *Sleep.* 1982;5 Suppl 2:S82–94.

Rollag MD, Berson DM, and Provencio I. Melanopsin, ganglion-cell photoreceptors, and mammalian photoentrainment. *J Biol Rhythms.* Jun 2003;18(3):227–234.

Roth T, Stubbs C, and Walsh JK. Ramelteon (TAK-375), a selective MT1/MT2-receptor agonist, reduces latency to persistent sleep in a model of transient insomnia related to a novel sleep environment. *Sleep.* Mar 1 2005;28(3):303–307.

Roth T, Wright KP, Jr., and Walsh J. Effect of tiagabine on sleep in elderly subjects with primary insomnia: A randomized, double-blind, placebo-controlled study. *Sleep.* Mar 1 2006;29(3): 335–341.

Rybarczyk B, Stepanski E, Fogg L, Lopez M, Barry P, and Davis A. A placebo-controlled test of cognitive-behavioral therapy for comorbid insomnia in older adults. *J Consult Clin Psychol.* Dec 2005;73(6):1164–1174.

Saper CB, Scammell TE, and Lu J. Hypothalamic regulation of sleep and circadian rhythms. *Nature.* Oct 27 2005;437(7063): 1257–1263.

Schafer T. Physiology of breathing during sleep. Basel: Karger 2006.

Shahar E, Redline S, Young T, et al. Hormone replacement therapy and sleep-disordered breathing. *Am J Respir Crit Care Med.* May 1 2003;167(9):1186–1192.

Spiegel R, Herzog A, and Koberle S. Polygraphic sleep criteria as predictors of successful aging: An exploratory longitudinal study. *Biol Psychiatry.* Feb 15 1999;45(4):435–442.

Speilman A and Glovinski P. *A behavioral perspective on insomnia treatment.* Vol 10;1987.

Stein MB. *Anxiety disorders*: Elsevier; 2005.

Stepanski EJ and Rybarczyk B. Emerging research on the treatment and etiology of secondary or comorbid insomnia. *Sleep Med Rev.* Feb 2006;10(1):7–18.

Stepnowsky CJ and Ancoli-Israel S. Sleep and its disorders in seniors. *Sleep Med Clin.* 2008;3(2):281–293.

Takimoto M, Hamada A, Tomoda A, et al. Daily expression of clock genes in whole blood cells in healthy subjects and a patient with circadian rhythm sleep disorder. *Am J Physiol Regul Integr Comp Physiol.* Nov 2005;289(5):R1273–1279.

Terzano MG, Rossi M, Palomba V, Smerieri A, and Parrino L. New drugs for insomnia: comparative tolerability of zopiclone, zolpidem and zaleplon. *Drug Saf.* 2003;26(4):261–282.

Touitou Y. Human aging and melatonin. Clinical relevance. *Exp Gerontol.* Jul 2001;36(7):1083–1100.

Valentinuzzi VS, Scarbrough K, Takahashi JS, and Turek FW. Effects of aging on the circadian rhythm of wheel-running activity in C57BL/6 mice. *Am J Physiol.* Dec 1997;273(6 Pt 2):R1957–1964.

van Coevorden A, Mockel J, Laurent E, et al. Neuroendocrine rhythms and sleep in aging men. *Am J Physiol.* Apr 1991;260(4 Pt 1): E651–661.

Van Cauter E, Leproult R, and Kupfer DJ. Effects of gender and age on the levels and circadian rhythmicity of plasma cortisol. *J Clin Endocrinol Metab.* Jul 1996;81(7):2468–2473.

Van Reeth O, Zhang Y, Zee PC, and Turek FW. Aging alters feedback effects of the activity-rest cycle on the circadian clock. *Am J Physiol.* Oct 1992;263(4 Pt 2):R981–986.

Verrier RL. *Cardiovascular disorders and sleep*: Hanley and Belfus; 2002.

Vitiello MV, Smallwood RG, Avery DH, Pascualy RA, Martin DC, and Prinz PN. Circadian temperature rhythms in young adult and aged men. *Neurobiol Aging.* Mar-Apr 1986;7(2):97–100.

Walsh JK and Erwin G. Subjective hypnotic efficacy of trazadone and zolpidem in DSM III-R primary insomnia. *Human Psychopharmacology.* 1998;13:191–197.

Walsh JK, Randazzo AC, Frankowski S, Shannon K, Schweitzer PK, and Roth T. Dose-response effects of tiagabine on the sleep of older adults. *Sleep.* Jun 1 2005;28(6):673–676.

Wang D, Teichtahl H, Drummer O, et al. Central sleep apnea in stable methadone maintenance treatment patients. *Chest.* Sep 2005;128(3):1348–1356.

White DP. *Central sleep apnea.* 4th ed: Elsevier; 2005.

Wilcox S, Brenes GA, Levine D, Sevick MA, Shumaker SA, and Craven T. Factors related to sleep disturbance in older adults experiencing knee pain or knee pain with radiographic evidence of knee osteoarthritis. *J Am Geriatr Soc.* Oct 2000;48(10):1241–1251.

Wilson S and Argyropoulos S. Antidepressants and sleep: A qualitative review of the literature. *Drugs.* 2005;65(7):927–947.

Wyatt JK. Delayed sleep phase syndrome: Pathophysiology and treatment options. *Sleep.* Sep 15 2004;27(6):1195–1203.

Yaggi HK, Concato J, Kernan WN, Lichtman JH, Brass LM, and Mohsenin V. Obstructive sleep apnea as a risk factor for stroke and death. *N Engl J Med.* Nov 10 2005;353(19):2034–2041.

Young T, Finn L, Austin D, and Peterson A. Menopausal status and sleep-disordered breathing in the Wisconsin Sleep Cohort Study. *Am J Respir Crit Care Med.* May 1 2003;167(9):1181–1185.

Young T, Peppard PE, and Gottlieb DJ. Epidemiology of obstructive sleep apnea: A population health perspective. *Am J Respir Crit Care Med.* May 1 2002;165(9):1217–1239.

48 Headache in the Elderly

Cynthia Bamford and MaryAnn Mays

Introduction

Headache is a common symptom with multiple causes. In adults age 65 and older, it is the 10th most common reported symptom in women and 14th most common symptom in men. In a study by Solomon and Kunkel, 8% of total outpatient population of 120,000 patients at the Cleveland Clinic in the year 1988 carried a diagnosis of headache and 4% of that headache population was 65 and older (Solomon 1990). Headaches can be classified as primary headache disorders or secondary headache disorders. Primary headaches occur without any other cause; these include migraine, tension-type headache, cluster headache, and new daily persistent headache. Secondary headache disorders are attributable to another disorder. After the age of 50, there is a decrease in incidence of primary headache disorders and an increase in secondary headaches caused by systemic disorders or structural lesions which account for approximately one-third of headache pain in the elderly (Solomon 1990)

New onset headaches, especially severe headaches, in patients over the age of 50 always warrant evaluation and testing to rule out secondary pathology. Testing would include imaging, CT scan or MRI, X-ray of the spine or chest, and laboratory tests including CBC, CMP, ESR, CRP, TSH, drug levels and lumbar puncture if appropriate. Treatment would depend on the underlying cause. Treatment of headache in the elderly can be challenging due to underlying comorbidities and multiple medications.

Evaluating the Patient with Headache

Headache diagnosis is based on a thorough history and general and neurologic examination with testing to exclude organic causes. A high index of suspicion should be maintained in patients over the age of 50 with new onset headache or a change in pattern of a chronic headache, even if the headache is not severe. The mnemonic, SNOOPP, is useful (Dodick 2003).

- Secondary risk factors—underlying disease, immunosuppression, malignancy

- Neurological symptoms or abnormal signs—confusion, alteration of consciousness, abnormal exam

- Onset—sudden, abrupt, split second (first or worst)

- Older—new onset and progressive, especially in age >50

- Pattern change—first headache or different from typical pattern

- Previous headache history—attack frequency, severity, and/or clinical features (Dodick 2003)

The International Classification of Headache Disorders (ICHD) second edition is an effort to classify headache disorders and provide diagnostic criteria for primary and secondary headache disorders as well as cranial neuralgias and central pain (The Headache Classification subcommittee of the IHS 2004). This is a useful tool for both the headache specialist as well as the general practitioner, especially when symptoms are not typical.

The Primary Headache Disorders

Migraine

Migraine is a common disorder affecting 12% of the population. The prevalence of migraine peaks around the age of 25 to 55 years and then declines, affecting 7.5% of women and 2.5% of men over the age of 60 years (Lipton et al. 2001). Despite this, more than half of patients with a prior diagnosis of migraine continue to have active disease past the age of 65 years. Approximately 2% of migraineurs will first begin to experience migraine headaches after the age of 60 years. Clinical characteristics of migraine headaches change with aging, becoming more atypical in presentation. Often reported to be shorter in duration, more often bilateral and diffuse, and the associated symptoms of photophobia, phonophobia, nausea, and vomiting are less problematic (Mazzotta 2003; Bigal et al. 2005; Martins et al. 2006). Individuals may have a family history of migraine, suggesting a genetic contribution. Migraine is divided into two major subtypes: migraine without aura and migraine with aura (Table 1).

Migraine without Aura

Migraine without aura is the commonest subtype. The headache experienced by the migraineur is typically unilateral, pulsating or throbbing in nature, and may be accompanied by nausea and/or vomiting, and/or phonophobia and/or photophobia. Some patients will have premonitory symptoms that occur minutes to days prior to the onset of headache, consisting of such symptoms as fatigue, impaired concentration, mood changes, or neck stiffness. A postdrome period may follow the resolution of the headache. During this time patients continue to experience disability due to residual effects such as cutaneous allodynia, fatigue, myalgias, and mood changes.

Migraine with Aura

Only 15–20% of migraineurs will experience aura prior to the onset of headache pain. Auras are a complex of neurological symptoms which are fully reversible that gradually develop over 5 to 20 minutes, lasting less than 60 minutes, followed within one hour by a headache. The most common auras consist of changes in vision (i.e. flickering lights, spots, zigzag lines, and scotoma), parasthesias and numbness, or speech dysphasia. A number of different auras may occur in succession. Patients that experience migraine with aura often experience migraine without aura as well. Rarely motor auras will present as paralysis. These migraine auras are now grouped separately as hemiplegic migraine. In basilar migraine, patients will experience

558 SECTION 7 DISEASE STATES IN THE ELDERLY

Table 1 ICHD-II Diagnostic Criteria: Migraine

Migraine without Aura	Migraine with Aura
≥5 attacks fulfilling criteria B-D	≥ 2 attacks fulfilling criteria B-D
HA lasting 4–72 h*	Aura: > 1 of the following but no motor weakness
≥2 of the following:	Fully reversible visual sx including (+) and/or (-) features
Unilateral	Fully reversible sensory sx including (+) and/or (-) features
Pulsating	Fully reversible dysphasic speech disturbance
Moderate or severe intensity	≥ 2 of the following:
Aggravation by or causing avoidance of routine physical activity	Homonymous visual sx and/or unilateral sensory sx
≥1 of the following:	1 aura and/or different auras in succession gradually develop over 5 min.
Nausea and/or vomiting	Each sx lasts ≥ 5 min and ≤ 60 min.
Photophobia and phonophobia	HA begins during or w/i 60 min of aura
Not attributable to another disorder	Not attributable to another disorder

HA, headache; sx, symptom; (+) positive; (-) negative; w/o, without; w/i, within
*Untreated or treated unsuccessfully

symptoms related to brainstem dysfunction. Hemiplegic and basilar migraines typically start during childhood or adolescence and cease during adulthood. With aging, those migraineurs with aura may begin to experience aura without migraine pain. Currently these are classified as typical aura without headache. When this occurs in a patient with a history of migraine aura and the aura symptoms are typical of previous auras, the diagnosis is not difficult. Auras may be typical in duration of minutes but may last for hours, tend to build up over time, and may progress from one type of aura to another. These features may clue the clinician to the diagnosis of typical aura without headache. In individuals with no prior history of migraine with aura, the diagnosis is one of exclusion. Evaluation should included neuroimaging of brain and carotid arteries, Holter monitor, echocardiogram, and possibly hypercoagulable panel or EEG.

Migraine Pathophysiology

Multiple mechanisms for generating migraine are likely to exist. Those individuals susceptible to migraine can be exposed to a variety of stimuli which trigger spreading cortical depression leading to neuronal dysfunction. Cortical spreading depression may then trigger vasodilation of cerebral blood vessels. The vasodilation stimulates the trigeminal nerve ending and a release of vasoactive neuropeptides. The release of neuropeptides produces inflammation and further vasodilation resulting in sensitization of peripheral meningeal pain receptors. Pain is transmitted along the trigeminal nerve to the trigeminal nucleus caudalis (TNC) in the brain stem where pain is processed and relayed to higher-order neurons in the thalamus and cortex, resulting in perception of pain. Migraine involves sensitization of both peripheral and central pain pathways, which are recruited sequentially. When pain is left untreated, a process of central sensitization occurs by which the TNC fires independent of any peripheral activation. Central sensitization contributes to the development of a full-blown migraine refractory to treatment.

Treatment of Migraine

Studies that have evaluated the efficacy of migraine medications have traditionally excluded the elderly. Despite this, most medications that are used in the younger population can be used successfully in the geriatric population, taking into account comorbid diseases and medication interactions as well as reduced metabolism of medications. Elderly patients often get inadequate treatment for their headaches due to these concerns; even when prescribed medications are offered, the elderly themselves may be reluctant to take additional medications. Treatment choice should be individualized and depend on attack frequency, disability, and associated symptoms, especially if nausea and vomiting are prominent. Intranasal or parenteral medication would be

more effective than an oral abortive in these individuals. Attention to the patient's previous response to medications and coexistent medical conditions must be taken into account; a strategy to utilize medications that may treat both the migraine and other co-existing disease conditions may be very useful. Conversely, avoiding medications that could potentially worsen an underlying condition is essential.

Preventive therapy should be considered when: 1) Patient experiences disabling migraines despite acute treatment; 2) frequent attacks (>2/week) thereby increasing the risk of acute medication overuse; 3) problems with acute treatment medications (ineffective, contraindicated, troublesome side effects, or overused); 4) patient preference; or 5) presence of uncommon migraine conditions such prolonged aura or migrainous cerebral infarct.

Non-pharmacologic Interventions

Patients should be instructed in a number of self-help techniques to manage their migraines. More than likely, a lifelong migraine suffer has identified their individual triggers. Aging individuals experience new stressful life experiences not previously encountered. Stress management with biofeedback, relaxation training, and cognitive behavioral therapy can assist in coping. Referral to a physical therapist can be very beneficial particularly for individuals with occipital headaches or associated neck pain. Acupuncture is an alternative therapy to consider, especially when a myofascial component exists with the headache.

Pharmacologic Interventions—Preventative Therapy

It is recommended that medications are started at a low dose and slowly titrated to therapeutic effect. A 2–3 month trial is recommended. Discontinue medications once migraine control has been achieved for 6–12 months. A realistic goal is a 50% reduction in headache frequency or severity. There are a variety of commonly used preventative therapies with the varying levels of efficacy including beta blockers, antidepressants, anticonvulsants, calcium channel blockers, and other agents including herbal supplements (Table 2). The US Headache Consortium determined the level of evidence for treatment efficacy based upon results of published studies and established goals for the treatment of migraine (Silberstein 2000).

Pharmacologic Interventions—Abortive Therapy

Early intervention increases the probability of achieving a pain-free response by treating a migraine attack while pain is still mild, rather than delaying treatment until pain has progressed to moderate or severe. To avoid medication overuse-induced chronic headaches, limit abortive medications to 2–3 days per week. Medication choices can depend on the severity of pain. For patients with mild to moderate pain, simple and combination analgesics can be effective.

Table 2 Prophylactic Migraine Therapy

Medication	Usual Effective Dose	Efficacy
Beta Blockers		High
Atenolol	25–100 mg/d	
Metoprolol	50–200 mg	
Nadolol	40–80 mg/d	
Propranolol	80–240 mg/d	
Timolol	10–30 mg /d	
Antidepressants		
TCAs		High
Amitriptyline	25–150 mg	
Doxepin	25–150 mg	
Nortriptyline	25–150 mg	
Protriptyline	5–60 mg/d	
SSRIs/SNRIs		Probably
Fluoxetine	20–80 mg/d	
Sertraline	50–150 mg/d	
Venlafaxine	75–225 mg/d	
Duloxetine	30–60 mg/d	
Other		
Mirtazapine	15–45 mg/d	
Anticonvulsants		
Valproate	500–1000 mg/d	High
Topiramate	100–200 mg/d	High
Neurontin	1800–2400 mg/d	Probably
Calcium Channel Blocker		
Verapamil	120–240 mg/d	Possibly
Amlodipine	2.5–10 mg/d	
Other		
NSAIDS	Various	Probably
Lisinopril	10–40 mg/d	Probably
Candesartan	8–32 mg/d	Probably
Botulinum toxin	100–200 units	Probably for CDH
CoQ10	150–300 mg/d	Probably
Feverfew	50–82 mg/d	Probably
Magnesium	400–800 mg/d	Probably
Riboflavin	400 mg/d	Probably
Petasites	75 mg bid	High
Methysergide	2–8 mg/d	High

Migraine-specific medications are indicated for patients experiencing moderate to severe pain, which include the triptans, dihydroergotamine, and ergotamine.

Simple analgesics including combination analgesics can be effective for patients with mild to moderate pain. These include agents such as aspirin, non-steroidal anti-inflammatories (NSAIDs), and APA/ASA/caffeine. Of the NSAIDs, commonly used agents with proven efficacy include diclofenac (50–75 mg bid–tid), flurbiprofen (100 mg bid), ibuprofen (800 mg tid), indomethacin (25–50 mg tid), ketoprofen (50 mg tid), ketorolac (30–60 mg IM), meclofenamate (100 mg bid), nabumetone (500–750 mg bid), and naproxen (500–1000 mg bid). Potential side effects include gastrointestinal side effects (nausea, gastritis, bleeding and GERD), renal dysfunction, peripheral edema, exacerbation of asthma or hypertension, and tinnitus. Acetaminophen is also likely effective for non-disabling migraines. Isometheptene/acetaminophen/dichloralphenalzone combination analgesic is effective for acute migraine of mild intensity.

Combination analgesics containing butalbital have commonly been used over the years but there is little evidence to support the effectiveness in the acute management of migraines, although this treatment is probably effective for nonspecific headaches. There is a risk of dependency and medication-overuse headache with frequent use and thus should be limited and patients carefully monitored. Opioids have greater evidence supporting their effectiveness but also have the risk of dependence and contribution to medication-overuse headache. These medications can be used for those patients with infrequent disabling headaches for which no alternative therapy can be found. Patients who have had bleeding peptic ulcers, are on Coumadin therapy, or have cerebrovascular, cardiovascular, or peripheral vascular disease are the most challenging for the clinician to find reasonable safe alternative therapies.

Antiemetics that are dopamine antagonists may be very useful in abortive treatment to help alleviate not only the pain, but also the nausea and gastroparesis associated with migraine. They may be used alone or as adjunctive therapy. They are available by various routes of administration including oral, rectal, IM, or IV, which make them a good option for those migraines that are most disabling or are associated with vomiting. Metoclopramide, prochlorperazine, promethazine, and chlorpromazine are most commonly used. Side effects include drowsiness and extrapyramidal effects, which occur with greater incidence in the elderly and thus frequent use should be discouraged. Due to potential for severe tissue injury associated with intravenous promethazine, parenteral use is not recommended.

Migraine-specific medications are indicated for patients experiencing moderate to severe pain. They include the triptans, dihydroergotamine (DHE), and ergotamine. The triptans are the preferred therapy due to better tolerability, although dihydroergotamine is a reasonable alternative in those that have failed triptans, have recurrence despite initial treatment success, or would benefit from the available routes of nasal, IM/SQ, or IV. Intravenous DHE is particularly useful for migraine status.

Table 3 lists the available triptans and recommended dosing. Triptans are 5-HT1B/1D receptors agonist. They produce vasoconstriction of meningeal blood vessels via the 5-HT1B receptor and prevent release of neuropeptides that produce neurogenic inflammation via the 5-HT1D receptor. Common adverse events include fatigue, dizziness, parasthesias, non-cardiac chest pain, and nausea. The Triptan Cardiovascular Safety Expert Panel found that while serious cardiovascular events have been reported after the use of triptans, their occurrence appears to be extremely low, on the order of less than one in one million. Recommendations suggest that patients at low risk of coronary heart disease (one or no risk factors: increasing age, abnormal cholesterol profiles, uncontrolled blood pressure, a diagnosis of diabetes, and smoking) can be prescribed triptans without the need for a more intensive cardiac evaluation. Patients with established coronary heart disease should not be prescribed triptans. Patients at intermediate risk of coronary heart disease (two or more risk factors) require cardiovascular evaluation before triptans can be prescribed (Dodick et al. 2004).

Tension-type Headache

Tension-type headache (TTH) is the most prevalent of the primary headache disorders, across all ages. Similar to migraine headaches, the peak prevalence occurs between 20–39 years and declines with age. TTHs affect females only slightly more than males (ratio of 4:5 male to female), whereas there is a preponderance of females in migraine (ratio of 1:3 or 1:2 following menopause) (Lisotto et al 2004). Although they are the most commonly encountered headache in the population, they have not been as well studied as migraine headaches. There is great variability in the clinical presentation amongst individuals. TTHs are generally mild to moderate in severity, bilateral, non-throbbing pain, and lack associated symptoms of photophobia, phonophobia,

Table 3 Triptans for Acute Migraine Therapy

Triptan	Dosing
Sumatriptan (Imitrex®)	PO: 100 mg: 1 po q 2 hour prn; Max 200 mg per day NS: 20 mg: 1 puff q 2 hour prn; Max 40 mg per day SQ: 4 or 6 mg: 1 SQ q 1 hr prn; Max 12 mg per day
Sumatriptan/ Naproxen (Treximet®)	PO: 1 po q 2 hour prn; Max 2 tablets per day
Zolmitriptan (Zomig®)	PO (oral tablet and dissolvable oral tablet ZMT): 5 mg: 1 po q 2 hour prn; Max 10 mg per day NS: 5 mg: 1 puff q 2 hour prn; Max 10 mg per day
Naratriptan (Amerge®)	PO: 2.5 mg q 4 hours prn; Max 5 mg per day Slower onset of action than other triptans but lower adverse effects and lower headache recurrence may offset slower onset of headache relief.
Rizatriptan (Maxalt®)	PO (oral tablet and dissolvable oral tablet MLT): 10 mg: 1 po q 2 hour prn; Max 30 mg per day
Almotriptan (Axert®)	PO: 12.5 mg: 1 po q 2 hour prn; Max 25 mg per day
Frovatriptan (Frova®)	PO: 2.5 mg: 1 po q 2 hour prn; Max 7.5 mg per day Slower onset of action than other triptans but lower adverse effects and lower headache recurrence may offset slower onset of headache relief.
Eletriptan (Relpax®)	PO: 40 mg: 1 po q 2 hour prn; Max 80 mg per day

Table 4 ICHD-II Diagnostic Criteria: Tension-Type Headache

Tension-type Headache

≥10 attacks fulfilling B-E
Number of days per month with such headache determines subtype
   < 1 day a month: infrequent episodic TTH
   1-14 days a month: frequent episodic TTH
   > 15 days a month: chronic TTH
HA lasting 30 min–7 days for episodic; hours or continuous for chronic TTH
≥2 of the following:
   Bilateral location
   Pressure/tightening (not pulsating)
   Mild or moderate intensity (may inhibit but not prohibit activities)
   Not aggravated by routine physical activity
Both of the following:
   No nausea or vomiting (anorexia may occur)
   No more than one of photophobia or phonophobia
Not attributable to another disorder

Treatment of Tension-type Headaches

There are far fewer studies evaluating medication treatments for TTH than there are for migraines. For this reason, most clinicians rely on what they use to treat other pain disorders including migraine. Those patients with low frequency may rely on simple analgesics, particularly non-steroidal anti-inflammatories, COX-2 inhibitor (celecoxib), or acetaminophen. Various peripheral acting muscle relaxers are used frequently but there is a lack of evidence to support their use. Tizanidine (6–12 mg/d), an α-adrenergic drug may have some benefit. Opioids are to be avoided. In those with frequent TTH, a tricyclic antidepressant such as amitriptyline has been found to be beneficial in TTH prevention. Other selective serotonin reuptake inhibitors and serotonin-norepinephrine re-uptake inhibitors have not proven beneficial except for mirtazapine (15–30 mg/d); this agent could be considered if the patient also suffers from depression. Botulinum toxin has been studied with mixed results; it may be more effective for those with chronic daily headache. Nonpharmocologic therapies such as relaxation training, biofeedback, and cognitive therapy and physical therapy are beneficial.

Cluster Headache

Cluster headaches are severe unilateral headaches, periorbital in location, with associated autonomic features such as lacrimation and nasal congestion. Men are much more often affected than women. Attacks tend to occur at night and last 15–180 minutes in duration. Attacks occur daily during a cluster cycle, followed by a period of remission. Cluster headaches can continue to be a problem for the elderly patient and may even occur for the first time after the age of 65 years. Although they often become less of a problem with time, manifesting with longer remissions as one ages, occasionally they may become chronic in nature. Typical preventative therapies include verapamil, topiramate, valproic acid, and lithium. Prednisone, which is helpful for cluster, must be used with caution in the elderly due to risk of osteoporosis, blood sugar elevation, and gastric ulceration. Although the triptans, dihydroergotamine, and ergotamine are effective for aborting cluster attacks, they would be contraindicated in patients with vascular disease due to their vasoconstrictive effects. Oxygen therapy is a safer, although less effective therapy.

Prognosis of Primary Headache Disorders

The prognosis for primary headaches is favorable with migraine as well as tension type headache. In one ten-year population study, 42% of

or nausea. (Table 4) There are three subtypes of tension type headache: infrequent episodic (<1 attack per month), frequent episodic (< 15 attacks per month), and chronic (>15 attacks per month) TTH. They are further subdivided into those with or without pericranial muscle tenderness. Patients with chronic TTH report more severe headaches than those with episodic TTH and are more likely to seek treatment from their physician. Patients with frequent TTH are at risk for developing CTTH due to medication overuse. Comorbid illnesses often co-exist including depression, anxiety, insomnia, and fibromyalgia, making the management of these patients all the more challenging.

Pathophysiology of Tension Headaches

The exact pathophysiology is not known for TTH and it is likely that there are different mechanisms of pathogenesis for episodic TTH and chronic TTH. In episodic TTH, it is likely that there are peripheral mechanisms responsible for pain. Increased pericranial muscle tenderness has been demonstrated which then activates peripheral nociceptosr. If the peripheral sensitization is frequent or prolonged, such as the case with frequent episodic TTH, then central sensitization of second order neurons occurs at the level of the spinal dorsal horn/trigeminal nucleus leading to facilitation and decreased inhibition of pain. Those individuals have a hypersensitivity to pain and thus develop the chronic TTH (Bendtsen 2000).

migraineurs experienced a remission, 38% had infrequent migraines, but 20% were found to have a poor outcome with more than 14 migraine days per year. No one in this study developed chronic migraines, although the prevalence in other studies is about 3%. For tension type headache, 45% had remission but 39% continued to have frequent episodic tension headaches, and 16% had chronic tension headaches (Lyngberg et al. 2005). These remission rates are similar to other studies. Factors such as high migraine frequency, younger age of onset (<20 years), and medication overuse are predictors of worse prognosis for migraineurs. Poorer outcome for tension type headaches has been associated with a number of factors including, older age at baseline, female gender, coexisting migraines, analgesic overuse, psychiatric disorders, sleep disorders, and stress.

Chronic Daily Headache

Chronic daily headaches (CDH) refer to headache disorders that occur on more than 15 days per month. Several prevalence studies have indicated that approximately 3% of individuals over the age of 65 will have CDH. Of these, 25% to 37.5% were attributed to medication overuse (Wang et al. 2000; Prencipe et al. 2001). Overuse of symptomatic medications greater than ten days per month puts one at greatest risk for CDH. Primary chronic daily headaches may be grouped into those that have headache durations greater than four hours duration or those with duration less than four hours. Those CDH of greater than four hours duration are chronic migraine, chronic tension-type headache, new daily persistent headache, and hemicrania continua. Those that are less than four hours duration include cluster headache, paroxysmal hemicrania, hypnic headache, idiopathic stabbing headache, and SUNCT (short-lasting, unilateral, neuralgiform headache attacks with conjunctival injection and tearing).

Of note is a rare headache disorder that is primarily seen in the elderly population known as hypnic headache. Just like cluster headaches, the pain can awaken the patient at about the same time each night. Due to the clockwork regularity of occurrence, it has also been termed "alarm clock" headache. The headache generally lasts for 1–2 hours and it is a dull pain of moderate intensity, often bilateral in location. Attacks occur on a near nightly basis (>15 times per month). There is a lack of autonomic features commonly seen with cluster headache attacks. Women tend to be more affected. Evaluation with an MRI and polysomnogram should be part of the evaluation of these patients. Patients respond well to nighttime use of lithium (300–600 mg qhs), caffeine (40–60 mg qhs), and indomethacin (75 mg qhs).

The Secondary Headache Disorders

There are numerous causes of secondary headaches, the most common and most worrisome will be highlighted. Table 5 lists the groups of secondary headaches in the ICHD-II, all of which may apply to the elderly. There are well over 100 secondary headache disorders listed in the ICHD-II. Table 6 lists the general diagnostic criteria for secondary headaches.

Headaches Attributed to Head and Neck Trauma

Falls are common in the elderly. A five-year prospective study of active ambulatory patients in an institutionalized setting revealed an annual fall rate of 668 incidents per 1,000 person-months (Gryfe 1977). In a study of elderly living in the community, the incidence rate for falls was 41.4 falls per 1,000 person-months (O'Loughlin 1993). Headache may occur with head trauma. Headaches may be acute and short lived, or chronic of greater than three months duration. Headache may also

Table 5 The ICHD-II Classes of Secondary Headache Disorders

Headache attributed to head and neck trauma

Headache attributed to cranial or cervical vascular disorder

Headache attributed to non-vascular intracranial disorder and other causes

Headache attributed to substances or their withdrawal

Headache attributed to infection

Headache attributed to disturbance of homeostasis

Headache or facial pain attributed to disorder of cranium, neck, eyes, ears, nose, sinuses, teeth, mouth, or other facial or cranial structures

Headache attributed to psychiatric disorder

be associated with whiplash injury and subdural hematoma. Typically, headache that occurs with concussion and whiplash can be readily diagnosed by the history. Headache can occur even with mild head injury. Occasionally, in approximately 1% of patients, headache will begin weeks after the injury. Headache attributed to head trauma has no particular distinguishing characteristics. Post-concussive syndrome includes symptoms of headache, dizziness, and mild cognitive impairment after a head injury. Evaluation would include neuroimaging, either CT or MRI of the brain and/or cervical spine. Treatment is symptomatic with mild analgesics such as acetaminophen or NSAIDs if not contraindicated.

The elderly are susceptible to tears of the intracranial bridging veins even with trivial trauma. Headache may be acute or progressive with a typical onset within 24–72 hours after development of the hematoma. The headache symptoms are nonspecific. Other symptoms may include confusion, decreased level of consciousness, and localizing symptoms including weakness, numbness, and gait disturbance. Neuroimaging is the test of choice. CT is excellent for detection of an acute subdural hematoma, but a subacute subdural hematoma is isodense on CT, and MRI would be a better choice to detect varying ages of blood products. Evacuation of hematoma may be necessary depending on the size and location of the subdural hematoma.

Headache and Vascular Disease

Headache may occur with cranial or cervical vascular disorders including ischemic stroke, intracranial hemorrhage, ruptured AVM, arteritis, carotid or vertebral artery dissection, and vasculitis. The symptoms and signs will typically lead to the diagnosis. Headache may occur with both thrombotic and embolic stroke. Pain may be ipsilateral to the stroke. It is debatable whether one can predict vascular territory by location of headache. Again the diagnosis is made by

Table 6 ICHD-II Diagnostic Criteria for Secondary Headaches

A. Headache with one (or more) of the following [listed] characteristics and fulfilling criteria C and D

B. Another disorder known to be able to cause headache has been demonstrated

C. Headache occurs in close temporal relation to the other disorder and/or there is other evidence of a causal relationship

D. Headache is greatly reduced or resolves within three months (this may be shorter for some disorders) after successful treatment or spontaneous remission of the causative disorder

the accompanying focal symptoms and signs which may include hemiparesis, aphasia, gait abnormality, or other localizing symptoms. Migraine may present with similar symptoms but that is a diagnosis of exclusion. Appropriate evaluation includes emergent imaging and treatment.

Intracranial hemorrhage presents as acute severe headache. With subarachnoid bleed due to ruptured cerebral aneurysm, headache is typically severe and accompanied by decreased level of consciousness and meningeal signs. Appropriate evaluation includes CT scan and if negative, lumbar puncture and neurosurgical consultation. Intraparenchymal hemorrhage due to hypertension may present with headache, confusion, and focal signs. Again, emergent imaging must be performed and management of blood pressure as well as reversal of anticoagulation if the patient is on warfarin therapy.

Temporal arteritis is a systemic inflammatory disorder affecting extracranial branches of the aorta including the carotid, vertebral, and coronary arteries. This occurs in people older than 50 years of age and most often 75–85 years of age with an incidence of 15–25 cases per 100,000 persons over the age of 50. In the study by Solomon and Kunkel, 16% of all elderly patients complaining of headache had temporal arteritis (Solomon 1990). Symptoms reflect the vascular territory involved which may include headache, jaw claudication, scalp tenderness, vertigo, loss of vision, transient ischemic attacks, and encephalopathy. Systemic symptoms include fever, night sweats, malaise, weight loss, and myalgias. Affected individuals may also have symptoms of polymyalgia rheumatica with shoulder and hip pain bilaterally. If untreated, temporal arteritis may result in partial loss of vision or blindness from ischemic optic neuropathy, myocardial infarction, and stroke.

An erythrocyte sedimentation rate (ESR) is usually elevated between 60–120 mm/hr, although 1% of patients may have normal ESR. An elevated C-reactive protein (CRP) and ESR may yield a higher degree of specificity. Temporal artery biopsy is necessary to confirm the diagnosis before committing a patient to 1–2 years of corticosteroid treatment. The pathology is a panarteritis with mononuclear infiltrates through all the arterial wall layers. This results in stenosis and then occlusion of the vessel (Weyand 2003).

If suspicion is high, corticosteroid treatment should be started immediately at 60 mg/day prior to the biopsy. Once the diagnosis is confirmed, the prednisone can be slowly tapered to the lowest effective dose and patients are typically treated from 1–2 years. Monitoring with ESR is the best method to ensure the steroid taper is not proceeding too quickly resulting in exacerbation of disease.

Headache and Neoplasm

Headache may occur with brain tumor. In a study by Schanklin et al., all inpatients with primary and metastatic CNS tumors from a large neurosurgical department in a university hospital (N=97) were recruited during the year 2002. Twelve were excluded due to lack of pathology or incomplete questionnaires. The histopathology of the remaining 85 patients included astrocytoma, glioblastoma multiforme, meningioma, and metastatic tumors from lung, breast, kidney, and malignant melanoma. Of the 85 subjects in the study, 60% had a headache at the time of the evaluation, 47.1% recalled history of headache, 54.1% had focal neurological deficits, 37.6% had neuropsychological signs, and 27.1% had symptomatic seizures. Blurred vision, nausea, vomiting, and tinnitus occurred in 36.5% of subjects. Only 2% of patients had headache as the only presenting symptom. The tumor headaches could be unilateral or bilateral, usually medium intensity, and dull in character. In half of all cases, headache did not last for >4 hours. Headache frequency varied from continuous, in 11.8% to daily in 29.4%, and less than once a week in 43.1%. In terms

of location of tumor, if headache was unilateral, only 61% of the time was the tumor located on the same side of the headache. Univariate analysis of risk factors for headache revealed that a positive family history of headache and pre-existing headache were positive factors for developing headache. There was no strong correlation with histopathology of tumor type and type of pain. Of interest, none of the patients in this study met criteria for ICHD-II headache attributable to neoplasm (Schanklin 2007).

The headaches described in ICHD-II are the "classic" tumor headache with symptoms of worsening in the morning, coughing or Valsalva maneuver, nausea and vomiting, and attributable to increased intracranial pressure either due to mass effect or hydrocephalus.

Headache and Medication

Headache can be an adverse effect to medication or due to medication overuse. Common medications that are used in the elderly that cause headache are caffeine, alcohol, antibiotics (trimethoprim-sulfamethoxozole, tetracycline), sedatives, stimulants, anti-parkinsonian drugs (amantadine, levodopa), vasodilators (dipyridamole), anti-hypertensives including beta-blockers and calcium channel blockers, anti-arrhythmics, NSAIDs, H2 blockers, bronchodilators, chemotherapeutics (tamoxifen, cyclophosphamide), hormones, and erectogenic agents. Elimination of the drug is the treatment of choice.

Cervicogenic Headache

The diagnosis of cervicogenic headache is controversial. This headache typically has features similar to tension type headache, a primary headache disorder. Pain occurs in the occiput and neck. It can be unilateral or bilateral. Cervicogenic headache may manifest as chronic TTH or migraine or hemicrania continua or occipital neuralgia. Many adults over the age of 50 have spondylosis of the cervical spine so an abnormal X-ray or MRI of the cervical spine does not make the diagnosis of cervicogenic headache. There are maneuvers that may exacerbate or precipitate pain but currently there are no standardized maneuvers that are specific or sensitive for diagnosing cervicogenic etiology. The ICHD-II criteria for cervicogenic headache are listed in Table 7. This includes diagnostic nerve blocks at C1–3 with 100% pain relief to confirm the diagnosis. Greater occipital nerve (GON) blocks are neither specific nor sensitive for cervicogenic headaches and patients with migraines, occipital neuralgia, or tension type headaches may respond

Table 7 ICHD-II Diagnostic Criteria for Cervicogenic Headache

Diagnostic Criteria:

A. Pain, referred from a source in the neck and perceived in one or more regions of the head and/or face, fulfilling criteria C and D

B. Clinical, laboratory and/or imaging evidence of a disorder or lesion within the cervical spine or soft tissues of the neck known to be, or generally accepted as, a valid cause of headache

C. Evidence that the pain can be attributed to the neck disorder or lesion based on at least one of the following:
   1. demonstration of clinical signs that implicate a source of pain in the neck
   2. abolition of headache following diagnostic blockade of a cervical structure or its nerve supply using placebo- or other adequate control

D. Pain resolves within three months after successful treatment of the causative disorder or lesion

to GON blocks. Other cervical causes of neck pain include developmental anomalies of the craniovertebral junction, tumors, osteomyelitis of upper cervical vertebra, RA of upper cervical spine, and ankylosing spondylitis. The history may reveal clues—pain is precipitated by certain movements and may have associated shoulder pain and pain radiating down the arm. Treatment options include nerve blocks, physical therapy, NSAIDs, tricyclic antidepressants, and muscle relaxants if not contraindicated.

Cervical dystonia may present with occipital pain and neck pain and examination will reveal the dystonia which may be subtle. Botox therapy is beneficial.

Other Secondary Causes of Headache

Coronary artery ischemia may manifest as an exertional headache also known as cardiac cephalgia. The headache typically resolves with rest or nitrates whereas migraines will worsen with nitrates. There may or may not be typically features of angina associated with this headache. A cardiac evaluation is required.

Headache can also be a referred pain from the mediastinum or lung through the vagus nerve. This may present as unilateral face, ear, or temporal pain. Pain may be a constant severe aching with sharp stabbing pains. A CXR is needed to look for an apical or mediastinal mass (Biondi 2000).

Ocular pain may be a referred pain as a symptom of a primary headache disorder but occasionally the eye may be the source of a headache. Acute primary angle closure glaucoma will cause severe boring pain, redness of the eye, nausea, vomiting, and diaphoresis. Blindness may occur. The pain is due to increased intraocular pressure and is typically periorbital with clouding of the eye or red eye; symptoms resolve with treatment. Refractive errors can cause eyestrain with symptoms of fatigue and discomfort in the eyes and in the frontal regions. Optic neuritis is associated with periorbital pain and pain with movement of the eye. Inflammatory disorders will also cause a painful red eye (Tomsak 2006).

There are numerous metabolic causes of headache. Hypothyroidism should be mentioned because this may cause a new onset daily headache. Thus a TSH is a useful screening tool. Review of symptoms in a patient with new onset headache should include questions about other symptoms of hypothyroidism—skin changes, hair loss, fatigue, weight gain, and constipation. Examination should include palpation of thyroid gland. Low thyroid hormone may have a pronociceptive effect, but the actual mechanism is not known.

Summary

Headache is a common symptom in the elderly. Primary headaches continue to occur in the elderly, but there is an increase in secondary headaches. A new headache or change in headache pattern in patients should be aggressively evaluated. Treatment approaches depend on the underlying cause. Treatment of both primary and secondary headache can be challenging due to multiple comorbidities and medications in the elderly, however it is as important to appropriately treat pain and improve quality of life as it is to exclude secondary pathology.

References

Bendtsen L. Central sensitization in tension-type headache-possible pathophysiological mechanisms. *Cephalalgia* 2000;20:486–508.

Bigal ME, Rapoport AM, Sheftell FD, et al. Chronic migraine is an earlier stage of transformed migraine in adults. *Neurology* 2005; 65:1556–1561.

Biondi D and Saper J. How to make the diagnosis and manage the pain. *Geriatrics* 2000; 55(12):40, 43–45, 48–50.

Dodick D, Lipton RB, and Vincent M. Consensus Statement: Cardiovascular safety profile of triptans (5-HT1B/1D Agonists) in the acute treatment of migraine. *Headache* 2004; 44(5):414–425.

Dodick D. Diagnosing headache: Clinical clues and clinical rules. *Adv Stud Med* 2003;3(2):87–92.

Haan J, Hollander J, and Ferrari MD. Migraine in the elderly: A review. *Cephalagia* 2006;27:97–106.

Headache classification subcommittee of the International Headache Society. The International Classification of the Headache Disorders: 2nd edition. *Cephalagia* 2004;24 (Suppl 1).

Edmeads JG and Wang, SJ. Headaches in the elderly. In Olesen J, Goadsby PJ, Ramadan N., eds. *The headaches*, 3rd edition. Lipincott Williams and Wilkins, 2006, 1105–1110.

Lipton RB, Steward WF, Diamond S, et al. Prevalence and burden of migraine in the United States: Data from the American Migraine Study II. *Headache* 2001; 41:646–657.

Lisotto C, Mainardi F, Maggioni F, et al. Headache in the elderly: A clinical study. *J Headache Pain*. 2004;5:36–41.

Lyngberg AC, Rasmussen BK, Jorgensen T et al. Prognosis of migraine and tension-type headache: A population-based follow-up study. *Neurology* 2005;65:580–585.

Martins KM, Bordini CA, Bigal ME, et al. Migraine in the elderly: A comparison with migraine in young adults. *Headache* 2006; 46:312–316.

Mazzotta G. Characteristics of migraine in an out-patient population over 60 years of age. *Cephalalgia* 2003; 23(10): 953–960.

Prencipe M, Casini AR, Ferretti C, et al. Prevalence of headache in elderly population: Attack frequency, disability and use of medication. *J Neurol Neurosurg Psychiatry* 2001;70:377–381.

Silberstein S. Practice parameter: Evidence-based guidelines for migraine headache (an evidence-based review) report of the Quality Standards Subcommittee of the American Academy of Neurology. *Neurology* 2000; 55:754–762.

Schankin CJ, Ferrari U, Reinisch VM, et al. Characteristics of brain tumor-associated headache. *Cephalalgia*. 2007; 27(8):904–11. Epub 2007 Jul 17.

Solomon GD, Kunkel RS, Jr., and Frame J. Demographics of headache in elderly patients. *Headache* 1990;30:273–276.

Tomsak, RL and Daroff, RB. Ocular Disorder. In Olesen J, Goadsby PJ, Ramadan N., eds. *The headaches*, 3rd edition. Lipincott Williams and Wilkins, 2006, 1013-1018.

Wang, SJ, Fuh, JL, Lu, SR, et al. Chronic daily headache in Chinese elderly: Prevalence, risk factors and biannual follow-up. *Neurology* 2000; 54:314–319.

Weyand, C and Goronzo, J. Medium- and large-vessel Vasculitis. *N Eng J Med* 2003;349:160–169.

49 Shingles and Postherpetic Neuralgia in the Elderly

Larry E. Davis and Molly K. King

Introduction

The story of shingles or herpes zoster begins with chickenpox and varicella-zoster virus (VZV), a childhood illness that occurs worldwide. Most cases occur in grammar school-aged children with an incubation period of 10–21 days and a prodrome of malaise and low-grade fever 1–2 days before the rash (Whitley 2005; LaRussa 2000). The rash is the hallmark of the infection and typically develops over most areas of skin, particularly on the chest. Five to ten millimeter maculopapules on an erythematous base appear over the trunk and face and spread centrifugally to other areas of the body. New vesicles appear over several days. The maculopapules develop into vesicles with a clear fluid that evolves into a pustule with whitish fluid containing inflammatory cells. The pustules rupture, crust, and the scabs fall off over 1–2 weeks. The illness is typically benign. However, there is an associated mortality of 2/100,000 cases (Whitley 2005) that mainly occur when chickenpox develops in immunocompromised individuals or adults.

Varicella-Zoster Virus (VZV) and Pathogenesis of Shingles

VZV is a member of the herpesvirus family and shares many common properties with herpes simplex virus. VZV contains double stranded DNA surrounded by a capsule containing glycoprotein spikes and replicates by budding from infected cells (Arvin 1996). VZV exclusively infects humans and thus has no natural reservoir or vector. Almost every vertebrate and invertebrate species has their own herpes family virus, suggesting the herpesviruses have been in evolution a very long time. The virus is very successful in infecting humans, and serological studies show that over 98% of healthy adults have previously been infected with the virus (Kilgore 2003) and now carry latent VZV.

Transmission of VZV among children typically occurs via respiratory spread (Whitley 2005). Other modes can occur from hand-oral spread from infected chickenpox or shingles vesicles or possibly from infected saliva in patients with shingles or chickenpox (Mehta 2008). The initial infection begins in cells of the nasopharyngeal tract with spread to tonsils (Dworkin 2007). Viral replication in the tonsils infects memory CD4+T cells, which are abundant in tonsils (Ku 2005). The infected T-cells re-enter the circulation and appear to have a tropism for skin epidermis and ganglia (Ku 2005). Several days later the T-cells infect areas of skin, allowing viral replication in epidermal cells. These foci of VZV infection become the vesicles that contain virus present mainly in the cells at the base of the vesicle. Uninfected T-cells attracted to the vesicles can become infected and further transmit the spread of the virus via viremia.

Spread of VZV to ganglia neurons occurs mainly by cell-free virus in the vesicle infecting sensory axons in that area of the skin. Virus then travels retrograde back to the neuron cell body located in a dorsal root ganglion or trigeminal ganglion where the virus establishes latency. For unknown reasons the virus virtually never continues its retrograde transmission back to the spinal cord dorsal root entry zone or brain. A second route of VZV transmission to ganglia occurs via infected memory T-cells entering ganglia and directly infecting neuron cell bodies. In this manner, sensory and autonomic nerve ganglia that are not connected with skin can be latently infected. Examples of such ganglia include autonomic ganglia around the heart, GI track, and inner ear (Pui 2001; Wackym 1997; Furuta 1997). Detailed information of how infected T-cells directly infect ganglia neurons is poorly understood.

Latency develops in sensory and autonomic ganglia neurons in a manner similar to that of herpes simplex virus. VZV DNA enters the nucleus but remains extrachromosomal, where it is circular and exists in the latent stage usually for the rest of the host's life (Gilden 2003). Latently infected ganglia neurons show restricted expression of six genes to messenger RNA which produces six proteins that move to the cytoplasm but not to the cell membrane where they could trigger a host immune response (Dworkin 2007). This combination of VZV RNAs and proteins somehow maintains latency. At present it is unclear how many dorsal root ganglia are latently infected in adults, but studies of the trigeminal ganglia demonstrated latent virus in 1–7% of the neurons with greater than ten copies of VZV DNA per neuron (Cohrs 2000; Levin 2003).

Decades later, something triggers the latent virus to break latency in presumably one neuron within one ganglion. Details of how that happens are unknown. With reactivation, the virus now replicates in the neuron, subsequently releasing virus within the ganglion which then infect other ganglion neurons. The ensuing ganglion infection triggers inflammatory cells that invade, resulting in sufficient inflammation to produce the prodromal symptoms seen in many patients. VZV from many infected ganglion neurons simultaneously travel anterograde down to the skin of the dermatome. The rash is distributed along the entire dermatome but not other dermatomes.

Once VZV reactivates in a ganglion neuron, several clinical events may occur besides shingles. (1). *Asymptomatic infection.* There is increasing evidence for the ability of the trigeminal ganglia to break latency and shed VZV into mouth saliva without producing shingles on the face. Astronauts on shuttle flights have been shown to release VZV DNA detected by PCR assay during and shortly after their shuttle flight without ever developing any shingles rashes (Mehta 2004). In addition, patients with shingles in any dermatome may shed VZV virions in their saliva without evidence of vesicles in the mouth or face (Mehta 2008). (2). *Zoster-sine-herpete.* Occasional patients may develop severe itching or deep pain along a dermatome for several weeks without developing a shingles rash in that dermatome (Gilden 1994). Diagnosis of this unusual infection has been difficult as most of the time the dermatomal pain is not from shingles. One study of 57 patients presenting with unilateral pain consistent with zoster-sine-herpete and carefully studied by the above methods for 28 days, found only two (4%) with evidence of VZV reactivation (McKendrick 1999). Methods to establish the diagnosis range from detection of VZV DNA by PCR assay in CSF, detection of circulating blood monocytes infected with VZV DNA by PCR, and establishing a 4-fold rise in VZV antibody titer from acute to convalescent serum (Gilden 1994). (3). *CNS VZV infections* (discussed under complications of shingles).

Shingles Epidemiology and Risk Factors

Shingles is the most common infection of the nervous system and develops in over 1 million individuals per year in the United States (Harpaz 2008). The lifetime incidence is as high as 30% but the incidence in individuals over the age of 85 years is 50% (Harpaz 2008). Increasing age and immunosuppression are the most important risk factors for the development of shingles. The incidence of shingles increases significantly in adults over 50–60 years (Hope-Simpson 1965; Ragozzino 1982). Many studies have reported the incidence for adults 60–69 years of age to be about six cases per 1,000 persons per year (Hope-Simpson 1965; Ragozzino 1982). Data for these incidence studies were derived from patients with the shingles rash visiting an emergency room or their physician. However, more recent data suggests the actual incidence is higher. The Shingles Prevention Study found an incidence of nine cases per 1,000 persons per year for those 60–69 years (Oxman 2005). Higher numbers have also been reported in self-report surveys of patients (Yih 2005) and health maintenance organization records (Jumaan 2005). The higher incidence comes from the detection of mild cases of shingles (minimal dermatomal rash and little discomfort proven by VZV PCR assay) in which the patient would not have sought medical attention. After age 80 years, the incidence climbs to 12 per 1,000 persons per year (Oxman 2005).

Immunocompromise, secondary to disease or drugs, is another important risk factor for shingles. Common immunodeficiency diseases include HIV with AIDS, hematologic malignancies, organ transplants, immunological diseases such as systemic lupus erythematous and rheumatoid arthritis, and administration of high dose corticosteroids, anticancer drugs, or drugs directed against components of the immune system (Schmader 2008). In patients with AIDS, the incidence of shingles increases about 15 fold. A third risk factor is trauma to a dermatome or irradiation involving dorsal root ganglia. Finally, there is some evidence that high level stress within the previous two months may also trigger shingles (Mehta 2004, Schmader 2008).

Shingles Clinical Features

Shingles is defined as an erythematous vesicular rash conforming to a dermatome with variable pain or itching due to varicella-zoster virus. The various components include:

Prodrome

Fifty percent of individuals develop a prodrome lasting 1–4 days before rash appearance (Schmader 2008). The prodrome is a deep aching pain or itching along the dermatome. It is not uncommon for the prodromal pain to be confused with angina, heart attack, cholecystitis, appendicitis, nephrolithiasis, or nerve root pain in an arm or leg.

Rash

The rash begins with macules and papules developing over an erythematous base scattered in clusters along a single dermatome (Figure 1). New vesicles often appear along the dermatome for the next 3–5 days. Similar to that described for chickenpox earlier, the clear vesicles soon become cloudy and pustulate, rupture, and crust

over 1–2 weeks (Schmader 2008). Healing of the rash commonly occurs over the next 2–3 weeks, but in the elderly it may continue for up to six weeks.

The rash may be broader than the dermatome described in textbooks due to sensory axons from that dermatome spreading slightly into the adjacent dermatomes. In thoracic or abdominal shingles, the extent of the rash in the back usually ends at the midline and circles somewhat downward ending within a few centimeters either side of the midline. The rash may be spotty along the dermatome.

The dermatomal distribution is not a random occurrence. Thoracic rashes develop in about 50%, facial rashes occur in 20% with the upper face predominating, cervical and lumbar dermatome rashes each develop in 13%, and a sacral dermatomal rash develops in 3% (Seiler 1949). The distribution of the rashes in shingles matches the distribution of vesicles in children with chickenpox, suggesting in adults there is more latent VZV in thoracic and abdominal dorsal root ganglia and trigeminal ganglia than other dermatomes.

Pain

Patients describe variable pain or itching along a distribution restricted to the dermatome. Itching is less common than pain and both may occur. The intensity of the pain varies from none or mild (40%), to moderate (35%), to severe (25%) (Dworkin 2001). There may be three characteristics to the pain of both shingles and postherpetic neuralgia. The most common pain is a burning sensation, like that of burning your fingers on a hot stove. This pain is accompanied by aching or throbbing sensations that can be very disagreeable. A second type of pain that some patients develop is brief stabbing or electric shock-like pains lasting seconds and radiating up or down the dermatome. The third type of pain is allodynia or painful sensations developing in affected areas of the dermatome from light touching of clothing, cold or warm temperatures placed on the skin, or breezes blowing over the skin. Allodynia may range from uncomfortable dysesthesias or paresthesias to intense painful sensations that prevent wearing of light

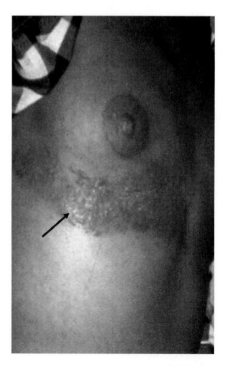

Figure 1 Right T5 acute shingles in adult. Courtesy of Michael Oxman, MD.

clothing that touches the involved skin. Intense allodynia is more common in postherpetic neuralgia than in shingles. Typically, the pain is most intense during the first two weeks of rash and then slowly subsides around the time of rash healing. Some patients may experience continued pain that slowly resolves for up to three months (Schmader 2008).

Severe herpetic pain occurs most commonly in patients with extensive epidermal denuding of their rash, secondary bacterial infection, and rashes occurring in sensitive skin such as face, eye, and genital areas.

Laboratory Findings

Abnormal CSF is frequent. Studies report the most common findings in immunocompetent individuals are leukocytosis in 46%, elevated protein in 26%, oligoclonal bands in 9%, VZV IgG antibody in 23% occurring on day two and persisting up to three months, and VZV DNA in 24% (Haanpaa 1998). MRI with gadolinium-contrast abnormalities have been reported in patients with facial shingles (enhancement of pons and/or trigeminal nerve) or cervical shingles (enhancement of cervical spinal cord) (Haanpaa 1988).

Diagnosis of Shingles

The appearance of a vesicular rash on an erythematous base corresponding to a unilateral dermatome is sufficiently distinctive that a clinical diagnosis of shingles is usually accurate. However, about 5% of such rashes are due to herpes simplex virus when cultured (Oxman 2005). In patients with "recurrent shingles," the rash usually is due to herpes simplex virus unless the interval has been more than ten years or the patient is immunocompromised. In atypical cases, laboratory confirmation of VZV can be established by several methods (Harpaz 2008). Tzanck smears are inexpensive and detect multinucleated giant cells in lesion specimens, but they do not distinguish between herpes simplex and VZV. Direct fluorescent antibody (DFA) staining of VZV-infected cells in a scraping of cells from the base of the lesion is rapid and sensitive. DFA and other antigen-detection methods can be used on biopsy material. Histopathology sections of lesions often demonstrate eosinophilic nuclear inclusions (Cowdry type A). PCR assays can detect VZV DNA rapidly and sensitively in properly-collected vesicle fluid, CSF, whole blood, white blood cells, or other tissues (Gnann 2002). Using different VZV DNA primers in the PCR assay can differentiate between wild VZV and vaccine VZV (Oxman 2005). Viral culture of specimens for VZV or a four-fold increase in VZV antibody titer between acute shingles and convalescence serum samples is diagnostic. All methods have sensitivities above 60% but the PCR assay is as high as 97% (Nahass 1992).

Shingles Management

Antiviral Drugs

Three antiviral drugs have been shown in prospective randomized, double-blind clinical trials to: 1) shorten the duration of new lesions by about one day, 2) reduce the total number of vesicles by 25%, 3) lessen the duration of viral shedding from the rash, 4) shorten the time to rash healing by a few days, 5) lessen the intensity and duration of acute pain during the rash in about 1/3 of patients, 6) reduce the risk of VZV dissemination in immunosuppressed patients, and 7) slightly reduce the risk of postherpetic neuralgia per meta-analysis studies (Dworkin 2007; Tyler 2007; Schmader 2007; Gnann 2002; Wood 1996). All randomized trials to date required the antiviral drugs to be given within the first 72 hours of rash. As such, the benefit of administering an antiviral drug late in the clinical course is unknown but is seldom done unless the patient is immunosuppressed or continues to develop new vesicles. Patients with mild shingles often do not require antiviral therapy unless it involves the upper face near the eye.

Famciclovir (500 mg orally 3 times daily for 7–10 days), valaciclovir (1,000 mg orally 3 times daily for 7–10 days), and acyclovir (800 mg orally 5 times daily for 7–10 days) are essentially equally effective (Tyring 2000; Beutner 1995; Tyring 1995; Ormrod 2000; Huff 1988). All three drugs are guanosine analogs that are phosphorylated by viral thymidine kinase and cellular kinases to a triphosphate molecule that inhibits VZV polymerase and hence interrupts viral replication. The three drugs are excreted by the kidneys so dosages must be adjusted downward for patients with renal insufficiency. In general, all have relatively few adverse effects that include headache and nausea.

Corticosteroid Adjunctive Therapy

There is controversy regarding the addition of high dose corticosteroids along with an antiviral drug. However, use of corticosteroids without concomitant administration of an antiviral drug carries a low but real risk of cutaneous dissemination of the rash even in healthy individuals (Whitley 1996). Two clinical trials of acyclovir with and without high dose corticosteroids for 21 days failed to demonstrate any additional benefit in preventing postherpetic neuralgia when given with acyclovir (Whitley 1996; Wood 1994). However, there was some evidence for slightly more rapid rash healing and less acute pain. Adverse effects were more frequent in the steroid groups.

Management of the Rash

Good hygiene of the rash is important to prevent secondary bacterial skin infections. The rash should be gently cleaned frequently with soap and water and kept as dry as possible (Davis 2003). Should the denuded skin develop pus and appear secondarily bacterially infected, topical antibiotics may be administered over the rash. Should the superficial infection worsen and become a cellulitis, bacterial cultures are needed along with systemic antibiotics. Prevention of bacterial infections is a challenge if the shingles are in a sacral dermatome. It should be noted that transmission of the virus to susceptible children or adults can occur from the rash during the first week. One study reported 16% of susceptible household contacts develop chickenpox (Seiler 1949).

Pain Control

Randomized placebo-controlled double-blinded trials of oral treatments for acute pain management in shingles are sorely lacking. As a general principle, pain management needs to be approached based on the individual patient's pain and underlying conditions with an eye toward treating aggressively and early. Another principle is to manage the pain consistently with scheduled around-the-clock dosing of analgesics rather than using as needed. Mild to moderate pain management starts with acetaminophen or NSAIDs. Weak opiates such as codeine or tramadol can be added if necessary. While there are various approaches available for moderate to severe zoster pain, opiates are the drug of choice. Short acting opiates (e.g. oxycodone) are used around the clock until the dose is titrated upward to effect. According to patient preference, this final dose can be converted to a long-acting opiate (e.g. extended release oxycodone or methadone) and the short acting types can be held in reserve for breakthrough pain if needed (Schmader 2008). Associated side effects need to be managed. Nausea and vomiting, constipation, and cognitive changes/sedation are the more common complaints. Pre-emptive management of the constipation with routine use of stool softeners and laxatives is advisable.

If moderate to severe pain is not adequately managed with the antiviral medications in combination with oral analgesics, adjuvant medications such as anticonvulsants (e.g., gabapentin (Berry 2005) or pregabalin) or tricyclic antidepressants (e.g., nortriptyline or desipramine) could be considered even though none have been evaluated in the acute setting in randomized, controlled trials. Gabapentin and pregabalin have been shown to relieve chronic neuropathic pain (Dworkin 2003). Dosing is typically started at night to minimize side effects and gradually increased to effect (three times daily schedule for gabapentin; two times daily schedule for pregabalin). As these are renally excreted, dose adjustments need to be considered where appropriate and patients warned of the more common side effects of sedation, dizziness, ataxia, and peripheral edema. Tricyclic antidepressants have been proven efficacious in relieving chronic neuropathic pain but side effects may preclude use. Nortriptyline and desipramine have fewer side effects than amitriptyline but all have varying amounts of anticholinergic side effects (Dworkin 2007). Electrocardiograms are recommended in all patients >50 years of age especially if they have known cardiac disease since this class can prolong the QT interval. Other potential effects include urinary retention, dry mouth, visual changes, cognitive impairment (a particular problem in dementia patients), constipation, and dizziness/orthostatic hypotension.

An experimental option in patients with severe, unremitting pain from herpes zoster is neural blockade. Hwang et al. (1999) showed the treatment group with intravenous acyclovir and an epidural blockade versus patients with intravenous acyclovir alone showed a reduction in acute pain and a significantly shorter duration of pain.

Complications of Shingles

Herpes zoster oticus or Ramsey Hunt syndrome: This syndrome is a peripheral facial palsy often accompanied by vestibulocochlear dysfunction due to VZV. Herpes zoster oticus is responsible for 2–10% of all cases of facial palsy and has an incidence of five cases per 100,000 population annually (Murakami 1997). Studies indicate that the VZV infection begins in the geniculate ganglion (sensory ganglion for the facial nerve) and spreads outward, causing paresis or paralysis of the facial nerve and a vesicular eruption mainly of the concha of the auricle but vesicles may also appear along the external auditory canal and roof of the mouth. The ear vesicles typically are present the day before or on the day of facial paralysis but their appearance can be delayed several days (Crabtree 1968). About 50% of patients also develop a variety of inner ear symptoms including tinnitus, ipsilateral hearing loss, vertigo, and occasionally other cranial nerve palsies (Sweeney 2001). About 2/3 of patients experience a complete facial nerve paralysis, which is higher than with the more common idiopathic Bell's palsy. Elderly or immunosuppressed patients are more likely to have severe disease.

In 50% of patients, MRI with gadolinium demonstrates enhancement in the geniculate ganglion, labyrinthine segments, and premeatal regions of the affected facial nerve (Wackym 1997). The pathology appears to be a geniculate ganglionitis with VZV DNA in the geniculate ganglia by PCR of autopsy specimens from patients previously experiencing herpes zoster oticus (Sweeney and Gilden 2001; Wackym 1997).

Currently, early treatment with any of the three antiviral drugs is felt to improve prognosis (Murakami 1997) but no careful randomized, double-blind study has been done (Uscategui 2008). There is weak anecdotal evidence that the addition of corticosteroids is beneficial (Muarakami 1997) but no randomized controlled trials have been done (Uscategui 2008). Two-thirds of patients with incomplete acute facial nerve paralysis make an excellent recovery while only 10–50% of patients with complete facial nerve paralysis make a full recovery (Sweeney and Gilden 2001). Eyelid or oral synkinesis is commonly seen late in those with complete facial paralysis. Fortunately, permanent

hearing loss is uncommon and the vertigo spontaneous resolves over a few weeks.

Herpes zoster ophthalmicus (HZO): About 20% of shingles affects the face and about half of those rashes affect the eye. Rashes involving the nasociliary branch of the ophthalmic division of cranial nerve V are important, as this nerve innervates the tip and the side of the nose, skin of both eye lids, conjunctiva, sclera, cornea, iris, choroid, and anterior and posterior ethmoid sinuses.

HZO usually begins with prodromal malaise, headache, and eye pain. Ocular involvement is variable, complex, and may include ocular damage from viral infection, inflammation, vasculitis, and neuritis (Liesegang 2008). Serious ocular disease manifestations include blepharoconjunctivitis, episcleritis, epithelial keratitis, dendritic keratitis, uveitis, acute retinal necrosis, and optic neuritis (Shaikh 2002). Patients usually have vesicles over the eyelids, ptosis with varying amounts of monocular loss of vision, and severe eye pain. Management consists of administration of any of the three oral antiviral drugs and immediate referral to an ophthalmologist for treatment of eye complications. Antiviral drugs have been shown to be of benefit in preventing or reducing conjunctivitis, superficial and stromal keratitis, and anterior uveitis (Shaikh 2002) but they may not prevent all complications, especially some of the late complications. Immunosuppressed patients tend to have more severe ocular infections that involve deeper layers of the eye (Vafai 2001).

Motor weakness in shingles: Historically, overt motor weakness is uncommon in shingles with an incidence of 1–5% of all cases (Hope-Simpson 1965). The weakness develops in the face, arms, or legs and involves myotome muscles of the cervical or lumbar dermatome with rash or the facial nerve from herpes zoster oticus. Interestingly, one study reported 21/40 (53%) of patients with shingles had evidence of myotome denervation by electromyography even if the patients did not report weakness (Haapaa 1997). Most of these patients had thoracic shingles where minor weakness of chest muscles would not be recognized. Unexpectedly, they also reported half of the patients developed bilateral myotome denervation by electromyography. Overall, the prognosis for full recovery is good.

Dissemination of shingles: Dissemination of VZV (more than 20 vesicles appearing in skin outside the affected or adjacent dermatomes) is rare in immunocompetent patients (Schmader 2008). However, in immunocompromised patients dissemination may develop with spread of the virus to other parts of the skin and to visceral organs (Gnann 2002; Vafai 2001). Visceral infections commonly involve the lung with pneumonia, liver with hepatitis, and central nervous system. Immunosuppressed patients with severe shingles may require intravenous acyclovir (10 mg/kg every 8 hours for 10–14 days) (Vafai 2001). Death occurs most commonly from pneumonia or encephalitis.

Central nervous system complications: Involvement of the CNS is rare when shingles occurs in healthy individuals but may include encephalitis, myelitis and a syndrome of delayed contralateral hemiparesis (Gilden 2000; Hilt 1983). The delayed contralateral hemiparesis occurs when a patient develops shingles over the upper face accompanied by a low-grade VZV arteritis of the ipsilateral middle cerebral, anterior cerebral, or carotid artery (Melanson 1996). The large vessel arteritis can trigger emboli to the brain or a thrombosis of the vessel producing contralateral hemiparesis weeks to a few months after the rash onset. Treatment with acyclovir is often successful but the morbidity is high.

In immunocompromised patients, VZV can directly invade the CNS to cause myelitis or small vessel arteritis to produce an encephalitis with white matter foci of demyelination and localized cerebral infarctions. VZV infection occurs in parenchymal blood vessels, cerebral neurons, and oligodendroglia (Gilden 2000). These CNS infections are difficult to treat with intravenous acyclovir so there is a high mortality rate.

A recent review of all VZV vasculopathies found that rash or even CSF pleocytosis was not required for the diagnosis but neuroimaging abnormalities were always present (Nagel 2008). There was often a delay of several months between those with rash and onset of CNS symptoms. The CSF usually contains VZV DNA by PCR assay.

Postherpetic Neuralgia (PHN)

PHN is a common dreaded complication of shingles with a prevalence in the United States as high as 1 million (Dworkin 2007). In most patients with shingles, the dermatomal pain slowly resolves over 2–12 weeks. Unfortunately, in a few patients the dermatomal pain either persists or subsides and then returns. Predisposing factors for PHN include advanced age, severity of shingles rash, severity of prodromal or shingles pain, immunosuppression, and development of a secondary bacterial infection (Jung 2004; Dworkin 2007). However, age is the most important risk factor. Early epidemiology studies used a definition of PHN as pain persisting past one month of any intensity and reported the incidence in the elderly to be as high as 50%. The current definition of PHN is dermatomal pain persisting longer than three months that is severe enough to interfere with activities of daily living (Oxman 2005). This change in definition results in a much lower incidence of PHN. The Shingles Prevention Study reported an incidence of PHN of 12.5% in subjects over 60 years who received the placebo and developed shingles (Oxman 2005; Oxman 2008).

Three types of neuropathic pain often develop in PHN that are similar to the pain types in shingles. Almost all patients experience a burning, aching pain. Some also experience brief lancinating pains, and many experience allodynia. It is the allodynia that often interrupts their quality of life. Light touch, hot or cold temperatures, and even breezes over areas trigger severe pain in the involved dermatome even in skin that has healed and appears normal. Some patients with allodynia cannot even tolerate having their shirt touch certain areas of their skin. While the pain in PHN may persistent indefinitely, it often subsides over months. Once it subsides, it does not return.

Evidence is growing that the pathogenesis of PHN is multifocal, involving both the peripheral and central nervous system. Peripheral nervous system involvement comes from both a sensory neuritis and the sensory ganglionitis. Shingles can cause a distal sensory neuritis, damaging nerve fibers near the skin that are depleted, demyelinated, or have damaged sensory endings (Watson 1991; Sakai 2006). These fibers are hyperexcitable, sending spontaneous pain signals to the spinal cord. Evidence exists that the initially involved ganglion may remain abnormal with scarring, ganglion neuron loss, or continued inflammation. Both the abnormal nerves and ganglion may allow ectopic firing of pain signals (Gilden 2003; Oaklander 2008). Evidence for a persistent ganglionitis comes from histologic evidence of continued inflammation in the ganglion (Watson 1991) and continued presence of VZV DNA within circulating blood monocytes, suggesting the ganglion mononuclear cells acquire VZV infection and leave to circulate in blood (Mahalingam 1995). In uncomplicated shingles, infected circulating monocytes subside by six weeks when the rash heals.

Evidence of central nervous system involvement comes from fibrosis in the spinal cord dorsal horns of the involved dermatome found at autopsy (Watson 1991) and gadolinium contrast enhancement of the pons in facial shingles and spinal cord in shingles of cervical dermatomes (Haanpaa 1998). Additional indirect evidence comes from the observations of neurosurgeons that cutting the involved sensory nerve at the root entry zone does not abolish PHN. Finally, there is evidence that unilateral PHN is associated with bilateral sensory

neuron damage (Oaklander 1998). It has been speculated that abnormal sensitivity of the thalamus in PHN may also occur. These multiple sites of pain origin are likely the reason it is so difficult to adequately control pain in these patients.

The management of pain in PHN is challenging, as often medications do not fully control the chronic pain. In addition, the elderly patient is more likely to suffer PHN and can be sensitive to medications and their side effects. In general, the management of PHN uses the same medications as pain management in acute zoster pain. Medication choices need to be based on the patient's pain level, comorbidities, and with anticipation of potential side effects.

Tricyclic antidepressants (Raja 2005) (nortriptyline or desipramine) are typically titrated up slowly to a total dose of 75 to 150 mg nightly. Amitriptyline can also be used but the anticholinergic effects (sedation, constipation, urinary retention, blurry vision) of this drug are particularly poorly tolerated in the elderly. Confusion can be prominent in the elderly and prolonged QT intervals have been associated with this drug class, warranting an electrocardiogram prior to the initiation of therapy.

Anti-epileptic medications include gabapentin 300 mg orally daily titrated up to a maximum of 2700 mg total daily dose (in three times daily dosing schedule) and pregabalin 75–150 mg orally twice daily (this may be titrated up to 200 mg po three times daily as the maximum dose) (Dworkin 2003). Both are renally excreted and may require dosage adjustment in patients with renal dysfunction.

Opiates, such as short-acting oxycodone, are used in moderate to severe PHN. Oxycodone is started at 5 mg four times daily and can be titrated upward to effect. Once the effective dose is found it can be converted to long-acting opiates such as extended release oxycodone or methadone with short-acting oxycodone for breakthrough pain. As in acute pain management sedation, constipation, nausea, tolerance, and abuse are potential side effects.

Lidocaine patches (5%) can be applied directly over the affected area for 12 hours at a time (Pei-Lin 2008). This not only acts as a physical barrier but drug delivery can reduce PHN. Up to three patches can be cut to size and used at any one time; local skin irritation seems to be the only potential adverse effect.

Other topical treatments such as capsaicin (0.025–0.075%) have been used three or four times daily with success in appropriately chosen patients.

Finally, a single study using intrathecal methylprednisolone for intractable PHN showed long-lasting benefit (Kotani 2000). However, potential complications were significant and the study has not yet been replicated.

Prevention of Shingles

As seen in Figure 2, the ability to prevent shingles also prevents PHN and all other complications of shingles. Currently there are three approaches that are being used to prevent shingles.

Preventing VZV from Becoming Latent in Ganglia through Childhood Vaccination with a VZV Vaccine

The concept is simple. Vaccinate children with a shingles vaccine in which the virus produces immune responses that protects against infection with wild VZV yet does not produce latency or produces latency that rarely reactivates. Since 1995 in the U.S., live attenuated VZV vaccines are in production aimed initially at preventing chickenpox and hopefully any subsequent shingles. Overall, these vaccines are quite safe and effective in preventing chickenpox either from the vaccine itself or from subsequent exposure to wild VZV. Multiple studies have demonstrated that VZV vaccine reduces the incidence of

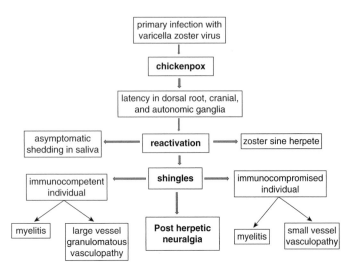

Figure 2 Schematic diagram of the pathogenesis of shingles. Modified from Gilden et al. 2003.

chickenpox by as much as 85% (Vazquez 2001; Hambleton 2005). Unfortunately, the vaccine can produce a transient viremia, which is sufficient to result in vaccine virus becoming latent in sensory ganglia. It is known that ganglia with latent vaccine VZV can occasionally reactivate, resulting in shingles (Galea 2008; Lawrence 1988). To date, shingles in vaccinated children have always been mild and primarily in individuals who were immunocompromised (Galea 2008; Lawrence 1988; Hardy 1991). Interestingly, the shingles mainly developed in the dermatome that the vaccine was initially administered (Galea 2008).

Currently for healthy children receiving the vaccine, the frequency of developing latency and the number of ganglia possessing latent virus is unknown. Also unknown is how often wild VZV can infect a vaccinated child or adult to produce a subclinical wild VZV infection and a subsequent latent infection in ganglia. If that occurs, then there is a risk of subsequent shingles from wild virus later in life.

There is a debate whether childhood vaccination programs may actually increase the risk of shingles in non-vaccinated adults. The concern centers on whether re-exposure to wild VZV during adulthood in immune adults boosts their immunity, which in turn lessens the risk of their subsequently reactivating latent virus and developing shingles. The concern is so far theoretical and based on epidemiology studies of special populations. Sixty-four percent of immune adults who had exposure to individuals with chickenpox developed increases in their VZV antibody and cell-mediated immunity without developing any rash or illness (Arvin 1983). Likewise, adults who raised children and had more exposure to chickenpox than other adults without children appear to have better protection against subsequently developing shingles (Brisson 2002; Thomas 2002). Amongst physicians, pediatricians have fewer cases of shingles than psychiatrists and dermatologists, presumably due to more exposure and subclinical infections with VZV (Solomon 1998).

These observations raise the possibility that as the incidence of chickenpox in society diminishes from widespread use of the varicella virus vaccine there will be less boosting of natural VZV immunity and thus an increase in the incidence of shingles in adults. Since the vaccine in the U.S. was only licensed in 1995, early studies on the incidence of shingles have varied regarding this question (Yawn 2007; Jumaan 2005). Time will tell if this becomes a problem. If so, it could be overcome by vaccinating adults with the adult form of the VZV vaccine.

Preventing Shingles when VZV Reactivates from Latency by Administering Antiviral Drugs to High-risk Individuals

The concept is to prevent shingles in very high-risk patients by administering antiviral drugs prophylactically. It is known that adults receiving transplants are at high risk of subsequently developing severe shingles in the first year post transplant (Ljungman 2001). In addition, markedly immunosuppressed patients are also at higher risk of developing severe shingles (Boeckh 2006). For allogenic hematopoietic cell transplantation the risk of shingles after transplantation is about 33% (Asano-Mori 2008; Kanda 2001). If high or lower dose acyclovir or valacyclovir is given daily for 6–12 months, the risk of shingles greatly reduces (Erard 2007; Kanda 2001). Unfortunately, following discontinuation of the prophylactic antiviral medication, the risk of shingles returns at a higher rate than similar-aged healthy adults (Erard 2007).

While prophylactic administration of antiviral medications is of benefit to some high-risk groups, it is impractical for the general older population. Currently even transplant programs are leaning more towards immunization of the transplant candidate before the transplantation with an inactivated shingles vaccine (Ljungman 2003; Hardy 1991).

Preventing VZV from Reactivating from a Latent Ganglia Infection by Immunization of Adults with Live VZV Attenuated Vaccine

The aim of this approach is to improve VZV immunity in the host to reduce the risk of VZV reactivation and shingles. The major challenge in preventing VZV from reactivating is to better understand what factors maintain latency. As noted above, we understand what VZV genes are responsible for maintaining latency but continue to have limited information on what host factors are responsible for maintaining the latency. Nevertheless, healthy individuals only get chickenpox once, so the immune system prevents symptomatic reinfection. Also, adults typically get only one episode of shingles in their lifetime since host cell-mediated immunity (CMI) and antibody to VZV both increase after an attack of shingles. Caveats to this rule are 20–30 years between the two shingles episodes or that the individual becomes immunocompromised.

Studies report that levels of serum antibody to VZV remain constant over time and do not correlate with the risk of developing shingles (Gershon 1981; Webster 1989). However, levels of CMI against VZV do correlate with protection (Dolin 1978). Levels of VZV CMI slowly diminish with age, reaching low levels around age 60 years. In addition, illnesses that affect host cellular immunity dramatically increase the risk of developing shingles. For example, patients with leukemia, lymphoma, and stem cell transplantation develop a risk of developing shingles from 20–50% in the first six months after transplantation (Sandherr 2006).

Based on the hypothesis that a high level of VZV CMI is an important factor in maintaining VZV latency in the host, a decision was made to identify methods to accomplish this. In the 1980s, VZV from a child in Japan with chickenpox was attenuated in tissue culture and became the basis for the varicella vaccine. From clinical trials in children, the vaccine was found to elicit both humoral and cellular immunity to VZV that was highly protective against developing chickenpox after exposure to the wild virus (Arvin 2008). It was later demonstrated that immunization with a modification of the vaccine increases VZV CMI without causing disease in the elderly (Levin 2008).

To test efficacy in preventing shingles in elderly adults, the Shingles Prevention Study was performed. This study was a placebo-controlled, double-blind, multicenter trial of 38,546 volunteer healthy elderly adults that received either the shingles vaccine (which contained about 19 times the live attenuated virus as the childhood vaccine) or placebo (Oxman 2005). Everyone was followed by monthly phone calls for a mean of 3.1 years. All suspicious rashes were evaluated by a clinical investigator to determine whether the rash followed a dermatomal pattern. Suspicious rashes were photographed and lesion scrapings were obtained for PCR assay to detect wild and vaccine VZV as well as herpes simplex virus. In addition, a viral culture or direct fluorescent antibody staining for VZV of lesion scrapings was often obtained. Patients diagnosed clinically as having shingles were treated with famciclovir and appropriate pain medications and followed regularly until the rash healed and the pain resolved.

The median age in both groups was 69 years and 7% of the subjects were 80 years or older. Remarkably, only 0.6% of subjects withdrew or were lost to follow up and 4% died before the end of the study. Use of the shingles vaccine reduced the incidence of shingles by 51% (P<0.001), reduced the incidence of postherpetic neuralgia by 67% (P<0.001), and reduced the burden of illness due to shingles by 61% (P<0.001). When volunteers 70 years or older were examined, the efficacy of the vaccine in preventing shingles fell to 38% but the efficacy in preventing postherpetic neuralgia remained high at 67%. The vaccine produced more mild local reactions than the placebo but there was no increase in serious adverse reactions. No cases of shingles were due to the vaccine. The shingles vaccine, now called Zostavax®, was approved by the FDA in 2006. In 2010, the vaccine is lyophilized and must be stored frozen at –20°C until being subcutaneously administered within a half hour of thawing and adding the diluent. However, a new refrigerator-stable formulation of the shingles vaccine produced by the company appears promising to replace the frozen vaccine (Gilderman 2008).

Summary

Virtually all adults today have been infected with wild VZV and carry latent VZV in their sensory ganglia. Thus, the hope of eradicating VZV from the world similar to what was done with variola, the smallpox virus, is impossible in the near future. Shingles will continue to occur frequently in the elderly and immunocompromised and occasionally in younger adults. The availability of good antiviral drugs for VZV does lessen the duration of the acute rash and pain by a few days and prevent viral dissemination in high risk patients. However, the rash is often still quite painful and antiviral drugs do little to reduce the risk of postherpetic neuralgia. The major hope of currently reducing both the incidence of shingles and postherpetic neuralgia lies with widespread use of the shingles vaccine but even then the incidence of shingles will only be reduced by half. As our population continues to age, the number of cases of shingles and postherpetic neuralgia may actually increase. It remains to be determined whether vaccination of children with the varicella vaccine will markedly reduce the incidence and severity of shingles as they grow into adulthood.

References

Arvin, A.M.: Varicella zoster virus. *Clin Microbiol Rev* 9:361–381, 1996.

Arvin, A.M.: Humoral and cellular immunity to varicella-zoster virus: An overview. *J Infect Dis* 197(suppl):S58–60, 2008.

Arvin, A.M., Koropchak, C.M., and Wittek, A.E.: Immunologic evidence of reinfection with varicella-zoster virus. *J Infect Dis* 148:200–205, 1983.

Asano-Mori, Y., Kanda, Y., Oshima, K., et al: Long-term ultra-low-dose acyclovir against varicella-zoster virus reactivation after allogeneic hematopoietic stem cell transplantation. *Am J Hematol* 83:472–476, 2008.

Berry JD and Petersen KL. A single dose of gabapentin reduces acute pain and allodynia in patients with herpes zoster. *Neurology* 655:444–447, 2005.

Beutner, KR., Friedman, D.J., Forszpaniak, C., et al: Valaciclovir compared with acyclovir for improved therapy for herpes zoster in immunocompetent adults. *Antimicrob Agents Chemother* 39:1546–1553, 1995.

Boeckh, M.: Prevention of VZV infection in immunosuppressed patients using antiviral agents. *Herpes* 13:60–65, 2006.

Brisson, M., Gay, N.J., Edmunds, W.J., and Andrews, N.J.: Exposure to varicella boosts immunity to herpes-zoster: Implications for mass vaccination against chickenpox. *Vaccine* 20:2500–2507, 2002.

Cohrs, R.J., Gilden, D.H., Kinchington, R.R., et al: Analysis of individual human trigeminal ganglia for latent herpes simplex virus type 1 and varicella-zoster virus nucleic acids using real-time PCR. *J Virol* 743:11464–11471, 2000.

Crabtree, J.A.: Herpes zoster oticus. *Laryngoscope* 78:1853–1878, 1968.

Davis, L.E. and King, M, K.: Shingles and postherpetic neuralgia in the elderly. *Clin Geriatr* 11:47–53, 2003.

Dolin, R., Reichman, R.C., Mazure, M.H., and Whitley, R.J.: NIH conference: Herpes zoster-varicella infections in immunosuppressed patients. *Ann Intern Med* 89:375–388, 1978.

Dworkin, R.H., Johnson, R.W., Breuer, J., et al: Recommendations for the management of herpes zoster. *Clin Infect Dis* 44(suppl1):S1–26, 2007.

Dworkin, R.H., Corbin A.E., Young Jr, A.P., et al: Pregabalin for the treatment of postherpetic neuralgia: A randomized, placebo-controlled trial. *Neurology* 60:1274–1283, 2003.

Erard, V., Guthrie, K.A., Varley, C., et al: One-year acyclovir prophylaxis for preventing varicella-zoster virus disease after hematopoietic cell transplantation: No evidence of rebound varicella-zoster virus disease after drug discontinuation. *Blood* 110:3071–3077, 2007.

Furuta, Y., Takasu, T., Suzuki, S., et al: Detection of latent varicella-zoster virus infection in human vestibular and spiral ganglia. *J Med Virol* 51:214–216, 1997.

Galea, S.A., Sweet, A., Beninger, P., et al: The safety profile of varicella vaccine: A 10-year review. *J infect Dis* 197(suppl 2):S165–169, 2008.

Gershon, A.A. and Steinberg, S.P.: Antibody responses to varicella-zoster virus and the role of antibody in host defense. *Am J Med Sci* 282:12–17, 1981.

Gnann, J.W. Jr. and Whitley, R.J.: Herpes zoster. *N Engl J Med* 347:340–346, 2002.

Gilden, D.H., Cohrs, R.J., Hayward, A.R., et al: Chronic varicella-zoster virus ganglionitis—a possible cause of postherpetic neuralgia. *J Neurovirol* 9:404–407, 2003.

Gilden, D.H., Cohrs, R.J., and Mahalingam, R.: Clinical and molecular pathogenesis of varicella virus infection. *Viral Immunol* 16:243–258, 2003.

Gilden, D.H., Kleinschmidt-DeMaster, B.K., LaGuardia, J.J., et al: Neurologic complications of the reactivation of varicella-zoster virus. *N Engl J Med* 342:635–645, 2000.

Gilden, D.H., Wright, R.R., Schneck, S.A., et al: Zoster sine herpete, a clinical variant. *Ann Neurol* 35:530–533, 1994.

Gilderman, L.I., Lawless, J.F., Nolen, T.M., et al: A double-blind, randomized, controlled, multicenter safety and immunogenicity study of a refrigerator-stable formulation of Zostavax. *Clin Vaccine Immunol* 15:314–319, 2008.

Haanpaa, M., Hakkinen, V., and Nurmikko, T.: Motor involvement in acute herpes zoster. *Muscle Nerve* 20:1433–1438, 1997.

Haanpaa, M., Dastidar, P., Weinberg, A., et al: CSF and MRI findings in patients with acute herpes zoster. *Neurology* 51:1405–1411, 1998.

Hambleton, S. and Gershon, A.A.: Preventing varicella-zoster disease. *Clin Microbiol Rev* 18:70–80, 2005.

Hardy, I., Gershon, A.A., Steinberg, S.P., and LaRussa, P.: The incidence of zoster after immunization with live attenuated varicella vaccine. A study in children with leukemia. Varicella Vaccine Collaborative Study Group. *N Engl J Med* 325:1545–1550, 1991.

Harpaz, R., Ortega-Sanchez, I.R., and Seward, J.F.: Prevention of herpes zoster: Recommendations of the Adult Committee on Immunization Practices (ACIP). *MMWR* 57:1–3, 2008.

Hilt, D.C., Bucholz, D., Krumholz, A., et al: Herpes zoster ophthalmicus and delayed contralateral hemiparesis caused by cerebral angiitis: Diagnosis and management approaches. *Ann Neurol* 14:543–553, 1983.

Hope-Simpson, R.E.: The nature of herpes zoster: A long term study and a new hypothesis. *Proc R Soc Med* 58:9–20, 1965.

Huff, J.C., Bean, B., Balfour, H.H., et al: Therapy of herpes zoster with oral acyclovir. *Am J Med* 85(suppl 2A):84–89, 1988.

Hwang, S.M., Kang, Y.C., Lee, Y.B., et al: The effects of epidural blockade on the acute pain in herpes zoster. *Arch Dermatol* 135:1359–1364, 1999.

Jumaan, A.O., Yu, O., Jackson, L.A., et al: Incidence of herpes zoster, before and after varicella-vaccination-associated decreases in the incidence of varicella, 1992-2002. *J Infect Dis* 191:2002–2007, 2005.

Jung, B.F., Johnson, R.W., Griffin, D.R.J., and Dworkin, R.H.: Risk factors for postherpetic neuralgia in patients with herpes zoster. *Neurology* 62:1545–1551, 2004.

Kanda, Y., Mineishi, S., Saito, T., et al: Long-term low-dose acyclovir against varicella-zoster virus reactivation after allogeneic hematopoietic stem cell transplantation. *Bone Marrow Transplant* 28:689–692, 2001.

LaRussa, P.: Clinical manifestations of varicella. In *Varicella-zoster virus.* (Arvin, A., Greshon, A. eds.). Cambridge University Press, Cambridge. 2000, pp206–219.

Levin, M.J., Cai, G.Y., Manchak, M.D., and Pizer, L.I.: Varicella-zoster virus DNA in cells isolated from human trigeminal ganglia. *J Virol* 77:6979–6987, 2003.

Levin, M.J., Oxman, M.H, Zhang, J.H., et al: Varicella-zoster virus—specific immune responses in elderly recipients of a herpes zoster vaccine. *J Infect Dis* 197(suppl):825–835, 2008.

Liesegang, T.J.: Herpes zoster ophthalmicus: Natural history, risk factors, clinical presentation and morbidity. *Ophthalmology* 115:S3–12, 2008.

Kilgore, P.E., Kruszon-Moran, D., Seward, J.F., et al: Varicella in Americans from NHANES III: Implications for control through routine immunization. *J Med Virol* 70(suppl1):S111–118, 2003.

Kotani, N., Kushikata, T., Hashimoto, H., et al: Intrathecal methylprednisolone for intractable postherpetic neuralgia. *N Engl J Med* 343:1514–1519, 2000.

Ku, C.C., Besser, J., Abendroth, A., et al: Varicella-zoster virus pathogenesis and immunobiology: New concepts emerging from investigations with the SCID hu mouse model. *J Virol* 79:2651–2658, 2005.

Lawrence, R., Gershon, A.A., Holzman, R., and Steinberg, S.P.: The risk of zoster after varicella vaccination in children with leukemia. *N Engl J Med* 318:543–548, 1988.

Ljungman, P.: Prophylaxis against herpesvirus infections in transplant patients. *Drugs* 61:187–196, 2001.

Ljungman, P., Wang, F.Z., Nilsson, C., et al: Vaccination of autologous stem cell transplant recipients with live varicella vaccine: A pilot study. *Support Care Cancer* 11:739–741, 2003.

Mahalingam, R., Wellish, M., Brucklier, J., and Gilden, D.H.: Persistence of varicella-zoster virus DNA in elderly patients with postherpetic neuralgia. *J Neurovirol* 1:130–133, 1995.

McKendrick, M.W., Care, C.C., Kudesia, G., et al: Is VZV reactivation a common cause of unexplained unilateral pain? Results of a prospective study of 57 patients. *J Infect* 39:209–212, 1999.

Mehta, S.K., Tyring, S, K., Gilden, D.H., et al: Varicella-zoster virus in saliva of patients with herpes zoster. *J Infect Dis* 197:654–657, 2008.

Mehta, S.K., Cohrs, R.J., Forghani, B., et al: Stress-induced subclinical reactivation of varicella zoster virus in astronauts. *J Med Virol* 72:174–179, 2004.

Melanson, M., Chalk, C., Georgevich, L., et al: Varicella-zoster virus DNA in CSF and arteries in delayed contralateral hemiplegia: Evidence for viral invasion of cerebral arteries. *Neurology* 47:569–570, 1996.

Murakami, S., Hato, N., Horiuchi, J., et al: Treatment of Ramsay Hunt syndrome with acyclovir-prednisone: Significance of early diagnosis and treatment. *Ann Neurol* 41:353–357, 1997.

Nagel, M.A., Cohrs, R.J., Mahalingam, R., et al: The varicella zoster virus vasculopathies: Clinical, CSF, imaging, and virologic features. *Neurology* 70:853–860, 2008.

Nahass, G.T., Goldstein, B.A., Zhu, W.Y., et al: Comparison of Tzanck smear, viral culture, and DNA diagnostic methods in detection of herpes simplex and varicella-zoster infection. *JAMA* 268:2541–2544, 1992.

Oaklander, A.L.: Mechanisms of pain and itch caused by herpes zoster (shingles). *J Pain* 9(suppl1):S10–18, 2008.

Oaklander, A.L., Romans, K., Horasek, S., et al: Unilateral postherpetic neuralgia is associated with bilateral sensory neuron damage. *Ann Neurol* 44:789–795, 1998.

Ormrod, D. and Goa, K.: Valaciclovir: A review of its use in the management of herpes zoster. *Drugs* 59:1317–1340, 2000.

Oxman, M.N., Levin, M.J., Johnson, G.R., et al: A vaccine to prevent herpes zoster and postherpetic neuralgia in older adults. *N Engl J Med* 352:2271–2284, 2005.

Oxman, M.N., Levin, M.J., and Shingles Prevention Group: Vaccination against herpes zoster and postherpetic neuralgia. *J Infect Dis* 197:S228–236, 2008.

Pei-Lin, Shou-Zen Fan, Chi-Hsaing Huang, et al: Analgesic Effect of Lidocaine Patch 5% in the treatment of acute herpes zoster: A double-blind and vehicle-controlled study. *Reg Anesth Pain Med* 33:320–325, 2008.

Pui, J.C., Furth, E.E., Minda, J., et al: Demonstration of varicella-zoster virus infection in the muscularis propria and myenteric plexi of the colon of an HIV-positive patient with herpes zoster and small bowel pseudo-obstruction (Ogilvie's syndrome). *Am J Gastroenterol* 96:1627–1629, 2001.

Ragozzino, M.W., Melton, L.J., Kurland, L.T., et al: Population-based study of herpes zoster and its sequelae. *Medicine* 61:310–316, 1982.

Raja SN, Haythornthwaite JA, Pappagallo M, et al. Opioids versus antidepressants in postherpetic neuralgia: A randomized trial. *Neurology* 51:1166–1171, 2005.

Sakai, T., Tomiyasu, S., Yamada, H., and Sumikawa, K.: Evaluation of allodynia and pain associated with postherpetic neuralgia using current perception threshold testing. *Clin J Pain* 22:359–352, 2006.

Sandherr, M., Einsele, H., Hebart, H., et al: Antiviral prophylaxis in patients with haematological malignancies and solid tumours: Guidelines of the Infectious Diseases Working Party (AGIHO) of the German Society for Hematology and Oncology (DGHO). *Annal Oncol* 17:1051–1058, 2006.

Schmader, K.: Herpes zoster and postherpetic neuralgia in older adults. *Clin Geriatr Med* 23:615–632, 2007.

Schmader, K.E. and Dworkin, R.H.: Natural history and treatment of Herpes Zoster. *J Pain* 9(suppl1):S3–9, 2008.

Schmader, K., Studenski, S., MacMillan, J., et al.: Are Stressful life events risk factors for herpes zoster? *J Am Geriatr Soc* 38:1188–1194, 1990.

Seiler, H.E.: A study of herpes zoster particularly in relation to chickenpox. *J Hyg* 47:253–262, 1949.

Shaikh, S. and Ta, C.N.: Evaluation and management of herpes zoster ophthalmicus. *Am Fam Physician* 66:1723–1732, 2002.

Solomon, B.A., Kaporis, A.G., Glass, A.T., et al: Lasting immunity to varicella in doctors study (L.I.V.I.D. study). *J Am Acad Dermatol* 38:763–765, 1998.

Sweeney, C.J. and Gilden, D.H.: Ramsay Hunt syndrome. *J Neurol Neurosurg Psychiatry* 71:149–152, 2001.

Thomas, S.L., Wheeler, J.G., and Hall, A.J.: Contacts with varicella or with children and protection against herpes zoster in adults: A case-controlled study. *Lancet* 360:678–682, 2002.

Tyler, K.L. and Beckham, J. D.: Management of acute shingles (herpes zoster). *Rev Neurol Dis* 4:203–208, 2007.

Tyring, S., Barbarash, R.A., Nahlik, J.E., et al: Famciclovir for the treatment of acute herpes zoster: Effects of acute disease and postherpetic neuralgia. *Ann Intern Med* 123:89–96, 1995.

Tyring, S.K., Beutner, K.R., Tucker, B.A., et al: Antiviral therapy for herpes zoster. Randomized, controlled clinical trial of valacyclovir and famciclovir therapy in immunocompetent patients 50 years and older. *Arch Fam Med* 9:863–869, 2000.

Uscategui, T., Doree, C., Chamberlain, I.J, and Burton, M.J.: Antiviral therapy for Ramsay Hunt syndrome (herpes zoster oticus with facial palsy). *Cochrane Database Syst Rev* Oct 8: 4):CD006851, 2008.

Uscategui, T., Doree, C., Chamberlain, I.J, and Burton, M.J.: Corticosteroids as adjuvant to antiviral treatment in Ramsay Hunt syndrome (herpes zoster oticus with facial palsy). *Cochrane Database Syst Rev* Jul 16:(3):CD006852.

Vafai, A. and Berger, M.: Zoster in patients infected with HIV: A review. *Am J Med Sci* 321:372–380, 2001.

Vazquez, M., LaRussa, P.S., Gershon, A.A., et al: The effectiveness of the varicella vaccine in clinical practice. *N Engl J Med* 344:955-960, 2001.

Wackym, P.A.: Molecular temporal bone pathology: II. Ramsay Hunt syndrome (herpes zoster oticus). *Laryngoscope* 107:1165–1175, 1997.

Watson, C.P.N., Deck, J.H., Morshead, C., et al: Post-herpetic neuralgia: Further post-mortem studies of cases with and without pain. *Pain* 44:105–117, 1991.

Webster, A., Grint, P., Brenner, M.K., et al: Titration of IgG antibodies against varicella zoster virus before bone marrow transplantation is not predictive of future zoster. *J med Virol* 27:117–119, 1989.

Whitley, R.J.: Varicella-zoster virus. In *Principles and practice of infectious diseases*, 6th Ed. (Mandell, G.L., Bennett,J.E., Dolin, R. Eds). Elsevier Churchill Livingstone, Philadelphia, 2005: pp1780–1786.

Whitley. R. J., Weiss, H., Gnann, J.W., et al: Acyclovir with and without prednisone for the treatment of herpes zoster. *Ann Intern Med* 125:376–383, 1996.

Wood M.J., Johnson, R.W., McKendrick, M.W., et al: A randomized trial of acyclovir for 7 days or 21 days with and without prednisolone for treatment of acute herpes zoster. *N Engl J Med* 330:896–900, 1994.

Wood, M.J., Kay, R., Dworkin, R.H., et al: Oral acyclovir therapy accelerates pain resolution in patients with herpes zoster: A meta-analysis of placebo-controlled trials. *Clin Infect Dis* 22:341–347, 1996.

Wu, C. L. and Raja, S. N.: An update on the treatment of postherpetic neuralgia. *J Pain* 9(suppl1):S19–30, 2008.

Yawn, B.P., Saddier, P., Wollan, P.C., et al: A population-based study of the incidence and complication rates of herpes zoster before vaccine introduction. *Mayo Clin Proc* 82:1341–1349, 2007.

Yih, W.K., Brooks, D.R., Lett, S.M, et al: The incidence of varicella and herpes zoster in Massachusetts as measured by the Behavioral Risk Factor Surveillance System (BRFSS) during a period of increasing varicella vaccine coverage, 1998–2003. *BMC Public Health* 5:68, 2005.

8

Neurological Therapeutics

50 Neurorehabilitation in the Elderly

Ricardo Cruz and Mike Reding

Neuroplasticity in the Aged Brain

Demonstration of neuroplasticity in the human adult brain, including aged brains, has been the source of renewed hope, interest and funding in the field of rehabilitation of stroke and neurologic injury. Initial studies as far back as the 1960s and 1970s by Scheibel (Scheibel et al. 1976), Rosenzweig (Rosenzweig et al. 1962), Coleman (Coleman and Riesen 1968), and others demonstrated beneficial effects of environmental enrichment on the aged brain. Aged rats housed in small groups were compared to those housed with young pups and presented each day with novel "toys" to explore. Histologic analysis of dendritic arborization showed significantly greater dendritic branching and cortical thickness for aged rats exposed to enriched environments. Studies by Merzenich (Merzenich, Nelson, and Stryker 1984) and others showed electrophysiologic evidence of cortical remodeling following digit amputation in squirrel monkeys. Areas previously responsive to stimulation from the amputated digits became responsive to sensory stimulation of the remaining adjoining digits. Nudo (Nudo et al. 1996) and others have used a squirrel monkey model to study the effects of stroke lesions placed over the motor cortex responsible for hand function. Adjacent cortex previously producing face and shoulder movements when electrically stimulated began producing hand movements in response to hand motor re-training protocols. Nudo's studies provide major support for the importance of motor training and motor learning as necessary and sufficient for the electrophysiologic changes observed.

Stroke is an age-related disorder, and recovery following stroke is a good example of neuroplasticity inherent in an aged brain. Functional magnetic resonance imaging (fMRI) and electrophysiologic studies in humans using transcranial magnetic stimulation (TMS) both provide strong evidence for neural plasticity in humans following stroke. Strokes affecting the motor cortex or sub-cortical white matter projections from the primary motor cortex are associated with increased fMRI activation of ipsi-lesional pre-motor cortex, and homologous contra-lesional primary motor cortex (Cramer et al. 1996). More severe strokes are associated with less ipsi-lesional pre-motor cortex and more prominent contra-lesional homologous motor cortex fMRI activation (Cramer et al. 2001). Ipsi-lesional pre-motor cortex activation may be beneficial, while contra-lesional motor cortex activation may be detrimental. Transcranial magnetic stimulation studies also support the ability of pre-motor cortex to effect movement in paretic muscles following stroke. This has been most convincingly described by Liepert et al. (Liepert et al. 1998) following a course of constraint induced therapy (CIT) focused on intensive training of the paretic hand following stroke.

Neuropharmacology, Molecular Neurobiology and Neurogenetics in Rehabilitation

There is increasing awareness that traditional neurorehabilitation techniques described below may be further enhanced by our understanding of the role of neurotransmitter systems on arousal, attention, motivation, cognition, behavior, and motor learning. Psycho-stimulant agents such as dextroamphetamine (Crisostomo et al. 1988), methylphenidate (Grade et al. 1998), amantadine (Barrett and Eslinger 2007) and modafinil have all been used to enhance arousal and attention following stroke and traumatic brain injury. They may also enhance motor learning and improve motor performance both in normal subjects and in patients with stroke or traumatic brain injury. Serotonergic agents such as the selective serotonin re-uptake inhibitors improve mood and motivation in depressed patients following stroke (Miyai and Reding 1998). Cholinesterase inhibitors and NMDA receptor blockers have shown benefit for cognitive impairment due to vascular dementia (Bowler 2004). Dopamine receptor blockers have a limited role in ameliorating psychotic behavior in patients with Alzheimer's disease, vascular dementia, and delirium following stroke or traumatic brain injury (Dervaux and Levasseur 2008).

Recent advances in molecular neurobiology suggest novel strategies which may limit initial neuronal injury, the neuro-inflammatory response to injury, or the apoptotic response produced by ischemic stroke, traumatic brain injury, or spinal cord injury. Key molecules or molecular pathways identified include: hypoxia inducible factor (HIF) (Ratan et al. 2007), tissue necrosis factor-alpha (TNF-α) (Jayaraman et al. 2005), Histone deacetylase (HDAC) inhibitors (Sinn et al. 2007), and PPAR-gamma agonists (Lee and Reding 2007). These have all been identified as potential targets for neuropharmacologic intervention. Knowing how and when to either inhibit or promote these molecular targets promises to add significantly to our ability to promote neuronal responsiveness to traditional rehabilitation techniques. Appropriate modulation of molecular mechanisms underlying neuronal survival and neuroplasticity should aid recovery of motor, perceptual, cognitive, and behavioral impairments in the future.

Neuro-genetic advances have shown that Apolipoprotein E (ApoE) polymorphisms may identify patient populations with differential susceptibility to Alzheimer's disease or differential recovery following traumatic brain injury (Abboud et al. 2008). Patients with one or more ApoE-2 allele are less likely to develop Alzheimer's disease, and they show better functional recovery following traumatic brain injury compared to patients with one or more ApoE-4 allele. Brain-derived neurotrophic factor (BDNF) polymorphisms involving valine/valine and methionine/methionine substitutions identify different functional recovery patterns following TBI and stroke (Siironen et al. 2007). The importance of brain-derived neurotrophic factor for neuronal survival and recovery is self-evident. Catechol-O-methyltransferase (COMT) polymorphisms involving valine and methionine substitutions are also relevant for recovery following brain injury (Bosia et al. 2007). The putative mechanism of action for different COMT polymorphisms involves their differential effect on mono-amine synthesis and indirectly their effect on enhancement of recovery. The challenge for clinicians will be to identify pharmacologic interventions that appropriately target and ameliorate the above mentioned dysfunctional genetic polymorphisms. With time, there will undoubtedly be many more genetic variations identified that predispose to development of neurodegenerative disorders, and inhibit recovery from neuronal injury.

Traditional Neurologic Rehabilitation

Rehabilitation is an effort to bring back lost function. Geriatric rehabilitation cannot hope to restore the functions of youth, but attempts to optimize the individual's ability to function given the constraints of the aging process. The World Health Organization (WHO) has advocated that we consider different aspects of loss of function: 1) impaired function at the level of a body organ, such as brain, heart, muscle, bone, etc.; 2) impaired function at the level of the organism such as being able to feed, dress, groom, bathe, walk, etc.; and 3) impaired function at a social level, being able to fulfill our roles as spouse, friend, worker, citizen etc. This three level WHO classification of functional loss is often summarized by using the terms respectively: **Impairment, Disability, Handicap** (Barbotte et al. 2001).

Aging is associated with loss of function in each organ system. The WHO classification of function is useful in organizing our approach to geriatric rehabilitation. This WHO classification helps focus rehabilitation efforts on conceptually distinct aspects of the geriatric patient's function.

Priority is placed on optimizing organ system **impairment**. If there is cognitive impairment, what strategies can retard or improve cognitive function? At present, this would lead one to consider prescribing an acetyl-cholinesterase inhibitor, or N-methyl dopamine antagonist. If there is congestive heart failure, what strategies can optimize cardiovascular impairment? Reviewing the patient's sodium intake, use of diuretic, beta blocker, and angiotensin converting enzyme inhibitor would be most important.

Once organ system impairments have been optimized, there may be need for additional strategies to ameliorate **disability** with self-care and mobility functions. Using the examples above, for the patient with cognitive impairment this might entail recommending use of a memory book, pill dispenser, or delivery of pre-cooked meals. For someone with CHF, prescribing a hospital bed with head elevation may help with orthopnea, moving bed and toilet facilities to the same level of the home, or using a bedside commode will help conserve energy.

Handicap issues are addressed by accessing services to help support the patient's independence in their home and community. Examples would be use of home care or daycare programs while family members are at work. For patients without a family caregiver, arrangements could be made for daily calls by a volunteer to check on the patient's well being and adherence to their medication regimen. Referral to other community services can provide transportation for health care appointments, or to attend rehabilitation or wellness programs.

Using the concepts of impairment, disability, and handicap, it is easy to categorize geriatric rehabilitation intervention strategies, and to some extent the skill set of the clinicians providing these services.

For addressing organ system impairments one would expect a physician with special expertise in the organ system affected to be most helpful. For ameliorating disability, a physiatrist (or other physician with special training in rehabilitation medicine), a rehabilitation nurse, occupational therapist, physical therapist, speech language pathologist, social worker, and psychologist are all likely to be able to provide useful treatment and advice. Handicap issues reflect dysfunction fulfilling accustomed social roles in the home or community and are usually addressed by a social worker or psychologist with referral for specific equipment or services as needed.

Rehabilitation care is evolving from a multi-disciplinary to a trans-disciplinary approach to patient management. The above discussion implies that each of the clinicians involved in geriatric rehabilitation has a special set of skills, and that the skill set is sufficiently broad as to be inadequately mastered by any one clinician. This concept of a multi-disciplinary approach to rehabilitation is changing to a trans-disciplinary concept of care. A trans-disciplinary approach recognizes that there is considerable overlap in many of our rehabilitation disciplines, and that clinicians should be encouraged to cross traditional boundaries compatible with their experience and care settings. Common examples of overlap treatment areas are occupational therapy addressing ambulation and transfer techniques to and from the tub and toilet, or addressing dysphagia-related food and liquid consistency modifications and swallowing strategies to improve deglutition. Ambulation is traditionally considered to be a physical therapy task and dysphagia a speech-language pathologist's treatment area. The trans-disciplinary approach encourages clinicians to focus on the patient's needs, and not on the clinician's job description.

Rehabilitation Strategies to Improve Organ System Impairments

This book is entitled Clinical Neurology of Aging. Its focus is on neurologic changes associated with aging. Many neurologic disorders, however, may be secondary to age-related changes in other organ systems, to altered metabolism or adverse effects of prescribed medications. Before focusing on specific neurologic impairments it is prudent to assess the patient's general medical condition, other organ system co-morbidities, and medication list for factors that may adversely affect neurologic function. Chapter 52 is specifically devoted to a review of neurologic side-effects of medications.

Cardiovascular changes are most obviously manifested as stroke. Chronic obstructive pulmonary disease may be associated with treatment-related steroid or xanthine oxidase inhibitor cognitive-behavioral side effects. More advanced pulmonary disease can lead to hypoxic encephalopathy or carbon dioxide narcosis. Age-related changes in gastrointestinal function may lead to B12, folate, and other vitamin and nutritional deficiencies giving rise to brain, peripheral nerve, and neuro-muscular wasting disorders. Details of age-related changes in brain-gut neuropeptide interactions involving leptin, grehlin, somatomedin, somatostatin, and cholecystokinin are yet to be elucidated. Renal-electrolyte abnormalities affecting neural function most commonly seen in the elderly are pre-renal azotemia and hypernatremia due to inadequate hydration. Hyponatremia may be due to diuretic use, inappropriate anti-diuretic hormone secretion, or to age-related renal dysfunction with resultant salt-wasting nephropathy. Age-related endocrine disorders with neural consequences are diabetes mellitus, thyroid, and parathyroid dysfunction. Many age-related myelodysplastic and neoplastic hematologic disorders predispose to stroke by causing either hyper or hypo-coagulable states with thrombocytosis, thrombocytopenia, or polycythemia.

Rehabilitation strategies to improve cognitive impairment have focused on pharmacologic interventions to enhance central acetylcholine availability by inhibition of acetylcholinesterase, or by inhibition of stimulatory neurotoxic effects of glutamate using N-methyl D-aspartate receptor blockade. Computer-based cognitive-linguistic exercises have not been shown to be useful. Teaching mnemonic techniques may help with list learning and recall in patients with mild cognitive impairment, but not in patients with significant dementia. Diagnosis and treatment of the dementing disorders are discussed in Chapters 16–21. Adaptive strategies to compensate for progressive cognitive impairment are discussed below under the heading of disability-related rehabilitation strategies.

Hemianopic visual impairment following stroke has been shown to have at least a transient response to use of prism adaptation. Prism glasses are worn for 10 to 15 minutes while performing reach-to-target tasks (Frassinetti et al. 2002). Prisms are worn so that objects appear to be displaced toward the intact visual field. When patients adapt to the prisms they are able to reach for the targets without error. The prisms are then removed with a compensatory after-effect biasing oculomotor and reaching behavior towards the side of visual-spatial neglect. Limited success has also been achieved with use of computerized visual field training devices. Presenting visual stimuli progressing from the intact to impaired visual field can be shown to improve visual perception in the hemianopic visual field. At least one such computerized visual perception training system is now commercially available (Poggel, Kasten, and Sabel 2004). It is supported by internet linkage between the patient, the visual perception therapist, and the manufacturer. On-line downloading of weekly performance from the patient's home computerized visual training system allows for regular scoring, and reinforcement of progress made. Based on results, visual perception, task presentation difficulty, and treatment goals can be revised. There appears to be sufficient data to document a 5 to 10 degree reduction of the hemianopic visual field as a result of several months' daily practice using such systems. The drawbacks of this computerized approach to visual field retraining are the limited 5 to 10 degree of visual field improvement, the cost of leasing the equipment, and the additional cost of therapist assistance to help incorporate improved visual perception into functional self-care, mobility, visual scanning, and reading comprehension tasks. However, this is a real-life example of the power of retraining a brain function utilizing the neuroplasticity of the residual brain tissue.

The speech language pathologist (SLP) is trained to address cognitive-linguistic deficits, dysphonia, aphasia, and dysphagia-related impairments, most commonly seen following stroke, but also related to many other neurologic disorders affecting the geriatric population. Cognitive-linguistic deficits are difficult to treat directly, but may improve by helping the patient avoid distraction, and use of the visual, spatial, and linguistic mnemonic techniques rehearsed above. These mnemonic techniques may help the patient follow the thought content of conversational speech. Aphasia, primarily expressive aphasia, can be improved by teaching cueing, pacing, and melodic intonation techniques (Belin et al. 1996). Vocal exercises can improve vocal volume and articulation. Vocal exercises have been used most successful in treatment of hypophonia due to Parkinson's disease (Sapir et al. 2007).

Most dysphagia treatment strategies use diet modifications or compensatory swallowing techniques to improve deglutition. These will be discussed under compensatory treatment techniques below. The Shaker neck flexion exercises stress the use of neck flexor muscle groups to ameliorate laryngeal elevation deficits associated with dysphagia following stroke (Shaker et al. 2002). Maximal activation of voluntary neck flexors is thought to produce over-flow activation of less voluntarily activated myo-hyoid and thyro-hyoid muscle groups to elevate the larynx during deglution. Strengthening of these muscle groups by voluntary exercise is thought to enhance more reflexive contractions seen during the "swallow reflex" (Kiger, Brown, and Watkins 2006). At least one functional electrical stimulation (FES) system is now available to assist with dysphagia due to inadequate timing or extent of laryngeal elevation during the swallowing reflex. It delivers functional electrical stimulation to the above muscle groups when manually triggered by the patient or their SLP therapist. This FES system is not intended to be in use during feeding, but is a reasonable treatment intervention to improve dysphagia associated with impaired laryngeal elevation. There are credible studies to support its efficacy in properly selected patients; this technique is in fairly widespread use clinically for post-stroke and brain injury rehabilitation.

Rehabilitation interventions that seek to improve neuromuscular strength and balance in the elderly have been tested in both community-based and in long-term care settings. The effects of aerobic exercise on gait, balance, walking endurance, falls prevention, depression, and osteoporosis in both community-based elders, and nursing home residents are positive and significant. The beneficial effects of aerobic conditioning, and tai-chi based balance and stretching exercises for the elderly are covered in Chapters 27, 28, and 54.

There is no evidence that one type of physical therapy rehabilitation technique is better than another for optimizing motor recovery following stroke. The oldest type of rehabilitation philosophy, often called traditional therapy, attempts to mobilize the patient with whatever devices or techniques are necessary. Knott and Voss described what they labeled a proprioceptive neuromuscular facilitation (PNF) approach for treatment of stroke-related neuromuscular impairments in 1956 (Knott M, Voss 1956). This therapeutic approach is based on their assessment of normal functional joint movements and stresses the need for rehearsing normal "spiral and diagonal" movements for recovery of upper and lower limb function. Additional techniques such as "rhythmic stabilization" and "dynamic reversal" are described and elaborated in a systematized approach to the hemiplegic patient. The Brunnstrom approach was described in 1970 (Brunnstrom 1970). Brunnstrom advocated the use of segmental and suprasegmental spinal cord reflexes to modulate flexor and extensor muscular tone in the hemiplegic arm and leg. Techniques were based upon segmental and supra-segmental motor reflex control systems. The head extension reflex of Magnus and de Kleijn was used to enhance the spastic tone of axial and paretic leg extensor muscle groups during the gait cycle. Flexor versus extensor tone of the paretic arm was modulated by tonic neck reflexes enhancing flexor muscle groups with head rotation toward the non-paretic limb. The upper limb crossed-flexor response and the lower limb reciprocal flexion-extension reflexes observed in inter-collicular transected vertebrates were also used as the basis for additional treatment techniques. Brunnstrom's physical therapy techniques are to be contrasted with the neuro-developmental techniques (NDT) advocated by Bobath in 1970 (Bobath 1970). From a philosophical perspective, the Brunnstrom and Bobath physical therapy techniques are diametrically opposed. The Brunnstrom approach attempts to facilitate movement in the paretic limbs by using techniques that either augment or inhibit the segmental and suprasegmental spinal cord reflexes previously described. The NDT approach views segmental and supra-segmental spinal cord movement patterns as abnormal movements that should always be inhibited and never used to elicit movement. Motor learning theory (MLT) is a relatively new approach advocated by Carr and Shepherd in 1982 (Carr and Shepherd 1982). Their approach stresses the results of more recent studies that show the value of "massed practice," "error free learning," and "minimizing training interference performing competing tasks during the same treatment session." There are six prospective randomized studies that do not show superiority of any one particular physical therapy approach over the others: traditional, PNF, NDT, or MLT. These studies involve small numbers of patients and have been scored by observers who were not blinded to the type of treatment given. Most therapists utilize various techniques from each approach based upon the patient's response, which may differ significantly depending upon the interval since stroke onset.

Selected neuropharmacologic agents have been studied for their ability to improve neurologic impairments following stroke and traumatic brain injury. L-dopa and dopamine agonists have been used to help improve expressive speech and language deficits. The initial studies, often with single subjects using ABA trial design, were encouraging. Subsequent studies with larger sample sizes have not shown these agents to have significant effects on speech fluency measures (Gupta et al. 1995). L-dopa and dopamine agonists have also been studied for their ability to help improve visual-spatial hemi neglect following unilateral parietal lobe stroke or traumatic brain injury (Fleet et al. 1987). Initial reports were encouraging but not supported by subsequent larger studies.

There are limited data suggesting that use of dextroamphetamine or methylphenidate may enhance motor recovery following stroke. The first controlled, double-blinded clinical study was performed in 1988 and showed a significant benefit of 10 mg dextroamphetamine given orally one hour prior to subsequent physical and occupational therapy focused on paretic upper and lower limb strengthening exercises (Crisostomo et al. 1988). Assessments of strength were performed the next day and seemed to imply a durable enhancement of motor scores. There were, however, only four dextroamphetamine subjects and four placebo controls. A subsequent double-blind, randomized control study of 21 stroke rehabilitation inpatients using daily doses of 10 mg dextroamphetamine at 9AM each morning prior to daily PT and OT therapy sessions for two weeks showed no benefit on motor strength scores, Barthel Activity Of Daily Living Scores, or Beck Depression Scores (Ratan et al. 2007). Lack of benefit with daily dosing suggested that patients may show a tachyphylactic response to daily dosing of dextroamphetamine, which has a seven hour half-life. Patients in the initial study who showed a beneficial dextroamphetamine effect were only 7 days post stroke, and in the subsequent study were 21 days post stroke at study entry. Most of the patients in the initial study had only motor paresis, while 70% of the subjects in the subsequent study had more extensive stroke-related impairments with hemiparesis, hemihypesthesia, and hemianopic visual deficits. Several subsequent dextroamphetamine studies have been performed, some showing benefit, others not. Methylphenidate, which has only a two hour half-life, was used on a daily basis in one study and showed improvement in motor scores compared to placebo (Martinsson, Wahlgren, and Hardemark 2003). It is possible that the short half-life of methylphenidate may allow sufficient time for withdrawal; that it may not show a tachyphylaxis response with daily dosing. Discrepant outcomes have focused debate on the need for more information concerning the effects of time post stroke, the severity of motor deficit, and dosing regimen on pharmacologic response. At present there is not sufficient evidence to advocate use of either dextroamphetamine or methylphenidate as a pharmacologic agent to enhance motor recovery following stroke.

More specialized interventions have been studied following acute neurologic disorders such as stroke, traumatic brain injury, spinal cord injury, and to a lesser extent in chronic progressive disorders such as Parkinson's disease and multiple sclerosis. Such treatment techniques include: constraint-induced therapy (CIT) (Grotta, Noser, and Ro 2004), Functional Tone Management (FTM) (Saebo Inc) upper limb orthotic devices, functional electrical stimulation (FES) (Ring and Rosenthal 2004), trans-cranial direct current (TCDC) (Fregni 2005) stimulation, robotic therapy (Stein et al. 2006), and partial body weight supported treadmill training (PBWSTT) (Kosak and Reding 2000). Applicability of these techniques to geriatric patients with deficits from stroke, Parkinson's disease, or traumatic brain injury has been documented.

The simplest approach for enhancing upper limb function of selected patients with arm and hand paresis following stroke is to force them to use their paretic hand by constraining the good hand in a sling or covering it with a boxing glove this is the technique of constraint-induced therapy (CIT). Use of a constraint on the unaffected hand is what gives this technique its name (Grotta, Noser, and Ro 2004). In order for patients to be appropriate for this training strategy, they must have at least 10 degrees of voluntary finger flexion/extension and 20 degrees of voluntary wrist extension. Given this degree of voluntary motor control it is possible to begin modeling the patient's movements so that they can practice progressively more complex hand functions. The protocol usually requires one-to-one patient-therapist interaction in massed practice sessions at least six hours a day five days per week for two weeks. Modifications of the protocol allow small group sessions with several patients working with one another, but always with constant occupational therapist supervision and facilitation. Selection of tasks must be challenging but not beyond the patient's capabilities, and modified as they show improvement in hand function. The constraint condition is used while the patient is awake for most of the day, even when not in therapy sessions for this two-week period. The patient may be allowed to remove the constraint condition for feeding, toileting, and bathing if necessary. CIT works best for patients with paresis plus superimposed learned non-use of the paretic hand. The concept is that because of the severity of their initial weakness, the patients gave up making the effort to use their plegic hand for daily self-care and other functional tasks. Severe weakness plus hemisensory or visual-spatial neglect are thought to further promote development of learned non-use. Most studies have validated CIT as a means of improving the patient's use of the paretic limb in daily activities. Outcome measures assessing muscle strength changes have shown less significant improvement. There is general consensus, however, that CIT is beneficial when used as described above.

Use of a Functional Tone Management orthotic device is a simple approach for improving grasp and release for selected patients with hemiparetic upper limbs following stroke (Saebo Inc) (see Figure 1). The orthotic is meant to be a training device allowing patients to practice grasp and release hand functions, initially with large diameter, but light, puff-ball type objects. As range of finger flexion-extension improves, the size and weight of objects manipulated can be altered to increase task difficulty. The natural recovery of hand function following stroke is for patients to have some ability to voluntarily flex the fingers. There may, however be no ability to extend the fingers, making it difficult to initiate grasp release. The FTM device is a simple exoskeleton fitting over the dorsum of the forearm, wrist, and hand. Finger cots resembling thimbles are placed over each finger and thumb, and are attached by springs to five struts mounted on the dorsally situated orthotic. Adjustments are made on the spring tension for each digit to allow the patient's voluntary finger flexor movements to just barely overcome the finger extensor tone provided by the spring-loaded finger extension force. The value of this device is provided by simple demonstration of hand function with use of the device versus without its use. Repetitive practice over time allows eventual discontinuation of the FTM orthotic as voluntary grasp and release improve. This device can be used to improve voluntary finger flexion-extension to

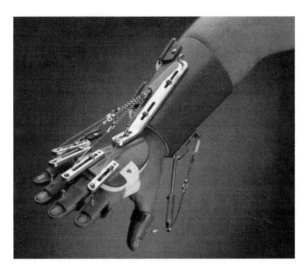

Figure 1 This functional tone management device helps overcome intrinsic post-stroke flexor tone. It allows the patient to open the hand sufficiently to grasp appropriately sized test objects. The device is a useful training tool for patients who have sufficient voluntary flexor strength to grasp the test object once the hand has been mechanically opened.

allow the patient to qualify for initiation of constraint-induced therapy as described above.

Functional electrical stimulation (FES) of the affected shoulder, arm, and hand has been shown to improve spasticity, shoulder subluxation, and motor strength scores in selected patients with hemiparesis post stroke. FES as a rehabilitation treatment tool has been available since the 1950s. Early FES used bulky equipment requiring a 115 volt current source, metal electrodes, and painful levels of stimulation current. Today we have compact portable multi-channel programmable battery-powered stimulators that deliver stimulation currents which are easily tolerated by patients. At least two FES systems are commercially available, each with a different electrode configuration design for stimulating appropriate muscle groups in the upper versus the lower limb (Ring and Rosenthal 2004; Stein et al. 2006) (see Figure 2). The devices are easily adjustable by an appropriately trained occupational or physical therapist to optimize electrode

placement, stimulation parameters, and comfort. The patient and caregiver are trained to apply the device themselves, and may purchase or lease it for daily use in their homes. Some of the devices can be manually triggered to provide stimulation of forearm finger flexors, thumb flexor, and forearm finger-extensor muscle groups to allow functional grasp and release. Some of these FES systems are designed to sense weak and ineffective surface EMG activity from voluntary muscle activation and use these patient-initiated EMG signals to trigger larger, more functional muscle contractions by the FES stimulator. The gains seen in motor scores, spasticity reduction, and secondary joint contractures, while statistically significant, have not been sufficiently robust to translate into improvements in self-care scores. These devices, like the FTM orthotic, may be used to improve voluntary finger flexion-extension to allow the patient to qualify for initiation of constraint-induced therapy as described above.

FES has also been shown to help improve foot-drop and functional gait while being worn on the hemiparetic leg by selected patients following stroke. As for the upper limb, the FES systems are fitted by the patient's therapist, adjusted to optimize quality of gait, then purchased or leased by patients for daily use in their homes (see Figure 3). The devices are battery powered, compact, and safe. Electrical stimulation parameters and timing are actuated by either an accelerometer in the device or foot-plate sensor placed in the sole of the patient's shoe. Surface-mounted electrodes under the FES device are held in place over the peroneal nerve by elastic straps. Use of FES for foot-drop following stroke may improve quality of gait and help strengthen foot dorsiflexors. This is in contrast to use of an ankle-foot orthosis, which if not used appropriately, may inhibit motor recovery.

Trans-cranial direct current (TCDC) stimulation is a new electrical stimulation technique that is gaining interest as more data supporting its mechanism of action and potential clinical effects becomes available. When direct current is passed through the brain, the threshold potential of cortical neurons is lowered under the anodal (+) electrode and it is raised under the cathodal (-) electrode. Clinical trials using

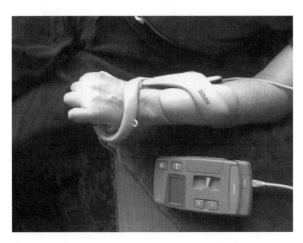

Figure 2 Functional electrical stimulation device which contains surface electrode pads that can be individually positioned for each patient. Appropriately timed stimulation-trains activate finger and thumb flexors and extensors allowing programmed grasp and release.

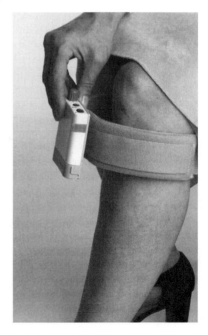

Figure 3 Functional electrical stimulation device with an elastic band containing surface electrodes over the peroneal nerve. Adjustment of the accelerometer-triggered device tailors stimulation timing and intensity to optimize the patient's foot-drop gait following stroke.

TCDC have been limited and initiated only in the past several years. It is too soon to speak about efficacy, but this new technique is receiving growing attention as a modulatory tool for facilitating recovery of speech and language, motor recovery, and for treatment of hemi-spatial visual neglect (Fregni 2005). Each of these neurologic impairments is thought to be modulated by competitive input to remaining ipsi-lesional cortex from homologous region of the contra-lesional hemisphere. There is now sufficient evidence to show that inhibition of recovery by the unaffected hemisphere does indeed occur. This evidence is based on functional magnetic resonance data and transcranial magnetic coil stimulation and inhibition studies. Given this information, it is reasonable to use TCDC to enhance neuronal function in affected ipsilesional cortex, and inhibit detrimental competing input from the homologous contralesional cortex. The neuroscience data supporting the potential value of TCDC as a new stroke and TBI treatment tool have generated considerable optimism and warrant thorough study.

There are now several robotic systems that are commercially available for use in upper limb motor recovery following stroke (Volpe, Krebs, and Hogan 2003; REO Therapy, Motorika USA Inc). They allow a robotic device to move the paretic arm or hand to follow visual cues on a video monitor (see Figure 4). They use different computer game protocols to present the patient with a movement task that requires the patient to move the cursor to specific targets. Initially the robot may be programmed to wait variable periods of time for the patient to respond. If there is no response, the robot begins the desired movement, carrying the patient's arm through the motion. As the patient's strength, speed and accuracy improve, the robot is programmed to provide less assistance. The programs also challenge patients by increasing target speed of presentation, and by providing either steady or random resistance to movement. In a 45 minute treatment session, the upper limb robot may be able to present the patient with more than a thousand goal-directed movements. The variability of video games and the responsiveness of the robot to patient performance keep the patient challenged and engaged in the task. Controlled studies have compared robotic upper extremity training with traditional occupational therapy in patients who are more than six months post stroke and who have reached a plateau in their upper limb motor scores. Such studies show an approximate 20% improvement in favor of robotic therapy compared to traditional occupational therapy. This improvement in motor score has not however translated into significant improvement in upper limb self-care scores. Use of robotic systems for enhancement of motor function is in its infancy. It is hoped that with more advanced systems, patients will be able to practice more functional tasks with robotic assistance provided across multiple joints.

Partial body weight supported treadmill training (PBWSTT) is now an established approach to help recover ambulation following stroke or incomplete spinal cord injury (Kosak and Reding 2000) (see Figure 5). Selected patients with significant weakness who are difficult for a therapist to mobilize using simpler techniques such as temporary bracing, quadruped cane, and hemi-bar are most likely to benefit. The body is fully supported by a parachute type harness that allows the patient to be supported over a moving treadmill. The patient's paretic or plegic leg is guided through the gait cycle from single stance, toe push, swing phase, and heel-strike by their therapist who is seated alongside the treadmill. The speed of the treadmill is steadily advanced as the patient's gait quality improves. Several of the difficulties of this technique are that the patient must be able to cooperate, and support 70% or more of their body weight. There must be at least this degree of patient participation to show a treatment effect. Due to gait dyspraxia and difficulties with pelvic weight shifting during the gait cycle, an additional therapist may be needed to model movement of the non-paretic leg, and another therapist may be needed to assist with pelvic shift during the gait cycle. The time spent placing the harness on the patient, and the need for additional therapists or therapist aides to assist with movement represent relative impediments to this form of assisted gait training. There are now two commercially available robotic gait trainers that provide all assistance needed for both leg movements and pelvic tilt. Their ease of use and need for less manpower are, however, offset by their initial cost and maintenance expense.

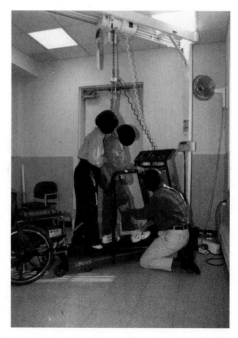

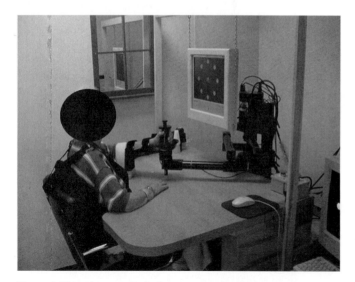

Figure 4 This robotic upper limb trainer may initially assist limb movement to reach for a target on the video screen. As the patient improves, the device is programmed to provide less assistance, and advance target speed to keep the video tasks challenging.

Figure 5 Partial body weight-supported treadmill training device allows the patient to practice walking while safely protected from falling by a body harness. The therapists can help control paretic leg movement and pelvic tilt during the gait cycle to allow the patient to practice "normal" walking.

Rehabilitation Strategies to Improve Disability with Self-care and Mobility

After attempts have been made to minimize the patient's neurologic impairments, using the strategies rehearsed above, one is often left with the need to help the patient adapt to the deficits that remain. Rehabilitation tools which are primarily adaptive in nature can be classified as compensatory techniques or adaptive devices. Techniques are taught that make living with residual neurologic impairments easier and safer. Devices are recommended that will help optimize ease and safety of specific self-care and mobility tasks.

Compensatory Techniques

The focus of this chapter is on geriatric neurologic rehabilitation. Many other considerations and options are appropriate for geriatric patients with orthopedic, rheumatologic, and cardio-pulmonary disabilities. Though quite important, they will not be addressed here.

Occupational therapists are specially trained to teach techniques for helping geriatric patients remain in the community as independently and safely as possible. To do this they must assess the impact of the patient's residual neurologic impairments: cognitive, perceptual, motor praxis, motor paresis, motor coordination, sensory deficits, balance, and gait. The most common cause of neurologic disability in the USA is stroke, followed by Alzheimer's disease, benign essential tremor, Parkinson's disease, and other neurodegenerative disorders.

Stroke victims with residual cognitive, perceptual, motor, sensory, and balance impairments serve as a common and extreme example of the difficulties involved in optimizing a patient's functional independence.

Patients with memory deficits can be taught mnemonic techniques based on visual, spatial, or linguistic strategies to enhance list learning, or recall of activity sequences needed to complete a motor task.

Visual search techniques can be taught to help patients with hemianopsia or unilateral visual neglect to properly scan their environment to finish the food on their plate, or find obstacles in their path before they attempt to transfer from bed to wheelchair, or before they stand to walk.

Urinary urge incontinence and constipation related to neurologic impairment can be ameliorated by teaching timed-prompted voiding techniques, and by appropriate use of dietary fiber modifications, stool softeners, and suppositories. These techniques are often rehearsed and reinforced by the rehabilitation nurse. Timed prompted voiding assumes that the patient has impaired awareness of bladder filling and impaired ability to voluntarily inhibit micturition. Adequate fluid intake is assured by encouraging 1.5 liters of fluid per day, consumed prior to 6PM. Timing voiding to half an hour after each meal and at two hour intervals between meals while awake acknowledges the need to void related to fluid intake at mealtime, the patient's unawareness of bladder filling, and their inability to inhibit automatic micturition. Geriatric patients in general and particularly following stroke are relatively immobile. Immobility is a risk factor for constipation and fecal impaction. Use of a 35 gram fiber diet, a stool softener such as docusate nightly, and bisacodyl suppository every other day if no bowel movement are reasonable approaches to prevent impactions, and allow the patient to time evacuation of stool. Placing the bisacodyl suppository may itself initiate the anal-colic reflex directly. There is also a direct stimulatory effect of bisacodyl on the smooth muscle of the rectal ampulla, further stimulating evacuation. The bowel and bladder management of geriatric patients is very important for quality of life. .

Residual hemiparesis may require the patient to learn to live their life one-handed. The simplest tasks such as grooming, bathing, feeding, dressing, and toileting can seem impossible for a hemiplegic patient. There are, however, specific techniques which can be taught that will help the patient accomplishing each of these tasks whether they involve use of the dominant or non-dominant hand. Managing trunk support and safety as one lifts under-clothing and pants may require learning how to dress while supine or while performing a hemiplegic sit-to-stand or stand-pivot transfer maneuver. This is accomplished by learning to stand, balance, and pivot using the unaffected leg. The hemiplegic dressing sequence starts with dressing of the paretic arm first. Different techniques are then taught for pullover versus front-buttoning clothing. Other tasks such as cooking, laundering, and home-making may need to be taught, depending upon their appropriateness for the patient's residual impairments and home environment.

The physical and/or occupational therapist may need to teach the hemiplegic patient how to prepare themselves for rising from the sit-to-stand position. Prior to stroke, this function would have been performed unconsciously. Following stroke, the patient may need to mentally rehearse the sequence to position the paretic leg parallel to the non-paretic leg, and "bring the nose over the toes." This assures proper positioning of the body's center of gravity in order to allow for safe sit-to-stand transfer. Hemiparetic gait sequencing must be taught to patients with need for cane and brace who are not able to safely swing the paretic leg from toe-push to heel strike in one fluid motion. This involves advancing the cane (held in the non-paretic hand), then advancing the paretic leg to the level of the cane, then finally advancing the non-paretic leg to the level of the cane. (See Figure 6) This three-part sequence, "cane, paretic leg, good leg" seems simple to learn, but may take the stroke victim a week or two of rehearsal before the movement sequence becomes relatively automatic. The hemi-paretic stair-climbing sequence is another technique which improves function and safety. Hemiparetic patients are taught to go "up with the good leg, and down with the bad." Using the unimpaired leg to raise the body's weight to the level of the next step is mechanically sound. Safely positioning the paretic leg in full extension on the descending stair provides maximum support of the patient's full weight as the non-paretic leg is brought to the same level. Some therapists are reluctant

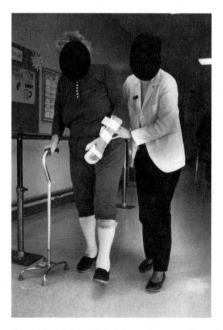

Figure 6 Traditional hemipleg gait training using a quadruped cane, and ankle-foot-orthosis with therapist assistance.

to use the term "bad leg" but "up with the good and down with the bad" is too easily remembered to be discarded.

Most dysphagia treatment strategies use diet modifications or compensatory swallowing techniques to improve deglutition. Diet modifications can provide an appropriate food consistency (puree, ground, chopped, or mechanical soft diet) to allow the patient with impaired motor control of lips and tongue to manage food appropriate for their level of buccal-labial-oral motor control. Lip function is important for maintaining lip-seal with liquids; tongue function is required for moving the food bolus in the mouth allowing for adequate mastication. Once the food is properly prepared for swallowing, the tongue must move the food bolus to the entrance to the oral pharynx. Once past the anterior faucial pillars, the food or liquid bolus normally triggers the swallow reflex. Liquids are particularly difficult to contain during the oral phase of deglutition, and may prematurely spill into the oral pharynx. The most common pharyngeal abnormality seen following stroke is delay of the swallow reflex, with delayed elevation of the larynx and inadequate protection of the airway. Elevation of the larynx plus posterior excursion of the tongue and eventration of the epiglottis are essential for closure of the laryngeal airway. Providing the patient with thickened liquids of either nectar or honey consistency is an appropriate strategy to help improve control of the liquid bolus in the mouth, and slow down the flow of liquid once it enters the pharynx, thereby lessening the risk of aspiration.

Multiple other compensatory dysphagia treatment strategies are also available. Their use is indicated if they can be shown to be helpful in improving functional deglutition by objective means such as videofluoroscopic modified barium swallow (VMBS) (Finestone et al. 2002) test or fiberoptic endoscopic evaluation of swallow with sensory stimulation (FEESST) (Rees 2006) study. Commonly used compensatory swallowing techniques include: head turn, chin-tuck, Mendelsohn maneuver, swallow-cough sequence, and supra-glottic swallow. The value of each is dependent upon objective demonstration in a particular patient; that use of the technique obviates laryngeal penetration or aspiration of the test material, or that it helps clear any spillage past the epiglottis into the laryngeal vestibule.

Functional Assist Devices

The most commonly used mobility assist devices are cane, walker, brace, and wheelchair. Canes are useful for stabilization of gait and for pelvic weight shifting during the gait cycle. They are useful for patients with hemiparesis, orthopedic back or lower limb joint limitations, or arthritic pain. Proper use of a cane requires that in double-stance phase of gait, the elbow of the hand holding the cane is slightly flexed 7 to 10 degrees. This allows for elbow extension, which can provide additional support without need to disturb shoulder-girdle and upper trunk balance. The cane chosen should provide the smallest base of support needed to meet the patient's needs. The progression is as follows: standard cane, bent-handle cane, tripod cane, quadruped cane. Tripod and quadruped canes can be either narrow based or wide based.

Walkers also help with balance and weight shift, but are more cumbersome and require two hands for manipulation. They are considered when use of a cane is not sufficient. Rolling walkers are easier to use but less supportive than platform walkers. Walkers are available that have additional features such as a seat if the patient becomes fatigued, and carrying basket to add functionality.

Use of an ankle brace may be appropriate for patients with an unstable ankle, foot-drop during the swing phase of gait, or knee buckling during the single-stance phase of gait. A flexible ankle-foot orthosis (AFO) or hinged-ankle AFO will help provide medial-lateral stability of a paretic ankle as well as dorsiflexion assistance during the swing-phase of gait. Fitting patients with a more supportive rigid-ankle AFO

can be used to inhibit knee buckling during the single stance phase of gait over the paretic leg. A prefabricated AFO intended for temporary use may be prescribed if likely to be needed only for a month or two. A custom molded AFO is appropriate if longer use is anticipated or if adequate fit and comfort cannot be obtained using a prefabricated brace. (See Figure 7)

Need for a wheelchair or motorized scooter implies more significant disability. If a patient is to spend more than an hour or two a day in a wheelchair or motorized scooter, it is important that they be tailored to the patient's size and needs. Wheelchair evaluations are commonly done by the occupational or physical therapist. There are over 100 options that need to be considered when ordering a wheelchair: seat height, seat width, chair weight, seat-cushion, back height, need for lateral support, headrest, legrest specifications, brake extension, etc. Motorized chairs and scooters are usually reserved for patients unable to self-propel a manual chair, or who need to be independent over longer distances at work or in the community. There is a cardio-pulmonary advantage associated with encouraging the patient to propel their own wheelchair. The main contraindications for use of a motorized chair are impaired cognition, judgment, or safety awareness due to hemi-spatial visual-field deficits. Patients may need both a motorized chair for the home and a light-weight transport wheelchair for use moving from home to car to the community.

The most common home safety devices prescribed are associated with improving safety in the bathroom while assisting with toileting and bathing. A raised toilet seat and armrests make rising from sit-to-stand easier and safer. Grab bars affixed to the wall can also help transitioning on and off the toilet or to the tub or shower. Tub bench and Showerall® allow the patient to bathe while seated using the hand-held shower-head. Ramps, doorway modifications, motorized chair lifts for managing stairs, etc., are all appropriate for selected individuals (see Figure 8). An occupational therapy review with the patient and family or a visit by the therapist to the home will help assure that the patient's home has been optimized for their safety. A home visit by the therapist may reveal fall hazards such as poorly organized furniture, throw rugs, etc., that impede ambulation or wheelchair use.

The occupational therapist and patient have access to catalogs full of devices that can help with every aspect of self care. Some of these devices may help the patient with bilateral rheumatologic hand deformities or hemiplegic patients with use of only one hand. These ADL device catalogs feature items that one without disability might

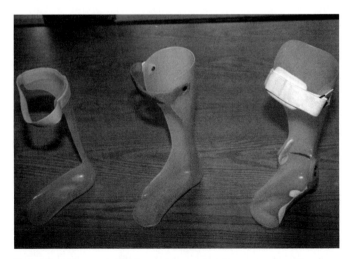

Figure 7 Alternative ankle-foot-orthoses used for treating foot-drop due to either central or peripheral motor control disorders. From left to right, flexible AFO, solid ankle AFO, hinged ankle AFO.

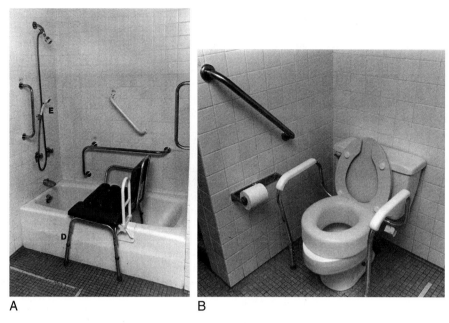

Figure 8 Bath and toilet assist devices. (A) Tub transfer bench, grab bars (multiple options shown for demonstration purposes only), hand held shower; (B) Raised toilet seat, and armrests.

not imagine. Examples include toothpaste dispensers, soap holders, button hooks, one-handed potato peelers, etc.

Rehabilitation Strategies to Minimize Handicap

Handicap within the World Health Organization classification signifies disability fulfilling the patient's accustomed interpersonal functions. These roles are multi-faceted such as within the family as spouse or parent, outside the family as a friend, member of a club or other organization, and at work if not retired. These social roles are usually managed ad-hoc by the individuals involved. While the patient still has adequate mental capacity it is important to encourage them to consider and sign a living will, health care proxy, and power of attorney which will be needed if should they become cognitively impaired in the future. These documents assure that their wishes and their best interests are pursued by who they designate. These arrangements are usually made by the patient and their family with legal advice if there is likelihood of anyone contesting these documents in the future. If there is question of the patient's capacity to make appropriate judgments, then formal neuropsychological assessment may be necessary. If there is impaired mental capacity and no designated health care proxy, or power of attorney, then referral to adult-protection services or other legal assistance will be required to initiate a competency hearing, with the final decision as to the patient's mental competence decided by a judge. Chapter 12 presents a more complete discussion of mental capacity, mental competence, and legal aspects of assisting geriatric patients with health care decisions. The theme that pervades these interactions is to balance the patient's need for self-determination with their need for a safe care environment.

Initial clinical social worker assistance may be in the form of arranging for home care through local visiting nurse services, or for further out-patient rehabilitation services. An illness sufficiently severe as to require hospitalization usually meets criteria for coverage of home-care services for several weeks by the Center for Medicare Services.

For a major illness such as stroke, this may include home visits by a nurse, several hours of home health aide assistance each week, speech-language pathologist visits for treatment of aphasia or dysphagia, and occupational therapist and physical therapist visits as appropriate.

The clinical social worker is expected to be aware of local community-based programs for the patient to provide socialization, a mid-day meal, and exercise-wellness programs to maintain optimum general health and well-being. The social worker can help arrange for handicapped transportation and parking services to facilitate participation in community activities.

Day care programs can be quite beneficial for the patient, and a welcome respite for the caregiver. The social worker is also expected to be aware of local caregiver support groups.

The clinical social worker is also a valuable resource for patient and family considering the need for more supervision and assistance, particularly appropriate for geriatric patients with progressive degenerative neurologic disorders. The social worker can discuss options such as hiring a part time or live-in home health aide, moving of the patient to an independent living facility, to an assisted living facility, or to a nursing home. Documentation of the patient's level-of-care needs can be formally evaluated by nursing, physical therapy, or occupational therapy assessments of self-care and mobility function. Such geriatric evaluation scales are discussed more fully in Chapter 13.

Many geriatric rehabilitation programs incorporate an assessment by a recreational therapist. The recreational therapist helps patients optimize their ability to resume accustomed recreational activities. Such activities are important for maintaining quality of life threatened by progressive impairments due to the many geriatric neurologic disorders covered in this book. Recreational activities may require modification to accommodate cognitive, perceptual, motor, or coordination deficits. Adaptive devices may be available to help overcome residual neurologic impairment: card holders, large print books, books on CD or iPod format, etc. The recreational therapist is often able to provide craft activities that extend the work of the physical therapist, occupational therapist, and speech therapist outside of regular therapy hours. Careful thought must be given to assure that such craft activities are compatible with the patient's interests and within the limits of their motor skills to complete. Recreational activities can also be designed to rehearse linguistic, cognitive, perceptual, and coordination skills.

Optimal Geriatric Neurologic Rehabilitation Outcomes: A Team Approach

This book discusses common problems encountered in geriatric neurology. Each reader will have a different perspective and interest depending upon their background as geriatrician, neurologist, internist, family physician, or other clinician. The above discussion of geriatric neurologic rehabilitation strategies for optimizing impairment, disability, and handicap is intended to stress the breadth of clinical skills currently available to optimize the patient's independence in their home and community.

It would be ideal but unrealistic to hope that each patient has access to a coordinated geriatric neurologic rehabilitation program in their area. Inability to create this ideal need not deter one from modeling the care delivery system as closely as possible to this goal within their practice setting.

The geriatric clinician usually has access to a nurse who can help with self-care and mobility assessments. Problems identified can be referred to a physical therapist or occupational therapist colleague in the community. Bracing needs can sometimes be met using prefabricated braces, but hinged ankle or custom molded braces will require referral to an orthotist. The geriatric nurse specialist is an appropriate person to discuss bowel and bladder care issues. General nutritional screening for body mass index, lipid panel, fasting glucose, renalelectrolyte balance, and serum pre-albumin might prompt referral for more formal nutritional evaluation and treatment. Aphasia and dysphagia would prompt referral to a collaborating speech-language pathologist.

Appropriate referrals can be made by the geriatric nurse or collaborating clinical social worker for problems with any of the above impairments, disabilities, or handicaps. These may require specific rehabilitation interventions, access to ongoing community meal delivery programs, wellness programs, home care programs, or day programs.

The geriatric neurologic rehabilitation clinic model need not take place within the same building. What is important is the communication, mutual respect, and follow-up that is practised among the multiple clinicians. With time and rehearsal, the several individual clinicians comprising this community-based team will learn to function as a unit. Each of the members will be encouraged to suggest alternative treatment strategies and know that their suggestions are being carefully considered.

The most difficult component of the geriatric neurologic rehabilitation clinic to reproduce in a community setting is the scheduling of face-to-face meetings of team members rehearsing the patient's current treatment plan, progress, and goals. Conference calls and HIPAAcompatible Internet communication may, however, help overcome this obstacle.

References

Abboud S, Viiri L, Lutjohann D, and Goebeler S, Associations of apolipoprotein E gene with ischemic stroke and intracranial atherosclerosis, *Eur J Hum Genet* 2008;16:955–960.

Barbotte E, Guillemin F, Chau N, and the Lorhandicap Group, Prevalence of impairments, disabilities, and handicaps and quality of life in the general population: A review of recent literature, *Bull of World Health Org* 2001;79:1047–1055.

Barrett A, Eslinger P, Amantadine for adynamic speech: Possible benefit for aphasia? *Am J Phys Med Rehabil* 2007;86:605–612.

Belin P, Van Eckhout Ph, Zilbovicius M, et al., Recovery from nonfluent aphasia after melodic intonation therapy: A PET study. *Neurology* 1996;47:1504–1511.

Bobath B, *Adult hemiplegia: Evaluation and treatment*, William Heinemann Medical Books, London, 1970.

Bosia M, Bechi M, Marino E, and Anselmetti S, Influence of Catechol-O-methyltransferase Val158Met polymorphism on neuropsychological and functional outcomes of classical rehabilitation, *Neurosci Lett* 2007;417:271–274.

Bowler J, Vascular cognitive impairment, *Stroke* 2004:35:386–388

Brunnstrom S, *Movement therapy in hemiplegia: A neurophysiological approach*, Harper & Row, Philadelphia, 1970.

Carr J and Shepherd R, A motor relearning programme for stroke, William Heinemann Medical Books, London, 1982.

Coleman P and Riesen A, Environmental effects on cortical dendritic fields, *J Anat* 1968;102:363–374.

Cramer S, Nelles G, Benson R, Kaplan J, Parker R, and Kwong K. A functional MRI study of subjects recovered from hemiparetic stroke. *Stroke* 1997:28:2518–2527.

Cramer S, Nelles G, Schaecter J, Kaplan J, Finklestein S, and Rosen B, A functional MRI study of three motor tasks in the evaluation of stroke recovery. *Neurorehabil Neural Repair* 2001;15:1–8.

Crisostomo E, Duncan P, Propst M, Dawson D, and Davis J, Evidence that amphetamine with physical therapy promotes recovery of motor function in stroke patients, *Ann Neurol* 1988;23:94–97.

Dervaux A and Levasseur M, Risperidone and valproate for mania following stroke, *J Neuropsychiatry Clin Nerosci* 2008;20:247.

Finestone H, Woodbury M, Foley N, Teasell R, and Greene-Finestone L, Tracking clinical improvement of swallowing disorders after stroke, *J Stroke Cerebrovasc Dis* 2002;11:23–27.

Fleet W, Valenstein E, Watson R, and Heilman K, Dopamine agonist therapy for neglect in humans, *Neurology* 1987;37:1765–1770.

Frassinetti F, Angeli V, Meneghello F, Avanzi S, and Ladavas E, Long-lasting amelioration of visuospatial neglect by prism adaptation, *Brain* 2002;125:608–623.

Fregni F, Transcranial direct current stimulation of the unaffected hemisphere in stroke patients, *Neuroreport* 2005;16:1551–1555.

Grade C, Redford B, Chrostowski J, Toussaint L, and Blackwell B, Methylphenidate in early poststroke recovery: A double-blind, placebo-controlled study, *Arch Phys Med Rehabil* 1998;79: 1047–50.

Grotta J, Noser E, and Ro T, Constraint-induced movement therapy. *Stroke* 2004;35:2699–2701.

Gupta S, Mlcoch A, Scolaro C, and Moritz T, Bromocriptine treatment of nonfluent aphasia, *Neurology* 1995;45:2170–2173.

Jayaraman T, Berenstein V, Li M, and Mayer J, Tumor necrosis factor alpha is a key modulator of inflammation in cerebral aneurysms, *Neurosurg* 2005;57:558–564.

Kiger M, Brown C, and Watkins L, Dysphagia management: An analysis of patient outcomes using VitalStim therapy compared to traditional swallow therapy, *Dysphagia* 2006;21:243–253.

Knott M and Voss D, *Proprioceptive neuromuscular facilitation: Patterns and techniques*, Harper & Row, New York, 1956.

Kosak M and Reding M, Comparison of partial body weight supported treadmill training versus aggressive bracing assisted walking post stroke, *Neurorehabil Neural Repair* 2000;14:13–19.

Lee J and Reding M, Effects of thiazolidinediones on stroke recovery: A case- matched controlled study, *Neurochem Res* 2007;32: 635–638.

Liepert J, Miltner W, Bauder H, Sommer M, Dettmers C, and Taub E, Motor cortex plasticity during constraint-induced movement therapy in stroke patients. *Neurosci Lett* 1998;250:5–8.

Martinsson L, Wahlgren N, and Hardemark H, Amphetamines for improving recovery after stroke (Cochrane Review). In: *The Cochrane Library, Issue 3,* 2003. Oxford: Update Software.

Merzenich M, Nelson R, and Stryker M. Somatosensory cortical map changes following digit amputation in adult monkeys, *J Comp Neurol* 1984;224:591–605.

Miyai I and Reding M, Effects of antidepressants on functional recovery following stroke: a double-blind study. *J Neuro Rehab* 1998;12:5–13.

Nudo R, Milliken G, Jenkins W, and Merzenich M, Use-dependent alterations of movement representations in primary motor cortex of adult squirrel monkeys. *J Neurosci* 1996;16:785–807.

Poggel D, Kasten E, and Sabel B, Attentional cueing improves vision restoration therapy in patients with visual field defects. *Neurology* 2004;63:2069–2076.

Ratan R, Siddiq A, Smirnova N, and Karpisheva K, Harnessing hypoxic adaptation to prevent, treat, and repair stroke. *J Mol Med* 2007;85:1331–1338.

Reding M, Solomon B, and Borucki S. Effect of dextroamphetamine on motor recovery after stroke. *Neurology* 1995;45(suppl 4):A222.

Rees C, Flexible endoscopic evaluation of swallowing with sensory testing, *Curr Opin Otolaryngol Head Neck Surg* 2006;14:425–430.

REO Therapy, Motorika USA Inc., 523 Fellowship Rd, Suite 228, Mount Laurel, NJ 08054.

Ring H and Rosenthal N, Controlled study of neuroprosthetic functional electrical stimulation in sub-acute post-stroke rehabilitation, *J Rehabil Med* 2004;26:1–6.

Rosenzweig, M, Krech, D, Bennett, E, and Diamond M, Effects of environmental complexity and training on brain chemistry and anatomy: A replication and extension, *J Comp Physiol Psychol* 1962;55:429–437.

#Saebo Inc. Six Lake Pointe Plaza, 2725 Water Ridge Pkwy Suite 320, Charlotte, NC 28217.

Sapir S, Spielman J, Ramig L, Story B, and Fox C, Effects of intensive voice treatment (the Lee Silverman Voice Treatment) on vowel articulation in dysarthric individuals with idiopathic Parkinson's disease, *J Speech Lang Hear Res* 2007;50:899–912.

Scheibel M, Lindsay R, Tomiyasu U, and Scheibel A, Progressive dendritic changes in the aging human limbic system. *Exp Neurol* 1976;53: 420–430.

Shaker R, Easterling C, Kern M, Nitschke T, and Massey B, Rehabilitation of swallowing by exercise in tube-fed patients with pharyngeal dysphagia secondary to abnormal UES opening, *Gastroenterol* 2002;122:1314–1321.

Siironen J, Juvela S, Kanarek K, and Vilkki J, The Met allele of the BDNF Val66Met polymorphism predicts poor outcome among survivors of aneurysmal subarachnoid hemorrhage, *Stroke* 2007;38:2858–2860.

Sinn D, Kim S, Chu K, and Jung K, Valproic acid mediated neuroprotection in intracerebral hemorrhage via histone deacetylase inhibition and transcriptional activation, *Neurobiol Dis* 2007;26: 464–472.

Stein R, Chong S, Everaert D, et al. A multicenter trial of a footdrop stimulator controlled by a tilt sensor. *Neurorehabil Neural Repair* 2006;20:371–379.

Volpe B, Krebs H, and Hogan N, Robot-aided sensorimotor training in stroke rehabilitation. *Adv Neurol* 2003;92:429–433.

51 Pain Management in the Elderly

Don H. Bivins

Introduction

It may seem trite to state that pain management issues in the elderly are problematic and pervasive. Few health care providers would disagree with that basic premise. With aggressive research and education of the medical community, the problems should lessen as baby boomers reach the benchmark 65 years of age, at which time the Federal Government considers them "elderly." Indeed, we are now divided into three groups: the younger old (age 65–74 years); the older old (age 75–84 years); and the oldest old (85+ years).

The health of the elderly is problematic due to the nearly obligatory polypharmacy, their multiplicity of interactive diseases, the numerous physicians involved in their care, and the metabolic changes peculiar to the elderly. Especially with regards to pain management, we unfortunately see a large number of physicians uncomfortable in managing pain disorders.

This chapter will attempt to succinctly address these issues, while providing clinical information readily useful in the practitioner's office. This chapter will not address headache in the elderly, as that has been reviewed in chapter 48 by Drs. Bamford and Mays, but this author will approach the subject of pain management with the assumption that the treating practitioner is already aware of their patients' diagnoses.

Epidemiology

Establishing accurate epidemiological data has been imperfect, as many clinical studies have examined only certain disease states, only nursing home patients, or only community dwelling elderly. Surprisingly, the best general data may be gleaned from 2000 US Census Bureau statistics. In 2000, 42% of the population 65 and older reported a physical disability. Within that category, 21.5% of the younger old cited a disability, 32.7% of the older old, and 53.1% of the oldest old. Similar percentage differences were documented for disabilities in blindness or deafness, activities of daily living, and mental disability (Deane and Smith 2008).

More directly to the point, the American Geriatrics Society Panel on Persistent Pain in Older Persons (2002) suggests approximately 20% of older Americans have unrelenting pain, and 18% of people over 65 take analgesics regularly (AGS 2002). Several other authors report on the prevalence of pain in the elderly, but their findings vary tremendously due to stated differences in study design, data collection, statistical analysis, or even if their elderly study subjects can or would admit to having pain. Actually, findings of some authors disagree as to the increase or decrease in pain prevalence as the population ages.

Despite discrepancies in available data, it is sufficient to state that pain, if acute or chronic, is a significant problem for the elderly. That 25% or so of those with unrelenting pain receive **no** analgesic treatment is an indictment. Equally sobering are reports that lower treatment rates are found for the oldest old and those with cognitive and communicative disorders (Maxwell 2008).

Without consideration of age, pain has unequivocal social consequences: impaired ambulation, anxiety, depression, sleep disturbance, decreased socialization, and increased health care utilization and costs (AGS 2002). These difficulties are more evident in the elderly, who are prone to them because of their changing social climate or their comorbid illnesses. Maxwell reported that daily pain is more likely seen in females having three or more comorbid conditions; using nine or more prescription and over the counter (OTC) drugs; having arthritis, osteoporosis, and/or cancer; exhibiting mild to moderate depressive symptoms; and less likely to have cognitive impairment or a communication disorder (Maxwell 2008). Common pain syndromes in the elderly include osteoarthritis, spinal and radicular disorders, neuralgias and neuropathies, rheumatoid arthritis, cancer, and fibromyalgia. This review will analyze these disorders primarily to explain the pathophysiology of pain.

Pathophysiology of Acute and Chronic Pain

Pain is often categorized as somatic, visceral, neuropathic, or sympathetically maintained (or, autonomic). Somatic refers to pain originating from the musculoskeletal system; and visceral from the visceral organs. Neuropathic pain (NpP) implies certain changes have occurred within either peripheral nerves or central tracts and neurons, creating a self-perpetuating pain. Disagreement continues as to the significance of sympathetically maintained pain, but there are now studies confirming its actuality even though we do not fully understand it. Its name implies that the sympathetic nervous system is involved in the transmission or maintenance of pain signals. Pains within these categories tend to have characteristic clinical features, but the underlying pathophysiology is similar within all categories.

Our understanding of the pathophysiology of pain should dictate our treatment decisions. In the elderly, acute pain is often secondary to trauma or surgery, creating injury in any number of bony or soft tissues, but the pathophysiology is generally the same in any tissue.

Myelinated Aδ and unmyelinated C-fibers carry the acute pain signals from the periphery to central sites, but there is more cellular and biomolecular activity at the injury site than just the transmission of an electrical impulse. Direct trauma to the nerve initiates the pain signaling, which would soon cease if the source of injury is quickly removed. However, acute pain persists after the injury due to the normal inflammatory responses accompanying the injury. Locally, histamine, substance P, prostaglandins, leukotrienes, excitatory amino acids, and free radicals are immediately released. Cytokines (interleukins, tumor necrosis factor [TNF]) and neurotrophins (nerve growth factor [NGF]) also accumulate at the injury site. Obviously, the intent of the inflammatory response is to produce healing of the injury, though any of the agents mentioned above may directly lower the threshold of nociceptors, simultaneously activitate those nociceptors, and increase the severity of the pain (Levin 2002). If the healing process proceeds normally, the inflammation diminishes, the tissues recover, the nociceptors reduce their transmission, and the pain subsides. Acute pain is thus self-limited though it may be present for several days.

There is consensus that chronic pain, by definition, is present for at least six months. Longstanding pain is possibly due to continued pain signaling from the unmyelinated C or other A-fiber types, implying ongoing tissue injury secondary to acute reactions. One could imagine a scenario of a cancerous or infectious lesion continuing to grow, or of osteoarthritis compressing or irritating nerves and other soft tissues, leading to persistent, acute inflammatory changes locally.

Absent such an expanding or irritative lesion, chronic pain arises from spontaneous, uncontrolled firing of injured peripheral fibers or dysfunctional central neurons. This is neuropathic pain, which arises from an abnormal response to the acute inflammatory reactions by a process known as sensitization. Obviously, the inflammatory response did not promote healing in this situation.

To better understand this aberrant course, let's re-examine the inflammatory response after acute injury.

At the moment of the acute injury (independent of its cause), macrophages and granulocytes are attracted to the site. Numerous genes become operational or at least upregulated, creating a host of biomolecular changes at the site of injury. As mentioned previously, histamine, substance P, prostaglandins, leukotrienes, excitatory amino acids, free radicals, interleukins, TNF-α, and NGF, among other substances, are released at or attracted to the injured tissue. This initially occurs over a matter of minutes but can continue for days. Activated macrophages and newly denervated Schwann cells cause an interruption of the blood-nerve barrier. Hyperemia and swelling occur in the area due to bradykinin, nitric oxide, and calcitonin gene-related peptide release. This "inflammatory soup" self-perpetuates for hours or days. Simultaneous with the production and attraction of these destructive agents, phagocytosis of the damaged material occurs so that Schwann cells can restructure and the injured axon or dendrite regrow. For reasons not always evident, instead of healing, a maladaptive process begins. Proinflammatory cytokines, TNF factors, and activated macrophages continue the destructive pattern at the site of the injured peripheral nerve.

Concurrently over a matter of days, even though remote to the injured peripheral fiber, macrophages and glial cells within the dorsal root ganglion (DRG) are activated. Upregulation of genes within the DRG occurs, leading to release of cytokines, TNF, and excitatory amino acids. DRG neurons respond to this injury with increased neuronal activity and spontaneous action potential discharges. As sodium and calcium ion channels increase in number and permeability, as N-methyl-D-aspartate (NMDA) receptors numerically increase, and as Toll-like receptors upregulate, the DRG's neurons' firing threshold is lowered significantly. Peripheral sensitization has now occurred. Therefore, instead of the patient having pain signals arising only from the injured peripheral nerve fiber, spontaneous pain signals now also arise from the DRG itself.

Occasionally the maladaptive process will arrest at this anatomical level. More often, though, the changes in the DRG are accompanied by T lymphocyte invasion, causing astrocytic changes in the ipsilateral spinal cord. The same inflammatory changes that have occurred in the periphery and the DRG now lead to glial activation that can proceed cephalad as far as the thalamus and possibly the parietal sensory cortex.

Once the ion channels and NMDA receptors are upregulated and the neuronal firing threshold is lowered, central sensitization has occurred (Devor 2002; Moalem 2006; White 2007). At that time, the brain is constantly bombarded by pain signals from the periphery, the DRG, and the central structures. Neuropathic pain—that unrelenting sharp, electrical, burning, throbbing agony—is now the self-perpetuating companion of our patients.

Genetic Contributions to Acute or Chronic Pain

While research in the biomolecular arena has proliferated in the past decade, genetic research is now coming to the fore and we have much to learn. We know well that genetic disorders such as Charcot-Marie-Tooth disease and rheumatoid arthritis are accompanied by chronic pain. However, this is not to say that patients so afflicted have specific genetic alterations that create the pain state. Instead, nerve injury, irritation, or inflammation inherent to the disorder causes the pain in the fashion described previously. The larger question needing exploration is whether certain individuals, families, or ethnic groups are genetically inclined to experience pain differently. We know from personal experience and formal studies that there is individual, racial, and ethnic variation in the experience of pain. But the influence of the environment must be removed to determine with some accuracy if the mentioned variations are indeed genetic.

Zubieta and colleagues demonstrated a functional polymorphism in the gene coding for catechol-o-methyltransferase, resulting in alterations of the functional responses of μ-opioid neurotransmitters in the central nervous system. This could result in the patient's inability to modulate pain signaling endogenously. Human genetic variation is also known to affect codeine metabolism due to polymorphisms in CYP2D6. Not only do these individuals have difficulty metabolizing codeine, they also exhibit a decreased basal pain tolerance. Candidate genes within the major histocompatibility complex are likely to predispose individuals to complex regional pain syndrome (MacGregor 2004). Some patients with fibromyalgia are known to have genetic alterations causing a dysfunctional serotonin transporting protein.

These are but a few examples of positive results in this genetic exploration. Since many groups are active in this investigation, the future holds promise in identifying specific gene abnormalities that actually create a pain disorder or a predisposition to heightened pain states. This may lead to developing novel treatments specific to those identified genes, a goal for the larger field of pharmacogenetics.

Clinical Presentation of Selected Disorders of Pain Occurring in the Elderly

We are all aware that the elderly can suffer from a multiplicity of diseases. The following diseases are reviewed since they are common and since they provide a platform from which treatment recommendations can be made based on the known pathophysiology.

Osteoarthritis

More than 80% of people older than 75 have clinical osteoarthritis (OA), which is a disease of the joint cartilage and bone typically affecting weight-bearing joints asymmetrically. Risk factors are multiple and complex. There is a female preponderance for the disorder, but the disease affects the genders differently. Women have more multiple joint involvement, especially of the hands, knees, ankles, and feet. The disease localizes in men more to the hips, wrists, and spine. OA of the hip is uncommon in African-Americans and in Indian / Pakistani groups. OA of the hand is rare in African-Americans and Malaysians. These and other gender or ethnic differences are considered genetic rather than environmental. Childhood and adolescent obesity predisposes one to OA, as does injury to any specific joint. Surprisingly, but nevertheless quite true, there is little correlation between the degree of radiographic change of an arthritic joint and the intensity of pain the patient ascribes to that joint.

Once thought to be a disorder of "degeneration" only, it is clear now that ongoing metabolic changes occur within the osteoarthritic joint. It is the breakdown of the cartilage that releases cytokines and other proinflammatory molecules. The release of interleukin-1 (IL-1) and interleukin-6 (IL-6) induces the production of cyclo-oxygenase (COX)-2 and inducible nitric oxide synthase (iNOS). These two enzymes amplify the production of prostaglandin E_2 (PGE_2) and nitric oxide (NO), both of which are strongly proinflammatory (Kean 2008). The degree of inflammation may vary from time to time, thus allowing the patient to experience more or less pain accordingly. As the cartilage and then the bone undergo degenerative remodeling, nociceptors are stimulated and pain ensues. OA is an example in which the pain may persist due to the low-grade ongoing inflammation with subsequent chronic C-fiber activation or due to neuropathic sensitization that leads to chronic NpP, despite the fact that the primary pathology is in the bones and cartilage of the joint. Since inflammation—albeit usually low grade—is a distinct feature of osteoarthritis, one can easily understand why patients with OA often report pain reduction with anti-inflammatory medicines.

Rheumatoid Arthritis

Rheumatoid arthritis (RA) is a multisystem, complex autoimmune disorder to which people are predisposed genetically and environmentally. Though several genetic markers exist, the most consistent one is the class II major histocompatibility complex antigen HLA DR4. The presence of this marker conveys a six fold increase in the relative risk of developing this disease. The prevalence varies considerably within countries or people groups; for instance, there is a lower prevalence in rural black groups than in urbanized blacks in Africa. Overall, the incidence and severity are decreasing (Jayson 2002).

Though RA is considered a multisystem disease, for the purposes of this chapter, we will consider only the skeletal changes. RA is a symmetrical, peripheral, inflammatory polyarthritis most often afflicting the small joints of the extremities, the knees, and the cervical spine. The predilection for these areas is unexplained. As discussed in the pathophysiology section above, RA typically demonstrates the cascade of release of histamine, prostaglandins, reactive species, and cytokines. This results in injury to the joints, ligaments, tendons, and visceral organs, and to the adjacent neural structures. Ongoing damage to somatic and visceral nerves causes acute pain, and the spontaneous neuronal discharging characteristic of the sensitized peripheral and central neural structures follows. Both types of pain can fluctuate from day to day in their intensity.

Spinal and Radicular Disorders

The intended brevity of this chapter does not allow a thorough appraisal of non-specific low back pain (LBP), which is surely one of the most common complaints in the elderly. In fact, up to 90% of patients of any age who have LBP do not have an identified specific etiology. This review will highlight only the pain associated with certain disorders of the spine and spinal (radicular) nerves.

Osteoarthritis of the spine occurs predominantly in the lumbar region, apparently due to its load bearing over the years. As the inflammation, bone remodeling, and disk disruption begin and persist, rather dramatic changes develop in the architecture of the spinal column. The normally well hydrated annulus pulposus begins to dry and the annulus fibrosus loses its elasticity and strength, resulting in loss of disk height. As the vertebral bodies move closer together, alterations subsequently occur in the anterior and posterior longitudinal spinal ligaments, the ligamenta flava, and the facet joints. The ligamentum flavum joins the lamina of one vertebral body to the adjacent body above and below. The facet joints are also known as zygapophysial joints, articulating surfaces between the transverse processes of the adjacent vertebrae. The facets now articulate abnormally, stimulating additional inflammatory changes and remodeling. Osteophytic lipping develops around the edges of the vertebral bodies and can become so severe that osteophytic bridges are created between adjacent vertebrae. As the vertebral disks and bodies lose height, the neural foramina become smaller, leading to nerve root (radicular) encroachment or compression. Sufficient loss of height participates in the creation of spinal canal stenosis in which the diameter of the canal is significantly reduced and nerve roots compressed. The changes in the longitudinal ligaments allow for the vertebral bodies to slip in an anteroposterior direction, resulting in spondylolysthesis. Usually, the more superior vertebral body slips forward in relation to the vertebra beneath. In so doing, the spinal canal and neural foramina are narrowed even further with subsequent radicular compromise.

Spinal stenosis produces pain symptoms known as neurogenic claudication. These patients will typically have a poorly localized ache in the low and mid back nearly constantly. Leaning forward, as in resting one's arms on the grocery cart handle while shopping, will often ease this back discomfort. When the patient walks a flight of stairs or takes a brisk walk for exercise, the pain becomes more intense and extends into the buttocks and/or upper legs. It is relieved by rest, only to recur more quickly once exercise is re-initiated. Depending on the vertebral level of the stenosis, the pain may localize more intensely to the buttocks, the inguinal area, or the upper legs. In opposition to the vascular variety, neurogenic claudication is less likely to extend to the calves.

It is well known that sensory symptoms of radicular compression include tingling, burning, stinging, and electric or knife-like pains within the distribution of a spinal nerve. Weakness may also develop in the myotome of the injured root. Health care providers often think of patients having just one nerve root compressed, as with a ruptured disk; but the elderly are particularly prone to polyradiculopathies secondary to the multiple changes occurring at multiple levels of the vertebral column.

Due to their propensity to falls and the weakness of the skeletal system, the elderly may suffer gradual vertebral height shortening or frank vertebral collapse. The former may be painless and simply lead to postural abnormalities. The latter most often occurs after trauma and is acutely painful. Whenever a vertebra collapses, especially if there is not a history of trauma, one must suspect other pathologic processes, such as a metastatic lesion. If the collapse has occurred traumatically, vertebroplasty may be indicated as long as an MRI scan shows persistent edema within the marrow at the fracture site.

Metastatic disease, discitis, and osteomyelitis of the spine may present as sharp, well localized pain or a more diffuse ache. For the latter, the physical exam may localize the lesion to a specific vertebra. For many years, researchers could not understand how pain could arise from a metastasis growing *inside* a bone if the periosteum was uninvolved. After all, anatomists thought that nociceptors were present only in the periosteum and pain had to be secondary to periosteal injury. Only fairly recently did we learn that nociceptors are indeed present within the bony matrix and thus understood the pain coming from a metastatic lesion buried well within a single bone. Metastatic lesions can cause both somatic and neuropathic pain.

It should be obvious that pain arising from such spinal disorders may be simply nociceptor stimulation, but could also occur in response to the inflammatory changes and neuronal sensitization seen in more chronic conditions. Therefore, treatment of the pain can be multifaceted.

Neuralgias and Neuropathies

Trigeminal and glossopharyngeal neuralgias are relatively well known to health care providers, and are recognized as intensely painful cranial nerve syndromes. Occipital neuralgia is a common cause of posterior head pain, though not as intense. The term "neuralgia" is commonly used to suggest an etiology that is unknown. However, these three syndromes now appear to be secondary to nerve fiber compression. The seminal discovery that the trigeminal nerve was often compressed by an adjacent vascular structure was instrumental in opening a new therapeutic field for such disorders. Herpes zoster can lead to acute or chronic facial pain, but for purposes of taxonomy is considered a neuropathy, implying a known etiology.

Neuropathies may affect cranial nerves (shingles), radicular nerves (shingles, Guillain-Barré syndrome), or peripheral nerves (carpal tunnel syndrome, diabetic polyneuropathy, Charcot-Marie-Tooth disease). Multiple etiologies are possible: trauma, infectious, metabolic, ischemic, compressive, tumor, toxic, or genetic (Pappagallo 2008). Since these are NpP, the symptoms are similar because of the category of pain within which they fall, not because of the underlying etiology. Thus the patient will report numbness, tingling, stinging, electric jolts, stabbing, or knife-like pains. They may be constant or intermittent; even changing position may influence the presence or intensity of the pain. There are far too many varieties of neuropathies to review individually here. The essential lesson is to understand that the nerves have been injured by whatever etiology, sensitization has occurred, and the neuropathy's pain is spontaneous and self-perpetuating.

Cancer Pain

With advances in medical care, life expectancies are extending, allowing more people to experience a variety of chronic illnesses for a longer portion of their lives. Cancer is a classic example. Regrettably, we must admit that cancer pain is not well controlled in our country, despite technological advances. Many cancer patients just expect to have pain as a normal consequence of their disease, so they may be less inclined to complain. Patients also fear "becoming addicted" and so use a minimum of their opiates to achieve a modicum of relief.

At the risk of sounding redundant, the pathophysiology of cancer pain has similar mechanisms as other chronic pains. There are nociceptive and neuropathic features. The nociceptive aspect may begin as the tumor expands, either compressing adjacent nerve endings or irritating the nociceptive fibers within the capsule of any organ. So the initial pain is typically somatic or visceral in origin, with acute pain signaling by way of C-fibers. Inflammation eventually occurs as the host's defenses begin their fight against the foreign tumor cells. The inflammation expectedly can adversely affect any normal adjacent viscera or neural tissue. The previously described cascade occurs and NpP is once again present (Delgado-Guay 2008).

Fibromyalgia

There is a misperception among some health care providers that fibromyalgia is a disorder affecting young women living in Westernized countries. Population studies have clearly shown this not to be true; it does reportedly have a female to male ratio of 7:1 but it is reported to occur in third-world countries, and a substantial number of patients

report symptom onset after the age of 50. Another misperception is that the disorder cannot be treated, resulting in thousands of patients having unnecessary unrelenting pain. There is little doubt that the disorder is notably overdiagnosed, but this unfortunately leaves a large cohort of patients with treatable diseases untreated or at least under managed.

For years, fibromyalgia was considered strictly of psychologic origin, and this stigma persists despite a wealth of data proving otherwise. Though disagreement exists if fibromyalgia is a true NpP, there is complete agreement that the nervous system is intimately involved in the origin and maintenance of the pain. For example, ample research demonstrates that patients have malfunctioning endogenous pain modulatory systems. This endogenous system performs by releasing amino acids and peptides that bear a striking functional resemblance to synthetic opioids. When serving the individual properly, this system reduces the pain signaling from the periphery and the patient indeed has less pain. However, in addition to this inhibitory arm of modulation, there is also a facilitative arm. This is not an aberrancy, but rather a protective mechanism to prevent additional injury to the individual; if I put my hand in a candle's flame, I remove it reflexively to prevent tissue injury. This facilitative endogenous system in fibromyalgia, however, reacts aberrantly, thus amplifying perceived pain. Patients describe this as their skin feeling hypersensitive to light touch or to mild changes in temperature.

Other data reveals disruption of the normal hypothalamic-pituitary-adrenal axis, blunted cortisol responses to stress, a well-defined genetic pattern in several families, abnormal blood flow to non-sensory portions of the brain, abnormal patterns of fMRI pain recognition and responsiveness, higher spinal fluid levels of substance P, elevated serum levels of IL-6 and IL-8, and an unusually high number of activated mast cells on skin biopsies of affected individuals. The synthesis of this data suggests that fibromyalgia is a neuroimmunoendocrine disorder with inflammatory characteristics (Perrot 2008). Of considerable interest is the possibility that the commencing of the pathology is within the cerebral substance with subsequent development of peripheral symptoms that strongly resemble NpP.

Pain Management Options

I have attempted to plainly distinguish acute somatic or visceral pain from chronic neuropathic pain, based on pathophysiologic mechanisms. It is from this basis that we can now consider specific treatment alternatives. Generally speaking, these treatment alternatives can be successfully applied to any pain disorder if one attempts to first understand the mechanism.

Acetaminophen

This agent is on the first rung of the World Health Organization (WHO) pain treatment ladder, and appropriately so. It is a relatively weak analgesic for most individuals, but does inhibit some aspects of prostaglandin synthesis and subsequently provides weak inhibition of the COX-2 pathway. Garcia-Rodriguez and Hernandez studied the risk of upper gastrointestinal (GI) bleeding and the risk of liver toxicity due to acetaminophen. At doses greater than 2000 mg/day, this agent exhibits a clear toxicity profile for both upper GI bleeding and hepatotoxicity. Thus, some argue that several of the non-steroidal anti-inflammatory drugs (NSAIDs) are a better choice for analgesia since the risks are the same or less, and the analgesic profile is better with the NSAID (Kean 2008).

Acetaminophen purchased OTC is probably the only instance when a patient uses this drug by itself. It is commonly used in prescribed combinations with hydrocodone, propoxyphene, and oxycodone.

However, many physicians are unaware of the quantity of acetaminophen in these formulated combinations. For example, providers often write "Darvocet N-100™, 1–2 tabs every 4 hours prn pain." This prescription allows the patient to use as many as 12 tablets in a 24 hour span. Those 12 tablets contain 7800 mg of acetaminophen! This is well above the toxic limit for acetaminophen. Needless to say, caution is advised.

NSAIDs

Depending on their mechanism of action, this class of analgesics is divided into two groups, COX-1 and COX-2 inhibitors. A few work by both mechanisms. The agents inhibit the cyclo-oxygenase pathway and thereby reduce the formation and release of prostaglandins. This mechanism is thus effective in reducing the inflammatory response at any site of injury, with a concomitant reduction in pain.

The COX-1 inhibitors generally have a 25–35% risk of adverse effects, with the elderly at greater risk. These adverse effects impact the homeostasis of the GI tract, renal and cardiovascular systems, liver, skin, and mucous membranes.

The COX-2 selective inhibitors are quite effective against inflammation, but their adverse effect profiles have radically reduced their utility and availability. Post-marketing analysis revealed little difference in the incidence of GI adverse effects between celecoxib, ibuprofen, and diclofenac. Additional work revealed that using a non-selective NSAID and a proton pump inhibitor (PPI) simultaneously had slightly fewer GI adverse effects than did using a celecoxib alone. COX-1 and COX-2 agents have similar adverse effects on the kidney: increased sodium reabsorption, decreased response to diuretics, fluid retention, induction of hypertension or reduced responsiveness to anti-hypertensive agents, hyperkalemia, renal tubular acidosis, congestive heart failure, and renal failure. The cardiac adverse effects have been well studied, though some of these effects were established post-marketing. Both classes increase platelet adhesiveness and increase arterial constriction, but the COX-2 agents are clearly more problematic. Interestingly, high doses of ibuprofen and diclofenac, but not naproxen, are also associated with a moderate risk of coronary or carotid vascular events.

It must be emphasized that NSAIDs should be used with caution in the elderly due to a multiplicity of adverse effects. Even if the elderly patient has no known cardiac or hypertensive disease and an NSAID is begun, the patient must be monitored carefully for cardiovascular adverse effects (Roberts 2002; Kean 2008).

The non-selective NSAIDs are divided into different chemical classes. It seems prudent that if the patient does not respond to an agent in one class, then a change to a different class might be an appropriate step—though most physicians simply switch to another NSAID with which they are familiar. Please refer to Table 1 for a listing of the NSAIDs by chemical class.

Tramadol

Tramadol is neither an NSAID nor an opiate, but is a synthetic analogue of codeine. It does not appear in the Food and Drug Administration (FDA) narcotic schedules. It binds weakly to μ receptors as if it were an opiate, but it also weakly inhibits the reuptake of serotonin and norepinephrine. Its primary metabolite is active and 2–4 times more potent than the parent molecule. It will be most helpful for acute somatic or visceral pain, though studies do reveal moderate effectiveness in some NpP. It is generally well tolerated, but can precipitate seizures, especially if taken in doses greater than 400 mg daily.

Tricyclic Anti-depressants

As a class, these agents are not efficacious for acute or inflammatory pain. Several studies demonstrate benefit in NpP, especially for

Table 1 Non-Selective Non-Steroidal Anti-Inflammatory Drugs Arranged by Chemical Class

Salicylic acid derivatives	Aspirin
	Sodium salicylate
	Salsalate
	Sulfasalazine
Para-aminophenol derivatives	Acetaminophen
Indole and indene acetic acids	Indomethacin
	Sulindac
	Etodolac
Heteroaryl acetic acids	Tolmetin
	Diclofenac
	Ketorolac
Arylpropionic acids	Ibuprofen
	Naproxen
	Ketoprofen
	Fenoprofen
Anthranilic acids (fenamates)	Mefenamic acid
	Meclofenamic acid
Enolic acids	Piroxicam
	Meloxicam
Alkanones	Nabumetone

amitriptyline and nortriptyline. Since a major side effect of the class is sleepiness, they are often prescribed at night as a sleep aid; their long half-lives provide pain control for up to 24 hours. They are primarily used adjunctively. Major adverse effects are related to their anticholinergic properties.

Selective Serotonin and Norepinephrine Reuptake Inhibitors

Both serotonin and norepinephrine are helpful in the control of pain based on receptor affinity. Substance P levels drop in the presence of serotonin, at least in the spinal fluid. As a class, they are not efficacious for acute or inflammatory pain. Multiple studies show their effectiveness in reducing NpP. Venlafaxine and duloxetine are the most promising in the class. Their "side effect" as anti-depressants is also of great use in the patient with pain; some patients also find them useful in correcting sleep disturbances. They are recognized for their GI and sexual adverse effects.

Neuromodulators

Most health care providers refer to this class as anticonvulsants. However, the wide range of therapeutic benefits clearly extends beyond seizure control. They can be very effective for NpP control and migraine headache prevention. So the moniker of neuromodulator has been applied instead. The mechanism of action of most neuromodulators is either γ-aminobutyric acid (GABA) potentiation, or sodium or calcium ion channel inhibition. In either role, they reduce the spontaneous firing present in the injured nerve. Gabapentin, lamotrigine, phenytoin, pregabalin, and topiramate have positive studies, though some agents are definitely more beneficial than others. Nevertheless, if one agent does not work, the provider should use another. All agents should be dosed to therapeutic blood levels, if levels can be obtained commercially, or to adverse effects. Potential adverse effects are multiple and usually self-limiting. Phenytoin, if used over years, can lead to facial cosmetic changes, osteoporosis and cerebellar degeneration. Cases of a life-threatening rash have been reported with lamotrigine.

Opiates

The FDA categorizes these medicines into four different schedules. The most potent agents are in schedule 2 and are the most controversial medicines in the treatment of pain disorders. Though not specifically anti-inflammatory, opiates can be used to treat inflammatory pain merely because of their analgesic properties. For years they were thought ineffectual in treating NpP, until quality studies revealed otherwise. They work primarily at the μ receptor (of which there is an assortment), though it appears that certain agents may be more efficacious at certain μ class receptors. The fact that different people have different numbers of various μ receptors leads us to understand why some patients respond better to certain opiates. Approximately 30% of Caucasians cannot metabolize codeine, which renders it useless as an analgesic for them, but causes many physicians to glance warily at the patient who makes such a claim. We can only dream for a rapid, inexpensive pharmacogenetic screen to assist in such a scenario.

Not inappropriately, the opiates are used with great caution by many providers. However, that caution may be driven more by fear of legal recrimination or by lack of education rather than fear of adverse effect. A majority of patients and providers do not grasp the truths of tolerance, physical dependence, and addiction. Tolerance indicates that some beneficial **or** adverse effect that used to be present at one dose is no longer present at that dose. Physical dependence indicates that withdrawal symptoms will occur if the medicine is abruptly discontinued, whether an opiate or corticosteroid. Addiction indicates that the patients is willing to do harm to himself or to others to obtain more of any substance—opiates, money, alcoholic beverages, or sex.

Space does not allow a full discussion of the utility and the concerns of the opiates. The practitioner is advised to start with the milder agents in the opiate naïve patient, to be on guard for acetaminophen toxicity in the formulated compounds, to always begin an appropriate bowel regimen for the patient as they will almost certainly become constipated, to be extremely careful in the writing of prescriptions and the maintenance of the patient's health records, and to rely on the patient's subjective report regarding the effectiveness of the opiate used. We must trust the patient to be honest with their subjective analysis, but that does not prevent us from careful monitoring with unannounced pill counts and urine toxicology screens. The opiates are available in every conceivable form of administration, and we know that some forms have much greater street value than do others. The transdermal preparations are most beneficial therapeutically when the agent can saturate the adipose tissue beneath the patch, allowing the medicine to be released gradually from that "reservoir." Thus, if the patient has little adipose tissue beneath the patch, absorption may be substantially limited.

Please see Table 2 for a listing of the opiates by FDA schedules.

Patches and Topicals

The sodium channel blocker lidocaine is available in a cream or as a patch and is directed against NpP. The patch can be trimmed to adjust to any particular area and can be worn for up to 18 hours without concern for toxicity. It can be quite beneficial when applied to an arthritic joint or to superficial trigger points. The opiate fentanyl is available in patches of differing doses and is usually worn for 72 hours. Some rapid metabolizers may need to change the patch every 48 to 60 hours. The NSAID diclofenac is now available as a patch. Clonidine is an α_2-selective adrenergic agonist, and apparently has some effect on sympathetically maintained pain and in reducing the effects of opiate withdrawal.

Compounded topical agents can be very effective for both somatic and neuropathic pain. Ketoprofen and other NSAIDs are often used in

Table 2 The Opiates According to FDA Schedules

Schedule 5	Codeine elixir
Schedule 4	Propoxyphene
Schedule 3	Buprenorphine
	Codeine tablets
	Hydrocodone
	Hydrocodeine
Schedule 2	Hydromorphone
	Fentanyl
	Meperidine
	Methadone
	Morphine
	Oxycodone
	Oxymorphone

combination with a neuromodulator such as gabapentin. Nortriptyline may be used alone or in combination with other agents. Ketamine, an NMDA receptor antagonist, is especially helpful against NpP. Generally, side effects are less with topical agents, though dosing ketamine must be done with considerable caution. Gloves should be worn by the person applying the topical. I strongly advise that practitioners use topicals compounded at pharmacies that have demonstrated experience in the process.

Intravenous Agents

Intravenous lidocaine (a sodium channel blocker) at a dose of 3–4 mg / kg given over 30 minutes can be very effective in reducing NpP for as long as 2–3 weeks. We do not understand why the effect can be so long lasting. Intravenous ketamine is often considered as a "last resort" but is extremely effective in reducing somatic or NpP. This drug is often used for conscious sedation in surgical procedures, but with proper dosing can be very effective in palliation.

Steroids

Oral dexamethasone is efficacious in reducing pain from bony metastases or from general NpP. It is assumed that pain control in the latter is due to the anti-inflammatory properties of dexamethasone. The practitioner must use appropriate caution regarding the numerous potential adverse effects of this drug class.

Steroids can be used effectively in reducing the pain from radicular lesions or spinal stenosis. If possible, for treating radicular lesions, transforaminal injections are preferred to injecting a bolus in the epidural space. Different steroid preparations are used for these injections; celestone is often the agent of choice due to the small size of its particulate matter. There are few quality studies demonstrating any clinical superiority for celestone otherwise.

For those elderly with significant radicular or spinal disease, multidisciplinary treatment is recognized to be the most efficacious approach, provided that significant neurological deficits are not present. If surgery must be undertaken, less is best. For example, when dealing with spinal stenosis, the minimally invasive surgical procedure X-stop™ may be just as beneficial to the patient's continued level of activity as would extensive decompression of the spine with subsequent instrument implantation. Several studies show that all age groups, after one year of non-surgical multidisciplinary treatment for radicular disease, have as much benefit as those with prompt surgery (Lavelle 2008). Decisions to use spinal cord stimulators or pumps should be made by physicians who deal with those patients and that technology frequently; this intervention should be avoided unless all other reasonable efforts fail. The risk of infection in both procedures causes concern.

Summary

In my introductory comments, I stated that pain management in the elderly is a serious clinical problem. Numerous studies of our elderly definitively reveal that they do not receive adequate pain management.

I postulate these reasons for poor pain management in our elderly:

1) The elderly believe that pain is to be expected as one ages, so why bother to remark on its presence?

2) Numerous comorbidities in the elderly force the patient to prioritize their complaints when they undergo their brief visit with their doctors, and pain is far down on the list.

3) The elderly have a particularly strong aversion to addiction, due largely to a misunderstanding of true addiction.

4) Health care providers have a particularly strong aversion to addiction, due largely to a misunderstanding of physical dependence, tolerance, and true addiction.

5) Health care providers are poorly trained in pain management.

6) Numerous comorbidities in the elderly force the health care provider to prioritize their time and conversation with the patient, and pain is far down on the list.

7) The health care provider believes that pain is to be expected as one ages, so why bother to inquire about its presence?

Without consideration for age, all humans have a right for reasonable efforts at pain control; physicians have a duty to attempt to assist the individual to manage the pain. The elderly do present medical challenges for us as we make these reasonable efforts, but the challenges can be overcome by a diligent and persistent practitioner. Though medical and technological advances will aid us as the future evolves to the present, this author aspires to think that this brief review may trigger us meanwhile to be the more diligent practitioners.

References

American Geriatrics Society Panel on Persistent Pain in Older Persons. 2002. The management of pain in older persons. *Journal of the American Geriatric Society* 50:1–20.

Deane, G. and Smith, H. 2008. Overview of pain management in older persons. *Clinics in geriatric medicine,* edited by Howard S. Smith, MD, 185–201. Saunders.

Delgado-Guay, M.O. and Bruera, E. Management of pain in the older person with cancer. *Oncology* 22 (1): 56–61. URL: www.cancernetwork.com/display/article/10165/1147001.

Devor, M. and Seltzer, Z. 2002. Pathophysiology of damaged nerves in relation to chronic Pain. *Textbook of pain,* edited by P. D. Wall and R. Melzack, 129–164. Churchill Livingstone.

Garcia-Rodriguez, L. A., Hernadez-Diaz, S. 2001. Relative risk of upper gastrointestinal complications among users of acetaminophen and non-steroidal anti-inflammatory drugs. *Epidemiology* 12 (5): 570–576.

Gutstein, H.B. and Akil, H. 2001. Opioid analgesics. *Goodman & Gilman's: The pharmacological basis of therapeutics,* edited by J. G. Hardman and L. E. Limbird, 569–620. McGraw Hill.

Jayson, M. I. V. 2002. Rheumatoid arthritis. *Textbook of pain,* edited by P. D. Wall and R. Melzack, 505–516. Churchill Livingstone.

Kean, W. F., Rainsford, K. D., and Kean, I. R. I. 2008. Management of chronic musculoskeletal pain in the elderly: Opinions on oral medication use. *Inflammopharmacology* 16: 53–75.

Lavelle, W. F., Lavelle, E. D., and Smith, H. S. 2008. Interventional techniques for back pain. *Clinics in Geriatric Medicine,* edited by Howard S. Smith, MD, 345–368. Saunders.

Levin, J. D. and Reichling, D. G.2002. Peripheral mechanisms of inflammatory pain. *Textbook of pain,* edited by P. D. Wall and R. Melzack, 59–84. Churchill Livingstone.

MacGregor, A. J. 2004. The heritability of pain in humans. *The genetics of pain,* edited by Jeffrey S. Mogil, PhD, 151–170. IASP Press.

Maxwell, C. J., Dalby, D. M., Slater, M. Patten, S. B., et al. 2008. The prevalence and management of current daily pain among older home care clients. *Pain* 138: 208–216.

Moalem, G., Tracey, D. J. 2006. Immune and inflammatory mechanisms in neuropathic pain. *Brain Research Reviews* 51: 240–264.

Pappagallo, M. and Werner, M. 2008. *Chronic pain: A primer for physicians.* Remedica.

Perrot, S., Dickenson, A. H., and Bennett, R. 2008. Fibromyalgia: Harmonizing science with clinical practice considerations. *Pain Practice.* 8(3): 177–189.

Roberts, L. J. and Morrow, J. D. 2002. Analgesic-antipyretic and anti-inflammatory agents and drugs employed in the treatment of gout. *Goodman & Gilman's: The pharmacological basis of therapeutics,* edited by J. G. Hardman and L. E. Limbird, 669–686.

White, F. A., Jung, H., Miller, R. J. 2007. Chemokines and the Pathophysiology of Neuropathic Pain. *Proceedings of the National Academy of Sciences.*104 (51): 20151–20158.

52 Pharmacotherapy Considerations in Geriatric Neurology

Melanie A. Dodd and Jessica Campaign

The Institute of Medicine report, "To err is human," identified drug-related problems as a major safety concern (Kohn, Corrigan, and Donaldson 1999). A cost-of-illness study estimated that morbidity and mortality related to drug-related problems in ambulatory patients cost $177.4 billion per year in the United States (Ernst and Grizzle 2001). Furthermore, elderly patients are at an increased risk for experiencing adverse drug reactions (ADRs). In a sample of 3,170 elderly residents, 10% reported an ADR in the previous year (Chrischilles, Segar, and Wallace 1992). Elderly patients are at an increased risk for ADRs for several reasons. In general, elderly patients use multiple medications, have multiple comorbidities, and have age-related changes in drug pharmacokinetics and pharmacodynamics.

Medication use in the elderly population is greater than in other age segments of the population. In a survey of an ambulatory population in the United States, 81% and 71% of women and men, respectively, 65 years or older had used at least one prescription medication the week prior to the survey (Kaufman et al. 2002). In contrast, only 46% and 29% of women and men, respectively, in the 18 to 44 year old age group had reported using at least one prescription medication. Additionally, 23% and 19% of women and men, respectively, 65 years or older reported using five or more different prescription medications during the last week. In contrast, only 3% and less than 1% of women and men, respectively, in the 18 to 44 years age group, used five or more prescription medications during the last week.

Nursing home resident medication use is even higher than use in noninstitutionalized patients. One study of 1,106 patients in 12 skilled-nursing facilities determined that on average, patients were prescribed 7.2 medications (Beers et al. 1992). An additional study in 12 intermediate-care nursing facilities of over 800 patients determined that on average, patients were prescribed 8.1 medications (Beers et al. 1988). This increase in drug utilization in the elderly makes drug interactions and ADRs more likely.

Pharmacokinetic and Pharmacodynamic Considerations in Older Adults

As the human body ages, changes in physiology may occur which impact drug pharmacokinetics, i.e., absorption, distribution, metabolism, and elimination, all of which may cause ADRs (Guay et al. 2003). Of the four pharmacokinetic parameters, absorption shows the least clinically significant change with aging. However, we do see changes in the gastrointestinal tract such as delayed gastric emptying and decreased intestinal blood flow with age, which may impact drug absorption. These changes may also occur in younger adults, related to chronic disease states such as diabetes and congestive heart failure. Hepatic blood flow decreases with age and is also correlated with decreased cardiac output. As a result of this decreased hepatic blood flow, medications with high hepatic extraction will have increased systemic bioavailability. Examples of medications that have high hepatic extraction include propranolol and lidocaine. In addition, the pH of the stomach may increase with age or as a result of use of acid-reducing medications such as antacids, histamine-2 receptor antagonists, and proton pump inhibitors. This change in pH may impact the absorption of acid-dependent medications such as ketoconazole and iron. Potential drug-drug interactions can also affect absorption. Concomitant administration of drugs that bind to each other, such as fluoroquinolones and divalent cations, e.g. calcium and iron, will prevent absorption of the medications. Therefore, it is recommended that they be given at least two hours apart.

Volume of distribution (Vd) describes the relationship between the serum drug concentration and the total amount of drug in the body. The percentage of body fat increases and the percentage of lean body mass decreases with increasing age. In addition, total body water decreases, and cardiac output declines with age, all of which may impact drug distribution. As a result of these changes in body composition with age, the Vd of lipophilic medications increases and the Vd of hydrophilic medications decreases. There is a direct relationship between Vd and half-life ($t_{1/2}$) of the drug as well as a direct relationship between the Vd and the clearance (Cl) of the drug as follows:

$$Vd = Cl \times t_{1/2}/0.693$$

Therefore, lipophilic medications like the benzodiazepine, diazepam, may have an increased $t_{1/2}$ in an older adult partially due to the increased Vd.

Another component that influences Vd is protein binding. Albumin binds with acidic drugs while alpha$_1$-acid glycoprotein binds with basic drugs. Older adults may have significant decreases in albumin, especially hospitalized and malnourished patients. Acidic medications that have significant protein binding (>90%) e.g., phenytoin, will have increased free-drug concentrations in individuals that have low serum albumin. Therefore, it is recommended that free drug concentrations be used instead of total drug concentrations when serum drug concentrations are used for monitoring purposes, as total drug concentrations can be misleading.

Drug metabolism occurs via two different types of reactions in the liver, phase I (oxidative reactions) and phase II (conjugative/synthetic reactions). The cytochrome P450 (CYP 450) mono-oxygenase enzymes mediate most phase I reactions. Age tends to decrease phase I metabolism (Guay et al. 2003; Cusack 2004). However, studies are not conclusive as to the exact mechanism. It may be due to changes in the sinusoidal endothelium, which may reduce the availability of oxygen for drug metabolism or it may be due to a reduction in the number of CYP 450 enzymes. In contrast, phase II reactions do not seem to be affected by age. Therefore, it is recommended that medications that are metabolized via phase II reactions be selected over medications metabolized via phase I reactions. For example, when selecting a benzodiazepine, those metabolized via phase II reactions such as lorazepam, oxazepam, or temazepam might be selected for an older adult instead of other options in the therapeutic class.

Changes in renal function that occur with aging such as reduction in renal mass, glomerular filtration rate (GFR), tubular secretion, and renal blood flow will result in decreased elimination of renally excreted medications and/or metabolites. The GFR is estimated to decrease by about 0.5% per year after age 20 years (Guay et al. 2003). This decline in GFR may result in increased toxicity of renally eliminated medications. The GFR has been found to be the most accurate estimate of kidney function. It is difficult and costly to measure GFR directly. Therefore, mathematical equations have been used to estimate creatinine clearance, a surrogate for GFR, using serum creatinine. Serum creatinine (SCr) alone should not be used as an estimation of renal function in older adults as it is an imperfect marker due to the decline in creatinine production due to the reduction in muscle mass. One equation that can be used to estimate creatinine clearance is the Cockcroft-Gault equation, which follows (Cockroft and Gault 1996):

$$CrCl = \frac{(140\text{-age}) \times (\text{total body weight in kg}) (\text{X } 0.85 \text{ for females only})}{72 \times \text{Scr in mg/dL}}$$

Recently, another equation has been developed for estimating kidney function, the Modification of Diet in Renal Disease (MDRD) (Levey et al. 1999). This equation was found to be more accurate for estimation of GFR in patients with chronic kidney disease. In one study, it was found that the specific dosage change for antimicrobials was different for 40% of the patients when using the Cockcroft-Gault versus the MDRD equation to estimate GFR (Hermsen et al. 2009). In another study, it was found that the specific dosage changes for the majority of patients and the majority of medications were not significantly different between the two equations (Stevens et al. 2009). It is currently recommended by the National Kidney Disease Education Program that either the Cockcroft-Gault or MDRD be used for medication dosing modification in patients with reduced renal function (NIH 2009).

Aging may also affect a drug's pharmacodynamics, i.e., the drug response (Guay et al. 2003). Elderly patients may have enhanced or reduced sensitivity to medications. They may also have altered physiologic or homeostatic mechanisms, such as autonomic nervous system dysfunction, reduced cognitive function reserve, and reduced number of receptors. These changes may increase adverse drug reactions (ADRs), such as falls, orthostatic hypotension, delirium, and constipation. It is therefore important to consider prescribing medications that have the least potential for causing ADRs in older adults.

Beers Criteria: Potentially Inappropriate Medications in Older Adults

There are a limited number of controlled studies of medication use in elderly patients. Therefore, it is difficult to use evidence-based medicine to identify medication-related problems. One technique which can be used to guide clinical practice when clinical information is lacking, is the development of consensus criteria. The Beers criteria for potentially inappropriate medication use in nursing home patients were developed by an expert consensus panel and published in 1991 (Beers et al. 1991). The Beers criteria were expanded to include all elderly patients 65 years or older, both nursing home and community-residing elderly, using the same consensus process in 1997 (Beers 1997). The Centers for Medicare & Medicaid Services (CMS) began including the 1997 criteria in nursing home regulations in July 1999.

The Beers criteria were most recently updated in 2003 (Fick et al. 2003). The criteria were developed using the same consensus panel process as the previous criteria. The criteria includes two lists; list one includes 48 medications to avoid in all older adults and list two includes 20 diseases or conditions and medications to be avoided in persons with these conditions. The lists include the concern with the medication and a severity ranking of high or low. An adverse outcome of high severity was given to 66 of the potentially inappropriate medications. Tables 1 and 2 highlight some of the high severity medications that should be avoided in older adults. The Beers criteria with some modifications are now incorporated into quality assurance criteria for several national organizations including the National Committee for Quality Assurance (NCQA) and the CMS.

The Beers criteria have been used by many researchers to determine the extent of inappropriate medication use in elderly populations. One publication reviewed articles which used the 1997 Beers criteria to assess inappropriate medication use in the elderly in the United States (Liu and Christensen 2002). This review found a range of 21.3% of community-dwelling elders to 40% of nursing home elders using at least one inappropriate medication. Using the 2000 National Ambulatory Medical Care Survey and the National Hospital Ambulatory Medical Care Survey, at least one Beers criteria medication was prescribed at 7.8% of elderly patients' ambulatory care visits (Goulding 2004). The number of inappropriate medications used in the elderly continues to be high, more than ten years since the first Beers criteria were published.

A few recent studies have quantified the extent of injuries related to the Beers criteria and other medications in the elderly. One study evaluated the number of drug-related problems (DRP) in older adults with at least one prescription for a Beers criteria medication versus those without any Beers criteria medications (Fick et al. 2008). It was found that 14.3% of those taking Beers criteria medications had a DRP compared with 4.7% in the non-Beers criteria group. In another study, it was found that of 177,504 emergency department visits for adverse drug events in older adults, 3.6% of those visits were related to Beers criteria medications (Budnitz et al. 2007). In addition, 33.3% of the visits were related to adverse events from three other medications: warfarin, insulin, and digoxin.

Anticholinergic Medications

A number of medications are included in the Beers criteria that have anticholinergic properties. These include antihistamines such as diphenhydramine, and an agent for urinary incontinence, immediate release oxybutynin. The blockage of the muscarinic receptors results in dry mouth, tachycardia, sweating, confusion, and urinary retention. Orthostatic hypotension, sedation, and blurring of vision are also associated with anticholinergic medications. These agents may additionally be associated with delirium symptoms and falls. In order to minimize these complications, it is suggested that agents with less anticholinergic activity be used. For treatment of allergy symptoms, medications such as nonsedating antihistamines or non-oral routes of administration could be considered. For treatment of urinary urge incontinence, nonpharmacologic methods such as scheduled toileting should be considered first. If a pharmacologic treatment is desired, a long-acting oral or transdermal formulation of oxybutynin may cause less dry mouth than immediate release oxybutynin (Anderson et al. 1999; Davila, Daugherty, and Sanders 2001).

The tricyclic antidepressants (TCAs) are used for treatment of depression and neuropathic pain. The TCAs are similar in efficacy for depression; however, they differ in their side effect profiles. The TCAs act at the noradrenergic and serotonergic receptors as well as several other

Table 1 Partial List of Potentially Inappropriate Medication Use in Older Adults: Independent of Diagnosis or Condition

Drug	Concern	Severity Rating
Analgesics:		
Meperidine (Demerol)	May cause confusion	High
Indomethacin (Indocin or Indocin-SR)	More CNS side effects than other NSAIDs	High
Ketorolac (Toradol)	Avoid immediate and long-term use-potential to produce GI bleeds	High
Longer half-life non-COX selective NSAIDs: naproxen (Naprosyn), oxaprozin (Daypro), piroxicam (Feldene)	Avoid long-term use of full dosage-potential to produce GI bleeds, renal failure, and high blood pressure	High
Propoxyphene	Offers few analgesic advantages over acetaminophen, yet has the adverse effects of other narcotic drugs	Low
Psychoactive Medications		
Long acting benzodiazepines: chlordiazepoxide (Librium), diazepam (Valium), chlorazepate (Tranxene)	Prolonged sedation and increased fall risk	High
Amitriptyline (Elavil), doxepin (Sinequan)	Strong anticholinergic and sedation properties	High
Daily fluoxetine (Prozac)	Long half-life, risk of producing CNS stimulation	High
Cardiac Medications		
Clonidine	Potential for orthostatic hypotension and CNS adverse effects.	Low
Doxazosin	Potential for hypotension, dry mouth, and urinary problems	Low
Ticlopidine (Ticlid)	No better than aspirin in preventing clotting and potentially more toxic	High

Adapted from Fick et al. 2003

receptors, which results in a number of adverse events. When considering use of TCAs in the elderly population, several issues should be considered as addressed in the Beers criteria. The side effect profile of the TCA class is of most concern when treating the elderly. Amitriptyline and doxepin have been determined to be rarely the antidepressant of choice due to their strong anticholinergic activity and sedating properties (Fick et al. 2003). Additionally, TCAs are not the drug of choice in patients with benign prostatic hypertrophy since they may impair micturation and cause obstruction. Also, use of TCAs in patients with arrhythmias should be considered with caution as they may induce arrhythmias. An additional concern is that TCAs will worsen constipation. Secondary amine agents such as desipramine and nortriptyline are a better choice due to their improved side effect profile including decreased anticholinergic activities, orthostatic hypotension, and sedation.

Elderly users of TCAs have been shown to have increased rates of falls. Postural hypotension and confusion from TCAs may lead to falls, which may result in serious complications. A population-based case–control study of hip fractures in persons ages 65 years or older identified 4,501 persons with a first hospitalization diagnosis of fracture of the proximal femur as well as 24,041 controls (Ray, Griffin, and

Malcolm 1991). After review of these patients' prescription records and controlling for several potential confounders, it was determined that current users of cyclic antidepressants had a 60% increased risk for hip fractures.

Two recent studies have compared the risk of hip fractures in elderly patients receiving TCAs versus selective serotonin–reuptake inhibitors (SSRIs) (Liu et al. 1998; Thapa et al. 1998). Liu and colleagues performed a case-control study of patients 66 years or older with a discharge diagnosis from an acute-care hospital of a hip fracture. The exposure to antidepressants before their hospitalization was examined. The antidepressants reviewed were divided into three classes, SSRIs, secondary-amine TCAs (nortriptyline, protriptyline, and desipramine), and tertiary-amine TCAs (amitriptyline, clomipramine, doxepin, imipramine, and trimipramine). The odds ratios for hip fractures associated with current use of antidepressants were significantly greater than one for all three classes. No significant difference in the risk of hip fracture was found between users of secondary-amine TCAs and SSRIs. Thapa and colleagues performed a retrospective cohort study of nursing home patients who were new users of TCAs, SSRIs, or trazodone, or nonusers of antidepressants (Thapa et al. 1998). The number of falls was determined during therapy and during a similar time-period for nonusers.

Table 2 Partial List of Potentially Inappropriate Medications in Older Adults: Considering Diagnoses or Conditions

Disease or Condition	Drug	Concern	Severity Risk
Heart failure	Disopyramide (Norpace)	Exacerbation of heart failure	High
Hypertension	Pseudoephedrine (Sudafed)	May produce elevation of blood pressure	High
Gastric or duodenal ulcers	NSAIDs and aspirin (>325 mg)	May exacerbate existing ulcers	High
Depression	Long-term benzodiazepine use	May produce or exacerbate depression	High
Syncope or falls	Short- to intermediate-acting benzodiazepines and tricyclic antidepressants	May produce ataxia, syncope, and additional falls	High

Adapted from Fick et al. 2003

The rate ratios for falls were calculated. A higher rate of falls was found for users versus nonusers even when adjusting for potential confounding factors. The rate of falls was highest for users of TCAs, but new users of SSRIs had a rate of falls that was 80% higher than the nonusers. This study suggests that the rate of falls is increased by TCAs or SSRIs.

When considering use of TCAs in the elderly population, altered pharmacokinetics need to be addressed. The TCAs are primarily hepatically metabolized, but the metabolites are renally excreted. The hydroxy metabolites are potentially cardiotoxic to the elderly with elevated plasma levels. Also of concern is the possibility of toxic TCA overdoses in suicidal patients. Therefore, elderly patients should be started on low doses of TCAs and slowly titrated upwards.

The TCAs are effective antidepressants in the elderly. However, many potential safety issues need to be considered. Adverse drug reactions including anticholinergic effects, orthostatic hypotension, and an increased risk for falls are of primary concern. Additionally, lower doses of TCAs need to be used in the elderly due to pharmacokinetic changes. If a TCA is being prescribed, secondary amine agents such as desipramine and nortriptyline should be considered first. However, caution should be utilized with all TCAs.

Analgesic Medications

As health care providers, we have reached a quandary regarding how we use nonsteroidal anti-inflammatory drugs, especially in older adults. The U.S. Food and Drug Administration (FDA) and the media have alerted the public to several potential safety issues regarding the use of the traditional nonsteroidal anti-inflammatory drugs (NSAIDs), e.g., naproxen, and cyclooxygenase-2 selective nonsteroidal anti-inflammatory inhibitors (COX-2 inhibitors), e.g., celecoxib and rofecoxib. The NSAIDs are known to increase the risk of gastrointestinal bleeds and renal impairment. Most recently, several COX-2 inhibitors have been removed from the U.S. market, including rofecoxib and valdecoxib due to increased cardiovascular (CV) toxicity. In April 2005, Pfizer, Inc. was asked by the FDA to voluntarily remove valdecoxib (Bextra®) from the U.S. market due to the risk of rare, but sometimes fatal skin reactions such as Stevens-Johnson syndrome as well as the increased risk of CV events. Currently, the only remaining COX-2 inhibitor on the U.S. market is celecoxib (Celebrex®).

The enzyme cyclooxygenase consists of two isoforms, COX-1 and COX-2. The COX enzymes are responsible for catalyzing the formation of prostaglandins, prostacyclins and thromboxane in the arachidonic acid pathway. The COX-1 enzyme is a constitutive enzyme that is found in most tissues. It is responsible for maintaining the gastric mucosal barrier, maintenance of renal perfusion, and is involved in thrombogenesis through promotion of platelet aggregation. The COX-2 enzyme is an inducible enzyme that is primarily found at inflammation sites. The nonselective NSAIDs inhibit both COX-1 and COX-2. Due to the inhibition of COX-1 and in turn the decreased production of the mucoprotective prostaglandins in the gastrointestinal (GI) tract by the NSAIDs, these agents increase the risk of GI bleeding. As a result of this risk and the discovery of the two isoforms of COX, the COX-2 selective inhibitors were developed. A hypothesis was developed that the COX-2 inhibitors would have the benefit of the traditional NSAIDs through selective inhibition of COX-2, without the increased GI bleeding caused by inhibiting COX-1. This hypothesis has been validated through several large trials. In clinical practice the COX-2 inhibitors have usually been used in patients at high risk for GI bleeding such as patients who use anticoagulants or chronic oral corticosteroids or who have a history of GI bleeding.

Some of the first concerns about CV risks with NSAIDs and COX-2 inhibitors originated with the VIGOR trial (Bombardier et al. 2000).

This trial compared rofecoxib 50 mg daily with naproxen twice daily in patients with rheumatoid arthritis for a median follow-up of nine months. The authors found a 0.1 percent and a 0.4 percent incidence, respectively, of acute myocardial infarction (AMI) in the naproxen and rofecoxib treatment groups (relative risk (RR) = 0.2, 95% confidence interval (CI), 0.1–0.7).

Celecoxib has also been associated with CV risk. The Adenoma Prevention with Celecoxib (APC) study compared two doses of celecoxib, 200 mg twice daily and 400 mg twice daily, with placebo in patients with a history of colorectal neoplasia to evaluate the efficacy of prevention of adenomatous polyps over approximately 3 years (Solomon et al. 2005). This study saw a dose-related increase in the incidence of CV death. The CV composite end point of death was 1.0% in the placebo group, 2.3% in the 200 mg group (HR=2.3, 95% CI, 0.9–5.5), and 3.4% in the 400 mg group (HR=3.4, 95% CI, 1.4–7.8). Due to these observations and other similar trends the study was discontinued early. In contrast, however, a similar trial, the Prevention of Spontaneous Adenomatous Polyps (PreSAP), did not replicate these results, with a HR of 1.1 for celecoxib 400 mg twice daily compared with placebo (U.S. FDA 2009).

Naproxen, a non-selective NSAID, may also increase the risk of CV and cerebrovascular events. The Alzheimer's Disease Anti-inflammatory Prevention Trial (ADAPT) was an Alzheimer's prevention trial comparing naproxen 220 mg twice a day, celecoxib, or placebo for up to three years (ADAPT Research Group 2006). The study was halted early due to preliminary data released from the study that suggested an increase in CV and cerebrovascular events in the naproxen group as well as the CV event data on celecoxib released from the APC study. A 3-year case-control study reviewed the incidence of first time hospitalization for AMI in NSAID and COX-2 inhibitor users and non-NSAID users in three counties in Denmark (Johnsen 2005). This study found that current users of rofecoxib had an increased risk of hospitalization for MI compared with nonusers of any category of nonaspirin NSAIDs (adjusted relative risk (ARR)=1.80, 95% CI, 1.47–2.21). A trend for increased risk of hospitalization for AMI was also seen in current users of celecoxib (ARR=1.25, 95% CI, 0.97–1.62), etodolac, meloxicam, and nabumetone (ARR=1.45, 95% CI, 1.09–1.93), naproxen (ARR=1.50, 95% CI 0.99–2.29), and other conventional nonaspirin NSAIDs (ARR=1.68, 95% CI, 1.52–1.85).

The FDA concluded that there is an increased risk of serious adverse CV events associated with the COX-2 selective NSAIDs, celecoxib, rofecoxib, and valdecoxib, compared with placebo (FDA Public Health Advisory 2009). They also concluded that the COX-2 selective NSAIDs do not have a greater risk of CV events than non-selective NSAIDs, based on long-term trials comparing COX-2 inhibitors with nonselective NSAIDs. Long-term placebo-controlled clinical trial data are not available to assess the CV risk of non-selective NSAIDs. With the exception of valdecoxib after CABG surgery, NSAIDs do not appear to increase the incidence of CV events when used short-term. The U.S. FDA concludes that the approved COX-2 inhibitors do reduce the incidence of GI ulcers compared with certain non-selective NSAIDs. However, they believe that the overall benefit is uncertain for reducing the risk of serious GI bleeding with COX-2 inhibitors. The benefit of other techniques for reducing GI bleeding with chronic NSAID use, such as concomitant proton pump inhibitors, remains uncertain as well according to the U.S. FDA. As a result of this data, the U.S. FDA has asked manufacturers of all prescription NSAIDs, including the COX-2 inhibitor celecoxib, to add a black box warning to the product labeling that highlights the potential for increased CV risk and serious, life-threatening bleeding associated with their use. The manufacturers of nonprescription NSAIDs have also been asked to revise their product labeling to include more specific information about the potential for CV and GI risks. In addition, the American Heart Association/American College of Cardiology 2007 ST elevation myocardial infarction (STEMI) and unstable angina/non-STEMI guidelines have recommended that NSAIDs with increasing degrees of COX2 selectivity not be used for management of musculoskeletal discomfort when acetaminophen, low dose opiates, nonacetylated salicylates, or nonselective NSAIDs provide adequate comfort (Antman et al. 2008; Fraker and Fihn 2007).

As health care providers and patients we are faced with a quandary regarding how to use the NSAIDs in treatment as we assess the risks and benefits. Until we have further long-term clinical data regarding the CV risks of the NSAIDs, it is important to carefully assess the risks and benefits of using a NSAID in every patient. Some questions that should be considered when assessing a patient include the following:

1) Does the patient need an anti-inflammatory or is acetaminophen or physical therapy or another nonpharmacologic approach more appropriate?

2) What are the patient's risks of GI bleeding, including prior history of GI bleeding, chronic oral corticosteroid or anticoagulation use?

3) What are the patient's CV risks? Can their CV risk be reduced by addressing issues such as smoking status or hyperlipidemia?

Overall, it is difficult to manage chronic pain in older adults as they may experience adverse reactions secondary to multiple pain medications. In addition to risks from the NSAIDs discussed above, older adults may also be at risk for sedation, fall, and fractures when using opiates. One meta-analysis showed a relative risk for fractures for patients using opiates of 1.38 (95% CI, 1.15–1.66) (Takkouche et al. 2007) The American Geriatric Society has recently updated their guidelines for management of persistent pain in older adults (AGS Panel on Persistent Pain in Older Persons 2009). The guidelines primarily address pharmacologic management of pain. It is suggested that the reader refer to these guidelines for suggestions for pain management in the older adult.

Anticonvulsant Medications

Anticonvulsant medications are frequently used in the elderly population. This is due in part to the increasing incidence of epilepsy with advancing age; one study in community-dwelling elderly reported an incidence of 25.8 cases per 100,000 person-years in those aged 60–74 and 101.1 cases per 100,000 person-years in those aged 75–89, versus 10.6 cases per 100,000 person-years in those aged 45–59 (Hussain et al. 2006). The incidence of epilepsy is even higher in patients who reside in nursing homes (Leppik 2007). Besides seizure disorders, some anticonvulsant medications are utilized to treat other conditions, including neuropathic pain and some psychiatric and mood disorders. In one survey of medication use in six nursing homes, 3.9% to 22% of residents over 65 years of age used at least one anticonvulsant medication (Cloyd, Lackner, and Leppik 1994). Pugh et al. found that the most commonly prescribed anticonvulsant medications in geriatric patients newly diagnosed with epilepsy in the Veteran Health Administration from 2000–2004 were: phenytoin (67%), gabapentin (11%), carbamazepine (8.5%), valproate (5.6%), phenobarbital (2.5%), levetiracetam (2.3%), lamotrigine (1.6%), topiramate (1%), and oxcarbazepine (0.6%) (n=9628) (Pugh et al. 2008). Many of these anticonvulsants, especially the older drugs (phenytoin, carbamazepine, valproate, and phenobarbital) can be associated with significant side effects and multiple drug interactions. Anticonvulsant side effects and interactions are of an even greater concern in the elderly population, due to presence of concomitant disease states, prevalence of

polypharmacy, and age-related changes in absorption, distribution, metabolism, and elimination of drugs. Therefore, it is important to be aware of the characteristics of these drugs and to closely monitor those patients who use them.

Side Effects

Cognitive and central nervous system (CNS) side effects are frequently associated with many of the anticonvulsants. Common symptoms include: somnolence, dizziness, lethargy, drowsiness, confusion/disorientation, decreased memory, decreased concentration, and cognitive slowing (Arif et al. 2009; Camfield and Camfield 2006). The elderly may be more sensitive to these effects than younger adults (Cloyd, Lackner, and Leppik 1994; Bergey 2004). These adverse effects can be compounded by concomitant use of other medications with CNS side effects, such as psychotropic medications and benzodiazepines.

Selection of anticonvulsant therapy depends on many factors, including efficacy and tolerability. Many of the newer anticonvulsants are associated with fewer side effects than the older drugs. Phenobarbital is associated with a large burden of side effects, and usually is not considered to be the most appropriate anticonvulsant in the elderly (Pugh et al. 2004; Smith et al. 1987). Consensus guidelines recommend against using phenytoin or phenobarbital as first-line agents for epilepsy, due in part to their unacceptable side effect profiles (Karceski, Morrell, and Carpenter 2001). In a study of over 1,100 patients, phenytoin and topiramate were associated with more cognitive side effects than gabapentin, carbamazepine, valproate, levetiracetam, or lamotrigine (Arif et al. 2009). A randomized, blinded study comparing gabapentin, lamotrigine, and carbamazepine for new-onset epilepsy in elderly patients demonstrated that patients taking lamotrigine or gabapentin experienced fewer adverse effects than those taking carbamazepine (Rowan et al. 2005). Whether frequent or infrequent, adverse effects can result from the use of any anticonvulsant medication, whether old or new. These effects may be significant and may lead to drug discontinuation in some patients. Side effects associated with selected anticonvulsant medications are presented in Table 3.

Monitoring

It is important to monitor elderly patients who use anticonvulsants, not only because these medications have a high propensity to cause adverse effects, but also because there is a great degree of variability in kinetic parameters of these agents in the elderly. As previously discussed, there are a number of age-related changes in the absorption, distribution, metabolism, and elimination of drugs in the elderly as compared to younger adults. Effects of anticonvulsants may not be predictable due to these variations, so it is important to monitor for efficacy and serum drug concentrations (for those drugs with established reference ranges) in addition to the appearance of side effects. This monitoring will enable the practitioner to tailor drug therapy to the individual to optimize quality of life and avoid toxicity.

Anticonvulsant medications exert their effects in the body in a concentration-dependent manner. Serum drug levels should be monitored in patients taking drugs with established reference ranges. Drug concentration monitoring is useful to determine if levels are subtherapeutic, therapeutic, or toxic, and to correlate levels with efficacy or toxicity in a given patient. In general, appropriate times to check serum drug concentration are: after treatment initiation, after change in dosage, after addition of concomitant medications that alter anticonvulsant distribution or metabolism, after treatment failure, and when there are signs of toxicity (Johannessen and Tomson 2006). Elderly patients are at risk for unpredictable variation in drug concentrations, due to alterations in body composition, low serum albumin, and

Table 3 Side Effects of Selected Anticonvulsants

Anticonvulsant	Side Effects
Phenytoin	CNS effects (sedation, drowsiness, lethargy, blurred vision, confusion, cognitive impairment, ataxia) Gastrointestinal discomfort Osteoporosis Rash (SJS/TEN rare)
Gabapentin	CNS effects (dizziness, nystagmus, ataxia) Pedal edema Weight gain
Carbamazepine	CNS effects (dizziness, drowsiness, diplopia, headache) Gastrointestinal discomfort Hyponatremia Osteoporosis Rash (SJS/TEN rare)
Valproate	CNS effects (sedation) Gastrointestinal discomfort Fine hand tremor Osteoporosis
Phenobarbital	CNS effects (sedation, drowsiness, fatigue, cognitive impairment, ataxia, depression) Behavior/mood changes Osteoporosis Rash (SJS/TEN rare)
Levetiracetam	CNS effects (sedation, fatigue, agitation)
Lamotrigine	CNS effects (sedation, dizziness, diplopia, headache) Gastrointestinal discomfort Rash—dose-related (SJS/TEN rare)
Topiramate	CNS effects (dizziness, confusion, abnormal thinking, impaired concentration, memory problems) Nephrolithiasis
Oxcarbazepine	CNS effects (sedation, dizziness, headache, ataxia) Gastrointestinal discomfort Hyponatremia Rash (SJS/TEN rare)

CNS= central nervous system; SJS/TEN = Stevens-Johnson syndrome/toxic epidermal necrolysis

Asconape 2002; Bergey 2004; Lacy et al. 2004; Ramsay, Rowan and Pryor 2004; Rowan et al. 2005; .

reduced hepatic and renal function (Cloyd 1997). Due to this variability, elderly patients may need lower doses and/or longer dosing intervals than younger adults.

Total blood concentration is not always the most appropriate level to monitor because it is only the "free fraction" or unbound drug in the serum that is active. For those anticonvulsants that are highly protein-bound (phenytoin, carbamazepine, and valproate), unbound fraction of drug can vary drastically in patients with low albumin, as is the case in many elderly patients (Willmore 1997). Elderly patients who use these drugs will have higher free concentrations than younger adults who take the same dose, even if their total serum concentrations are equal. Also, highly protein-bound drugs given in combination can displace each other from plasma proteins, causing a further increase in the free fraction of each. This necessitates close monitoring of unbound drug levels for highly protein-bound anticonvulsants in the elderly, because total serum concentrations are not reflective of the true levels of active drug.

An additional issue with phenytoin is its saturable, non-linear metabolism. Phenytoin dose adjustments result in disproportionate changes in serum concentration, where a minute increase in dose can cause a massive increase in concentration (Willmore 1997). These changes are not easily predictable, and there is significant interpatient variability of serum concentration in response to dose (Bauer and Blouin 1982). In addition, concentrations can vary considerably over time in an individual patient, even with no changes in dose (Birnbaum et al. 2003). For these reasons, phenytoin dosing must always be individually tailored and closely monitored, and dose adjustments must be made cautiously and in small increments, to avoid toxicity (Cloyd, Lackner, and Leppik 1994).

Elderly patients may require slower dose titration of anticonvulsants than younger patients (Stephen 2003). In addition, it has been suggested that therapeutic ranges for some of these medications in the elderly may actually be lower than those ranges generally accepted for younger adults (Bauer and Blouin 1982; Stephen 2003). The astute practitioner must recognize that one cannot tailor therapy based on numbers alone, and that the entire clinical situation of the individual patient must be taken into account when making therapeutic decisions. As with any drug monitoring, one should take steps to ensure that the appropriate labs are drawn at the appropriate times. These precautions will help to avoid inappropriate dose changes based on levels.

Many medications have the potential to interact with anticonvulsant drugs. In a series of over 11,000 patients with epilepsy who used anticonvulsants, patients over 65 years of age used a mean of at least six concomitant prescription medications (Gidal et al. 2009). Concomitant use of medications that inhibit metabolism of anticonvulsants increase the risk of anticonvulsant-related side effects and toxicity. Conversely, use of medications that induce metabolism of anticonvulsants lowers the levels of anticonvulsants in the body, increasing the risk for treatment failure. Some anticonvulsants also have the ability to induce changes in drug-metabolizing enzymes themselves, presenting opportunities for toxicity or treatment failure of other drugs. As mentioned previously, highly protein-bound drugs can compete for binding sites on plasma proteins, increasing free fractions of each. For elderly patients who are prescribed multiple medications, it is prudent to be aware of the potential for interactions between the agents. Compared to the older anticonvulsants, many of the newer agents have a much lower potential for drug interactions. Examples of potential drug interactions can be viewed in Table 4.

Multiple opportunities for side effects and drug interactions highlight the importance of monitoring in elderly patients who are prescribed anticonvulsants.

General Prescribing Principles

As you can see, medication use in the elderly is an area that should be carefully monitored. Following are some general principles to consider when prescribing medications to older adults:

- Obtain a complete medication history
  - Include all prescription, over-the-counter, herbal, and alternative medications
  - Include a complete medication allergy and adverse event history
  - Note discontinued medications
  - Encourage patients to maintain a complete list of medications by generic name and bring to all health care appointments
  - Start low, go slow, but go! (consider titrating medications as appropriate)

Table 4 Drug Interaction Potential of Selected Anticonvulsants

Anticonvulsant	Potential for Drug Interactions	Reasons
Phenytoin	High	• Significant hepatic metabolism • Strongly induces multiple hepatic enzymes • High protein binding
Gabapentin	Low	• No hepatic metabolism • No protein binding
Carbamazepine	High	• Strongly induces multiple hepatic enzymes • High protein binding
Valproate	High	• Hepatic metabolism • Inhibits multiple hepatic enzymes • High protein binding
Phenobarbital	High	• Significant hepatic metabolism • Strongly induces multiple hepatic enzymes
Levetiracetam	Low	• Minimal metabolism • No protein binding
Lamotrigine	Moderate	• Hepatic metabolism
Topiramate	Moderate	• Hepatic metabolism • Mildly induces/inhibits some hepatic enzymes
Oxcarbazepine	Moderate	• Induces/inhibits some hepatic enzymes

Adapted in part from Asconape 2002 and Johannessen 2006.

◆ Avoid the prescribing cascade

  ◆ Medication adverse effects should always be included in your differential diagnoses

  ◆ Avoid prescribing a second medication for management of the side effects from the first medication. Consider modifying the first medication.

◆ Avoid starting or stopping more than one medication at a time if possible

  ◆ If a medication adverse effect occurs, it is easier to identify

It is important that health care providers utilize techniques such as the Beers criteria to reduce the number of inappropriate medications that elderly patients receive, which will potentially reduce the number of ADRs. It is also important to carefully assess use of those medications that have specific monitoring requirements. Finally, it is important to consider pharmacokinetic and pharmacodynamic changes that occur with age and adopt general prescribing principles for older adults in order to reduce ADRs.

References

ADAPT Research Group. Cardiovascular and cerebrovascular events in the randomized, controlled Alzheimer's Disease Anti-Inflammatory Prevention Trial (ADAPT). *PLoS Clin Trials* 2006 17;1(7):e33.

AGS Panel on Persistent Pain in Older Persons. Pharmacological management of persistent pain in older persons. American Geriatrics Society. *J Am Geriatr Soc* 2009;57(8): 1331–1346.

Anderson RU, Mobley D, Blank B, et al. OROS Oxybutynin Study Group. Once daily controlled versus immediate release oxybutynin chloride for urge urinary incontinence. *J Urol* 1999;161(6):1809–12.

Antman EM, Hand M, Armstrong PW, et al. 2007 focused update of the ACC/AHA 2004 guidelines for the management of patients with ST-elevation myocardial infarction: A report of the American College of Cardiology/American Heart Association Task Force on Practice Guidelines (Writing Group to Review New Evidence and Update the ACC/AHA 2004 guidelines for the management of patients with ST-elevation myocardial infarction). *Circulation* 2008;117: 296–329.

Arif H, Buchsbaum R, Weintraub D, et al. Patient-reported cognitive side effects of antiepileptic drugs: Predictors and comparison of all commonly used antiepileptic drugs. *Epilep Behav* 2009;14:202–9.

Asconape JJ. Some common issues in the use of antiepileptic drugs. *Semin Neurol* 2002;22(1):27–39.

Bauer LA and Blouin RA. Age and phenytoin kinetics in adult epileptics. *Clin Pharmacol Ther* 1982;31:301–4.

Beers MH. Explicit criteria for determining potentially inappropriate medication use by the elderly. *Arch Intern Med* 1997;157:1531–36.

Beers M, Avorn J, Somerai SB, et al. Psychoactive medication use in intermediate-care facility residents. *JAMA* 1988;260:3016–20.

Beers MH, Ouslander JG, Rollingher I, et al. Explicit criteria for determining inappropriate medication use in nursing home residents. UCLA Division of Geriatric Medicine. *Arch Intern Med* 1991;151(9):1825–32.

Beers MH, Ouslander JG, Fingold SF, et al. Inappropriate medication prescribing in skilled-nursing facilities. *Ann Intern Med* 1992;117:684–9.

Bergey GK. Initial treatment of epilepsy: Special issues in treating the elderly. *Neurology* 2004;63(Suppl 4):S40–8.

Birnbaum A, Hardie NA, Leppik IE, et al. Variability of total phenytoin serum concentrations within elderly nursing home residents. *Neurology* 2003;60:555–9.

Bombardier C, Laine L, Reicin A, et al. Comparison of upper gastrointestinal toxicity of rofecoxib and naproxen in patients with rheumatoid arthritis. *N Engl J Med* 2000;343:1520–8.

Budnitz DS, Shebab N, Kegler SR, and Richards CL. Medication use leading to emergency department visits for adverse drug events in older adults. *Ann Intern Med* 2007;147:755–765.

Camfield P and Camfield C. Monitoring for adverse effects of antiepileptic drugs. *Epilepsia* 2006;47(Suppl 1):31–4.

Chrischilles EA, Segar ET, and Wallace RB. Self-reported adverse drug reactions and related resource use: A study of community-dwelling persons 65 years of age and older. *Ann Intern Med* 1992;117: 634–40.

Cockroft DW and Gault MH. Prediction of creatinine clearance from serum creatinine. *Nephron* 1976;16:31-41.

Cloyd J. Commonly used antiepileptic drugs: Age-related pharmacokinetics. In: Rowan AJ, Ramsay RE, eds. *Seizures and epilepsy in the elderly.* Boston: Butterworth-Heinemann. 1997: 219–28.

Cloyd JC, Lackner TE, and Leppik IE. Antiepileptics in the elderly. Pharmacoepidemiology and pharmacokinetics. *Arch Fam Med* 1994;3:589–98.

Cusack BJ. Pharmacokinetics in older persons. *Am J Geriatr Pharmacother* 2004;2:274–302.

Davila GW, Daugherty CA, and Sanders SW; Transdermal Oxybutynin Study Group. A short-term, multicenter, randomized double-blind dose titration study of the efficacy and anticholinergic side effects of transdermal compared to immediate release oral oxybutynin treatment of patients with urge urinary incontinence. *J Urol* 2001; 166(1):140–5.

Ernst FR and Grizzle AJ. Drug-related morbidity and mortality: Updating the cost-of-illness model. *J Am Pharm Assoc* 2001;41:192–9.

FDA Public Health Advisory—FDA announces important changes and additional warnings for COX-2 selective and non-selective non-steroidal anti-inflammatory drugs (NSAIDs). Available at: http://www.fda.gov/Drugs/DrugSafety/PostmarketDrugSafetyInformationforPatientsandProviders/ucm150314.htm. Accessed on September 7, 2009.

Fick DM, Cooper JW, Wade WE, et al. Updating the Beers criteria for potentially inappropriate medication use in older adults: Results of a US consensus panel of experts. *Arch Intern Med* 2003;163(22):2716–24.

Fick DM, Mion LC, Beers MH, and Waller JL. Health outcomes associated with potentially inappropriate medication use in older adults. *Res Nurs Health* 2008;31(1):42–51.

Fraker TD Jr and Fihn SD, writing on behalf of the 2002 Chronic Stable Angina Writing Committee. 2007 chronic angina focused update of the ACC/AHA 2002 guidelines for the management of patients with chronic stable angina: A report of the American College of Cardiology/American Heart Association Task Force on Practice Guidelines Writing Group to Develop the Focused Update of the 2002 guidelines for the management of patients with chronic stable angina. *Circulation* 2007;116:2762–2772.

Gidal BE, French JA, Grossman P, et al. Assessment of potential drug interactions in patients with epilepsy: Impact of age and sex. *Neurology* 2009;72:419–25.

Guay DRP, Artz MB, Hanlon JT, and Schmader K. The pharmacology of aging. In: Tallis RC, Fillit HM, editors: *Brocklehurst's textbook of geriatric medicine and gerontology, 6th edition.* Churchill Livingstone, Spain, 2003;155-61.

Goulding MR. Inappropriate medication prescribing for elderly ambulatory care patients. *Arch Intern Med* 2004;164:305-12.

Hermsen ED, Maiefski M, Florsecu MC, et al. Comparison of the modification of diet in renal disease and cockcroft-gault equations for dosing antimicrobials. *Pharmacotherapy* 2009;29(6):649–655.

Hussain SA, Haut SR, Lipton RB, et al. Incidence of epilepsy in a racially diverse, community-dwelling, elderly cohort: Results from the Einstein aging study. *Epilep Res* 2006;71:195–205.

Johannessen SI and Tomson T. Pharmacokinetic variability of newer antiepileptic drugs: When is monitoring needed? *Clin Pharmacokinet* 2006;45(11):1061–75.

Johnsen SP, Larsson H, Tarone RE, et al. Risk of hospitalization for myocardial infarction among users of rofecoxib, celecoxib, and other NSAIDs: A population-based case-control study. *Arch Intern Med* 2005;165:978–84.

Karceski S, Morrell M, and Carpenter D. The expert consensus guideline series: Treatment of epilepsy. *Epilepsy Behav* 2001;2(6):A1–50.

Kaufman DW, Kelly JP, Rosenberg L, et al. Recent patterns of medication use in the ambulatory adult population of the United States. *JAMA* 2002;287:337–44.

Kohn L, Corrigan J, and Donaldson M. Committee on Quality of Health Care in America, Institute of Medicine. *To err is human: Building a safer health system.* Washington, DC, National Academy of Sciences, 1999.

Lacy CF, Armstrong LL, Goldman MP, et al, eds. *Drug information handbook* (12th Ed). Hudson, Ohio: Lexi-Comp. 2004.

Leppik IE. Epilepsy in the elderly: Scope of the problem. *Int Rev Neurobiol* 2007;81:1–14.

Levey AS, Bosch JP, Lewis JB, et al, for the Modification of Diet in Renal Disease Study Group. A more accurate method to estimate glomerular filtration rate from serum creatinine: A new prediction equation. *Ann Intern Med* 1999;130:461–70.

Liu B, Anderson G, Mittmann N, et al. Use of selective serotonin–reuptake inhibitors or tricyclic antidepressants and risk of hip fractures in elderly people. *Lancet* 1998;351:1303–7.

Liu GG and Christensen DB. The continuing challenge of inappropriate prescribing in the elderly: An update of the evidence. *J Am Pharm Assoc* 2002;42:847–57.

National Institutes of Health, National Kidney Disease Education Program. *CKD and drug dosing: Information for providers. Estimation of kidney function for prescription medication dosage in adults. 2009.* Available from: http://www.nkdep.nih.gov/professionals/drug-dosing-information.htm. Accessed September 7, 2009.

Pugh MJV, Cramer J, Knoefel J, et al. Potentially inappropriate antiepileptic drugs for elderly patients with epilepsy. *J Am Geriatr Soc* 2004;52:417–22.

Pugh MJV, Van Cott AC, Cramer JA, et al. Trends in antiepileptic drug prescribing for older patients with new-onset epilepsy: 2000–2004. *Neurology* 2008;70(Part 2):2171–8.

Ramsay RE, eds. *Seizures and epilepsy in the elderly.* Boston: Butterworth-Heinemann. 1997:229–37.

Ramsay RE, Rowan AJ, and Pryor FM. Special considerations in the treatment of elderly patients with epilepsy. *Neurology* 2004;62 (Suppl 2):S24–9.

Ray WA, Griffin MR, and Malcolm E. Cyclic antidepressants and the risk of hip fracture. *Arch Intern Med* 1991;151:754–6.

Rowan AJ, Ramsay RE, Collins JF, et al. New onset geriatric epilepsy. A randomized study of gabapentin, lamotrigine, and carbamazepine. *Neurology* 2005;64:1868–73.

Smith DB, Mattson RH, Cramer JA, et al. Results of a nationwide Veterans Administration cooperative study comparing the efficacy and toxicity of carbamazepine, phenobarbital, phenytoin, and primidone. *Epilepsia* 1987;28(suppl 3):S50–8.

Solomon SD, McMurray JJV, Pfeffer MA, et al. Cardiovascular risk associated with celecoxib in a clinical trial for colorectal adenoma prevention. *N Engl J Med* 2005;352:1071–80.

Stephen LJ. Drug treatment of epilepsy in elderly people. *Drugs Aging* 2003;20(2):141–52.

Stevens LA, Nolin T, Richardson M, et al. Comparison of drug dosing recommendations based on measured GFR and kidney function estimating equations. *Am J Kid Dis* 2009;54(1):33–42.

Takkouche B, Montes-Martinez A, Gill SS, et al. Psychotropic medications and the risk of fracture: A meta-analysis. *Drug Safety* 2007;30 (2):171–184.

Thapa PB, Gideon P, Cost TW, et al. Antidepressants and the risk of falls among nursing home residents. *N Engl J Med* 1998;339:875–82.

Unpublished data presented to the U.S. FDA at the February 16–18, 2005 FDA meeting of the Arthritis Advisory Committee and the Drug Safety and Risk Management Advisory Committee. Available at http://www.fda.gov/ohrms/dockets/ac/cder05.html#ArthritisDrugs. Accessed on September 7, 2009.

Willmore LJ. Commonly used antiepileptic drugs: age-related efficacy. In: Rowan AJ, Ramsay RE, eds. *Seizures and epilepsy in the elderly.* Boston: Butterworth-Heinemann. 1997:229–37.

53 Cognitive Enhancement in the Elderly
David Q. Beversdorf

As our population ages, there is increasing interest in discovering ways to enhance cognition in the setting of aging or at least delaying the onset of any cognitive decline. Agents utilized to affect cognition in a clinical setting, such as the anticholinergics typically used in Alzheimer's disease and stimulants used in attention deficit disorder, are not the primary agents of choice in the healthy aging population, although stimulants are increasingly popular for cognitive enhancement among younger individuals. Their cost as well as their availability being limited through prescription serves to limit their use, as well as the consideration that they may not have a preventative role. However, a number of other strategies are being explored for cognitive enhancement and prevention of cognitive decline. We will review these strategies, the evidence behind them, and other agents that may soon enter into the discussion.

Mental Activity

A number of studies have suggested that mental activity plays a protective role against the development of cognitive decline. In a meta-analysis of 22 studies on this topic from 1996 to 2004, presence of higher brain reserve (defined by education, occupation, premorbid intelligence, and mental activities) decreased risk of dementia by 46% in a median follow-up of 7.1 years across 29,000 subjects (Valenzuela and Sachdev 2006). More recently, though, postmortem examination in the Rush Memory and Aging Project demonstrated no protective effect of cognitive activity for the neuropathology of Alzheimer's, despite confirming the previous findings of a reduced clinical incidence of mild cognitive impairment and slower decline in cognitive function (Wilson et al. 2007). This begins to suggest that mental activity serves to delay the onset of cognitive decline by augmenting compensatory strategies rather than affecting pathology itself. In fact, Alzheimer's pathology occurs earliest in the brain regions involved in the 'default network,' the regions with the greatest baseline metabolic activity (Buckner et al. 2005), which could suggest that mental activity may even increase pathology. One recent study suggests that cognitive activity delays the onset of Alzheimer's disease, but once the disease does manifest, it can progress more rapidly (Wilson et al. 2010). This raises the possibility that one potential role of cognitive activity is to enhance compensatory ability to maintain function during the early pathology of Alzheimer's disease. Future work will need to disentangle these competing possibilities of compensatory benefits of mental activity and the putative negative effects of greater metabolic activity. Furthermore, decreased mental activities in midlife may be a reflection of early subclinical effects of cognitive changes rather than a potentially modifiable risk factor (Friedland et al. 2001). However, the overall decreased risk of cognitive decline associated with mental activity does appear to be a consistent finding. Furthermore, several studies are beginning to suggest that cognitive training does offer some benefit in healthy aging individuals (Acevedo and Lowenstein 2007). Cognitive enrichment early in life appears to be particularly beneficial for delaying later cognitive decline, but the protective effects are more robust for crystallized intelligence rather than fluid intelligence (Milgram et al. 2006). Thus, mental activity could play some role in cognitive enhancement in the elderly.

Physical Activity

As physical activity is another readily modifiable variable, research has examined whether it may also play a role in prevention of cognitive decline. Several studies have demonstrated the potential for such an effect. In the Honolulu-Asia Aging Study, greater daily distance walked in physically capable aged men was associated with a decreased risk of dementia in subsequent years (Abbott et al. 2004). Similarly, in the Nurses' Health Study, a similar association between greater levels of physical activities as well as walking and decreased cognitive decline was found among older women (Weuve et al. 2004). The Group Health Cooperative in Seattle also found regular exercise to be associated with subsequent decreased dementia risk among older individuals (Larson et al. 2006). However, one cannot determine with certainty based on this evidence whether physical activity represents a modifiable risk factor or whether it may relate to the premorbid changes that could be associated with the decline into dementia.

Significant animal data does support potential mechanisms whereby physical activity might affect cognition. In a transgenic mouse model of Alzheimer's disease, mice allowed long term access to a running wheel had fewer amyloid-β plaques and better performance on the Morris water maze (Adlard et al. 2005), where mice are placed in an opaque pool of water and must swim to find a platform submerged and therefore hidden at a fixed location, which assesses learning and memory as the mice must learn the location through extramaze cues despite being placed in the pool at varying locations. Increased neurogenesis in the dentate gyrus of the hippocampus has also been reported in aged mice with access to a running wheel (van Praag et al. 2005; Kramer et al. 2006). Exercise in rodent models has also been associated with enhanced long-term potentiation and increased hippocampal expression of the NR2B subunit of the N-methyl-D-aspartate receptor (Farmer et al. 2004), increased hippocampal brain-derived neurotrophic factor (Cotman and Berchtold 2002; Garza et al. 2004; Neeper et al. 1995) which continues beyond the end of the exercise period (Berchtold et al. 2010), and beneficial effects on the serotonergic (Bloomstrand et al. 1989) and cholinergic systems (Fordyce and Farrar 1991), and on GABAergic neurons (Berchtold et al. 2002). Exercise is also associated with attenuated dopamine loss in hemi-parkinsonian rodents as well (Poulton and Muir 2005). Therefore, the animal literature does suggest that physical activity could represent, at least in part, a modifiable risk factor rather than acting solely as a marker of premorbid decline. However, in some cases, this benefit is not sustained if exercise is discontinued, at least for cerebral blood flow and learning in monkeys (Rhyu et al. 2010).

Evidence from controlled trials has also begun to emerge supporting a clinical effect of exercise and fitness training on cognition in aging (Kramer et al. 2006). A meta-analysis of earlier trials of various aerobic fitness training programs (1966–2001) demonstrated a beneficial effect on cognition with a modest effect size (0.48), with the greatest cognitive effects observed for executive control processes, more benefit when accompanied by strength and flexibility training, and a greater effect in women (Colcombe and Kramer 2003). Controlled trials have also demonstrated that walking three times a week for 45 minutes for six months resulted in better performance on an attentional task and increased frontal and parietal activity on functional MRI and less need for compensatory anterior cingulate activity with this task among the healthy elderly (Colcombe et al. 2004). Another trial of a six-month aerobic training program resulted in increased gray matter volume in the frontal lobes and superior temporal lobes with semiautomated image segmentation analysis of high resolution MRI data in the elderly (Colcombe et al. 2006).

Therefore, physical activity may be a modifiable risk factor for cognitive changes with aging. Other aspects of the effects of physical activity on aging will be discussed in the subsequent chapter. Furthermore, physical activity may also affect cognition in aging indirectly by its effects on cardiovascular factors, which are also known to affect the aging brain as will be discussed further later in this chapter. In general, interactions between these major categories of contributors to cognitive health in aging may become increasingly important as we better understand their individual effects.

Stress and Inflammation

Several lines of evidence suggest an effect of stress on cognitive decline. The Religious Orders Study found that individuals with the greatest tendency (top 10%) to experience psychological distress were twice as likely to develop Alzheimer's disease as individuals with the least tendency (bottom 10%) to experience psychological distress in an average of five years of follow-up (Wilson et al. 2003). In subsequent work with the Religious Orders Study, chronic psychological distress was similarly associated with an increased risk of mild cognitive impairment in up to 12 years of follow-up (Wilson et al. 2007). As further evidence of the role of stress, a recent study demonstrated that dementia risk is greater in caregivers of dementia patients (Norton et al. 2010). Long-term exposure to high levels of endogenous glucocorticoids, due to activation of the hypothalamic-pituitary-adrenal (HPA) axis in response to stress, is associated with memory impairments and atrophy of the hippocampus in aging (Lupien et al. 2005). Sustained glucocorticoid elevations affect behaviors related to the prefrontal cortex as well as the hippocampus, in addition to the anatomical effects detected on neurons in these areas (Sotiropoulos et al. 2008). Furthermore, transgenic mice with overexpression of glucocorticoid receptors in the forebrain develop an accelerated cognitive decline with aging without exposure to stress, along with acceleration of a number of other age-related neuroendocrine changes (blunted response to restraint stress and delayed turn-off of the stress response), suggesting that glucocorticoids are critical to this effect of stress on aging rather than some other aspect of the stress response (Wei et al. 2007).

Furthermore, corticotropin-releasing factor receptors, also a critical component of the HPA axis stress response, appear to be critical to the mechanism by which stress induces phosphorylation of tau, a key event in the development of neurofibrillary tangles in Alzheimer's disease (Rissman et al. 2007). Genetic polymorphisms in the interleukin-6 gene promoter (-572C/G) are also associated with the risk of sporadic Alzheimer's disease (He et al. 2010), further supporting a relationship between inflammation and Alzheimer's disease.

A long literature has demonstrated a relationship between stress and inflammation in a range of settings, with a particularly significant impact in the elderly (Kiecolt-Glaser et al. 2007). Inflammation is a well-known feature of Alzheimer's disease (Yasojima et al. 2000) and has been purported as a risk factor for Alzheimer's disease (Engelhart et al. 2004). In the Framingham Heart Study, increased presence of inflammatory biomarkers was found to be associated with greater brain atrophy in aging, an effect which was greatest in males (Jefferson et al. 2007). The relationship between inflammation and Alzheimer's disease, though, will also be important as a contributor to risks associated with a number of other subsequent factors in this chapter, aside from stress, such as cardiovascular disease, fatty acids, and antioxidants. Inflammation will therefore be readdressed in subsequent sections as it relates to those topics. However, it does appear that stress and potentially inflammation, which is affected by stress, may both ultimately represent modifiable risk factors for cognitive changes in aging.

Support

Psychosocial and socioeconomic environments, which contain elements of mental and physical activity as well as stress and the component of social interaction, have been independently studied for their effects on Alzheimer's disease. Case-control studies have shown in a logistic regression analysis of dementia patients and healthy controls that greater psychosocial networks (number of confidants, sports activities, and cultural activities) were associated with decreased presence of dementia, and in one particular study, when the data was adjusted for the effect of the psychosocial network, the protective effect of greater education for dementia was neutralized (Seidler et al. 2003). However, the relationship between social factors and Alzheimer's disease is complex, and in need of further study. When subjects were assessed for the presence of the apolipoprotein (APOE) 4 allele, which confers a higher risk for Alzheimer's disease, a synergistic relationship was found between presence of this gene and growing up in a lower socioeconomic household, based on census records, for risk of dementia (Moceri et al. 2001). A wide range of social factors will need to be studied to better understand these effects, and to disentangle them from more basic issues, such as nutrition, stress, and mental and physical activities, before we can understand how psychosocial support and other related social factors might represent a modifiable risk factor for cognitive changes in aging.

Sleep

Disordered sleep has also been associated with cognitive decline in the elderly. The best studied disorder of sleep in this setting is sleep apnea syndrome. Sleep apnea can be due to obstructive sleep apnea, where snoring, repetitive apnea during sleep, and daytime sleepiness occur often due to upper airway obstruction resulting from obesity or craniofacial abnormalities (Banno and Kryger 2007; Norman and Loredo 2008), or due to central sleep apnea with breathing cessation due to decreased central respiratory drive from heart failure or neurological disease (Banno and Kryger 2007). Obstructive sleep apnea may contribute to depression as well as impairments in memory, attention, and learning (Naegele et al. 1995), and has been associated with axonal dysfunction, frontal white matter myelin changes, and executive function impairments (Kales et al. 1985), with some cognitive aspects (attention, visuospatial learning, and motor performance) demonstrating a response to continuous positive airway pressure (CPAP) (Ferini-Strambi et al. 2003). Other studies have found improvements in the delayed reaction times, divided attention deficits, and the increased number of accidents on simulated driving tests in sleep apnea patients with CPAP treatment (Mazza et al. 2006), and also improved attention and vigilance on cognitive testing with such treatment (Aloia et al. 2004), as well as improved depression, fatigue, and health-related quality of life (McMahon et al. 2003). The sleep disruption inherent in sleep apnea appears to be the major contributor to these impairments, which leads to the implication that adequate sleep appears to be important in healthy cognitive aging, and assessment for treatable sleep disturbances should be undertaken if suspected.

Cardiovascular Factors

Recent evidence has supported an association between a range of cardiovascular factors and the development of dementia. Cardiovascular health factors such as hypertension, dyslipidemia, and diabetes, as well as cardiovascular lifestyle issues such as lack of exercise, obesity, and smoking are all associated with cognitive decline and dementia. Adequate treatments for these conditions imply an improved chance for optimal cognitive health in aging (Duron and Hanon 2008; Fillit et al. 2008). The related association with fatty acids and statins will be discussed later in this chapter.

Metabolic syndrome consists of a group of five cardiovascular risk factors: abdominal obesity, hypertriglyceridemia, low high-density lipoprotein levels, hypertension, and hyperglycemia. Each alone results in a slight increase in risk of cardiovascular disease and diabetes, but are synergistic together; when at least three of the five are present, the risk for disease dramatically increases and the patient is considered to have the metabolic syndrome. Recent evidence also demonstrates that metabolic syndrome, itself, is associated with accelerated cognitive decline, particularly when in combination with elevated serum inflammatory markers (Yaffe 2007).

Diets high in trans and saturated fats adversely affect cognition while those high in fruits, vegetables, cereals, and fish are associated with a lower risk of dementia (Parrott and Greenwood 2007). Several studies have indicated that adherence to the Mediterranean diet, rich in vegetables, legumes, fruits, cereals, unsaturated fats (mostly from olive oil), and fish, with moderate alcohol (mostly wine) and dairy (mostly cheese and yogurt), and low intake of poultry and other meats and saturated fats in general, is associated with a lower risk of Alzheimer's disease as well as a decreased risk of Alzheimer's disease-related mortality (Scarmeas et al. 2006; Scarmeas et al. 2007).

One particular area of recent interest related to diet and cardiovascular risk factors and their effects on cognitive health has been calorie restriction. After initial success in rodent models, recent studies have demonstrated that a 30% calorie reduction in rhesus monkeys yields better maintenance of gross and fine motor performance with aging, fewer age-related changes in brain imaging markers (Ingram et al. 2007) and decreased iron deposition (Kastman et al. 2010). At least some of this effect is believed to be due to anti-inflammatory effects of dietary restriction (Morgan et al. 2007).

Overall, evidence thus far suggests that dietary changes and reduction of cardiovascular risk factors in general show some promise as modifiable risk factors for optimization of cognition with aging.

Fatty Acids

Recent evidence has demonstrated that in large community studies, greater fish consumption is associated with a slower cognitive decline with age, believed to be due to the high content of omega-3 fatty acids in fish (Morris et al. 2005). Among the omega-3 fatty acids, docosahexaenoic acid (DHA) in the brain appears to be important in regulation of cerebral glucose uptake (Freemantle et al. 2006). Dietary DHA and docosapentaenoic acid were found to decrease amyloid-beta and tau pathology by affecting presenilin 1 levels in a transgenic mouse model exhibiting both amyloid-beta and tau pathologies (Green et al. 2007). DHA alone was also observed to reduce amyloid burden in a transgenic mouse Alzheimer model (Lim et al. 2005). DHA appears to decrease dendritic pathology in mouse models of Alzheimer's disease (Calon et al. 2004). The increased amount of omega-6 fatty acids in proportion to the omega-3 fatty acids in the Western diet is also believed to be a significant contributor to neurodegeneration (Borsonelo and Galduróz 2008). Early randomized controlled trials of omega-3 fatty acids in Alzheimer's disease have not yet yielded benefit (Freund-Levi et al. 2006), but some have reported benefit in a small sample of mild cognitive impairment patients with a combination of DHA and arachidonic acid (Kotani et al. 2006).

Earlier epidemiological studies have suggested that use of cholesterol-lowering statins reduces the risk of developing Alzheimer's disease (Jick et al. 2000; Wolozin et al. 2000; Rockwood et al. 2002). This effect is believed to be mediated at least in part by anti-inflammatory effects, as statins have been shown to reduce beta-amyloid-induced microglial inflammatory responses (Cordle and Landreth 2005). Some early studies from clinical trials have shown promise for the use of statins in mild to moderate Alzheimer's disease (Sparks et al. 2005). A recent larger trial, though, failed to show a beneficial effect from statins in mild to moderate Alzheimer's disease (Feldman et al. 2010).

Utilization of statins and omega-3 fatty acids in optimization of cognition in aging continue to be active areas of research interest.

Antioxidant Vitamins

One earlier study suggested that high doses of vitamin E (2000 IU daily) decreased the risk of Alzheimer's disease in a two-year double-blind, placebo-controlled trial (Sano et al. 1997). Subsequent retrospective studies suggested that such doses of vitamin E worked well in combination with cholinesterase inhibitors, as well (Klatte et al. 2005). However, subsequent studies did not demonstrate a protective effect from vitamin E in the progression from mild cognitive impairment to Alzheimer's disease, while detecting such an effect with cholinesterase inhibitors (Petersen et al. 2005). Furthermore, a meta-analysis of all of the early high dose vitamin-E studies suggested an increase in all cause mortality with doses above 400 IU (Miller et al. 2004). A subsequent study countered this, though, showing no increased mortality, but rather a 29% reduction in mortality risk with 2000 IU of vitamin E daily in a retrospective study of 847 Alzheimer's disease patients (Pavlik et al. 2009) Therefore, the role of vitamin E is still under investigation.

To further complicate the picture, regression analysis of a large clinical population suggests that a combination of various forms of tocopherol, rather than the isolated alpha-tocopherol, which is the usual form administered in vitamin E capsules as is utilized in the aforementioned studies, may be important in the vitamin E protective effect with Alzheimer's disease (Morris et al. 2005). This would be in agreement with earlier epidemiological studies suggesting a benefit from vitamin E obtained from food in reducing Alzheimer's disease risk among those with the APOE ε4 allele (Morris et al. 2002) and a protective effect of high dietary vitamin E and vitamin C reported for Alzheimer's disease (Engelhart et al. 2002; Zandi et al. 2004). Other studies, though, have not supported a protective effect from vitamin C for risk of dementia (Gray et al. 2008). Previous reports have suggested a tolerable range for vitamin C intake, with patients taking 1 g or more at greater risk of adverse consequences (Levine et al. 1999). This may be an important consideration for future studies. Recent evidence from a canine model of aging has suggested a significant benefit from dietary antioxidants when combined with environmental enrichment for both cognition and brain pathology (Head 2007). Therefore, the roles of the antioxidant vitamins in the optimization of cognition in aging remains unclear and needs more study.

B Vitamins

Early studies revealed an association between low blood levels of folate, vitamin B12, and elevated total serum homocysteine levels and histologically confirmed Alzheimer's disease in a case-control study (Clarke et al. 1998); increased plasma homocysteine has also been found to be a strong independent risk factor for development of dementia in the Framingham Study (Seshadri et al. 2002). In the MacArthur studies of successful aging, increased plasma homocysteine was associated with cognitive decline, but this was largely accounted for by the presence of low folate levels (Kado et al. 2005), as folate, B12, and homocysteine are highly metabolically interrelated.

Studies examining the effects of B vitamin supplementation are conflicting, though, with examples including higher folate intake being associated with a lower risk of Alzheimer's disease independent of other B vitamins in a food frequency questionnaire including supplements following 965 elderly individuals without dementia at the outset (Luschinger et al. 2007), but dietary folate, B6 and B12 were not associated with development of Alzheimer's disease in follow-up of 1041 elderly individuals without dementia at the outset (Morris et al. 2006). Some have raised the question of whether low B vitamin levels and elevated homocysteine levels are risk factors or just markers for the development of Alzheimer's disease (Seshadri 2006). Recent evidence does suggest that higher B6 and B12 intake spares the decline in gray matter observed during aging (Erickson et al. 2008). Therefore, the roles of B vitamins in the optimization of cognition in aging remain under investigation.

Other Agents

Numerous other substances have received attention regarding their potential for cognitive enhancing or neuroprotective effects.

Earlier studies suggested a modest benefit from Ginkgo biloba in Alzheimer's disease (Le Bars et al. 1997), but no benefit has been observed in more recent studies (DeKosky et al. 2008). Several epidemiological studies have suggested a protective effect from nonsteroidal anti-inflammatory drugs, in particular ibuprofen (in't Veld et al. 2001; Vlad et al. 2008) and aspirin (Anthony et al. 2000), but as of yet no clinical trials have yielded benefit.

Epidemiological studies also suggested that estrogen replacement therapy might be protective for Alzheimer's disease (Zandi et al. 2002), but the Women's Health Initiative study has actually suggested that such treatment might, for some formulations, increase the risk of dementia in a randomized trial (Shumaker et al. 2003). Some investigators, though, believe that the conflict may be due to existence of a critical time window for beneficial administration of estrogen, which may warrant further investigation (Sherwin 2006). However, lower testosterone has consistently been associated with Alzheimer's disease in men (Paoletti et al. 2004), and spatial and verbal memory improvements have been observed with testosterone administration in healthy older men (Cherrier et al. 2001). Pilot studies suggest a beneficial effect in Alzheimer's disease and mild cognitive impairment as well (Cherrier et al. 2005; Lu et al. 2006).

Small amounts of alcohol appear to be protective against future dementia according to a recent meta-analysis of earlier studies (Peters et al. 2008). Furthermore, high levels of polyphenols in red wine may offer a neuroprotective effect (Sun et al. 2002). There is an increased interest overall in phytochemicals, or plant-derived foods, due to their high content of combinations of flavonoids and other polyphenols (Lila 2007; Carlson et al. 2008). One recent study showed a delay in Alzheimer's disease associated with fruit and vegetable juices despite no association with vitamins E, C, or beta-carotene, or tea consumption (Dai et al. 2006). The green tea polyphenol extract epigallocatechin-3-gallate has been found to favorably affect amyloid precursor protein cleavage to reduce cerebral amyloidosis in an Alzheimer transgenic mouse model (Rezai-Zadeh et al. 2005). Green tea catechins were also found to prevent age-related spatial learning and memory decline in otherwise healthy mice through their impact on the hippocampal cyclic AMP-response element binding protein (CREB) signaling cascade (Li et al. 2009). Resveratrol, a specific polyphenol found in high concentrations in grapes and red wine, has shown early promise in neurotoxicity models such as excitotoxic damage induced by kainic acid in animals (Wang et al. 2004). Benefits have also been reported with blueberry supplementation in a rodent model of Alzheimer's disease, an effect also believed to be related to polyphenols (Joseph et al. 2003).

A number of agents that affect the mitochondrial system have also been explored for cognitive preservation, and are also considered to be antioxidants. Several lines of evidence have suggested alpha-lipoic acid may be helpful for neurodegenerative diseases due to beneficial effects on the mitochondrial system (Liu 2008). Another mitochondrial agent, coenzyme Q10, decreases beta-amyloid pathology in mice with an Alzheimer presinilin 1 mutation (Yang et al. 2008). Apocynin, derived from the rhizome of the Himalayan medicinal herb Picrorhiza kurroa, has also demonstrated neuroprotective effects in animal models (Wang et al. 2006); it is believed to act on the NADPH oxidase system critical in neurodegeneration (Sun et al. 2007). Curcumin also appears to be neuroprotective in animal models, decreasing lipid peroxidation and mitochondrial dysfunction (Wang et al. 2005). L-carnitine decreased 1-Methyl-4-phenylpyridinium ion (MPP+) induced apoptosis in an animal model (Wang et al. 2007). Creatine has demonstrated some neuroprotective effects, inducing reduced caspase-3 activation and cytochrome c release resulting in decreased infarct size in an animal ischemia model (Zhu et al. 2004); it has recently been demonstrated to benefit cognition in elderly humans in a pilot study (McMorris et al. 2007).

Finally, much recent attention has been raised by the neuroprotective effect of cannabinoids, by blocking microglial activation (Ramírez et al. 2005), and with the anti-inflammatory effects of the cannabinoid agonist WIN-55212-2 (Marchalant et al. 2007).

Whereas all of these agents and interventions are of significant interest for their role in optimization of cognition in aging, all are in significant need of further investigation before a recommendation for general consumption can be made.

Further Notes

A wide range of agents and strategies have been considered for optimization of cognition in the aged. Many of these measures show intriguing promise, but none have conclusive evidence for their benefit. Further study is necessary for all of them. Many of the prospective studies thus far have been carried out in patients with cognitive decline or in patients at high risk. As many of these agents are proposed to play a preventative role in cognitive decline, introducing them at this stage may be too late, with the pathology already well established and accelerating. This may explain the frequent discrepancies between clinical trials and the more favorable epidemiological and animal data. However, trials at a sufficiently early stage would be difficult to implement, due to the large sample sizes and the very long follow-up period that would be required for such studies.

Understanding of how these agents interact is also critical. The importance of this has already been demonstrated for cardiovascular risk factors in the metabolic syndrome (Yaffe 2007). An integrated treatment approach including antidepressants, cholinesterase inhibitors, supplements (multivitamins, vitamin E, alpha-lipoic acid, omega-3 fatty acids, and coenzyme Q10), and lifestyle modifications (diet and exercise) has shown promise in a pilot trial in mild dementia patients with depression, resulting in improvements in cognitive performance reported to persist out to 24 months (Bragin et al. 2005). A more recent pilot trial examining a combination intervention including omega-3 fatty acids, phospholipids, choline, B-vitamins, and antioxidants has also shown promise in mild Alzheimer's disease (Scheltens et al. 2010). Furthermore, more sensitive measures will be helpful in identifying more subtle changes in cognition, such as more sensitive memory tasks (Blackwell et al. 2004; Swainson et al. 2001), and tests of problem-solving ability which may incorporate subtle executive function and attentional impairments (Beversdorf et al. 2007).

Agents for maintaining and optimizng cognition in the elderly are a major area of current study, and much further research needs to be done. Continued study in this area is critical. The potential implications of success would be tremendous for our aging society.

References

Abbott RD, White LR, Ross GW, Masaki KH, Curb JD, and Petrovitch H. Walking and dementia in physically capable elderly men. *J Am Med Assoc* 2004;292:1447–1453.

Acevedo A and Lowenstein DA. Nonpharmacological cognitive interventions in aging and dementia. *J Geraitr Psychiatry Neurol* 2007;20:239–249.

Adlard PA, Perreau VM, Pop V, and Cotman CW. Voluntary exercise decreases amyloid load in a transgenic model of Alzheimer's disease. *J Neurosci* 2005;25:4217–4221.

Aloia MS, Arnedt JT, Davis JD, Riggs RL, and Byrd D. Neuropsychological sequelae of obstructive sleep apnea-hypopnea syndrome: A critical review. *J Int Neuropsychol Soc* 2004;10:772–785.

Anthony JC, Breitner JC, Zandi PP, et al. Reduced prevalence of AD in users of NSAIDs and H2 receptor antagonists: The Cache County Study. *Neurology* 2000;54:2066–2071.

Banno K and Kryger MH. Sleep apnea: Clinical investigations in humans. *Sleep Med* 2007;8:400–426.

Berchtold NC, Castello N, and Cotman CW. Exercise and time-dependent benefits to learning and memory. *Neurosci* 2010;167:588-597.

Berchtold NC, Kesslak JP, and Cotman CW. Hippocampal brain-derived neurotrophic factor gene regulation by exercise and the nedial septum. *J Neurosci Res* 2002;68:511–521.

Beversdorf DQ, Ferguson JLW, Hillier A, et al. Problem solving ability in patients with mild cognitive impairment. *Cog Behav Neurol* 2007;20:44–47.

Blackwell AD, Sahakian BJ, Vesey R, Semple JM, Robbins TW, and Hodges JR. Detecting dementia: Novel neuropsychological markers of preclinical Alzheimer's disease. *Dement Geriatr Cogn Disord* 2004;17:42–48.

Bloomstrand E, Perret D, Parry-Billings M, and Newsholme EA. Effect of sustained exercise on plasma amino acid concentrations on 5-hydroxytryptamine metabolism in six different brain regions in the rat. *Acta Physiol Scand* 1989;136:473–481.

Borsonelo EC and Galduróz JCF. The role of polyunsaturated fatty acids (PUFAs) in development, aging, and substance abuse disorders: Review and propositions. *Prostoglandins Leukot Essent Fatty Acids* 2008;78:237–245.

Bragin V, Chemodanova M, Dzhafarova N, Bragin I, Czerniawski JL, and Aliev G. Integrated treatment approach improves cognitive function in demented and clinically depressed patients. *Am J Alzheimers Dis Other Demen* 2005;20:21–26.

Buckner RL, Snyder AZ, Shannon BJ, et al. Molecular, structural, and functional characterization of Alzheimer's disease: Evidence for a relationship between default activity, amyloid, and memory. *J Neurosci* 2005;25:7709–7717.

Calon F, Lim GP, Yang F, et al. Docosahexaenoic acid protects from dendritic pathology in an Alzheimer's disease mouse model. *Neuron* 2004;43:633–645.

Carlson S, Peng N, Prasain JK, and Wyss JM. Effects of botanical dietary supplements on cardiovascular, cognitive, and metabolic function in males and females. *Gender Med* 2008;5(supplA):S76–S90.

Cherrier MM, Asthana S, Plymate S, et al. Testosterone supplementation improves spatial and verbal memory in healthy older men. *Neurology* 2001;57:80–88.

Cherrier MM, Matsumoto AM, Amory JK, et al. Testosterone improves spatial memory in men with Alzheimer disease and mild cognitive impairment. *Neurology* 2005;64:2063–2068.

Clarke R, Smith AD, Jobst KA, Refsum H, Sutton L, and Ueland PM. Folate, vitamin B12, and serum total homocysteine levels in confirmed Alzheimer disease. *Arch Neurol* 1998;55:1449–1455.

Colcombe SJ, Erickson KI, Scalf PE, et al. Aerobic exercise training increases brain volume in aging humans. *J Gerontol* 2006;61A:1166–1170.

Colcombe S and Kramer AF. Fitness effects on the cognitive function of older adults: A meta-analytic study. *Psychol Sci* 2003;14:125–130.

Colcombe SJ, Kramer AF, Erickson KI, et al. Cardiovascular fitness, cortical plasticity, and aging. *Proc Natl Acad Sci USA* 2004;101:3316–3321.

Cordle A and Landreth G. 3-hydroxy-3-methylglutaryl-coenzyme A reductase inhibitors attenuate β-amyloid-induced microglial inflammatory responses. *J Neruosci* 2005;25:299–307.

Cotman CE and Nerchtold NC. Exercise: A behavioral intervention to enhance brain health and plasticity. *Trends Neurosci* 2002;25:295–301.

Dai Q, Borenstein AR, Wu Y, Jackson JC, and Larson EB. Fruit and vegetable juices and Alzheimer's disease: The Kame Project. *Am J Med* 2006;119:751–759.

DeKosky ST, Williamson JD, Fitzpatrick AL, et al. Ginkgo biloba for prevention of dementia: A randomized controlled trial. *J Am Med Assoc* 2008;300:2253–2262.

Duron E and Hanon O. Hypertension, cognitive decline and dementia. *Arch Cardiovasc Dis* 2008;101:181–189.

Engelhart MJ, Geerlings MI, Meijer J, et al. Inflammatory proteins in plasma and the risk of dementia: The Rotterdam Study. *Arch Neurol* 2004;61:668–672.

Engelhart MJ, Geerlings MI, Ruitenberg A, et al. Dietary intake of antioxidants and risk of Alzheimer disease. *J Am Med Assoc* 2002;287:3223–3229.

Erickson KI, Suever BL, Prakash RS, Colcombe SJ, McAuley E, and Kramer AF. Creater intake of vitamins B6 and B12 spares gray matter in healthy elderly: Avoxel-based morphometry study. *Brain Res* 2008;1199:20–26.

Farmer J, Zhao X, van Praag H, Wodtke K, Gage FH, and Christie BR. Effects of voluntary physical activity on synaptic plasticity and gene expression in the dentate gyrus of adult-male Sprague-Dawley rats in vivo. *Neurosci* 2004;124:71–79.

Feldman HH, Doody RS, Kivipelto M, et al. Randomized controlled trial of atorvastatin in mild to moderate Alzheimer disease: LEADe. *Neurology* 2010;74:956–964.

Ferini-Strambi L, Baietto C, di Gioia MR, et al. Cognitive dysfunction in patients with obstructive sleep apnea (OSA): Partial reversibility after continuous positive airway pressure (CPAP). *Brain Res Bull* 2003;61:87–92.

Fillit H, Nash DT, Rundek T, and Zuckerman A. Cardiovascular risk factors and dementia. *Am J Geriatr Pharmacother* 2008;6:101–118.

Fordyce DE and Farrar RP. Enhancement of spatial learning in F344 rats by physical activity and related learning-associated alterations in hippocampal and cortical cholinergic functioning. *Behav Brain Res* 1991;46:123–133.

Freemantle E, Vandal M, Tremblay-Mercier J, et al. Omega-3 fatty acids, energy substrates, and brain function during aging. *Prostoglandins Leukot Essent Fatty Acids* 2006;75:213–220.

Freund-Levi Y, Eriksdotter-Jönhagen M, Cederholm T, et al. ω-3 fatty acid treatment in 174 patients with mild to moderate Alzheimer disease: OmegAD study, a randomized double-blind trial. *Arch Neurol* 2006;63:1402–1408.

Friedland RP, Fritsch T, Smyth KA, et al. Patients with Alzheimer's disease have reduced activities in midlife compared with healthy control-group members. *Proc Natl Acad Sci USA* 2001;98: 3440–3445.

Garza AA, Ha TG, Garcia C, Chen MJ, and Russo-Neustadt AA. Exercise, antidepressant treatment, and BDNF mRNA expression in the aging brain. *Pharmacol Biochem Behav* 2004;77:209–220.

Gray SL, Anderson ML, Crane PK, et al. Antioxidant vitamin supplement use and risk of dementia or Alzheimer's disease in older adults. *J Am Geriatr Soc* 2008;56:291–295.

Green KN, Martinez-Coria H, Khashwji H, et al. Dietary docosahexaenoic acid and docosapentaenoic acid ameliorate amyloid-β and tau pathology via a mechanism involving presenilin 1 levels. *J Neurosci* 2007;27:4385–4395.

He M, Yang Y, Zhang M. et al. Association between interleukin-6 gene promoter -572C/G polymorphism and the risk of sporadic Alzheimer's disease. *Neurol Sci* 2010;31:165–168.

Head E. Combining an antioxidant-fortified diet with behavioral enrichment leads to cognitive improvement and reduced brain pathology in aging canines: Strategies for healthy aging. *Ann N Y Acad Sci* 2007;1114:398–406.

Ingram DK, Young J, and Mattison JA. Calorie restriction in nonhuman primates: assessing effects on brain and behavioral aging. *Neuroscience* 2007;145:1359–1364.

in't Veld BA, Ruitenberg A, Hofman A, et al. Nonsteroidal antiinflammatory drugs and the risk of Alzheimer's disease. *New Engl J Med* 2001;345:1515–1521.

Jefferson AL, Massaro JM, Wolf PA, et al. Inflammatory biomarkers are associated with total brain volume: The Framingham Heart Study. *Neurology* 2007; 68: 1032–1038.

Jick H, Zornberg GL, Jick SS, Seshadri S, and Drachman DA. Statins and the risk of dementia. *Lancet* 2000;356:1627–1631.

Joseph JA, Denisova NA, Arendash G, et al. Blueberry supplementation enhances signaling and prevents behavioral deficits in an Alzheimer disease model. *Nutr Neurosci* 2003;6:153–162.

Kado DM, Karlamangla AS, Huang MH, et al. Homocysteine versus the vitamins folate, B6, and B12 as predictors of cognitive function and decline in older high-functioning adults: MacArthur Studies of Successful Aging. *Am J Med* 2005;118:161–167.

Kales A, Caldwell AB, Cadieux RJ, Vela-Bueno A, Ruch LG, and Mayes SD. Severe obstructive sleep apnea-II: Associated psychopathology and social consequences. *J Chronic Dis* 1985;38:427–434.

Kastman EK, Willette AA, Coe CL, et al. A calorie-restricted diet decreases brain iron accumulation and preserves motor performance in old rhesus monkeys. *J Neurosci* 2010:30:7940–7947.

Kiecolt-Glaser JK, Belury MA, Porter K, Beversdorf DQ, Lemeshow S, and Glaser R. Depressive symptoms, omega-6:omega-3 fatty acids, and inflammation in older adults. *Psychosomat Med* 2007;69:217–224.

Klatte ET, Scharre DW, Nagaraja HN, Davis RA, and Beversdorf DQ. Combination therapy of donepezil and vitamin E in Alzheimer disease. *Alzheimer Dis Assoc Disord* 2005;17:113–116.

Kotani S, Sakaguchi E, Warashina S, et al. Dietary supplementation of arachidonic and docosahexaenoic acids improves cognitive dysfunction. *Neurosci Res* 2006;56:159–164.

Kramer AF, Erickson KI, and Colcombe SJ. Exercise, cognition, and the aging brain. *J Appl Physiol* 2006;101:1237–1242.

La Bars PL, Katz MM, Berman N, Itil TM, Freedman AM, and Schatzberg AF. A placebo-controlled, double-blind, randomized trial of an extract of Ginkgo biloba for dementia: North American EGb Study Group. *J Am Med Assoc* 1997;278:1327–1332.

Larson EB, Wang L, Bowen JD, et al. Exercise is associated with reduced risk for incident dementia among persons 65 years of age or older. *Ann Intern Med* 2006;144:73–81.

Levine M, Rumsey SC, Daruwala R, Park JB, and Wang Y. Criteria and recommendations for vitamin C intake. *J Am Med Assoc* 1999;281:1415–1423.

Li Q, Zhao HF, Zhang ZF, et al. Long-term administration of green tea catechins prevents age-related spatial learning and memory decline in C57BL/6 J mice by regulating hippocampal cyclic AMP-response element binding protein signal cascade. *Neurosci* 2009;159:1208–1215.

Lila MA. From beans to berries and beyond: teamwork between plant chemicals for protection of optimal human health. *Ann N Y Acad Sci* 2007;1114:372–380.

Lim GP, Calon F, Morihara T, et al. A diet enriched with the omega-3 fatty acid docosahexaenoic acid reduces amyloid burden in an aged Alzheimer mouse model. *J Neurosci* 2005;25:3032–3040.

Liu J. The effects and mechanisms of mitochondrial nutrient -lipoic acid on improving age-associated mitochondrial and cognitive dysfunction: an overview. *Neurochem Res* 2008;33:194–203.

Lu PH, Masterman DA, Mulnard R, et al. Effects of testosterone on cognition and mood in male patients with mild Alzheimer disease and health elderly men. *Arch Neurol* 2006;63:177–185.

Lupien SJ, Fiocco A, Wan N, Maheu F, Lord C, Schramek T, and Tu MT. Stress hormones and human memory function across the lifespan. *Psychoneuroendocrinology* 2005;30:225–242.

Marchalant Y, Rosi S, and Wenk GL. Anti-inflammatory property of the cannabinoid agonist WIN-55212-2 in a rodent model of chronic brain inflammation. *Neurosci* 2007;144:1516–1522.

Mazza S, Pepin JL, Naegele B, et al. Driving ability in sleep apnoea patients before and after CPAP treatment: Evaluation of a road safety platform. *Eur Respir J* 2006;28:1020–1028.

McMahon JP, Foresman BH, and Chisholm RC. The influence of CPAP on the neurobehavioral performance of patients with obstructive sleep apnea hypopnea syndrome: A systematic review. *WMJ* 2003;102:36–43.

McMorris T, Mielcarz G, Harris RC, Swain JP, and Howard A. Creatine supplementation and cognitive performance in elderly individuals. *Aging Neuropsychol Cogn* 2007;14:517–528.

Milgram NW, Siwak-Tapp CT, Araujo J, and Head E. Neuroprotective effects of cognitive enrichment. *Ageing Res Rev* 2006;5:354–369.

Miller ER III, Pastor-Barriuso R, Dalal D, Riemersma RA, Appel LJ, and Guallar E. Meta-analysis: high-doseage vitamin E supplementation may increase all-cause mortality. *Ann Intern Med* 2004;142:37–46.

Moceri VM, Kukull WA, Emanual I, et al. Using census data and birth certificates to reconstruct the early-life socioeconomic environment and the relationship to the development of Alzheimer's disease. *Epidemiology* 2001;12:383–389.

Morgan TE, Wong AM, and Finch CE. Anti-inflammatory mechanisms of dietary restriction in slowing aging processes. *Interdiscpl Top Gerontol* 2007;35:83–97.

Morris MC, Evans DA, Tangney CC, Bienias JL, and Wilson RS. Fish consumption and cognitive decline with age in a large community study. *Arch Neurol* 2005;l62:1849–1853.

Morris MC, Evans DA, Bienias JL, et al. Dietary intake of antioxidant nutrients and the risk of incident Alzheimer disease in a biracial community study. *J Am Med Assoc* 2002;287:3230–3237.

Morris MC, Evans DA, Tangney CC, et al. Relation of the tocopherol forms to incident Alzheimer disease and to cognitive change. *Am J Clin Nutr* 2005;81:508–514.

Naegele B, Thouvard V, Pepin JL, et al. Deficits of cognitive executive functions in patients with sleep apnea syndrome. *Sleep* 1995;18: 42–52.

Neeper S, Gomez-Pinilla F, Choi J, and Cotman JC. Exercise and brain neurotrophins. *Nature* 1995;373:109.

Norman D and Loredo JS. Obstructive sleep apnea in older adults. *Clin Geriatr Med* 2008;24:151–165.

Norton MC, Smith KR, Østbye T, et al. Greater risk of dementia when spouse has dementia? The Cache County Study. *J Am Geriatr Soc* 2010;58:895–900.

Paoletti AM, Congia S, Lello S, et al. Low androgenization index in elderly women and elderly men with Alzheimer's disease. *Neurology* 2004;62:301–303.

Parrott MD and Greenwood CE. Dietary influences on cognitive function with aging: From high-fat diets to healthful eating. *Ann N Y Acad Sci* 2007;1114:389–397.

Pavlik VN, Doody RS, Rountree SD, and Darby EJ. Vitamin E use is associated with improved survival in an Alzheimer's disease cohort. *Dement Geriatr Cogn Disord* 2009;28:536–540.

Peters R, Peters J, Warner J, Beckett N, and Bulpitt C. Alcohol, dementia and cognitive decline in the elderly: A systematic review. *Age Ageing* 2008;37:505–512.

Petersen RC, Thomas RG, Grundman M, et al. Vitamin E and donepezil for the treatment of mild cognitive impairment. *New Engl J Med* 2005;352:2379–2388.

Poulton NP and Muir GD. Treatmill training ameliorates dopamine loss but not behavioral deficits in hemi-parkinsonian rats. *Exp Neurol* 2005;193:181–197.

Ramírez BG, Blazquez C, Gomez del Pulgar T, Guzman M, and de Ceballos ML. Prevention of Alzheimer's disease pathology by cannabinoids: Neuroprotection mediated by blockade of microglial activation. *J Neurosci* 2005;25:1904–1913.

Rezai-Zadeh K, Shytle D, Sun N, et al. Green tea epigallocatechin-3-gallate (EGCG) modulates amyloid precursor protein cleavage and reduces cerebral amyloidosis in Alzheimer transgenic mice. *J Neurosci* 2005;25:8807–8814.

Rhyu IJ, Bytheway JA, Kohler SJ, et al. Effects of aerobic exercise training on cognitive function and cortical vascularity in monkeys. *Neurosci* 2010;167:1239–1248.

Rissman RA, Lee K-F, Vale W, and Sawchenko PE. Corticotropin-releasing factor receptors differentially regulate stress-induced tau phosphorylation. *J Neurosci* 2007;27:6552–6562.

Rockwood K, Kirkland S, Hogan DB, et al. Use of lipid-lowering agents, indication bias, and the risk of dementia in community-dwelling elderly people. *Arch Neurol* 2002;59:223–227.

Sano M, Ernesto C, Thomas RG, et al. A controlled trial of selegiline, alpha-tocopheraol, or both as treatment for Alzheimer's disease. *New Engl J Med* 1997;336:1216–1222.

Scarmeas N, Luschinger JA, Mayeux R, and Stern Y. Mediterranean diet and Alzheimer disease mortality. *Neurology* 2007;69:1084–1093.

Scarmeas N, Stern Y, Tang MX, Mayeux R, and Luschinger JA. Mediterranean diet and risk for Alzheimer's disease. *Ann Neurol* 2006;59:912–921.

Scheltens P, Kamphuis PJGH, Verhey FRJ, et al. Efficacy of a medical food in mild Alzheimer's disease: a randomized controlled trial. *Alzheimers Dement* 2010; 6:1–10.

Seidler A, Bernhardt T, Nienhaus A, and Frölich L. Association between the psychosocial network and dementia—a case-control study. *J Psychiatr Res* 2003;37:89–98.

Seshadri S. Elevated plasma homocysteine levels: Risk factor or risk marker for the development of dementia and Alzheimer's disease. *J Alzheimers Dis* 2006;9:393–398.

Seshadri S, Beiser A, Selhub J, et al. Plasma homocysteine as a risk factor for dementia and Alzheimer's disease. *New Engl J Med* 2002;356:476–483.

Sherman BB. The critical period hypothesis: Can it explain discrepancies in the oestrogen-cognition literature? *J Neruoendocrinol* 2006;19:77–81.

Shumaker SA, Legault C, Rapp SR, et al., for the WHIMS Investigators. Estrogen plus progestin and the incidence of dementia and mild cognitive impairment in postmenopausal women. *J Am Med Assoc* 2003;289:2651–2662.

Sotiropoulos I, Cerqueria JJ, Catania C, Takashima A, Sousa N, and Almeida OFX. Stress and glucocorticoid footprints in the brain-the path from depression to Alzheimer's disease. *Neurosci Biobehav Rev* 2008;32:1161–1173.

Sparks DL, Sabbagh MN, Connor DJ, et al. Atorvastatin for the treatment of mild to moderate Alzheimer disease. *Arch Neurol* 2005;62:753–757.

Sun AY, Simonyi A, and Sun GY. The 'French Paradox' and beyond: Neuroprotective effects of polyphenols. *Free Radical Biol Med* 2002;32:314–318.

Sun GY, Horrocks LA, and Farooqui AA. The roles of NADPH oxidase and phospholipases A2 in oxidative and inflammatory responses in neurodegenerative diseases. *J Neurochem* 2007;103:1–16.

Swainson R, Hodges JR, Galton CJ, et al. Early detection and differentiatial diagnosis of Alzheimer's disease and depression with neuropsychological tasks. *Dement Geriatr Cogn Disord* 2001;12:265–280.

Valenzuela MJ and Sachdev P. Brain reserve and dementia: A systematic review. *Psychol Med* 2006;36:441–454.

van Praag H, Shubert T, Zhao C, and Gage FH. Exercise enhances learning and hippocampal neurogenesis in the adult mouse dentate gyrus. *J Neurosci* 2005;25:8680–8685.

Vlad SC, Miller DR, Kowall NW, and Felson DT. Protective effects of NSAIDs on the development of Alzheimer disease. *Neurology* 2008;70:1672–1677.

Wang Q, Sadovova N, Ali HK, et al. L-carnitine protects neurons from 1-methyl-4-phenylpyridinium-induced neuronal apoptosis in rat forebrain culture. *Neurosci* 2007;144:46–55.

Wang Q, Sun AY, Simonyi A, et al. Neuroprotective mechanisms of curcumin against cerebral ischemia-induced neuronal apoptosis and behavioral deficits. *J Neurosci Res* 2005;82:138–148,

Wang Q, Thompkins KD, Simonyi A, Korthuis RJ, Sun AY, and Sun GY. Apomycin protects against global cerebral ischemia-reperfusion-induced oxidative stress and injury in the gerbil hippocampus. *Brain Res* 2006;1090:182–189.

Wang Q, Yu S, Simonyi A, Rottinghaus G, Sun GY, and Sun AY. Resveratrol protects against neurotoxicity induced by kainic acid. *Neurochem Res* 2004;29:2105–2112.

Wei Q, Hebda-Bauer EK, Pletsch A, et al. Overexpressing the glucocorticoid receptor in forebrain causes an aging-like neuroendocrine phenotype and mild cognitive dysfunction. *J Neurosci* 2007;27:8836–8844.

Weuve J, Kang JH, Manson JE, Breteler MMB, Ware JH, and Grodstein F. Physical activity, including walking, and cognitive function in older women. *J Am Med Assoc* 2004;292:1454–1461.

Wilson RS, Barnes LL, Aggarwal NT, Boyle PA, Hebert LE, Mendes de Leon CF, and Evans DA. Cognitive activity and the cognitive morbidity of Alzheimer disease. *Neurology* 2010;75: 990–996.

Wilson RS, Evans DA, Bienias JL, Mendes de Leon CF, Schneider JA, and Bennett DA. Proneness to psychological distress is associated with risk of Alzheimer's disease. *Neurology* 2003;61:1479–1485.

Wilson RS, Scherr PA, Schneider JA, Tang Y, and Bennett DA. Relation of cognitive activity to risk of developing Alzheimer disease. *Neurology* 2007;69:1911–1920.

Wilson RS, Schneider JA, Boyle PA, Arnold SE, Tang Y, and Bennett DA. Chronic distress and incidence of mild cognitive impairment. *Neurology* 2007;68:2085–2092.

Wolozin B, Kellman W, Ruosseau P, Celesia GG, and Siegel G. Decreased prevalence of Alzheimer disease associated with 3-hydroxy-3-methyglutaryl coenzyme A reductase inhibitors. *Arch Neurol* 2000;57:1439–1443.

Yaffe K. Metabolic syndrome in cognitive disorders. Is the sum greater than its parts? *Alzheimer Dis Assoc Disord* 2007;21:167–171.

Yang X, Yang Y, Li G, Wang J, and Yang ES. Coenzyme Q10 attenuates -amyloid pathology in the aged transgenic mice with Alzheimer presinilin 1 mutation. *J Mol Neurosci* 2008;34: 165–171.

Yasokima K, Schwab C, McGeer EG, and McGeer PL. Human neurons generate C-reactive protein and amyloid P: Upregulation in Alzheimer's disease. *Brain Res* 2000;887:80–89.

Zandi PP, Anthony JC, Khachaturian AS, et al. Reduced risk of Alzheimer disease in users of antioxidant vitamin supplements. *Arch Neurol* 2004;61:82–88.

Zandi PP, Carlson MC, Plassmen BL, et al. Hormone replacement therapy and incidence of Alzheimer's disease in older women: The Cache County Study. *J Am Med Assoc* 2002;288:2123–2129.

Zhu S, Li M, Figueroa BE, et al. Prophylactic creatine administration mediates neuroprotection in cerebral ischemia in mice. *J Neurosci* 2004;24:5909–5912.

54 Cognitive and Physical Benefits of Exercise in the Aging

Krupa Shah and Dennis T. Villareal

Introduction: Physical and Cognitive Changes with Aging

Aging is a progressive and dynamic process which often causes changes in the structure and function of various physiological systems that ultimately reduce an individual's ability to adapt to the environment, thereby increasing the vulnerability to the onset of pathological processes. Aging causes a progressive decline in physical function, and leads to frailty, loss of independence, disability, and increased nursing home admissions (Frontera et al. 1991; Holloszy and Kohrt 1995). As one's strength, endurance, speed, and coordination decrease, the risk of disability and injurious falls increases. To put this in perspective, one third of community-dwelling elderly persons experience falls each year and this number is even higher in older adults living in nursing homes (Tinetti, Speechley, and Ginter 1988). It should be noted that falls in older adults are associated with an elevated risk of hospitalization, institutionalization, and mortality (Tinetti and Williams 1998; Gill et al. 2004; Campbell et al. 1990). Therefore, fall prevention interventions in older people remain a major health care priority. This topic is addressed in detail in chapter 26.

The effects of aging on aerobic capacity and skeletal muscle function are frequently the focus of attention in the musculoskeletal system. After age 30, aerobic capacity, often measured as peak oxygen uptake (VO_{2peak}) (Rogers et al. 1990), declines with age and contributes to a decrease in the older adult's ability to perform activities of daily living (ADL) (Cress et al. 1996). This is largely due to three major causes 1) a decline in the ability of the cardiopulmonary system to deliver O_2, 2) a decline in the ability of the working muscle to extract O_2, and 3) a decline in metabolically active muscle mass and parallel increase in metabolically inactive fat mass (Fletcher et al. 2001; Lambert and Evans 2005). There are significant changes in body composition with aging that influence physical function (Villareal et al. 2005). Although an older individual may maintain the same body weight over several years, it is likely that his or her percentage of body fat has increased, while the percent of lean body mass has decreased. It has been reported that isometric and dynamic strength of the quadriceps increases until age 30, and decreases after age 50 (Larsson, Grimby, and Karlsson 1979). A 30% reduction in strength between 50 and 70 yr of age is generally found, with muscle strength losses being most dramatic after age 70 (Larsson 1978). Most of the decline in strength can be explained by selective atrophy of type II muscle fibers and the loss of neuronal activation (Larsson 1983). In addition, balance and postural control begins to decline from middle age on and poor balance function has also been associated with increased risk of fall and injury (Era and Heikkinen 1985; Woollacott and Shumway-Cook 1990). Along with the musculoskeletal system, the vestibular, somatosensory, and visual systems all show decline with aging and may contribute to postural instability (Woollacott 2000).

Likewise, the central nervous system (CNS), and consequently cognitive functioning, undergoes changes as people grow older. In the course of normal aging the human brain begins to lose tissue in the third decade of life. On average there is a loss of approximately 15% of the cerebral cortex and 25% of the cerebral white matter from ages 30 to 90, with disproportionately high losses in the frontal, parietal, and temporal cortices (Jernigan et al. 2001). This pattern is linked to declines in cognitive performance (Silbert et al. 2003).

Cognitive function comprises numerous components, including memory, language, executive function, judgment, perception, and attention. However, not all components decline at the same time or at the same rate. In studies of healthy, community-dwelling older adults, the decline occurs at distinctly different rates across various domains of cognitive capability (Salthouse 1996; Singer et al. 2003; Schaie et al. 1998). Recent studies suggest that executive function is first to decline with normal aging (Bherer, Belleville, and Hudon 2004). Such changes in executive function preceded declines in memory and other cognitive domains with consequent impairment in the ability to perform instrumental ADL. The age-related changes in cognition are multidimensional, progress over a broad range of severity and occur over many decades. Efforts to moderately improve an individual's competence on various cognitive functions or to reduce the rate of functional decline across cognitive abilities could produce great benefits in the long term to allow the individual to maintain independence, delay the onset of dementia, and improving quality of life. The prevalence of dementia rises exponentially after age 65, and affects approximately 50% of people older than 80 (Larson and Langa 2008; Kukull et al. 2002). In the U.S., dementia remains one of the leading causes of years of life lost due to disability (Wimo, Jonsson, and Winblad 2003). The pursuit for factors that may delay or prevent the onset of dementia has become an important public health problem.

Thus a typical aging curve suggests that most physiological functions improve from birth through the late teens, and then level off in the mid-20s to 30s. For the most part, it is downhill from there. Everyone ages differently, and the rate of change is not equal among individuals. What is clear is that there are several modifiable mediating factors on the aging curve. One of the most important modifiable factors is physical activity. It is estimated that only 31% of persons 65 to 74 years of age regularly engage in moderate physical activity for 20 minutes or more a day three days a week. This rate drops to 20 percent when one reaches 75 years of age (CDC 2000). These trends have not improved over the past decade. The sedentary lifestyle is a major contributor to the leading causes of death among adults in the United States (Chakravarthy and Booth 2004). It is estimated that 15% of the 1.6 million chronic health conditions that are newly diagnosed each year are due to a sedentary lifestyle alone, independent of other risk factors (Booth, Chakravarthy, and Gordon 2002).

It is projected that by the year 2030, the number of individuals 65 years of age and over will more than double to 71.5 million in the U.S. alone, and those who are 85 years of age and older will be the fastest growing segment of the population (U.S. Department of Health and Human Services 2003). Therefore, as more individuals live longer, it is imperative to determine interventions that can improve health, quality of life, and independence.

Effect of Exercise on Physical Function

The American College of Sports Medicine has published a report on exercise and activity for older adults (American College of Sports Medicine Position Stand 1998). It concluded that exercise reduces and prevents a number of functional declines in aging. The current literature overwhelmingly points to a positive effect of exercise on falls risk reduction and prevention, a major cause of morbidity and mortality in the elderly. Older individuals at any age can generally adapt and respond to both aerobic and resistance training (Lambert and Evans 2005) (Table 1). Aerobic exercise improves cardiovascular function by increasing VO_{2peak} and stroke volume, reducing heart rate and blood pressure both at rest and during near peak exercise, and increasing maximal exercise times (Rogers et al. 1990; Lambert and Evans 2005; Ehsani et al. 1991; Seals et al. 1984). On the other hand, resistance training has a greater impact on muscle mass and function (Hunter, McCarthy, and Bamman 2004). Resistance training programs can prevent strength loss well into older age (Frontera et al. 1988) and could demonstrate an improvement in strength, which corresponds with that in younger persons (Fiatarone et al. 1994). Resistance training can be an important adjunct to weight loss interventions in the elderly obese persons as it can efficiently increase energy expenditure, decrease body fat mass, and maintain metabolically active muscle mass in healthy older persons (Villareal et al. 2005). Both aerobic and resistance exercises also result in improvements in postural stability, increase flexibility, and improve overall levels of physical activity (Lambert and Evans 2005). In particular, tai chi has been shown to improve dynamic balance and fall risk reduction in older adults (Harmer and Li 2008). A meta-analysis examining the role of exercise in reducing the risk of falling showed that even short term (10–36 weeks) exercise training (in one or more aerobic, resistance, flexibility, and Tai Chi exercises) is beneficial in reducing the risk of falls when follow-up was obtained for up to 2–4 years (Province et al. 1995).

A longitudinal (13 year follow-up) study examined the development of disability in a large cohort of elderly men and women who were members of a running club. They were compared to age-matched, community-based individuals who were of comparable health but not runners. Among the runners, for both genders, there was a lower rate of increased disability scores as compared to those who did not

exercise on a regular basis (Wang et al. 2002). Numerous studies now support the American College of Sports Medicine's recommendations that older persons stay active. This evidence includes data from randomized clinical trials (RCT). In one RCT, the prevention of disabilities in response to exercise was examined in older persons with knee osteoarthritis (Penninx et al. 2001). The exercise program consisted of 3 months of supervised aerobics or resistance exercise, followed by a 15-month home-based program. After 18 months, there was a higher risk of developing ADL disability in the controls compared with the exercisers. The greater maintenance of ability to perform ADLs was similar in the aerobic and resistance exercise intervention groups. In fact, an intensive multi-component exercise training program can ameliorate frailty in frail older persons. In one clinical trial, older adults who had impairments in physical performance and VO_{2peak} were randomized to nine-month intensive exercise training or a low intensity home exercise program. The adults who had intensive training had significant improvements in physical function and preclinical disability (Binder et al. 2002).

In an RCT in frail obese older adults, a weight-loss program was combined with a multi-component exercise (aerobic, resistance, and flexibility) training intervention (Villareal et al. 2006). The combined weight loss and exercise program resulted in significant improvements in physical function and quality of life. In particular, the improvements in objective measures of function, such as VO_{2peak}, strength, gait, and balance, were accompanied by subjective improvements in the ability to function. Importantly, exercise training prevented weight-loss induced reduction in lean mass in these older participants. The Lifestyle Interventions and Independence for Elders (LIFE) pilot study demonstrated that physical activity of even moderate intensity resulted in a clinically meaningful improvement of physical performance as assessed by using the Short Physical Performance Battery (a series of tests including walking, balance, and chair stands tests that predict mobility disability, institutionalization, and death) (Pahor et al. 2006). This study also presented promising evidence on the effectiveness of exercise in the prevention of the disability in walking as assessed by the capacity to complete a 400-meter walk.

Exercise can also improve physical function in dementia patients. A recent meta-analysis showed that cognitively impaired individuals who participate in exercise rehabilitation programs have similar positive outcomes in response to resistance and aerobic training as age and gender-matched cognitively intact persons and therefore impaired persons should not be excluded from exercise rehabilitation programs (Heyn, Johnson, and Kramer 2008).

Recommendations

A structured exercise program to improve physical function in older adults is recommended (American College of Sports Medicine Position Stand 1998). The goals of exercise in older persons are to increase aerobic ability, strength, balance and flexibility; therefore, a multi-component exercise program that includes stretching, aerobic activity, and strength exercises is generally recommended (Table 2) (Haskell et al. 2007). Even very old or frail persons can participate in these activities.

The exercise program should be at least three to five times per week, for 30 to 45 minutes, at an intensity that is vigorous enough to raise the pulse rate to 70–80% of the maximal heart rate. The exercise program should be individualized according to an older individual's medical conditions and disability. The program should start at a low-to-moderate intensity, duration, and frequency to promote compliance and avoid musculoskeletal injuries. If possible, the program should be gradually advanced over a period of several weeks or months to a longer, more frequent, and more vigorous effort. Older persons may require

Table 1 Type of Exercises

Aerobic Exercises	Resistance Exercises
Exercise that uses large muscle groups, and is maintained for a long periods and is rhythmic in nature. Examples: cycling/biking, running, swimming, cross-country skiing, playing basketball, jumping rope, roller skating, walking briskly, and dancing.	Exercise routine that builds strength by contraction of muscle against force. Examples: lifting on weight machines, hand weights, bar bells, dumb bells, and stretching bands.

Table 2 Exercise Recommendations

Aerobic Exercise

Moderate to vigorous activity enough to raise the pulse rate to 70–80% of the maximal heart rate. Activity performed for a minimum 20–30 minutes at least three days per week.

Resistance Exercise

The progressive training program should involve all major muscle groups of the upper and lower extremities and trunk.

A single set of 10–15 repetitions using eight to 8-10 different exercises, performed 2–3 nonconsecutive days per week.

Flexibility and Balance Exercise

Stretch major muscle groups after exercise. Flexibility activities should be performed on all days that aerobic or muscle-strengthening activity is performed.

Balance training exercises 2–3 times per week.

longer warm-up periods and cool down periods as their cardiovascular systems adjust to the work and adjust back to the resting state.

The American College of Sports Medicine states that older adults do not require medical consultation before starting a moderate-intensity program. However, those individuals who are sedentary, and have multiple cardiac risk factors should see a physician before starting a vigorous program. For these individuals, an exercise stress test is usually recommended prior to starting the exercise program. They should be advised that if they develop symptoms with moderate exercise they must discontinue and see their physician. Persons with known disease and other complications should be examined and given suitable advice. Nevertheless, most individuals can start at least a moderate level program without the need for extensive medical testing.

It is worth mentioning that changes in the lifestyle habits of older persons may present special challenges. Multiple medical problems, depression, sensory impairments, and cognitive dysfunction may make it difficult to change lifestyle. The increase in chronic disabilities with aging reduces physical activity and exercise capacity. To facilitate lifestyle change, program participation by spouse or caregivers should be encouraged. In addition, special consideration should be given to hurdles faced during learning by older adults, such as impaired vision and hearing, orthopedic conditions, multiple comorbidities, and limited financial resources.

Effect of Exercise on Cognitive Function

Animal models which focus on the relationship between exercise and brain health indicate that exercise targets many aspects of brain function and has positive effects on brain health. These effects are related by a chain of cellular and molecular cascades, including increased capillary density, increased length and number of the dendritic interconnections between neurons, and increased neurogenesis in the hippocampus (Van, Kempermann, and Gage 1999). These effects likely result from increases in growth factors such as brain-derived neurotrophic factor and insulin-like growth factor. The final result of these structural changes is that a better interconnected brain is more plastic and adaptive to change (Cotman and Berchtold 2002). In addition to central mechanisms, exercise reduces several systemic risk factors for dementia such as diabetes, hypertension, and cardiovascular disease. A common mechanism between many of these peripheral risk factors and cognitive decline is inflammation. A chronic inflammatory state can potentially cause brain dysfunction and neurodegeneration by interfering with growth factor signaling. Thus, through regulation of growth factors and

reduction of inflammation, exercise probably improves brain health and function (Cotman, Berchtold, and Christie 2007).

Numerous observational studies have found that people who are physically active seem less likely than sedentary persons to experience cognitive decline and dementia in later life. According to the Nurses' Health Study, women who exert higher levels of physical activity over a two-year period have higher cognitive scores (Weuve et al. 2004). Similarly, men who walk at least two miles a day are 1.8 times less likely than sedentary men to develop dementia over a six-year follow-up period (van Gelder et al. 2004). Another prospective cohort study showed that elderly subjects who performed exercise ≥3 times a week have a 32% reduced risk of developing dementia compared to subjects who performed exercise ≤3 times a week. These results were after adjusting for numerous confounding factors, such as depression, cardiovascular disease, APOE genotype, and functional status (Larson et al. 2006). Furthermore, the greater protective effect of exercise was observed among the participants with lower functional status, thereby emphasizing the protective relationship between functional and cognitive status. These findings suggest a temporal relationship between exercise and cognitive decline, and indicate that moderate exercise reduces the risk of cognitive decline and dementia. However, other cohort studies have failed to establish a relationship among exercise, cognitive decline, and dementia (Broe et al. 1998; Ravaglia et al. 2008). The observational design of these studies does not allow us to establish with certainty a causal relationship between exercise, cognitive decline, and dementia. The problem of inverse causality and the confounding effect of factors that were not measured cannot be excluded. Therefore, definitive results need to be achieved from randomized controlled clinical trials.

The effects of exercise on cognitive function have been examined in some randomized clinical studies. Nevertheless, the results obtained from these studies are mixed. Although some studies showed improvement of the cognitive function associated with exercise (Dustman et al. 2004; Kramer et al. 1999; Rikli and Edwards 1991), others failed to report this effect (Hill et al. 1993; Madden et al. 1989). A meta-analysis combining the data from the interventional studies (Kramer, Erickson, and Colcombe 2006) underscores the effectiveness of exercise in improving cognitive functions. In particular, the benefit of exercise appeared to be clear in the cognitive domain of executive function, which is more susceptible to age-related cognitive decline. Furthermore, this meta-analysis revealed a greater benefit of exercise based on trials of longer duration (> 6-months) or those that utilized a multi-component exercise program than trials that used either brief duration or examined aerobic exercise only. The majority of prospective intervention studies of exercise and cognition to date have focused on aerobic-based exercise training. However, it has been suggested that other types of exercise training, such as resistance training, may also benefit cognition (Liu-Ambrose and Donaldson 2008). In one study, a resistance training program has also shown equally beneficial effect on cognitive function (Cassilhas et al. 2007). Moreover, we must be cautious to draw definitive conclusions because of the methodological limitations of some of these studies. For example, these studies generally have a small sample size using a program of exercise with short duration, with varying degree of intensity and frequency of exercise.

There is a paucity of research investigating the mechanism of cognitive improvement with exercise training in humans. One study demonstrated that exercise training is associated with increased blood perfusion of brain regions that regulates attention (Colcombe et al. 2006). After a six-month period, study participants in the aerobic exercise group showed significantly greater task-related activity in executive control areas (e.g. the middle frontal gyrus, the superior frontal gyrus, superior parietal lobule). More importantly, the grey matter losses in these areas were substantially reduced as a function of aerobic fitness.

The cognitive effects of physical activity among people with cognitive impairment and dementia have been systematically reviewed (Heyn, Abreu, and Ottenbacher 2004). This meta-analysis demonstrated modest treatment effect of exercise training on cognition, and suggested that exercise is associated with improved cognitive function in older adults with cognitive impairment or dementia. The definition of physical activity in the studies included in this meta-analysis was unique to each study as were the cognitive outcomes. In a recent study, a group at high risk for cognitive decline and dementia (older patients complaining of memory impairment) was randomly assigned to receive either usual care or a 24-week home-based program of increased physical activity (Lautenschlager et al. 2008). At the 18-month follow-up period, the trial showed a fairly small statistically significant improvement in cognitive test scores. This improvement was not clinically significant as neither the family nor the patients appreciated any improvement.

Exercise has many beneficial effects, however, adherence to exercise is among the lowest for any of the commonpreventive health recommendations (Larson 2008). However, the pervasive fear of Alzheimer disease may help stimulate older individuals and society to become more physically active. The findings point to the need to learn more about exercise as an intervention to prevent cognitive decline and Alzheimer disease. The optimal dose, duration, and potency of the exercise training to achieve cognitive benefits need to be thoroughly investigated. Future larger clinical trials across a broad range of physical characteristics such as age, ethnicity, obesity etc., especially including persons older than 70 years, could test the effect of different fitness training protocols on measures of brain structure and function.

Conclusion

In conclusion, health advances of the past century have led more people to survive to extreme old age, when their risk of functional and cognitive decline increases substantially. Based upon the current evidence, participation in a regular exercise program is an effective intervention to prevent and reduce a number of functional declines associated with aging. Aerobic training can help maintain and improve various aspects of cardiovascular function and endurance, whereas resistance training helps counteract the loss in muscle mass and strength normally associated with aging. Together, these training adaptations greatly improve the physical functional capacity of older men and women, thereby improving the quality of life in this population. Exercise also appears to have a protective affect on late life brain health and cognition. However, there is a need for larger and longer-term randomized clinical trials in older persons that can confirm the relationship between exercise and cognition in the elderly.

References

American College of Sports Medicine Position Stand. Exercise and physical activity for older adults. *Med Sci Sports Exerc.* 1998;30(6):992–1008.

American College of Sports Medicine Position Stand. The recommended quantity and quality of exercise for developing and maintaining cardiorespiratory and muscular fitness, and flexibility in healthy adults. *Med Sci Sports Exerc.* 1998;30(6):975–991.

Bherer L, Belleville S, and Hudon C. [Executive function deficits in normal aging, Alzheimer's disease, and frontotemporal dementia]. *Psychol Neuropsychiatr Vieil.* 2004;2(3):181–189.

Binder EF, Schechtman KB, Ehsani AA. et al. Effects of exercise training on frailty in community-dwelling older adults: Results of a randomized, controlled trial. *Journal of the American Geriatrics Society.* 2002;50(12):1921–1928.

Booth FW, Chakravarthy MV, Gordon SE, and Spangenburg EE. Waging war on physical inactivity: Using modern molecular ammunition against an ancient enemy. *J Appl Physiol.* 2002;93(1):3–30.

Broe GA, Creasey H, Jorm AF, et al. Health habits and risk of cognitive impairment and dementia in old age: A prospective study on the effects of exercise, smoking and alcohol consumption. *Aust N Z J Public Health.* 1998;22(5):621–623.

Campbell AJ, Borrie MJ, Spears GF, Jackson SL, Brown JS, and Fitzgerald JL. Circumstances and consequences of falls experienced by a community population 70 years and over during a prospective study. *Age Ageing.* 1990;19(2):136–41.

Cassilhas RC, Viana VA, Grassmann V, et al. The impact of resistance exercise on the cognitive function of the elderly. *Med Sci Sports Exerc.* 2007;39(8):1401–1407.

Centers for Disease Control. *Physical inactivity for U.S. men and women, 2000. Behavioral risk factor surveillance survey.* Centers for Disease Control and Prevention, National Center for Chronic Disease Prevention and Health Promotion. http://www.cdc.gov/brfss/. 2008. Ref Type: Electronic Citation

Chakravarthy MV and Booth FW. Eating, exercise, and "thrifty" genotypes: Connecting the dots toward an evolutionary understanding of modern chronic diseases. *J Appl Physiol.* 2004;96(1):3–10.

Colcombe SJ, Erickson KI, Scalf PE, et al. Aerobic exercise training increases brain volume in aging humans. *J Gerontol A Biol Sci Med Sci.* 2006;61(11):1166–1170.

Cotman CW and Berchtold NC. Exercise: A behavioral intervention to enhance brain health and plasticity. *Trends Neurosci.* 2002;25(6):295–301.

Cotman CW, Berchtold NC, and Christie LA. Exercise builds brain health: Key roles of growth factor cascades and inflammation. *Trends Neurosci.* 2007;30(9):464–472.

Cress ME, Buchner DM, Questad KA, Esselman PC, deLateur BJ, and Schwartz RS. Continuous-scale physical functional performance in healthy older adults: A validation study. *Arch Phys Med Rehabil.* 1996;77(12):1243–1250.

Dustman RE, Ruhling RO, Russell EM, et al. Aerobic exercise training and improved neuropsychological function of older individuals. *Neurobiol Aging.* 1984;5(1):35–42.

Ehsani AA, Ogawa T, Miller TR, Spina RJ, and Jilka SM. Exercise training improves left ventricular systolic function in older men. *Circulation.* 1991;83(1):96–103.

Era P and Heikkinen E. Postural sway during standing and unexpected disturbance of balance in random samples of men of different ages. *J Gerontol.* 1985;40(3):287–295.

Fiatarone MA, O'Neill EF, Ryan ND et al. Exercise training and nutritional supplementation for physical frailty in very elderly people. *N Engl J Med.* 1994;330(25):1769–1775.

Fletcher GF, Balady GJ, Amsterdam EA et al. Exercise standards for testing and training: A statement for healthcare professionals from the American Heart Association. *Circulation.* 2001;104(14): 1694–1740.

Frontera WR, Hughes VA, Lutz KJ, and Evans WJ. A cross-sectional study of muscle strength and mass in 45- to 78-yr-old men and women. *J Appl Physiol.* 1991;71(2):644–650.

Frontera WR, Meredith CN, O'Reilly KP, Knuttgen HG, and Evans WJ. Strength conditioning in older men: Skeletal muscle hypertrophy and improved function. *J Appl Physiol.* 1988;64(3):1038–1044.

Gill TM, Allore HG, Holford TR, and Guo Z. Hospitalization, restricted activity, and the development of disability among older persons. *JAMA.* 2004;292(17):2115–2124.

Harmer PA and Li F. Tai Chi and falls prevention in older people *Med Sport Sci.* 2008;52:124–134.

Haskell WL, Lee IM, Pate RR, et al. Physical activity and public health: Updated recommendation for adults from the American College of Sports Medicine and the American Heart Association. *Med Sci Sports Exerc.* 2007;39(8):1423–1434.

Heyn P, Abreu BC, and Ottenbacher KJ. The effects of exercise training on elderly persons with cognitive impairment and dementia: A meta-analysis. *Arch Phys Med Rehabil.* 2004;85(10):1694–1704.

Heyn PC, Johnson KE, and Kramer AF. Endurance and strength training outcomes on cognitively impaired and cognitively intact older adults: A meta-analysis. *J Nutr Health Aging.* 2008;12(6):401–409.

Hill RD, Storandt M, and Malley M. The impact of long-term exercise training on psychological function in older adults. *J Gerontol.* 1993;48(1):12–17.

Holloszy JO and Kohrt WM. *Handbook of physiology - Aging.* London: Oxford University Press. 1995.

Hunter GR, McCarthy JP, and Bamman MM. Effects of resistance training on older adults. *Sports Med.* 2004;34(5):329–348.

Jernigan TL, Archibald SL, Fennema-Notestine C, et al. Effects of age on tissues and regions of the cerebrum and cerebellum. *Neurobiol Aging.* 2001;22(4):581–594.

Kramer AF, Erickson KI, and Colcombe SJ. Exercise, cognition, and the aging brain8. *J Appl Physiol.* 2006;101(4):1237–1242.

Kramer AF, Hahn S, Cohen NJ, et al. Ageing, fitness and neurocognitive function. *Nature.* 1999;400(6743):418–419.

Kukull WA, Higdon R, Bowen JD, et al. Dementia and Alzheimer disease incidence: A prospective cohort study. *Arch Neurol.* 2002;59(11):1737–1746.

Lambert CP, Evans WJ. Adaptations to aerobic and resistance exercise in the elderly. *Rev Endocr Metab Disord.* 2005;6(2):137–143.

Larsson L. Morphological and functional characteristics of the ageing skeletal muscle in man. A cross-sectional study *Acta Physiol Scand Suppl.* 1978;457:1–36.

Larson EB. Physical activity for older adults at risk for Alzheimer disease. *JAMA.* 2008;300(9):1077–1079.

Larson EB and Langa KM. The rising tide of dementia worldwide. *Lancet.* 2008;372(9637):430–432.

Larson EB, Wang L, Bowen JD, et al. Exercise is associated with reduced risk for incident dementia among persons 65 years of age and older. *Ann Intern Med.* 2006;144(2):73–81.

Larsson L, Grimby G, and Karlsson J. Muscle strength and speed of movement in relation to age and muscle morphology. *J Appl Physiol.* 1979;46(3):451–456.

Lautenschlager NT, Cox KL, Flicker L, et al. Effect of physical activity on cognitive function in older adults at risk for Alzheimer disease: A randomized trial. *JAMA.* 2008;300(9):1027–1037.

Liu-Ambrose T and Donaldson M. Exercise and cognition in older adults: Is there a role for resistance training programs? *Br J Sports Med.* 2008.

Madden DJ, Blumenthal JA, Allen PA, and Emery CF. Improving aerobic capacity in healthy older adults does not necessarily lead to improved cognitive performance. *Psychol Aging.* 1989;4(3):307–320.

Pahor M, Blair SN, Espeland M, et al. Effects of a physical activity intervention on measures of physical performance: Results of the lifestyle interventions and independence for Elders Pilot (LIFE-P) Study. *J Gerontol A Biol Sci Med Sci.* 2006;61(11):1157–1165.

Penninx BW, Messier SP, Rejeski WJ, et al. Physical exercise and the prevention of disability in activities of daily living in older persons with osteoarthritis. *Arch Intern Med.* 2001;161(19):2309–2316.

Province MA, Hadley EC, Hornbrook MC, et al. The effects of exercise on falls in elderly patients. A preplanned meta- analysis of the FICSIT Trials. Frailty and Injuries: Cooperative Studies of Intervention Techniques. *JAMA.* 1995;273(17):1341–1347.

Ravaglia G, Forti P, Lucicesare A, et al. Physical activity and dementia risk in the elderly: Findings from a prospective Italian study. *Neurology.* 2008;70(19 Pt 2):1786–1794.

Rikli RE and Edwards DJ. Effects of a three-year exercise program on motor function and cognitive processing speed in older women. *Res Q Exerc Sport.* 1991;62(1):61–67.

Rogers MA, Hagberg JM, Martin WH, III, Ehsani AA, and Holloszy JO. Decline in VO2max with aging in master athletes and sedentary men. *J Appl Physiol.* 1990;68(5):2195–2199.

Salthouse TA. The processing-speed theory of adult age differences in cognition. *Psychol Rev.* 1996;103(3):403–428.

Schaie KW, Maitland SB, Willis SL, and Intrieri RC. Longitudinal invariance of adult psychometric ability factor structures across 7 years. *Psychol Aging.* 1998;13(1):8–20.

Seals DR, Hagberg JM, Hurley BF, Ehsani AA, and Holloszy JO. Endurance training in older men and women. I. Cardiovascular responses to exercise. *J Appl Physiol.* 1984;57(4):1024–1029.

Silbert LC, Quinn JF, Moore MM, et al. Changes in premorbid brain volume predict Alzheimer's disease pathology. *Neurology.* 2003;61(4):487–492.

Singer T, Verhaeghen P, Ghisletta P, Lindenberger U, and Baltes PB. The fate of cognition in very old age: Six-year longitudinal findings in the Berlin Aging Study (BASE). *Psychol Aging.* 2003;18(2):318–331.

Tinetti ME, Speechley M, and Ginter SF. Risk factors for falls among elderly persons living in the community *N Engl J Med.* 1988;319(26):1701–1707.

Tinetti ME and Williams CS. The effect of falls and fall injuries on functioning in community-dwelling older persons. *J Gerontol A Biol Sci Med Sci.* 1998;53(2):M112–M119.

U.S. Department of Health and Human Services, Administration on Aging. Profile of older Americans. 2003. http://www.aoa.gov/prof/Statistics/ profile/2003/2003profile.pdf. 2008. Ref Type: Electronic Citation

van Gelder BM, Tijhuis MA, Kalmijn S, Giampaoli S, Nissinen A, and Kromhout D. Physical activity in relation to cognitive decline in elderly men: The FINE Study. *Neurology.* 2004;63(12): 2316–2321.

van PH van, Kempermann G, and Gage FH. Running increases cell proliferation and neurogenesis in the adult mouse dentate gyrus. *Nat Neurosci.* 1999;2(3):266–270.

Villareal DT, Apovian CM, Kushner RF, and Klein S. Obesity in older adults: Technical review and position statement of the American Society for Nutrition and NAASO, The Obesity Society. *Obes Res.* 2005;13(11):1849–1863.

Villareal DT, Banks M, Sinacore DR, Siener C, and Klein S. Effect of weight loss and exercise on frailty in obese older adults. *Arch Intern Med.* 2006;166(8):860–866.

Wang BW, Ramey DR, Schettler JD, Hubert HB, and Fries JF. Postponed development of disability in elderly runners: A 13-year longitudinal study. *Arch Intern Med.* 2002;162(20):2285–2294.

Weuve J, Kang JH, Manson JE, Breteler MM, Ware JH, and Grodstein F. Physical activity, including walking, and cognitive function in older women. *JAMA.* 2004;292(12):1454–1461.

Wimo A, Jonsson L, and Winblad B. An estimate of the worldwide prevalence and direct costs of dementia in 2003. *Dement Geriatr Cogn Disord.* 2006;21(3):175–181.

Woollacott MH. Systems contributing to balance disorders in older adults. *J Gerontol A Biol Sci Med Sci.* 2000;55(8):M424–M428.

Woollacott MH and Shumway-Cook A. Changes in posture control across the life span—a systems approach. *Phys Ther.* 1990;70(12):799–807.

55 Palliative Care and Neurological Illness: An Approach to Long-term Neurological Conditions and Catastrophic Illness

Mark Stillman and Patricia Scripko

Introduction

In the half century following the aftermath of the Second World War, the field of medicine has made remarkable advances. The world has witnessed the medical sciences emerging from a position of unsubstantiated folk remedies, distorted theories on the genetics of races, and therapeutic impotence in the face of bacterial hordes to one where life can be prolonged on artificial life support systems in critical care units and the human genetic code has been sequenced in its entirety! In spite of such miraculous discoveries and the exponential growth of knowledge, human life remains finite, and man is condemned to the same mortal fate as his earliest hominid ancestors. The exuberant optimism greeting the quantum leaps in scientific knowledge has been accompanied by a glaring myopia and inability to anticipate long-term human needs associated with longevity, advancing age, and the chronic illness that has come to replace infectious diseases as the major cause of mortality.

Death due to such infectious epidemic illnesses as influenza, cholera, tuberculosis, and smallpox has been supplanted by mortality from cancer, atherosclerosis, and degenerative diseases. Included among these diseases are neurological conditions, such as mitochondrial disorders, Parkinson's disease and related movement disorders, the dementing illnesses, neurological malignancies, and progressive neuromuscular diseases. In addition, current (limited) ability to artificially prolong life has introduced clinical situations unimagined before the advent of intensive care units in the late 1950s, leaving clinicians the task of confronting irreversible and catastrophic sequelae of brain injury and stroke.

This chapter will address the therapeutic and ethical challenges to these problems with the understanding that we cannot affect a cure. At best, clinicians can provide comfort for the patient and his caregiver as death approaches. This discussion will also provide an overview of the therapeutic approach to long-term neurological conditions (LTNCs) and will use amyotrophic lateral sclerosis (ALS) as the signature disease to demonstrate the spectrum of care.

Any valid discussion would be incomplete without incorporating the ethical issues involved in care at the end of life. To many, ethics may seem more of a chess game played out in the courts of law, but the field of bioethics abides by universally accepted guidelines which hold the best interests of the patient as an inviolable goal. The astute reader will likely recognize among the ethical blueprints the same principles taught to medical students for generations.

What is Palliative Care?

The World Health Organization defines palliative care as the care offered by a multidisciplinary team of doctors, nurses, social workers, therapists, clergy, and volunteers and describes it as: "The active total care of patients whose disease is not responsive to curative treatment. Control of pain, of other symptoms, and of psychological, social, and spiritual problems is paramount. The goal of palliative care is the achievement of the best quality of life for patients and their families …. Palliative care … affirms life and regards dying as a normal process, … neither hastens nor postpones death, … provides relief from distressing symptoms, … integrates the psychological and the spiritual aspects of care, … offers a support system to help the family cope during the patient's illness and in their own bereavement" (Sepulveda et al. 2002: WHO 1990).

Multidisciplinary refers to the continually interactive nature of care, with patients and caregivers as the focus. Care is coordinated preferably by a team member central to all of the involved services so that care is integrated and as seamless as possible, and the clinical services have numerous opportunities to communicate and interact. The components of a typical palliative care service are listed in Table 1. In the United States, palliative care is predominantly, but not exclusively, a home-based system of care, and its development and refinement have been fostered by the Medicare Hospice Benefit, written into law by Congress in 1982. Regardless of which component of palliative care establishes first contact with a patient with a LTNC, the goals and principles of care are the same: to treat the patient and family, using an approach of interacting services, for the purpose of comfort and symptom relief and to improve quality of life for as long as feasible.

Many medical practitioners and lay people equate palliative care with hospice care, failing to realize that hospice is only one—usually the final—component of palliative care. At least in the United States, and as written into the Medicare Hospice Benefit mentioned above, hospice care is a form of home-based palliative care that a patient and family elect when life expectancy is limited to six months or less and the patient is home-bound. Among thought leaders in the field, palliative care is considered the management of both anticipated and unanticipated complications of a disease during a serious disease's entire course or trajectory (Doyle 1998; American Academy of Neurology Ethics and Humanities Subcommittee 1996; Foley and Carver 2001). Moreover, palliative care techniques and personnel should be involved as soon as a serious illness is diagnosed, whether or not cure is a possibility (Doyle 1998). This approach applies to the diagnosis of LTNCs, metastatic cancer, chronic lung disease and refractory cardiac disease, among other diagnoses. Using this construct, hospice is merely the last movement of the palliative care 'symphony' at the end of a patient's life.

A more recent controversy involves whether palliative medicine, the board-certified specialty that practices palliative care, should be a freestanding consultative service or whether competency training should be required for certification in internal medicine and other medical fields directly involved in the care of the critically ill (Reyners, Peters, and van Minnen 2007; Turner-Stokes et al. 2007). Should palliative care be the domain of a specialist or should it be one facet of integrated care within a primary care specialty? An argument can be made that

Table 1 Components of a Palliative Care Service

1. Hospice
   (a) Home-based
   (b) Inpatient or residential
2. Inpatient acute care facility for the management of acute medical or symptom control issues that cannot be managed as an outpatient
3. Inpatient palliative care consultation service for consultation of patients with palliative care issues on surgical and medical services
4. Outpatient consultation services

the complex integration of all the ancillary services required in palliative care can best be served by the initial or primary care service and that reliance on consulting a specialized medical service to oversee home-based, nursing home, or hospital-based palliative care fractures continuity of care (Reyners, Peters, and van Minnen 2007). One study by Turner-Stokes demonstrated the difficulty and seeming reluctance of neurologists, physiatrists, and palliative care specialists to enlist the help of colleagues in each other's particular specialty. The authors suggested the remedy to this might be cross training and the use of nurse specialists with expertise in end-of-life care and management of LTNCs (Turner-Stokes et al. 2007).

Closer scrutiny of this study, done in the United Kingdom, where, by most standards, palliative medicine is a mature and well-organized specialty, reveals perceived deficiencies in end-of-life care. The three signature specialties found close coordination of care to be rare. In particular, neurologists and rehabilitation specialists noted a shortage of palliative care facilities, limited access to palliative care consultation other than phone consultation, insufficient number of therapists in hospice or palliative care wards, or a lack of interest on the part of palliative care specialists in patients with non-cancer diagnoses. In their own right, the palliative care clinicians perceived a lack of adequate training and resources in management of LTNCs. Physiatrists felt palliative care specialists were lacking in skills for managing the more gradual decline of health in LTNCs. And all specialties saw inadequate support for neurology patients in the community with regards to nursing and social care, rehabilitation support, and residential domiciliary placement (Turner-Stokes et al. 2007).

Palliative Care in the U.S.

Palliative care in the United States was designed to aid patients and their caregivers in the dying process, preferably in the comfort of the home. In its nascent stage, palliative care was synonymous with hospice and the patients almost always carried the diagnosis of cancer. Curative modes of care were abandoned or rejected and a hospice liaison, usually a home-care or hospice nurse, served as the manager of all comfort care needs, with the medical and prescriptive back-up of a physician. As designed, the nurse, however, was an intermittent visitor, while the main day-to-day caregiver was either a family member or a surrogate (a hired nurse, nurse's aide, or a significant other). This caregiver's workload could be supplemented at times, when respite was required, by a nurse's aide from the hospice or palliative care team.

The field witnessed greater expansion in the 1980s with the development of hospital-based and residential palliative care programs at a handful of institutions, eventually growing in time to exceed 1200 such sites by the year 2000. Perhaps reflecting financial difficulties among

the population or a more pervasive breakdown of the nation's social safety net, the palliative care community had recognized the need to create residential or domiciliary units for those patients without a home or competent caregivers.

Long-term Neurological Conditions

In recent years there has been a trend for cancer patients to be joined by non-cancer patients with such irreversible diseases as refractory heart failure, chronic lung disease, and long-term neurological conditions. To this, another group of patients (and caregivers/family members) has been added: patients with irreversible acute neurological diseases such as coma, locked-in syndrome, and persistent vegetative state. While not classified as long-term neurological conditions, these afflictions warrant the particular skills and ethical training of palliative care practitioners. They will be discussed separately. A list of all of the neurological disorders under discussion in this chapter can be found in Table 2 (Turner-Stokes et al. 2006; Birch and Draper 2008; Klager and Duckett 2008; Gillick and Volandes 2008; Mitchell 2007; Volicer, McKee, and Hewitt 2001; Owens and Flom 2005; Ben-Zacharia and Lublin 2001).

In contrast to Europe, where the origins of hospice care can be traced to the Crusades, the United States is a latecomer. In Europe, medical schools have established departments of palliative medicine, whereas palliative medicine only became an American board-certified medical subspecialty in the late 1990s. Educators in medical and nursing schools are only now fully recognizing the role of palliative care as a field of medicine dedicated to patients with advanced disease and their caregivers. In comparison to another relative newcomer and related specialty—the field of pain management—palliative medicine remains relatively neglected if one peruses its coverage in standard nursing and medical textbooks as a gauge of its importance (Neatherlin and Fox 2006; Ferrell, Viran, and Grant 1996).

In the area of evidence based medicine (EBM) the field possesses obvious deficiencies and limitations. This is particularly true when comparing outcome research on care for LTNCs to that of cancer, where the crux of palliative care research appears to have been focused. These deficiencies appeared to be anchored to limitations in the applicability of research techniques to LTNCs compared with those applied to acute medical illnesses and non-neurological terminal illnesses. This fact can be explained by the following characteristics of LTNCs: (1) different and more protracted medical outcomes; (2) limited availability of outcome metrics; (3) difficulties with long-term outcome prognostication; and (4) different disabilities resulting from the particular neurological illnesses (Turner-Stokes et al. 2006).

Core Services Provided by a Palliative Care Service

Whether provided in the home, the hospital, or a different residential setting, palliative care should provide a spectrum of services. This is incorporated in the Medicare Hospice Benefit in the U.S. and is relatively uniform in countries where hospice and palliative care are practiced (Foley and Carver 2001). Table 3 itemizes these core services as adapted from Turner-Stokes et al. who more specifically address the care needs of patients with LTNCs (Turner-Stokes et al. 2007).

Naturally, the team approach to a patient, his family and caregivers, and his disease will differ from patient to patient and situation to situation. This individualized approach is one of the strengths of the multidisciplinary or interdisciplinary approach to care. It allows the interplay of different opinions and approaches to a problem. With LTNCs, the various presentations and trajectories of disease progression allow for a

Table 2 Long-term Neurological Conditions and Illnesses Amenable to Palliative Care

I. Progressive and degenerative illnesses

  a. Dementias—cortical and subcortical

    i. Alzheimer's disease

    ii. Frontotemporal dementias

    iii. Creutzfeld-Jacob disease and other spongiform encephalopathies

    iv. Huntington's disease

    v. Spinocerebellar degenerations

    vi. Paraneoplastic encephalitis and other encephalopathies related to cancer and its treatment

  b. Neuromuscular diseases

    i. Amyotrophic lateral sclerosis and other motor neuron diseases

    ii. Progressive and inherited neuropathies

    iii. Progressive muscular dystrophies and myopathies

  c. Basal ganglial disease and movement disorders

    i. Parkinson's disease

    ii. Lewy body disease

    iii. Multiple systems atrophy and syndromes of autonomic failure

    iv. Dystonic disorders

  d. Mitochondrial disorders

  e. Nervous system neoplastic disorders

    i. Glioblastoma and gliomatosis

    ii. Meningial carcinomatosis

    iii. Paraneoplastic disorders

    iv. Neurofibromatosis

    v. Primary CNS lymphoma

  f. CNS infections

    i. HIV-AIDS

    ii. Prion diseases

II. 'Static' neurological illnesses and the sequelae of catastrophic neurological events

  a. Coma—traumatic and non-traumatic

  b. Persistent vegetative state

  c. Locked-in syndrome

wide array of approaches clinically. Clinical care of end-stage dementias, for example, is more often than not reduced to end-of-life care of a patient with a severely depressed mental status. In such a situation, the palliative care team more closely resembles an ICU team dealing with catastrophic neurological injury, such as anoxic brain injury or a massive intracerebral bleed with herniation, than a geriatric or other chronic care team. The similarities are apparent enough that the issue

of medical futility and supervised withdrawal of care is applicable to both groups of patients and will be discussed in a later section.

In contrast, the approach to the neuromuscular LTNCs, where cerebral degeneration plays less of a role, demands different skills. ALS stands out in this respect as an invariably fatal illness sparing cognition and the patient's decision making capacity. That is not to say palliative care of the ALS patient comes without ethical dilemmas. Quite the contrary, ALS will be used as a model in exercising a specific plan of palliative care. It will complement the approach to the comatose and cognitively damaged patient, with its own ethical issues.

ALS as an Example of an LTNC

What has been written about palliative management of ALS has been derived from small studies, but the work is thoughtful and applicable to LTNCs as a whole. Certain principles of care—universal principles of care for any patient population—have been published by several concerned organizations, including the American Academy of Neurology and Promoting Excellence in the End-of-Life Care, and are itemized here (American Academy of Neurology Ethics and Humanities Subcommittee 1996; Completing the Continuum of ALS Care 2004; Miller et al. 1996).

- Open communication between health care practitioners with patient and family

- Good nursing care, with particular attention paid to body positioning to prevent skin breakdown in the bed-bound patient

- Awareness that most ALS patients have a normal mental status even when they are unable to communicate

- Special attention to facilitation of communication, swallowing, and breathing

- Anticipation of consequences of immobility: constipation, pain, anxiety and depression, insomnia, fatigue, bedsores, and urinary retention.

It cannot be overemphasized that recipients of care include not only the persons with ALS but also their family and primary caregivers. Considering that the progression of ALS implies an inevitable dependence in toileting, eating, and such seemingly mundane tasks as changing position in bed or even scratching an itch, failure to recognize the physical and psychological stresses on the caregiver is an egregious oversight (McDonald et al. 1994; Norris, Smith, and Denys 1985; O'Brien, Kelly, and Saunders 1992; Chio et al. 2005; Rabkin, Wagner,

Table 3 Core Services for Patients with LTNCs

1. Clinical assessment and diagnosis

2. Control of disease, progression, and prevention of medical complications

3. Symptom management

4. Physical and occupational therapy

5. Provision of physical aids and equipment to maintain activities of daily living

6. Coordination of support services

7. Social and psychological support

8. Spiritual support

9. Management of the dying process

10. Bereavement of surviving caregiver(s) and family

(After Turner-Stokes et al. 2007)

and Del Bene 2000; Goldstein et al. 2006). The inclusion of psychiatric social workers, specially trained nurses, home health aides, volunteers, and respite time (brief hospital admissions to allow a family under stress a period of rest) in the benefit package under the Medicare Hospice Benefit indicates that the hospice–palliative care approach anticipates such problems.

Communicating with the Patient and Caregiver

Like any seriously ill patient, the person with ALS is in danger of sudden fatal deterioration resulting from respiratory failure or intercurrent medical complications. The family needs to be informed of this from the outset in order to make an informed decision about the level of care in such a circumstance. Involved in this decision is a consideration of cardiopulmonary resuscitation and placement of an endotracheal tube for ventilation, as well as the the possibility of surgical insertion of a breathing tube (tracheostomy) for long-term respiratory support if desired by the patient. Some ALS patients choose to have a tracheostomy to help them breathe when diaphragmatic and chest wall muscles weaken to the point that independent breathing is no longer possible. Failure to anticipate such emergencies can lead to the imposition of unwanted treatment by emergency medical staff.

Symptom control

Table 4 lists the symptoms that most commonly plague the patient with ALS and that present a challenge to the palliative care or hospice team. These will be discussed briefly below, with references for the interested reader.

Pain

Although classic neurology textbooks regard pain as an uncommon symptom of ALS, the fact is that as many as two-thirds of all patients may experience pain. The pain is described as aching, cramping, or burning, and it may be attributed to either muscle cramps, abnormal stress on the musculoskeletal system from immobility (e.g., bedsores, stiff joints), or spasticity (increased muscle tone) from involvement of the upper motor neuron tracts.

Clearly, good nursing care is important, with frequent positioning and passive mobilization of joints. That may be all that is needed for some patients, but pain medications are necessary for others. The pharmacologic treatment of spasticity and stiffness is limited. Baclofen and tizanidine both work in the spinal cord to inhibit spasticity and muscle stiffness around a joint, but they do so at the expense of sedation and weakness. For those patients who rely on their spasticity to walk, the drug-induced weakness can be a problem. Diazepam and other muscle relaxants may be tried for spasticity but are probably better used for muscle cramps. However, their side effects and cost make them a second choice to baclofen. Other medications such as

Table 4 Symptoms Common to Patients with ALS

- Pain
- Dysphagia
- Drooling
- Dyspnea
- Weakness
- Bedsores
- Inability to sleep
- Anxiety and depression
- Constipation

dantrolene sodium have been used for ALS-related muscle spasms and spasticity, but they are used less frequently because of side effects.

When specific attempts to treat the pain fail, the use of pain medications should follow the guidelines established by the World Health Organization for cancer pain and acute pain (Miaskowski et al. 2005; Jacox et al. 1994). The "stepladder" approach, as it has come to be known, started with the recognition of pain and the initiation of treatment with a drug suited to the type of pain the patient described. Mild pain was treated with low doses of an opioid medication or an appropriately strong non-opioid analgesic. As the pain increased, either a stronger opioid replaced the initial weaker analgesic or a larger dose of the opioid was added (Jacox et al. 1994). This sequential step approach has more recently been supplanted by a stratified care approach that does not rely on sequential therapeutic trials before advancing to stronger opioid analgesics; it attempts to match the pain as the patient describes it at the bedside to the appropriately potent opioid with as little delay as possible. This is especially important for situations where quality time is limited.

The successful management of pain depends on the clinician's familiarity and understanding of the mechanism of pain and the appropriate use of analgesics, frequently in combinations. The use of opioids requires the experience and skill to balance beneficial effects with side effects, and is described, in detail, in the above mentioned references (Miaskowski et al. 2005; Jacox et al. 1994) and in this book in Chapter 51.

It is essential to mention that the use of opioid analgesics in practice, particularly in patients with compromised respiratory status, requires a working knowledge and familiarity with drug interactions, and opioid pharmacokinetics and pharmacodynamics. When asked how to treat the patient with ALS suffering from pain, any seasoned pain practitioner would invariably stress the importance of starting "low and going slow," with frequent observations at time of peak effect for analgesia and adverse effects but aggressive titration of the dose to the pain. If the primary care physician has any concerns or doubt, it is always advisable to err on the side of patient safety and ask for help from someone who is more experienced, especially in the situation where respiratory compromise is a possibility.

Dysphagia

Dysphagia is a common symptom of ALS and occasionally is the presenting symptom. The problem extends not only to foods but also to a patient's own secretions, resulting in the embarrassment of drooling. Weakness of the striated muscle—the tongue, pharyngeal muscles, and the upper esophagus—makes chewing and propulsion of food to the back of the throat and the esophagus increasingly difficult, leading to pooling of secretions and foodstuffs. Liquids, in particular, follow the quickest and most direct route directed by gravity, leading to aspiration down the trachea, and followed by reflexive coughing ("choking"). As a consequence, oral intake decreases and weight loss ensues because of the fear of choking or exhaustion from coughing spells (Newall, Orser, and Hunt 1996).

There are several approaches to this problem. The first and simplest approach is to alter the texture of the food under the guidance of a dietitian who is familiar with swallowing disorders. Under the Medicare Hospice Benefit, a speech pathologist trained to evaluate swallowing disorders should be available on an as-needed basis. Blenderized food or food thickened with starch will enable many people to get the liquid and calories needed to maintain weight, initially. Other options are now available. Previously, nasogastric tubes were placed into the stomach for feeding purposes, but patients found them uncomfortable, they were frequently dislodged and brought with them the risk of aspiration. Several procedures to deal with the problem of feeding people who cannot swallow have been developed in the past 15 years, including percutaneous endoscopic gastrostomy (PEG) and, less commonly, percutaneous endoscopic jejunostomy (PEJ). Feedings with clear liquids can safely commence within 24 to 48 hours of endoscopic (fiberoptic) tube placement through the abdominal wall, gradually building up to 100% supplementation of caloric needs through the use of commercial liquid diets (Mathus-Vliegen et al. 1994).

The widespread use of the PEG/PEJ tube feeding has led to symptomatic improvement in the population with ALS—less "choking" to be certain—but has not led to prolongation of survival when compared with NG feeding. Moreover, the procedure of inserting the tube is not without complications, and there may be abdominal wall pain severe enough to warrant opioid therapy for the first 24 to 48 hours. Even in the most experienced hands, there is a 1% to 4% 24-hour postoperative mortality resulting from pulmonary complications; postprocedural pain leads to abdominal splinting and places patients at great risk for developing pneumonia, pulmonary embolus, and respiratory failure. As a result, it is recommended that patients be considered candidates for PEG tube placement *earlier* rather than later—when weight loss approaches 5% and bulbar symptoms (dysphagia, dysarthria, or aspiration of oral secretions) first develop. Patients should have preoperative pulmonary function tests to document enough reserve lung function to mount an adequate cough.

The patient's and family's reluctance to submit to a surgical procedure in favor of more natural feeding methods frequently delays this procedure. When the patient finally agrees, it often is too late to reverse the weight loss or avoid the perioperative complications. Every effort should therefore be made to perform placement of a percutaneous feeding tube relatively early in the course of the disease if the patient and his family are willing.

Drooling

Drooling is an embarrassing and distressing symptom that results from a patient's inability to swallow saliva often enough to prevent oral overflow. Beyond the obvious use of a handkerchief, control of drooling requires drying out or suppressing the salivary glands. Surgical and radiotherapeutic control of salivation has been attempted, but medicinal manipulation is usually just as effective. A number of drugs may be useful.

Anticholinergic agents such as scopolamine hydrochloride and medications with anticholinergic side effects are frequently used to control drooling. A scopolamine patch used to treat motion sickness provides a convenient way to dry the mouth without the need to ingest yet another pill. This 1-mg patch is placed on the skin, usually behind the ear (but can be placed on any glabrous skin), and is left in place for three days. Anticholinergic antidepressants such as amitriptyline, nortriptyline, or desipramine predictably cause dry mouth as a side effect, even in doses as low as 10 mg per day. These agents have additional benefits such as pain relief, appetite stimulation, and the treatment of depression. Two other useful agents are propranolol and lithium.

An important caveat is that saliva is essential not only for food ingestion but also for dental maintenance and health. The loss of the protective effect of salivary antibodies against bacteria increases the risk of tooth decay; good dental hygiene is therefore essential.

Dyspnea and Respiratory Compromise

The sensation of shortness of breath is a serious and feared symptom in ALS. In general medical practice, there are numerous causes of dyspnea, including pneumonia, chronic lung disease (e.g., emphysema, chronic bronchitis), congestive heart failure, venous thromboembolism, and asthma. Although a person with ALS can have any of these, the progressive muscle weakness that accompanies the disease causes patients with ALS to develop restricted ability to breath. Simply stated, they neither have the chest wall strength nor mobility to take deep breaths. Portions of the lung may therefore collapse and pneumonia may develop. Patients describe a force or a weight restricting their ability to take a deep breath or to fully empty their lungs. The great fear is "choking" or "suffocating" to death.

Initial medical management should be directed at correcting any potentially reversible cause. This should include (a) controlling secretions and preventing regurgitation of tube feedings; (b) optimizing the patient's position in bed to minimize any chance of aspiration and maximize the ability of the diaphragm to function properly; (c) providing oxygen when needed; and (d) treating lung infections, bronchitis, or asthma. When these options fail or do not exist, the only therapeutic choices are to provide mechanical ventilation for the patient or to suppress the symptoms of breathlessness medicinally (i.e., palliative management).

The ultimate consequence of respiratory failure is death as a result of elevated carbon dioxide level (hypercapnea) and decreased oxygen level (hypoxia). If the symptoms accompanying dyspnea—agitation, anxiety, and air hunger—can be controlled, death can be peaceful, with the patient quietly entering a coma. Any agitation can be suppressed with sedative hypnotics. The alternative—the prolongation of life on mechanical ventilation after tracheostomy—is viewed as heroic therapy by many patients, families, and clinicians, merely forestalling the inevitable progression of the disease. It is therefore essential that families and caregivers of patients with ALS be aware of the natural history of ALS from the outset (Completing the Continuum of ALS Care 2004; Miller et al. 1999).

Symptoms indicating the approaching need of ventilatory support include disrupted sleep, orthopnea, daytime sleepiness, dyspnea with exertion, ineffective cough, and less than 50% of the predicted ability to exhale (forced vital capacity, FVC). All too often patients and families confront impending respiratory failure without prior knowledge of treatment options. In particular, they may not be aware that the patient can receive breathing support from a closely fitting mask, an endotracheal tube, or even a tracheostomy. A patient who is mechanically ventilated with an endotracheal tube for more than two weeks will eventually need a tracheostomy because the trachea's endothelium develops necrosis from the tamponade pressures of the endotracheal tube's balloon cuff for longer periods. One recent study found that 92% of patients who were on mechanical ventilator machines after tracheostomy had not decided in advance to undergo intubation and artificial respiration. Almost one-third were not satisfied with their quality of life as respirator-dependent patients. Sadly, many patients would not have opted for mechanical ventilation if they had known of the financial and social burdens placed on their families or if they had known they would have to go to a skilled nursing unit (Moss et al. 1993).

The alternative to tracheostomy and ventilation is noninvasive ventilation (NIV) using a tight-fitting nasal mask or face mask (Moss et al. 1993; Cazzolli and Oppenheimer 1996). This is an adequate option if the patient can tolerate the mask, has no problems managing secretions, and does not aspirate. Patients who have poor airway protection are at risk of aspiration with this ventilation technique.

Nasal NIV is therefore indicated for willing patients who do not have brain stem dysfunction (i.e., altered swallowing mechanisms) and who do not need suction. It is covered under the Medicare Hospice Benefit, costs less, and is associated with less complex care than mechanical ventilation and tracheostomy. More than 90% of patients are able to stay at home on NIV (Cazzolli and Oppenheimer 1996).

Symptomatic Treatment of Dyspnea

There are well-described techniques for the relief of dyspnea, borrowed from intensive care medicine, where these approaches are routinely used for people with cardiac or pulmonary dysfunction. The benefits of opioid analgesics have been amply demonstrated for the treatment of air hunger of cardiac pulmonary edema (severe heart failure). When given in small intravenous injections, morphine reduces shortness of breath and the inflated filling pressures of a flooded heart in heart failure. Oral preparations of morphine sulfate and morphine-related narcotics have been used in a similar manner and given on a round-the-clock basis for constant shortness of breath. The few studies that confirm the utility of opioids in dyspneic patients have demonstrated improved exercise tolerance for patients suffering from chronic obstructive lung disease.

Recent interest in inhaled or nebulized opioids has led to their increased use for patients with end-stage disease and associated breathlessness. The benefit of nebulized or aerosolized drug is its direct delivery to the sites (and presumably the receptors) where it is needed. Systemic absorption and side effects are limited (Floral et al. 2004). Despite few data in ALS, and the official recommendation not to use opioids for this purpose without more valid confirmatory studies, morphine sulfate and other drugs are being used in handheld nebulizers at the bedside with seemingly good results (Westphal and Campbell 2002). Even with nebulized drugs, there are concerns about side effects, especially respiratory depression in patients with impaired ventilatory function and there have been anecdotal reports of respiratory depression with nebulized morphine. In cases where nebulized morphine has been associated with wheezing, fentanyl or hydromorphone have been used successfully.

Other medications have been useful in treating dyspnea and associated anxiety. Sedative hypnotics have been used for years in the intensive care unit to treat agitated ventilated patients when the agitation interferes with ventilation. Benzodiazepines (diazepam, lorazepam, midazolam) and barbiturates have all been used in this situation. There has been recent interest in the phenothiazines, a class of drugs designed for the treatment of agitated psychoses. Their use has now been extended to the agitation caused by dyspnea.

Bedsores

Bedsores, or decubitus ulcers, are a common complication of immobility, although they are relatively rare in patients with ALS. Frequent turning and positioning in bed is needed to prevent them from developing, and special beds using airflow or continuously moving pellets have been designed for patients with ALS, spinal cord injury, and Guillain-Barré syndrome. Once a decubitus ulcer develops, however, meticulous attention must be paid to keeping pressure off the wound so that blood flow returns and airflow around the wound is maximized. Dead tissue must be removed and infection treated with dressing changes and wound cleaning; only in this way can new skin grow in and surgical grafting be avoided.

Constipation

Constipation is common in ALS, even though the disease does not affect the smooth muscle function in the bowel wall. Immobility and drugs such as opioids induce constipation. When this problem is combined with the patient's inability to self-toilet, it can create exceedingly unpleasant, painful and humiliating situations. As for patients without ALS, the treatment of constipation should follow a stepped approach starting with the maintenance of bowel hydration through the use of food fiber and adequate liquids as well as the institution of a set pattern of bowel elimination. A daily rectal suppository or a phosphosoda enema may help regulate the bowels, and stool softeners such as docusate should be used daily. For more severe constipation, cathartics

such as magnesium compounds (milk of magnesia or magnesium citrate) or senna pills may be started on a regular basis. If persistent constipation is anticipated, especially with the use of opioid analgesics, the addition of other agents may be necessary. Osmotic agents that induce bowel motions, such as lactulose or 70% sorbitol, can be very effective for the most resistant cases of drug-induced constipation.

Insomnia

Many people with ALS complain of an inability to fall asleep. The first task is to correct any reversible causes such as pain and dyspnea. Many agents are now available for the treatment of depression and anxiety. Once again, the tricyclic antidepressants are effective agents for depression, and their side effects of sedation, dry mouth, and appetite stimulation can be useful. Their efficacy surpasses that of the new agents in the selective serotonin reuptake inhibitor (SSRIs; fluoxetine, citalopram, paroxetine, and sertraline) and selective norepinephrine reuptake inhibitor classes (SNRIs; venlafaxine and duloxetine), which tend to interfere with sleep in non-depressed patients. The antipsychotic chlorpromazine, along with the newer atypical antipsychotic agents (olanzepine and quetiapine) are excellent medications for inducing sleep as well as relieving agitation, nausea, and vomiting.

Depression in Patients and Caregivers

It comes as no surprise that delivery of a diagnosis of ALS exacts an enormous emotional toll, affecting the psychological, somatic, and existential well-being of the patient (Chio et al. 2005; Rabkin, Wagner, and Del Bene 2000; Goldstein et al. 2006). Recent attention has been paid to the effect of ALS on the patient's primary caregiver, with some interesting revelations. One would expect patients with ALS to bear the major brunt of receiving the diagnosis of an incurable disease, but surprisingly, one study found a relatively low level of depression among the patients. However, there was a high correlation between depression in the patients' caregivers and depression in the patients themselves, suggesting that more attention paid to the caregivers' mental health would be rewarded in improvements in the patient with ALS. What determined the level of distress in the caregiver happened to be the appreciation of deteriorating quality of life in the patient and the perception of isolation and a loss of social support (Goldstein et al. 2006).

Recent major advances in the drug therapy for depression promise benefit to both groups. The SSRIs have few side effects and work relatively quickly and the SNRIs not only provide rapid treatment of depression but also analgesia. However, drugs alone are frequently not the answer, and the multidisciplinary approach of palliative medicine and hospice anticipates the impact of serious illness, not only on the patient but also on the family. Built into the services provided, particularly under the Medicare Hospice Benefit, are social work, clergy, respite care, home health care while the patient is alive, and bereavement counseling during the illness and for a full year after death.

Once again, the major benefit of a multidisciplinary approach, embodied in palliative medicine and hospice care, is total care, including mental health care, of the patient and his caregiver(s) during the trajectory of the illness.

Palliative Care, Biomedical Ethics, and the Care for the Patient with a Catastrophic Neurological Illness

Any chapter on the palliative care of long-term neurological conditions would be incomplete without a discussion of the issues surrounding the management of the individual with an irreparably damaged brain. There are several reasons for this. First, as mentioned above, many of the LTNCs in both adults and children exhibit clinical courses that inevitably reduce the patient to a vegetative state, with no hopes of recovery to an independent functioning state. Secondly, the approach clinicians must take to keep the LTNC patient and his caregivers informed requires the same skills and acumen physicians use to inform loved ones in critical care situations. Finally in palliative care, clinicians and caregivers must frequently confront difficult bioethical decisions regarding futility and withdrawal of aggressive medical approaches. Another way of looking at it, critical care illness (Intensive Care Unit, Trauma Unit) clinicians adopt palliative care techniques and principles in catastrophic situations where death is imminent or has occurred, but unlike palliative care physicians, they do not have the same 'luxury' of time to establish a working relationship with the family.

The four governing bioethical principles are (Randall and Downie 1996):

♦ Patient autonomy and right to decide
♦ Beneficence
♦ Nonmaleficence
♦ Distributive justice.

The principle of **patient autonomy** is the ethical equivalent to the legal right to self determination. It includes the right to request or refuse life sustaining treatment, and must abide by the doctrine of informed consent and refusal. This, in turn, includes the conveyance of adequate information to the patient by the clinician, the ability to decide (i.e., the competence of the patient), and the freedom from coercion or undue outside influence. Competency, or the medical ability to make an informed decision, is determined by a psychiatrist or a neurologist (Westphal and Campbell 2002; Randall and Downie 1996). In cases where the patient is deemed incompetent, such as a comatose, confused (encephalopathic), or demented patient or a patient in a persistent vegetative state, surrogates are authorized to act on behalf of the patient in providing directives for life sustaining treatments.

Beneficence is the principle of looking out for the patient's best interests. This principle dates back to Hippocrates in Greek times and the Knights Hospitallers of the Crusades in the eleventh century. **Nonmaleficence** refers to the directive to do no harm to the patient, or perform any service which in the clinician's opinion provides more potential harm than good. Finally, **distributive justice** dictates that no patient should be denied (the fair distribution of) services or access to care (Floral et al. 2004).

Advance Directives, Living Wills, and Durable Power of Attorney

In the palliative care and critical care unit population, where patients are frequently incapable of making decisions, there are alternative ways for patients to indicate treatment preferences. Advance directives are written documents that permit patients to communicate their preferences should they lose competency later in life. Advance directives were conceptually conceived in 1969 (Bernat 2001). Regrettably, state-to-state variability in legal regulation of directives has created confusion, begging for efforts to not only publicize, but to also standardize, the collection and use of advance directives (Stanley 1992). A federal statute, the Patient Self-Determination Act, mandating that covered medical institutions actively distribute, collect, and honor information on their protocol for handling advance directives, has not been sufficient, suggesting a need for efforts aimed at fixing the protocol, not just publicizing it (Brown 2003). Towards this end, the Uniform Health-Care Decisions Act of 1993 presented a replicable effort worth attention (Daroff 2006). This act clarified the proper collection and

use of advance directives, consent, advance directives, and appointment of durable power of attorneys in a manner that was likely to promote the patient's presumed wishes. Both the AARP and the American Bar Association endorsed this act, but only a fraction of states have adopted it (Stanley 1992).

An alternative to advance directives, albeit an inadequate one, is a living will or terminal care document. In general, a living will is activated only in terminal illness and not in temporary incapacity, but the appointment of a durable power of attorney for health care is more useful. The patient may assign this position to a certain individual; otherwise it is assigned to the patient's legal guardian or spouse and if this position is vacant, then to the oldest adult child.

Defining Human Life and Death at the Bedside

In the late twentieth and early twenty-first century, the media, national and state legislatures, and particularly the clergy have been engrossed in the debate concerning human life's beginning and its end. To the lay audience, defining life's beginnings and its end has proved difficult and the arguments have been based more on religious doctrine than fact and in an open society it is not difficult to see how nonscientific teachings can influence law and social opinion.

In neurology, the controversy in bedside brain death criteria originates from a general disagreement of what is necessary and sufficient to declare one a living human. Although the terminology is misleading, in the U.S. and most European countries *brain death* legally equates to death of the person, not simply the death of the brain in an otherwise living person. The ambiguous nomenclature is a manifestation of historical changes in what may be clinically observed (Daroff 2006). Prior to the nineteenth century, human death was recognized by cessation of breathing, changing in the 1800s to cessation of a heartbeat audible with the recently invented stethoscope. Once mechanical ventilation and resuscitation were introduced, allowing for the previously life-defining cardiopulmonary functions to continue without any integrated neurological input, the concept of brain death as physical death arose (Daroff 2006; Hacke 2006; Mohandas and Chou 1971). Clarified by the Harvard Commission in 1968 (Ad Hoc Committee of the Harvard Medical School 1968), and altered slightly on multiple occasions since (Mohandas and Chou 1971; US Collaborative Study 1997; U.S. President's Commission 1981; Conference of Medical Royal Colleges 1976; Conference of Medical Royal Colleges—Lancet 1976; American Academy of Neurology 1995) (see Daroff 2006 for review), brain death criteria have typically included the following: coma, or total unawareness to external and internal stimuli; cranial arreflexia, no spontaneous breathing (apnea); and a flat EEG, all observed with the exclusion of alternative explanations for the state, including intoxication, metabolic disorders, or hypothermia. (The American Academy of Neurology [1995] requires the absolute finding of the first three abovementioned criteria and their reproducibility after at least 6 hours; it does not require the presence of a flat EEG, as initially described [Ad Hoc Committee of the Harvard Medical School 1968].)

This clinical definition is in accordance with whole brain theorists, who believe the irreversible cessation of both higher and lower brain function is necessary and together sufficient to declare someone a deceased human. Higher and lower brain functions are defined, respectively, as the "capacity to think, to perceive and to respond," (cortical function) and the capacity to "integrate bodily functions" (brain stem function) (Veith et al. 1977). While higher brain theorists argue against the necessity of brain stem function to declare a person living, whole brain criteria remains the gold standard due to both the practical ease of testing brainstem reflexes, in contrast to higher corti-cal function, and to an ethically-seated fear that a less conservative definition may result in misdiagnoses of persons as brain dead who are actually transitioning to an improved neurological state (Bartlett and Youngner 1988; Brierly et al. 1971). In order to fulfill whole brain cri-teria, destruction of neuronal tissue must be so widespread that there is no doubt that the person's state is "irreversible," so that the ethical principle of non-maleficence is upheld (Bernat 2006).

Legal definitions depend on medical criteria, using vague terminol-ogy to provide room for these criteria to change without contradicting the law. The American Bar Association wrote,"for all legal purposes, a human body with irreversible cessation of total brain function….shall be considered dead," leaving medicine to elaborate on the specifics of what constitutes "irreversible" "total" and "function" (Am Bar Assoc Journal 1975).

Technology's Impact on the Definition of (a Valuable) Life

As medical progress creates technology capable of defying death, our understanding of life and death is questioned. Ventilators and resusci-tation machines, dialysis, and more recently organ transplantation, were first introduced into intensive care units in the 1950s and 1960s (Daroff 2006). Since that time, questioning has arisen regarding what defines life from death, and specifically whether machine-dependent life can be considered human life, or at least, a valuable human life. While formulated brain death criteria offered consensus on the defini-tion of death in modern 'high-tech' ICU (Ad Hoc Committee of the Harvard Medical School 1968; Conference of Medical Royal Colleges—Lancet 1976; American Academy of Neurology 1995), these criteria did not offer a consensus on what constitutes a *valuable* life. They left the question, "Is a machine-dependent life worth living?" unanswered.

A valuable human life has been more problematic to define than simply human life, in part because "valuable" is a term with a dichoto-mous meaning. Physicians use it interchangeably with "meaningful" to denote a life below a very high threshold of either suffering or dete-riorated function. For example, a patient with complete loss of higher brain function, in coma or a persistent vegetative state, is considered by most physicians and the prominent representative medical socie-ties, -including the American Academy of Neurology and the American Medical Association- to not be a living a valuable or meaningful life (The Quality Standards Subcommittee of the American Academy of Neurology 1995; Larriviere and Bonnie 2006), accordingly (Ad Hoc Committee of the Harvard Medical School 1968; Conference of Medical Royal Colleges—Lancet 1976; American Academy of Neurology 1989; Council on Scientific Affairs and Council on Ethical and Judicial Affairs 1990).

The first such article was the Ad Hoc Committee of the Harvard Medical School, a seminal article in the history of modern medical bioethics in that it recognized "irreversible coma" as a new criterion for death (Ad Hoc Committee of the Harvard Medical School 1968). However, to some in the lay population and to certain religious groups, it is unacceptable to suggest that *any* human life lacks value, as these groups of religious believers and individuals, unlike physicians, equate a valuable life with "human dignity," something all humans carry from life through death.

Futility and Withdrawal of Care

Futility refers to medical measures that attempt to reverse either an irreversible state of disease or disability in life or an irrevocable pro-gression to death. Such measures cannot sufficiently improve the qual-ity or quantity of life. In accordance with the bioethical principles discussed above, the physician is not ethically obligated to provide these measures (AAN Position Statement 1988), and providing futile care may be seen as antithetical to the wellbeing of others in need of such resources (Truog R and Burns 2007; Truog, Nrett, and Frader 1992). Looking at it in another light, providing care that is futile vio-lates the principle of non-maleficence in many instances. On palliative care services where a "do not resuscitate," status has not been clearly established, providing chest percussion with cardiopulmonary resusci-tation to the patient with widely disseminated bone metastases or a myelophthisic disorder will clearly produce more harm than benefit and is not in the best interests of the patient.

There is reluctance on the part of the general public to accept the reality of futility, in large part due to the lack of a consensus on a prac-tical definition of states or measures that signal futility. This was recently illustrated by the much publicized controversy over the Terri Schiavo case (Racine et al. 2008). Differences in these practical defini-tions are often dependent on the religious beliefs and cultural practices that assign particular restrictions, definitions and priorities to life, death, and medical intervention. Pope John Paul II's late statement in 2004 that artificial nutrition and hydration *is* a basic necessity of life to which all have a right, rather than a medical treatment, as the AAN stated (AAN Position Statement 1988), no doubt impacted the opin-ions of many who ascribe to Catholicism internationally, even though this statement contradicted previously held Catholic views (http://www.ncbcenter.org/JP2-PVS.pdf). In contrast to Catholic convention, it is imbedded in American culture to seek the newest, most expensive new tool, even before it has proven itself effective, and to use this tech-nology to combat death as a disease rather than fate (Callahan 1995). Due to wide variances in religiously and culturally-based views of life, death, and medical intervention, it is necessary for physicians to engage in conversation with patients and families to elicit these beliefs (Koenig and Gates-Williams 1995; O'Connell 1995).

In the practice of palliative medicine today, artificial nutrition and hydration are considered futile efforts in specific circumstances. The American Academy of Neurology (AAN Position Statement 1988) and the American Medical Association (Council on Scientific Affairs and Council on Ethical and Judicial Affairs 1990) have endorsed position statements that relieve physicians of any obligation to provide artificial nutrition and hydration in addition to ventilation, medicine and other medical treatments when such treatments are deemed futile (specifi-cally in the case of PVS patients) by the clinicians attending to the case. The three considerations for physicians, set forth by the AAN in their statement regarding futile care, are as follows (AAN Position Statement 1988):

1. A patient's right to self-determination is central to the medical, ethical and legal principles relevant to medical treatment decisions;

2. A physician must also attempt to promote the patient's well-being, either by relieving suffering or addressing or reversing a pathologic process. Where medical treatment fails to promote a patient's well-being, there is no longer an ethical obligation to provide it; and

3. Treatments which provide no benefit to the patient or the family may be discontinued. Medical treatment, including the medical provision of artificial nutrition and hydration (ANH), provide no benefit to patients in a persistent vegetative state, once the diagnosis has been established to a high degree of medical certainty.

For the patient's family, further complicating this difficult decision are the guilt and self-doubt embodied in the withdrawal of such basics as food and fluids For instance, those relatives and friends consider-ing withdrawal of artificial food and hydration must understand that dying patients do not experience hunger when food and hydration are withdrawn, but rather pass peacefully days to weeks later from metabolic disturbances of potassium, sodium, and chloride (The Quality Standards Subcommittee of the American Academy of Neurology 1995; Larriviere and Bonnie 2006). The Schiavo case, in particular, highlights the public's general misperception of dying by dehydration.

The Principle of Double Effect and Euthanasia: Action Beyond Withdrawal

The doctrine of double effect is an ethically sound concept that is well-understood and accepted in palliative medicine. Simply stated, it addresses the fact that medication, most commonly opioid analgesics, selected for purposes of pain relief, may secondarily lead to respiratory cessation and premature death (Boyle 2004). In the best of worlds this should be discussed with the patient or his medical power of attorney (should the patient not be competent) to attain their consent before potentially lethal doses are given. As such, **the unintentional death of the dying patient as a consequence of aggressive pain and symptom management** (the double effect) is not a form of euthanasia, and is accepted practice in all fifty states.

With acceptance of the double effect and a skillful practitioner, patients may be provided with a significant element of control over their symptoms and suffering, including power over the decision to risk respiratory cessation and death. The physician's duty is to describe the risks and benefits of opioid analgesics and other potentially lethal medications used for palliation of symptoms, documenting the patient's or his proxy's response to this information. In the current medico-legal environment, using the principle of double effect, both patient and family can be left unbridled by the guilt and specter of suicide. In fact, the prudent use of both the principle of double effect and the withdrawal of care considered futile enable the dying individual and/or his family to govern a *patient-assisted death.*

Euthanasia and Patient-assisted Suicide (PAS)

Euthanasia, or mercy killing, is the deliberate attempt to end a patient's life in order to relieve the patient of pain and suffering (Wilkinson 1998). Nowhere in the United States has it been legalized. However, as mentioned above, there are now two states where physician-assisted suicide (PAS) has been legalized as a result of initiatives promoted by the lay community. While a discussion of the benefits and risks of allowing patients to successfully schedule a "pleasant" or "good" death, under the auspices of a primary care physician, is beyond the scope of this chapter, several points can be made.

PAS describes the procedure in which a patient requests, or has requested by virtue of an advance directive, the means to end his life. The primary care physician provides the medications necessary to (peacefully and painlessly) terminate life. In no way is the physician allowed to administer the medication, as this would encompass voluntary euthanasia, which is a crime (Wilkinson 1998). As written into the Oregon law (Or.Rev.Stat. S127.800-879), to initiate the process, the patient must have:

1. A terminal illness with a life expectancy of six months or less, in the opinion of the attending physician (Oregon licensed MD or DO) and another consultant;

2. Intact decision-making capacity, which requires emotional stability, cognitive competence, understanding of the patient's options, and understanding of the diagnosis. This also requires informed consent concerning the risks and benefits of the prescribed

medication. (For an in-depth discussion of competency, the interested reader is directed to Chapter 12.).

3. Freedom from coercion, in the judgment of the attending physician; and

4. Age 18 years or older and a resident of Oregon (http://egov.oregon.gov/DHS/ph/pas/ors.shtml).

There have been concerns by the medical community that PAS would be over-utilized or abused. The difficulties with the legalization of PAS, critics claimed, included:

1. difficulties in prognosticating a survival of six months or less;

2. resorting to PAS without or before earnest attempts at palliative care/hospice;

3. failing to recognize depression or other psychiatric disorder; and

4. coercion by an outside party or family member to opt for PAS.

To many clinicians, these deficiencies in the process fueled a strong ethical argument against PAS unless very strict safeguards were observed. Now more than 15 years after the law's passage, and careful record keeping by the state (mandated by law) (http://egov.oregon.gov/DHS/ph/pas/ors.shtml), these fears have not been realized. However, careful scrutiny of the record has unearthed a small number of cases where patients were depressed, were 'successfully' administered PAS, but had never received formal psychiatric intervention (Ganzini, Goy, and Dobscha 2008). This occurred in spite of the mandatory confirmatory second consultation, driving home the fact that primary care clinicians are regrettably all too often inadequately trained to recognize mental disorders, including depression (Stillman and Rybicki 2001; Chochinov et al. 1995).

The discussion, then, returns to ALS where patients have both a debilitating, terminal disease and usually the cognitive competence to make decisions regarding end-of-life care. The records from Oregon, not surprisingly, document a large percentage of patients with ALS requesting PAS (http://egov.oregon.gov/DHS/ph/pas/ors.shtml; Ganzini et al. 1998). This, of course, comes as no surprise to many; as recently as 1998, a large survey showed that 56% of patients with ALS admitted to considering assisted suicide, and nearly 90% would reconsider it if it were legalized. Three-fourths of all caregivers concurred (Ganzini et al. 1998). With ALS and other LTNCs, approaching patients and families about the options for care, limited though they may be, will test the interpersonal and communication skills as well as the cultural awareness and sensitivity of the practitioner.

Communicating with the Patient and Family: Disclosing Diagnosis, Prognosis and Deciding on Treatment and Palliative Options

Two discordant views dominate the literature concerning communicating bad news. The first, "titratable disclosure," attempts to maintain the patient's hope by not disclosing poor prognostic information, whereas the second, referred to as "necessary collusion," attempts to honor what remains of the patient's abilities to make an informed decision.

Hope provides an important means to improve patients' well-being by mitigating worry and stress. Iatrogenic hopelessness is perceived by some in the field to be so damaging as to justify withholding information in certain cases (Da Silva et al. 2003; Helft 2005). The experienced oncologist will readily admit, when dealing with malignant disease, no population statistic is an accurate predictor of an individual patient's disease trajectory and attempts at prognosticating the timing of a patient's death are fraught with error. By offering hope, the physician may prevent emotionally harmful responses to stress that come from knowing the truth, among them alterations of hormones, such as cortisol, growth hormone, sex steroids, leptin, and others, in addition to neurotransmitters. Furthermore, prolonged stress can result in situational depression and markedly decreased life span and quality of life.

Complete disclosure of information, done for the sake of preserving patient autonomy, is considered ethically sound practice (Kirkland 2007). Clinical honesty ensures that decisions are based on the individual's wishes. Few argue this point, except to note two things: first that full disclosure may not be necessary to make informed decisions, and that the importance of hope outweighs the potential loss of hope that follows full disclosure (Kutner et al. 1999; Gold 2004). Kutner et al. showed that patients and families value honesty from their health care providers, but this varied in the extent of detailed prognostic information they wished to receive, fueling arguments over maintaining hope versus providing full, honest prognostic information (Kutner et al. 1999). Importantly, patients' perceptions of hope and honesty are culturally-dependent, behooving the clinician to thoroughly familiarize himself with his patients and their backgrounds (Koenig and Gates-Williams 1995; Gold 2004).

A bridge may be constructed between honesty in disclosure and hope. This bridge, which we call "titratable disclosure," varies in quantity, quality, and temporal characteristics based on the patient's desires and needs. An example of this method is as follows: The physician begins by delivering the diagnosis of ALS and telling a patient of his duty as physician to inform the patient about the disease so that the patient can properly make medical and life decisions. Then, the physician follows this statement with a question to the patient as to how much and what type (i.e., general, statistical, etc) of information he currently would like. Since ALS is a slowly progressive disease with a known outcome, not all information must be disclosed at the time of diagnosis, as treatment decisions need not be made immediately. Eventually, however, the patient will receive all prognostic information, and the physician will fulfill his duty and encourage disclosure and discussion (Da Silva et al. 2003; Kodish and Post 1995).

Similar to "titratable disclosure," is the method of "necessary collusion," as espoused by Helft (Helft 2005). In this model, the physician provides information only when directed to do so by the patient, and it assumes that the patient who does not specifically inquire may wish not to know. Necessary collusion, unlike the method of titratable disclosure, does not require that all information eventually be disclosed. Similar to a "Don't ask, don't tell" policy, necessary collusion is problematic since patients may want more information than they have asked for. Kutner et al. found that 21% of patients only wanted information regarding their prognosis if they asked directly (Kutner et al. 1999). This left 79% of patients in this study wanting prognostic information beyond the physician's responses to their direct inquiries, making such a policy insufficient to meet patients' needs (Kutner et al. 1999).

Both necessary collusion and titratable disclosure permit information to surface gradually, at a speed consistent with a patient's ability to cope. In doing this, a physician may also employ techniques that modify the way information is portrayed. For instance, the technique of "forecasting" in the delivery of bad news, as explained by the sociologist Douglas Maynard (Maynard 1996) may be used. This method results in "deeply collaborative, orderly achievement," making the bad news more tolerable to the receiver, the patient. Essentially, the patient is being desensitized to poor prognosis. In sum, physicians and patients must engage in a cooperative relationship that allows information to be portrayed in such a way that the patient is provided time to cope,

provided a means to understand and decide, and most importantly, provided support from the physician as their ally.

Conclusion

The march of progress in medical therapeutics has ushered in an era where patients are surviving illnesses they would have died from a half century ago. But cheating death comes with a heavy cost. Neurologists now find themselves capable of salvaging patients from diseases after the pathological process has exacted an enormous toll on quality of life. This leaves the patient with disabilities that family and caregivers frequently find catastrophic. It is neurologists' shared desire that our field of medicine discover effective therapies to successfully abort and reverse the pathological process and spare patients both morbidity and mortality.

Since we are not there yet, neurologists will continue to find themselves the stewards of desperately ill patients who are rapidly approaching death. The best we have to offer is palliation of symptoms and emotional support for both caregivers and patients. This chapter attempted to review the methods of palliative care for long-term neurological conditions. At the same time, it reviewed the bioethics involved in dealing with end-of-life issues. Virtually all neurologists will deal with these issues at some time during their careers, and experience proves to be the greatest teacher. What we have tried to do is introduce the reader to the major concepts so that he may avoid many of the mine fields.

References

http://www.ncbcenter.org/JP2-PVS.pdf Or.Rev.Stat. S127.800–879.

http://egov.oregon.gov/DHS/ph/pas/ors.

AAN Position Statement adopted on April 21, 1988. Available online at http://www.aan.com/about/ethics/109556.pdf.

Ad Hoc Committee of the Harvard Medical School. A definition of irreversible coma. *JAMA*. 1968. 205:337–340.

American Academy of Neurology. Practice parameters for determining brain death in adults. *Neurology* 1995;45:1012–1014.

American Academy of Neurology Ethics and Humanities Subcommittee. Palliative care in neurology. *Neurology* 1996;46:870–872.

American Academy of Neurology. The Quality Standards Subcommittee of the American Academy of Neurology. Practice parameters: Assessment and management of patients in the persistent vegetative state (summary statement). *Neurology* 1995; 45:1015–1018.

American Academy of Neurology. Position of the American Academy of Neurology on certain aspects of the care and management of the persistent vegetative state patient. Adopted by the Executive Board, American Academy of Neurology, April 21, 1988, Cincinnati, Ohio. *Neurology*. 1989;39:125–126.

Bartlett E and Youngner S. Human death and the destruction of the neocortex. In: Zaner RN (ed.), *Death: Beyond whole-brain criteria*. Dordrecht: Kluwer Academic Publishers. 1988. pp 199–215.

Beauchamp T and Childress J. 2001. *Principles of biomedical ethics*. 5th edition. New York: Oxford University Press.

Ben-Zacharia A and Lublin FD. Palliative care in patients with multiple sclerosis. *Neurol Clin* 2001;19:801–827.

Bernat J. How do physicians prove irreversibility in the determination of death? In: Sorondo, MS (ed.) *The signs of death: The proceedings of the working group*. Rome: Scripta Varia 110. Pontificia Academia Sciantiarum 2006. pp 159–176.

Bernat JL. Ethical and legal issues in palliative care. *Neurol Clin* 2001;19:969–987.

Birch D, and Draper J. A critical literature review exploring the challenges of delivering effective palliative care to older people with dementia. *J Clin Nursing* 2008;17:1144–1163.

Brierly JB, Adams JH, Graham DL, and Simpson JA. Neocortical death after cardiac arrest. *Lancet.* 1971; 2:560–565.

Brown BA. The history of advance directives: A literature review. *Journal of Gerontological Nursing*, 2003;29:4–14.

Callahan D. American culture and death. *West J Med.*1995;163: 226–230.

Cazzolli P and Oppenheimer E. Home mechanical ventilation for amyotrophic lateral sclerosis: Nasal compared to tracheostomy intermittent-positive pressure ventilation. *J Neurol Sci.* 1996;139(Suppl):123–128.

Chio A, Gauthier A, Calvo A, et al. Caregiver burden and patients' perception of being a burden in ALS. *Neurology.* 2005;64:1780–1782.

Chochinov HM, Wilson KG, Enns M, Mowchun N, Lander S, Levitt M, and Clinch JJ. Desire for death in the terminally ill. *Am J Psychiatry* 1995; 152:1185–1191.

Completing the Continuum of ALS Care: A consensus document. Missoula, Montana: Promoting Excellence in End-of-Life Care, a national program of The Robert Wood Johnson Foundation; 2004. http://www.promotingexcellence.org/als/als_report.

Conference of Medical Royal Colleges and their Faculties. Diagnosis of brain death. Statement issued by the honorary secretary of the Conference of Medical Royal Colleges and their Faculties in the United Kingdom on 11 October 1976.*Br Med J* 1976;2(6045): 1187–1188.

Council on Scientific Affairs and Council on Ethical and Judicial Affairs. Persistent vegetative state and the decision to withdraw or withhold life support. *JAMA.* 1990;263:426–430.

Daroff, R. The historical evolution of brain death from former definitions of death: The Harvard Criteria to the present. In: Sorondo MS (ed.) *The signs of death: The proceedings of the working group.* Rome: Scripta Varia 110. Pontificia Academia Sciantiarum 2006. pp 217–221.

Da Silva CH, Cunha RL, Tonaco RB, et al. Not telling the truth in the patient-physician relationship. *Bioethics.* 2003;17:417-424.

Diagnosis of brain death. Lancet. 1976;2(7994):1069–1070.

Doyle D. The provision of palliative care. In: Doyle D, Hanks GWC, MacDonald N (eds): *Oxford textbook of palliative medicine,* ed. 2. Oxford: Oxford University Press; 1998, pp.7–13.

Ferrell BR, Viran R, and Grant M. Analysis of end-of-life content in nursing textbooks. *Nursing Forum* 1996;26:869–876.

Foley KM and Carver AC. Palliative care in neurology: An overview. *Neurol Clin* 2001;19:789–799.

Foral PA, Malesker MA, Huerta G, and Hilleman DE. Nebulized opioids use in COPD. *Chest.* 2004;125:691–694.

Ganzini L, Goy ER, and Dobscha SK. Prevalence of depression and anxiety in patients requesting physicians' aid in dying: Cross sectional survey. *BMJ* 2008;337:a1682.

Ganzini L, Johnston W, MacFarland BH, et al. Attitudes of patients with amyotrophic lateral sclerosis and their care givers toward assisted suicide. *N Engl J Med.* 1998;339:967–973.

Gillick MR and Volandes AE. The standard of caring: Why do we still use feeding tubes in patients with advanced dementia? *J Am Med Dir Assoc* 2008;9:364–367.

Gold M. Is honesty always the best policy? Ethical aspects of truth telling. *Intern Med J.* 2004 Sep-Oct;34(9–10):578–580.

Goldstein LH, Atkins L, Landau S, Brown R, and Leigh PN. Predictors of psychological distress in careers of people with amyotrophic lateral sclerosis: A longitudinal study. *Psychol Med.* 2006;36:865–875.

Hacke W. Brain death - An artifact created by critical care medicine or the death of the brain has always been the death of the individual. In: Sorondo, MS (ed.) *The signs of death: The proceedings of the working group.* Rome: Scripta Varia 110. Pontificia Academia Sciantiarum. 2006. pp 84–91.

Helft PR. Necessary Collusion: Prognostic communication with advanced cancer patients. *Journal of Clinical Oncology.* 2005;23:3146–150.

House of Delegates redefines death, urges redefinition of rape, and undoes the Houston Amendments. *Am Bar Assoc J.* 1975; 61: 463–4.

Gold M. Is honesty always the best policy? Ethical aspects of truth telling. *Intern Med J.* 2004 Sep-Oct;34(9-10):578–580.

Jacox A, Carr DB, Payne R, Berde CB, Breitbart W, and Cain JM. *Management of cancer pain. Clinical practice guideline no. 9* (AHCPR Publication No. 94-0592) Rockville MD: Agency for Health Care Policy and Research. Department of Health and Human Services, Public Health Service, 1994.

Kirkland D. Truth telling, autonomy and the role of metaphor. *J Med Ethics.* 2007 Jan;33(1):11–14.

Klager J, Duckett A, Sandler S, and Moskowitz C. Huntington's disease: A caring approach at the end of life. *Care Manage J* 2008;9:75–81.

Kleinman A and Benson. Culture, moral experience and medicine. *Mt Sinai J Med.* 2006 Oct;73:834–839.

Kodish E and Post SG. Oncology and hope. *J Clin Oncol.* 1995 Jul;13:1817.

Koenig B and Gates-Williams J. Understanding cultural difference in caring for dying patients. *West J Med.* 1995;163:244–249.

Kutner JS, Steiner JF, Corbet KK et al: Information needs in terminal illness. *Soc Sci Med.* 1999. 48:1341–1352.

Larriviere D and Bonnie RJ. Terminating artificial nutrition and hydration in persistent vegetative state patients: Current and proposed state laws. *Neurology* 2006;6:1624-1628.

Mathus-Vliegen L, Louwerse L, Merkus MP, et al. Percutaneous endoscopic gastrostomy in patients with amyotrophic lateral sclerosis and impaired pulmonary function. *Gastrointest Endosc.* 1994;40:463–469.

Maynard DW. On "realization" in everyday life: The forecasting of bad news as a social relation. *Am Sociological Rev* 61:109–131, 1996.

McDonald E, Wiedenfeld S, Hillel A, et al. Survival in amyotrophic lateral sclerosis: The role of psychological factors. *Arch Neurol.* 1994;5: 17–23.

Miaskowski C, Cleary J, Burney R, et al. *Guideline for the management of cancer pain in adults and children. APS clinical practice guidelines series, No. 3.* Glenview IL: American Pain Society, 2005.

Miller RG, Rosenberg JA, Gelinas DF, et al. Practice parameter: The care of the patient with amyotrophic lateral sclerosis (an evidence–based review): Report of the Quality Standards Subcommittee of the American Academy of Neurology. *Neurology* 1999;52:1311.

Mitchell SL. A 93-year old man with advanced dementia and eating problems. *JAMA* 2007;298:2527–2536.

Mohandas A and Chou SN. Brain death—A clinical and pathologic study. *J Neurosurg* 1971;35:211–218.

Moss A, Casey P, Stocking CB, et al. Home ventilation for amyotrophic lateral sclerosis patients: Outcome, costs, and patient, family, and physician attitudes. *Neurology.* 1993;43:438–443.

Neatherlin JS and Fox S. End-of-life care concepts in the Journal of Neuroscience Nursing. *J Neuroscience Nursing* 2006;38:342–353.

Newall A, Orser R, and Hunt M. The control of oral secretions in bulbar ALS/MND. *J Neuro Sci.* 1996;139(Suppl):43–44.

Norris F, Smith R, and Denys E. Motor neurone disease: Towards better care. *Br Med J* 1985;291:259–262.

O'Brien T, Kelly M, and Saunders C. Motor neurone disease: A hospice perspective. *Br Med J* 1992;304:471–473.

O'Connell LJ. Religious dimensions of dying and death. *West J Med.*1995; 163: 231–235.

Boyle J. Medical ethics and double effect: The case of terminal sedation. *Theor Med Bioeth.* 2004;25:51–60.

Owens D and Flom J. Integrating palliative and neurological critical care. *AANC Clinical Issues* 2005;16:542–550.

Rabkin J, Wagner G, and Del Bene M. Resilience and distress among amyotrophic lateral sclerosis patients and caregivers. *Psychosom Med.* 2000;62:271–279.

Racine E, Amaram R, Seidler M, Karczewska M, and Illes J. Media coverage of the persistent vegetative state and end-of-life decision-making. *Neurology.* 2008;71:964–965.

Randall F and Downie RS. Ethics and aims in palliative care. In: Randall F and Downie RS: *Palliative care ethics. A good companion.* Oxford: Oxford University Press;1996, pp.1–24.

Reyners AKL, Peters FT, and van Minnen CA. Palliative care: For whom and by whom? *Lancet Oncol* 2007;8:573-574.

Sepulveda C, Marlin A, Yoshida T, and Ullrich A. Palliative care: The World Health Organization's global perspective. *J Pain Symptom Manage* 2002;24:91–96.

Sorondo, MS (ed.) *The signs of death: The proceedings of the working group.* Rome: Scripta Varia 110. Pontificia Academia Sciantiarum. 2006. pp 159–176.

Stanley JM. The Appleton International Conference: Developing guidelines for decisions to forgo life-prolonging medical treatment. *J Med Ethics* 1992;18(Supp):1–22.

Stillman MJ and Rybicki L: The Bedside Confusion Scale (BCS): Development of a reproducible, portable test for confusion in medically ill patients. *J Palliative Med* 3(4): 449–456, 2001

Truog R and Burns J. Futility: A concept in evolution. *Chest.* 2007 Dec. 132(6):1987–1993.

Truog R, Nrett A, and Frader J. The problem with futility. *N Engl J Med* 1992;326:1560–1564.

Turner-Stokes L, Harding R, Sergeant J, Lupton C, and McPherson K. Generating the evidence base for the National Service Framework for Long Term Conditions: A new research typology. *Clin Med,* 2006;6:91–97.

Turner-Stokes L, Sykes N, Silber E, Khatri A, Sutton L, and Young E. From diagnosis to death: Exploring the interface between neurology, rehabilitation and palliative care in managing people with long-tern neurological conditions. *Clin Med* 2007;7:129–136.

U.S. Collaborative Study. An appraisal of the criteria of cerebral death. *JAMA* 1977. 237: 982–986.

U.S. President's Commission. Guidelines for the determination of death. *JAMA* 1981; 246:2184–2186.

Veith FJ, Fein JM, Tendler MD, Veatch RM, Kleiman MA, and Kalkines G. Brain death: A status report of medical and ethical considerations. *JAMA* 1977. 238: 1651–1655.

Volicer L, McKee A, and Hewitt S. Dementia. *Neurol Clin* 2001;19:867–885.

Westphal CG and Campbell ML. Nebulized morphine for terminal dyspnea. *Am J Nurs.* 2002;Suppl:11–15.

Wilkinson J. Ethical issues in palliative care. In: Doyle D, Hanks GWC, MacDonald N (eds): *Oxford textbook of palliative medicine, ed. 2.* Oxford: Oxford University Press; 1998, pp.495–504.

World Health Organization. Cancer Pain Relief and Palliative Care. Geneva: WHO, p.11, 1990.

Index